Cancer Chemotherapy and Biotherapy: Principles and Practice

FIFTH EDITION

Bruce A. Chabner, MD

Director of Clinical Research
Massachusetts General Hospital Cancer Center
Professor of Medicine
Harvard Medical School
Boston, Massachusetts

Dan L. Longo, MD

Division of Hematology
Brigham and Women's Hospital
Deputy Editor
New England Journal of Medicine
Boston, Massachusetts

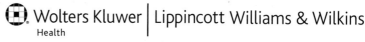

Wolters Kluwer | Lippincott Williams & Wilkins
Health

Philadelphia · Baltimore · New York · London
Buenos Aires · Hong Kong · Sydney · Tokyo

Senior Executive Editor: Jonathan W. Pine Jr.
Senior Product Manager: Emilie Moyer
Vendor Manager: Alicia Jackson
Senior Manufacturing Manager: Benjamin Rivera
Senior Marketing Manager: Angela Panetta
Creative Services Director: Doug Smock
Production Service: SPi Technologies

Library of Congress Cataloging-in-Publication Data
Cancer chemotherapy and biotherapy : principles and practice / editors, Bruce A. Chabner, Dan L. Longo. —5th ed.
      p. ; cm.
   Includes bibliographical references and index.
   Summary: "Updated to include the newest drugs and those currently in development, Cancer Chemotherapy and Biotherapy, Fifth Edition is a comprehensive reference on the preclinical and clinical pharmacology of anticancer agents. Organized by drug class, the book provides the latest information on all drugs and biological agents—their mechanisms of action, interactions with other agents, toxicities, side effects, and mechanisms of resistance. Chapters emphasize pharmacology and mechanisms of action at the molecular and cellular levels, followed by clinical activity and toxicity, both acute and delayed. The authors explain the rationale for use of drugs in specific schedules and combinations and offer guidelines for dose adjustment in particular situations. The previous edition was one of "Doody's Core Titles 2009." This edition's introduction includes timely information on general strategies for drug usage, the science of drug discovery and development, economic and regulatory aspects of cancer drug development, and principles of pharmacokinetics. Eight new chapters have been added and more than twenty have been significantly revised"—Provided by publisher.
   ISBN 978-1-60547-431-1 (hardback : alk. paper)
   1. Cancer—Chemotherapy. 2. Cancer—Immunotherapy. 3. Antineoplastic agents. 4. Biological response modifiers.
I. Chabner, Bruce. II. Longo, Dan L. (Dan Louis), 1949–
   [DNLM: 1. Neoplasms—drug therapy. 2. Antineoplastic Agents—therapeutic use. 3. Biological Products—therapeutic use. QZ 267 C21515 2011]
   RC271.C5C32219   2011
   616.99′4061—dc22   2010023843

Care has been taken to confirm the accuracy of the information presented and to describe generally accepted practices. However, the authors, editors, and publisher are not responsible for errors or omissions or for any consequences from application of the information in this book and make no warranty, expressed or implied, with respect to the currency, completeness, or accuracy of the contents of the publication. Application of the information in a particular situation remains the professional responsibility of the practitioner.

The authors, editors, and publisher have exerted every effort to ensure that drug selection and dosage set forth in this text are in accordance with current recommendations and practice at the time of publication. However, in view of ongoing research, changes in government regulations, and the constant flow of information relating to drug therapy and drug reactions, the reader is urged to check the package insert for each drug for any change in indications and dosage and for added warnings and precautions. This is particularly important when the recommended agent is a new or infrequently employed drug.

Some drugs and medical devices presented in the publication have Food and Drug Administration (FDA) clearance for limited use in restricted research settings. It is the responsibility of the health care provider to ascertain the FDA status of each drug or device planned for use in their clinical practice.

To purchase additional copies of this book, call our customer service department at (800) 638-3030 or fax orders to (301) 223-2320. International customers should call (301) 223-2300.

Visit Lippincott Williams & Wilkins on the Internet: at LWW.com. Lippincott Williams & Wilkins customer service representatives are available from 8:30 am to 6 pm, EST.

10 9 8 7 6 5 4 3 2 1

Many devoted people made possible this Fifth Edition of *Cancer Chemotherapy and Biotherapy: Principles and Practice* published under the Lippincott Williams & Wilkins banner. Jonathan W. Pine Jr, Senior Executive Editor, and Molly Ward, Senior Managing Editor, provided constant encouragement, monitored outstanding manuscripts, and watched the calendar, keeping us on track as never before. They were greatly helped by our Editorial Assistants, Renee Johnson, Laura Collins, and Pat Duffey, whose diligence and spreadsheets kept us on time and under budget. We want to thank the contributing authors, who were extraordinarily conscientious, making our editorial task much easier. We all felt a sense of mission about this book, as we do about our field in general.

There are others we wish to recognize. Our many fellows and colleagues in the field of medical oncology, many of whom have contributed to this book, have always been the sustaining force behind our work and have only added to our passion to cure this disease. We were fortunate to share this passion with our close colleagues in the Medicine Branch, National Cancer Institute, Bob Young, Vince DeVita, and George Canellos, and with our fellow faculty members at the Massachusetts General Hospital and Harvard, and at the National Institutes of Health, many of whom have become contributors. Our patients give us the courage to continue seeking better treatments, in spite of failures and disappointments. With the benefit of decades of experience, we have seen remarkable progress, but for most of those patients, the benefits came too late.

Finally and most importantly, we owe much to our wives, children, and grandchildren, who admire and support what we do, and despite their own careers and family concerns, recognize that it is much more than a job.

Carmen J. Allegra, MD
Chief, Oncology and Hematology
Department of Medicine
University of Florida
Gainesville, Florida

Kenneth C. Anderson, MD
Kraft Family Professor of Medicine
Harvard Medical School
Director, Jerome Lipper Multiple Myeloma Center
Department of Medical Oncology
Dana-Farber Cancer Institute
Boston, Massachusetts

Steven D. Averbuch, MD
Vice-President Oncology Transition Strategy & Development
Head, Pharmacodiagnostics Global Clinical Research
Bristol-Myers Squibb
Princeton, New Jersey

Tracy T. Batchelor, MD
Associate Professor of Neuro-Oncology
Department of Neurology
Harvard Medical School
Executive Director
Department of Neuro-Oncology
Massachusetts General Hospital
Boston, Massachusetts

Susan E. Bates, MD
Senior Investigator
Medical Oncology Branch
Center for Cancer Research
National Cancer Institute
Bethesda, Maryland

Angela R. Bradbury, MD
Assistant Professor
Clinical Genetics
Fox Chase Cancer Center
Philadelphia, Pennsylvania

Alina D. Bulgar, PhD
Case Comprehensive Cancer Center
Case Western Reserve University
Cleveland, Ohio

Helen X. Chen, MD
Associate Chief
Investigational Drug Branch
Cancer Therapy Evaluation Program
National Cancer Institute
Bethesda, Maryland

Monica G. Chiaramonte, PhD
Clinical Research Scientist
Technical Resources International, Inc
Bethesda, Maryland

Curtis R. Chong, MD
Instructor in Medicine
Harvard Medical School
Resident, Internal Medicine
Massachusetts General Hospital
Boston, Massachusetts

Jeffrey W. Clark, MD
Associate Professor of Medicine
Harvard Medical School
Medical Director, Clinical Trials
Massachusetts General Hospital Cancer Center
Boston, Massachusetts

Jerry M. Collins, PhD
Associate Director for Developmental Therapeutics
Division of Cancer Treatment and Diagnosis
National Cancer Institute, NIH
Bethesda, Maryland

Brian A. Costello, MD, MS
Assistant Professor
Department of Oncology
Mayo Clinic
Rochester, Minnesota

Brendan D. Curti, MD
Director, Genitourinary Oncology Research
Robert W. Franz Cancer Research Center
Earle A. Chiles Research Institute
Portland, Oregon

Shannon Decker, JD, MPH
Health Program Director
Marlene & Stewart Greenebaum Cancer Center
University of Maryland
Baltimore, Maryland

Robert B. Diasio, MD
Professor of Pharmacology
Mayo Clinic College of Medicine
Director
Mayo Clinic Cancer Center
Rochester, Minnesota

James H. Doroshow, MD
Director, Division of Cancer Treatment and Diagnosis
National Cancer Institute
Bethesda, Maryland

L. Austin Doyle, MD
Senior Investigator
Investigational Drug Branch
Cancer Therapy Evaluation Program
National Cancer Institute
Bethesda, Maryland

Charles Erlichman, MD
Chair, Department of Oncology
Deputy Director for Clinical Affairs
Mayo Clinic
Rochester, Minnesota

Igor Espinoza-Delgado, MD
Senior Clinical Investigator
Cancer Therapy Evaluation Program
Division of Cancer Treatment and Diagnosis
National Cancer Institute
Rockville, Maryland
Senior Medical Staff
Division of Cancer Treatment
National Institute of Health Clinical Center
Bethesda, Maryland

Jeanne Fourie Zirkelbach, PhD
Clinical Pharmacology Reviewer
U.S. Food and Drug Administration
Center for Drug Evaluation and Research
Office of Clinical Pharmacology
Division of Clinical Pharmacology V
Silver Spring, Maryland

Henry S. Friedman, MD
James B. Powell, Jr. Professor of Neuro-Oncology
Department of Surgery
Duke University Medical Center
Durham, North Carolina

Alison M. Friedmann, MD, MSc
Harvard Medical School
Assistant Professor of Pediatrics
Faculty, Pediatric Hematology/Oncology
Massachusetts General Hospital
Boston, Massachusetts

Ken-ichi Fujita, PhD
Assistant Professor
Department of Medical Oncology
Saitama Medical University
Hidaka, Japan

Stanton L. Gerson, MD
Director, Case Comprehensive Cancer Center
Case Western Reserve University
Director, Ireland Cancer Center
University Hospitals Case Medical Center
Cleveland, Ohio

Paul A. Glare, MBBS, FRACP, FACP
Professor
Department of Medicine
Weill Medical College
Cornell University
Chief, Pain and Palliative Care Services
Department of Medicine
Memorial Sloan Kettering Cancer Center
New York, New York

Jacob Glass, MD, PhD
Resident in Medicine
Weill-Cornell Medical College
New York, New York

François Goldwasser, MD, PhD
Professor of Medical Oncology
Paris Descartes University
Head of the Department of Medical Oncology
Cochin Teaching Hospital
Paris, France

Paul E. Goss, MD, PhD
Professor
Department of Medicine
Harvard Medical School
Physician
Department of Hematology and Oncology
Massachusetts General Hospital
Boston, Massachusetts

William J. Gradishar, MD
Professor of Medicine
Director, Maggie Daley Center for Women's Cancer Care
Program Director, Hematology-Oncology Fellowship
  Training Program
Robert H. Lurie Comprehensive Cancer Center
Northwestern University Feinberg School of Medicine
Northwestern Memorial Hospital
Chicago, Illinois

Jean L. Grem, MD
Professor of Medicine
University of Nebraska Medical Center
Associate Director for Translational Research
University of Nebraska Eppley Cancer Center
Omaha, Nebraska

Kenneth R. Hande, MD
Professor of Medicine and Pharmacology
Vanderbilt/Ingram Cancer Center
Vanderbilt University School of Medicine
Nashville, Tennessee

Teru Hideshima, MD, PhD
Principal Associate in Medicine
Harvard Medical School
Jerome Lipper Myeloma Center
Dana Farber Cancer Institute
Boston, Massachusetts

Melinda Hollingshead, DVM, PhD
Chief, Biological Testing Branch
Developmental Therapeutics Program
National Cancer Institute
Frederick, Maryland

S. Percy Ivy, MD
Associate Chief
Investigational Drug Branch
Cancer Therapy Evaluation Program
Division of Cancer Treatment and Diagnosis
National Cancer Institute
Bethesda, Maryland

Richard P. Junghans, MD, PhD
Associate Professor of Surgery and Medicine
Department of Surgery
Boston University School of Medicine
Chief, Division of Surgical Research
Department of Surgery
Roger Williams Medical Center
Providence, Rhode Island

Joseph G. Jurcic, MD
Associate Member, Memorial Hospital
Department of Medicine
Memorial Sloane-Kettering Cancer Center
Associate Attending Physician
Department of Medicine
Memorial Hospital for Cancer and Allied Diseases
New York, New York

Henry B. Koon, MD
Assistant Professor of Medicine
Case Western Reserve University
Director, Medical Oncology Cutaneous Malignancy Program
Ireland Cancer Center
Cleveland, Ohio

Ian E. Krop, MD, PhD
Assistant Professor of Medicine
Department of Medicine
Harvard Medical School
Associate Physician
Department of Medical Oncology
Dana-Farber Cancer Institute
Boston, Massachusetts

Nicole M. Kuderer, MD
Assistant Professor of Medicine
Division of Hematology, Oncology, and Cellular Therapy
Duke Comprehensive Cancer Center
Duke University Medical Center
Durham, North Carolina

Joanne Kurtzberg, MD
Professor of Pediatrics
Director, Carolinas Cord Blood Bank
Chief, Division of Pediatric Blood and Marrow Transplantation
Duke University Medical Center
Durham, North Carolina

David J. Kuter, MD, DPhil
Professor of Medicine
Harvard Medical School
Director of Clinical Hematology
Massachusetts General Hospital
Boston, Massachusetts

Jacob Laubach, MD, MPP
Instructor in Medicine
Department of Internal Medicine
Harvard Medical School
Instructor in Medicine
Department of Medical Oncology
Dana Farber Cancer Institute
Boston, Massachusetts

Richard J. Lee, MD, PhD
Instructor
Department of Medicine
Harvard Medical School
Assistant Physician
Department of Medicine
Massachusetts General Hospital
Boston, Massachusetts

Gary H. Lyman, MD, MPH, FRCP (Edin)
Professor of Medicine
Department of Medicine
Duke University
Durham, North Carolina

David F. McDermott, MD
Assistant Professor of Clinical Medicine
Harvard University
Clinical Director
Biologic Therapy Program
Beth Israel Deaconess Medical Center
Boston, Massachusetts

Constantine S. Mitsiades, MD, PhD
Instructor in Medicine
Department of Medical Oncology
Dana-Farber Cancer Institute
Department of Medicine
Harvard Medical School
Boston, Massachusetts

Beverly Moy, MD, MPH
Assistant Professor
Department of Medicine
Harvard Medical School
Assistant Physician
Department of Hematology/Oncology
Massachusetts General Hospital
Boston, Massachusetts

Maciej M. Mrugala, MD, PhD, MPH
Assistant Professor of Neurology and Neurological Surgery
Division of Neuro-Oncology
University of Washington School of Medicine
Fred Hutchinson Cancer Research Center
Seattle, Washington

Joel W. Neal, MD, PhD
Assistant Professor
Department of Medicine
Division of Medical Oncology
Stanford University
Staff Physician
Department of Medicine
Division of Oncology
Stanford Cancer Center
Stanford, California

Ian N. Olver, MD, PhD
Clinical Professor
Sydney Medical School
University of Sydney
Chief Executive Officer
Cancer Council Australia
Sydney, New South Wales, Australia

Richard L. Piekarz, MD, PhD
Medical Officer
Cancer Therapy Evaluation Program
Division of Cancer Treatment and Diagnosis, National Cancer
    Institute, National Institutes of Health
Rockville, Maryland
Medical Officer
National Institutes of Health Clinical Center
Bethesda, Maryland

Yves Pommier, MD, PhD
Chief, Laboratory of Molecular Pharmacology
National Cancer Institute
Bethesda, Maryland

Fahd Rahman, MD
National Institutes of Health
Bethesda, Maryland

Eddie Reed, MD
Professor
Mitchell Cancer Institute
University of South Alabama
Clinical Director
Mitchell Cancer Institute
University of South Alabama Hospitals
Mobile, Alabama

Paul Richardson, MD
Associate Professor of Medicine
Harvard Medical School
Clinical Director
Jerome Lipper Center for Multiple Myeloma
Dana-Farber Cancer Institute
Boston, Massachusetts

Thomas G. Roberts Jr., MD, M Soc Sci
Partner
Farallon Capital Management
San Francisco, California

Robert W. Robey
Medical Oncology Branch
Center for Cancer Research
National Cancer Institute
Bethesda, Maryland

Todd L. Rosenblat, MD
Assistant Member
Department of Medicine
Memorial Sloan-Kettering Cancer Center
Assistant Attending
Department of Medicine
Memorial Hospital for Cancer and Allied Diseases
New York, New York

Rachel P. Rosovsky, MD, MPH
Instructor
Harvard Medical School
Assistant Physician
Department of Hematology and Oncology
Massachusetts General Hospital
Boston, Massachusetts

Eric K. Rowinsky, MD
Adjunct Professor
Department of Medicine
New York University
New York, New York

David P. Ryan, MD
Associate Professor of Medicine
Harvard Medical School
Clinical Director
Massachusetts General Hospital Cancer Center
Boston, Massachusetts

Edward A. Sausville, MD, PhD, FACP
Professor of Medicine
Greenebaum Cancer Center
University of Maryland, Baltimore
Associate Director for Clinical Research
Greenebaum Cancer Center
University of Maryland Medical Center
Baltimore, Maryland

Philip J. Saylor, MD
Instructor
Department of Medicine
Division of Hematology-Oncology
Harvard Medical School
Assistant Physician
Department of Medicine
Division of Hematology and Oncology
Massachusetts General Hospital Cancer Center
Boston, Massachusetts

David A. Scheinberg, MD, PhD
Professor and Chair
Molecular Pharmacology and Chemistry Program
Memorial Sloan-Kettering Cancer Institute
Member, Department of Medicine
Memorial Hospital for Cancer and Allied Diseases
New York, New York

Richard L. Schilsky, MD
Professor and Chief
Section of Hematology/Oncology
Department of Medicine
University of Chicago
Chicago, Illinois

Lecia V. Sequist, MD, MPH
Assistant Professor of Medicine
Harvard Medical School
Massachusetts General Hospital Cancer Center
Boston, Massachusetts

George Sgouros, MD
Professor
Department of Radiology
Johns Hopkins University School of Medicine
Head, Radiopharmacuetical Dosimetry
Johns Hopkins Medical
Baltimore, Maryland

Robert Shoemaker, PhD
Chief, Screening Technologies Branch
Developmental Therapeutics Program
National Cancer Institute
Frederick, Maryland

Matthew R. Smith, MD, PhD
Associate Professor
Department of Medicine
Harvard Medical School
Physician
Department of Medicine
Massachusetts General Hospital
Boston, Massachusetts

Alex Sparreboom, PhD
Associate Member
Pharmaceutical Sciences
Saint Jude Children's Research Hospital
Memphis, Tennessee

Jeffrey G. Supko, PhD
Associate Professor
Department of Medicine
Harvard Medical School
Director
Department of Clinical Pharmacology Laboratory
Massachusetts General Hospital
Boston, Massachusetts

Richard D. Swerdlow, PhD
Clinical Research Scientist
PSI International
Bethesda, Maryland

Mario Sznol, MD
Professor of Internal Medicine
Yale Cancer Center/Yale New Haven Hospital
Yale University
New Haven, Connecticut

Naoko Takebe, MD, PhD
Senior Investigator
Investigational Drug Branch
Cancer Therapy Evaluation Program
National Cancer Institute
Bethesda, Maryland

William C. Timmer, PhD
Program Director
Clinical Grants and Contracts Branch
Cancer Therapy Evaluation Program
Division of Cancer Treatment and Diagnosis
National Cancer Institute
National Institutes of Health
Bethesda, Maryland

Sara M. Tolaney, MD, MPH
Instructor in Medicine
Department of Medicine
Harvard Medical School
Staff Physician
Department of Medical Oncology
Dana-Farber Cancer Institute
Boston, Massachusetts

Raymond C. Wadlow, MD
Instructor
Department of Medicine
Harvard Medical College
Assistant in Medicine
Department of Medicine
Massachusetts General Hospital
Boston, Massachusetts

Lachelle D. Weeks, BA
Cancer Biology Training Program
Department of Pathology
Case Comprehensive Cancer Center
Case Western Reserve University
Cleveland, Ohio

Eric P. Winer, MD
Professor of Medicine
Harvard Medical School
Chief Division of Women's Cancers
Director, Breast Oncology Center
Thompson Senior Investigator in Breast Cancer Research
Dana-Farber Cancer Institute
Boston, Massachusetts

Kari B. Wisinski, MD
Assistant Professor of Medicine
Department of Hematology/Oncology
University of Wisconsin Carbone Cancer Center
Assistant Professor of Medicine
Department of Hematoloy/Oncology
University of Wisconsin Hospital and Clinics
Madison, Wisconsin

John J. Wright, MD, PhD
Associate Branch Chief
Investigational Drug Branch
National Cancer Institute
Bethesda, Maryland

Cassian Yee, MD
Member, Clinical Research Division
Fred Hutchinson Cancer Research Center
Professor, Department of Medicine
University of Washington
Seattle, Washington

William C. Zamboni, PharmD, PhD
Associate Professor
Division of Pharmacotherapy and Experimental Therapeutics
University of North Carolina
Eshelman School of Pharmacy
Director of GLP Analytical Facility and Translational Oncology
Nanoparticle Drug Development Inititiative Lab
Molecular Therapeutics Program
University of North Carolina Lineberger Comprehensive Cancer Center
Chapel Hill, North Carolina

been associated with resistance to methotrexate,[14] as is a failure to transport or polyglutamate the drug.[15] High intratumoral levels of the DNA repair enzyme methylguanine methyl transferase predict resistance to nitrosoureas, dacarbazine, and temozolomide, all of which damage DNA by alkylating the O^6 position of guanine.[16] Mutations in mismatch DNA repair (the *MSH6* gene) are associated with resistance to methylating agents, to 6-mercaptopurine, and to cisplatin and carboplatin.[17] However, these molecular/biochemical tests have not been tested prospectively to prove their value in selecting treatment with cytotoxic drugs, and routine laboratory tests are not available.

Molecularly targeted discovery offers the hope of identifying new drugs tailored to specific receptors and intracellular enzymes critical for cell signaling and for maintaining viability and growth of tumors. Targeted drugs are effective against subsets of human malignancy. One such target, the *bcr-abl* tyrosine kinase, results from a translocation specific for chronic myelogenous leukemia (CML), and virtually all CML patients have this translocation at diagnosis. Imatinib, an inhibitor of the kinase, has striking activity in chronic and blastic phases of CML, and has limited toxicity for normal bone marrow cells.[18] Because imatinib also inhibits the *c-kit* tyrosine kinase, it is effective against gastrointestinal stromal tumors (GIST). Most patients with GIST express a mutated and activated form of *c-kit*. Pretreatment sequencing of the *c-kit* gene provides important prognostic information and allows appropriate selection of patients for treatment with imatinib (exon 11 mutations), sunitinib (exon 9 mutations), or other experimental drugs.[19]

Genetic tests to select patients for specific targeted therapies may dramatically improve response rates to these drugs. Activating mutations in the EGFR gene identify non–small cell lung cancer (NSCLC) patients who have a 70% response rate to gefitinib as first line therapy. Tumors lacking such mutations do not show clinical tumor regression, although some may derive benefit from a slowing of their growth.[20] The test for EGFR mutations should be performed in any nonsmoking patient with unresectable NSCLC.

The list of molecularly targeted agents, discussed further in various chapters of this book, is constantly growing. Effective agents targeting the *EML4-ALK* mutation in non–small cell lung cancer, the *ret* mutation in medullary thyroid cancer, and polyadenosyl ribose phosphatase (PARP) DNA repair function in breast and ovarian cancer[7] have shown evidence of dramatic efficacy in patients selected for the presence of mutations. Monoclonal antibodies (trastuzumab and cetuximab) are proving effective in combination with cytotoxic agents and as components of adjuvant therapies.[21] These results give hope that in the future, cancer treatment will be much more grounded in individualized treatment selection based on the molecular profile of the specific tumor. To do so would eliminate the waste of time and dollars and the needless toxicity of ineffective treatment, and would hasten drug approval.

Pharmacokinetic Determinants of Response

Although the outcome of cancer treatment depends in large part on the inherent sensitivity of the tumor being treated, the chances for success can be compromised by the oncologist's failure to consider important pharmacokinetic factors such as drug absorption,

metabolism, elimination, and drug interactions in designing experimental regimens and in clinical practice.

The pharmacokinetics of a given schedule of administration are subject to significant interindividual pharmacokinetic variability.[22] The origin of this variability is uncertain. Clearly, pharmacogenetics (polymorphisms in expression of drug-metabolizing enzymes) plays an important role in determining the rate of elimination and thus the toxicity of some drugs, including irinotecan hydrochloride (glucuronyl transferases), 6-mercaptopurine (TPMT), and 5-FU (dihydropyrimidine dehydrogenase).[23] In addition, variability in hepatic P-450 isoenzyme activity, protein binding of drug, and age-related changes in renal tubular function all contribute to variability of clearance. As a result, in a patient population with normal renal and hepatic function, measurement of drug levels in plasma will reveal at least a one log range of drug concentration at any given time point, and an equal interindividual variability in area under the curve (AUC) for a given dose of drug.[22]

Pharmacokinetic factors are important not only in general protocol design but also in determining specific modifications of dosage in individual patients. Dosage may be increased or decreased based on observed patterns of toxicity (neutrophil count following cytotoxic drug, acneform rash after EGFR inhibitor therapy) or lack thereof. If a pharmacokinetics laboratory is available, changes in dose may be based on direct drug concentration measurements. Drug levels are routinely measured in only a few settings: to identify patients at high risk of toxicity in regimens employing high-dose methotrexate, and to adjust dosage to achieve optimal blood levels in children receiving methotrexate for acute lymphocytic leukemia (ALL) (see Chapter 9). Studies of 5-FU pharmacokinetics have shown that response rates improve and episodes of extreme toxicity are rare when drug levels are monitored and doses adjusted to reach prespecific pharmacokinetic end points.[24] However, monitoring of 5-FU drug levels is not accepted as a routine practice, and the assay is not available in many cancer centers.

Most drugs are cleared through hepatic metabolism or renal excretion. Depending on the drug, either renal or hepatic dysfunction may delay drug elimination and result in overwhelming toxicity. To avoid such toxicity, doses of certain agents must be modified based on estimates of renal or hepatic function, as will be discussed in the individual drug chapters.

Reliable assays are available for virtually all antineoplastic agents and are primarily used for research purposes in conjunction with clinical trials. These methods are based on drug separation and quantitation by high-pressure liquid chromatography linked to mass spectrometry.

Combination Chemotherapy

Rationale for Combination Chemotherapy

Although the first effective drugs for treating cancer were brought to clinical trial in the 1940s, initial therapeutic results were disappointing. Impressive regressions of acute lymphocytic leukemia and adult lymphomas were obtained with single agents such as nitrogen mustard, antifolates, corticosteroids, and the vinca alkaloids, but responses were only partial and of short duration. When complete remissions were obtained, as in acute lymphocytic leukemia, they

TABLE
1.4   *Mechanisms of resistance*

Mechanism of resistance	Drug involved	Pharmacologic defect
Decreased drug uptake	Methotrexate sodium	Decreased expression of the folate transporter
Decreased drug activation	Cytosine arabinoside, fludarabine phosphate, cladribine	Decreased deoxycytidine kinase
	Methotrexate	Decreased folylpolyglutamyl synthetase
Increased drug target	Methotrexate	Amplified DHFR
	5-Fluorouracil	Amplified TS
	Imatinib	Amplified bcr-abl kinase
Altered drug target	Etoposide	Altered topo II
	Doxorubicin	
	Imatinib	Altered bcr-abl kinase
Increased detoxification	Alkylating agents	Increased glutathione or glutathione transferase
Enhanced DNA repair	Alkylating agents, platinum analogs	Increased nucleotide excision repair
	Nitrosoureas, procarbazine, temozolomide	Increased O^6-alkyl-guanine alkyl transferase
Defective recognition of DNA adducts	Cisplatin, 6-mercaptopurine	Mismatch repair defect
Increased drug efflux	Doxorubicin, etoposide, vinca alkaloids, paclitaxel, topotecan	Increased MDR expression or MDR gene amplification
Defective checkpoint function and apoptosis	Most anticancer drugs	*p53* mutations

DHFR, dihydrofolate reductase; MDR, multidrug resistance; topo II, topoisomerase II; TS, thymidylate synthase.

lasted a few months, and relapse was invariably associated with drug resistance. The introduction of cyclic combination chemotherapy for acute lymphocytic leukemia of childhood in the late 1950s marked a turning point in the effective treatment of neoplastic disease. Such combinations are now standard for treating cancer. The superior results of combination chemotherapy compared with single-agent treatment derive from the following considerations. Resistance to any given single agent is virtually certain to emerge, even for the most responsive tumors; for example, in patients with Hodgkin's disease, the complete response rate to alkylating agents or procarbazine does not exceed 20%, and virtually all patients thus treated relapse with resistant disease. Studies of imatinib resistance in CML have verified the long-standing hypothesis that initially responsive tumors harbor spontaneously resistant cells that are selected through exposure to the drug. Secondly, anticancer drugs and radiation therapy increase the rate of mutation to resistance in experimental studies, as does hypoxia.[25] The use of multiple agents, each with cytotoxic activity in the disease under consideration but with different mechanisms of action, allows independent cell killing by each agent. Cells resistant to one agent might still be sensitive to the other drugs in the regimen. The presence of multiple drugs discourages the outgrowth of malignant clones resistant to any single agent.

Patterns of crossresistance must be taken into consideration in formulating drug combinations. Resistance to many agents may result from unique and specific mutations, for example as may occur in the target enzymes of antimetabolites (such as dihydrofolate reductase or thymidylate synthase) or imatinib (bcr-abl kinase).[11] Mutations that alter binding of inhibitors of topoisomerase II, an enzyme that promotes DNA strand breaks in the presence of anthracyclines and epipodophyllotoxins, may mediate cross resistance to other members of this class of drugs.[26] In other cases, a single mutational change may lead to multidrug resistance. Table 1-4 describes crossresistance patterns for some of the well-defined mechanisms of multidrug resistance.

The most thoroughly studied and undoubtedly one of the more important mechanisms of multidrug resistance is increased expression of the *MDR-1* gene. This gene codes for the P-170 membrane glycoprotein, which promotes the efflux of vinca alkaloids, anthracyclines, taxanes, actinomycin D, epipodophyllotoxins, other natural products, and even small molecules that target tyrosine kinases. This protein occurs constitutively in many normal tissues, including most stem cells, and mature epithelial cells of the kidney, colon, and adrenal gland,[27] and has been identified in tumors derived from these tissues. It is prominently expressed in many tumors recurring after chemotherapy, including lymphomas, myeloid leukemias, multiple myeloma, and other cancers.[28] P-170–mediated resistance, and the associated decrease in intracellular drug levels, can be reversed experimentally by administration of calcium-channel blockers, amiodarone, quinidine, various steroid hormones, and cyclosporine analogues. Results of clinical trials investigating the use of agents reversing multidrug resistance have been confounded by pharmacokinetic interactions of the reversing agents and cancer drugs, and thus far have been inconclusive.

A second class of efflux transporters, the multidrug-resistance proteins (MRPs), may also confer complex patterns of crossresistance. In experimental tumors, these efflux pumps promote drug efflux and confer resistance to anthracyclines, etoposide, and vinca alkaloids. Members of the MRP family may also mediate efflux of methotrexate, 6-mercaptopurine, and camptothecin derivatives.[29]

The MRP family of genes is widely expressed in epithelial tumors,[27] and their potential for mediating multiagent resistance deserves further study.

Finally, classic alkylating agents (cyclophosphamide, melphalan hydrochloride, nitrogen mustard) may share crossresistance related to enhanced DNA repair mediated by nucleotide excision repair enzymes and by increased levels of intracellular nucleophilic thiols, such as glutathione. Increased expression of nucleotide excision repair (NER) components correlates with a poor outcome in ovarian cancer treated with platinum-based regimens.[30] Not all alkylating agents share crossresistance. As mentioned earlier, resistance to the nitrosourea, procarbazine, dacarbazine, and other methylating alkylators is mediated by increased levels of a different enzyme, methyl guanine methyl transferase. Thus, there is a clear rationale for combining different types of alkylators in a single regimen. While increased expression of NER components may mediate resistance to bis-chloroethyl alkylators, an intact mismatch repair complex, which recognizes areas of altered DNA duplex pairing and activates apoptosis, *is required* for sensitivity to methylating drugs and platinating agents. A single mutation in one component of this system, *MSH6*, confers resistance to platinating drugs and methylating agents, as well as 6-mercaptopurine.

The acquisition of drug resistance is believed to result from random mutations in a tumor cell population, although it is obvious that cancer drugs, as mutagens, increase mutation frequency. A corollary to this hypothesis is the concept that the probability of de novo drug resistance in any tumor population increases with increasing number of cells and the number of cell divisions.[31] Goldie et al. proposed a mathematical model based on the random-mutation hypothesis. It suggested several important considerations in protocol design to minimize treatment failure due to acquired drug resistance: (a) treatment should begin when the malignant cell population is at its smallest. (b) To avoid selection of doubly resistant mutants by sequential chemotherapy, use multiple mutually non–crossresistant drugs. (c) To achieve maximal kill of both sensitive and moderately resistant cells, administer drugs as frequently as possible and in maximally tolerated doses. The Goldie-Coldman model serves to explain the success of combination therapies against hematologic malignancies such as non-Hodgkin's lymphoma and Hodgkin's disease.[32] However, randomized trials comparing new and more elaborate regimens, based on the Goldie-Coldman hypothesis, with older, empirically designed four-drug regimens, have failed to demonstrate any improvement in the cure rates of lymphomas.[33,34] Although these studies do not negate the basic tenants of Goldie-Coldman, they do suggest that the assumptions underlying the formal mathematical modeling missed important aspects of human tumor biology. For instance, the model assumes that resistance develops to individual agents, one at a time, and thus does not take into account multidrug resistance, as conferred by inactivation of *p53* or defects in apoptosis, or by multidrug-resistance transporters. An additional consideration beyond drug resistance supports combination chemotherapy. If drugs have nonoverlapping patterns of normal organ toxicity, each can be used in full doses, and the effectiveness of each agent will be fully maintained in the combination. Drugs such as vincristine sulfate, prednisone, bleomycin sulfate, L-asparaginase, high-dose methotrexate/leucovorin, and biological agents all lack bone marrow toxicity and are par-

ticularly valuable in combination with traditional myelosuppressive agents. Based on these principles, combinations have been devised to cure diseases not curable with single-agent treatment, including acute lymphocytic leukemia (vincristine, prednisone, doxorubicin, and L-asparaginase), Hodgkin's disease (mechlorethamine, vincristine, procarbazine, and prednisone [MOPP] and doxorubicin [adriamycin], bleomycin, vinblastine, and dacarbazine [ABVD]), diffuse large cell lymphoma (the combination of R-CHOP: rituximab, cyclophosphamide, doxorubicin, vincristine, and prednisone), and testicular carcinoma (bleomycin, etoposide, and cisplatin, BEP). Monoclonal antibodies and targeted agents can be added to drugs without increasing toxicity, but with enhanced results.

The entry of targeted drugs onto the therapeutic horizon led to the successful use of traztuzumab with taxanes for breast cancer, bevacizumab with 5-flourouracil and oxaliplatin for colon cancer, and cetuximab (erbitux) with irinotecan for colon cancer. This success is attributed to several mechanisms: (a) the ability of bevacizumab to normalize blood flow and improve cytotoxic drug delivery to otherwise poorly perfused tumors, and (b) the proapoptotic effects of receptor inhibitors such as traztuzumab and cetuximab, which block the antiapoptotic signaling from mutated or amplified tyrosine kinases. Unfortunately, not all targeted drugs have proven synergy or even additive in combination with chemotherapy. For no obvious reasons, trials of small molecular weight inhibitors of EGFR and VEGFR with chemotherapy in lung and breast cancer have failed, as have the small molecules that inhibit VEGFR in colon cancer. The reasons for the greater effectiveness of monoclonal antibodies in combination therapy may relate to their additional ability to mobilize components of the immune response, such as complement mediated cytotoxicity or T cell–mediated effects. A further step in targeted therapy will be the use of targeted agents in rational combinations to block parallel pathways that account for resistance to single agents. This issue is more fully discussed in Chapter 29 and in relevant reviews.[35]

Schedule Development in Combination Therapy: Kinetic and Biochemical Considerations

The detailed scheduling of drugs in multidrug regimens was based initially on both practical and theoretical considerations. Intermittent cycles of treatment permit periods of recovery for host bone marrow, gastrointestinal tract, and immune function, with the expectation that recovery of the tumor cell population would be slower than that of the injured normal tissues. A commonly used strategy is to incorporate myelotoxic agents on day 1 of each cycle, while delivering nonmyelosuppressive agents, such as bleomycin, vincristine, prednisone, or high-dose methotrexate with leucovorin rescue, during the period of bone marrow suppression (e.g., on day 8 of a 21-day cycle) to provide continuous suppression of tumor growth while allowing maximum time for marrow recovery.

Cytokinetic considerations also influence the specific sequencing of drugs in combination regimens. S-phase–specific drugs, such as cytosine arabinoside and methotrexate, are capable of killing cells only when they are present during the period of DNA synthesis. Experimentally, these agents are most effective if administered during the period of rapid recovery of DNA synthesis that follows a period of cytoreduction with drugs that are not cell-cycle-phase–specific, such as the bifunctional alkylating agents. Although most of the common anticancer drugs are administered as bolus infusions, continuous infusions provide longer exposure to chemotherapy above the threshold for cytotoxicity and may improve or change the toxicity profile for normal tissues. The R-EPOCH (rituximab, etoposide, prednisone, vincristine, cytoxan, doxorubicin) regimen, in which chemotherapy drugs are given as a 96-hour infusion, has produced impressive rates of long-term disease free survival in Burkitt's lymphoma and other large B cell lymphomas, but with diminished nausea, vomiting, bone marrow suppression, and cardiotoxicity as compared to bolus regimens (CHOP).[36] Similar extended infusion regimens have improved therapeutic ratios for several drugs, including 5-FU, etoposide, ifosfamide, and cytosine arabinoside when these are given as prolonged infusions.[37,38] Constant exposure of cells to cell-cycle-phase–specific agents such as cytosine arabinoside allows a greater fraction of the tumor cell population to be exposed to drug during the sensitive S-phase of the cell cycle, as compared to the more limited exposure after intermittent bolus therapy.[39] The same prolongation of exposure can be achieved by designing prodrugs that are slowly metabolized to the active parent, as accomplished by the capecitabine, an orally administered fluoropyrimidine, or by changing the formulation of the drug, as with liposomal encapsulation of doxorubicin in the doxil formulation.[40] As an added benefit, the cardiotoxicity associated with anthracyclines, which is more closely correlated with the peak concentration than with AUC, is lessened by liposomal preparations of doxorubicin and daunorubicin. These formulations provide the same advantage as prolonged infusion of these drugs, namely low peak concentrations, and decreased cardiotoxicity.

Additional Considerations in Combination Chemotherapy: Overcoming Drug Resistance

Resistance is a complex process involving multiple mechanisms (defective recognition of DNA strand breaks and signaling of apoptosis, drug transporters) that may emerge in parallel or in series. Drug discovery efforts are aimed at taking advantage of these changes in repair or apoptosis. For example, defective DNA double-strand break repairs the fundamental lesion in patients with inherited forms of breast cancer due to mutations in BRCA 1 and BRCA 2. An inhibitor of the PARP-mediated repair of double-strand breaks has significant activity against breast and ovarian cancers in early trials.[7]

Apoptosis is an active, energy-requiring, and protein synthesis–dependent process whereby cells, in response to specific signals, undergo an orderly, programmed series of intracellular events that lead to death. This process is a necessary component of normal development in all multicellular organisms and is required for the maintenance of normal function of many proliferating or renewable tissues such as the lymphatic system. Suppression of apoptosis is a common feature of neoplastic transformation. It may be the direct result of mutation or overexpression of antiapoptotic genes such as bcl-2, as in lymphomas, or indirectly, through activation of growth factor pathways such as the PI3 kinase and epidermal growth factor (EGF) pathways in epithelial cancers or HER-2-neu in breast cancer. Translocation and overexpression of bcl-2 is to the pathogenesis of follicular B-cell lymphomas,[41] but the same gene is commonly overexpressed in epithelial tumors. Activation of other protective factors such as NF-K$_B$ and the PI-3 kinase pathway in response to DNA damage suppresses cytotoxicity of chemotherapy drugs and radiation.[42] Lowe et al.[43] elegantly demonstrated that, in the presence of normal p53, transformation of normal mouse embryo fibroblasts (MEF) with the adenovirus E1A transforming gene (functionally equivalent to loss of c-myc regulation) created a cell line with supersensitivity to doxorubicin, 5-FU, and etoposide, as well as x-irradiation, and that the cells died through the process of apoptosis. MEF cells lacking the p53 gene were resistant to doxorubicin, 5-FU, and etoposide, as well as x-irradiation. This experiment may explain the selectivity of chemotherapeutic agents for malignant cells over nonmalignant cells with similar proliferative rates. It reinforces the results of other studies linking loss of cell-cycle control to resistance to chemotherapeutic agents[44] and offers an explanation for the high rate of inherent resistance of many p53-mutated solid tumors to chemotherapeutic agents (Fig. 1-1). Furthermore, these results suggest potential targets for effectively bypassing the elaborate defense machinery available to the cancer cell. Drugs are currently in development that activate apoptosis (TRAIL receptor agonists), or attack antiapoptotic proteins, such as survivin, XIAP, NFkB, HIF-1 alpha, and the BH3 domain proteins. A drug that inhibits the antiapoptotic bcl-2 has shown activity in treating chronic lymphocytic leukemia.[45]

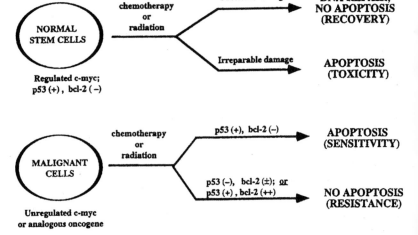

Figure 1-1 Effect of c-myc regulation, p53, and bcl-2 on sensitivity of normal and malignant cells proliferating at comparable rates. (The dose of drug or radiation causing apoptosis of normal stem cells with regulated c-myc is much higher than the dose causing apoptosis of malignant cells with normal p53, but unregulated c-myc or analogous oncogene activation.)

Dose-Intensification Strategies

Dose intensification has received increasing emphasis in recent years as a strategy for overcoming resistance to chemotherapy. Citron et al.[46] have shown that the intensity of conventional treatment, that is, the dose per time unit, correlates with decreased recurrence rates in adjuvant therapy of breast cancer. By decreasing the interval between treatments, using a "dose-dense" regimen, they found improvement in relapse-free survival. Drug-responsive tumors have a steep dose-response curve, a finding that underlies the importance of delivering maximum tolerated doses as rapidly as possible has been emphasized repeatedly. The concept of *dose intensity*, defined as the milligram per square meter of delivered drug per week of therapy, was introduced by Levin and Hryniuk.[47] They retrospectively analyzed the dose intensity of different chemotherapeutic regimens in breast cancer, colon cancer, and ovarian cancer trials and found a correlation between dose intensity and response rates for 5-FU in colon cancer, doxorubicin in breast cancer, and cisplatin in ovarian cancer. Similarly, retrospective analyses of MOPP or related regimens in Hodgkin's disease have concluded that delivered doses of vincristine, alkylators and procarbazine correlate with response rates and disease-free intervals.[48] These studies have been criticized because they are retrospective[47] and because the authors made the arguable assumption that the individual drugs in different regimens made equal contributions to the efficacy of the regimens.

The dose-response relationships discerned from acute leukemia trials[49] constitute strong evidence supporting the role of dose intensity. This concept has been invoked to explain the poorer survival of postadolescent patients with ALL, who often received less intensive therapy than children with the same disease.[49] Thus, while readily tolerable ("standard") doses of combination chemotherapy drugs are sufficient for patients with sensitive tumors, greater dose intensity may be necessary for the subset of patients with less favorable pharmacokinetics or with drug-resistant tumors. The challenge is to develop reliable de novo predictive tumor markers (such as, potentially, *bcl-2* overexpression or mutations in *p53* or k-*ras* genes) or pharmacokinetic parameters that identify patients who will benefit from more intensive therapy. In the absence of such markers, the only alternative is to treat every potentially curable patient with maximally tolerated doses, as established by the published or experimental protocol. The following dosing principles underlie the treatment of Hodgkin's disease,[50] but are broadly applicable to other curable cancers: (a) Do not modify planned doses or schedules of chemotherapy in anticipation of toxicity that has not yet happened, nor for short-term, non–life-threatening toxicity, such as emesis or mild neuropathy. (b) Because significant individual variation may exist in the pharmacokinetics of drugs or in the sensitivity of the bone marrow (and other normal organs) to drug-related toxicity, the granulocyte count should be used as an in vivo biologic assay of the individual dosage limits of myelotoxic agents. In some protocols, dose escalation is built into some protocols to achieve a target nadir of the granulocyte count (usually $<1,000/mm^3$). An alternative strategy for dose intensification is to shorten the interval between courses, as has been done in breast cancer chemotherapy.[46]

Recombinant hematopoietic growth factors can mitigate the bone marrow toxicity of chemotherapy. Granulocyte colony-stimulating factor is effective in decreasing the duration of granulocyte nadir after myelotoxic chemotherapy. Agonists of the thrombopoietin receptor are approved for other indications, and may eventually find a useful role in preventing or reversing thrombocytopenia. However, erythropoietin preparations decrease survival in most settings and should only be used to correct chemotherapy induced anemia with $Hg < 10/mm^3$ in symptomatic patients (see Chapter 38).

High-Dose Chemotherapy

Marrow-ablative dosages of chemotherapy represent the ultimate extrapolation of the dose intensity concept. In practice, it is possible to rescue the host with either autologous bone marrow or peripheral blood stem cells, or with stem cells or marrow from an allogeneic but histocompatible donor. During the past 40 years, this approach has been investigated in many centers as salvage therapy for patients relapsing after primary treatment for leukemias, Hodgkin's and non-Hodgkin's lymphomas, other hematologic malignancies, and testicular cancers. Rescue with marrow from a human leukocyte antigen (HLA)-compatible donor has the advantage of the marrow product being free of malignant cells. Marrow donated by an allogeneic donor also contains T lymphocytes, which generate a beneficial, if not curative graft versus tumor response. The drugs used in these programs cause prolonged myelosuppression as their primary dose-limiting toxicity, but in the setting of marrow transplantation, extramedullary toxicities become limiting. Alkylators such as busulfan, ifosfamide, and cyclophosphamide are prominent in most ablative regimens because characteristically their extramyeloid toxicity becomes dose limiting at twofold to sevenfold higher dosage than the myeloablative dosage. *High-dose regimens exaggerate the extramyeloid toxicities of each drug and introduce new sites of organ damage.* Virtually every organ in the body, including heart, lungs, liver, gastrointestinal epithelium, and the nervous system may suffer significant acute and/or chronic toxicity during high-dose chemotherapy, and the specific patterns of such toxicity, and their reversibility are discussed in relevant chapters.

Randomized trials comparing high-dose regimens with best conventional therapy generally have not proven the value of dose escalation in patients with metastatic solid tumors with the possible exception of relapsed testicular cancer.[51] High-dose regimens with allogeneic bone marrow transplant are curative in approximately 40% to 50% of patients (<65) with acute myeloid leukemia, whereas autologous bone marrow transplant or peripheral blood stem cell transplant regimens are equally effective in drug-responsive Hodgkin's disease in first or second relapse and in intermediate-grade and high-grade non-Hodgkin's lymphoma in first relapse. One should remember that both the acute and the late toxicities of high-dose chemotherapy in both autologous and allogeneic bone marrow transplant regimens are formidable.[52] Opportunistic infection, acute gastrointestinal and pulmonary toxicity, and veno-occlusive disease of the liver result from drug damage to bone marrow, epithelial tissue, and vascular endothelium, respectively, and contribute to acute mortality of high-dose regimens. Later, patients cured of lymphoma may develop chemotherapy-induced acute leukemia and myelodysplasia.[53] Finally, graft versus host disease causes both acute and chronic toxicity, and a fatal outcome, in allograft patients. The overall risk of treatment-related death from allogeneic programs may be as high as 15% to 30%, depending on the age and underlying health of the patient, and the level of match of the donor and host.

Drug Interactions in Combination Chemotherapy: Pharmacokinetic Interactions and Overlapping Toxicity

Specific drug interactions, both favorable and unfavorable, must be considered in developing combination regimens. These interactions may take the form of pharmacokinetic, cytokinetic, or biochemical effects of one drug that influences the pharmacokinetic or pharmacodynamic properties of a second component of a combination. Patterns of overlapping toxicity are a primary concern. Drugs that cause renal toxicity, such as cisplatin, must be used cautiously in combination with other agents (such as methotrexate, the purine analogues, or bleomycin) that depend on renal elimination as their primary mechanism of excretion. It is important to monitor renal function in regimens that incorporate cisplatin with other drugs that are cleared by the kidney, as dose adjustment of the second agent may be necessary to avoid toxicity. The sequence of drug administration may be critical; in many experimental systems, administration of paclitaxel before cisplatin gives additive or synergistic results, whereas the opposite sequence yields antagonism and increased toxicity.[54] Paclitaxel (taxol) delays the clearance of doxorubicin and increases the risk of cardiotoxicity.[55] Traztuzumab and doxorubicin cause incremental cardiac toxicity. Induction of P-450–dependent metabolism by phenytoin or phenobarbital accelerates the clearance of irinotecan, paclitaxel, vincristine, imatinib, and many other "targeted" drugs, and may render standard doses of the cancer drugs ineffective (see Chapter 21). The opposite effect, a diminished clearance of the cancer drugs, results from their combined use with inhibitors of P450, such as ketoconazole. The potential for important interactions between cancer drugs and other medications must always be kept in mind during the routine care of cancer patients.

Biochemical interactions between cancer drugs also may be important considerations in determining the choice of agents and their sequence of administration. Both synergistic and antagonistic interactions have been described. A chemotherapeutic drug may be modulated by a second agent that has no antitumor activity in its own right but that enhances the intracellular activation or target binding of the primary agent or inhibits the repair of lesions produced by the primary drug. The best example of this synergy is the use of leucovorin (5-formyltetrahydrofolate), which itself has no cytotoxic effect but which enhances the affinity of the binding of 5-FU to its target enzyme, thymidylate synthase, by forming a ternary complex among the enzyme, 5-dFUMP, and folate.[56] This combination is more effective clinically than 5-FU alone in colorectal cancer. Other such interactions are described in greater detail in subsequent chapters.

Combination of Chemotherapy with Radiotherapy

A further innovation in the use of antineoplastic drugs is to combine drugs with irradiation. Many clinical protocols have been designed to take advantage of the well-documented synergy between irradiation and drugs with radiosensitizing properties (cetuximab, cisplatin, paclitaxel, hydroxyurea, and 5-FU). The mechanism of synergy differs for each drug and is discussed in detail in specific chapters.

The design of integrated chemotherapy-radiotherapy combinations presents special problems because of the synergistic effects of the two therapies on both normal and malignant tissue. The normal tissue of greatest concern is the bone marrow, although intestinal epithelium, heart, lungs, and brain may also be affected by such interactions.[57] Radiation given to the pelvic or midline abdominal areas produces a decline in blood counts, and a decrease in bone marrow reserve. This can severely compromise the ability to deliver myelotoxic chemotherapy, even months or years after the radiation. Conformal irradiation, administered through multiple portals, narrows the irradiation field around the tumor and preserves a greater portion of the marrow-bearing tissue. For some toxicities, the sequence of administration of drugs and irradiation may be crucial. For example, mediastinal irradiation after combination chemotherapy for massive mediastinal Hodgkin's disease has proven to be practicable and effective. Because the initial chemotherapy results in significant shrinkage of the mediastinal tumor, smaller radiation portals can be used to encompass the residual tumor completely, with proportionately less radiation to lungs and heart. In small cell carcinoma of the lung confined to the thorax, simultaneous administration of radiotherapy and chemotherapy has produced better results than either therapy alone or in sequence.[58] Similarly, simultaneous radiation and chemotherapy is superior to radiotherapy alone in adjuvant therapy for head and neck cancer (with cisplatin and 5-FU), anal cancer (with mitomycin or 5-FU), cervical cancer (with hydroxyurea or cisplatin),[59] and rectal cancer (with 5-FU).[60] Thus, although it is important to consider the cumulative toxicities of chemotherapy and radiation on bone marrow and other vulnerable tissues in the radiation field, the therapeutic benefits of simultaneous irradiation and chemotherapy often outweigh the disadvantages.

Many chemotherapeutic agents greatly potentiate the effects of irradiation and may lead to unacceptable toxicity for organs usually resistant to radiation damage. Doxorubicin sensitizes both normal and malignant cells to radiation damage, possibly because both doxorubicin and x-rays produce free-radical damage to tissues. Doxorubicin adjuvant chemotherapy given in conjunction with irradiation to the left chest wall increases the risk of intense skin reactions and increased cardiac toxicity.[61] Extreme care must be taken in treatment planning to keep the heart out of the radiation field. Similarly, bleomycin and radiation cause synergistic pulmonary toxicity, as does gemcitabine with abdominal irradiation.

A final consideration in the combined use of radiotherapy and chemotherapy is the carcinogenicity of both modalities. Among patients who are cured of their primary tumors, their greatest fear, next to relapse, is a secondary malignancy. In studies of patients cured of Hodgkin's disease, the risk for secondary solid tumors increases significantly after 10 years and into the second and third decades. The cumulative risk for all secondary radiation-induced (i.e., occurring within the radiation portal) solid tumors is approximately 15% at 15 years and may be as high as 20% at 25 years.[62] On the other hand, little evidence exists that concomitant chemotherapy with radiation therapy increases this risk of secondary solid tumors, above the risk caused by radiation alone. The most important chemotherapy-related second malignancy is leukemia due to DNA alkylating or methylating agents. Among the most potently leukemogenic agents are the mustard-type alkylators, nitrosoureas, and procarbazine. The risk for leukemia increases with cumulative dose of alkylators, a fact that must be considered when long-term or high-dose alkylator use is contemplated. Leukemia has been reported after chemotherapy for Hodgkin's disease, non-Hodgkin's lymphoma, breast cancer (adjuvant therapy), ovarian cancer, multiple myeloma, and virtually every kinds of cancer treated with drugs (see Chapter 5). Not all regimens are equally leukemogenic. The risk for myeloid leukemia is not increased after ABVD therapy for Hodgkin's disease. A qualitatively different type of secondary nonlymphocytic leukemia is associated with topoisomerase II inhibitors, including etoposide, teniposide, and doxorubicin.[63] Characteristically, acute myelogenous leukemia associated with topoisomerase II inhibitor therapy has a much shorter latency period (1 to 4 years) than does alkylator-induced leukemia (3 to 7 years), is frequently of the myelomonocytic or monocytic FAB subtypes (M-4 or M-5, respectively), and is associated with reciprocal chromosomal translocations involving the *MLL* gene at chromosome band 11q23. The risk of this type of leukemia is associated with higher total cumulative dose of the topoisomerase II inhibitor and with a weekly or twice-weekly schedule. In addition, the risk may be increased when the topoisomerase II agent is combined with high-dose alkylators or with agents that inhibit DNA repair.

In summary, cancer chemotherapeutic agents have had a profoundly beneficial effect on the well being and survival of patients with cancer. Because these agents have the potential for causing severe or disabling toxicity and yet must be used at maximal dosages to ensure full therapeutic benefit, the physician is literally walking a therapeutic tightrope and must constantly balance gain against likely toxicities. In this effort, every advantage afforded by the physician's knowledge of the patient, the disease, and the drugs must be used to achieve maximum benefit. The foregoing discussion emphasizes that an intimate knowledge of drug action, drug disposition, and drug interactions, as well as late drug effects, is essential to the design and application of effective cancer chemotherapy. Most recently, research is moving the chemotherapy field very rapidly in the direction of personalizing therapy: understanding the biology of each tumor at the molecular level will add highly relevant information, but additional complexity to the challenge of selecting appropriate therapy for individual patients.[7] The essential information for this task is presented in the following chapters on individual drugs and is summarized in the initial tables that describe key features of each agent. This information can only enhance the chances of success in the difficult but rewarding task of treating cancer.

References

1. Greco FA, Vaughn WK, Hainsworth JD. Advanced poorly differentiated carcinoma of unknown primary site: recognition of a treatable syndrome. Ann Intern Med 1986;104:547–553.
2. Kwiatkowski DJ, Harpole DH, Godleski J, et al. Molecular-pathologic substaging in 244 stage I non-small cell lung cancer patients: clinical implications. J Clin Oncol 1998;16:2468–2477.
3. Lynch TJ, Bell DW, Sordella R, et al. Activating mutations in the epidermal growth factor receptor underlying responsiveness of non-small-cell lung cancer to Gefitinib. N Engl J Med 2004;350:2129–2139.
4. Sotiriou C, Pusztai L. Gene-expression signatures in breast cancer. N Engl J Med 2009;360:790–800.
5. Shaw AT, Yeap B, Mino-Kenudson M, et al. Clinical features and outcome of patients with non-small-cell lung cancer harboring EML4-ALK. JCO 2009;27:4232–4235

6. Holleman A, Cheok MH, Den Boer ML, et al. Gene-expression patterns in drug-resistant acute lymphoblastic leukemia cells and response to treatment. N Engl J Med 2004;351:533–542.
7. Chabner BA. Three favorites at ASCO. Oncologist 2009, in press.
8. Skipper HE, Schabel FM Jr, Mellett LB, et al. Implications of biochemical, cytokinetic, pharmacologic, and toxicologic relationships in the design of optimal therapeutic schedules. Cancer Chemother Rep 1970;54:431–450.
9. Fialkow PJ. Clonal origin of human tumors. Biochim Biophys Acta 1976;458:283–321.
10. Chin L, Gray JW. Translating insights from the cancer genome into clinical practice. Nature 2008;452:553–563.
11. Deininger MW, Druker BJ. SR Circumventing imatinib resistance. Cancer Cell 2004;6:108–110.
12. Diehn M, Cho RW, Lobo NA, et al. Association of reactive oxygen species levels and radioresistance in cancer stem cells. Nature 2009;458:780–783.
13. Gurubhagavatula S, Liu G, Park S, et al. XPD and XRCC1 genetic polymorphisms are prognostic factors in advanced non-small-cell lung cancer patients treated with platinum chemotherapy. J Clin Oncol 2004;22:2594–2601.
14. Curt GA, Carney DN, Cowan KH, et al. Unstable methotrexate resistance in human small-cell carcinoma associated with double-minute chromosomes. N Engl J Med 1983;308:199–202.
15. Gorlick R, Goker E, Trippett T, et al. Defective transport is a common mechanism of acquired methotrexate resistance in acute lymphocytic leukemia and is associated with decreased reduced folate carrier expression. Blood 1997;89:1013–1018.
16. Scudiero DA, Meyer SA, Clatterbuck BE, et al. Sensitivity of human cell strains having different abilities to repair O6-methyl guanine in DNA to inactivation by alkylating agents including chloroethyl nitrosoureaus. Cancer Res 1984;44:2467–2474.
17. Hunter C, Smith R, Cahill DP, et al. A hypermutation phenotype and somatic *MSHG* mutations in recurrent human malignant gliomas after alkylator chemotherapy. Cancer Res 2006;66:3987–3991.
18. Druker B. Perspectives on the development of a molecularly targeted agent. Cancer Cell 2002;1:31–36.
19. Gajiwala KS, Wu JC, Christensen J, et al. KIT kinase mutants show unique mechanisms of drug resistance to imatinib and sunitinib in gastrointestinal stromal tumor patients. PNAS 2009;106:1542–1547.
20. Sequist LV, Lynch TJ. EGFR tyrosine kinase inhibitors in lung cancer: an evolving story. Annu Rev Med 2008;59:429–442.
21. Cunningham D, Humblet Y, Siena S, et al. Cetuximab monotherapy and cetuximab plus irinotecan in irinotecan-refractory metastatic colorectal cancer. N Engl J Med 2004;351:337–345.
22. Hande K, Messenger M, Wagner J, et al. Inter- and intrapatient variability in etoposide kinetics with oral and intravenous drug administration. Clin Cancer Res 1999;5(10):2742–2747.
23. Watters JW, Kraja A, Meucci MA, et al. Genome-wide discovery of loci influencing chemotherapy cytotoxicity. PNAS 2004;101:11809–11814.
24. Gamelin E, Delva R, Jacob J, et al. Individual fluorouracil dose adjustment based on pharmacokinetic follow-up compared with conventional dosage: results of a multicenter randomized trial of patients with metastatic colorectal cancer. J Clin Oncol 2008;26:2099–2105.
25. Rice GC, Hoy C, Schimke RT. Transient hypoxia enhances the frequency of DHFR gene amplification in Chinese hamster ovary cells. Proc Natl Acad Sci U S A 1986;83:5978–5982.
26. Sugimoto Y, Tsukahara S, Oh-hara T, et al. Decreased expression of DNA topoisomerase I in camptothecin-resistant tumor cell lines as determined by monoclonal antibody. Cancer Res 1990;50:6925–6930.
27. Ross DD, Doyle LA. Mining our ABCs: pharmacogenomic approach for evaluating transporter function in cancer drug resistance. Cancer Cell 2004;6:105–107.
28. Marie JP, Zittoun R, Sikic BI. Multidrug resistance (mdr1) gene expression in adult acute leukemias: correlation with treatment outcomes and in vitro drug sensitivity. Blood 1991;78:586–592.
29. Lee K, Belinsky MG, Bell DW, et al. Isolation of MOAT-B, a widely expressed multidrug resistance-associated protein/canalicular multispecific organic anion transporter-related transporter. Cancer Res 1998;58:2741–2747.

30. Taniguchi T, Tischkowitz M, Ameziane N, et al. Disruption of the Fanconi anemia-BRCA pathway in cisplatin-sensitive ovarian tumors. Nat Med 2003;9:568–574.

31. Goldie JH, Coldman AJ, Gudanskas GA. Rationale for the use of alternating non-cross-resistant chemotherapy. Cancer Treat Rep 1982;66:439–449.

32. DeVita VT, Hubbard SM, Longo DL. The chemotherapy of lymphomas: looking back, moving forward—The Richard and Hinda Rosenthal Foundation Award Lecture. Cancer Res 1987;47:5810–5824.

33. Gordon LI, Harrington D, Andersen J, et al. Comparison of a second-generation combination chemotherapeutic regimen (m-BACOD) with a standard regimen (CHOP) for advanced diffuse non-Hodgkin's lymphoma. N Engl J Med 1992;327:1342–1349.

34. Connors JM, Klimo P, Adams G, et al. Treatment of advanced Hodgkin's disease with chemotherapy—comparison of MOPP/ABV hybrid regimen with alternating courses of MOPP and ABVD: a report from the National Cancer Institute of Canada clinical trials group. J Clin Oncol 1997;15:2762.

35. Kwak EL, Clark JW, Chabner BA. Targeted agents: the rules of combination. Clin Cancer Res 2007;13:5232–5237.

36. Wilson WH, Dunleavy K, Pittaluga S, et al. Phase II study of dose-adjusted EPOCH and Rituximab in untreated diffuse large B-Cell lymphoma with analysis of Germinal Center and Post-Germinal Center biomarkers. J Clin Oncol 2008;26:2717–2724.

37. Anderson H, Hopwood P, Prendiville J, et al. A randomized study of bolus versus continuous pump infusion of ifosfamide and doxorubicin with oral etoposide for small cell lung cancer. Br J Cancer 1993;67:1385–1390.

38. De Gramont A, Bosset JF, Milan C, et al. Randomized trial comparing monthly low-dose leucovorin and fluorouracil bolus with bimonthly high-dose leucovorin and fluorouracil bolus plus continuous infusion for advanced colorectal cancer: a French intergroup study. J Clin Oncol 1997;15:808–815.

39. Lai GM, Chen YN, Mickley LA, et al. P-glycoprotein expression and schedule dependence of adriamycin cytotoxicity in human colon carcinoma cell lines. Int J Cancer 1991;49:696–703.

40. Cowens JW, Creaven PJ, Greco WR, et al. Initial clinical (phase I) trial of TLC-D-99 (doxorubicin encapsulated in lyposomes). Cancer Res 1993;53:2796–2802.

41. Korsmeyer SJ. Bcl-2 initiates a new category of oncogenes: regulators of cell death. Blood 1992;80:879–886.

42. Green DR, Bissonnette RP, Cotter TG. Apoptosis and cancer. Important Adv Oncol 1994;8:37–52.

43. Lowe SW, Ruley HE, Jacks T, et al. p53-dependent apoptosis modulates the cytotoxicity of anticancer agents. Cell 1993;74:957–967.

44. Kohn KW, Jackman J, O'Connor PM. Cell cycle control and cancer chemotherapy. J Cell Biochem 1994;54:440–452.

45. Denicourt C, Dowdy SF. Medicine: targeting apoptotic pathways in cancer. Science 2004;305:1411–1413.

46. Citron ML, Berry DA, Cirrincione C, et al. Randomized trial of dose-dense versus conventionally scheduled and sequential versus concurrent combination chemotherapy as postoperative adjuvant treatment of node-positive primary breast cancer: first report of Intergroup Trial C9741/Cancer and Leukemia Group B Trial 9741. J Clin Oncol 2003;21:2226.

47. Levin L, Hryniuk WM. Dose intensity analysis of chemotherapy regimens in ovarian carcinoma. J Clin Oncol 1987;5:756–767.

48. Longo DL, Young RC, Wesley M, et al. Twenty years of MOPP therapy for Hodgkin's disease. J Clin Oncol 1986;4:1295–1306.

49. Moghrabi A, Levy DE, Asselin B, et al. Results of the Dana-Farber Cancer Institute ALL Consortium Protocol 95-01 for children with acute lymphoblastic leukemia. Blood 2007;109:896–904.

50. Kaufman D, Longo DL. Hodgkin's disease. Crit Rev Oncol Hematol 1992;13:135–187.

51. Droz J-P, Kramar A, Biron P, et al. Failure of high-dose cyclophosphamide and etoposide combined with double-dose cisplation and bone marrow support in patients with high-volume metastatic nonseminomatous germ-cell tumours: mature results of a randomised trial. Eur Urol 2007;51:739–748.

52. Socié G, Stone JV, Wingard JR, et al. Long term survival and late deaths after allogeneic bone marrow transplantation. N Engl J Med 1999;341:14–21.

53. Howe R, Micallef INM, Inwards DJ, et al. Secondary myelodysplastic syndrome and acute myelogenous leukemia are significant complications following autologous stem cell transplantation for lymphoma. Bone Marrow Transplant 2003;32:317–324.

54. Liebmann J, Fisher J, Teague D, et al. Sequence dependence of paclitaxel (Taxol®) combined with cisplatin or alkylators in human cancer cells. Oncol Res 1994;6:25–31.

55. Holmes FA, Rowinsky EK. Pharmacokinetic profiles of doxorubicin in combination with taxanes. Semin Oncol 2001;28(Suppl 12):8–14.

56. Sotos GA, Grogan L, Allegra CJ. Preclinical and clinical aspects of biomodulation of 5-fluorouracil. Cancer Treat Rev 1994;20:11–49.

57. Pihkala J, Saarinen UM, Lundstrom U, et al. Myocardial function in children and adolescents after therapy with anthracyclines and chest irradiation. Eur J Cancer 1996;32A:97–103.

58. Bunn PA, Lichter AS, Makuch RW, et al. Chemotherapy alone or chemotherapy plus chest radiation therapy in limited-stage small-cell lung cancer. Ann Intern Med 1987;106:655–662.

59. Rose PG, Bundy BN, Watkins EB, et al. Concurrent cisplatin-based chemoradiation improves progression-free and overall survival in advanced cervical cancer: results of a randomized Gynecologic Oncology Group study. N Engl J Med 1999;340:1144–1153.

60. Fisher B, Wolmark N, Rockette H, et al. Postoperative adjuvant chemotherapy or radiation therapy for rectal cancer: results from NSABP protocol R-01. J Natl Cancer Inst 1988;80:21–29.

61. Shapiro CL, Harrigan Hardenbergh P, Gelman R, et al. Cardiac effects in adjuvant doxorubicin and radiation therapy in breast cancer patients. J Clin Oncol 1998;16:3493–3501.

62. Lavey RS, Eby NL, Prosnitz LR. Impact on second malignancy risk of the combined use of radiation and chemotherapy for lymphomas. Cancer 1990;66:80–88.

63. Pui CH, Ribeiro RC, Hancock ML, et al. Acute myeloid leukemia in children treated with epipodophylotoxins for acute lymphoblastic leukemia. N Engl J Med 1991;321:1682–1687.

Target Identification and Drug Discovery

Shannon Decker, Melinda Hollingshead, Robert Shoemaker, and Edward A. Sausville

This chapter provides an overview of three stages of the preclinical development of an anticancer drug. The first stage is the identification of a drug target. Numerous approaches for target identification exist ranging from biologically based ones to newer chemogenomics- and RNA interference–based techniques. The second stage is the discovery of an active drug candidate with therapeutic potential and the selection of the optimal candidate or limited set of candidates for further evaluation. These studies would also ideally allow an assessment of how the new molecule differs from currently available therapeutic agents. In the third stage, early preclinical development is directed at increasing confidence that the drug lead will actually function as a useful therapeutic agent in humans. These studies focus predominantly on eliciting activity in animal models of cancer and ideally correlate the degree of antitumor activity with the pharmacology of the drug.

Cancer Drug Target Selection

Within the past 15 years, the approach to the discovery and development of cancer drugs has undergone a marked change, from focusing classically on empirical antiproliferative activity as a basis for initial interest in a compound, to selecting drug candidates on the basis of their capacity to modulate molecular targets that are important in cancer pathophysiology. Modern approaches to identifying targets include specific departure from our understanding of cancer cell biology, efforts to "retrofit" active molecules for which target knowledge is uncertain, and approaches derived from newer techniques such as chemogenomics and RNA interference.

Biologically Based Approaches

Our current view of the cancer cell leads to the view that by the time a cancer is clinically manifest in a patient, a number of genetic lesions have occurred in the tumor, resulting in discrete sets of abnormalities that may differ in detail from tumor to tumor, but exist as categories of molecular defects common to essentially all tumor types. This idea, articulated elegantly by Hanahan and Weinberg,[1] points to deregulated proliferation-control pathways, loss of tumor suppressor gene function, loss of functions that would promote tumor cell programmed death (apoptosis), acquisition of limitless replication potential through telomere-replicating strategies, activation of host angiogenesis, and the capacity to invade into normal stroma as attributes of all tumors. To these features must be added the capacity of tumors to thwart the host immune system (e.g., Uttenhoeve et al.[2]). Of special importance to cancer drug discovery is the existence of different degrees of deregulated DNA repair processes, perhaps as a way of tolerating mutational events in the life history of a particular tumor. The result is a potential vulnerability to DNA-damaging agents. This is exemplified by increased susceptibility of cells with lesions in the ERCC1 (excision repair nucleus) to platinum.[3] Each of the specific molecules or pathways creating the altered cellular state that underlies tumor cell biology as compared to the normal cell could conceivably be a target for cancer drug discovery and development.

Those molecules consistently mutated in the course of the development of cancer in patients can be thought of as defined by nature as important in the pathophysiology of that tumor and can be characterized as *pathogenic targets*. These molecules may come to attention not only by point mutations in their coding sequence but also by their proximity to frequently observed chromosomal breaks points or regions of DNA amplification in tumors. Examples of molecules of this type that have been already validated as cancer drug targets include the p210[bcr/abl] oncoprotein of chronic myelogenous leukemia[4] and the *HER-2-neu* tyrosine kinase[5] that is frequently detected by genomic amplification in breast carcinoma. Approved drugs directed at these targets include imatinib and the monoclonal antibody trastuzumab, respectively. In validation of this way of thinking, patients enjoying the best clinical response to the epidermal growth factor receptor tyrosine kinase inhibitors erlotinib and gefitinib possess a mutated, activated form of the agent's target kinase.[6-8] Alternatively, the drug target could be downstream of a mutationally activated oncoprotein. This is exemplified by the observations of Settleman et al. that among cell lines highly sensitive to inhibitors of B-raf are not only the expected B-raf mutant bearing lines but also those with amplified N-ras.[9] In either event, mutational activation of a pathway defines a state of "oncogene addiction" that is the basis for strategic design of approaches to intervene pharmacologically by inhibitor design.[10]

Ontologic targets relate to the normal tissue of origin of the tumor. Examples of validated targets of this type include the estrogen or androgen receptors in breast or prostate cancer, respectively, and the CD20 cell surface determinant of non-Hodgkin's lymphoma. *Pharmacologic* targets relate to the pharmacokinetic or pharmacology names of a drug itself. For example, dihydropyrimidine dehydrogenase is a target whose degree of activity modulates susceptibility and toxicity of fluorinated pyrimidines, or dexrazoxane modulates levels of free iron, a "target" that modulates the cardiotoxic potential of anthracyclines. *Stromal or microenvironmental* targets include the large array of molecules responsible for sculpting tumor stroma and supporting cell framework including mediators of angiogenesis.

The regulatory approval of bevacizumab, a monoclonal antibody to vascular endothelial growth factor (VEGF),[11] presaged the intense clinical trials activities leading to the approval of the "small" molecule multitarget kinase inhibitors such as sorafenib and sunitinib that also target VEGF-R signaling. Immunologic strategies, including immunomodulating cytokines or even vaccines, might be considered as special cases ultimately directed at the tumor microenvironment.

Another concept that is potentially important in the identification of targets is that of "synthetic lethality," which has been well articulated by Kaelin.[12] In essence, mirroring findings from yeast genetics, two genes are "synthetic lethal" if mutation of both genes results in cell death even though mutation of either alone is compatible with cell viability. This approach envisions the identification of target genes that are synthetic lethal to a mutation relevant only to cancer cells, leaving normal cells viable. Synthetic lethal screening may also allow the identification of compounds with selective toxicity to cells bearing mutational or other silencing of genes, particularly relevant to modulators of tumor suppressor gene pathways, frequently deregulated in cancer through loss of the tumor suppressor loci. Synthetic lethal screening has become an important concept in RNA interference screening techniques discussed below.

The many approaches to target identification defined above derive from a growing understanding of cancer cell biology and have actually created a wealth of potential cancer drug targets. Indeed, extensive efforts to define potential targets with altered expression pattern in tumors have been made available through publicly funded (e.g., the Cancer Genome Anatomy Project; see http://cgap.nci.nih.gov/) and privately maintained databases. A major question is, how might these targets be prioritized?

The argument for a particular target is strengthened when a phenotype related to tumor behavior can be modulated in cell models (antisense, small interfering RNA, dominant negatives, or ribozyme approaches) or in animal models (knock-outs or transgenics) by genetic approaches to altering the presence or function of a tumor target. For example, topoisomerase IIIβ knock-out mice exhibit premature senescence, which suggests that the use of a topoisomerase poison, specific for that isoform, would drive tumor cells toward senescence.[13]

Other practical criteria that influence the suitability for selection of a molecular target for a drug discovery campaign include the availability (and cost) of reagents to allow screening of leads and the identification of an assay format that is amenable to high-throughput screening (HTS). Finally, the size of the patient population (market) and availability of effective treatments for a particular cancer are usually considered before investing resources toward a new target.

"Retrofitting" Active Molecules

Rather than starting from the tumor cell to find a target and a drug affecting the target, some have approached target identification by starting from or "retrofitting" active molecules. For example, geldanamycin and other benzoquinone ansamycins had been known for many years to have activity in empirical antiproliferative assays. Neckers et al. prepared a solid-phase immobilized geldanamycin derivative and used affinity precipitation in a search for molecular targets, ultimately identifying the heat-shock protein 90 (HSP90).[14] Not only did this identify a target for the geldanamycins, but this work also helped spawn further drug discovery efforts for other HSP90 inhibitors. Similarly, the immunosuppressive drug rapamycin was known to interfere with the progression from G1 to S phase, but the pathway was not known. Sabers et al. used an affinity matrix of glutathione-S-transferase, rapamycin's intracellular receptor FKBP12, and rapamycin in the isolation of mammalian targets of rapamycin (mTOR), the biology of which has now been extensively studied and exploited for drug discovery efforts.[15] The fumagillin derivative TNP-470 was the subject of intense efforts to develop an effective antiangiogenic agent, although little was known of its molecular mechanism of action. Human umbilical venous endothelial cells were incubated with a fumagillin derivative complexed with biotin to test the hypothesis that fumagillin was forming an adduct with a cellular protein, from which efforts the methionyl aminopeptidases were identified as targets.[16]

In addition to efforts to identify targets for single active agents, computational methods have also been employed for target identification. As described later in this chapter, in the National Cancer Institute (NCI) 60 cell line screen, various pattern recognition algorithms have been used to compare the patterns of activity of known active compounds with the levels of expression of various molecular targets in the cell lines. The identified putative targets associated with a compound's action can then serve as a starting point to deconvolute the basis for compound action for further drug discovery efforts. A more modern successor to this approach uses even larger groups (e.g., 500) of cell lines,[9] but they are ones which screen for compound activity in a way that annotates target or target pathway activation status.

Newer Technologies

Newer technologies such as chemogenomics and RNA interference have also come to the forefront for target identification. These techniques also have potentially broad utility for other aspects of drug discovery and lead into the discussion of screening strategies.

Chemogenomics has been described by some as discovery and association of all possible drugs with all possible drug targets,[17] involving the combination of modern genomic technologies with the effects of compounds on biological targets.[18] A chemical genetics application would use small molecules to probe the functions of proteins by adding a library of small molecules to cells, selecting the molecules producing the desired phenotype and identifying the protein bound by the molecules.[19] This technique can also be reversed to use the small molecules to further understand the identified protein. The Broad Institute of Harvard and MIT is home to the NCI-funded Initiative for Chemical Genetics, a public access research facility whose data utilizing several aspects of this approach are deposited into the ChemBank web site (http://chembank.broad.harvard.edu/).

RNA interference was first recognized after seeking to define mechanisms for regulating gene expression in model invertebrate systems such as worms, flies, or plants. More detailed discussions of the mechanisms related to RNA interference are summarized elsewhere.[20,21] Briefly (Fig. 2-1), expression of a double-stranded "short interfering RNA" (siRNA), one strand of which has homology to a target sequence in the mRNA of a gene of interest, allows a complex to be formed with the target cellular RNA and act as a degradation mechanism through engagement of the RNA-induced

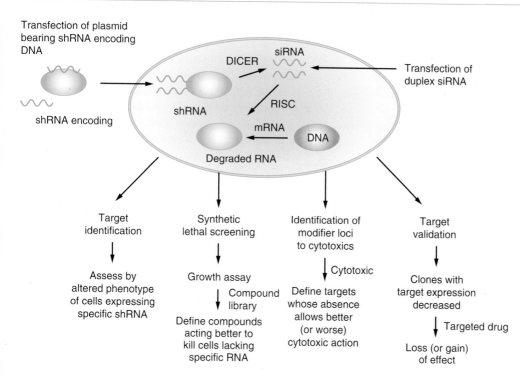

Transfection of plasmid bearing shRNA encoding DNA

shRNA encoding

siRNA

DICER

Transfection of duplex siRNA

shRNA

RISC

mRNA

DNA

Degraded RNA

Target identification

Assess by altered phenotype of cells expressing specific shRNA

Synthetic lethal screening

Growth assay

Compound library

Define compounds acting better to kill cells lacking specific RNA

Identification of modifier loci to cytotoxics

Cytotoxic

Define targets whose absence allows better (or worse) cytotoxic action

Target validation

Clones with target expression decreased

Targeted drug

Loss (or gain) of effect

FIGURE 2-1 siRNA and its potential applications.

silencing complex (RISC), to result in loss of mRNAs bearing the target sequence. SiRNAs may be introduced directly into cells, or result from cleavage from "short hairpin RNAs" (shRNAs) arising from introduced plasmid DNA sequences and acted upon by cellular RNAses to cleave a spacer RNA forming the hairpin between the two stretches of complementary RNA. RNA interference technology has utility in virtually all aspects of cancer drug discovery, and is a basis for many recent innovative screening strategies, specifically reviewed in Iorns et al.[22] Specific uses include target identification, synthetic lethal screening, exploration of drug sensitization or resistance mechanisms, and target validation.

For target identification, a single siRNA, or libraries of siRNAs representing a variety of potential targets, alters a cellular phenotype, for example, proliferative state, invasive capacity, survival, etc. and discloses whether the target(s) altered after expression or action of the siRNA(s) modulates the phenotype. In that event, screening strategies to define modulators of target function can then be designed. This effort can result in an assessment of targets in a particular disease context. For example, utilizing siRNA-based technology, Woo et al. identified "driver genes" in hepatocellular carcinoma, each of which might now be considered in a campaign to define hepatocellular carcinoma-related drugs.[23] Specific targets relevant to the action of specific candidate drugs can also be usefully highlighted by siRNA technology. For example, Tetsu and McCormick utilized siRNAs to cyclin-dependent kinase 2 (CDK2) to reveal little impact of removing that target, and offered the point of view therefore that CDK2 might not be a suitable cancer drug target.[24] This outcome actually reveals a limitation of siRNA screening, as target classes such as CDKs with redundancy of function in different family members might not be highlighted as potentially valuable target classes if only a single representative of the class is targeted. In contrast, for example, Ludwig et al. utilized siRNA-based approaches to validate that NSC73306 is a putative first in class multidrug-resistance targeted agent that actually depends for its action on the expression of mdr1.[25] A particularly important

aspect of this strategy is the design of control or "counterscreens" to assure that the siRNA is functioning as a specific indicator of target action across a range of cellular contexts related to eventual use of the drug candidate.

The concept of "synthetic lethality" in cancer drug screening was discussed generally above. In approaches of this type utilizing RNA interference, siRNA-mediated downmodulation of a target can result in the acquisition of sensitivity to drug action, therefore linking the action of the drug to the presence of the target. A classical demonstration of the relevance of siRNA-related synthetic lethal screens emerged from the observation that cells deficient in BRCA-1 were highly sensitive to concomitant poly(ADP-ribose) polymerase (PARP) inhibition,[26] owing to the inability to repair DNA lesions utilizing homologous recombination. This logically leads to potential value of utilizing cells deficient in various DNA repair enzymes and repair-related signaling systems to identify additional determinants of sensitivity to PARP inhibitors.[27,28] Other examples of this application relate to the definition of target alliance to newly defined compound action, such as the recent demonstration that apoptosis was mediated by Candida spongiolide protein kinase R function.[29] In a variation of this approach, modulation of a pathway's activation by specific siRNAs may either be mimicked by a compound or a compound class, thus identifying the compound as mechanistically involving the pathway in its action. Exemplifying this approach, Gaither et al. identified siRNAs that conveyed resistance to the "second mitochondrial-derived activator of caspases" (Smac) mimetic compound LBW242 (a putative modulator of apoptotic effect), and found that entities conveying such resistance were members of the TNF-α pathway as well as X-linked inhibitors of apoptosis (XIAP).[30]

Synthetic lethal screening can also focus on pathways that are modulated by the action of a siRNA or, more commonly, libraries of siRNAs. Alternatively, as also reviewed comprehensively by Gaither,[18] synthetic lethal screens may provide critical information about genes or set of genes modulated by the novel compound.

SiRNA-based screening approaches can also be used to define pathway members that in a specific disease context serve as a basis for maintaining disease phenotype and therefore could serve as putative targets for drug discovery, as exemplified by modulation of the NFκB pathway in large B-cell lymphoma activated B-cell phenotype as defined by Ngo et al.[31]

Conceptually allied to synthetic lethal screening in "discovery" campaigns, siRNA-related screens have defined important aspects of drug sensitization or resistance mechanisms related to the use of established agents in a way that could lead to a more focused use of the agent. For example, Whitehurst et al. identified numerous genes apparently conveying greatly enhanced sensitivity to paclitaxel.[32] Bartz et al. analogously defined genes conveying enhanced sensitivity to cisplatin, gemcitabine, and paclitaxel.[33]

Of critical importance to industrial prioritization in drug discovery and development campaigns is target validation, the clear demonstration that a potential target has relevance to disease mechanisms in vivo. Classical xenograft models discussed elsewhere in this chapter are frequently ambiguous in conveying enthusiasm for the development of a compound class. However, siRNA-based approaches can be utilized to create in vivo models that convey forcefully the importance of target function. For example, Hoeflich et al. demonstrated in melanoma models in mice that shRNAs to mutated B-raf,[34] in this case expressed through tetracycline-responsive promoter elements, impaired growth of the model, a finding that certainly encouraged discovery of B-raf inhibitors.

Defining an Active Drug Candidate

Initial recognition of a lead compound can come from a purely molecularly targeted screen, directed against a purified enzyme or a cell engineered to overexpress or underexpress a particular target, or through a chemogenomic or siRNA-based activity described above, or from a cell- or animal-model–based antiproliferative screen, against naturally occurring or engineered tumor cells. Each screening model has its distinct advantages and disadvantages. The molecular targeted approach may yield a drug candidate with clear selectivity for a particular target, but then target modulation must be documented in a cellular context, hopefully with evidence of

useful antitumor activity. Ideally, constant evidence of effects "on target" can be an important aid to lead optimization. Cell-based screens have the advantage that drug candidates defined by this route have the ability to distribute across plasma membranes and survive in the intracellular milieu. On the other hand, their mechanism of action must be determined prior to efficient lead optimization, and cell-based screens are less frequently amenable to high-throughput approaches. In contrast, pure in vitro biochemical molecular targeted screens have the attraction of being very amenable to the screening of large collections of molecules.

Figure 2-2 illustrates the generic process of high-throughput, molecular targeted screening (HTS). The process requires initial identification and validation of a target, followed by development and characterization of an assay suitable for HTS. This assay is then used to screen chemical collections or "libraries" to identify active samples that are the focus of additional testing to establish potency, selectivity, and other features important for further development. Screening is typically conducted in a "campaign" mode, with primary screening data from a particular library evaluated after the whole library has been tested. Criteria for activity are frequently established such that a "hit rate" on the order of 1% is obtained. Thus, for a library of 100,000 samples, 1,000 of the most active samples would be selected for the confirmatory testing. Efficient testing has often demanded that the primary screen is conducted at a single concentration, although some researchers are now popularizing quantitative high-throughput screening ("qHTS") testing multiple concentration on 384- and 1,536-well plates.[35] Confirmatory testing may be done using the same protocol or may be done in a more traditional concentration-response fashion to facilitate subsequent consideration of screening leads in the context of potency.

Sources of Diversity for Lead Identification

A crucial issue in any screening project for new anticancer drugs is the acquisition of compound libraries. Whether the initial screen is a target-directed biochemical screen or an empirical antiproliferation screen, the greater the structural diversity in the set of molecules examined, the more likely a novel inhibitor will be identified. Historically, natural products, defined here as extracts from plants, microbial, and animal sources, have provided an excellent source of bioactive molecules with novel structures and mecha-

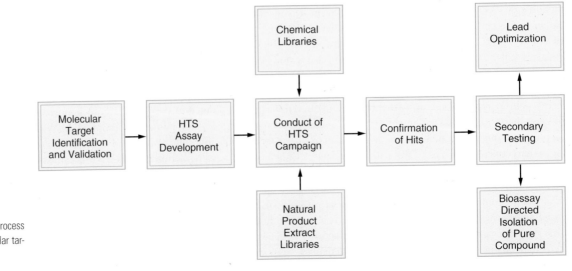

FIGURE 2-2 Generic process for high-throughput molecular targeted drug discovery.

nisms of action. In cancer treatment, natural products constitute several major therapeutic classes including the vinca alkaloids, camptothecins, and taxanes. Natural product extracts as sources for cancer drug discovery have been extensively reviewed[36-38] and are not discussed further here. More recently, collections or libraries of synthetic compounds have gained prominence in anticancer drug discovery efforts.

Again, there are distinct advantages to each type of compound source. Synthetic compound libraries consist of easily identified single compounds and are usually amenable to assignment of activity to a unique chemical structure by a facile deconvolution algorithm. On the other hand, they are limited by the pharmacophore(s) around which the library has been constructed. Although natural product extracts have the possibility of remarkable diversity and stereochemically unique scaffolds, in some cases they require reacquisition from rather exotic ecological niches, optimization of fermentation or extraction approaches, and deconvolution of the active molecule(s) in the extract before the lead can be meaningfully pursued. The first step is the assignment of a structure for the active principle, often a tedious and challenging process. These strengths and limitations must be carefully considered when evaluating sources for screening endeavors.

The number and variety of synthetic compounds available for screening endeavors has been magnified by the use of combinational chemistry. The method of deliberately synthesizing more than one compound as a result of a single reaction began approximately 25 years ago with the synthesis by Geysen et al.[39] of multiple peptides on polyethylene rods. These early endeavors, confined to the synthesis of small peptide libraries, were of limited value to cancer drug discovery because peptides tend not to enter cells and generally are not suitable drug candidates. Subsequent advances in the field included development of more efficient ways to track the compounds, use of a greater number of scaffolds on which to construct libraries, and use of a wider variety of reagents and amenable reaction conditions. Now, combinatorial chemistry provides an efficient method of exploring chemical space in a focused manner and, when applicable, an excellent means of rapidly defining structure activity relationships around active compounds. A somewhat newer trend is the use of "fragment libraries" where chemical fragments with potentially drug-like properties are screened at high concentrations to find scaffolds that are then chemically elaborated to increase potency.[40,41]

Advances in computer-based analysis of the physical properties and interactions of a novel, active compound have provided powerful tools for the pursuit of new anticancer drugs. Medicinal chemists traditionally have used parameters such as steric bulk, hydrogen-bonding ability, and hydrophobic interactions in the design of new drugs. The target pharmacophore now can be further refined by supplementing the information from these physical properties with biologic factors such as the crystal or solution structure of the target enzyme or receptor, the nature of the ligand, and the mechanism of the target-ligand (or target-inhibitor) interaction. Moreover, computer programs can create "virtual libraries," which can be evaluated for exploring biochemical, functional space and the fit of proposed structure into that space. The use of computer models to design and filter novel structures can be a very efficient mechanism to increase the odds of identifying a potent and selective inhibitor of a well-defined target as recently exemplified by Keiser et al.[42]

Compound Libraries

Over the years, collections of pure compounds and natural product extracts coalesced into libraries, arrayed into 96-well plates or 384-well plates suitable for HTS. Popular commercial libraries are available from ChemBridge Corp. (San Diego, CA), Maybridge (Cornwall, England), and Sigma-Aldrich (St. Louis, MO; notably the Library of Pharmacologically Active Compounds or LOPAC), many of which may be cost prohibitive for academic researchers. Additional smaller collections of compounds are commercially available from an assortment of other suppliers. The NCI Open Source Repository (OSR) of approximately 250,000 samples is the publicly available subset of the compounds obtained by the NCI Developmental Therapeutics Program (DTP) over the past 50 years for use in anticancer drug screening (http://dtp.nci.nih.gov). Smaller subsets of the DTP collection, including diversity sets and collections of approved oncology agents, are also available; for both nonprofit and small business entities (costs are limited to shipping).

A major challenge for all suppliers of compounds is authentication of the structure and quantification of the purity of library materials. For the costlier commercial collections, one can expect suppliers to have undertaken appropriate quality control measures. Most compound sets derived from historical libraries of compounds show evidence of the toils of time, storage conditions, and questionable provenance. Most samples in the NCI compound repository were donated by academic chemists or industrial organizations, were accepted without further chemical characterization, and were stored at room temperature unless other conditions were specified by the supplier. As a result, the samples in this collection range in quality from those with a very high degree of sample integrity (purity and authenticity of structure) to those with little or none of the substance indicated by the supplier actually in the bottle. For such collections, verifying the structure and purity of selected "active" compounds may be easier than characterizing the entire library.

Numerous algorithms exist by which the diversity of a set of compound structures can be measured; however, little agreement is found regarding the best approach. In general, software programs partition libraries into a uniform array of blocks or cells on the basis of descriptor coordinates, and the number of cells is proportional to the level of diversity. Some algorithms define atom pair fingerprints, which indicate the presence or absence of pairs of atom types separated by a defined number of bonds, and use them to describe and differentiate each structure. Other algorithms cluster structures into groups; the Jarvis-Patrick clustering algorithm requires that each member of a cluster have in common a predefined number of chemical neighbors.[43] The similar Hodes clustering model has been used by the NCI to assess structural novelty of new compounds submitted for screening.[44] Often, the goal of these computer algorithms is to define a library of the smallest number of compounds that covers the greatest diversity of "molecular space." Using these approaches, large collections of compounds can be winnowed into smaller sublibraries. However, detractors point out that by using these, for the most part, unproven tools and limiting the compounds screened, one risks decreasing the chance of finding drug leads. On the other hand, the economics of HTS calls for prudent use of reagents and encourages the use of such approaches.

A detailed analysis of the NCI OSR was conducted, with special emphasis on the uniqueness of the library relative to commercial libraries and other databases.[45] Substantial chemical diversity is present in the NCI repository, which has generated a subset of the OSR containing approximately 140,000 compounds arrayed into multi-well plates. The inventory for most of the remaining compounds is simply too small for these compounds to be provided for routine screening campaigns. Notwithstanding, the plated version of the NCI OSR is a unique publicly available (see http://dtp.nci.nih.gov) resource that includes many unique compounds. In an attempt to provide the structural diversity of the OSR in a smaller package, further subsets of the compounds (Diversity Sets I and II) have been selected based on an attempt to span the entire map of structural space.[46] The original Diversity Set has found application in pilot-scale screening to support HTS assay development and has yielded interesting lead compounds from a variety of molecular targeted screens.[47–49]

High-Throughput Screening Assay Design

To screen for inhibitors or activators of a given molecular target, the activity of the target protein or other system (cells, pathways in cells, etc.) must be linked to a readily detectable readout. Commonly used types of screening assays can be loosely divided into two categories: separation based, in which starting material must be removed before the product can be detected, and homogeneous, in which separation of the starting material and the product is not required. Examples of separation-based protocols include filter-binding assays in which the product is selectively retained by the filter (usually an ion-exchange media) and precipitation assays during which one component is selectively precipitated and removed by a glass fiber filter. When used as a screening assay, enzyme-linked immunosorbent assays are generally considered to be separation based. Some techniques that are classified as homogeneous assays include fluorescence polarization, fluorescent resonance energy transfer, scintillation proximity, and luminescent proximity (APLHA Screen). Other homogeneous assays measure changes in light absorbance (UV/vis), in the activity of luciferase, or in the expression of green fluorescent or other related proteins. In general, the throughput of samples with homogeneous assays is much higher than with separation-based assays because the latter require secondary manipulation of the samples.

Within these categories, the assays can be further divided into cell based and in vitro (cell free). Cell-based assays measure the ability of a compound to affect a target within the milieu of an intact cell, whereas cell-free assays measure interaction with a purified protein. A strength of cell-based assays is the ability to detect inhibitors of an entire targeted pathway (as opposed to a particular step in a pathway). Limitations of cell-based assays include the need to subsequently define the identity of the actual target within the pathway, interference from toxic compounds, and inability to test compounds that cannot penetrate the cell (although this latter feature can also be viewed as an advantage). In comparison, cell-free screening assays are limited neither by cell permeability of compounds nor by nontargeted compound toxicity. As an initial assay, aimed at identifying a lead "hit," a cell-free assay is usually preferred. When possible, it can be very informative to screen a selected target in both cell-based and in vitro assay systems because their strengths are complementary.

Common Issues in High-Throughput Screening Implementation

A major restriction to the development of new HTS assays has been the acquisition and standardization of reagents. Even with substantial miniaturization, many molecularly targeted screens require much more target protein (and/or many more cells) than is needed for basic research on the target. It is essential that sufficient reagents are available for the entire screening effort to avoid batch-to-batch variation. Also, many of the newer, highly sensitive technologies, although affordable on a small scale, become prohibitively expensive when screening large libraries. The availability and cost of reagents can be pivotal factors in deciding whether to screen a selected target.

An ideal assay plate design includes untreated, negative control well and wells with compound or condition known to affect the target (positive controls). These provide clear definition of the maximum and minimum signal on an individual plate and, therefore, the window in which compound activity can be measured. However, when studying a newly identified and incompletely characterized target, a specific inhibitor (or activator) may not be known. For some targets, a more generic method of inhibition can be used in the absence of a specific inhibitor (e.g., ethylene diamine tetraacetic acid [EDTA] inhibits most metal-dependent enzymes). The reproducibility among the control wells within a plate and the reproducibility of the control wells among the plates within a set are indicative of the quality of the screen. Once a new screening assay has been designed and standardized, it is important to characterize its performance by completing pilot-scale screens. For example, application of a consistent set of "training compounds" of different structural types can provide a quantitative measure of the reproducibility of the assay, sometimes even leading to the identification of intriguing lead.[46,49] In establishing a cell-free screening system, it is necessary to define the biochemical features of the target, including the kinetics of interaction with natural substrates, cofactor requirements, pH optima, and reaction product.

Chemoinformatics: Lead Identification

The goal of any molecularly targeted screen is to identify inhibitors (or activators, in some cases) of a particular protein or pathway, and it is a sine qua non of such exercises to distinguish real "hits" from false positives. Two primary factors to consider are the overall quality of the screening data and the definition of a hit. The most common metric to quantify the suitability or quality of the assay is known as Z' and is defined by the following equation[50]:

$$Z' = \frac{1 - [(3\sigma_\mathrm{p} - 3\sigma_\mathrm{n})]}{\mu_\mathrm{p} - \mu_\mathrm{n}}$$

In this equation, μ is the mean value of the positive and negative controls for the assay and σ is the standard deviation of these values. Assays for which $Z' > 0.5$ are considered acceptable for HTS.

There are three commonly used strategies for selecting active compounds for secondary analysis: (a) to select all compounds displaying a particular level, or range of activity; (b) to select all compounds with activity that falls outside a designated level of deviation from the mean; and (c) to select a particular number of compounds

Intravenous Tumor (Disseminated Tumor)

Disseminated tumor models in which intravenously injected tumor cells colonize the lungs and other tissues offer another method for evaluating agents effective in the later stages of metastasis. One of the most widely used of the disseminated tumor models is the murine melanoma, B16-BL6.[95] The B16-BL6 melanoma is able to metastasize from a primary subcutaneous site as well as following intravenous injection. Thus, the same tumor cell can be used to assess both upstream and downstream events in the metastatic process. This model has been utilized successfully to evaluate a matrix metalloproteinase inhibitor designed to inhibit basement membrane degradation.[96] Although not as well characterized as B16-BL6, other human xenograft models cells produce disseminated disease in immune-deficient mice, particularly SCID mice. Examples of human tumor cell lines producing this effect are LOX melanoma, SK-MEL-28 melanoma, K562 chronic myelogenous leukemia, AS-283 AIDS-related lymphoma, and A549 lung tumor.[97] Problems with the disseminated models include the need for reproducible intravenous inoculations in rodents and the inability to identify the exact cause for reduction in lung or other organ colonization.

Antiangiogenic Agents

Recognition of the important role of angiogenesis on tumor growth and metastasis has led to the development of specific antiangiogenic assays. Various in vitro assays can assess the impact of a therapeutic agent on endothelial cell proliferation, migration, and cord formation.[98] These assays help delineate the mechanism of action for a potential therapeutic, but they may not show activity with all agents. Compounds whose effects are mediated through a secondary mechanism, such as cytokine induction, would not demonstrate effects in these in vitro assays. For in vivo studies, many laboratories use the chicken chorioallantoic membrane as a substrate to assess antiangiogenic agents.[99] This is a more complex assay than the in vitro assays, but it still lacks several features of human neoplasia. These differences include (a) it is not mammalian, (b) it is embryonic, (c) it does not emulate the tumor angiogenesis microenvironment, (d) it is only semiquantitative, and (e) it may not measure clinically relevant activity.

Various in vivo models are described that measure the growth of blood vessels into an exogenous substrate. Although various substrates have been described,[98] the most commonly used is Matrigel to which various angiogenic agents, for example, VEGF, basic fibroblast growth factor (bFGF), have been added.[100] Matrigel (BD Biosciences, San Jose, CA) is a basement membrane extract in which new blood vessels develop following injection into the subcutaneous tissue of rodents. By quantitating the number of vessels and/or the hemoglobin content, the angiogenesis response can be defined. Matrigel can be used to support xenogeneic tumor cells for injection into mice because it protects the tumor cells, provides a physiologic support, and may provide a medium into which vascular components can migrate.

The corneal angiogenesis assay provides another tumor-independent assay.[101,102] For this assay, controlled-release pellets containing angiogenic agents, for example, bFGF or VEGF, are placed into corneal micropockets and vessel growth is quantified in the presence or absence of treatment with putative antiangiogenic agents. This approach was used in the initial assessment of the antiangiogenic potential of TNP-470 and thalidomide.

Molecular Targets and Transgenic Animals

Transgenic animals expressing targets of interest, or lacking classical tumor suppressor genes have been used for confirmation of drug action. Intrinsic limitations to their use include variability in penetrance and latency of the phenotype of the altered genetic change. However, the impact of chemotherapeutic agents on tumor development and growth may be assessed following treatment at various times relative to the predicted tumor's natural history in a (usually) immunologically intact host. The range of models available has recently been reviewed.[103] As an example of their value, Barrington et al.[104] reported that L-744,832, a farnesyltransferase inhibitor, is *p53* independent utilizing transgenic mice expressing one or more oncogenes in the presence or absence of *p53*. These transgenic mice offer an exciting approach to manipulating potential treatment targets; however, their use for routine in vivo screening is often limited by the time required for tumor development and the amount of compound necessary to treat for a protracted period of time. Additionally, the number of mice developing tumors may be <50%, so extremely large treatment groups are necessary to obtain statistically relevant results. For example, a transgenic model in which only 30% of mice develop tumors may require hundreds of test animals to achieve statistical validity. In such cases, a statistician should be consulted to aid in determining the appropriate treatment group size for a given tumor model prior to embarking on a chemotherapy trial.

Acknowledgments

Paula Krosky contributed to a prior edition of this chapter.

References

1. Hanahan D, Weinberg RA. The hallmarks of cancer. Cell 2000;100:57–70.
2. Uttenhoeve C, Pilotte L, Théate I, et al. Evidence for a tumoral immune resistance mechanism based on tryptophan degradation by indoleamine 2, 3-dioxygenase. Nat Med 2003;9:1269–1274.
3. Olaussen KA, Dunant A, Fouret P, et al. DNA repair by ERCC1 in non-small-cell lung cancer and cisplatin-based adjuvant chemotherapy. N Eng J Med 2006;355:983–991.
4. O'Brien SG, Guilhot F, Larson RA, et al. Imatinib compared with interferon and low-dose cytarabine for newly diagnosed chronic myelogenous leukemia. N Eng J Med 2003:348:994–1004.
5. Vogel CL, Cobleigh MA, Tripathy D, et al. Efficacy and safety of trastuzumab as a single agent in first-line treatment of HER2-overexpressing metastatic breast cancer. J Clin Oncol 2002;20:719–726.
6. Paez JG, Janne PA, Lee PC, et al. EGFR mutations in lung cancer: correlation with clinical response to gefitinib therapy. Science 2004;304:1458–1461.
7. Lynch TJ, Bell DW, Sordella R, et al. Activating mutations in the epidermal growth factor receptor underlying responsiveness of non-small-cell lung cancer to gefitinib. N Engl J Med 2004;350:2129–2139.
8. Shepherd FA, Rodrigues Pereira J, Ciuleanu T, et al. Erlotinib in previously treated non-small cell lung cancer. N Eng J Med 2005;353:123–132.
9. McDermott U, Sharma SV, Dowell L, et al. Identification of genotype-correlated sensitivity to selective kinase inhibitors by using high-throughput tumor cell line profiling. Proc Natl Acad Sci U S A 2007;104:19936–19941.
10. Weinstein IB. Cancer. Addiction to oncogenes—the Achilles heel of cancer. Science 2002;297:63–64.

11. Hurwitz H, Fehrenbacher L, Novotny W, et al. Bevacizumab plus irinotecan, fluorouracil, and leucovorin for metastatic colorectal cancer. N Eng J Med 2004;350:2335–2342.

12. Kaelin WG Jr. The concept of synthetic lethality in the context of anticancer screening. Nat Rev Cancer 2005;5:689–698.

13. Kwan KY, Wang JC. Mice lacking DNA topoisomerase IIIbeta develop to maturity but show a reduced mean lifespan. Proc Natl Acad Sci U S A 2001;98:5717–5721.

14. Whitesell L, Mimnaugh EG, De Costa B, et al. Inhibition of heat shock protein HSP90-pp60^{v-src} heteroprotein complex formation by benzoquinone ansamycins: essential role for stress proteins in oncogenic transformation. Proc Natl Acad Sci U S A 1994;91:8324–8328.

15. Sabers CJ, Martin MM, Brunn GJ, et al. Isolation of a protein target of the FKBP12-rapamycin complex in mammalian cells. J Biol Chem 1995;270:815–822.

16. Sin N, Meng L, Wang MQW, et al. The anti-angiogenic agent fumagillin covalently binds and inhibits the methionine aminopeptidase, MetAP-2. Proc Natl Acad Sci U S A 1997;94:6099–6103.

17. Caron PR, Mullican MD, Mashal RD, et al. Chemogenomic approaches to drug discovery. Curr Opin Chem Biol 2001;5:464–470.

18. Gaither LA. Chemogenomics approaches to novel target discovery. Expert Rev Proteomics 2007;4:411–419.

19. Stockwell BR. Chemical genetics: ligand-based discovery of gene function. Nat Rev Genet 2000;1:116–125.

20. Fire A, Xu SQ, Montgomery MK, et al. Potent and specific genetic interference by double-stranded RNA in Caenorhabditis elegans. Nature 1998;391:806–811.

21. Tuschl T, Zamore PD, Lehmann R, et al. Targeted mRNA degradation by double-stranded RNA in vitro. Genes Dev 1999;13:3191–3197.

22. Iorns E, Lord CJ, Turner N, et al. Utilizing RNA interference to enhance drug discovery. Nat Rev Drug Discov 2007;6:556–568.

23. Woo HG, Park ES, Lee JS, et al. Identification of potential driver genes in human liver carcinoma by genomewide screening. Cancer Res 2009;69:4059–4066.

24. Tetsu O, McCormick F. Proliferation of cancer cells despite CDK2 inhibition. Cancer Cell 2003;3:233–245.

25. Ludwig JA, Szakács G, Martin SE, et al. Selective toxicity of NSC73306 in MDR1-positive cells as a new strategy to circumvent multidrug resistance in cancer. Cancer Res 2006;66:4808–4815.

26. Farmer H, McCabe N, Lord CJ, et al. Targeting the DNA repair defect in BRCA mutant cells as a therapeutic strategy. Nature 2005;434:917–921.

27. Lord CJ, McDonald S, Swift S, et al. A high-throughput RNA interference screen for DNA repair determinants of PARP inhibitor sensitivity. DNA Repair (Amst) 2008;7:2010–2019.

28. Turner NC, Lord CJ, Iorns E, et al. A synthetic lethal siRNA screen identifying genes mediating sensitivity to a PARP inhibitor. EMBO 2008;27:1368–1377.

29. Trisciuoglio D, Uranchimeg B, Cardellina JH, et al. Induction of apoptosis in human cancer cells by candidaspongiolide, a novel sponge polyketide. J Natl Cancer Inst 2008;100:1233–1246.

30. Gaither A, Porter D, Yao Y, et al. A Smac mimetic rescue screen reveals roles for inhibitor of apoptosis proteins in tumor necrosis factor-alpha signaling. Cancer Res 2007;67:11493–11498.

31. Ngo VN, Davis RE, Lamy L, et al. A loss-of-function RNA interference screen for molecular targets in cancer. Nature 2006;441:106–110.

32. Whitehurst AW, Bodemann BO, Cardenas J, et al. Synthetic lethal screen identification of chemosensitizer loci in cancer cells. Nature 2007;446:815–819.

33. Bartz SR, Zhang Z, Burchard J, et al. Small interfering RNA screens reveal enhanced cisplatin cytotoxicity in tumor cells having both BRCA network and TP53 disruptions. Mol Cell Biol 2006;26:9377–9386.

34. Hoeflich KP, Gray DC, Eby MT, et al. Oncogenic BRAF is required for tumor growth and maintenance in melanoma models. Cancer Res 2006;66:999–1006.

35. Inglese J, Auld DS, Jadhav A, et al. Quantitative high-throughput screening: a titration-based approach that efficiently identifies biological activities in large chemical libraries. Proc Natl Acad Sci U S A 2006;103:11473–11478.

36. Cragg GM, Newman DJ. Antineoplastic agents from natural sources: achievements and future directions. Expert Opin Investig Drugs 2000;9:2783–3797.

37. Cragg GM, Grothaus PG, Newman DJ. Impact of natural products on developing new anti-cancer agents. Chem Rev 2009;109:3012–3043.

38. Newman DJ, Cragg GM. Natural products as sources of new drugs over the last 25 years. J Nat Prod 2007;70:461–477.

39. Geysen HM, Meloen RH, Barteling SJ. Use of peptide synthesis to probe viral antigens for epitopes to resolution of a single amino acid. Proc Natl Acad Sci U S A 1984;81:3998–4002.

40. Rees D, et al. Fragment-based lead discovery. Nat Rev Drug Discov 2004;3:660–672.

41. Zartler ER, Shapiro MJ, ed. Fragment-Based Drug Discovery: A Practical Approach. Chichester: Wiley, 2009.

42. Keiser MJ, Setola V, Irwin JJ, et al. Predicting new molecular targets for known drugs. Nature 2009;462:175–181.

43. Jarvis RA, Patrick EA. Clustering using a similarity measure based on shared near neighbors. IEEE Trans Comput 1973;C22:1025–1034.

44. Hodes L. Clustering a large number of compounds. 1. Establishing the method on an initial sample. J Chem Inf Comput Sci 1989;29:55–71.

45. Voigt JH, Bienfait B, Wang S, et al. Comparison of the NCI open database with seven large chemical structural databases. J Chem Inf Comput Sci 2001;41:702–712.

46. Shoemaker RH, Scudiero DA, Melillo G, et al. Application of high-throughput, molecular targeted screening to anticancer drug discovery. Curr Top Med Chem 2002;2:229–246.

47. Stephen AG, Worthy KM, Towler E, et al. Identification of HIV-1 nucleocapsid protein: nucleic acid antagonists with cellular anti-HIV activity. Biochem Biophys Res Commun 2002;296:1228–1237.

48. Lazo, JS, Aslan DC, Soutwick EC, et al. Discovery and biological evaluation of a new family of potent inhibitors of the dual specificity protein phosphatase Cdc25. J Med Chem 2001;44:4042–4049.

49. Rapisarda A, Uranchimeg B, Scudiero DA, et al. Identification of small molecular inhibitors of hypoxia-inducible factor 1 transcriptional activation pathway. Cancer Res 2002;62:4316–4324.

50. Zhang JH, Chung TD, Oldenburg KR. A simple statistical parameter for use in evaluation and validation of high throughput screening assays. J Biomol Screen 1999;4:67–73.

51. Hajduk PJ, Huth JR, Fesik SW. Druggability indices for protein targets derived from NMR-based screening data. J Med Chem 2005;48:2518–2525.

52. Wendt MD, Shen W, Kunzer A, et al. Discovery and structure-activity relationship of antagonists of B-cell lymphoma 2 family proteins with chemopotentiation activity in vitro and in vivo. J Med Chem 2006;49:1165–1181.

53. Tsai J, Lee JT, Wang W, et al. Discovery of a selective inhibitor of oncogenic B-Raf kinase with potent antimelanoma activity. Proc Natl Acad Sci U S A 2008;105:3041–3046.

54. Galkin AV, Melnick JS, Kim S, et al. Identification of NVP-TAE684, a potent, selective, and efficacious inhibitor of NPM-ALK. Proc Natl Acad Sci U S A 2007;104:270–275.

55. Soda M, Takada S, Takeuchi K, et al. A mouse model for EML4-ALK-positive lung cancer. Proc Natl Acad Sci U S A 2008;105:19893–19897.

56. Shoemaker RH, Sausville EA. New drug development. In: Souhami RI, Tannock I, Honenberger P, et al., eds. Oxford Textbook of Oncology. Oxford: Oxford University Press, 1999:781–788.

57. Holbeck SL. Update on NCI in vitro drug screen utilities. Eur J Cancer 2004;40:785–793.

58. Shoemaker RH. The NCI60 human tumour cell line anticancer drug screen. Nat Rev Cancer 2006;6:813–823.

59. Paull KD, Shoemaker RH, Hodes L, et al. Display and analysis of patterns of differential activity of drugs against human tumor cell lines: development of mean graph and COMPARE algorithm. J Natl Cancer Inst 1989;81:1088–1092.

60. Rabow AA, Shoemaker RH, Sausville EA, et al. Mining the National Cancer Institute's tumor screening database: identification of compounds with similar cellular activities. J Med Chem 2002;45:818–840.

61. Yamori T, Matsunaga A, Sato S, et al. Potent antitumor activity of MS-247, a novel DNA minor groove binder, evaluated by an in vitro and in vivo human cancer cell line panel. Cancer Res 1999;59:4042–4049.

62. Stegmaier K, Ross KN, Colavito SA, et al. Gene expression-based high-throughput screening (GE-HTS) and application to leukemia differentiation. Nat Genet 2004;36:257–263.

63. McDermott U, Ames RY, Iafrate AJ, et al. Ligand-dependent platelet-derived growth factor receptor (PDGFR)-alpha activation sensitizes rare lung cancer and sarcoma cells to PDGFR kinase inhibitors. Cancer Res 2009;69:3937–3946.

64. Plowman J, Dykes DJ, Hollingshead MG, et al. Human tumor xenograft models in NCI drug development. In: Teicher BA, ed. Anticancer Drug Development Guide: Preclinical Screening, Clinical Trials, and Approval. Totowa, NJ: Humana Press, 1997:101–125.

65. le Coutre P, Mologni L, Cleris L, et al. In vivo eradication of human BCR/ABL-positive leukemia cells with an ABL kinase inhibitor. J Natl Cancer Inst 1999;91:163–168.

66. Luo FR, Yang Z, Camuso A, et al. Dasatinib (BMS-354825) pharmacokinetics and pharmacodynamic biomarkers in animal models predict optimal clinical exposure. Clin Cancer Res 2006;12:7180–7186.

67. Adams J, Kauffman M. Development of the proteosome inhibitor Velcade. (Bortezomib). Cancer Invest 2004;2:304–311.

68. El-Rayes BF, LoRusso PM. Targeting the epidermal growth factor receptor. Br J Cancer 2004;91:418–424.

69. Johnson JI, Decker S, Zaharevitz D, et al. Relationships between drug activity in NCI preclinical in vitro and in vivo models and early clinical trials. Br J Cancer 2001;84:1424–1431.

70. Peterson JK, Houghton PJ. Integrating pharmacology and in vivo cancer models in preclinical and clinical drug development. Eur J Cancer 2004;40:837–844.

71. Jänne PA, Gray N, Settleman J. Factors underlying sensitivity of cancers to small-molecule kinase inhibitors. Nat Rev Drug Discov 2009;8:709–723.

72. Kinders RJ, Hollingshead M, Khin S, et al. Preclinical modeling of a phase 0 clinical trial: qualification of a pharmacodynamic assay of poly (ADP-ribose) polymerase in tumor biopsies of mouse xenografts. Clin Cancer Res 2008;14:6877–6885.

73. Kummar S, Kinders R, Gutierrez ME, et al. Phase 0 clinical trial of the poly (ADP-ribose) polymerase inhibitor ABT-888 in patients with advanced malignancies. J Clin Oncol 2009;27:2705–2711.

74. Hollingshead MG, Alley MC, Camalier RF, et al. In vivo cultivation of tumor cells in hollow fibers. Life Sci 1995;57:131–141.

75. Decker S, Hollingshed M, Bonomi CA, et al. The hollow fiber model in cancer drug screening: the NCI experience. Eur J Cancer 2004;40:821–826.

76. Zhang G-J, Chen T-B, Hargreaves R, et al. Bioluminescence imaging of hollow fibers in living animals: its application in monitoring molecular pathways. Nat Protoc 2008;3:891–899.

77. Zhang G-J, Safran M, Weil W, et al. Bioluminescent imaging of Cdk2 inhibition in vivo. Nat Med 2004;10:643–648.

78. Hall LA, Krauthauser CM, Wexler RS, et al. The hollow fiber assay: continued characterization with novel approaches. Anticancer Res 2000;20(2A):903–911.

79. Waud WR. Murine L1210 and P388 leukemias. In: Teicher BA, ed. Anticancer Drug development Guide: Preclinical Screening, Clinical Trials, and Approval. Vol 40. Totowa, NJ: Humana Press, 1997:802–820.

80. Corbett T, Valeriote F, LoRusso P, et al. In vivo methods for screening and preclinical testing use of rodent solid tumors for drug discovery. In: Teicher BA, ed. Anticancer Drug Development Guide: Preclinical Screening. Clinical Trials and Approval. Totowa, NJ: Humana Press, 1997:74–99.

81. Fiebig HH, Maier A, Burger AM. Clonogenic assay with established human tumour xenografts: correlation of in vitro to in vivo activity as a basis for anti-cancer drug discovery. Eur J Cancer 2004;40:802–820.

82. Giovanella BC, Stehlin JS. Heterotransplantation of human malignant tumors in "nude" thymusless mice. I. Breeding and maintenance of "nude" mice. J Natl Cancer Inst 1973;51:615–619.

83. Leonessa F, Green D, Licht T, et al. MDA435/LCC6 and mDA435/LCC6-MDR1: ascites models of human breast cancer. Br J Cancer 1996;73:154–161.

84. McLemore TL, Abbott BJ, Mayo JG, et al. Development and application of new orthotopic in vivo models for use in the US National Cancer Institute's drug screening program. In: Wu B-Q, Zheng J, eds. Immune-Deficient Animals. Basel: Karger, 1989:334–343.

85. Clarke R. Issues in experimental design and endpoint analysis in the study of experimental cytotoxic agents in vivo in breast cancer and other models. Breast Cancer Res Treat 1997;1:311–326.

86. Fine DL, Shoemaker R, Gazdar A, et al. Metastasis models for human tumors in athymic mice: useful models for development. Cancer Detect Prev Suppl 1987;1:291–299.

87. Hoffman RM. Patient-like models of human cancer in mice. Curr Perspect Mol Cell Oncol 1992;1:311–326.

88. Fidler IJ, Wilmanns C, Staroselsky A, et al. Modulation of tumor cell response to chemotherapy by the organ environment. Cancer Metastasis Rev 1994;13:20–49.

89. Fidler IJ. Rationale and methods for the use of nude mice to study the biology and therapy of human cancer metastasis. Cancer Metastasis Rev 1986;5:29–49.

90. Giavazzi R. Metastatic models. In: Boven E, Winograd B, eds. The Nude Mouse in Oncology Research. Boca Raton, FL: CRC Press, 1991:117–132.

91. Dickson RB, Johnson MD, Maemura M, et al. Anti-invasion drugs. Breast Cancer Res Treat 1996;39:121–132.

92. Fidler IJ. Selection of successive tumour lines for metastasis. Nat New Biol 1973;242:148–149.

93. Zetter BR. Angiogenesis and tumor metastasis. Ann Rev Med 1998;49:407–424.

94. Wang Y, Iyer M, Annala A, et al. Noninvasive indirect imaging of vascular endothelial growth factor gene expression using bioluminescence imaging in live transgenic mice. Physiol Genomics 2006;24:173–180.

95. Talmadge JE, Fidler IJ. Cancer metastasis is selective or random depending on the parent tumour population. Nature 1982;297:593–594.

96. Chirivi RG, Garofalo A, Crimmin MJ, et al. Inhibition of the metastatic spread and growth of B16-BL6 murine melanoma by a synthetic matrix metalloproteinase inhibitor. In J Cancer 1994;58:460–464.

97. Guilbaud N, Kraus-Berhier L, Sant-Dizier D, et al. Antitumor activity of S 16020-2 in two orthotopic models of lung cancer. Anticancer Drugs 1997;8:276–282.

98. Taraboletti G, Giavazzi R. Modeling approaches for angiogenesis. Eur J Cancer 2004;40:881–889.

99. Schlatter P, Konig MF, Karlsson LM, et al. Quantitative study of intussusceptive capillary growth in the chorioallantoic membrane (CAM) of the chicken embryo. Microvasc Res 1997;54:65–73.

100. Passaniti A, Taylor RM, Pili R, et al. A simple quantitative methods for assessing angiogenesis and antiangiogenic agents using reconstituted basement membrane, heparin, and fibroblast growth fact. Lab Invest 1992;67:519–528.

101. Mutyhukkaruppan V, Auerbach R. Angiogenesis in the mouse cornea. Science 1979;205:1416–1418.

102. Kenyon BM, Voest EE, Chen CC, et al. A model of angiogenesis in the mouse cornea. Invest Ophthalmol Vis Sci 1996;37:1625–1632.

103. Hansen K, Khanna C. Spontaneous and genetically engineered animal models: use in preclinical cancer drug development. Eur J Cancer 2004;40:858–880.

104. Barrington RE, Saubler MA, Rands E, et al. A farnesyltransferase inhibitor induced tumor regression in transgenic mice harboring multiple oncogenic mutations by mediating alterations in both cell cycle control and apoptosis. Mol Cell Biol 1998;18:85–92.

105. Johnson LN. Protein kinase inhibitors: contributions from structure to clinical compounds. Q Rev Biophys 2009;42:1–40.

106. Harris PA, Boloor A, Cheung M, et al. Discovery of 5-[[4-[(2,3-dimethyl-2H-indazol-6-yl)methylamino]-2-pyrimidinyl]amino]-2-methyl-benzenesulfonamide (Pazopanib), a novel and potent vascular endothelial growth factor receptor inhibitor. J Med Chem 2008;51:4632–4640.

Clinical Drug Development and Marketing Approval

Thomas G. Roberts, Jr.

In the fourth quarter of 2009, there were more than 800 agents in clinical trials for the treatment of cancer,[1] more than the number in any other therapeutic drug class.[2] The hematology/oncology therapeutic category comprises more than one third of all drug development candidates by some estimates.[2] Compared to many areas of medicine, the opportunity to identify additional novel molecular targets for cancer appears especially promising. To date, 350 cancer genes have been identified. It is possible, however, that researchers applying advanced DNA-sequencing techniques will identify more than 2,000 cancer genes, each offering a potential for multiple new agents.[3]

The Challenge of Cancer Drug Development

The sponsor of each new investigational agent ultimately seeks approval by major regulatory agencies, including the U.S. Food and Drug Administration (FDA), to market their product for at least one indication. However, only 2 to 7 new drugs and biologics for the treatment of cancer attain this goal per year. Marketing approval represents the final hurdle that sponsors must clear in their time-consuming efforts to discover and optimize lead compounds, test new drugs in animals, and conduct clinical studies in man. Without this license, the effort to develop a new drug, which may have consumed hundreds of millions of dollars and spanned more than a decade, could go in vain.[4,5] Small companies that concentrate on cancer drug development and which fail to attain marketing approval for at least one of their agents will eventually lose access to capital and will be forced to wind down operations or solicit an offer to be acquired. The impact of failures at larger companies is typically less extreme, but there is still a steep opportunity cost of failure that sponsors seek to avoid.

Companies face low odds, high expense, and long planning cycles in their quest to develop new agents. Fewer than one in ten investigational agents that enter phase 1 trials ultimately gain marketing approval.[6] The low odds of success is a major contributor to the expense and risk associated with cancer drug development.[7,8] The most recent published estimate of the average total cost (i.e., preclinical plus clinical costs) of developing a representative new cancer drug from concept to FDA approval is $1,042 million (in $2,000).[8,9] This figure accounts for the cost of developing other drugs that fail as well as the opportunity cost of capital. The average cost to develop a new oncology drug exceeds the mean of other

therapeutic classes by approximately 20% and is almost twice the cost of a drug for HIV/AIDS.[10] The higher costs to develop cancer drugs compared with other therapeutic classes are due in part to a greater frequency of late-stage failures and longer development times.[5,10] Sponsors can generally develop highly active cancer products quickly, but many compounds are not highly active and require time and careful planning to demonstrate their potential. It takes 14 years, on average, for a company to take a new anticancer agent along the path from preclinical testing through phase 3 human trials, with approximately half of the time spent in clinical development.[5,6,8]

Developing cancer drugs has always proven to be a challenging undertaking. The combination of an incomplete understanding of cancer biology, poorly predictive animal models, and frequently uninformative phase 2 trials has limited the speed of advancement over much of the last 50 years. The era of molecularly targeted therapies has brought not only enormous optimism and opportunities for advancement but also additional challenges. There is now an appreciation of genetic heterogeneity among most populations of cancer patients, yet investigators have encountered scientific and logistical impediments in their attempts to use biomarkers to enrich trials for patient subsets most likely to respond to the new agents. There has also been lack of consistent agreement on the definition of clinical benefit, which in turn has created uncertainty for sponsors and required ongoing collaborative input from multiple stakeholders. In some instances, the understanding of the transformation process and cancer phenotype is now greater than the ability of clinical researchers to evaluate efficiently the clinical potential of new drugs.[11] Some researchers have even suggested that drug development principles that evolved with traditional cytotoxic agents may not apply in the era of targeted therapy, since the newer agents possess different mechanisms of action and antineoplastic effects and have a different spectrum of toxicity.[12] It seems more appropriate, however, to build on the established principles and development platform, modifying them where necessary to account for methods of patient enrichment and adding new tools to assess biological and clinical activities of the new agents.

The Commercial Opportunity

Despite the risk and complexity, cancer drug development efforts have attracted substantial amounts of public and private funding, driven by the continued unmet medical need of cancer patients and potential for blockbuster success. In 2008, the worldwide market for cancer drugs was approximately $68 billion.[13] Over the 20-year period from 1987 to 2008, worldwide sales of cancer drugs grew at an annualized rate of 11%, exceeding by a wide margin the growth in sales of other major therapeutic categories in medicine. The growth in cancer therapies continues to be among the highest in the major therapeutic classes. The widespread adoption of the newer targeted agents has driven much of the market growth. Anticancer products like imatinib mesylate (Gleevec), bevacizumab (Avastin), and rituximab (Rituxan) now rank among the top-selling prescription agents across all drug categories, with 2008 worldwide sales of $3.7 billion, $5.0 billion, and $5.6 billion, respectively.[13] Research analysts predict that the size of the oncology market will grow to approximately $90 billion by 2014. This growth will likely make the oncology sector the largest therapeutic market within 5 years, overtaking sales of cardiovascular medicines. Every large pharmaceutical company and countless smaller biotech companies have major efforts in cancer drug development. Analysts estimate that monoclonal antibodies and oral tyrosine kinase inhibitors alone will reach $22 billion in worldwide sales by 2012.

Spending on cancer drug development has also grown more quickly than overall spending on biomedical research, which itself has more than doubled in real terms over the last 10 years.[6] Some analysts predict that companies will advance more than 500 anticancer agents into clinical development within the next 10 years,[14] consuming billions of dollars in public and private research capital in addition to patient resources. Pursuing efficient clinical development strategies is therefore not only an important issue for sponsoring companies but also a matter of public interest. This chapter will review various stages and strategies for the development of cancer drugs as well as regulatory hurdles for their marketing approval.

The Process of Cancer Drug Development

Clinical investigators and sponsors collaborate to develop cancer drugs in a stepwise process of discrete clinical phases, each with their own endpoints and milestones (Fig. 3-1). Cancer researchers have built the development process over many years to establish safe dosing, assess efficacy, and determine relative effectiveness compared to reference regimens. The process continues to evolve as investigators recognize the need to adapt clinical development paths to the more targeted nature of the newer agents. Over the past 5 years, clinical trial designs have become more flexible and innovative and have begun to utilize tissue genotyping and other biomarkers to select for patients who are most likely to receive a clinical benefit. These changes reflect the types of drugs under investigation. Until recently, almost all anticancer drugs were cytotoxic or hormonal. Since 2005, more than 60% of cancer drugs approved by the FDA have been molecularly targeted therapies.[15] The targeted therapies have thus far fallen into three major categories. Of the 169 targeted agents either on the market or in late-stage clinical development, 84 (50%) are small molecule kinase inhibitors, 30 (18%) are small molecule inhibitors of other types of enzymes implicated in cell growth, and 55 (32%) are large molecule biologics, including monoclonal antibodies.[15] There is reason to believe that sponsors will continue to adapt the process of cancer drug development to the types of agents under investigation. The biotech industry, comprising smaller, more focused firms, now accounts for the majority (68%) of cancer drugs in clinical development. These firms tend to display more flexibility in their development strategies and may face more scrutiny and pressure by investors to develop the agents as quickly and as efficiently as possible.

Sponsors decide whether to advance an investigational agent into clinical testing on the basis of overall interest in the agent's target, the strength of preclinical data in cell lines and animal models, and the attractiveness of the agent's pharmaceutical properties. Most companies will also perform some analysis to determine whether

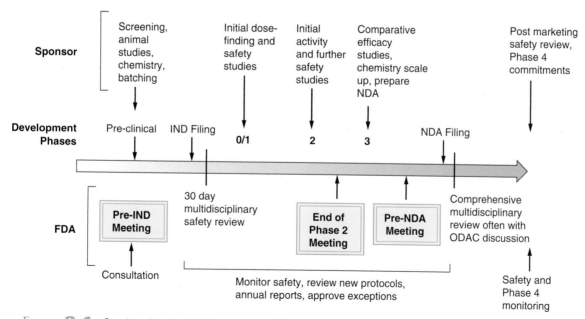

FIGURE 3-1   Overview of the drug development process. The multiple interactions between drug sponsors and the FDA reflect the convergence of the duties and responsibilities throughout the phases of development. IND, initial new drug application; NDA, new drug application; ODAC, Oncologic Drug Advisory Committee.

the expected return on investment exceeds a predetermined hurdle-rate, which is often similar to the firm's estimated cost of capital. A broad discussion of the preclinical problem of target validation and assessment is beyond the scope of this chapter (see Chapter 2). However, if the target is not essential to growth, spread, or survival of the tumor, or if pathway redundancy exists that allows the tumor to escape from single pathway inhibition, the potential therapy is not likely to produce a clinical benefit.[5,16]

Once a sponsor has decided to pursue clinical development, a number of regulatory and scientific review steps must be completed prior to initiating clinical trials. These requirements can prove onerous for many sponsors, but they help to protect research subjects participating in trials, focus the research effort, and, if successfully employed, may improve data quality.[17] In their planning, sponsors collaborate with academic investigators, the FDA, and in some cases, the National Cancer Institute (NCI) to decide on the optimal patient populations to study, appropriate trial endpoints and designs, and potential for combination regimens with other approved or investigational agents.[18] The number of permutations of possible developmental strategies available to a sponsor for any given investigational agent is enormous, but a thorough understanding of the underlying biology can help clarify the overall development path and avoid unnecessary detours and delays.

Phase 0

Clinical investigators, FDA, and the NCI have all recognized that a major weakness inherent in the cancer drug development process is the preclinical/clinical transition.[5] Most agents fail in clinical testing because animal studies fail to predict their behavior in humans. Tumor-bearing mice have been useful in determining antitumor activity of target inhibitors, comparing drug analogues, and optimizing dose and schedule of administration. Unfortunately, however, the mouse does not predict reliably for success in the clinic. Drug disposition is in general faster, tolerance for toxicity greater, and growth of tumors more rapid in the mouse, all of which tend to make drugs more effective in mice. Although extensively employed in preclinical drug testing, neither human tumors grown in immunodeficient mice nor spontaneous murine solid tumors have reliable predictive value for human tumors.[19] Often single animal or xenograft tumors are subjected to testing, but the results have unclear relevance to the diversity of molecule subtypes encompassed by a single pathological category (colon cancer) in humans.

Up to 25% of investigational cancer agents that enter phase 1 trials will be discontinued prior to phase 2 studies.[6] About half of these early discontinuations are due to undesirable pharmacokinetic (PK) characteristics that are inconsistent with the predictions made from preclinical animal models.[11] It would therefore be helpful if investigators had access to additional PK and pharmacodynamic (PD) data early in the development effort to help ensure that the investigational agents are interacting with the desired targets and in the appropriate concentrations prior to initiating more expensive and time-consuming phase 1 and 2 trials. When sponsors do not know until well into the phase 2 effort whether an investigational agent displays the desired biological activity or interacts with the intended target, resources may be spent on programs with little promise, displacing the opportunity for more worthwhile investments.

In 2004, the FDA undertook an effort to modernize the clinical trials process called the Critical Path Initiative. As one of the first changes under the Critical Path, the FDA introduced new guidelines for early exploratory drug studies in order to improve the preclinical/clinical transition. A 2006 guidance document[20] provides specific recommendations regarding safety testing, manufacturing, and clinical approaches to be used in very early clinical studies, sometimes called *exploratory* or *phase* 0 trials. The goal of phase 0 studies is to establish quickly whether an investigational agent displays biological activity in humans before large numbers of patients receive exposure to potentially inactive agents.[14] The phase 0 strategy requires fewer preclinical animal studies than a typical phase 1 trial and allows sponsors to make smaller batches of an experimental drug.[21] To mitigate safety issues that may arise in exploratory testing, researchers limit these early human tests to a few patients (10 or fewer), shorten the time of drug exposure (e.g., 7 days or less), and reduce the doses of medicines than would be employed in a typical phase 1 trial (e.g., <1% of what researchers expect would be the agent's standard dose).[14] Types of phase 0 trials include microdose studies evaluating PK or functional imaging modalities as well as trials evaluating mechanisms of action related to efficacy. Phase 0 studies may evaluate and compare a series of related compounds.[11] Functional imaging studies or target measures in normal tissues may be useful when repeat biopsies before and after dosing are not possible or logistically difficult. Importantly, phase 0 trials are neither intended to replace the traditional dose escalation, safety, and tolerance studies that are required in phase 1 testing nor intended to evaluate clinical benefit.

It would be inappropriate for researchers to employ a phase 0 trial for each new agent. First, a small dose of an investigational agent may not provide meaningful information in the absence of a validated biomarker. At present, most new investigational agents do not have a validated biomarker that can predict tumor activity with sufficient accuracy at the start of clinical development to make optimal use of a phase 0 trial.[21] Second, researchers must be sure that the drug's mechanism of action is defined by that target to avoid misleading data.[14] Sorafenib, for example, was originally tested in clinical trials as a B-Raf kinase inhibitor, but its primary mechanism of action in renal cell carcinoma may be the result of other "off-target" effects on angiogenesis. Third, the PK inferences drawn from very small doses of drugs are reliable only if the drug displays linear or first-order pharmacokinetics (the plasma concentration of drug at a given time after dosing is directly proportional to the administered dose). The majority of clinically used cancer agents display linear PK; however, those that are eliminated by a potentially saturable process such as active tubular secretion or enzymatic metabolism are unlikely to be good candidates for phase 0 testing. Therefore, the ideal agent for phase 0 testing has a target that can be monitored, a biomarker that can be assayed with validity and reproducibility, and kinetics that appear linear.

The recent trial involving ABT-888, an orally bioavailable inhibitor of poly (ADP-ribose) polymerase (PARP), provides an excellent example of a phase 0 trial.[22] PARP inhibitors may hold particular promise as chemotherapy and radiation sensitizers since PARP is involved in DNA repair via poly (ADP-ribosyl)ation of histones and DNA repair enzymes. The primary endpoint of the trial was PD, specifically target modulation in human samples. The effort was successful: within 5 months of starting the phase 0 trial, strongly supportive data were available including the molecular proof-of-target inhibition by ABT-888, as well as PK and PD data that could serve as the foundation for subsequent combination studies of ABT-888 with DNA-damaging agents. Specifically, the data demonstrated that a twice-daily schedule for ABT-888 was appropriate, and, based on significant inhibition of PARP in tumor biopsies at 25 mg, the authors recommended that the phase 1 dose of ABT-888 in combination with DNA-damaging agents should be 10 mg BID. ABT-888 was an appropriate candidate for testing in a phase 0 trial because its preclinical data demonstrated that PARP inhibition was indeed the target for ABT-888, and there was a validated assay before the initiation of phase 1 trials. Additionally, researchers demonstrated that PARP inhibition, needed for preclinical antitumor activity, occurred at doses and exposures well below those associated with toxicity.[11]

This example highlights several important points about phase 0 trials. First, the rapid completion of complex, early-phase clinical trials requires an integrated, multidisciplinary research team capable of performing PK and PD studies in real time. The authors of the ABT-888 accomplished their studies in 48 hours or less after sample acquisition. Second, researchers must pay particular attention to ensure that biopsy procedures are performed only after careful validation of the assay procedures. The authors of the ABT-888 study made efforts to ensure that that they could draw statistically and scientifically meaningful inferences from a limited number of biopsy samples. Finally, researchers should make efforts to avoid unnecessarily invasive studies if possible. The authors of the ABT-888 study found that there was a strong correlation between the effects of ABT-888 in peripheral blood mononuclear cells (PBMCs) versus tumor samples, which may obviate the need for biopsies in future clinical research. It is possible that examples such as this one will drive the adoption and broader uptake of carefully conceived, PD-driven driven early-phase clinical trials in oncology.[22]

Several sponsors such as Novartis, Merck, and Pfizer have registered phase 0 clinical trials in the ClinicalTrials.gov database. They are using these trials to explore PK and PD primary objectives as well as positioning backup compounds. At the very least, phase 0 trials may help clinical investigators choose among several potentially promising compounds before sponsors are required to undertake the requisite small and large animal preclinical work.[11] Whether or not sponsors choose to incorporate phase 0 trials, researchers should generate sufficient preclinical data prior to phase 1 in order to (a) establish the molecular target of the novel drug; (b) determine the effect of the drug on normal and malignant cells; and (c) explore the relationship between the agent's dose/schedule and its antitumor effects, target effects, PK measures, and toxicology.[12] This work will help to define the optimal biological dose in phase 1 and may allow investigators to incorporate analytically validated assays into early phase trials of the agent to assess for target modulation.[18]

Phase 1

There are more than 1,000 phase 1 intervention studies open worldwide according to ClinicalTrials.gov, and the numbers are steadily increasing as more products from the biopharmaceutical industry reach the clinic.[23] Traditionally, phase 1 trials have represented the first testing of investigational agents in humans. The two major objectives of these trials are to characterize the agent's toxicity profile and determine a dose and schedule appropriate for phase 2 testing. Under the standard phase 1 design, investigators enroll successive cohorts of 3 to 6 patients at increasing doses of an experimental therapy with the goal of determining dose-limiting toxicity and then

backing down to a dose appropriate for phase 2 testing.[24] Phase 1 trials in most other areas of medicine enroll healthy participants, whereas phase 1 trials in oncology typically enroll patients who have advanced cancer and who have exhausted standard treatment options. A second difference among oncology-focused phase 1 trials is that sponsors and physicians also seek to evaluate the potential for therapeutic benefit, usually as a secondary endpoint.[24–26] Such observance for therapeutic benefit in phase 1 is appropriate from a development standpoint, given the positive correlation found between response rates (RRs) in phase 1 and ultimate FDA approval.[24]

The more recent focus on modern molecularly targeted agents has drawn into question several aspects of traditional phase 1 trials. Toxicity has been the classical primary endpoint used to determine the recommended dose for phase 2. The basis for recommending the maximum tolerated dose (MTD) for phase 2 testing focuses on the assumption that the therapeutic effect and the associated toxic effects are correlated and that the mechanism of action of the therapeutic and that of the associated toxic effects are correlated. Such an assumption may not be appropriate for the new generation of targeted agents.[18] These agents often have a wider therapeutic index; the proposed mechanism of therapeutic versus toxic effects could differ due to off-target effects; they may require prolonged doses at relatively low levels to provide clinical benefit; and they may not cause impressive tumor shrinkage as single agents.[18] Some investigators have even expressed a view that the key point in phase 1 trials for targeted therapies should evolve from the current idea of MTD in normal tissue to a more suitable endpoint of the dose required to maximally inhibit the relevant target in tumor tissue.[27] Moreover, most sponsors now realize that demonstrating that a novel compound has the target effect for which it was designed may be an equally important aspect of phase 1, particularly if such target validation was not achieved prior to a phase 1 effort.[12]

Use of Biomarkers in Phase 1

One of the more controversial trends in phase 1 trials is the inclusion of biomarker assays. Goulart et al. found that of 2,458 abstracts of phase 1 clinical trials submitted to the American Society of Clinical Oncology (ASCO) annual meetings from 1991 to 2002, approximately 20% (503 of 2,458) included at least one biomarker study as part of the phase 1 trial. This proportion increased over time (14% of the abstracts reported inclusion of biomarkers in 1991 compared with 26% of the abstracts in 2002).[28] Trials focusing on large-molecule biologics and those sponsored by the NCI were more likely to include a biomarker study as part of the trial. Biomarkers contributed to dose and schedule selection in only 13% and 8%, respectively, and in only one instance out of 87 trials did a biomarker contribute to dose selection independent of clinical (i.e., MTD) data. However, biomarkers played a more substantive role in confirming mechanism of action (39% of the trials) and in helping to select patients for future studies (22%). Biopsies of either normal or tumor tissue were more likely to confirm mechanism of action compared to serum-or imaging-based biomarkers. Similar findings were seen in a review of phase 1 trial designs for solid tumor studies that focused exclusively on targeted, noncytotoxic agents.[29] Of the 60 studies reviewed, 36 used toxicity data and 8 used PK data as endpoints for selection of the recommended phase 2 dose. Biomarker studies provided the basis for dose selection in only one trial that evaluated an epidermal growth factor receptor (EGFR) antibody. Drug effects on surrogate tissue (e.g., PBMC or buccal mucosa) provided the primary basis for the recommended phase 2 dose in only one study, which evaluated a Raf kinase inhibitor. In ten (17%) of the trials, however, biomarker studies in surrogate tissue did provide supplementary data supporting dose selection. Information from functional imaging studies was included in six trials, and it provided the basis for a recommended phase 2 dose in one trial.

The phase 1 trial of the PARP inhibitor AG014699 in combination with temozolomide provides an example of the potential promise and limitations of including biomarker studies in phase 1 trials.[30] Preclinical evidence demonstrated that inhibiting PARP potentiates the effects of cytotoxics, particularly alkylating agents and topoisomerase 1 inhibitors. Investigators were able to establish, within the context of the phase 1 trial, the dose of AG014699 that effectively inhibited PARP in peripheral blood leukocytes and confirmed the inhibition in tumor deposits from melanoma. They then used the PD endpoint of PARP inhibition, rather than the more classic toxicity or PK variables, to define the dose recommended for phase 2 trials. Although successful, this trial also demonstrated the potential limitations of using blood-based tissue to establish a PD-defined dose. For example, the investigators found no evidence of increased PARP inhibition between the dose levels of 12 and 18 mg/m^2 AG014699 in the surrogate PD tissue (PBMC), whereas they did observe a trend toward a dose-dependent increase in inhibition in tumor biopsies. Second, many targets for cancer such as PARP are overexpressed in malignant tissues, so it is possible that doses sufficient to inhibit PARP in surrogate tissue may not be high enough to do so effectively in tumor tissue. Another recent example of a biomarker that was studied in phase 1 is the translocation of the EML4-ALK gene, which appears to predict treatment response to a kinase inhibitor targeting ALK. A phase 1 study reported that ten out of 19 (53%) patients with the translocation had a significant response to treatment with a targeted oral drug that inhibits ALK receptor kinase (PF-02341066). This very promising finding, which defines a new subset of patients with non–small-cell lung cancer (NSCLC), awaits confirmation in more advanced trials.[31] The ALK receptor kinase trial demonstrates that when investigators apply effective biomarkers in phase 1, the inferences gained from these early trials may be equal to or exceed what can be produced from traditional phase 2 studies.

In 2007, investigators from the NCI and the NCI of Canada Clinical Trials Group led a task force along with other academic researchers to review design issues in phase 1 studies of targeted anticancer agents.[12] The group specifically addressed whether toxicity (i.e., MTD) and PK data should remain the focus of phase 1 testing. They concluded that both toxicity and PK remain appropriate endpoints to establish the dosing range for novel compounds, advising that investigators establish dose ranges with the upper limit defined by toxic effects, particularly if toxic effects are mechanism based. If no toxic effects are seen, the group recommended other factors to consider including biomarker measurements, PK measures, and feasibility of delivery of the dose. The task force concluded that the recommended dose should be the highest safe dose unless there is a clear biological rational otherwise.

The group also addressed the issue of whether investigators should routinely include biomarker studies in phase 1 trials, and in general they raised a number of cautions.[12] In particular, they recommended that any planned biomarker assays should be developed

and fully validated before the start of the phase 1 study and that such studies should preferentially be focused in patients enrolled at potentially therapeutic doses so that they may be helpful in establishing a "biological active" dose range. Finally, the group cautioned that potentially hazardous/uncomfortable procedures should not be mandated unless essential to the endpoint of the study, despite evidence that tumor biopsies can be performed safely in most instances in the context of phase 1 trials.[27] They suggested that when molecular proof of principle appears important for subsequent development decisions, clinical investigators should consider expanding one or more cohorts after the conclusion of the escalation phase, or designing a separate study to confirm that the doses identified on the basis of toxicity in fact are able to affect the molecular target.[12]

It would be ideal to have obtained evidence of antitumor effect and to have identified a biomarker at the completion of phase 1 to help inform phase 2 trials. However, whether or not biomarker tests are employed, the phase 1 effort should have determined a phase 2 dose recommendation, a range of doses that appear biologically active if future combination studies are planned, and a decision whether to proceed with further development based on prespecified criteria that may include evidence of intended biological activity).[29] Table 3-1 presents a proposed generalized prephase 3 clinical development plan for antineoplastic agents.

TABLE 3.1 Generalized prephase 3 clinical development plan for antineoplastic agents

Phase 1

Explore does range up to MTD unless limited by formulation or bioavailability

Include as heterogeneous a patient population as can be ethically justified

Define relationship of dose to toxicity and PKs

Observe for mechanism-related toxicity (e.g., skin rash with EGFR inhibitors) as a readily observable biomarker

Consider inclusion of biomarker studies on readily accessible tissue (e.g., peripheral mononuclear cells) to assess mechanism of action and minimal potential effective dose

Consider use of tumor biopsies at highest dose if results are to be used to make "Go/No Go" decision

Phase 2a

Unless anticipated evidence of benefit is partial response, consider conducting dose-ranging randomized trials to detect activity, including use of novel endpoints

Consider crossover design to allow for use of placebo when possible

Consider analysis of previously collected diagnostic material to correlate with activity

Phase 2b

Consider studies of predictive biomarkers (including tumor biopsies) once drug is shown to be active

Adapted from Ratain MJ, Glassman RH. Biomarkers in phase I oncology trials: signal, noise, or expensive distraction? Clin Cancer Res 2007; 13(22 Pt 1):6545–6548.

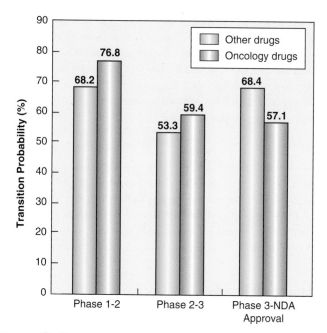

FIGURE 3-3 Clinical phase transition probabilities for investigational oncology and all compounds for the 20 largest firms by 2005 pharmaceutical sales for compounds that first entered clinical testing during 1993 to 2002. NDA, new drug application. (Adapted from DiMasi JA, Grabowski HG. Economics of new oncology drug development. J Clin Oncol 2007;25(2):209–216.)

studies or studies comparing two dose levels without an active comparator).[59] Phase 3 trials still provide the basis for most regulator approvals. Of the 51 oncology-related NDAs approved from 1995 to 2008, phase 3 trials supported efficacy findings for 75% of regular approvals versus 26% of AAs.[60]

Some investigators have questioned the practice of approving cancer drugs after phase 2,[61] but a recent review of the ultimate fate of oncology drugs approved by the FDA without a randomized trial produced reassuring findings.[62] The review found that from 1973 to 2006, the FDA approved 31 of 68 (46%) oncology drugs (excluding hormone therapy and supportive care) without a randomized trial, most commonly using objective response as the approval endpoint. Sponsors conducted a median of two clinical studies per drug to obtain approval (range, 1 to 7 clinical trials), and the median number of patients studied per drug approval was 79 (range, 40 to 413 patients). The approved agents produced a median RR of 33% (range, 11% to 90%). Of the 31 agents approved without a randomized trial, the FDA has restricted marketing for only one agent, gefitinib, and even this agent is being considered for reintroduction after showing efficacy in the first-line treatment of patients with NSCLC whose tumors have EGFR mutations.[63] Nineteen of the thirty-one (61%) approved agents demonstrated enough data to have additional uses listed in major treatment guidelines, and 11 (35%) of the agent received additional FDA approval. Finally, no drug approved without a randomized trial has demonstrated safety concerns significant enough to restrict marketing.

Biomarker-Based Registration Strategies

Compared to phases 1 and 2, investigators have made fewer phase 3 design modifications to accommodate the evaluation of targeted agents. One area, however, that has attracted considerable interest is whether sponsors should attempt to use biomarker-based

registration strategies in the phase 3 evaluation of targeted agents. Historically, investigators have sought to achieve a clinically homogenous population by defining specific inclusion criteria, but it has become clear that patients with seemingly similar clinical characteristics may have tumors with markedly different molecular features.[50] Researchers have used tools such as immunohistochemistry, fluorescence in situ hybridization (FISH), high-dimensional microarrays, and proteomic-based classifiers to successfully stratify patient subsets. If the drug is only effective in subsets of patients with certain molecular features, investigators may need to enroll large sample sizes to detect small differences for the entire cohort. The concern with this approach is that a positive treatment effect in a small minority of patients may drive a statistically significant finding, which may lead to a new marketing indication for the entire group of patients, despite the reality that only a small group of patients will experience a benefit.[50] Alternatively, a negative study may lead to the therapy being discarded despite offering real benefit to a specific subpopulation of patients, as exemplified by gefitinib in NSCLC.[64]

Even large trials may not be able to overcome the dilutive effect of nonresponsive subsets. If the sponsor of trastuzumab would have attempted to develop it in combination with chemotherapy without preselecting for patients with HER-2/neu-positive cancer, such a study would have required up to 24,000 randomly assigned patients to demonstrate an absolute 1-year survival improvement of 2.4%.[50] Instead, the sponsor used an enrichment strategy, enrolling only HER-2/neu-positive patients. The trial, which included only 469 patients, demonstrated an 11% absolute improvement in 1-year survival (from 67% to 78%) for trastuzumab combined with paclitaxel following treatment with an anthracycline-based regimen.[47] The trastuzumab example is also instructive because researchers identified HER-2/neu overexpression as a biomarker relatively early in the development process. During preclinical studies, researchers noted that antagonists to the 185-kDa transmembrane glycoprotein receptor of HER-2/neu were only effective at inhibiting growth of tumors and transformed cells that expressed high levels of the receptor.[65] By the time investigators began to plan phase 2 trials, they had decided to restrict enrolment to those patients with metastatic breast cancer whose tumor overexpressed HER-2/neu.[66,67] The failure of trastuzumab to improve outcomes in a phase 3 study of HER-2/neu non-overexpressors appears to validate this decision.[68]

In evaluating biomarker-based registration strategies, sponsors must try to balance the commercial impact of an indication that is restricted to a particular subset versus the risk of failure in a broader study population. Several guidelines may help sponsors make this decision. First, a biomarker-based strategy should be favored when the following conditions prevail: (a) there is an underlying true predictive marker that has been identified; (b) the prevalence of the marker is low; (c) the treatment is unlikely to produce a benefit in patients whose tumors do not possess the marker; and (d) the methods for determining the marker status are well established. If one or more of these conditions fail to be met, the randomize-all design is recommended (with possible retrospective testing for overall and within-marker treatment effect).[69] Investigators may also consider the toxicity of the agent (the more toxicity present the more an enrichment design is favored) and whether an unselected design is ethically impossible based on previous studies.[70] One group recently created a model to evaluate the economic trade-offs of a stratified approach versus randomize-all approach to oncology drug development. The authors found that biomarker-based approaches need only to increase phase 3 success rates modestly in order to justify their application from an economic perspective.[71]

At present, researchers are unable to identify a biomarker with enough scientific basis and supporting clinical data to permit prospectively defined, biomarker-based phase 3 registration trials for the majority agents under investigation (though the situation may improve as better targeted drugs and more clear subsets of patients are identified). It is therefore important to consider the requirements for a valid retrospective assessment of predictive biomarkers. One group has suggested that retrospective analyses should meet the following criteria: (a) the underlying outcomes data are derived from a well-conducted randomized controlled trial; (b) samples are available for a large majority of patients to avoid selection bias; (c) the hypothesis is prospectively stated; and (d) the investigators use a predefined and standardized assay and scoring system.[70] One example of a marker that has been successfully validated using data collected from previous phase 3 trials is KRAS mutation as a predictor of lack of efficacy for panitumumab and cetuximab in advanced colorectal cancer.

In addition to identifying markers that predict for primary benefit (or lack of benefit), researchers have been able to use such retrospective approaches to identify biomarkers, and the underlying mechanisms, of resistance. There are at least four possible factors that control for resistance to molecular targeted therapies: (a) increased transcriptional expression of the target because of gene amplification; (b) the presence of mutations downstream from the intended target (e.g., KRAS); (c) the emergence of additional mutations in the target (e.g., secondary mutations in exon 20 [T790M] of EGFR that confers resistance after initial response to EGFR tyrosine kinase inhibitors in NSCLC); and (d) activation of other pathways (e.g., insulin-like growth factor receptor 1 activation may mediate resistance to anti-EGFR therapy).[18] Researchers are actively working to identify additional markers of resistance,

but the underlying science is often complex. It is not only the presence but also the type of mutation that can confer resistance. For example, the response to sunitinib in imatinib-resistant GIST correlates with the type of KIT and PDGFRA mutations. In one study, those patients with either a primary KIT exon 9 mutation or wild-type KIT/PDGFRA enjoyed greater PFS and overall survival compared to those with KIT exon 11 mutations.[18]

Phase 4

Phase 4 trials are performed in the postmarketing period, often undertaken by the sponsor in order to seek additional marketing indications. The FDA may also require a phase 4 confirmatory trial as part of the conditions set forth under an AA in order to provide evidence of clinical benefit and collect additional safety data.[45] A detailed discussion of phase 4 trials is beyond the scope of this chapter.

Regulatory Review

Provided that completed clinical studies produce promising data, sponsors usually choose to advance their investigational agent to regulatory review (the final premarketing phase). The sponsor carefully prepares and submits a *new drug application* (NDA) or *biological licensing application* (BLA) containing all relevant preclinical and clinical data to the agencies that regulate approval in each jurisdiction for which marketing approval is sought (e.g., FDA, the European Medicines Agency, and Japanese Ministry of Health). The sponsor may choose to submit their NDA or BLA to multiple countries simultaneously. Commonly, however, they make their submissions in sequence given the interjurisdictional differences in approval requirements that exist despite efforts at international harmonization. Regulatory review represents only 5% to 10% of total clinical development time for most new oncology products (Fig. 3-4).[58]

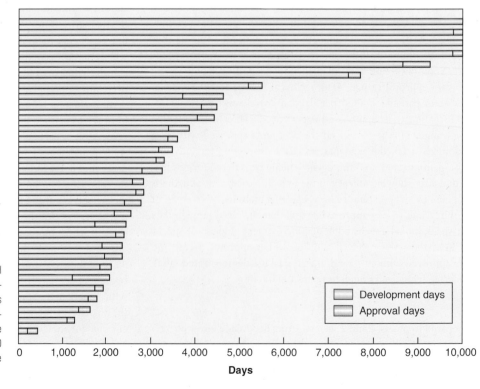

FIGURE **3-4** Development and approval times for NMEs approved 1995 to 2002. Regulatory review time (approval period) now represents approximately 5% to 10% of total clinical development time for most new oncology products. The fastest quintile of approvals occurs within 2,000 days (5.5 years) of beginning clinical trials. The data are from the FDA.

Legend: Development days / Approval days

X-axis: Days (0 to 10,000)

This proportion has decreased over time, from 33% in the 1960s, to approximately 25% in the 1980s, and to approximately 15% in the early 1990s.[72]

The FDA

In the United States, the FDA participates in the regulation of almost every step of clinical development. This regulation includes the oversight of clinical research, the evaluation of marketing claims for drugs seeking approval, and the monitoring of postmarketing activity for safety.[58] Over time, the FDA has evolved its approach to these regulatory activities. During the last 10 years in particular, decisions by the FDA have become more transparent and the relationship between the agency and the pharmaceutical industry has become more collaborative. Sponsors now consult with the agency throughout all stages of development, particularly in defining endpoints, selecting indications, and designing clinical trials. The FDA has also shown flexibility with respect to its approval and review policies. This flexibility has been especially evident with respect to drugs intended to treat serious or life-threatening illnesses such as cancer and AIDS and for indications that fulfill unmet medical needs. In response to criticism about the pace of drug development and FDA review, programs such as *Fast Track Designation*, *Priority Review*, and *Accelerated Approval* have been brought forward to allow patients suffering from cancer and other life-threatening illnesses to receive new medicines at relatively early stages of development.

The FDA derives its authority and direction from laws originating in the United States Congress (e.g., the Food and Drug Administration Modernization Act of 1997) and from multiple *regulations*. Regulations, which are published in the Code of Federal Regulations, do not require Congressional action but are subjected to a period of public review and scrutiny. When finalized, they are binding until revised or withdrawn. The FDA regulations stipulate that, "The purpose of conducting clinical investigations of a drug is to distinguish the effect of a drug from other influences, such as spontaneous change in the course of the disease, placebo effect, or biased observation."[73] The regulations specify further that reports of "adequate and well-controlled investigations" are required to provide the primary basis for determining whether there is "substantial evidence" to support the claims of effectiveness for new drugs.

In addition to the laws and regulations governing the agency, the FDA itself can issue *guidance documents* to reflect its current thinking. These documents are not binding, but they can be helpful to industry in its interpretation of the laws and regulations. Some examples of FDA guidance documents include, "Guidance on Providing Clinical Evidence of Effectiveness for Human Drug and Biological Products," issued in May 1998, and a series of documents issued in conjunction with the International Conference on Harmonization on the conduct and analysis of clinical studies. When issues arise that require greater clarification, the Federal Advisory Committee Act provides the FDA authority to consult a panel of outside experts to solicit advice and recommendations on policy.[58] The relevant panel for cancer is the Oncologic Drugs Advisory Committee (ODAC) that has a committee chairperson and 12 voting members, each serving staggered terms. At least one of the members is a patient representative and another is a statistician. Some members may abstain from voting due to potential conflicts of interest. The FDA typically follows the advice of the ODAC in response to questions addressed to the committee. However, the agency does not present all reviews for licensing applications to this committee and renders approval decisions based on the totality of the evidence, of which ODAC opinions represent a part. Two recent examples of FDA decisions that differed from ODAC recommendations include the approvals of bevacizumab in combination with paclitaxel in advanced breast cancer and gemcitabine (Gemzar) in combination with carboplatin in advanced ovarian cancer. In both instances, the FDA approved the indication despite an ODAC vote recommending against approval (by 5 to 4 in the negative for bevacizumab and 9 to 2 in the negative for gemcitabine). The FDA can also consider appointing an independent expert, at the request of a sponsor, to assist in the design of pivotal phase 3 protocols.

Interactions Between the FDA and Sponsors

The FDA possesses formal mechanisms to communicate with sponsors throughout the drug development process (Fig. 3-1). Prior to the initiation of clinical testing of an investigational agent, a drug sponsor must file an investigational new drug (IND) application and the FDA must grant permission to proceed with clinical studies. The IND application must include a copy of the protocol for each proposed study; a description of the physical, chemical, and biological characteristics of the agent; information on absorption, distribution, metabolism, and excretion; and an integrated summary of animal toxicology data.[74] IND filing is also required for the use of approved products that a sponsor wants to study in new populations or in regimens for which the risks are unknown. The IND approval process provides federal oversight of clinical investigations and is designed to protect potentially vulnerable research subjects.

The optimal times for the sponsor to solicit FDA input occur when particular landmarks are reached in the development process. Prior to filing a formal IND application, it can be helpful to the sponsor to request a pre-IND Meeting to solicit FDA advice regarding requirements for preclinical studies and to discuss clinical development scenarios, particularly for new molecular entities (NMEs). After the completion of phase 1 trials, a sponsor may request an end of phase 1 meeting to help in the planning of phase 2 trials, but such meetings are not universally sought. Once data are available from phase 2 studies, however, sponsors almost always request a meeting to discuss approaches to formally establishing efficacy of their investigational agents. In this critical end of phase 2 meeting, sponsor can discuss clinical trial design and analysis plans for proposed registration studies. The goal of the end of phase 2 meeting is to design and complete a trial or group of trials that will produce the relevant data from which a marketing claim may be made and labeling established. One analysis of NME approvals demonstrated that agents that were discussed in pre-IND and end of phase 2 conferences had shorter development times compared to those which were not discussed.[75] Table 3-2 outlines the many issues that sponsors must consider as they design and execute these pivotal studies.

At the conclusion of the end of phase 2 meeting, the sponsor can submit a detailed proposal for their critical phase 3 trial. This proposal is submitted for *Special Protocol Assessment* (SPA), with a legally mandated FDA review time of 45 days. In their assessment of the protocol, the FDA responds to specific questions the sponsor may have and provides general comments. If the FDA concurs with the

<table>
<tr><td>TABLE
3.2</td><td>*Key questions that sponsors must consider in the planning of registration trials*</td></tr>
</table>

What are the key endpoints?

Is the expectation to prolong life or make it better (or both)?

Is the nature of the anticipated benefit clinically meaningful?

Is the benefit measured directly or through a surrogate? Is the surrogate validated?

Is the data analysis plan stated in advance?

Does the analysis plan address the endpoints appropriately?

Is the comparator for a controlled study reasonable and appropriate?

Is the target patient population representative of people with the disease or condition?

What is the burden of visits and tests?

Is AA (using a surrogate) considered?

If AA is considered, what is the proposed follow-up study?

protocol, then a commitment exists to accept the design and size of the study as acceptable to support approval, but the agency makes no commitment for ultimate approval, which ultimately depends on the data. FDA agreement on a SPA does not necessarily indicate that the particular study alone will be a sufficient basis for licensing approval. Additional meetings are often scheduled before filing for an NDA or BLA to address particular chemical and manufacturing concerns (Product Meetings) and to seek input on the organization and format of the licensing application and the product labeling.

FDA Programs with Special Relevance to Oncology

The regulatory review process has undergone significant evolution since 1980, prompted by concerns that patients lacked access to innovative therapies and were impacted negatively by a lengthy review process.[76-78] Table 3-3 presents some of the major reform programs introduced since 1980 with particular relevance to cancer, including *Orphan Drug Designation* and the *"Fast Track"* programs.

In 1983, The U.S. Congress enacted the Orphan Drug Act, allowing the FDA to provide incentives and grants for certain drugs intended to treat diseases with a prevalence of less than 200,000 people in the United States, or those that affect more than 200,000 people, but for which there is no reasonable expectation that the costs of development would be recovered from sales in the United States. Orphan designation qualifies the sponsor for a longer period of marketing exclusivity (7 years starting on the approval date compared to 5 years); a 50% tax credit for money spent on clinical trials for the orphan indication; exemptions from application filing user fees; and the option to compete for FDA development grants.[79] Cancer drugs and biologics have comprised about 20% of all orphan drug approvals since its introduction. Among the 68 new oncology compounds approved by the FDA from 1990 to 2005, nearly half of the oncology drugs were initially approved with an orphan drug indication, while less than one in five other drugs had orphan drug status at first approval.[6] Examples of approved products with orphan designation include pemetrexed (Alimta) in the treatment

<table>
<tr><td colspan="3">TABLE
3.3   *FDA policy changes relevant to cancer*</td></tr>
<tr><td>Year(s)</td><td>Action</td><td>Result</td></tr>
<tr><td>1980s</td><td>Multiple guidance documents</td><td>Efficacy is defined as a demonstration of prolongation of life, a better life, or an established surrogate for at least one of these.</td></tr>
<tr><td>1983</td><td>Orphan Drug Act</td><td>Enables FDA to promote research and marketing of drugs for rare diseases (prevalence <200,000 in the United States), providing tax credits for clinical research and allowing 7 y of postapproval marketing exclusivity (compared to 5 y for regular approvals).</td></tr>
<tr><td>1991</td><td>Joint FDA/NCI proposal</td><td>Disease-free survival is allowed as a valid end point in the adjuvant setting if a large proportion of recurrences are symptomatic. Tumor RRs may be taken into consideration along with response duration, drug toxicity, and relief of tumor-related symptoms.</td></tr>
<tr><td>1992</td><td>Prescription Drug User Fee Act is enacted and Subpart H is added</td><td>*AA* is allowed for serious or life-threatening diseases when the new drug appears to provide benefit over available therapy, but when the demonstrated benefit does not meet the standard for regular approval; RRs alone may provide basis for AA when they are "reasonably likely surrogates" for clinical benefit. *Priority review* is instituted for those products that provide significant improvements in safety or efficacy in treating, diagnosing, or preventing serious disease; the FDA is required to review 90% of priority-related drug applications within 6 mo of filing date. Payment of *user fees* by sponsors is tied to a series of FDA performance goals that commit the agency to accelerating the review process.</td></tr>
<tr><td>1997</td><td>FDA Modernization Act</td><td>Allows the FDA to consider data from "one adequate and well-controlled clinical investigation" with confirmatory evidence if data are sufficient to establish effectiveness. Codifies the *fast track processes* for speeding the development of drugs that address unmet needs.</td></tr>
</table>

NCI, National Cancer Institute.

of malignant pleural mesothelioma, bortezomib (Velcade) in the treatment of multiple myeloma, and rituximab in the treatment of non-Hodgkin's B-cell lymphoma. The Orphan Drug Program was not designed to address either the criteria for approval nor establish new target goals for FDA review times.

Over the period from 1992 to 1997, the U.S. Congress enacted two laws, the Prescription Drug User Fee Act of 1992 (PDUFA) and the FDA Modernization Act of 1997 (FDAMA), which together have had a major impact on the process that the agency uses for reviewing and approving cancer drugs.[80] The three programs introduced over this time period with the greatest impact include *Fast Track designation*, *Accelerated Approval*, and *Priority Review*. The Fast Track mechanism represents a formal structure by which sponsors may interact with the FDA. As described in the FDAMA, Fast Track designation can be granted to the combination of a product and a claim that addresses an unmet medical need for a serious or life-threatening illness. The benefits of Fast Track designation, if granted, include scheduled meetings to seek FDA input into development plans; the option of submitting an NDA in sections rather than all components simultaneously; and the option of requesting evaluation of studies using surrogate endpoints. For the most part, these interactions were already available to sponsors prior to the FDAMA, but the Fast Track mechanism formalized the approach for a subset of drugs.

Accelerated Approval

Of the programs that have been designed to expedite the drug development process, none has had more impact or has generated more public commentary than AA. The AA regulations were added in 1992 (under Subpart H for drugs and under Subpart E for biologics). These provisions allow the FDA to approve agents intended to treat serious or life-threatening illnesses before the clinical benefit necessary to meet the standard for regular approval has been demonstrated. Using AA, the FDA can grant a provisional approval on the basis of a reasonably likely surrogate measure of clinical benefit (e.g., tumor shrinkage) if the treatment is considered superior to available therapy for a serious or life-threatening illness.[81] The regulatory standard for an AA can be less challenging than the standard for regular approval because regular approval is predicated on the demonstration of a clinical benefit (e.g., prolonged survival or an improved quality of life) and not on a surrogate endpoint. The FDA grants the approval and receives the sponsor's agreement to complete confirmatory phase 4 trials to demonstrate the clinical benefit in a timely manner during the postapproval period. If these trials do not confirm a clinical benefit, the drug can be withdrawn from the market. Congress passed legislation in 2007 that grants the FDA authority to impose fines on sponsors and to limit drug distribution if postmarketing commitments are not completed.[60]

The FDA granted the first oncology-related AA in 1995. From 1995 to 2008, the FDA granted marketing approval for a total of 51 NMEs: 32 with regular approvals and 19 with AA.[60] Table 3-4 lists oncology agents approved using the AA through 2008. Through the end of 2008, eleven of 19 (63%) oncology NMEs granted AA had clinical benefit confirmed in confirmatory trials and have been granted regular aproval.[60] One review of the AA program from 1992 through 1997 estimated that access to the program shortened overall development time by as much as 4 years in some instances.[72] The FDA and others in the medical community have expressed concern over the failure of sponsors to complete confirmatory phase 4 studies,[61,82] prompting a focus on the issue during the March 2003 meeting of the ODAC.

There is some evidence that it has become more difficult to obtain FDA approval with the AA process.[60] The FDA has granted fewer approvals of oncology-related NMEs using the AA mechanism versus regular approval over the past several years. In the early 2000s, 78% of oncology NMEs received AA versus 22% regular approval. However, since 2004, only 32% of oncology NMEs received AA versus 68% regular approval. This reduction is coincident with the failure of gefitinib to demonstrate clinical benefit in its confirmatory phase 3 trial and with concern expressed by FDA officials at ODAC meetings in 2003 and 2005 that sponsors failed to complete agreed-upon confirmatory trials. FDA officials have encouraged sponsors to file initial applications for AA on surrogate outcomes reported in interim analyses of phase 3 trials rather than on final analyses of phase 2 trials, a policy, which is similar to what is typically followed in agents used to treat HIV infection.[60]

Priority Review

The final FDA program highlighted in this chapter is *Priority Review*. Priority Review is relevant only after a claim has been submitted to the FDA for review. As described in the PDUFA and the FDAMA, the FDA designates reviews for NDAs as either standard or priority. A standard designation sets the target date for the agency to complete all aspects of a review and to take action on the application (i.e., approve or not approve) at 10 months after the date of NDA filing. In comparison, a priority designation sets the target date for the FDA action at 6 months. Similar to the Fast Track program, priority review is intended for those products that address unmet medical needs. Of the 68 compounds approved by the FDA from 1990 to 2005, 71% of the oncology drug approvals were given a priority review rating by the FDA, in contrast to 40% for new drugs in other therapeutic categories.[6] Among the quickest priority reviews to date have been imatinib mesylate for the treatment of chronic myelogenous leukemia (CML) and oxaliplatin (Eloxatin) in combination with 5-fluorouracil and leucovorin for the treatment of relapsed or refractory colorectal cancer, receiving approval after just 10 and 7 weeks of FDA review, respectively.

Despite more often obtaining regulatory advantages from programs to speed clinical development and regulatory review of marketing applications, U.S. clinical development times and total times from the start of U.S. clinical testing to marketing approval were longer (1.5 years), on average, for oncology drugs than for other drugs approved from 1990 to 2005. The recent efforts by the FDA to establish new approaches to assess the efficacy and safety of investigational drugs through its Critical Path Initiative hold the promise of shorter development times for oncology and other drugs.[6] Of particular relevance for oncology drugs is the Critical Path Initiative's goal to find and validate new biomarkers.

Approval Strategies

The FDA does not approve a drug but rather approves a claim about the use of a drug.[58] However, it is common after approval for oncologists to use agents for other than the approved claim.[83] A sponsor can take multiple pathways to achieve approval for the first marketing claim of its drug or biologic agent. A major decision

TABLE

3.4 *Oncology NMEs that received accelerated FDA approval from 1995 through 2008*

	Indication	Date of FDA approval	Primary end point	Trials that support approval		No. of patients included in trials	Subpart H completion date
				Phases	No. of trials		
Orphan drug indication							
Denileukin diftitox	Cutaneous T-cell lymphoma	2/5/99	RR	I/II, III		106	10/15/08
Temozolomide	Anaplastic astrocytoma/high-grade glioma with radiation therapy	8/11/99	RR	II		162	3/15/05
Gemtuzumab	CD33+ AML	5/17/00	RR	II	3	142	Pending
Alemtuzumab	B-cell CLL, treated with alkylating agents, failed fludarabine	5/7/01	RR	II		93	9/19/07
Imatinib	Ph-positive CML in AP, CP after failure of IFN, blast crisis	5/10/01	RR	II	3	1,027	12/8/03
Ibritumomab tiuxetan	Relapsed, refractory, low-grade follicular or transformed NHL	2/19/02	RR	II, III		197	Pending
Bortezomib	Refractory multiple myeloma	5/13/03	RR	II	2	256	3/25/05
Tositumomab	Rituximab-naïve follicular NHL	6/27/03	RR	II		40	9/19/07
Cetuximab	EGFR-positive metastatic colorectal cancer in second-line combination with irinotecan	2/12/04	RR	II	3	524	10/2/07
Clofarabine	Pediatric ALL	12/28/04	CR	I, II	2	86	Pending
Nelarabine	T-cell ALL/lymphoma	10/28/05	RR	II	2	67	Pending
Nilotinib	CP and AP Ph-positive CML	10/29/07	RR	II		337	Pending
Non–orphan drug indication							
Docetaxel	Metastatic breast cancer	5/14/96	RR	II	3	134	6/22/98
Irinotecan	Metastatic colorectal cancer	6/14/96	RR	II	3	304	10/22/98
Capecitabine	Metastatic breast cancer	4/30/98	RR	II		163	9/7/01
Oxaliplatin	Metastatic colorectal cancer	8/9/02	RR, TTP	III		463	1/9/04
Gefitinib	Single-agent therapy for refractory NSCLC	5/5/03	RR	II		142	6/17/05
Sunitinib	Advanced renal cell carcinoma	1/26/06	TTP	III		312	2/2/07
Panitumumab	Third-line treatment of EGFR-expressing metastatic colon cancer, progression after other chemotherapy	9/27/06	PFS	III		463	Pending

FDA, U.S. Food and Drug Administration; RR, response rate; AML, acute myeloid leukemia; CLL, chronic lymphocytic leukemia; CML, chronic myelogenous leukemia; ALL, acute lymphocytic leukemia; AP, acute progression; CP, chronic progression; IFN, interferon; NHL, non-Hodgkin's lymphoma; EGFR, epidermal growth factor receptor; CR, complete response; Ph-positive, Philadelphia chromosome positive; TTP, time to progression; NSCLC, non–small-cell lung cancer; PFS, progression-free survival. Data are from Richey EA, Lyons EA, Nebeker JR, et al. Accelerated approval of cancer drugs: improved access to therapeutic breakthroughs or early release of unsafe and ineffective drugs? J Clin Oncol 2009.

that sponsors must make is for what line of treatment they will seek approval. A common approach is to begin therapeutic development with the use of a new single-agent as second- or third-line therapy for relapsed or refractory disease, a setting in which there may be no effective treatment. The assumption is that activity in treatment-experienced patients will translate into clinical benefit for treatment-naïve patients. The phase 2 trials of gefitinib (Iressa) for the treatment of advanced NSCLC after failure of platinum- and docetaxel-based chemotherapies illustrate this approach since the data from these trials initially supported an AA of gefitinib in the third-line setting.[84,85] In comparison, first-line approvals tend to be more difficult to achieve since the new agent must prove at least as good as the best treatment available. In order to either show an outcome difference or establish noninferiority, trials supporting first-line approvals will typically require more patients and longer follow-up than single-arm trials in refractory or relapsed populations, unless the new agent is impressively superior to available therapy. First-line approvals are also less likely to earn an AA because there is at least one first-line regimen established for most cancers, and AA requires a demonstration of superiority if a standard therapy exists.

Despite the risks associated with seeking a first-line indication, the effort can be worthwhile because a first-line approval will apply to a larger treatment population. A common strategy in the first-line setting is to examine whether a new agent adds any benefit (or risk) to an established regimen. The registration trial of bevacizumab provides an example of this strategy: previously untreated patients with metastatic colorectal cancer were randomly assigned to receive irinotecan, bolus fluorouracil, and leucovorin (IFL) plus bevacizumab versus IFL alone.[86]

A second decision that sponsors must make is how many registration studies to undertake. In general, the FDA regards results of a single trial supporting approval as inadequate evidence.[87] However, a single study may be considered adequate for licensing when the study is a well designed, large multicenter study; when the implementation is of unquestionable quality; when the findings appear clinically important; when the results are statistically persuasive and internally consistent; and when the confirmation of the results would present ethical or logistical hurdles. Often single large trials are supported by multiple phase 2 studies.

Over the past 15 years, the oncology market has provided an attractive arena for drug development compared to many other areas of medicine. In most of the large-market indications, standard of care chemotherapeutic regimens have not extended beyond second-line treatments.[15] This situation has created a relatively straightforward path for the many of the more tolerable targeted therapeutic agents that have reached the market supported by either third-line trial data in large indications or by first-line data in indications where standards of care are either absent or clearly inadequate. As indications have filled over the past several years, sponsors will likely have to pursue more creative, costly, and lengthy development of the newer targeted agents in combination with existing standards of care.[15]

General Approval Considerations

The FDA has approved approximately 110 agents for the treatment of cancer, and there has been a steady trend over the past several decades toward more frequent approvals.[15] At the most fundamental level, the agency must determine if there are differences between the treatment and control groups and then determine if the differences are due to the intervention under review. Establishing an appropriate control is therefore critical because it is often difficult to determine efficacy without a control unless the results are close to miraculous. Controls can either be historical or concurrent, and sponsors using the AA mechanism have usually employed historical controls in their phase 2 trials that support approval. However, concurrent controls have multiple advantages. Specifically, concurrent controls ensure consistency of diagnosis, uniform techniques and frequency of clinical assessments of response and toxicity, a common level of supportive care, and consistency of administration of an intervention. Concurrent controls also allow for the possibility of reducing bias through blinding, although it is often difficult to blind cancer trials because of side effects.

The regulations guide the overall process of FDA approval, but the steps and the sequence of steps that the agency can take in this process are not completely standardized and therefore allow for some flexibility. During a review of a licensing application, the separate disciplines at the FDA review all primary data. The agency determines the nature of the claim, prepares a survey of available therapies that address the same problem (focusing on the nature and duration of the treatment effect of each therapy), and reconstructs what data and analysis would support a new claim. The FDA then identifies the key elements of the submission that provide the data to support the claim. The agency reviews the study protocols (focusing on eligibility, endpoints, measured variables, and planned analysis) and conducts its own analysis with regard to each patient meeting eligibility, having the requisite measurements, and completing the study. The treatment effect is then determined, and the FDA analysis is compared to the sponsor's planned and submitted analyses.

If the FDA analysis demonstrates that the efficacy of the experimental treatment is either inferior to a control or cannot be distinguished from placebo effect, then there is no need for further analysis, and the application is denied. If the agency determines that the efficacy of the treatment is either superior to or at least not inferior to an active control, and if dropouts and censored patients can be adequately accounted for, the FDA proceeds with a safety analysis for each study to determine an estimate of the risk-to-benefit ratio (Fig. 3-5). Although a discussion of noninferiority is beyond the scope of this chapter, the factors that are critical in

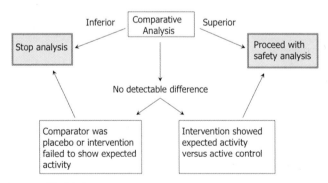

FIGURE **3-5**   Flow diagram of the initial FDA review process. The first step is to determine if the intervention showed its expected activity. If the expected activity is not demonstrated, the analysis is stopped without proceeding to a safety analysis. If the expected activity is demonstrated, the agency proceeds with a safety analysis, and the intervention may be eligible for approval if a favorable risk-to-benefit ratio is found.

the design and analysis of a noninferiority study are the magnitude and reproducibility of the active control effect, defining the acceptable margin of retaining the active control effect, and describing in detail the analytic plan including provisions for missing data and censoring. After completing its analysis, the agency compares the efficacy data and safety data to the proposed marketing claims and then, if approval can be made, adjusts the claims in alignment with the conclusions supported by the data.

Assessment of Benefit and Risk

The assessment of risk is reasonably standard for oncology studies. The FDA evaluates toxicity in the context of the organ systems involved, severity, and reversibility of adverse events, using the same principles of a graded scale (e.g., NCI Common Toxicity Criteria) that are applied in other areas of medicine. The assessment of benefit on the other hand is less standardized (Table 3-5) and is often the subject of considerable dialogue and discussion.

Response Rates

In the 1970s and early 1980s, the FDA approved oncology drugs on the basis of RR alone. By the mid 1980s the ODAC advised the FDA against using RR as the sole basis for approval since the possible benefit of a response may be outweighed by toxicity. Moreover, the correlation between RR and survival benefit had not been established for most solid tumors.[88] In response to this recommendation, the FDA adopted a new position calling for an improvement in survival or patient symptoms as the standard for regular approval.[89] Guidance documents promulgated in the 1980s specified further that the requirement for efficacy should be demonstrated by prolongation of life, a better life (e.g., relief of symptoms), or an established surrogate for at least one of these.[81]

In 1991, the NCI and FDA jointly examined the potential of various endpoints to demonstrate clinical benefit and again considered the issue of whether RRs could be used as a valid endpoint for drug approval. The two agencies concluded that complete responses of reasonable duration, particularly in acute leukemia, could be a potentially valid endpoint, as long as they correlated with clinical benefits such as reduced transfusion requirements. Partial responses

TABLE

3.5   *Types of endpoints used in clinical oncology*

Survival
   Overall
   Disease-free
Progression
   Tumor (usually based on imaging results)
   Onset or worsening of disease-related symptoms
Response
   Tumor (usually based on imaging results)
   Patient benefit (palliation, improvement in symptoms)
Protection against adverse events with no decrease in survival
Reduction in the risk of disease
   From initial onset in a high-risk population
   From recurrence in adjuvant setting

were also considered as possibly valid endpoints, but only after considering their duration, the associated toxicity, and the potential to relieve tumor-related symptoms.[90]

A summary of the endpoints used in studies to support licensure for 90 separate claims for a variety of indications between 1985 and 2003 is shown in Table 3-6. The data show that most applications have multiple endpoints, and in most cases, the determination of approving a claim for marketing was made on the totality of the evidence and not on a single endpoint. If several endpoints indicate the same trend, the support for considering approval is usually increased. Table 3-7 presents a tabulation of the endpoints from Table 3-6 to indicate their frequency in the aggregate of all 90 approved claims. The data show that few endpoints were used as sole criteria for marketing approval, but RR was used most frequently, appearing in 60% of all claims and about 75% of AAs. In the hematologic malignancies, complete responses of a predetermined duration can be considered beneficial to patients due to absence of disease complications such as bleeding, need for transfusions, or infections. Overall survival was used as a component of 27% of all claims, but as a single criterion in only 5% of claims—twice for first-line colorectal cancer, once for first-line glioblastoma multiforme, and once each for second-line NSCLC and glioblastoma multiforme. The frequency of use of overall survival and time to disease progression are quite similar. Disease-free survival and recurrence rate have been primarily used in the adjuvant setting.

The difficulty in establishing a coherent policy on the use of RRs to support approval relates to the lack of a documented relationship between tumor response and clinical benefit for most tumors. This relationship has been evaluated adequately in only a few tumor types and often with conflicting results. For example, Buyse et al. performed a meta-analysis of 25 trials in colorectal cancer involving fluoropyrimidines and concluded that tumor response was a significant independent predictor of survival.[91] In contrast, Chen et al. did not find a significant correlation of phase 2 RRs with median survival times in phase 3 trials of the same regimen in small cell lung cancer.[92] RRs may provide a reasonable surrogate for survival but only in certain diseases and with certain drugs. At present, the FDA continues to approve agents on the basis of RRs, but most of these approvals only meet the standard for AA, and therefore require confirmatory trials that employ clinical benefit endpoints. Finally, some investigators have suggested reporting efficacy as a continuous variable (percent change in tumor size) rather than as response versus nonresponse since the threshold for a partial response is necessarily arbitrary.[64]

Progression-Free Survival

Some agents, particularly those with mechanisms of actions that are not cytotoxic, may produce clinical benefit by delaying tumor progression, with relatively low RRs. For these agents, time to tumor progression (TTP) or PFS may be a more appropriate surrogate endpoint than response. TTP or PFS is typically defined as the time from enrollment to documented progression of tumor size based on imaging tests (and not on biochemical tumor markers). The difference between TTP and PFS is that in the latter, death is considered progression. Two major benefits of using progression include the potential need for smaller sample sizes and shorter follow-up times than for overall survival studies. Delayed progression in conjunction with RRs have been considered adequate surrogates for clinical

TABLE

3.6 *Endpoints for approvals of oncology drug marketing applications January 1, 1985 to November 1, 2003*

Disease indication	Line(s) of treatment	Accelerated approval?	Endpoint(s)	No. of claims	Percent of total claims (%)
Acute lymphocytic leukemia	First, second		CR	3	3
AIDS-related Kaposi's sarcoma	First		RR, TTP	2	2
AIDS-related Kaposi's sarcoma	Second	YES	RR	1	1
AIDS-related Kaposi's sarcoma	Second		RR	2	2
Acute myelogenous leukemia	Second	YES	CR	1	1
Acute myelogenous leukemia	First, second		CR	8	9
B-cell chronic lymphocytic leukemia	Second	YES	RR	1	1
B-cell chronic lymphocytic leukemia	Second		RR	1	1
Bladder cancer	Second		RR	1	1
Central nervous system cancer	First		OS	1	1
Central nervous system cancer	Second		OS	1	1
Central nervous system cancer	Second	YES	RR	1	1
Breast cancer	Adjuvant	YES	DFS	1	1
Breast cancer	Adjuvant		DFS, OS	5	6
Breast cancer, metastatic	First		RR, TTP, 1-y survival	3	3
Breast cancer, metastatic	Second	YES	RR	2	2
Breast cancer, metastatic	Second		RR, TTP	6	7
Chronic myelogenous leukemia	First	YES	CR	1	1
Chronic myelogenous leukemia	Second	YES	CR	1	1
Chronic myelogenous leukemia	Second		CR	1	1
Colorectal cancer	Adjuvant		Recurrence rate	1	1
Colorectal cancer, metastatic	First		OS	2	2
Colorectal cancer, metastatic	Second	YES	RR, TTP	2	2
Colorectal cancer, metastatic	Second		RR, OS	1	1
Cutaneous T-cell lymphoma	Second		RR	3	3
Esophageal cancer	Palliative		Symptom benefit	1	1
Lymphoma, follicular	Second	YES	RR	1	1
Lymphoma, follicular	Second		RR	1	1
Gastrointestinal stromal tumor	First, second	YES	RR	1	1
Hairy cell leukemia	First		CR, RR, TTP	3	3
Hairy cell leukemia	Second		CR	1	1
Lung cancer, nonsmall cell	First		OS, RR, TTP	4	4
Lung cancer, nonsmall cell	Second		OS	1	1
Lung cancer, nonsmall cell	Third	YES	RR	1	1
Lung cancer, nonsmall cell	Palliative		Symptom benefit	1	1
Lung cancer, small cell	First		OS, RR	2	2
Lung cancer, small cell	Second		RR, symptom benefit	1	1
Lymphoma, non-Hodgkin's	Second	YES	RR	2	2
Lymphomatous meningitis	Second	YES	RR	1	1
Melanoma	Adjuvant		DFS, OS	1	1
Multiple myeloma	Third	YES	RR	1	1
Multiple myeloma	Third		RR	1	1
Osteosarcoma	First		RR	1	1
Ovarian cancer	First		OS, RR	2	2
Ovarian cancer	Second	YES	RR	1	1
Ovarian cancer	Second		RR, TTP, OS	3	3
Pancreas cancer	First, second		OS, symptom benefit	1	1
Pleural effusion, malignant	Palliative		Recurrence rate	2	2
Prostate cancer	Palliative		Symptom benefit	2	2
Testicular cancer	Third		RR, DFS	2	2

CR, complete response; RR, response rate; TTP, time to tumor progression, DFS, disease-free survival; OS, overall survival.
Data are from the FDA.

TABLE

3.7 *Tabulation of registration study endpoints that supported marketing claims from January 1, 1985 to November 1, 2003*

Endpoint	Regular approval (%)	Accelerated approval (%)	Total[a] (%)
CR	3	18	21
RR	17	43	60
TTP	2	23	26
OS	0	27	27
DFS	1	9	10
1-y survival rate	0	3	3
Recurrence rate	0	3	3
Symptom benefit	0	7	7

[a]Totals exceed 100% because most applications included multiple endpoints.
CR, response rate; RR, response rate; TTP, time to tumor progression; OS, overall; DFS, disease-free survival.
Data are from the FDA.

benefit in evaluating hormonal treatments for breast cancer, supporting regular approvals for exemestane, toremifene, anastrozole, letrozole, and fulvestrant in randomized trials comparing each of these with tamoxifen or with another approved hormonal agent.[81] It seems to be a more appropriate endpoint for hormonal or other targeted agents that have a cytostatic effect.

The ODAC has expressed concern with PFS as an endpoint for a number of submissions outside of the adjuvant setting.[93] Their negative assessments relate to the general limitations of using PFS an endpoint. First, PFS can only be evaluated reliably in the context of randomized trials, due to the difficulty of comparing results from historical controls in which assessment of tumor status post therapy is not consistent across trials. In addition, there are few historical control databases that have used PFS as an endpoint. Second, even within randomized trials, PFS outcomes may be influenced by the frequency of obtaining imaging studies. If effective blinding is not performed, investigator bias may influence decisions regarding the timing of imaging studies and the interpretation of clinical data. FDA officials have suggested during a recent ODAC meeting that a large effect on PFS may compensate for these limitations. Despite these concerns, the use of PFS in appropriate disease settings remains an attractive endpoint to sponsors because of the shorter time frame to assess results compared to overall survival and the absence of potential confounding of survival effect by subsequent therapy.

Surrogate Endpoints

The Biomarkers Definitions Working Group defined biomarkers as "a characteristic that is objectively measured and evaluated as an indicator of normal biological processes, pathologic processes, or pharmacologic responses to a therapeutic intervention."[94] A subset of biomarkers that can potentially substitute for a clinical endpoint can be denoted as surrogate endpoints.[49] The FDA has issued guidance for industry on pharmacogenomic biomarkers and their degree of validity: exploratory biomarkers, probably valid biomarkers,

and known valid biomarkers. An example of an exploratory biomarker includes the use of gene panels in preclinical studies. For an exploratory biomarker to achieve the status of a probably valid biomarker, it needs to be "measured in an analytic test system with well-established performance characteristics and for which there is an established scientific framework or body of evidence that elucidates the physiologic, toxicologic, pharmacologic, or clinical significance of the test results."[95] Advancing from "probably valid" to "known valid" status requires the achievement of a broad consensus in cross-validation experiments.[95] Investigators and the FDA will likely focus increasingly on surrogate markers as the science underlying the use of biomarkers progresses, as discussed earlier in the chapter.

Relief of Tumor-Related Symptoms

Relief of tumor-related symptoms has been used as a primary or supportive basis for licensing in six applications for antitumor products between 1985 and 2003 (Table 3-6). Examples of symptom benefit supporting licensure include the approval of mitoxantrone in combination with corticosteroids as initial chemotherapy for the treatment of patients with pain related to advanced hormone-refractory prostate cancer; the predefined "clinical benefit response," a composite endpoint of pain, weight gain, and performance status, that provided support for the approval of gemcitabine for the treatment of locally advanced or metastatic pancreatic cancer, even though a small but significant improvement in survival was the primary basis for approval; changes in respiratory symptoms in small cell lung cancer associated with topotecan use; and changes in respiratory symptoms in NSCLC associated with the use of porfimer sodium in the photodynamic treatment of endobronchial lesions.

Survival

Of all of the possible endpoints to assess benefit, survival is the least prone to bias and the least controversial in terms of its ability to support an FDA approval. All other endpoints used to support approval must not have a negative impact on survival.[58] Survival as an endpoint, however, is not without its limitations. The accurate recording of survival times requires long follow-up and potentially large sample sizes depending upon the magnitude of drug effect. Subsequent treatments after progression can also confound or mitigate the interpretation of survival effect, particularly in crossover study designs. In part due to these limitations, overall survival has contributed to the basis for approval for only about a quarter of claims (Table 3-7).

Conclusion

The availability of molecular diagnostics and the focus on targeted therapies have created enormous opportunities and challenges for investigators and sponsors. There are more investigational agents, more effective lines of therapy, more diseases, and more complex regulatory hurdles. However, the new oncology drugs that have been approved in recent years have been novel and commercially successful. Approved oncology drugs have been more often first-in-class and diffused more widely to major international markets than has been the case for drugs in other classes.[6] Nonetheless, there is a need for new therapies for cancer that are effective and safe. The incentives and scientific opportunities to develop highly effective oncology drugs in the future will depend critically on public-sector investment in basic research, developments in translational medicine, and regulatory reforms that advance drug-development science.[6]

What will it take? A recent plenary talk from a prominent investigator and ASCO President may have summed it up the best. It will take, "a biospecimen from every patient, a validated assay run in a Clinical Laboratory Improvement Amendments (CLIA)-certified laboratory with acceptable turnaround time, a drug that hits the target, a regulatory system willing to approve drugs and companion diagnostics with greater flexibility, reimbursement and regulatory incentives to develop molecular diagnostics, a drug industry willing to trade widespread, short-term drug use for chronic therapy in more limited populations, and doctors and patients who are willing and able to participate in clinical trials."[55] Ultimately, investigators will need a more complete understanding of the biology underlying cancer to enhance the pace of development. Investigators will need to continue to work collaboratively with sponsors to design controlled trials that most efficiently screen and test new agents. In order for these collaborative efforts to prove most successful, investigators will increasingly require reproducible assays to assess for the presence and activity of critical targets as well as reliable surrogate markers to assess for benefit.

Note: The views presented in this chapter represent independent work and do not necessarily represent those of Noonday Asset Management or its affiliates.

Acknowledgment

The author would like to thank Steven Hirschfeld, MD, PhD of the National Institutes of Health for his participation in helpful discussion on a previous version of this chapter.

Additional Resources

U.S. Food and Drug Administration Development and Approval Process (Drugs): http://www.fda.gov/Drugs/Development ApprovalProcess/default.htm

U.S. Food and Drug Administration Development Office of Oncology Drug Products: http://www.fda.gov/AboutFDA/Centers Offices/CDER/ucm091745.htm

U.S. Food and Drug Administration Critical Path Initiative: http://www.fda.gov/ScienceResearch/SpecialTopics/Critical PathInitiative/default.htm

References

1. Pharmaceutical Research and Manufacturers of America. Medicine in Development for Cancer. Washington, DC: Pharmaceutical Research and Manufacturers of America, 2009.
2. IMS LifeCycle, R&D focus. In: Parexel's Pharmaceutical R&D Statistical Sourcebook 2006/2007. Walthan, MA: Parexel.
3. Downing JR. Cancer genomes—continuing progress. N Engl J Med 2009;361(11):1111–1112.
4. Dimasi JA. New drug development in the United States from 1963 to 1999. Clin Pharmacol Ther 2001;69(5):286–296.
5. Roberts TG Jr, Lynch TJ Jr, Chabner BA. The phase III trial in the era of targeted therapy: unraveling the "go or no go" decision. J Clin Oncol 2003;21(19):3683–3695.
6. DiMasi JA, Grabowski HG. Economics of new oncology drug development. J Clin Oncol 2007;25(2):209–216.
7. Von Hoff DD. There are no bad anticancer agents, only bad clinical trial designs—twenty-first Richard and Hinda Rosenthal Foundation Award Lecture. Clin Cancer Res 1998;4(5):1079–1086.
8. DiMasi JA, Hansen RW, Grabowski HG. The price of innovation: new estimates of drug development costs. J Health Econ 2003;22(2):151–185.
9. Vernon JA, Golec JH, Dimasi JA. Drug development costs when financial risk is measured using the Fama-French three-factor model. Health Econ 2009;19(8):1002–1005.
10. Adams CP, Brantner VV. Estimating the cost of new drug development: is it really 802 million dollars? Health Aff (Millwood) 2006;25(2):420–428.
11. Eliopoulos H, Giranda V, Carr R, et al. Phase 0 trials: an industry perspective. Clin Cancer Res 2008;14(12):3683–3688.
12. Booth CM, Calvert AH, Giaccone G, et al. Endpoints and other considerations in phase I studies of targeted anticancer therapy: recommendations from the task force on Methodology for the Development of Innovative Cancer Therapies (MDICT). Eur J Cancer 2008;44(1):19–24.
13. Cowen and Company. Therapeutic Categories Outlook: Comprehensive Study. New York, NY: Cowen and Company, 2009:791.
14. LoRusso PM. Phase 0 clinical trials: an answer to drug development stagnation? J Clin Oncol 2009;27(16):2586–2588.
15. Canaccord Adams. Life Sciences—Emerging Therapeutics: Targeted Therapeutics in Oncology. New York, NY: George Farmer & Laura Ekas.
16. Schilsky RL. Target practice: oncology drug development in the era of genomic medicine. Clin Trials 2007;4(2):163–166; discussion 173–177.
17. Abrams JS, Mooney M, Goldberg J, et al. Bringing new agents to market: navigating the regulatory requirements for investigators. AACR Educ Book 2005:211–216.
18. Gutierrez ME, Kummar S, Giaccone G. Next generation oncology drug development: opportunities and challenges. Nat Rev Clin Oncol 2009;6(5):259–265.
19. Johnson JI, Decker S, Zaharevitz D, et al. Relationships between drug activity in NCI preclinical in vitro and in vivo models and early clinical trials. Br J Cancer 2001;84(10):1424–1431.
20. US Food and Drug Administration. Guidance for industry, investigators, and reviewers: exploratory IND studies. This is a Guidance by the FDA available at http://www.fda.gov/downloads/Drugs/GuidanceComplianceRegulatory Information/Guidances/ucm078933.pdf. Rockville, MD: U.S. Food and Drug Administration, January 2006.
21. Twombly R. Slow start to phase 0 as researchers debate value. J Natl Cancer Inst 2006;98(12):804–806.
22. Kummar S, Kinders R, Gutierrez ME, et al. Phase 0 clinical trial of the poly (ADP-ribose) polymerase inhibitor ABT-888 in patients with advanced malignancies. J Clin Oncol 2009;27(16):2705–2711.
23. ClinicalTrials.gov: A Service of the US National Institutes of Health, Developed by the National Library of Medicine. http://www.clinicaltrials.gov/. Accessed October 29, 2009.
24. Roberts TG Jr, Goulart BH, Squitieri L, et al. Trends in the risks and benefits to patients with cancer participating in phase 1 clinical trials. JAMA 2004;292(17):2130–2140.
25. Meropol NJ, Weinfurt KP, Burnett CB, et al. Perceptions of patients and physicians regarding phase I cancer clinical trials: implications for physician-patient communication. J Clin Oncol 2003;21(13):2589–2596.
26. Daugherty C, Ratain MJ, Grochowski E, et al. Perceptions of cancer patients and their physicians involved in phase I trials. J Clin Oncol 1995;13(5):1062–1072.
27. Dowlati A, Haaga J, Remick SC, et al. Sequential tumor biopsies in early phase clinical trials of anticancer agents for pharmacodynamic evaluation. Clin Cancer Res 2001;7(10):2971–2976.
28. Goulart BH, Clark JW, Pien HH, et al. Trends in the use and role of biomarkers in phase I oncology trials. Clin Cancer Res 2007;13(22 Pt 1):6719–6726.
29. Parulekar WR, Eisenhauer EA. Phase I trial design for solid tumor studies of targeted, non-cytotoxic agents: theory and practice. J Natl Cancer Inst 2004;96(13):990–997.
30. Plummer R, Jones C, Middleton M, et al. Phase I study of the poly(ADP-ribose) polymerase inhibitor, AG014699, in combination with temozolomide in patients with advanced solid tumors. Clin Cancer Res 2008;14(23):7917–7923.

31. Petrelli NJ, Winer EP, Brahmer J, et al. Clinical cancer advances 2009: major research advances in cancer treatment, prevention, and screening—a report from the American Society of Clinical Oncology. J Clin Oncol 2009;27(35):6052–6069.

32. Michaelis LC, Ratain MJ. Phase II trials published in 2002: a cross-specialty comparison showing significant design differences between oncology trials and other medical specialties. Clin Cancer Res 2007;13(8):2400–2405.

33. Roberts TG Jr, Lynch TJ Jr, Chabner BA. Identifying agents to test in phase III clinical trials. In: Figg WD, ed. Pharmacokinetics and Pharmacodynamics of Anti-cancer Drugs. Totowa, NJ: Humana Press, 2004.

34. Tufts Center for the Study of Drug Development Impact Report (September/October 2007). Despite more cancer drugs in R&D, overall U.S. approval rate is 8%. Boston, MA. Vol 9, Number 5.

35. Rubinstein L, Crowley J, Ivy P, et al. Randomized phase II designs. Clin Cancer Res 2009;15(6):1883–1890.

36. Eisenhauer EA, Therasse P, Bogaerts J, et al. New response evaluation criteria in solid tumours: revised RECIST guideline (version 1.1). Eur J Cancer 2009;45(2):228–247.

37. Vickers AJ, Ballen V, Scher HI. Setting the bar in phase II trials: the use of historical data for determining "go/no go" decision for definitive phase III testing. Clin Cancer Res 2007;13(3):972–976.

38. Simon R. Optimal two-stage designs for phase II clinical trials. Control Clin Trials 1989;10(1):1–10.

39. Ratain MJ, Humphrey RW, Gordon GB, et al. Recommended changes to oncology clinical trial design: revolution or evolution? Eur J Cancer 2008;44(1):8–11.

40. Zia MI, Siu LL, Pond GR, et al. Comparison of outcomes of phase II studies and subsequent randomized control studies using identical chemotherapeutic regimens. J Clin Oncol 2005;23(28):6982–6991.

41. Goffin J, Baral S, Tu D, et al. Objective responses in patients with malignant melanoma or renal cell cancer in early clinical studies do not predict regulatory approval. Clin Cancer Res 2005;11(16):5928–5934.

42. El-Maraghi RH, Eisenhauer EA. Review of phase II trial designs used in studies of molecular targeted agents: outcomes and predictors of success in phase III. J Clin Oncol 2008;26(8):1346–1354.

43. Parmar MK, Barthel FM, Sydes M, et al. Speeding up the evaluation of new agents in cancer. J Natl Cancer Inst 2008;100(17):1204–1214.

44. Booth CM, Calvert AH, Giaccone G, et al. Design and conduct of phase II studies of targeted anticancer therapy: recommendations from the task force on methodology for the development of innovative cancer therapies (MDICT). Eur J Cancer 2008;44(1):25–29.

45. Roberts TG Jr, Chabner BA. Beyond fast track for drug approvals. N Engl J Med 2004;351(5):501–505.

46. Druker BJ, Talpaz M, Resta DJ, et al. Efficacy and safety of a specific inhibitor of the BCR-ABL tyrosine kinase in chronic myeloid leukemia. N Engl J Med 2001;344(14):1031–1037.

47. Slamon DJ, Leyland-Jones B, Shak S, et al. Use of chemotherapy plus a monoclonal antibody against HER2 for metastatic breast cancer that overexpresses HER2. N Engl J Med 2001;344(11):783–792.

48. Chung KY, Shia J, Kemeny NE, et al. Cetuximab shows activity in colorectal cancer patients with tumors that do not express the epidermal growth factor receptor by immunohistochemistry. J Clin Oncol 2005;23(9):1803–1810.

49. Ratain MJ, Glassman RH. Biomarkers in phase I oncology trials: signal, noise, or expensive distraction? Clin Cancer Res 2007;13(22 Pt 1):6545–6548.

50. Bergh J. Quo vadis with targeted drugs in the 21st century? J Clin Oncol 2009;27(1):2–5.

51. Fu P, Dowlati A, Schluchter M. Comparison of power between randomized discontinuation design and upfront randomization design on progression-free survival. J Clin Oncol 2009;27(25):4135–4141.

52. Ratain MJ, Eisen T, Stadler WM, et al. Phase II placebo-controlled randomized discontinuation trial of sorafenib in patients with metastatic renal cell carcinoma. J Clin Oncol 2006;24(16):2505–2512.

53. Stadler WM, Rosner G, Small E, et al. Successful implementation of the randomized discontinuation trial design: an application to the study of the putative antiangiogenic agent carboxyaminoimidazole in renal cell carcinoma—CALGB 69901. J Clin Oncol 2005;23(16):3726–3732.

54. Simon R. Randomized clinical trials in oncology. Principles and obstacles. Cancer 1994;74(9 Suppl):2614–2619.

55. Schilsky RL. Personalizing cancer care: American Society of Clinical Oncology presidential address 2009. J Clin Oncol 2009;27(23):3725–3730.

56. Kola I, Landis J. Can the pharmaceutical industry reduce attrition rates? Nat Rev Drug Discov 2004;3(8):711–715.

57. Elias T, Gordian M, Singh N, et al. Why products fail in phase III. In Vivo. April 2006. Available at http://www.mckinsey.com/clientservice/pharmaceuticalsmedicalproducts/pdf/why_products_fail_in_phase_III_in_vivo_0406.pdf

58. Hirschfeld S, Pazdur R. Oncology drug development: United States Food and Drug Administration perspective. Crit Rev Oncol Hematol 2002;42(2):137–143.

59. Dagher R, Johnson J, Williams G, et al. Accelerated approval of oncology products: a decade of experience. J Natl Cancer Inst 2004;96(20):1500–1509.

60. Richey EA, Lyons EA, Nebeker JR, et al. Accelerated approval of cancer drugs: improved access to therapeutic breakthroughs or early release of unsafe and ineffective drugs? J Clin Oncol 2009;27(26):4398–4405.

61. Schilsky RL. Hurry up and wait: is accelerated approval of new cancer drugs in the best interests of cancer patients? J Clin Oncol 2003;21(20):3718–3720.

62. Tsimberidou AM, Braiteh F, Stewart DJ, et al. Ultimate fate of oncology drugs approved by the US food and drug administration without a randomized Trial. J Clin Oncol 2009;27(36):6243–6250.

63. Mok TS, Wu YL, Yu CJ, et al. Randomized, placebo-controlled, phase II study of sequential erlotinib and chemotherapy as first-line treatment for advanced non-small-cell lung cancer. J Clin Oncol 2009;27(30):5080–5087.

64. Stewart DJ, Kurzrock R. Cancer: the road to Amiens. J Clin Oncol 2009;27(3):328–333.

65. Harwerth IM, Wels W, Schlegel J, et al. Monoclonal antibodies directed to the erbB-2 receptor inhibit in vivo tumour cell growth. Br J Cancer 1993;68(6):1140–1145.

66. Baselga J, Tripathy D, Mendelsohn J, et al. Phase II study of weekly intravenous recombinant humanized anti-p185HER2 monoclonal antibody in patients with HER2/neu-overexpressing metastatic breast cancer. J Clin Oncol 1996;14(3):737–744.

67. Cobleigh MA, Vogel CL, Tripathy D, et al. Multinational study of the efficacy and safety of humanized anti-HER2 monoclonal antibody in women who have HER2-overexpressing metastatic breast cancer that has progressed after chemotherapy for metastatic disease. J Clin Oncol 1999;17(9):2639–2648.

68. Seidman AD, Berry D, Cirrincione C, et al. Randomized phase III trial of weekly compared with every-3-weeks paclitaxel for metastatic breast cancer, with trastuzumab for all HER-2 overexpressors and random assignment to trastuzumab or not in HER-2 nonoverexpressors: final results of Cancer and Leukemia Group B protocol 9840. J Clin Oncol 2008;26(10):1642–1649.

69. Hoering A, Leblanc M, Crowley JJ. Randomized phase III clinical trial designs for targeted agents. Clin Cancer Res 2008;14(14):4358–4367.

70. Mandrekar SJ, Sargent DJ. Clinical trial designs for predictive biomarker validation: theoretical considerations and practical challenges. J Clin Oncol 2009;27(24):4027–4034.

71. Goren A. Assessing the economic case for stratified medicine. Masters of Science in Biomedical Enterprise Dissertation, Massachusetts Institute of Technology, 2007.

72. Shulman SR, Wood-Armany MJ. Accelerating access to cancer drugs. J Biolaw Bus 1999;2(2):38–44.

73. CFR Title 21 Part 314—Subpart D—Section 126.

74. Food and Drug Administration. Content and Format of Investigational New Drug Applications (INDs) for Phase 1 Studies of Drugs, Including Well-Characterized, Therapeutic, Biotechnology-Derived Products. Rockville, MD: Food and Drug Administration, 1995.

75. DiMasi JA, Manocchia M. Initiatives to speed new drug development and regulatory review: the impact of FDA-sponsor conferences. Drug Info J 1997;31(3):771–788.

76. Reichert JM. Trends in development and approval times for new therapeutics in the United States. Nat Rev Drug Discov 2003;2(9):695–702.

77. Lasagna L. Congress, the FDA, and new drug development: before and after 1962. Perspect Biol Med 1989;32(3):322–343.

78. Anderson LF. Cancer and AIDS groups push for changes in drug approval process. J Natl Cancer Inst 1989;81(11):829–831.

79. Milne CP. Orphan products—pain relief for clinical development headaches. Nat Biotechnol 2002;20(8):780–784.

80. Milne C-P. Fast track designation under the food and drug administration: the industry experience. Drug Info J 2001;35(1):71–83.

81. Johnson JR, Williams G, Pazdur R. End points and United States food and drug administration approval of oncology drugs. J Clin Oncol 2003; 21(7):1404–1411.

82. Mitka M. Accelerated approval scrutinized: confirmatory phase 4 studies on new drugs languish. JAMA 2003;289(24):3227–3229.

83. Laetz T, Silberman G. Reimbursement policies constrain the practice of oncology. JAMA 1991;266(21):2996–2999.

84. Kris MG, Natale RB, Herbst RS, et al. Efficacy of gefitinib, an inhibitor of the epidermal growth factor receptor tyrosine kinase, in symptomatic patients with non-small cell lung cancer: a randomized trial. JAMA 2003;290(16):2149–2158.

85. Fukuoka M, Yano S, Giaccone G, et al. Multi-institutional randomized phase II trial of gefitinib for previously treated patients with advanced non-small-cell lung cancer. J Clin Oncol 2003;21(12):2237–2246.

86. Hurwitz H, Fehrenbacher L, Novotny W, et al. Bevacizumab plus irinotecan, fluorouracil, and leucovorin for metastatic colorectal cancer. N Engl J Med 2004;350(23):2335–2342.

87. Food and Drug Administration. Providing Clinical Evidence of Effectiveness of Human Drugs and Biological Products. Rockville, MD: Food and Drug Administration, 1998.

88. Pazdur R. Response rates, survival, and chemotherapy trials. J Natl Cancer Inst 2000;92(19):1552–1553.

89. Johnson JR, Temple R. Food and Drug Administration requirements for approval of new anticancer drugs. Cancer Treat Rep 1985;69(10):1155–1159.

90. O'Shaughnessy JA, Wittes RE, Burke G, et al. Commentary concerning demonstration of safety and efficacy of investigational anticancer agents in clinical trials. J Clin Oncol 1991;9(12):2225–2232.

91. Buyse M, Thirion P, Carlson RW, et al. Relation between tumour response to first-line chemotherapy and survival in advanced colorectal cancer: a meta-analysis. Meta-Analysis Group in Cancer. Lancet 2000;356(9227): 373–378.

92. Chen TT, Chute JP, Feigal E, et al. A model to select chemotherapy regimens for phase III trials for extensive-stage small-cell lung cancer. J Natl Cancer Inst 2000;92(19):1601–1607.

93. Hirschfeld S, Ho PT, Smith M, et al. Regulatory approvals of pediatric oncology drugs: previous experience and new initiatives. J Clin Oncol 2003;21(6):1066–1073.

94. Biomarkers Definitions Working Group. Biomarkers and surrogate endpoints: preferred definitions and conceptual framework. Clin Pharmacol Ther 2001;69(3):89–95.

95. Chau CH, Rixe O, McLeod H, et al. Validation of analytic methods for biomarkers used in drug development. Clin Cancer Res 2008;14(19):5967–5976.

Principles of Pharmacokinetics

Jerry M. Collins and Jeffrey G. Supko

It is generally accepted that the biologic effects of a drug are related to the time course of the concentration of the administered compound or an active metabolite in the bloodstream. The realization of this association has evolved through advances in the discipline of pharmacokinetics. This discipline is defined as the study of rate processes involved in the absorption of drug from the administration site into the bloodstream, its subsequent distribution to extravascular regions throughout the body, and its eventual elimination from the body. From a broader perspective, pharmacokinetics may be thought of as the effect that the body has on a drug, whereas the pharmacologic effects that a drug has on the body are the realm of pharmacodynamics (PDs).

In anticancer chemotherapy, the general goal of killing tumor cells or inhibiting their proliferation and metastasis is clearly defined. However, in most cases, we are severely limited by an inability to deliver drugs in a manner that separates antitumor effects from normal tissue toxicity. Much remains to be learned about the exploitable differences between normal and tumor tissues. Thus, although pharmacokinetics is a tool that can be used to evaluate the feasibility of a drug delivery strategy based on intended pharmacodynamic effects, it does not replace knowledge of exploitable differences between host and tumor.

Studies to characterize the pharmacokinetic behavior of a drug have become integral to the preclinical and clinical development of new anticancer agents. One group[1] has even suggested that "it is now inconceivable to perform clinical research in cancer chemotherapy without obtaining adequate pharmacokinetic data." The objectives for undertaking a pharmacokinetic study in the context of a phase I or II clinical trial in cancer patients include (a) initial characterizing of the pharmacokinetic behavior of new chemotherapeutic agents in humans, (b) assessing whether or not an administration schedule provides a potentially effective pattern of systemic exposure to drug, (c) determining the magnitude of intrapatient and interpatient variability in pharmacokinetic parameters, (d) assessing the influence of patient characteristics on drug disposition, (e) establishing predictive correlations between biologic effects and pharmacokinetic parameters, and (f) determining whether combining drugs results in pharmacokinetic interactions. In addition, pharmacokinetic drug level monitoring has been used to improve therapy through dose individualization, to evaluate patient compliance during chronic therapy, and to assess whether alterations in drug disposition or metabolism are associated with the development of toxicity or the lack of effect.

The fundamental obstacle to greater success in the application of pharmacokinetics and clinical drug level monitoring to anticancer therapy is our limited knowledge of pharmacodynamics. A complete understanding of the actions of a drug necessarily requires discerning the nature of the association between its pharmacokinetic behavior and pharmacodynamic effects. Relationships between pharmacokinetics and the severity of toxicity have been established for many anticancer drugs. However, pharmacokinetic associations accounting for the therapeutic effects of a chemotherapeutic agent are more difficult to establish because of the multiplicity of factors involving the host and tumor that influence response, as noted above, as well as the time lapse from initiating treatment to the first indications of a therapeutic response. In succeeding chapters, these relationships are discussed for individual agents. Nevertheless, elucidating the pharmacokinetic behavior of an anticancer drug may benefit efforts to determine the dose, route of administration, and schedule that maximize the therapeutic potential while minimizing serious toxic effects.

The intention of this chapter is to provide readers with a fundamental understanding of clinical pharmacokinetics and its practical application to the development and use of anticancer chemotherapy. Numerous texts with widely varying levels of complexity and focus are available for those interested in a more comprehensive discourse of the subject, ranging from easily understood introductions to the discipline[2] to more advanced texts with a mathematical approach.[3]

Acquisition and Analysis of Pharmacokinetic Data

Sample Collection and Drug Concentration Measurement

Pharmacokinetic studies involve collecting serial specimens of blood and other biologic fluids, such as urine, at predetermined time intervals from subjects following administration of the drug. Plasma is the blood component in which drugs are most commonly measured during pharmacokinetic studies, although determinations are also made in serum and, less frequently, in whole blood. The concentration of drug present in the study samples is measured using an appropriate bioanalytical method. Technical advances in separation and detection methods, especially the maturation of high-performance liquid chromatography coupled to mass spectrometry into a technique suitable for routine use, have provided a greatly improved basis for drug concentration measurement during the past decade. Review articles surveying the current techniques used for assaying drugs in biologic fluids regularly appear in the literature.[4]

Many anticancer drugs are difficult to measure because of inherent instability, either spontaneously degrading in solution or being degraded by enzymes in blood or tissues. It is therefore important to recognize that the quality of data derived from any pharmacokinetic study ultimately depends on the reliability of the assay used to measure the drug as well as the manner by which samples were processed and stored prior to analysis. The majority of bioanalytical methods used for pharmacokinetic studies measure the total concentration of drug, that is, free drug plus that which is reversibly associated with plasma proteins. However, the reversible binding of a drug to plasma proteins, such as albumin and α_1-acid glycoprotein, needs to be considered in the interpretation of total drug concentrations.[5] Only the free or unbound drug is pharmacologically active. Protein binding is usually assessed experimentally by ultrafiltration or equilibrium dialysis.

The Plasma Concentration-Time Profile

Except for cases in which a drug is given by bolus intravenous injection, the plasma concentration-time ($C \times T$) profile of any drug exhibits an initial region of increasing concentration, the achievement of a peak or maximum concentration (C_{max}), followed by a continual decline in concentration (Fig. 4-1A). The concentration of drug in plasma increases as long as the rate of input into systemic circulation exceeds the rate of loss due to distribution into other extracellular fluids, intracellular spaces, and tissues throughout the body, and elimination from the body. The C_{max} is achieved when the rate of drug input is equivalent to the rate of loss from plasma, a time point that occurs at the instant that an intravenous injection or short infusion is terminated. During a continuous intravenous infusion, plasma levels of the drug increase at a progressively decreasing rate and eventually become constant, indicative of achieving steady-state conditions, if the infusion is continued for a sufficiently long time (Fig. 4-1C).

Figure 4-1 shows the same $C \times T$ data plotted on graphs with semilog axes (panel A) and rectangular coordinate axes (panel B). Presenting pharmacokinetic drug $C \times T$ profiles on semilog graphs provides a better visual depiction of the entire data set than a coordinate plot because plasma levels of a drug frequently differ by several orders of magnitude during the course of the observation period. Furthermore, the concentration of many drugs in systemic circulation decays in an apparent first-order manner, exemplified by a terminal region in the plasma profile in which the logarithm of the drug concentration is a linear function of time. Thus, a semilog plot provides some immediate inferences regarding the nature of the pharmacokinetic behavior of a drug.

The pattern of decay in the plasma concentration of a drug that exhibits first-order kinetics comprises one or more exponential phases. In the case of a plasma profile with drug concentrations that decline in a single log-linear phase, the entire body appears to be kinetically homogenous. In this case, the equilibrium of the drug between plasma and other fluids or tissues into which it distributes is very rapidly achieved, before the first blood specimen has been acquired. Polyexponential behavior results from distinguishable differences in the reversible transfer of drug from plasma to various regions or compartments of the body. Thus, for example, the presence of two exponential decay phases implies that the body behaves as if it is composed of two kinetically distinct compartments: the

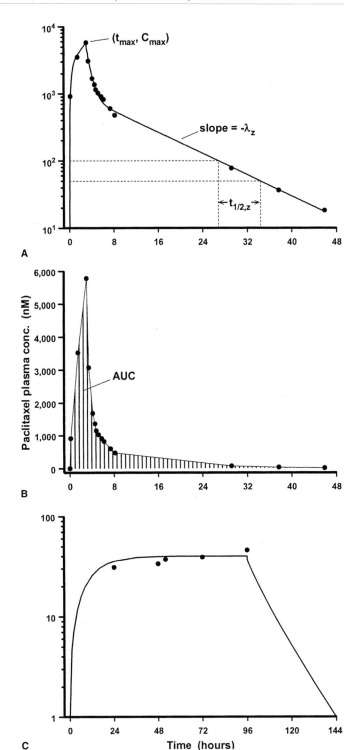

Figure 4-1 A. Plasma $C \times T$ profile for a 175 mg/m² dose of paclitaxel administered as a 3-hour continuous intravenous infusion shown on a graph with log-linear axes. Pharmacokinetic variables that can be estimated by visual inspection are indicated: maximum drug concentration (C_{max}), the time at which the peak concentration (t_{max}) occurs, and the biological half-life ($t_{1/2,z}$). **B.** Presentation of the same data shown in the upper panel on rectangular coordinate axes. The shaded area corresponds to the area under the curve (AUC). **C.** Time course of paclitaxel in plasma when given as a 96-hour continuous intravenous infusion at a rate of 25 mg/m²/d. The steady-state plasma concentration of the drug is approximately 40 nM.

first comprising plasma and tissues with which equilibrium is rapidly established and the second "deeper" compartment comprising all other regions of the body into which drug distributes more slowly.

For some purposes, a mathematical equation or model is necessary to interpret pharmacokinetic data, but often questions may be answered without a formal model construction. Recently, there has been a growing trend toward analyzing pharmacokinetic data by empirical approaches that consider only the concentration of drug in the sampled fluid and require few assumptions about model structure. In these techniques, which include model-independent analysis[6] and noncompartmental analysis,[7] the various exponential decay phases are usually referred to simply as the initial, intermediate, and terminal disposition phases. Regardless of the particular method of analysis employed, the ultimate objective is the same, which is to estimate values of descriptive pharmacokinetic parameters from the $C \times T$ data.

Physiologic Pharmacokinetic Models

For pharmacologists interested in developing an understanding of drug disposition in individual tissue compartments, models that incorporate physiologic compartments are of considerable interest. These models require measurements of actual physiologic parameters, such as volumes and blood flow rates, as well as drug concentrations in various compartments, and therefore are based primarily on data from experimental animals. Entry into specific areas such as the central nervous system may be of critical importance in the use of drugs, and physiologic models can allow comparisons of $C \times T$ profiles for various schedules and routes of administration. Physiologic models have been constructed for many anticancer drugs. Models have been published for the most important drugs in clinical practice, among which are methotrexate (MTX),[8] 5-fluorouracil (5-FU),[9] cisplatin,[10] and doxorubicin.[11]

In the most general form, physiologic pharmacokinetic models are overly complex and require too large a database for routine clinical use. However, they provide a basis for understanding a drug's kinetic behavior that can be incorporated into simpler models, either physiologic or hybrid, assimilating both empiric observations and physiologic information. Physiologic modeling goes beyond the usual goals of empiric pharmacokinetic modeling to allow for incorporation of data obtained in other species or in vitro. The compartments comprising a physiologic pharmacokinetic model have an anatomic basis, and the transfer processes in the model have a physiologic or pharmacologic identity. Each organ is modeled separately; then, the model connections are provided by blood flow. The structure for the physiologic model for cytarabine is presented in Figure 4-2.[12]

Pharmacokinetic Parameters

Area Under the Curve

Noncompartmental analysis is considerably simpler than any equation-defining method of pharmacokinetic data analysis. All calculations and data manipulations can be performed by most spreadsheet software programs. The observed plasma $C \times T$ data are numerically integrated, most commonly by the trapezoidal method. In its

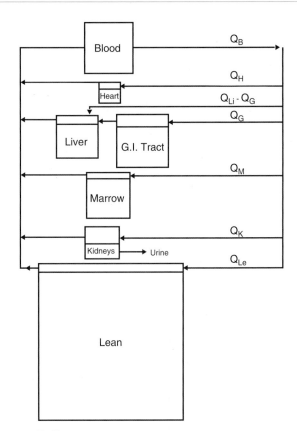

Figure 4-2 Physiologic pharmacokinetic model for cytosine arabinoside. GI, gastrointestinal. (Reprinted from Dedrick RL, Forrester DD, Cannon JN, et al. Pharmacokinetics of 1-β-D-arabinofuranosylcytosine (ARA-C) deamination in several species. Biochem Pharmacol 1973;22:2405–2417, with permission.)

simplest application, each successive set of data points, beginning with time zero, is used to define a trapezoid, the area of which is readily calculated. The cumulative sum of the areas of all such trapezoids affords an estimation of the area under the $C \times T$ curve to the last sample with a measurable drug concentration ($[C_t] \mathrm{AUC}_{0 \to t}$). The slope of the terminal log-linear phase of the $C \times T$ profile ($-\lambda_z$) is then determined by linear regression using log-transformed concentration values (see Fig. 4-1A). The area under the curve from time zero to infinity (AUC) can then be calculated as

$$\mathrm{AUC} = \mathrm{AUC}_{0 \to t} + C_t / \lambda_z \qquad [4.1]$$

Although the AUC is not a pharmacokinetic parameter per se, because its magnitude depends on the administered dose of drug, it represents an important quantitative measure of total systemic drug exposure, as illustrated in Figure 4-1B. In addition, knowledge of the AUC is required to calculate values of pharmacokinetic parameters, as described in the following section.

Total Body Clearance

The total body clearance (CL) of a drug is formally defined as the volume of plasma from which drug is completely removed per unit time. It is readily calculated as

$$\mathrm{CL} = D_{iv} / \mathrm{AUC} \qquad [4.2]$$

where D_{iv} is the dose of the drug given by intravenous injection or infusion. CL reflects the combined contribution of all processes by which drug is removed from the body, as represented by the equation

$$CL = CL_R + CL_{NR} \qquad [4.3]$$

where CL_R and CL_{NR} designate renal and nonrenal clearance, respectively.[13] Renal clearance is usually the only route of drug elimination that can be directly and quantitatively determined in patients by noninvasive procedures. All other mechanisms of drug elimination that cannot be readily estimated, including biliary excretion of unchanged drug, metabolism, nonenzymatic irreversible reactions with endogenous molecules, and spontaneous chemical degradation, are grouped together as CL_{NR}. CL has units of volume per time (e.g., milliliters per minute, liter per hour) and is frequently normalized to the body weight or body surface area of subjects (e.g., milliliters per minute per kilogram, liter per hour per square meter) under the presumption of minimizing interpatient variability in the magnitude of the parameter. However, this practice has recently become a topic of considerable controversy because the underlying presumption of a relationship between unnormalized clearance values and body surface area does not exist for a significant number of anticancer drugs.[14] The CL values are often compared with glomerular filtration rate and hepatic blood flow, average values of which are approximately 125 mL/min (4.6 L/h/m²) and 1,500 mL/min (56 L/h/m²), respectively, in normal adults.[15,16] Although often informative, these comparisons can be extremely misleading unless the extent of plasma protein binding has been taken into account because only the free fraction of drug that is not bound to plasma proteins is usually subject to organ-mediated excretion or metabolism.

Apparent Volume of Distribution

The total body apparent volume of distribution, V_z, is strictly a proportionality constant relating the total amount of drug in the body to plasma concentration. It may be calculated by the equation

$$V_z = CL / \lambda_z \qquad [4.4]$$

and has units of volume, typically expressed in terms of milliliters or liters normalized to body weight or body surface area (e.g., milliliters per kilogram, liters per square meter). V_z is designated as an apparent volume because it is a hypothetical value that is not directly related to any real physiologic space. Nevertheless, it is an informative parameter, providing an indication of the relative extent of drug distribution from plasma. Specifically, for a given amount of drug in the body, the fraction present in plasma decreases as its distribution into peripheral tissues increases, leading to greater values of V_z.[17] Therefore, the effective lower limit of V_z is the plasma volume, which is approximately 4.5% of body weight (i.e., 45 mL/kg, 1.7 L/m²) for a normal adult. There really is no upper limit, as V_z can assume extremely large values in cases where the half-life of the terminal disposition phase is long relative to that of the preceding disposition phase, and drug levels decrease by several orders of magnitude before the terminal phase is achieved. For example, some anticancer agents, such as the anthracyclines, have V_z values exceeding 1,000 L/m² (27 times body weight).

Biologic Half-Life

The biologic half-life of a drug ($t_{1/2,z}$) is the time required for its plasma concentration to decrease by 50% any time during the terminal log-linear phase in the $C \times T$ profile (see Fig. 4-1A). It is only applicable to drugs that exhibit apparent first-order pharmacokinetics (see later discussion). As indicated by the relationship,

$$t_{1/2,z} = 0.693 \cdot V_z / CL \qquad [4.5]$$

$t_{1/2,z}$ reflects both the ability of the body to eliminate the drug as well as the extent to which the drug distributes throughout the body. Nevertheless, there is a recurrent tendency in the anticancer drug literature to place undue emphasis on the value of $t_{1/2,z}$ as an indicator of drug elimination. The $t_{1/2,z}$ has an important practical application in that steady-state conditions during administration of a drug by continuous intravenous infusion or a multiple dosing regimen are achieved when the duration of treatment exceeds four times the value of $t_{1/2,z}$.

Linear and Nonlinear Pharmacokinetics

The majority of clinically used anticancer agents exhibit linear or first-order pharmacokinetics, whereby plasma concentrations of the drug decline in an exponential manner following intravenous administration. A distinguishing and defining characteristic of linear pharmacokinetics is that the plasma concentration of drug at a given time after dosing is directly proportional to the administered dose. Thus, the AUC increases proportionately with the dose and values of the pharmacokinetic parameters (i.e., CL, V_z) are independent of the dose. When a drug is predominantly eliminated by a potentially saturable process, such as hepatic metabolism or active tubular secretion, departures from linear pharmacokinetic behavior may become evident if sufficiently high doses can be administered to patients. As illustrated in Figure 4-3, classic nonlinear pharmacokinetics is indicated by a change in the appearance of the plasma profile from exponential character at lower doses to the appearance of a distinct downward curvature in the semilog plot of the plasma profile at higher doses.[18] In addition, the apparent CL exhibits a progressive decrease in magnitude as the dose is escalated. A clear

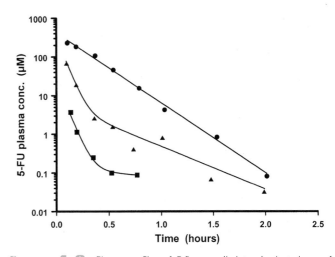

FIGURE 4-3 Plasma profiles of 5-flourouracil determined at doses of 25 mg/m² (■), 125 mg/m² (▲), and 375 mg/m² (●) illustrating the effect of classic nonlinear pharmacokinetics. Values of the apparent total body clearance decreased progressively from 142 L/h/m² for the 25 mg/m² dose to 47 L/h/m² at 125 mg/m² and 30 L/h/m² at 375 mg/m². There would be no significant difference between the clearance determined at different doses if the pharmacokinetic behavior of the drug was linear.

example of this phenomenon was reported recently for high-dose cytarabine given by continuous intravenous infusions in which small changes in the infusion rate produced disproportionately large increases in the steady-state drug concentration in plasma.[19]

Drug Elimination

Renal and Hepatic Excretion

Establishing the major pathways of drug elimination in patients is also an important objective of clinical pharmacokinetic studies. Disease states that compromise the function of a major drug-eliminating organ, such as the kidneys or liver, can enhance a patient's sensitivity to the toxic effects of the drug as a result of increased drug exposure. For this reason, patients with significant organ impairment are usually excluded from initial phase I studies to avoid possibly confounding sources of toxicity.

Renal excretion is a quantitatively significant route of elimination for many relatively small compounds, with molecular weights less than about 300, that are also highly to moderately hydrophilic,[20] if they are not substantially metabolized. Larger compounds and those with a more lipophilic character tend to be predominantly eliminated by biliary excretion, either directly or after metabolism. Determining CL_R involves measuring the amount of unchanged drug present in the urine (A_e) collected during one or more defined time intervals (Δt) following intravenous drug administration. It may be calculated by either of the following equations

$$CL_R = A_e / AUC_{0 \to t} \qquad [4.6]$$

$$CL_R \approx (\Delta A_e / \Delta D_t) / C_{mid} \qquad [4.7]$$

depending on whether urine has been continuously collected and pooled from the beginning of dose administration throughout the time that plasma specimens were obtained, or during one or more discrete time intervals after dosing. In the second equation, C_{mid} is the plasma concentration of drug at the midpoint of the urine collection interval. The amount of unchanged drug in feces cannot be taken as a direct indication of biliary excretion because of the potential for drug metabolism by the gastrointestinal microflora.[21]

In cases in which renal or biliary excretion is a significant pathway of drug elimination, a predictive correlation may exist between clinical indicators of renal or hepatic function, such as serum creatinine and bilirubin levels, respectively, and CL. Establishing these relationships serves as the basis for defining guidelines pertaining to the minimal organ function required for patient eligibility in phase II studies and devising an empirical algorithm for dosage adjustment, including those documented in Table 4-1[22] (see also "Organ Dysfunction and its Effect on Drug Clearance").

Drug Metabolism

Metabolism represents a quantitatively important route of elimination for most anticancer agents. Xenobiotic biotransformation reactions may be broadly categorized into two classes, designated phase I and phase II. The principal phase I reactions are oxidation, reduction, and hydrolysis. Phase II reactions involve the conjugation or coupling of endogenous molecules, including glucuronide, sulfate, amino acid, methyl and glutathione moieties to the parent drug

TABLE 4.1	Predominant elimination mechanisms and dose adjustment recommendations for anticancer drugs	
Major route of elimination	**Anticancer agent**	**Dose adjustment for organ dysfunction**[a]
Renal excretion	Bleomycin	b
	Carboplatin, cisplatin	b
	Etoposide	b
	Fludarabine	b
	Hydroxyurea	b
	Methotrexate	b
	Pentostatin	b
	Topotecan	b
Hepatic metabolism CYP450	Busulfan	c
	Chlorambucil	No
	Cyclophosphamide[b]	No
	Ifosfamide[b]	No
	Imatinib	e
	Irinotecan	No
	Paclitaxel	c
	Thio-TEPA	No
	Vinca alkaloids	c
Conjugation	Etoposide	c
	SN-38	
Ubiquitous enzymes	Cytarabine	No
	Gemcitabine	No
	6-Mercaptopurine	d
Nonenzymatic hydrolysis	BCNU[b]	No
	Mechlorethamine	No
	Melphalan	No
Biliary excretion	Doxorubicin	No
	Irinotecan	No
	Vinca alkaloids	c

[a]b, decrease dose in proportion to the reduction in creatinine clearance below 60 mL/min; c, serum bilirubin: 1.5 to 3.0 mg/100 mL, 50% dose reduction; >3.0 mg/100 mL, 75% dose reduction; d, patients with S-methyl transferase deficiency; e, insufficient data to determine if dose reduction is necessary in hepatic dysfunction.
[b]Enzymatic or spontaneous chemical reactions required for drug activation.

or a precursory phase I metabolite. Hepatic oxidation mediated by the cytochromes P450 (CYP450), a large family of heme-containing isozymes, undoubtedly plays the greatest overall role in drug metabolism among the phase I reactions.[23] The CYP450 enzymes are most abundantly expressed in the liver, but they are also present in the kidney, lung, and gastrointestinal epithelium. The predominant enzyme in this family, CYP3A4, catalyzes the oxidation of a multitude of structurally diverse compounds.[24–26] These include imatinib, gefitinib (and most other synthetic inhibitors of tyrosine kinases), docetaxel, etoposide, ifosfamide, vincristine, and paclitaxel. In addition to hepatic metabolism, some important phase I reactions are mediated by ubiquitous enzymes found in virtually all tissues of the body, such as dihydropyrimidine dehydrogenase, which catalyzes the reduction of 5-FU, and cytidine deaminase, which inactivates cytarabine.[27,28] Glucuronide conjugation catalyzed by uridine diphosphate glucuronosyl-transferases (UGT) is the most commonly encountered phase II reaction. In contrast to phase I metabolism, which may yield a biologically active product, glucuronidation almost exclusively represents a detoxification mechanism that inactivates a compound and facilitates its excretion through enhanced hydrophilicity and recognition by biliary canicular efflux proteins.[29] Glucuronidation is a clinically important route of elimination for 7-ethyl-10-hydroxycamptothecin (SN-38), the active metabolite of irinotecan, as the extent of its glucuronidation has been associated with the risk of severe diarrhea for the weekly treatment schedule of irinotecan.[30]

Chemical Degradation

Chemical degradation can be a significant elimination mechanism for drugs that are susceptible to hydrolysis or conjugation with sulfhydrils, such as many of the alkylating agents. Nonenzymatic reactions between drugs and endogenous molecules can also contribute prominently to elimination. For example, platinum-alkylating agents form covalent adducts with serum albumin and with small molecular weight sulfhydrils such as glutathione.[31]

Factors Contributing to Pharmacokinetic Variability

Obtaining an indication of interpatient variability in the values of pharmacokinetic parameters and related variables is an important objective of phase I trials. This information has considerable practical utility with regard to clinical drug development. These findings provide the basis for assessing the ability to reliably predict the C_{max} and AUC of a drug following the administration of any given dose to patients who have not been previously studied. The recommended dose of cytotoxic anticancer drugs is typically close to the maximum tolerated dose, and dose-limiting toxicities are often related in some manner to the levels of drug achieved in plasma. Thus, the margin of safety of these agents very much depends on the consistency of their pharmacokinetic behavior between patients. Conversely, the existence of a high degree of interpatient pharmacokinetic variability can result in unpredictable episodes of toxicity at the maximum tolerated dose, which may make it difficult to establish a potentially effective and safe dose. Although rarely employed in these circumstances, drug level monitoring to establish the optimal dosing regimen in individual patients may be warranted.

Patient Characteristics

Clinically significant associations between CL and patient characteristics such as age, sex, and race have been identified for many anticancer drugs. For example, it has been shown that the CL of 5-FU in females is significantly lower than in males and that formation of the glucuronide metabolite of SN-38 by UGT is subject to pharmacogenetic variations related to both race and gender.[32,33] These factors are now being examined extensively during the clinical evaluation of new anticancer drugs.

Currently, more than half of all cancers occur in patients over 65. However, relatively few elderly patients are entered into early-stage clinical trials because of referral patterns, physiological limitations such as renal or hepatic function, or investigator bias. As a consequence, the pharmacokinetic behavior of most anticancer drugs has not been adequately characterized in elderly patients.[34] Older cancer patients display considerable heterogeneity in their handling of drugs as a result of age-related changes in body composition, including decreased muscle mass, increasing adipose tissue, and decreased renal function. Aging is accompanied by a 25% to 35% decrease in liver volume and a 35% to 40% decrease in hepatic blood flow.[35,36] Thus, the CL of drugs with a high hepatic extraction ratio, which is limited by liver blood flow, may be decreased in the elderly.[37,38] Age-associated decreases in the function of some drug-metabolizing enzymes have been identified but their clinical significance remains uncertain.[39,40]

At the other end of the age spectrum, experience has shown that safe and effective doses of anticancer agents for children very often cannot be determined by scaling down from adult doses, using body weight or body surface area.[41] Age-related changes are profoundly responsible for drug elimination and can have a profound effect on pharmacokinetics.[42] Thus, the rational use (alone or in combination) of drug eliminated by hepatic metabolism in adults requires the thorough characterization of pharmacokinetics and metabolism in children.

Organ Dysfunction and its Effect on Drug Clearance

Physiologic conditions that affect hepatic or renal function, including blood flow to the liver or kidneys, can have a dramatic effect on the pharmacokinetic behavior of a drug in individual patients.[43] Powis[44] reviewed the effects of both renal and hepatic dysfunction for anticancer drugs. The estimation of creatinine clearance from serum creatinine concentration is a conveniently measured indicator of renal function. Hepatic function is more difficult to quantify. Serum transaminase and bilirubin concentrations provide indirect but somewhat useful information on hepatic function. Empirical guidelines for dose reduction in patients with underlying renal or hepatic dysfunction are devised by establishing relationships between these biochemical parameters and CL. In general, these adjustments would be expected to be less precise than adjustments based on drug-level measurements. Occasionally, there is a close relationship between a renal function indicator and plasma pharmacokinetics. Egorin et al.[45] have elegantly applied such correlations for dose adjustments of carboplatin (Fig. 4-4) and other agents.[46] In fact, individualizing the dose of carboplatin to target a specific AUC value based on estimated creatinine clearance in patients has become a routine clinical practice.[47] Table 4-1 summarizes the recommended dose modifications for the standard anticancer drugs.

Drug Interactions

Essentially all treatment protocols include combinations of drugs, encompassing two or more anticancer drugs, as well as various other drugs related to general symptomatic and supportive therapy of the patient. Many adjuvant medications that are routinely used in the management of cancer patients can potentially affect the pharmacokinetics of chemotherapeutic agents by either inhibiting

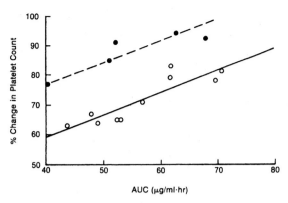

FIGURE **4-4** Relationship between thrombocytopenia and plasma levels of carboplatin. AUC, area under the concentration × time curve. (Reprinted from Egorin MJ, Van Echo DA, Olman EA, et al. Prospective validation of a pharmacologically based dosing scheme for the *cis*-diamminedichloroplatinum(II) analog diamminecyclobutanedicarboxylatoplatinum. Cancer Res 1985;46:6502–6506, with permission.)

or enhancing metabolic elimination (Table 4-2). Because cytotoxic anticancer drugs are usually administered at their maximum tolerated doses, there is a substantially greater risk for pharmacokinetic interactions resulting in clinically significant toxicity than exists with drugs for most other indications. Accordingly, whenever possible, physicians should avoid administration of an anticancer agent together with another drug that modulates (induces or inhibits) the activity of an enzyme required for elimination of the first agent. Another important consideration is the highly variable pharmacokineticsof drugs predominantly eliminated by hepatic metabolism.[48] It is becoming increasingly apparent that genetic polymorphisms and mutations affecting key drug-metabolizing enzymes, including the cytochrome P450 enzymes, may account for aberrant pharmacokinetics in some patients, or an otherwise high degree of interpatient variability (see Chapter 6).[49]

The serious adverse reactions caused by administration of ketoconazole to patients taking terfenadine,[50] which had been widely used and considered to be a relatively safe antihistamine, provide a cautionary note for potential interactions with anticancer drugs because of their much narrower therapeutic index. Another common drug, cimetidine, is reported to inhibit the metabolism of cyclophosphamide[51] and hexamethylmelamine.[52] On the other hand, anticancer drugs interfere with the absorption of noncancer drugs, such as digoxin.[53] Balis[54] has reviewed the literature of drug interactions related to anticancer drugs. When evaluating drug-drug interactions, recent findings with paclitaxel illustrate the difficulties generated by interspecies differences in metabolic pathways.[55] Thus, animal studies may yield inaccurate predictions of drug interactions and metabolic pathways in humans.

Chemotherapeutic agents that are metabolized by the hepatic CYP450 system, especially members of the CYP3A subfamily, are particularly prone to pharmacokinetic interactions from the multitude of drugs and compounds of dietary origin that are inhibitors or inducers of CYP450.[56] A particularly serious example is the use of the dietary supplement, St. John's wort. This product induces drug-metabolizing enzymes and produces lack of drug efficacy.[57] Repeated daily administration of glucocorticoids, commonly used as antiemetics, can induce the expression of hepatic CYP450 and thereby enhance the CL of anticancer drugs that are CYP3A4 substrates.[58] In addition to hepatic drug-metabolizing enzymes, there are examples of pharmacokinetic interactions resulting from effects directed on other enzyme systems, excretory pathways, and even drug absorption. Salicylates can reduce the renal tubular secretion of MTX.[59,60] Morphine and its derivatives can alter the rate and extent of absorption of orally administered cytotoxic drugs by reducing gastrointestinal motility.[61] As discussed in a subsequent chapter, antiseizure drugs (dilation and Phenobarbital) often used in brain tumor patients enhance the clearance of many anticancer agents by inducing CYP450 enzymes.

TABLE

4.2 *Clinically significant pharmacokinetic drug interactions involving anticancer agents*

Chemotherapeutic agent	Interacting drug	Effect on clearance of anticancer agent	Probable mechanism
Cyclophosphamide	Phenobarbital	↑	CYP450 enzyme induction
Doxorubicin	Cyclosporin A	↓	Inhibits biliary excretion
Etoposide	Phenytoin	↑	CYP450 enzyme induction
Irinotecan		↑	
Paclitaxel		↑	
6-Mercaptopurine	Allopurinol	↓	Inhibits xanthine oxidase
	Methotrexate	↓	
Methotrexate	Aspirin	↓	Inhibits tubular secretion
	Probenecid	↓	
Paclitaxel	Verapamil	↓	Inhibits CYP450 metabolism or biliary excretion
Topotecan	Cisplatin	↓	Inhibits tubular secretion
Vinblastine	Erythromycin	↓	Inhibits CYP450 metabolism

Dose Individualization

The existence of a high degree of interpatient pharmacokinetic variability can result in unpredictable episodes of toxicity and make it difficult to establish a potentially effective and safe dose for the population. For the individual, clinical monitoring and pharmacokinetics offer the possibility of tailoring drug delivery to the particular patient's needs. The standard doses derived from group studies do not allow for interindividual variability. However, doses may be adjusted on the basis of direct measurements of drug concentration in the individual patient, indicators of renal or hepatic dysfunction, or interactions of the anticancer drug with concomitant medications. Under these circumstances, it may also be beneficial to individualize doses of the drug based on plasma levels of the compound afforded by a test dose or a biochemical parameter that is predictive of CL.[62] Although this technique is rarely employed, dose individualization has significantly improved the outcome and minimized toxicity for children with B lineage acute lymphocytic leukemia (ALL) treated with MTX.[63]

Dosing Regimens

For the average patient, or the general population, pharmacokinetics can help answer the fundamental questions in delivery of drugs: (a) What route of administration? (b) How much to give (dose)? (c) How often to administer (schedule)? These questions are answered using empiric observation (what works best in an experimental or clinical setting) as well as biochemical, cell kinetic, and pharmacokinetic considerations.

Routes of Drug Administration

The choice of drug administration *route* is based primarily on the ability to formulate an acceptable dose preparation for intravenous, oral, intramuscular, intrathecal, or subcutaneous use and pharmacokinetic assessment of the pattern of systemic drug exposure that they provide. Although current trends point toward the preferential development of orally administered drugs, cytotoxic anticancer drugs are still most commonly given by the intravenous route as this provides complete control over the actual dosage delivered to the systemic circulation and the rate at which it is presented. This results in maximum safety because the variability in systemic drug exposure between and within patients achieved with direct intravenous administration is typically much lower than that resulting from oral administration. Furthermore, for agents given by continuous intravenous infusion, drug delivery can be readily terminated, if necessary, because of the occurrence of an acute adverse reaction during administration.

All routes of administration other than intravenous, including oral, subcutaneous, intramuscular, intraperitoneal, and intrathecal delivery, involve an absorption process whereby dissolved drug molecules are transferred from the site of administration into the vasculature. Accordingly, drug given by an extravascular route is conceptualized as being outside the body until gaining access to the systemic circulation. Oral dosage forms are presently available for an increasing number of anticancer drugs including hydroxyurea, MTX, etoposide, idarubicin, flutarabine, and many of the receptor tyrosine kinase inhibitors. In the future, oral administration will

undoubtedly attain greater prevalence from the clinical development of cytostatic antiproliferative agents that require chronic dosing for efficacy.

The bioavailability of a drug given by any extravascular route is defined as the rate and extent of absorption into systemic circulation. The absolute systemic availability (F) of a drug is ascertained by determining the AUC in the same patient following intravenous and extravascular administration of the agent, with an adequate time interval period between the two treatments. For the same dose given intravenously and extravascularly,

$$F = (AUC_{ev} / AUC_{iv}) \cdot (D_{iv} / D_{ev})$$ [4.8]

where D is the dose. In studies where an agent is administered exclusively by the oral route, CL and F are indeterminable, as explicitly indicated by the relationship

$$D_{ev} / AUC_{ev} = CL / F$$ [4.9]

Many factors influence oral bioavailability, including release of the drug from the dosage form, dissolution of drug within the gastrointestinal tract, drug stability under conditions encountered in the gastrointestinal tract, transport of dissolved drug across the intestinal epithelium into the vasculature, and the extent of first-pass hepatic metabolism. Mercaptopurine is an example of a drug with very low and erratic bioavailability,[64] whereas imatinib is a drug with consistently high bioavailability.[65]

Absorption through the lipid-bilayer cell membrane of the intestinal mucosa is determined by molecular size, lipid solubility, and the presence of transport systems. As cancer chemotherapy shifts increasingly toward oral drug delivery, the importance of many general carrier systems, such as the "ABC" transporters, is becoming more widely appreciated alongside such specialized carriers as the folate transport mechanisms for antifolates. The physiologic state of the intestinal tract may be affected adversely by disease or by previous drug therapy. Vomiting induced by chemotherapeutic drugs such as cisplatin may lead to loss of a major portion of an oral dose. In addition to intestinal absorption, presystemic metabolism and biliary excretion may prevent orally administered drugs from reaching the systemic circulation in an active form. Presystemic metabolism, also known as the "first-pass effect," is a unique concern for the oral route because a drug is exposed to metabolism both in the gastrointestinal mucosa and in the liver, which it enters through the portal vein before returning to the heart.[66]

A tumor may grow in a region of the body, such as the central nervous system, that is not penetrated readily by systemically administered drugs. Accordingly, several unusual routes of administration have been implemented to maximize delivery of drugs to the site of the tumor and to reduce the deleterious effects associated with ordinary systemic administration. At least two of these routes have become accepted therapeutic practice: intrathecal delivery for meningeal leukemia[67] and intravesical delivery for transitional-stage bladder carcinoma. As discussed in detail in Chapter 21, intrathecal administration has been used primarily to obtain adequate drug levels in the cerebrospinal fluid to eradicate cancer cells that are otherwise protected from effective therapy. Intra-arterial drug administration, especially hepatic arterial delivery, is another route that has been actively investigated but has not emerged as standard therapy.

Peritoneal dialysis continues to be evaluated as a delivery vehicle for anticancer drugs when disease is localized to the abdomen.[68] The pharmacokinetic rationale suggests that tumor tissue may be exposed to high local concentrations, whereas systemic levels are no greater than normally encountered with intravenous therapy. In an analogous fashion to intrathecal delivery, only cells in close contact with the peritoneal fluid will benefit from this mode of drug delivery. The intraperitoneal route has been the subject of many pilot studies and formal phase I and phase II trials by our group and others. Some promising pharmacologic results have been obtained and more definitive therapeutic trials are in progress. Three randomized phase III trials totaling approximately 3,000 patients with ovarian cancer have shown an advantage for intraperitoneal delivery compared with intravenous delivery for both time to disease recurrence/progression[69,70] and survival.[69,71] Pharmacokinetic analysis can help to evaluate the potential usefulness of these approaches. Of course, the pharmacokinetic advantage of achieving greater drug exposure is not always associated with improved responses.

Dose

Dose is usually determined by an empiric phase I trial using a fixed treatment schedule, with stepwise evaluation of toxicity at progressively higher doses. In certain circumstances, dose also may be determined by setting pharmacologic objectives, such as a target drug concentration in a specific body compartment such as plasma, cerebrospinal fluid, or ascites. This type of regimen planning requires pharmacokinetic design and verification by drug level monitoring and has been used in only a few clinical oncologic settings, such as intrathecal chemotherapy with MTX and intraperitoneal therapy with MTX and 5-FU. Additional information on the relationship of drug concentration to tumor cell kill, as provided by in vitro assays, may provide a basis for more precise pharmacokinetic adjustment of dosage.

Pharmacologically guided dose escalation was developed as an alternative to the predetermined escalation procedures such as the modified Fibonacci method for phase I trials.[72] After the first group of patients has been treated with the starting dose in a phase I clinical trial, the rate of dose escalation is determined by the plasma levels of drug relative to target plasma levels measured in mice at the maximum tolerated dose. With this approach, investigators can estimate the difference between the target concentration and plasma levels produced by the current dose level. Such information provides the opportunity to intervene at an early stage in the phase I trial. Cautious escalation may be indicated if it is determined that plasma levels of the drug are close to the target. If the current plasma levels are substantially below the targeted value, then a more rapid escalation of the dose could generate considerable savings in time and clinical resources, and fewer patients will be exposed to doses that have little potential of being therapeutically effective. Although this procedure is conceptually attractive and found support in Europe and Japan, as well as the United States,[73–75] it has not been widely used, primarily because of logistical difficulties in its implementation.

Administration Schedule

The route and frequency of administration evaluated in the initial phase I trial of a cytotoxic anticancer agent are generally derived from the schedule that produces an optimal therapeutic effect against preclinical in vivo tumor models. There is an increasing interest in assessing the use of noncytotoxic compounds, such as cytostatic, differentiation-inducing, and antiangiogenic agents in the treatment of neoplastic diseases. However, accepted preclinical models to evaluate and refine in vivo efficacy for many classes of candidate noncytotoxic antiproliferative drugs do not presently exist. Under these circumstances, it would be reasonable to base the treatment schedule evaluated in initial phase I trials on that required to achieve the pattern of systemic exposure to drug in laboratory animals that best approximates the concentration and duration of exposure necessary for optimal in vitro activity.

Past experience has repeatedly demonstrated that impressive preclinical antitumor activity is not a reliable predictor of clinical efficacy. A reasonable argument can also be advanced to support the hypothesis that a candidate drug has little likelihood of being therapeutically effective unless a clinically tolerable dosing regimen provides a pattern of systemic exposure to the drug that is at least comparable with that required for activity against appropriate in vivo or in vitro preclinical models. Accordingly, when considered together with toxicologic and physiologic response factors, pharmacokinetic data acquired during phase I studies can facilitate efforts to optimize dosing regimens. Alternatively, withdrawing an agent from continued clinical development may be an option that warrants serious consideration in situations in which the plasma concentrations achieved in patients treated at the maximum tolerated dose are considerably lower than target levels, given the availability of limited clinical resources and ethical considerations of entering patients into a phase II trial of a compound that has little prospect of being therapeutically effective.

The *schedule* of drug administration depends highly on pharmacokinetic considerations and requires a choice of the duration of administration (e.g., bolus intravenous injection versus prolonged intravenous infusion), frequency of repeated dosing, and the sequencing of multiple drugs or drugs and other treatment modalities such as radiation. Bolus intravenous injection provides maximal peak drug levels in plasma but a rapid decline thereafter as the drug is eliminated from the plasma compartment by metabolism or excretion. This very convenient dosing method is appropriate for drugs that are not cell cycle-phase dependent and therefore do not have to be present during a specific phase of the cell cycle. Examples are the alkylating agents, such as chloroethylnitrosoureas, nitrogen mustards, and procarbazine, as well as other drugs that chemically interact with DNA.

Administration by prolonged intravenous infusion (i.e., 6 to 120 hours) is advantageous for agents that act preferentially in discrete phases of the cell cycle, such as S-phase–specific drugs (e.g., cytarabine, MTX, camptothecins), particularly if the drug is rapidly cleared from systemic circulation. Prolonged infusions have the additional advantage of providing a specific and constant plasma concentration of the drug, a desirable feature if information regarding the chemosensitivity of the tumor is available, as determined experimentally by various in vitro tests. Intermediate-length infusions (i.e., 1 to 4 hours) may provide a means to overcome the acute toxicities that are produced by exposing host organs to high peak drug levels. Particularly for acutely neurotoxic or cardiotoxic compounds, rapid intravenous infusions may present unacceptable dangers, but intermediate-length infusions may reduce peak drug levels adequately while retaining some of the convenience of bolus dosing.

It may be desirable to achieve the steady-state concentration rapidly for a drug given as a continuous intravenous infusion, in which case a *loading dose* may be given by bolus injection at the same time that the infusion is started. This is now standard practice for the administration of 5-FU (see Chapter 6). The bolus dose is usually selected to achieve an initial concentration near the steady-state target value. In this way, the time lag to achieve the plateau in the $C \times T$ profile, which may be considerable for some drugs, is eliminated. As an alternative to administering a drug by continuous intravenous infusion, it may be possible to maintain reasonably constant plasma levels using a repeated bolus injection dosing regimen. There is an approach to steady-state conditions in which the peak and trough plasma concentrations increase successively during repeated doses before becoming constant. As with the continuous intravenous infusion, steady state can be reached immediately with the proper choice of loading dose. The most common such schedule targets the peak concentration as twice the trough concentration. This design requires dosing once each half-life. An initial dose of twice the successive (maintenance) doses abolishes the time lag. As the dosing frequency increases, the ratio of peak-to-trough concentrations approaches 1, and the $C \times T$ curve appears more like that of a constant infusion. These same scheduling considerations also apply to the timing of oral drug delivery.

Pharmacokinetic-Pharmacodynamic Relationships

The toxicities of anticancer drugs are often better correlated with a pharmacokinetic variable than the administered dose. Relationships between the severity of toxicity and the AUC are most commonly encountered. However, other variables such as the C_{max} and duration of time that the drug concentration in plasma exceeds a particular threshold level are also predictive of toxicity. For example, the time interval that plasma levels of paclitaxel remain above 50 nM is better correlated with neutropenia, the principal dose limiting toxicity, than either C_{max} or AUC.[76] The nature of these relationships can often be described by a sigmoidal E_{max} model, but they may appear linear unless patients have been evaluated across a sufficiently broad range of doses.[77]

As previously indicated, therapeutic response ultimately depends on the delivery of drug from the bloodstream to the tumor in such a way that malignant cells are exposed to biologically effective concentrations of the active form of the agent for an adequate duration of time. The rate processes associated with drug distribution and elimination depend on the physicochemical properties of the drug and numerous physiologic factors. As is the case with any specific organ or tissue, the time course of the concentration of a compound within a solid tumor cannot be defined from experimental data restricted to measurements made in plasma, serum, or whole blood. Although there is undoubtedly some temporal relationship between drug concentrations in plasma and the tumor, elucidating the tumor $C \times T$ profile requires physical measurement of drug levels within the tumor itself. Whereas this cannot be easily accomplished in solid tumors, in most cases, hematologic malignancies are considerably more amenable to such studies because the cancer cells reside within the bloodstream itself, bone marrow or lymphatic tissues, which are considerably more accessible to drug. Consequently, efforts to determine whether adequate concentrations of the active form of a drug are achieved in cancer cells should be considered an important objective of phase I trials to evaluate new anticancer drugs in hematologic malignancies. The availability of this information will better facilitate the rational selection of drugs warranting further clinical evaluation. The emergence of noninvasive imaging techniques and studies of circulating tumor cells undoubtedly will enlighten pharmacokinetic-pharmacodynamic (i.e., PK-PD) relationships in solid tumors.

Conclusions

There are numerous reasons for acquiring pharmacokinetic data during various stages in the clinical development of anticancer drugs. The therapeutic indices of many drugs used in the treatment of cancer are inherently narrow because they are used at doses close to the upper limit of tolerability. Furthermore, cancer patients frequently exhibit increased sensitivity to many medications due to compromised organ function or diminished overall tolerance due to their underlying disease state, augmenting the potential for an undesirable pharmacokinetic interaction with the host of concurrent medications used in the clinical management of cancer patients. The chances for an adverse event resulting from inappropriate dosing of a chemotherapeutic agent to a cancer patient are, therefore, considerably greater than experienced with most other patient groups. Since the dose-limiting toxicities of a chemotherapeutic agent are very often related to some measure of systemic exposure to the drug, the margin of safety of a potentially effective dose is dependent upon the consistency of its pharmacokinetic behavior among patients.

Pharmacokinetics can also serve a useful role in the process of drug development by assisting the overall integration of data between preclinical testing and early clinical trials.[78] Initial human studies rely heavily on toxicologic and pharmacologic data obtained in mice and dogs, and pharmacokinetics provides a convenient approach to comparative analysis.

The ultimate goal of pharmacokinetics is to assist in the optimization of therapy. Although progress has been made in pharmacokinetic areas, the limiting step for optimization of therapy is inadequate knowledge of the relationship between drug $C \times T$ profiles and drug effects. Pharmacokinetics can serve as a useful tool to help elucidate pharmacodynamic relationships by determining which profiles are feasible and by helping design administration strategies. Also, because overall drug effect results from both kinetic and dynamic variables, studies can be designed to adjust doses individually so that kinetic differences between patients can be minimized and attention can be focused solely on drug dynamics.

Our ability to find useful relationships between drug exposure and clinical outcomes is greatest for drugs that offer substantial benefits for patients. The success of imatinib in patients with chronic myeloid leukemia (CML) and gastrointestinal stromal tumors (GIST) has provided immediate tangible benefits for these individuals. This success has also provided a major boost to the field of drug development. In the domain of pharmacokinetics, oral delivery of imatinib and other drugs presents substantial challenges in areas such as patient adherence to dosing regimens, erratic drug absorption, and drug-drug interactions. The rationale for efforts to emphasize improvement in these areas must be driven by solid indications of concentration-response relationships.

The demonstration of associations between plasma concentrations of imatinib and both complete cytogenetic response and major molecular response in CML supplies the impetus for further exploration.[79] Similarly, the report of associations in GIST between plasma concentrations of imatinib and both overall objective benefit and time to tumor progression provides additional incentive.[80] Although observational studies are not as powerful as prospective interventional studies, these strong signals have been replicated by other groups. Thus, research into the possibility of improving therapy via pharmacokinetic monitoring of plasma concentrations should be a high priority for continuing to optimize the use of imatinib in CML and GIST.

References

1. Donelli MG, D'Incalci M, Garattini S. Pharmacokinetic studies of anticancer drugs in tumor-bearing animals. Cancer Treat Rep 1984;68:381–400.
2. Notari RE. Biopharmaceutics and Clinical Pharmacokinetics. New York, NY: Marcel Dekker, 1987.
3. Gilbaldi M, Perrier D, eds. Pharmacokinetics. 2nd ed. New York, NY: Marcel Dekker, 1982.
4. Timmerman PM, de Vries R, Ingelse BA. Tailoring bioanalysis for PK studies supporting drug discovery. Curr Top Med Chem 2001;1:443–462.
5. Wright JD, Boudinot FD, Ujhelyi MR. Measurement and analysis of unbound drug concentrations. Clin Pharmacokinet 1996;30:445–462.
6. Dunne A. An iterative curve stripping technique for pharmacokinetic parameter estimation. J Pharm Pharmacol 1986;38:97–101.
7. Gillespie WR. Noncompartmental versus compartmental modelling in clinical pharmacokinetics. Clin Pharmacokinet 1991;20:253–262.
8. Dedrick RL, Myers CE, Bungay PM, et al. Pharmacokinetic rationale for peritoneal drug administration in the treatment of ovarian cancer. Cancer Treat Rep 1978;62:1–11.
9. Speyer JL, Sugarbaker PH, Collins JM, et al. Portal levels and hepatic clearance of 5-fluorouracil after intraperitoneal administration in humans. Cancer Res 1981;41:1916–1922.
10. Farris FF, King FG, Dedrick RL, et al. Physiologic model for the pharmacokinetics of cis-dichlorodiammineplatinum(II) (DDP) in the tumored rat. J Pharmacokinet Biopharm 1985;13:13–39.
11. Chan KK, Cohen JL, Gross JF, et al. Prediction of adriamycin disposition in cancer patients using a physiologic, pharmacokinetic model. Cancer Treat Rep 1978;62:1161–1171.
12. Dedrick RL, Forrester DD, Cannon JN, et al. Pharmacokinetics of 1-β-D-arabinofuranosylcytosine (ARA-C) deamination in several species. Biochem Pharmacol 1973;22:2405–2417.
13. Rowland M, Benet LZ, Graham GG. Clearance concepts in pharmacokinetics. J Pharmacokinet Biopharm 1973;1:123–136.
14. Sawyer M, Ratain M. Body surface area as a determinant of pharmacokinetics and drug dosing. Invest New Drugs 2001;19:171–177.
15. Carlisle KM, Halliwell M, Read AE, et al. Estimation of total hepatic blood flow by duplex ultrasound. Gut 1992;33:92–97.
16. Cockcroft DW, Gault MH. Prediction of creatinine clearance from serum creatinine. Nephron 1976;16:31–41.
17. Gibaldi M, McNamara PJ. Apparent volumes of distribution and drug binding to plasma proteins and tissues. Eur J Clin Pharmacol 1978;13:373–380.
18. Collins JM, Dedrick RL, King FG, et al. Nonlinear pharmacokinetic models for 5-fluorouracil in man: intravenous and intraperitoneal routes. Clin Pharmacol Ther 1980;28:235–246.
19. Donehower RC, Karp JE, Burke PJ. Pharmacology and toxicity of high-dose cytarabine by 72-hour continuous infusion. Cancer Treat Rep 1986;70:1059–1065.
20. Besseghir K, Roch-Ramel F. Renal excretion of drugs and other xenobiotics. Ren Physiol 1987;10:221–241.
21. Ilett KF, Tee LB, Reeves PT, et al. Metabolism of drugs and other xenobiotics in the gut lumen and wall. Pharmacol Ther 1990;46:67–93.
22. Balis FM, Holcenberg JS, Bleyer WA. Clinical pharmacokinetics of commonly used anticancer drugs. Clin Pharmacokinet 1983;8:202–232.
23. Glue P, Clement RP. Cytochrome P450 enzymes and drug metabolism—basic concepts and methods of assessment. Cell Mol Neurobiol 1999;19:309–323.
24. von Moltke LL, Greenblatt DJ, Schmider J, et al. Metabolism of drugs by cytochrome P450 3A isoforms. Implications for drug interactions in psychopharmacology. Clin Pharmacokinet 1985;29:33–43.
25. Gillum JG, Israel DS, Polk RE. Pharmacokinetic drug interactions with antimicrobial agents. Clin Pharmacokinet 1993;25:450–482.
26. Kivisto KT, Kroemer HK, Eichelbaum M. The role of human cytochrome P450 enzymes in the metabolism of anticancer agents: implications for drug interactions. Br J Clin Pharmacol 1995;40:523–530.
27. Chabot GG, Bouchard J, Momparler RL. Kinetics of deamination of 5-aza-2′-deoxycytidine and cytosine arabinoside by human liver cytidine deaminase and its inhibition by 3-deazauridine, thymidine or uracil arabinoside. Biochem Pharmacol 1983;32:1327–1328.
28. Milano G, McLeod HL. Can dihydropyrimidine dehydrogenase impact 5-fluorouracil-based treatment? Eur J Cancer 2000;36:37–42.
29. Clarke DJ, Burchell B. The uridine diphosphate glucuronosyltransferase multigene family: function and regulation. In: Kauffman FC, ed. Handbook of Experimental Pharmacology, Conjugation-Deconjugation Reactions in Drug Metabolism and Toxicity. Berlin: Springer-Verlag, 1994:3–43.
30. Ratain MJ. Insights into the pharmacokinetics and pharmacodynamics of irinotecan. Clin Cancer Res 2000;6:3393–3394.
31. Ivanov AI, Christodoulou J, Parkinson JA, et al. Cisplatin binding sites on human albumin. J Biol Chem 1998;273:14721–14730.
32. Milano G, Etienne MC, Cassuto-Viguier E, et al. Influence of sex and age on fluorouracil clearance. J Clin Oncol 1992;10:1171–1175.
33. Innocenti F, Iyer L, Ratain MJ. Pharmacogenetics of anticancer agents: lessons from amonafide and irinotecan. Drug Metab Dispos 2001;29:596–600.
34. Lichtman SM, Skirvin JA. Pharmacology of antineoplastic agents in older cancer patients. Oncology 2000;14:1743–1752.
35. Geokas M, Haverback B. The aging gastrointestinal tract. Am J Surg 1969;117:881–892.
36. Bender A. the effect of increasing age on the distribution of peripheral blood flow in man. J Am Geriatr Soc 1965;13:192–198.
37. Bach B, Hansen J, Kampmann J, et al. Disposition of antipyrine and phenytoin correlated with age and liver volume in men. Clin Pharmacokinet 1981;6:389–396.
38. Durnas C, Loi C, Cusack BJ. Hepatic drug metabolism and aging. Clin Pharmacokinet 1990;19:359–389.
39. Baker SD, Grochow LB. Pharmacology of cancer chemotherapy in the older person. Clin Geriatr Med 1997;13:169–183.
40. Kinirons MT, O'Mahony MS. Drug metabolism and ageing. Br J Clin Pharmacol 2004;57:540–544.
41. Anderson GD. Children versus adults: pharmacokinetic and adverse-effect differences. Epilepsia 2002;43(Suppl 3):53–59.
42. Hammerlein A, Derendorf H, Lowenthal DT. Pharmacokinetic and pharmacodynamic changes in the elderly. Clinical implications. Clin Pharmacokinet 1998;35:49–64.
43. Barre J, Houin G, Brunner F, et al. Disease-induced modifications of drug pharmacokinetics. Int J Clin Pharmacol Res 1983;3:215–226.
44. Powis G. Effect of human renal and hepatic disease on the pharmacokinetics of anticancer drugs. Cancer Treat Rev 1982;9:85–124.
45. Egorin MJ, Van Echo DA, Olman EA, et al. Prospective validation of a pharmacologically based dosing scheme for the cis-diamminedichloroplatinum(II) analogue diamminecyclobutanedicarboxylatoplatinum. Cancer Res 1985;45:6502–6506.
46. Egorin MJ, Sigman LM, Van Echo DA, et al. Phase I clinical and pharmacokinetic study of hexamethylene bisacetamide (NSC95580) administered as a five-day continuous infusion. Cancer Res 1987;47:617–623.
47. van den Bongard HJ, Mathot RA, Beijnen JH, et al. Pharmacokinetically guided administration of chemotherapeutic agents. Clin Pharmacokinet 2000;39:345–367.

48. Shimada T, Yamazaki H, Mimura M, et al. Interindividual variations in human liver cytochrome P-450 enzymes involved in the oxidation of drugs, carcinogens and toxic chemicals: studies with liver microsomes of 30 Japanese and 30 Caucasians. J Pharmacol Exp Ther 1994;270:414–423.

49. Watters JW, McLeod HL. Cancer pharmacogenomics: current and future applications. Biochim Biophys Acta 2003;1603:99–111.

50. Peck CC, Temple R, Collins JM. Understanding consequences of concurrent therapies. JAMA 1993;269:1550–1552.

51. Dorr RT, Soble MJ, Alberts DS. Interaction of cimetidine but not ranitidine with cyclophosphamide in mice. Cancer Res 1986;46:1795–1799.

52. Hande K, Combs G, Swingle R, et al. Effect of cimetidine and ranitidine on the metabolism and toxicity of hexamethylmelamine. Cancer Treat Rep 1986;70:1443–1445.

53. Bjornsson TD, Huang AT, Roth P, et al. Effects of high-dose cancer chemotherapy on the absorption of digoxin in two different formulations. Clin Pharmacol Ther 1986;39:25–28.

54. Balis FM. Pharmacokinetic drug interactions of commonly used anticancer drugs. Clin Pharmacokinet 1986;11:223–235.

55. Jamis-Dow CA, Klecker RW, Katki AG, et al. Metabolism of taxol by human and rat liver in vitro: a screen for drug interactions and interspecies differences. Cancer Chemother Pharmacol 1995;36:107–114.

56. van Meerten E, Verweij J, Schellens JH. Antineoplastic agents. Drug interactions of clinical significance. Drug Saf 1995;12:168–182.

57. Markowitz JS, Donovan JL, DeVane CL, et al. Effect of St John's wort on drug metabolism by induction of cytochrome P450 3A4 enzyme. JAMA 2003;290:1500–1504.

58. McCune JS, Hawke RL, LeCluyse EL, et al. In vivo and in vitro induction of human cytochrome P4503A4 by dexamethasone. Clin Pharmacol Ther 2000;68:356–366.

59. Bannwarth B, Pehourcq F, Schaeverbeke T, et al. Clinical pharmacokinetics of low-dose pulse methotrexate in rheumatoid arthritis. Clin Pharmacokinet 1996;30:194–210.

60. Evans WE, Christensen ML. Drug interactions with methotrexate. J Rheumatol 1985;12(Suppl 12):15–20.

61. Wood M. Pharmacokinetic drug interaction in anaesthetic practice. Clin Pharmacokinet 1991;21:285–307.

62 Kerr IG, Jolivet J, Collins JM, et al. Test dose for predicting high-dose methotrexate infusions. Clin Pharmacol Ther 1983;33:44–51.

63. Evans WE, Relling MV, Rodman JH, et al. Conventional compared with individualized chemotherapy for childhood acute lymphoblastic leukemia. N Engl J Med 1998;338:499–505.

64. Zimm S, Collins JM, Riccardi R, et al. Variable bioavailability of oral mercaptopurine: is maintenance chemotherapy in acute lymphoblastic leukemia being optimally delivered? N Engl J Med 1983;308:1005–1009.

65. Peng B, Dutreix C, Mehring G, et al. Absolute bioavailability of imatinib (Glivec) orally versus intravenous infusion. J Clin Pharmacol 2004;44:158–162.

66. Rubin GM, Tozer TN. Theoretical considerations in the calculation of bioavailability of drugs exhibiting Michaelis-Menten elimination kinetics. J Pharmacokinet Biopharm 1984;12:437–450.

67. Blasberg R, Patlak CS, Fenstermacher JD. Intrathecal chemotherapy: brain tissue profiles after ventriculocisternal perfusion. J Pharmacol Exp Ther 1975;195:73–83.

68. Myers CE, Collins JM. Pharmacology of intraperitoneal chemotherapy. Cancer Invest 1983;1:395–407.

69. Markman M, Bundy BN, Alberts DS, et al. Phase III trial of standard-dose intravenous cisplatin plus paclitaxel versus moderately high-dose carboplatin followed by intravenous paclitaxel and intraperitoneal cisplatin in small-volume stage III ovarian carcinoma: an intergroup study of the Gynecologic Oncology Group, Southwestern Oncology Group, and Eastern Cooperative Oncology Group. J Clin Oncol 2001;19:921–923.

70. Alberts DS, Markman M, Armstrong D, et al. Intraperitoneal therapy for stage III ovarian cancer: a therapy whose time has come! J Clin Oncol 2002;20:3944–3946.

71. Alberts DS, Liu PY, Hannigan EV, et al. Intraperitoneal cisplatin plus intravenous cyclophosphamide versus intravenous cisplatin plus intravenous cyclophosphamide for stage III ovarian cancer. N Engl J Med 1996;335:1950–1955.

72. Collins JM, Zaharko DS, Dedrick RL, et al. Potential roles for preclinical pharmacology in phase I trials. Cancer Treat Rep 1986;70:73–80.

73. EORTC Pharmacokinetics and Metabolism Group. Pharmacokinetically guided dose escalation in phase I clinical trials. Eur J Cancer Clin Oncol 1987;23:1083–1087.

74. Fuse E, Kobayashi S, Inaba M, et al. Application of pharmacokinetically guided dose escalation with respect to cell cycle phase specificity. J Natl Cancer Inst 1994;86:989–996.

75. Collins JM, Grieshaber CK, Chabner BA. Pharmacologically guided phase I trials based upon preclinical development. J Natl Cancer Inst 1990;82:1321–1326.

76. Gianni L, Kearns CM, Giani A, et al. Nonlinear pharmacokinetics and metabolism of paclitaxel and its pharmacokinetic/pharmacodynamic relationships in humans. J Clin Oncol 1995;13:180–190.

77. Holford NH. Clinical pharmacokinetics and pharmacodynamics of warfarin. Understanding the dose-effect relationship. Clin Pharmacokinet 1986;11:483–504.

78. Collins JM. Pharmacology and drug development. J Natl Cancer Inst 1988;80:790–792.

79. Larson RA, Druker BJ, Guilhot F, et al. Imatinib pharmacokinetics and its correlation with response and safety in chronic-phase chronic myeloid leukemia: a subanalysis of the IRIS study. Blood 2008;111:4022–4028.

80. Demetri GD, Wang Y, Wehrle E, et al. Imatinib plasma levels are correlated with clinical benefit in patients with unresectable/metastatic gastrointestinal stromal tumors. J Clin Oncol 2009;27:3141–3147.

Delivering Anticancer Drugs to Brain Tumors

Maciej M. Mrugala, Jeffrey G. Supko, and Tracy T. Batchelor

There were an estimated 51,140 new primary brain tumors diagnosed in the United States in 2007.[1] Malignant gliomas (anaplastic astrocytoma and glioblastoma) are the most common malignant primary brain tumors and represent the most frequent indication for cytotoxic chemotherapy in neuro-oncology. The goal of adjuvant chemotherapy for malignant glioma is eradication of the residual macroscopic and microscopic tumor felt to be the reason for surgical and radiation failure. Temozolomide (TMZ), an orally administered alkylating agent, significantly extends progression-free and overall survival when administered concurrently with radiation in patients with newly diagnosed glioblastoma.[2] This positive effect is particularly pronounced in patients with methylated O_6-methylguanine-DNA methyltransferase (MGMT) promoter and can be maintained for a prolonged period of time.[3,4] In addition, locally delivered chemotherapy in the form of 1,3-bis(2-chloroethyl)-1-nitrosourea (carmustine; BCNU) polymers also extends survival slightly in patients with malignant glioma when applied at the time of the initial debulking procedure.[5] A humanized monoclonal antibody against the vascular endothelial growth factor (VEGF) ligand, bevacizumab, extends progression-free survival in recurrent glioblastoma patients relative to historical controls when given alone or in combination with irinotecan.[6,7] Bevacizumab was approved as monotherapy for recurrent glioblastoma by the United States Food and Drug Administration in 2009. However, the survival benefit of adjuvant chemotherapy for patients with malignant gliomas is modest as demonstrated by an absolute increase in one-year survival of 6% in one meta-analysis of 12 randomized clinical trials.[8]

Mechanisms of chemotherapy resistance of brain tumors include factors common to other tumors such as multidrug resistance and increased efficiency of DNA damage repair systems.[9] In addition, treating malignant brain tumors represents a unique challenge for oncologists due to the presence of the blood-brain barrier (BBB), a physiologic impediment between the circulatory system of the brain and that of the body. The accessibility of many anticancer drugs to brain tumors is at least partially constrained by the BBB. Therefore, difficulty in achieving adequate and sufficiently sustained levels of the cytotoxic moiety at the tumor site is a significant factor contributing to the failure of systemic chemotherapy for malignant brain tumors.[10,11] Accordingly, the development of treatment strategies for brain tumors has emphasized techniques that are intended to overcome this barrier and improve drug delivery to these tumors. In addition, the multiplicity of ancillary agents used in the medical management of brain tumor patients, particularly glucocorticoids and enzyme-inducing antiseizure medications, increases the risk for drug interactions that may impact the efficacy or toxicity of chemotherapy. This chapter reviews the current state of approaches for delivering anticancer drugs to brain tumors, the various techniques that are available for assessing drug distribution to brain tumors, and important pharmacologic interactions that may affect both the accessibility of anticancer drugs to the CNS and the systemic pharmacokinetics of the anticancer agent.

Blood-Brain Barrier

Three main factors influence the extent to which a systemically administered anticancer agent distributes into the brain and brain tumors: (a) the plasma concentration-time profile of the drug; (b) regional blood flow; and (c) transport of the agent through the BBB and blood tumor barrier (BTB). The two former considerations are common to all solid tumors, whereas the latter is specific to brain tumors.[10] Erhlich was the first to propose the concept of the BBB at the beginning of this century. On administering the dye Trypan blue to rats by intravenous injection, he observed that all body organs were stained except for the brain and spinal cord.[12] The anatomic basis of the BBB was determined three decades ago with the introduction of the electron microscope. It results from a modification of the normal vascular endothelium whereby a sheet of cells is connected by tight junctions on a basement membrane (Fig. 5-1). The area of the exchange surface is 12 m^2 and the physiologic role of the BBB is assumed to include maintenance of a constant biochemical content of the interstitial milieu and protection of the brain from foreign and undesirable molecules.[13] Low hydraulic conductance, low ionic permeability, and high electrical resistance contribute to the very low permeability for hydrophilic nonelectrolytes in the absence of a membrane carrier.[14] These properties, together with the lack of intracellular fenestrations and pinocytotic vesicles, and the presence of a thicker basal lamina, create a physiologic barrier that is relatively impermeable to many water-soluble compounds.[15,16]

Some drugs use specific transport mechanisms present in the endothelial cell to traverse the BBB.[17] However, most cytotoxic drugs that gain access to the CNS, as exemplified by the chloroethylnitrosourea alkylating agents, cross the BBB by passive diffusion. Aside from pharmacokinetic properties, the main factors that influence the extent to which these compounds distribute into the CNS include lipid solubility, molecular mass, charge, and plasma protein binding. Specifically, small organic compounds with a molecular weight less than 200 that are lipid soluble, neutral at physiologic pH, and not highly bound to plasma proteins readily cross the BBB.[14]

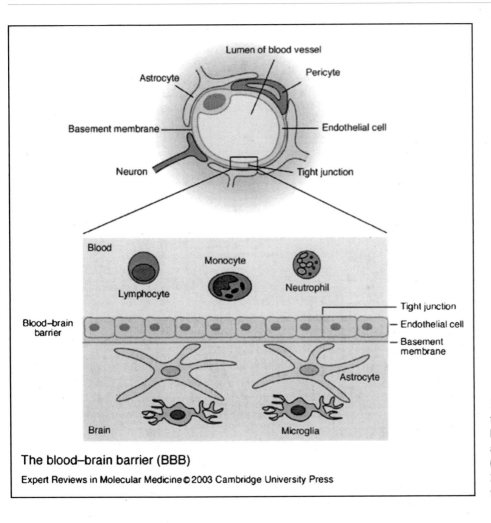

Lumen of blood vessel

Astrocyte

Pericyte

Basement membrane

Endothelial cell

Neuron

Tight junction

Blood

Monocyte

Lymphocyte

Neutrophil

Tight junction

Blood–brain barrier

Endothelial cell

Basement membrane

Astrocyte

Brain

Microglia

The blood–brain barrier (BBB)

Expert Reviews in Molecular Medicine © 2003 Cambridge University Press

FIGURE 5-1 Schematic representation of the normal intracerebral capillary. Crucial elements building Blood-Brain Barrier (basement membrane and endothelial tight junctions are visualized). (*Expert Reviews in Molecular Medicine*. Vol. 5; 23 May 2003. Cambridge University Press. http://www.expertreviews.org/, with permission.)

A second component of the BBB is the expression of P-glycoprotein (Pgp) on the luminal surface of brain capillary endothelial cells.[18] The presence of P-glycoprotein has been implicated in the active efflux of many chemotherapeutic drugs from the brain, including the vinca alkaloids and doxorubicin. Expression of P-glycoprotein has also been reported in malignant gliomas and may serve as another mechanism of chemotherapy resistance.[19,20] Multidrug resistance–related protein 1 (MRP1) and P-glycoprotein are differentially expressed in high- and low-grade gliomas. MRP1 overexpression appears to be more common in high-grade gliomas (WHO grade IV) while low-grade tumors (WHO grade II) exhibit greater Pgp expression. These findings may have potential therapeutic implications.[21] Agents that reverse the function of P-glycoprotein, such as verapamil, may increase passage of doxorubicin across the BBB.

The normal physiologic structure of the BBB is disrupted in vasculature within and adjacent to brain tumors. The barrier is usually more permeable in the center of a malignant tumor as opposed to the well vascularized and infiltrating edge that exhibits variable degrees of BBB integrity.[22] Figure 5-2 contrasts the normal BBB with the disrupted barrier found in a brain tumor. Vick and colleagues identified junctional clefts in the endothelial cells of capillaries adjacent to brain tumors.[23] These clefts correlated with the density of infiltrating tumor cells and were present in brain capillaries not in direct contact with the tumor. Evidence also exists that the microvasculature of these tumors lacks the properties of a normal BBB and has greater permeability as a result. Morphologic studies

have demonstrated that the BTB differs anatomically from the normal BBB, with open tight junctions, gap junctions, fenestrations, and numerous intracellular vesicles.[10,24] The increased permeability of these blood vessels forms the basis of contrast enhancement of brain tumors on CT and MRI scans. Iodinated, water-soluble

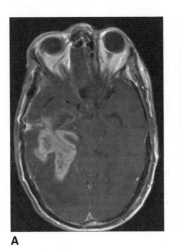 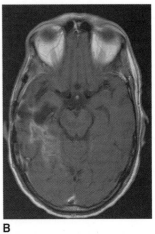

A   **B**

FIGURE 5-2 Response to antiangiogentic therapy. Contrast-enhanced MRI of the brain from a patient with recurrent glioblastoma in the right temporal area (**A**). Following administration of anti-VEGF agent (bevacizumab) in combination with carboplatin, dramatic decrease in the area of enhancement can be seen. In addition, significant reduction of surrounding vasogenic edema can be observed (**B**).

contrast agents do not penetrate areas of the brain with an intact BBB but are able to penetrate brain tumors.[25] These alterations in permeability are highly variable between tumors and within the same tumor.[26] For example, low-grade gliomas and proliferating edges of malignant gliomas seem to have a normally functioning, selective BBB and, consequently, do not typically show contrast enhancement on CT and MRI studies. A large variation in the enhancement patterns of malignant brain tumors on CT scans is common.[27,28] Approximately 30% of patients with anaplastic astrocytoma, a type of malignant glioma, are reported to have nonenhancing lesions.[27] A novel MRI technology for assessment of cerebral blood flow, cerebral blood volume and blood-brain-barrier leakage was recently developed and refined. Both dynamic susceptability contrast MRI (DSC-MRI) and T1-weighted dynamic contrast-enhanced MRI (DCE-MRI) allow for precise measurement of these paramenters. In additon, DCE-MRI can estimate the degree of BBB leakage.[29] Finally, positron emission tomography (PET) studies have shown that alterations in permeability usually occur in the central part of large tumors, whereas the periphery is intact.[30] The presence of a selective, normal BBB near the proliferating edge of a brain tumor may result in variable delivery of water-soluble drugs in this region and may contribute significantly to the high local failure rate of conventional anticancer drugs.

The central role hypothesized for the BBB in the resistance of brain tumors to chemotherapy has been questioned by some authorities. It has been suggested that because the BBB adjacent to tumors and the BTB lack the normal properties of an intact BBB,

drug delivery to these areas should not be compromised.[23] Indirect support for this argument comes from the observation that brain tumors occasionally respond to cytotoxic drugs that would not be expected to cross the BBB due to their physicochemical properties. A more consistent observation, however, has been that the most effective classes of antineoplastic drugs against malignant brain tumors are lipid-soluble molecules that can easily penetrate an intact BBB. Moreover, in addition to the existence of normal BBB at the proliferating edge of brain tumors, PET studies have demonstrated that, whereas the BBB and BTB may be abnormal at the time of diagnosis, these structures may become normalized on subsequent treatment.[31] These latter observations support a pivotal role for the BBB and BTB in the resistance of brain tumors to systemically administered chemotherapy. Novel anti-VEGF (vascular endothelial growth factor) agents were recently introduced to glioma therapy.[32,33] Through their mechanism of action these agents influence both BBB and BTB and can produce striking imaging results, frequently leading to either partial or complete disappearance of the contrast-enhancing tumors from MRI scans (Fig. 5-3).

Vascular Normalization

The vascular network formed by high-grade brain tumors is abnormal and is characterized by dilated vessels, increased permeability, and abnormally thickened basement membranes. These morphological changes are associated with the formation of vasogenic brain edema and contribute to the hypoxic tumor microenvironment and increased interstitial fluid pressure (IFP).[34] Vasogenic brain

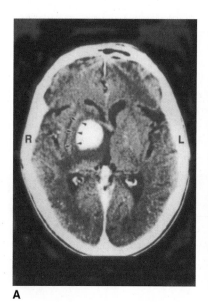
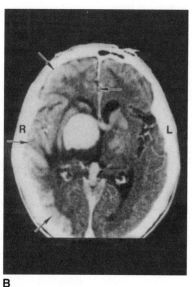
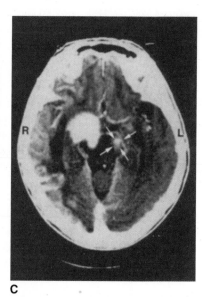

A   **B**   **C**

FIGURE **5-3** Heterogenicity of the blood-brain barrier. Contrast-enhanced CT scans of the basal ganglia of a 61-year-old woman with a primary CNS lymphoma, indicating that the permeability of the blood-tumor barrier is inconsistent for a given patient or even a given tumor nodule. **A.** CT scan demonstrating a bright, uniformly enhancing lesion in the right basal ganglia. The surrounding hypodense signal in the brain tissue around the tumor (*arrowheads*) should be noted. **B.** CT scan obtained after contrast agent administration. Contrast material was administered immediately after osmotic blood-brain barrier disruption (BBBD) and CT scans were obtained 30 minutes after the first BBBD treatment, to confirm and assess the grade of BBBD. The patient underwent right internal carotid artery disruption in the anterior and middle cerebral artery distributions (*arrows*). Opening of the brain tissue around the tumor in the area of the peritumoral hypodense signal evident in the CT scan in A should be noted. **C.** CT scan obtained after blood-brain barrier disruption (BBBD) in a patient with a right hemiparesis that was unexplained, because the only visible tumor was in the right cerebrum (**A**). BBBD the day after the CT scan in (**A**) extended into the posterior circulation via the posterior communicating artery. A left-side brainstem lesion not apparent in pre-BBBD imaging studies was noted. The right hemiparesis was thus attributable to a brainstem tumor (*arrows*) on the left that was not apparent on pre-BBBD MRI scans (intact BBB and no edema). (Courtesy of Edward A. Neuwelt, M.D., Oregon Health Sciences University. *Neurosurgery* 2004;54:131–142, with permission.)

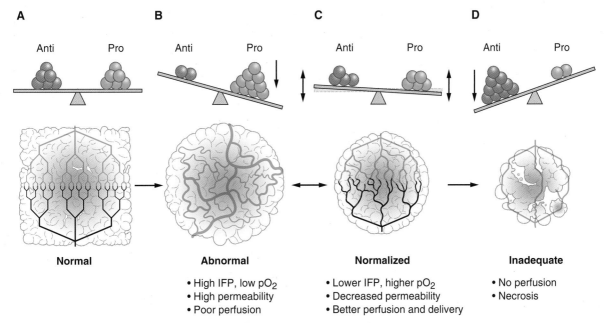

FIGURE 5-4 Schematic diagram to illustrate the process of vascular normalization. **A.** In healthy organs, there is a balance of proangiogenic and antiangiogenic molecules, which maintains an organized and efficient vascular supply. **B.** Tumors produce proangiogenic factors (*various shades of green*) that induce an abnormal, inefficient vascular network. **C.** Judiciously administered anti-VEGF therapy can restore the balance of proangiogenic and antiangiogenic signals and normalize the vascular network, potentially improving drug delivery and efficacy. **D.** However, if anti-VEGF therapy is continued, it can destroy the network totally, impeding delivery of oxygen and nutrients, and ultimately depriving the tumor of essential molecules for growth. In preclinical models, **panel C** usually progresses toward **panel D** (*single arrow*) with currently approved anti-VEGF agents. However, in human tumors, **panel C** commonly reverts to **panel B** after a "window of normalization" (*double arrow*). Anti, antiangiogenic molecules; IFP, interstitial fluid pressure; pO_2, tissue oxygen level; Pro, proangiogenic molecules. (From Jain RK, et al. Angiogenesis in brain tumours. Nat Rev Neurosci 2007;8(8):610–622, with permission.) (Ref. 194.)

edema is a cause of significant neurological morbidity in the brain tumor patient population and may decrease efficacy of cytotoxic therapies. Corticosteroids, also known to downregulate VEGF,[35] have been used as the primary therapy for brain edema for over 50 years. However, these agents cause significant toxicity in brain tumor patients. Anti-VEGF agents, by reducing vessel permeability and "normalizing" the brain tumor vascular network, may represent a new class of agents with antiedema properties. According to the vascular normalization hypothesis, the morphological and physiological effects of anti-VEGF agents on the tumor vasculature may also improve the efficacy of cytotoxic therapies by reducing the hypoxic fraction within the tumor and by improving delivery of therapeutic agents into the tumor mass[36] (Fig. 5-4). Preclinical and clinical observations have demonstrated that reduction in tumor hypoxia, improved delivery of therapeutics, and enhanced efficacy, all features consistent with the vascular normalization hypothesis, can be achieved with anti-VEGF therapy.[37–39]

Drug Delivery Methods

Following the administration of an anticancer drug by the intravenous or oral routes, the BBB can effectively impede the distribution of drug molecules from systemic circulation into the CNS. Consequently, considerable effort has been expended to develop drug delivery strategies that either entirely circumvent the BBB or modulate the permeability of the barrier to enhance the extent drug distribution into the brain from systemic circulation. These techniques include intra-arterial administration, BBB disruption with hyperosmolar solutions[40] or biomolecules, high-dose chemotherapy (HDCT), intrathecal (IT) injection, and local delivery by direct intratumoral injection of free drug or implantation of drug embedded in a controlled-release biodegradable delivery system. Even when drugs have crossed the BBB, however, their migration to tumor cells may be hindered by increased intercapillary distances, greater interstitial pressure, lower microvascular pressure, and the sink effect exerted by normal brain tissue.[41]

Intra-arterial Administration

The theoretical advantage for delivering anticancer drugs by the intra-arterial route is related to the ratio of systemic to regional blood flow. In comparison to intravenous injection, a considerably higher local drug concentration can be achieved with intra-arterial injection, thereby increasing the amount of the agent driven across the BBB. This has been confirmed experimentally, there was a two- to threefold increase in tumor concentration of cisplatin and a chloroethylnitrosourea, respectively, in the brains of animals after intra-arterial administration as compared to intravenous administration.[42] With this technique, sufficient local drug concentrations can be achieved with smaller than conventional doses so that systemic side effects are minimized.[43] The pharmacokinetic advantages of intra-arterial administration occur only during the first passage through the CNS, because the drug then enters venous circulation and the plasma profile is indistinguishable from that afforded by intravenous administration.

This approach has been clinically evaluated in various settings, including neoadjuvant and adjuvant therapy and recurrent malignant glioma.[44,45] Thus far, clinical trials of intra-arterial chemotherapy for malignant gliomas have not demonstrated improvement in survival over conventional intravenous therapy. A phase III study involving 315 patients with malignant gliomas failed to show any advantages of adjuvant intra-arterial BCNU over intravenous infusion of the same drug.[46] Moreover, subjects in the intra-arterial BCNU arm of this trial experienced significant treatment-related toxicities. 10% developed leukoencephalopathy and 15% developing ipsilateral blindness. Two randomized clinical trials compared intra-arterial and intravenous ACNU (nimustine). There was no significant difference in the progression-free survival and overall survival in each treatment arm. However, toxicity associated with intra-arterial ACNU was modest. No cases of leukoencephalopathy and only one case of transient visual impairment were reported.[47,48]

Potential disadvantages of the intra-arterial route include local complications related to catheterization (thrombosis, bleeding, infection) and neurological sequela (orbital and cranial pain, retinal toxicity, leukoencephalopathy, or cortical necrosis).[44,46,49] In addition, prodrugs requiring hepatic activation, such as cyclophosphamide, procarbazine and irinotecan, are not suitable for use by the intra-arterial route. One factor that partly explains the unique toxicities associated with intra-arterial administration is the "streaming" effect.[50] Infusion of drug into the high pressure, rapidly moving arterial bloodstream results in incomplete mixing of the drug and plasma and great variability in the amount of drug reaching different regions of the vascular territory. Depending on the characteristics of the distribution pattern, higher concentrations of drug might be achieved in normal brain, whereas lower amounts reach the tumor. Different strategies have been attempted to minimize the streaming effect, including rapid infusion,[50] superselective cannulation of the feeding artery,[49,51] diastole-phased pulsatile infusion,[52,53] and local blood flow adjusted dosage.[51] All of these techniques were combined in a phase I trial involving 21 brain tumor patients treated with intra-arterial carboplatin. The neurologic side effects were minor, and a two-fold escalation of the dose beyond the conventional intra-arterial dose was achieved with promising results.[51] Despite its serious limitations, there have been a few reports of promising results in patients receiving intra-arterial therapy for primary brain tumors. Intra-arterial carboplatin and etoposide were demonstrated to be safe and useful in the treatment of progressive optic-hypothalamic gliomas in children.[54] Safety and efficacy of intra-arterial chemotherapy with multiple agents in conjunction with osmotic disruption of the BBB were established.[55,56] It seems that intra-arterial chemotherapy, with all its current limitations, is slowly moving forward and may achieve wider applications. Perfection of the delivery techniques and development of newer less toxic compounds should increase its efficacy and safety.

Blood-Brain Barrier Disruption

BBB disruption involves the use of hyperosmolar solutions or biomolecules to increase the permeability of the BBB and improve drug delivery to brain tumors. The specific mechanisms underlying osmotic opening of the BBB and BTB are not entirely understood. Preliminary explanations suggested that a hyperosmotic environment caused endothelial cell shrinkage with resultant separation of tight junctions.[57] In addition to cellular shrinkage, osmotic stress releases biologically active molecules from endothelial cells, including serine proteases, that could potentially degrade the collagen matrix of the endothelial basement membrane. Finally, cellular shrinkage may also trigger second messenger signals and calcium influx, which could affect the integrity of tight junctions.[13]

Methods for disrupting the BBB involving both intravenous and intra-arterial administration have been developed for use in brain tumor patients.[57] The results of nonrandomized studies have been encouraging for certain brain tumor subtypes, especially primary CNS lymphoma.[58] Potential advantages of this method include increased tumor delivery of drug and lack of systemic toxicity from cytotoxic chemotherapy. Another possible advantage of this technique is avoiding the sink effect seen with other procedures used for delivering chemotherapy to brain tumors. The *sink effect* refers to the selective achievement of higher concentrations of a drug in areas of disrupted BBB in the tumor than to the rest of the brain. As a result of this concentration gradient, the drug rapidly diffuses out of the tumor into the surrounding brain and compromises tumor exposure time. Because BBB disruption theoretically affects the endothelium of both normal brain and brain tumor, a nonselective increase in drug delivery into both areas occurs, and no concentration gradient is established. Despite these potential advantages, the technique of BBB disruption is complex and requires transfemoral angiography and general anesthesia. Moreover, an attendant risk of stroke and a high frequency of seizures are associated with this method. These factors have limited the application of this technique.[57,59]

Tumor location and vascular supply determine the arterial circulation that is catheterized and infused. Most commonly, one major artery (left carotid, right carotid, left or right vertebral) is cannulated and treated. Some have advocated that documentation of BBB disruption with iodinated contrast agents be obtained before chemotherapy administration. Given the technical requirements of this procedure, it has not been widely adopted, and no definitive conclusions about the efficacy of the technique can be derived from the results of clinical trials that have been published to date. Other, less invasive techniques of BBB disruption are being investigated. It was recently shown that focused ultrasound exposure, when applied in the presence of preformed gas bubbles, can cause MRI-proven reversible opening of BBB in rabbits.[60,61] There is also interest in evaluating the use of biological agents to increase permeability of the BBB. Experimental data have demonstrated the effectivness of vasoactive compounds, including histamine, leukotriene C4, β-interferon, tumor necrosis factor-α, and bradykinin. The bradykinin analog RMP-7 (Cereport) selectively increases delivery of radiolabeled carboplatin to brain tumor in animal xenograft models and improves survival. However, a recent randomized double-blind, placebo controlled phase II study showed that RMP-7 does not improve efficacy of carboplatin in patients with recurrent malignant glioma.[62]

High-Dose Chemotherapy

Considering that the BBB is a major factor in brain tumor resistance to chemotherapy and that diffusion across this barrier depends on the concentration-time profile of the free fraction of drug (i.e., drug that is not bound to plasma proteins), the assumption has been that increasing the administered dose would drive more drug across the BBB.[10] The rationale for HDCT was derived from the relatively linear in vitro dose-response curve exhibited by the classic alkylating agents and the assumption that intrinsic cellular resistance could be overcome by increasing the dose. In the context of treating brain tumors, HDCT could overcome the previously mentioned sink effect and provide higher drug concentrations in the tumor for sustained periods. A number of phase I and II studies have been undertaken to evaluate this approach.[63] Despite the theoretical advantages, HDCT for recurrent malignant glioma has not made a significant impact on patient survival, although anecdotal cases of long-term survival have been observed. Among patients with newly diagnosed tumors, the median survival achieved using HDCT with bone marrow or stem cell rescue is comparable to that with conventional-dose chemotherapy (12 to 26 months versus 10 to 12 months, respectively). Treatment-related morbidity and mortality have been high, however, with a mortality rate as great as 27% in one early study. More recently, HDCT with autologous stem cell rescue was used with apparent success in treatment of medulloblastoma and malignant astrocytic tumors in children.[64] Adult patients with recurrent medulloblastoma do not seem to benefit from HDCT.[65] Safety and efficacy of HDCT were also addressed by investigators in the treatment of recurrent CNS germinomas and malignant astrocytomas in adults.[66,67] HDCT in conjunction with stem cell rescue achieved prolonged tumor control in the treatment of newly diagnosed anaplastic oligodendroglioma.[68] The strategy of HDCT followed by stem cell rescue may become an effective treatment strategy for potentially chemosensitive brain tumors such as anaplastic oligodendroglioma and primary CNS lymphoma (PCNSL). The best overall survival data achieved for patients with PCNSL have been reported after HDCT.[68–73]

Intrathecal Administration

IT chemotherapy involves the direct injection of drug into the CSF and is an obvious way to bypass the BBB. It is accomplished by injecting drug into the lumbar subarachnoid space, the cerebral ventricles, or the basal cisterns, with or without the use of catheters, pumps, or ventricular reservoirs.[74] The rationale is that the cells lining the fluid spaces of the brain are permeable, which results in a free exchange of molecules from extracellular fluid (ECF) to CSF and vice versa. Relatively small doses of a drug given by IT injection can achieve high local concentrations, due to the low volume of CSF (~150 mL), which thereby minimizes systemic toxicity. Furthermore, because of the intrinsically low levels of enzymes in the CSF, agents that are subject to rapid metabolism in blood, such as cytosine arabinoside (ara-C), remain in the active form in CNS for a longer periods of time. The three drugs administered most commonly in this manner are methotrexate sodium, ara-C, and thiotepa (thiotriethylene phosphoramide). These agents have been used mainly for the treatment of leptomeningeal metastases from systemic cancer.[75] Other agents that have been tested in the clinical setting via IT route include topotecan,[76,77] trastuzumab,[78–80] and rituximab.[81,82]

IT drug administration has disadvantages, including the necessity to establish access to the CSF compartment. The drug can be administered via lumbar route by performing a satndard lumbar puncture or through a ventricular catheter (Fig. 5-5). A ventricular

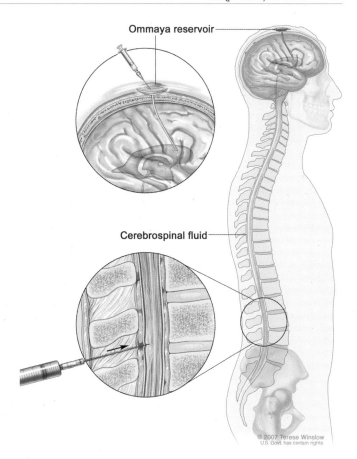

FIGURE 5-5 Different approaches to IT delivery of drugs. (From National Cancer Institute and Universtiatsklinikum Bonn; www.meb.uni-bonn.de, with permission.) (Please see Color Insert.)

access device is usually implanted in the frontal horn of the lateral ventricle to facilitate the administration of drug and minimize patient discomfort. This entails a small surgical risk of hemorrhage and infection. Moreover, the catheter may malfunction over time and require replacement.[83] IT drug administration also has numerous pharmacokinetic limitations. Among these, the drug must overcome bulk flow of CSF to penetrate the cisterns and ventricles (Fig. 5-6). In addition, the flow of interstitial fluid produced by brain cells and microvessels from ECF to CSF counteracts the diffusion of drug from CSF to ECF. Estimates are that CSF is completely renewed every 6 to 8 hours; thus, the concentration of a drug injected into the CSF is diluted continuously as a consequence of this process. This dilution can only be overcome by a continuous infusion or sustained-release system to maintain a clinically relevant concentration. Development of a liposomal form of ara-C allows sustained release of this drug into CSF and increases the effective half-life of the agent in the CSF by almost 50-fold.[84]

Another pharmacologic disadvantage of the IT route is the fact that production of CSF by the choroid plexus and its elimination into the venous circulation may be altered by the tumor itself, which disturbs bulk flow and modifies drug distribution and diffusion. For example, the clearance of methotrexate from CSF is decreased in the presence of leukemic meningitis.[85,86] Moreover, diffusion in the ventricular space is heterogeneous[87] and may result in uncertain and potentially toxic local concentrations in CSF, even if continuous-infusion devices are used.[74] Finally, and most important,

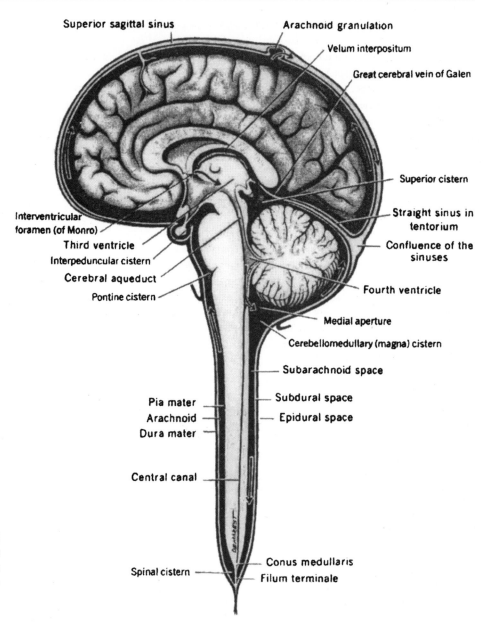

FIGURE **5-6** The subarachnoid spaces and cisterns of the brain and spinal cord. Schematic representation of cerebrospinal fluid pathways (*arrows*). (Reprinted from Fix J. High-Yield Neuro-anatomy, 2nd ed. Lippincott Williams & Wilkins, 2000:9, with permission.)

brain tumors are often in locations not adjacent to the ventricular system and may require diffusion of drug from CSF to tumor over a distance of several centimeters, which impairs the ability to achieve cytotoxic concentrations of the drug at the site of the tumor. In the case of methotrexate, the concentration of drug has been calculated to be no more than 0.1% of the CSF concentration 1 cm from the ependymal edge 48 hours after IT administration.[88] However, the relationship is quite complex. Whereas compounds with greater lipophilicity will access the ECF more effectively, they will also be subject to a higher rate of removal by the vascular and cellular compartments, thereby limiting the extent of drug penetration into brain tissue.[89] Therefore, at this point in time, IT chemotherapy is not feasible for brain tumors and is restricted to the treatment and prevention of leptomeningeal metastases.[90]

Intratumoral Administration

The simplest and most direct way to guarantee that a cytotoxic drug reaches its target is to deliver it directly into the tumor or into the cavity left after tumor resection. As with IT injection, this bypasses most of the previously mentioned obstacles pertaining to systemic drug administration for treating brain tumors. Systemic toxicity may also be reduced because substantially lower doses of drug may be given, and only a relatively small amount of drug distributes from the CNS to the bloodstream. A particularly attractive advantage of this strategy is that anticancer drugs (hydrophilic, high molecular weight) that are normally impeded by the BBB may be used. Conceptually, the low permeability of the BBB to such compounds should promote their retention within the CNS by inhibiting distribution into the bloodstream. Due to the high local drug concentrations that can be achieved, better distribution of drug may be provided within the tumor by diffusion and convection driven by the hydrostatic pressure of the tumor. The two techniques that have been most commonly used for directly introducing chemotherapeutic agents into brain tumors are parenteral delivery as either a bolus injection or continuous infusion through a cannula and implantation of drug embedded in a slow-release carrier system.

The feasibility of intratumoral infusion has been demonstrated in a number of clinical trials involving approximately ten different anticancer agents.[91] These studies, however, have not shown a clear survival advantage or direct evidence of increased drug delivery within the tumor. Furthermore, toxicity has been observed with this technique, including nervous system injury and infection.[91] Even if intratumoral infusion does avoid some obstacles to drug delivery, it does not circumvent the sink effect or problems associated with drug stability. Indeed, drug molecules released into the ECF must penetrate the brain interstitial tissue to reach tumor cells.[41] Before reaching its target, the compound could be inactivated by binding to normal tissue, by metabolism, by chemical degradation, or by elimination via the microvascular circulation.[92] Finally, tissue debris may obstruct the catheter.[91,92]

Controlled-release methods using polymer, microsphere, and liposomal carriers have been studied extensively in vitro and in vivo.[11] The goal of this strategy is to provide constant delivery of a cytotoxic drug into the tumor using a matrix that also protects the unreleased drug from hydrolysis and metabolism. A solid polymeric matrix facilitates the delivery of chemotherapeutic agents directly to brain tumors and has potential advantages. Biodegradable carriers have been developed that are unaffected by interstitial pH and provide near zero-order release of drug, with minimal inflammatory response.[93] Potential disadvantages include (1) drug release cannot be controlled once the device has been implanted, (2) unpredictable diffusion, (3) stability of the device and drug in the aqueous milieu, and (4) the possibility that the polymer may not release the drug as intended.

A biodegradable polyanhydride solid matrix, poly[bis(p-carboxyphenoxy)propane-sebacic acid] or p(CPP-SA), has been developed that releases drug by a combination of diffusion and hydrolytic polymer degradation.[94] Preclinical studies have demonstrated that this system is biocompatible and results in reproducible and sustained continuous release of BCNU. More than 300 patients with recurrent[95,96] and newly diagnosed[5,97–99] malignant gliomas have been treated with the BCNU polymer in phase I–IIIclinical studies. A phase III study in patients with recurrent malignant glioma demonstrated that intratumoral implantation of a 3.85% BCNU polymer was safe and resulted in minimal systemic side effects from BCNU. Median survival was significantly longer in subjects with glioblastoma who received the active polymer than in those who did not, even after adjustment for known prognostic factors.[95] A phase III randomized placebo controlled trial examining BCNU polymer application in glioblastoma patients at the time of primary surgical resection also showed survival benefit.[5,97] A phase I study designed to increase the amount of BCNU in the polymer (up to 20%) demonstrated that at the highest doses, BCNU plasma levels were significantly (500-fold) lower than those associated with systemic BCNU toxicity. As a result, no BCNU-related systemic toxicity was seen.[100] However, the risk of local neurotoxicity may be increased at higher BCNU concentrations in the polymer. Other studies of this delivery strategy are assesing use of the BCNU polymer in combination with systemic chemotherapy and incorporating other anticancer drugs into the polymer.[101] A clinical trial to evaluate intratumoral implantation of 5-fluorouracil-releasing microspheres has been initiated.[102,103] TMZ was incorporated into biodegradable polymers and tested in glioma-bearing rats. The active drug was released over 80 hours and in vivo biodistribution demonstrated

that the intracranial concentrations of TMZ increased threefold compared with orally delivered TMZ. Animals treated with TMZ polymer had improved survival compared to those treated with systemic TMZ.[104]

Nonchemotherapeutic approaches involving intratumoral administration are also being investigated. A fusion protein consisting of interleukin 13 (IL-13) linked to a mutated form of *Pseudomonas* exotoxin (IL-13 PE38QQR) that is administered by convection-enhanced delivery (CED) (see below) has entered phase I/II trials.[105–107] In addition, intratumoral delivery of chimeric proteins of transforming growth factor (TGF-α) linked to mutated *Pseudomonas* exotoxin PE-38 (TP-38) and directed against the epidermal growth factor receptor (EGFR) is being studied.[102]

Direct administration of therapeutic agents into the surgical cavity after tumor resection has also been investigated. The cavity, harboring the catheter with an external reservoir, analogous to the Ommaya system, can be intermittently filled with therapeutic agents. ^{131}I-labeled chlorotoxin (TM-601) was given in this fashion. In an uncontrolled, randomized trial, this approach was safe and resulted in prolonged progression-free survival in patients with recurrent malignant gliomas.[108]

Convection-Enhanced Delivery

Experimental evidence has demonstrated that properties of the brain parenchyma may impede delivery of drugs to the site of a brain tumor. Therefore, the BBB may not be the only obstacle that must be overcome for successful delivery of a cytotoxic drug to a brain tumor. Diffusion barriers intrinsic to brain tissue may also be important in limiting drug delivery to tumors. The hydrostatic pressure of brain tissue and the solubility of the drug are important factors that determine the diffusion of drug into surrounding tissue. CED is a pressure gradient–dependent method developed to overcome these potential barriers and consists of a direct infusion of drug solution through a catheter surgically implanted in the brain tumor.[109] Experimental studies of CED have demonstrated that drug delivery with this method is dependent on the anatomic site of the catheter. Infusion into gray matter results in spherical distribution of the drug, whereas infusion into white matter results in distribution along white matter fiber pathways. Therefore, the specific anatomic location of the brain tumor may be an important determinant of drug delivery.

Studies of the delivery of ara-C to rat brain after intravenous, IT, intraventricular administration or CED have been conducted.[110] Quantitative autoradiographic analysis revealed that drug concentration in brain tissue after CED was 4,000-fold higher than after intravenous administration. Moreover, the volume of distribution was ten-fold higher after CED than after IT or intraventricular administration. Experience with the use of CED in the treatment of patients with brain tumors has been limited. In a phase I study involving 18 patients with recurrent malignant gliomas, a high-flow interstitial microinfusion of a conjugated form of diphtheria toxin was conducted.[111] In 9 of 15 evaluable patients, at least a 50% regression of tumor was apparent on MRI, and two complete responses were observed. The treatment was well tolerated, and no treatment-related deaths or systemic toxicity occurred. The dose-limiting toxicity was local brain injury, which may have been the result of endothelial damage to cerebral capillaries.

Assessing Drug Delivery to the Brain

The clinical effectiveness of chemotherapy ultimately depends upon exposing tumor cells to adequate concentrations of the biologically active form of anticancer drugs for a sufficient duration of time. Distribution of drug from the administration site to the tumor and its subsequent elimination from the body are dependent upon the physicochemical properties of the drug and numerous physiological factors. Penetration of the BBB or BTB is an additional complexity in the use of parenterally or orally adminstered anticancer agents against tumors residing within the CNS that is not a consideration for treating hematological malignancies or solid tumors.[10,41,112] Characterizing the exposure of brain tumors to chemotherapeutic agents presents an extremely challenging problem. As is the case with any organ or tissue, the time course of the concentration of a drug or active metabolite within a tumor cannot be discerned from experimental data limited to measurements made in plasma, serum, or whole blood. Although some temporal relationship undoubtedly exists between drug concentrations in plasma and those in tumor, elucidating the tumor concentration-time profile necessarily requires measuring drug levels within the tumor itself.

Determining whether adequate concentrations of the active form of a drug reach the target tissue is extremely important in the context of phase I trials to evaluate the efficacy of new anticancer drugs for treating brain tumors. Because objective antitumor responses occur infrequently in phase I studies, the availability of data regarding the extent to which a chemotherapeutic agent reaches a brain tumor would provide a rational basis for selecting drugs that warrant further clinical evaluation. As described in this section, the principal techniques that are less invasive and potentially more informative than tissue biopsy studies for assessing the pharmacokinetics of anticancer drugs in the CNS and brain tumors include CSF sampling, microdialysis, and noninvasive imaging. Although no single method can be uniformly applied for monitoring drugs in human tissues in vivo, these techniques nevertheless are becoming increasingly important to the clinical development of anticancer drugs for the treatment of brain tumors.

Direct Measurment in Tumor Tissue

The traditional method for evaluating drug distribution to a solid tumor by directly measuring its concentration in tissue has numerous deficiencies. Subjecting brain cancer patients to the risks of an intracranial surgical procedure, that may have little or no direct benefit to the treatment of their disease, raises ethical concerns. It may be possible to circumvent this problem by obtaining tissue when a biopsy was diagnostically indicated or during a necessary tumor debulking procedure. Nevertheless, measuring the concentration of drug in a single biopsy specimen provides very limited information unless the tissue is obtained while drug is being given in a manner that provides continuous systemic exposure to the agent. Otherwise, the most appropriate time to obtain a single biopsy specimen relative to drug administration is speculative, at best, as the presence or absence of a measurable drug concentration has little interpretive value. Acquiring serial tumor specimens from the same patient presents even greater practical constraints than conducting a single biopsy, and the effect of prior procedures

on altering the transport of drug to and from the tumor represents a significant confounding factor. Conceivably, as part of a phase II study in which a moderately sized cohort of patients with comparable disease characteristics are treated with the same dose of drug, single biopsies of the tumor and adjacent peritumoral tissue could be performed in different patients over a range of times relative to drug administration, allowing a composite or pooled tissue concentration-time course to be constructed.

Cerebrospinal Fluid

Pharmacologic studies of anticancer agents directed against brain tumors often include the determination of drug or drug metabolite concentrations in the CSF as a surrogate for tumor levels and as a measure of drug delivery beyond the BBB. An understanding of the composition and normal physiology of CSF is important to discern the significance of drug level monitoring in this compartment. The most distinctive difference between CSF and plasma is the substantially lower concentration of proteins in CSF. Because of this, the total concentration of compounds that are poorly soluble in water or that bind avidly to proteins would be expected to be lower in CSF than in plasma or brain tissue, although the free concentration may be increased. In addition, CSF is slightly more acidic than plasma (pH of 7.32 versus 7.40), and this differential could conceivably influence the transport and retention of a drug in CSF, as well as its chemical stability relative to that in plasma, for compounds that have a functional group with a pK_a in the 7 to 8 range.

Figure 5-6 depicts the normal process involved in CSF formation and flow. The volume of CSF contained within the ventricles, cisterns, and subarachnoid space of a normal adult is approximately 150 mL.[113] Approximately 500 mL of CSF is produced every 24 hours, predominantly by the choroid plexus within the cerebral ventricles; therefore, the entire CSF volume is replenished three times during the course of a day. CSF formed in the lateral ventricles flows into the third ventricle and then to the fourth ventricle. Upon exiting from the fourth ventricle, it passes into the basal cisterns and the cerebral and spinal subarachnoid spaces, descending through the posterior aspect of the spinal cord and returning through the anterior aspect. Ascending CSF passes over the cerebral hemispheres toward the major dural sinuses, where absorption of CSF into the venous system occurs at the arachnoid villi. The presence of a brain tumor can significantly diminish both the formation and flow of CSF.[114]

Concentration gradients between the ventricular and lumbar regions exist for endogenous constituents of CSF as well as for xenobiotics that have gained access to the CSF. The concentration of systemically administered drugs is generally higher in CSF collected from the ventricles than from the lumbar region as drug distribution in the CNS follows CSF flow.[115] Because drug levels are often determined in CSF acquired by lumbar puncture, it should be recognized that this may significantly underestimate the concentrations in the ventricular region. Similarly, drug administered directly into lumbar CSF is poorly distributed to the ventricles.[87,116] Although patients cannot be subjected to frequently repeated lumbar punctures, ventricular access devices such as the Ommaya reservoir may be used to facilitate the serial acquisition of CSF specimens for drug level monitoring in the brain. Therefore, the specific space from which CSF samples were collected must be taken into account whenever drug concentrations reported in different

CNS and brain tumors for these settings would be desirable but present technical difficulties.

Conclusion

Treatment strategies for the most common type of primary brain tumor, malignant glioma, are rapidly expanding. The persistence of normal BBB near the proliferating edge of the tumor coupled with normalization of other areas of the BBB with treatment emphasizes the importance of strategies aimed at improving drug delivery across the BBB and to the tumor. In addition to the methods discussed in this review, cytotoxic drugs specifically designed for BBB penetration represent an important class of therapies to be assessed in the future. Methods for evaluating the success of these strategies are under development. Pharmacokinetic studies have assumed great importance in the development of antineoplastic therapy for hematologic and solid malignancies. Although application of the same principles to studies of brain tumor therapies is a relatively recent development and represents a unique set of challenges, these correlative studies add valuable information in the assessment of new brain tumor therapies. Moreover, with the emergence of cytostatic therapies for cancer, the traditional radiographic end points are insufficient, and these evaluative methods are likely to become surrogate end points in future clinical trials of these therapies. New response criteria for high-grade gliomas are currently being developed. Finally, drug interactions have assumed great importance in brain tumor clinical trials with the recognition that many common supporting medications used in this patient population affect the metabolism of cytotoxic drugs through induction of the CYP450 enzyme family. The development of noninvasive methods that more readily facilitate evaluation of drug distribution and accumulation in local tissue and tumor is a fundamental challenge for the future. The availability of such techniques will allow efficient assessment of promising agents for the treatment of malignant gliomas.

References

1. Central Brain Tumor Registry of the United States (CBTRUS). Statistical report: Primary brain tumors in the United States, 2007–2008. http://www.cbtrus.org/index.html

2. Stupp R, et al. Radiotherapy plus concomitant and adjuvant temozolomide for glioblastoma. N Engl J Med 2005;352(10):987–996.

3. Stupp R, et al. Effects of radiotherapy with concomitant and adjuvant temozolomide versus radiotherapy alone on survival in glioblastoma in a randomised phase III study: 5-year analysis of the EORTC-NCIC trial. Lancet Oncol 2009;10(5):459–466.

4. Hegi ME, et al. MGMT gene silencing and benefit from temozolomide in glioblastoma. N Engl J Med 2005;352(10):997–1003.

5. Westphal M, et al. A phase 3 trial of local chemotherapy with biodegradable carmustine (BCNU) wafers (Gliadel wafers) in patients with primary malignant glioma. Neuro Oncol 2003;5(2):79–88.

6. Vredenburgh JJ, et al. Bevacizumab plus irinotecan in recurrent glioblastoma multiforme. J Clin Oncol 2007;25(30):4722–4729.

7. Friedman HS, et al. Bevacizumab alone and in combination with irinotecan in recurrent glioblastoma. J Clin Oncol 2009;27(28):4733–4740.

8. Stewart LA. Chemotherapy in adult high-grade glioma: a systematic review and meta-analysis of individual patient data from 12 randomised trials. Lancet 2002;359(9311):1011–1018.

9. Phillips PC. Antineoplastic drug resistance in brain tumors. Neurol Clin 1991;9(2):383–404.

10. Greig NH. Optimizing drug delivery to brain tumors. Cancer Treat Rev 1987;14(1):1–28.

11. Sipos EP, Brem H. New delivery systems for brain tumor therapy. Neurol Clin 1995;13(4):813–825.

12. Pardridge WM, et al. Blood-brain barrier: interface between internal medicine and the brain. Ann Intern Med 1986;105(1):82–95.

13. Zlokovic BV, Apuzzo ML. Strategies to circumvent vascular barriers of the central nervous system. Neurosurgery 1998;43(4):877–878.

14. Crone C. The blood-brain barrier: a modified tight epithelium. In: Suckling AJ, Rumsby MG, Bradbury MWB, eds. The Blood-Brain Barrier in Health and Disease. Chichester, UK: Ellis Horwood, 1986.

15. Muldoon LL, et al. A physiological barrier distal to the anatomic blood-brain barrier in a model of transvascular delivery. Am J Neuroradiol 1999;20(2):217–222.

16. Fishman R. Cerebrospinal Fluid in Diseases of the Nervous System. Vol. 43. Philadelphia: WB Saunders, 1992.

17. Greig NH, et al. Facilitated transport of melphalan at the rat blood-brain barrier by the large neutral amino acid carrier system. Cancer Res 1987;47(6):1571–1576.

18. Henson JW, Cordon-Cardo C, Posner JB. P-glycoprotein expression in brain tumors. J Neurooncol 1992;14(1):37–43.

19. Fenart L, et al. Inhibition of P-glycoprotein: rapid assessment of its implication in blood-brain barrier integrity and drug transport to the brain by an in vitro model of the blood-brain barrier. Pharm Res 1998;15(7):993–1000.

20. Tsuji A. P-glycoprotein-mediated efflux transport of anticancer drugs at the blood-brain barrier. Ther Drug Monit 1998;20(5):588–590.

21. de Faria GP, et al. Differences in the expression pattern of P-glycoprotein and MRP1 in low-grade and high-grade gliomas. Cancer Invest 2008;26(9):883–889.

22. Neuwelt EA. Mechanisms of disease: the blood-brain barrier. Neurosurgery 2004;54(1):131–140; discussion 141–142.

23. Vick NA, Khandekar JD, Bigner DD. Chemotherapy of brain tumors. Arch Neurol 1977;34(9):523–526.

24. Waggener JD, Beggs JL. Vasculature of neural neoplasms. Adv Neurol 1976;15:27–49.

25. Steinhoff H, et al. Axial transverse computerized tomography in 73 glioblastomas. Acta Neurochir (Wien) 1978;42(1–2):45–56.

26. Blasberg RG, Groothuis DR. Chemotherapy of brain tumors: physiological and pharmacokinetic considerations. Semin Oncol 1986;13(1):70–82.

27. Chamberlain MC, Murovic JA, Levin VA. Absence of contrast enhancement on CT brain scans of patients with supratentorial malignant gliomas. Neurology 1988;38(9):1371–1374.

28. DeAngelis LM. Cerebral lymphoma presenting as a nonenhancing lesion on computed tomographic/magnetic resonance scan. Ann Neurol 1993;33(3):308–311.

29. Sourbron S, et al. Quantification of cerebral blood flow, cerebral blood volume, and blood-brain-barrier leakage with DCE-MRI. Magn Reson Med 2009;62(1):205–217.

30. Brooks DJ, Beaney RP, Thomas DG. The role of positron emission tomography in the study of cerebral tumors. Semin Oncol 1986;13(1):83–93.

31. Ott RJ, et al. Measurements of blood-brain barrier permeability in patients undergoing radiotherapy and chemotherapy for primary cerebral lymphoma. Eur J Cancer 1991;27(11):1356–1361.

32. Desjardins A, et al. Bevacizumab plus irinotecan in recurrent WHO grade 3 malignant gliomas. Clin Cancer Res 2008;14(21):7068–7073.

33. Vredenburgh JJ, et al. Experience with irinotecan for the treatment of malignant glioma. Neuro Oncol 2009;11(1):80–91.

34. Boucher Y, et al. Interstitial fluid pressure in intracranial tumours in patients and in rodents. Br J Cancer 1997;75(6):829–836.

35. Heiss JD, et al. Mechanism of dexamethasone suppression of brain tumor-associated vascular permeability in rats. Involvement of the glucocorticoid receptor and vascular permeability factor. J Clin Invest 1996;98(6):1400–1408.

36. Gerstner ER, et al. VEGF inhibitors in the treatment of cerebral edema in patients with brain cancer. Nat Rev Clin Oncol 2009;6(4):229–236.

37. Tong RT, et al. Vascular normalization by vascular endothelial growth factor receptor 2 blockade induces a pressure gradient across the vasculature and improves drug penetration in tumors. Cancer Res 2004;64(11):3731–3736.

38. Winkler F, et al. Kinetics of vascular normalization by VEGFR2 blockade governs brain tumor response to radiation: role of oxygenation, angiopoietin-1, and matrix metalloproteinases. Cancer Cell 2004;6(6):553–563.

39. Lee CG, et al. Anti-Vascular endothelial growth factor treatment augments tumor radiation response under normoxic or hypoxic conditions. Cancer Res 2000;60(19):5565–5570.

40. Rapoport SI, et al. Quantitative aspects of reversible osmotic opening of the blood-brain barrier. Am J Physiol 1980;238(5):R421–R431.

41. Jain RK. Transport of molecules in the tumor interstitium: a review. Cancer Res 1987;47(12):3039–3051.

42. Yamada K, et al. Distribution of radiolabeled 1-(4-amino-2-methyl-5-pyrimidinyl)methyl-3-(2-chloroethyl)-3-nitros ourea hydrochloride in rat brain tumor: intraarterial versus intravenous administration. Cancer Res 1987;47(8):2123–2128.

43. Bullard DE, Bigner SH, Bigner DD. Comparison of intravenous versus intracarotid therapy with 1,3-bis(2-chloroethyl)-1-nitrosourea in a rat brain tumor model. Cancer Res 1985;45(11 Pt 1):5240–5245.

44. Fine HA, et al. Meta-analysis of radiation therapy with and without adjuvant chemotherapy for malignant gliomas in adults. Cancer 1993;71(8):2585–2597.

45. Larner JM, et al. A phase 1–2 trial of superselective carboplatin, low-dose infusional 5-fluorouracil and concurrent radiation for high-grade gliomas. Am J Clin Oncol 1995;18(1):1–7.

46. Shapiro WR, et al. A randomized comparison of intra-arterial versus intravenous BCNU, with or without intravenous 5-fluorouracil, for newly diagnosed patients with malignant glioma. J Neurosurg 1992;76(5):772–781.

47. Kochii M, et al. Randomized comparison of intra-arterial versus intravenous infusion of ACNU for newly diagnosed patients with glioblastoma. J Neurooncol 2000;49(1):63–70.

48. Imbesi F, et al. A randomized phase III study: comparison between intravenous and intraarterial ACNU administration in newly diagnosed primary glioblastomas. Anticancer Res 2006;26(1B):553–558.

49. Tamaki M, et al. Parenchymal damage in the territory of the anterior choroidal artery following supraophthalmic intracarotid administration of CDDP for treatment of malignant gliomas. J Neurooncol 1997;35(1):65–72.

50. Blacklock JB, et al. Drug streaming during intra-arterial chemotherapy. J Neurosurg 1986;64(2):284–291.

51. Cloughesy TF, et al. Intra-arterial carboplatin chemotherapy for brain tumors: a dose escalation study based on cerebral blood flow. J Neurooncol 1997;35(2):121–131.

52. Saris SC, et al. Intravascular streaming during carotid artery infusions. Demonstration in humans and reduction using diastole-phased pulsatile administration. J Neurosurg 1991;74(5):763–772.

53. Gobin YP, et al. Intraarterial chemotherapy for brain tumors by using a spatial dose fractionation algorithm and pulsatile delivery. Radiology 2001;218(3):724–732.

54. Osztie E, et al. Combined intraarterial carboplatin, intraarterial etoposide phosphate, and IV Cytoxan chemotherapy for progressive optic-hypothalamic gliomas in young children. Am J Neuroradiol 2001;22(5):818–823.

55. Doolittle ND, et al. Safety and efficacy of a multicenter study using intraarterial chemotherapy in conjunction with osmotic opening of the blood-brain barrier for the treatment of patients with malignant brain tumors. Cancer 2000;88(3):637–647.

56. Fortin D, et al. Enhanced chemotherapy delivery by intraarterial infusion and blood-brain barrier disruption in malignant brain tumors: the Sherbrooke experience. Cancer 2005;103(12):2606–2615.

57. Kroll RA, Neuwelt EA. Outwitting the blood-brain barrier for therapeutic purposes: osmotic opening and other means. Neurosurgery 1998;42(5):1083–1099; discussion 1099–1100.

58. Angelov L, et al. Blood-brain barrier disruption and intra-arterial methotrexate-based therapy for newly diagnosed primary CNS lymphoma: a multi-institutional experience. J Clin Oncol 2009;27(21):3503–3509.

59. Neuwelt EA, et al. Therapeutic efficacy of multiagent chemotherapy with drug delivery enhancement by blood-brain barrier modification in glioblastoma. Neurosurgery 1986;19(4):573–582.

60. Sheikov N, et al. Cellular mechanisms of the blood-brain barrier opening induced by ultrasound in presence of microbubbles. Ultrasound Med Biol 2004;30(7):979–989.

61. Wang F, et al. Focused ultrasound microbubble destruction-mediated changes in blood-brain barrier permeability assessed by contrast-enhanced magnetic resonance imaging. J Ultrasound Med 2009;28(11):1501–1509.

62. Prados MD, et al. A randomized, double-blind, placebo-controlled, phase 2 study of RMP-7 in combination with carboplatin administered intravenously for the treatment of recurrent malignant glioma. Neuro Oncol 2003;5(2):96–103.

63. Fernandez-Hidalgo OA, et al. High-dose BCNU and autologous progenitor cell transplantation given with intra-arterial cisplatinum and simultaneous radiotherapy in the treatment of high-grade gliomas: benefit for selected patients. Bone Marrow Transplant 1996;18(1):143–149.

64. Perez-Martinez A, et al. High-dose chemotherapy with autologous stem cell rescue for children with high risk and recurrent medulloblastoma and supratentorial primitive neuroectodermal tumors. J Neurooncol 2005;71(1):33–38.

65. Gururangan S, et al. Efficacy of high-dose chemotherapy or standard salvage therapy in patients with recurrent medulloblastoma. Neuro Oncol 2008;10(5):745–751.

66. Modak S, et al. Thiotepa-based high-dose chemotherapy with autologous stem-cell rescue in patients with recurrent or progressive CNS germ cell tumors. J Clin Oncol 2004;22(10):1934–1943.

67. Chen B, et al. Safety and efficacy of high-dose chemotherapy with autologous stem cell transplantation for patients with malignant astrocytomas. Cancer 2004;100(10):2201–2207.

68. Abrey LE, et al. High-dose chemotherapy with stem cell rescue as initial therapy for anaplastic oligodendroglioma. J Neurooncol 2003;65(2):127–134.

69. Colombat P, et al. High-dose chemotherapy with autologous stem cell transplantation as first-line therapy for primary CNS lymphoma in patients younger than 60 years: a multicenter phase II study of the GOELAMS group. Bone Marrow Transplant 2006;38(6):417–420.

70. Soussain C, et al. Intensive chemotherapy followed by hematopoietic stem-cell rescue for refractory and recurrent primary CNS and intraocular lymphoma: Societe Francaise de Greffe de Moelle Osseuse-Therapie Cellulaire. J Clin Oncol 2008;26(15):2512–2518.

71. Abrey LE, et al. Intensive methotrexate and cytarabine followed by high-dose chemotherapy with autologous stem-cell rescue in patients with newly diagnosed primary CNS lymphoma: an intent-to-treat analysis. J Clin Oncol 2003;21(22):4151–4156.

72. Soussain C, et al. Results of intensive chemotherapy followed by hematopoietic stem-cell rescue in 22 patients with refractory or recurrent primary CNS lymphoma or intraocular lymphoma. J Clin Oncol 2001;19(3):742–749.

73. Illerhaus G, et al. High-dose chemotherapy with autologous stem-cell transplantation and hyperfractionated radiotherapy as first-line treatment of primary CNS lymphoma. J Clin Oncol 2006;24(24):3865–3870.

74. Bakhshi S, North RB. Implantable pumps for drug delivery to the brain. J Neurooncol 1995;26(2):133–139.

75. Pinkel D, Woo S. Prevention and treatment of meningeal leukemia in children. Blood 1994;84(2):355–366.

76. Gammon DC, et al. Intrathecal topotecan in adult patients with neoplastic meningitis. Am J Health Syst Pharm 2006;63(21):2083–2086.

77. Groves MD, et al. A multicenter phase II trial of intrathecal topotecan in patients with meningeal malignancies. Neuro Oncol 2008;10(2):208–215.

78. Stemmler HJ, et al. Application of intrathecal trastuzumab (Herceptintrade mark) for treatment of meningeal carcinomatosis in HER2-overexpressing metastatic breast cancer. Oncol Rep 2006;15(5):1373–1377.

79. Stemmler HJ, et al. Intrathecal trastuzumab (Herceptin) and methotrexate for meningeal carcinomatosis in HER2-overexpressing metastatic breast cancer: a case report. Anticancer Drugs 2008;19(8):832–836.

80. Ferrario C, et al. Intrathecal trastuzumab and thiotepa for leptomeningeal spread of breast cancer. Ann Oncol 2009;20(4):792–795.

81. Rubenstein JL, et al. Phase I study of intraventricular administration of rituximab in patients with recurrent CNS and intraocular lymphoma. J Clin Oncol 2007;25(11):1350–1356.

82. Antonini G, et al. Intrathecal anti-CD20 antibody: an effective and safe treatment for leptomeningeal lymphoma. J Neurooncol 2007;81(2):197–199.

83. Chamberlain MC, Kormanik PA, Barba D. Complications associated with intraventricular chemotherapy in patients with leptomeningeal metastases. J Neurosurg 1997;87(5):694–699.

84. Chamberlain MC, et al. Pharmacokinetics of intralumbar DTC-101 for the treatment of leptomeningeal metastases. Arch Neurol 1995;52(9): 912–917.

85. Ettinger LJ, et al. Pharmacokinetics of methotrexate following intravenous and intraventricular administration in acute lymphocytic leukemia and non-Hodgkin's lymphoma. Cancer 1982;50(9):1676–1682.

86. Bleyer WA, Drake JC, Chabner BA. Neurotoxicity and elevated cerebrospinal-fluid methotrexate concentration in meningeal leukemia. N Engl J Med 1973;289(15):770–773.

87. Shapiro WR, Young DF, Mehta BM. Methotrexate: distribution in cerebrospinal fluid after intravenous, ventricular and lumbar injections. N Engl J Med 1975;293(4):161–166.

88. Blasberg RG, Patlak C, Fenstermacher JD. Intrathecal chemotherapy: brain tissue profiles after ventriculocisternal perfusion. J Pharmacol Exp Ther 1975;195(1):73–83.

89. Blasberg RG. Methotrexate, cytosine arabinoside, and BCNU concentration in brain after ventriculocisternal perfusion. Cancer Treat Rep 1977;61(4):625–631.

90. Chamberlain MC. Leptomeningeal metastases: a review of evaluation and treatment. J Neurooncol 1998;37(3):271–284.

91. Walter KA, et al. Intratumoral chemotherapy. Neurosurgery 1995;37(6): 1128–1145.

92. Mak M, et al. Distribution of drugs following controlled delivery to the brain interstitium. J Neurooncol 1995;26(2):91–102.

93. Wu MP, et al. In vivo versus in vitro degradation of controlled release polymers for intracranial surgical therapy. J Biomed Mater Res 1994;28(3): 387–395.

94. Leong KW, et al. Bioerodible polyanhydrides as drug-carrier matrices. II. Biocompatibility and chemical reactivity. J Biomed Mater Res 1986;20(1): 51–64.

95. Brem H, et al. Placebo-controlled trial of safety and efficacy of intraoperative controlled delivery by biodegradable polymers of chemotherapy for recurrent gliomas. The Polymer-brain Tumor Treatment Group. Lancet 1995;345(8956):1008–1012.

96. Brem H, et al. Interstitial chemotherapy with drug polymer implants for the treatment of recurrent gliomas. J Neurosurg 1991;74(3):441–446.

97. Westphal M, et al. Gliadel wafer in initial surgery for malignant glioma: long-term follow-up of a multicenter controlled trial. Acta Neurochir (Wien) 2006;148(3):269–275; discussion 275.

98. Brem H, et al. The safety of interstitial chemotherapy with BCNU-loaded polymer followed by radiation therapy in the treatment of newly diagnosed malignant gliomas: phase I trial. J Neurooncol 1995;26(2):111–123.

99. Valtonen S, et al. Interstitial chemotherapy with carmustine-loaded polymers for high-grade gliomas: a randomized double-blind study. Neurosurgery 1997;41(1):44–48; discussion 48–49.

100. Olivi A, Barker F, Tatter S, et al. Toxicities and pharmakokinetics of interstittail BCNU administered vua wafers: results of phase I study in patients with recurrent malignant glioma. Proc Am Soc Clin Oncol 1999;18:142a.

101. Limentani S, Asher A, Fraser R, et al. A phase I trial of surgery, Gliadel and carboplatin in combination with radiation therapy for anaplastic astrocytoma (AA) or glioblastoma multiforme (GBM). Proc Am Soc Clin Oncol 1999;18:151a.

102. Mrugala MM, et al. Therapy for recurrent malignant glioma in adults. Expert Rev Anticancer Ther 2004;4(5):759–782.

103. Menei P, et al. Local and sustained delivery of 5-fluorouracil from biodegradable microspheres for the radiosensitization of malignant glioma: a randomized phase II trial. Neurosurgery 2005;56(2):242–248; discussion 242–248.

104. Brem S, et al. Local delivery of temozolomide by biodegradable polymers is superior to oral administration in a rodent glioma model. Cancer Chemother Pharmacol 2007;60(5):643–650.

105. Kunwar S. Convection enhanced delivery of IL13-PE38QQR for treatment of recurrent malignant glioma: presentation of interim findings from ongoing phase 1 studies. Acta Neurochir Suppl 2003;88:105–111.

106. Kioi M, et al. Convection-enhanced delivery of interleukin-13 receptor-directed cytotoxin for malignant glioma therapy. Technol Cancer Res Treat 2006;5(3):239–250.

107. Vogelbaum MA, et al. Convection-enhanced delivery of cintredekin besudotox (interleukin-13-PE38QQR) followed by radiation therapy with and without temozolomide in newly diagnosed malignant gliomas: phase 1 study of final safety results. Neurosurgery 2007;61(5):1031–1037; discussion 1037–1038.

108. Fiveash J, Nabors LB, Badie B, et al. A Randomized Phase II study of intra-cavitary 131-I TM601 in the Treatment of Recurrent Malignant Glioma. New Orleans, LA: Society for Neuro-Oncology Meeting, 2009.

109. Groothuis DR. The blood-brain and blood-tumor barriers: a review of strategies for increasing drug delivery. Neuro Oncol 2000;2(1):45–59.

110. Groothuis DR, et al. Comparison of cytosine arabinoside delivery to rat brain by intravenous, intrathecal, intraventricular and intraparenchymal routes of administration. Brain Res 2000;856(1–2):281–290.

111. Laske DW, Youle RJ, Oldfield EH. Tumor regression with regional distribution of the targeted toxin TF-CRM107 in patients with malignant brain tumors. Nat Med 1997;3(12):1362–1368.

112. de Lange EC, et al. Methodological considerations of intracerebral microdialysis in pharmacokinetic studies on drug transport across the blood-brain barrier. Brain Res Brain Res Rev 1997;25(1):27–49.

113. Cserr HF. Physiology of the choroid plexus. Physiol Rev 1971;51(2): 273–311.

114. Fishman R. Cerebrospinal Fluid in Disease of the Nervous System. Vol. 23. Philadelphia: WB Saunders, 1992.

115. Zamboni WC, et al. A four-hour topotecan infusion achieves cytotoxic exposure throughout the neuraxis in the nonhuman primate model: implications for treatment of children with metastatic medulloblastoma. Clin Cancer Res 1998;4(10):2537–2544.

116. Blaney SM, et al. Effect of body position on ventricular CSF methotrexate concentration following intralumbar administration. J Clin Oncol 1995;13(1):177–179.

117. Donelli MG, Zucchetti M, D'Incalci M. Do anticancer agents reach the tumor target in the human brain? Cancer Chemother Pharmacol 1992;30(4): 251–260.

118. Stewart DJ. A critique of the role of the blood-brain barrier in the chemotherapy of human brain tumors. J Neurooncol 1994;20(2):121–139.

119. Johansen MJ, Newman RA, Madden T. The use of microdialysis in pharmacokinetics and pharmacodynamics. Pharmacotherapy 1997;17(3):464–481.

120. Mary S, et al. A new technique for study of cutaneous biology, microdialysis. Ann Dermatol Venereol 1999;126(1):66–70.

121. Groth L. Cutaneous microdialysis. Methodology and validation. Acta Derm Venereol Suppl (Stockh) 1996;197:1–61.

122. Ungerstedt U, Pycock C. Functional correlates of dopamine neurotransmission. Bull Schweiz Akad Med Wiss 1974;30(1–3):44–55.

123. Muller M, et al. 5-fluorouracil kinetics in the interstitial tumor space: clinical response in breast cancer patients. Cancer Res 1997;57(13):2598–2601.

124. Hamani C, Luer MS, Dujovny M. Microdialysis in the human brain: review of its applications. Neurol Res 1997;19(3):281–288.

125. Landolt H, Langemann H. Cerebral microdialysis as a diagnostic tool in acute brain injury. Eur J Anaesthesiol 1996;13(3):269–278.

126. Benveniste H, Hansen AJ, Ottosen NS. Determination of brain interstitial concentrations by microdialysis. J Neurochem 1989;52(6):1741–1750.

127. Major O, et al. Continuous monitoring of blood-brain barrier opening to Cr51-EDTA by microdialysis following probe injury. Acta Neurochir Suppl (Wien) 1990;51:46–48.

128. Westergren I, et al. Intracerebral dialysis and the blood-brain barrier. J Neurochem 1995;64(1):229–234.

129. Hogan BL, et al. On-line coupling of in vivo microdialysis sampling with capillary electrophoresis. Anal Chem 1994;66(5):596–602.

130. Chen A, Lunte CE. Microdialysis sampling coupled on-line to fast microbore liquid chromatography. J Chromatogr A 1995;691(1–2):29–35.

131. de Lange EC, et al. Application of intracerebral microdialysis to study regional distribution kinetics of drugs in rat brain. Br J Pharmacol 1995;116(5):2538–2544.

132. Deviveni D, Klein-Szanto A, Gallo JM. In vivo microdialysis to characterize drug transport in brain tumors: analysis of methotrexate uptake in rat glioma-2 (RG-2)-bearing rats. Cancer Chemother Pharmacol 1996;38(6):499–507.

133. El-Gizawy SA, Hedaya MA. Comparative brain tissue distribution of camptothecin and topotecan in the rat. Cancer Chemother Pharmacol 1999;43(5):364–370.

134. Zamboni WC, et al. Relationship between tumor extracellular fluid exposure to topotecan and tumor response in human neuroblastoma xenograft and cell lines. Cancer Chemother Pharmacol 1999;43(4):269–276.

135. Palsmeier RK, Lunte CE. Microdialysis sampling in tumor and muscle: study of the disposition of 3-amino-1,2,4-benzotriazine-1,4-di-N-oxide (SR 4233). Life Sci 1994;55(10):815–825.

136. Ekstrom O, et al. Evaluation of methotrexate tissue exposure by in situ microdialysis in a rat model. Cancer Chemother Pharmacol 1994; 34(4):297–301.

137. Blakeley JO, et al. Effect of blood brain barrier permeability in recurrent high grade gliomas on the intratumoral pharmacokinetics of methotrexate: a microdialysis study. J Neurooncol 2009;91(1):51–58.

138. Portnow J, et al. The neuropharmacokinetics of temozolomide in patients with resectable brain tumors: potential implications for the current approach to chemoradiation. Clin Cancer Res 2009;15(22):7092–7098.

139. Blochl-Daum B, et al. Measurement of extracellular fluid carboplatin kinetics in melanoma metastases with microdialysis. Br J Cancer 1996;73(7):920–924.

140. Ronquist G, et al. Treatment of malignant glioma by a new therapeutic principle. Acta Neurochir (Wien) 1992;114(1–2):8–11.

141. He Q, et al. Proton NMR observation of the antineoplastic agent Iproplatin in vivo by selective multiple quantum coherence transfer (Sel-MQC). Magn Reson Med 1995;33(3):414–416.

142. Rodrigues LM, et al. In vivo detection of ifosfamide by 31P-MRS in rat tumours: increased uptake and cytotoxicity induced by carbogen breathing in GH3 prolactinomas. Br J Cancer 1997;75(1):62–68.

143. Wolf W, Waluch V, Presant CA. Non-invasive 19F-NMRS of 5-fluorouracil in pharmacokinetics and pharmacodynamic studies. NMR Biomed 1998; 11(7):380–387.

144. Findlay MP, Leach MO. In vivo monitoring of fluoropyrimidine metabolites: magnetic resonance spectroscopy in the evaluation of 5-fluorouracil. Anticancer Drugs 1994;5(3):260–280.

145. Presant CA, et al. Association of intratumoral pharmacokinetics of fluorouracil with clinical response. Lancet 1994;343(8907):1184–1187.

146. Maxwell RJ. New techniques in the pharmacokinetic analysis of cancer drugs. III. Nuclear magnetic resonance. Cancer Surv 1993;17:415–423.

147. Presant CA, et al. Human tumor fluorouracil trapping: clinical correlations of in vivo 19F nuclear magnetic resonance spectroscopy pharmacokinetics. J Clin Oncol 1990;8(11):1868–1873.

148. Kristjansen PE, et al. Intratumoral pharmacokinetic analysis by 19F-magnetic resonance spectroscopy and cytostatic in vivo activity of gemcitabine (dFdC) in two small cell lung cancer xenografts. Ann Oncol 1993;4(2):157–160.

149. Wolf W, Waluch V, Presant CA, et al. Pharmacokinetic imaging of gemcitabine in human tumors using non invasive ¹⁹F-MRS. Proc Am Assoc Cancer Res 1999;40:384.

150. Kissel J, et al. Pharmacokinetic analysis of 5-[18F]fluorouracil tissue concentrations measured with positron emission tomography in patients with liver metastases from colorectal adenocarcinoma. Cancer Res 1997;57(16):3415–3423.

151. Tilsley DW, et al. New techniques in the pharmacokinetic analysis of cancer drugs. IV. Positron emission tomography. Cancer Surv 1993;17:425–442.

152. Rubin RH, Fischman AJ. Positron emission tomography in drug development. Q J Nucl Med 1997;41(2):171–175.

153. Meikle SR, et al. Pharmacokinetic assessment of novel anti-cancer drugs using spectral analysis and positron emission tomography: a feasibility study. Cancer Chemother Pharmacol 1998;42(3):183–193.

154. Tyler JL, et al. Pharmacokinetics of superselective intra-arterial and intravenous [11C]BCNU evaluated by PET. J Nucl Med 1986;27(6):775–780.

155. Diksic M, et al. Pharmacokinetics of positron-labeled 1,3-bis(2-chloroethyl)nitrosourea in human brain tumors using positron emission tomography. Cancer Res 1984;44(7):3120–3124.

156. Ginos JZ, et al. [13N]cisplatin PET to assess pharmacokinetics of intra-arterial versus intravenous chemotherapy for malignant brain tumors. J Nucl Med 1987;28(12):1844–1852.

157. van Meerten E, Verweij J, Schellens JH. Antineoplastic agents. Drug interactions of clinical significance. Drug Saf 1995;12(3):168–182.

158. McLeod HL. Clinically relevant drug-drug interactions in oncology. Br J Clin Pharmacol 1998;45(6):539–544.

159. Kivisto KT, Kroemer HK, Eichelbaum M. The role of human cytochrome P450 enzymes in the metabolism of anticancer agents: implications for drug interactions. Br J Clin Pharmacol 1995;40(6):523–530.

160. Tanaka E. Clinically significant pharmacokinetic drug interactions between antiepileptic drugs. J Clin Pharm Ther 1999;24(2):87–92.

161. Baker DK, et al. Increased teniposide clearance with concomitant anticonvulsant therapy. J Clin Oncol 1992;10(2):311–315.

162. Rodman JH, et al. Altered etoposide pharmacokinetics and time to engraftment in pediatric patients undergoing autologous bone marrow transplantation. J Clin Oncol 1994;12(11):2390–2397.

163. Villikka K, et al. Cytochrome P450-inducing antiepileptics increase the clearance of vincristine in patients with brain tumors. Clin Pharmacol Ther 1999;66(6):589–593.

164. Chang SM, et al. Phase I study of paclitaxel in patients with recurrent malignant glioma: a North American Brain Tumor Consortium report. J Clin Oncol 1998;16(6):2188–2194.

165. Zamboni WC, et al. Phenytoin alters the disposition of topotecan and N-desmethyl topotecan in a patient with medulloblastoma. Clin Cancer Res 1998;4(3):783–789.

166. Gilbert MR, et al. Phase I clinical and pharmacokinetic study of irinotecan in adults with recurrent malignant glioma. Clin Cancer Res 2003;9(8): 2940–2949.

167. Liddle C, et al. Separate and interactive regulation of cytochrome P450 3A4 by triiodothyronine, dexamethasone, and growth hormone in cultured hepatocytes. J Clin Endocrinol Metab 1998;83(7):2411–2416.

168. Chang TK, et al. Enhanced cyclophosphamide and ifosfamide activation in primary human hepatocyte cultures: response to cytochrome P-450 inducers and autoinduction by oxazaphosphorines. Cancer Res 1997;57(10):1946–1954.

169. Brain EG, et al. Modulation of P450-dependent ifosfamide pharmacokinetics: a better understanding of drug activation in vivo. Br J Cancer 1998;77(11):1768–1776.

170. Yu LJ, et al. In vivo modulation of alternative pathways of P-450-catalyzed cyclophosphamide metabolism: impact on pharmacokinetics and antitumor activity. J Pharmacol Exp Ther 1999;288(3):928–937.

171. Marre F, et al. Hepatic biotransformation of docetaxel (Taxotere) in vitro: involvement of the CYP3A subfamily in humans. Cancer Res 1996;56(6):1296–1302.

172. Kamataki T, et al. Preclinical approach for identifying drug interactions. Cancer Chemother Pharmacol 1998;42(Suppl):S50–S53.

173. Levin VA, et al. The effect of phenobarbital pretreatment on the antitumor activity of 1,3-bis(2-chloroethyl)-1-nitrosourea (BCNU), 1-(2-chloroethyl)-3-cyclohexyl-1-nitrosourea (CCNU) and 1-(2-chloroethyl)-3-(2,6-dioxo-3-piperidyl)-1-nitrosourea (PCNU), and on the plasma pharmacokinetics and biotransformation of BCNU. J Pharmacol Exp Ther 1979; 208(1):1–6.

174. Reid AC, Teasdale GM, McCulloch J. The effects of dexamethasone administration and withdrawal on water permeability across the blood-brain barrier. Ann Neurol 1983;13(1):28–31.

175. Ziylan YZ. Effect of dexamethasone on transport of alpha-aminoisobutyric acid and sucrose across the blood-brain barrier. J Neurochem 1988;51(5):1338–1342.

176. Ziylan YZ, et al. Regional alterations in blood-to-brain transfer of alpha-aminoisobutyric acid and sucrose, after chronic administration and withdrawal of dexamethasone. J Neurochem 1989;52(3):684–689.

177. Hedley-Whyte ET, Hsu DW. Effect of dexamethasone on blood-brain barrier in the normal mouse. Ann Neurol 1986;19(4):373–377.

178. Shapiro WR, et al. Temporal effects of dexamethasone on blood-to-brain and blood-to-tumor transport of 14C-alpha-aminoisobutyric acid in rat C6 glioma. J Neurooncol 1990;8(3):197–204.

179. Jarden JO, et al. The time course of steroid action on blood-to-brain and blood-to-tumor transport of 82Rb: a positron emission tomographic study. Ann Neurol 1989;25(3):239–245.

180. Jarden JO, et al. Positron emission tomographic measurement of blood-to-brain and blood-to-tumor transport of 82Rb: the effect of dexamethasone and whole-brain radiation therapy. Ann Neurol 1985;18(6):636–646.

181. Yeung WT, et al. Effect of steroids on iopamidol blood-brain transfer constant and plasma volume in brain tumors measured with X-ray computed tomography. J Neurooncol 1994;18(1):53–60.

182. Andersen C, Astrup J, Gyldensted C. Quantitation of peritumoural oedema and the effect of steroids using NMR-relaxation time imaging and blood-brain barrier analysis. Acta Neurochir Suppl (Wien) 1994;60:413–415.

183. Ostergaard L, et al. Early changes measured by magnetic resonance imaging in cerebral blood flow, blood volume, and blood-brain barrier permeability following dexamethasone treatment in patients with brain tumors. J Neurosurg 1999;90(2):300–305.

184. Matsukado K, et al. Steroids decrease uptake of carboplatin in rat gliomas—uptake improved by intracarotid infusion of bradykinin analog, RMP-7. J Neurooncol 1997;34(2):131–138.

185. Straathof CS, et al. The effect of dexamethasone on the uptake of cisplatin in 9L glioma and the area of brain around tumor. J Neurooncol 1998;37(1):1–8.

186. Neuwelt EA, et al. Effects of adrenal cortical steroids and osmotic blood-brain barrier opening on methotrexate delivery to gliomas in the rodent: the factor of the blood-brain barrier. Proc Natl Acad Sci U S A 1982;79(14):4420–4423.

187. Jain RK. Normalization of tumor vasculature: an emerging concept in anti-angiogenic therapy. Science 2005;307(5706):58–62.

188. Trnovec T, Kallay Z, Bezek S. Effects of ionizing radiation on the blood brain barrier permeability to pharmacologically active substances. Int J Radiat Oncol Biol Phys 1990;19(6):1581–1587.

189. d'Avella D, et al. Radiation-induced blood-brain barrier changes: pathophysiological mechanisms and clinical implications. Acta Neurochir Suppl 1998;71:282–284.

190. Mima T, et al. Early decrease of P-glycoprotein in the endothelium of the rat brain capillaries after moderate dose of irradiation. Neurol Res 1999;21(2):209–215.

191. Remsen LG, et al. Decreased delivery and acute toxicity of cranial irradiation and chemotherapy given with osmotic blood-brain barrier disruption in a rodent model: the issue of sequence. Clin Cancer Res 1995;1(7):731–739.

192. Qin DX, et al. Influence of radiation on the blood-brain barrier and optimum time of chemotherapy. Int J Radiat Oncol Biol Phys 1990;19(6):1507–1510.

193. Riccardi R, et al. Cranial irradiation and permeability of blood-brain barrier to cytosine arabinoside in children with acute leukemia. Clin Cancer Res 1998;4(1):69–73.

194. Jain RK, et al. Angiogenesis in brain tumours. Nat Rev Neurosci 2007;8(8):610–622.

Pharmacogenetics

Curtis R. Chong, Jeanne Fourie Zirkelbach, Robert B. Diasio, and Bruce A. Chabner

Patients with cancer often demonstrate a variety of responses and side effects to chemotherapy. While some of these differences are due to underlying medical problems, age, sex, and organ function, genetic factors play a key role. Pharmacogenetics is the study of the host genetic contribution to variations in drug efficacy, metabolism, and toxicity. Pharmacogenomics, a term often used interchangeably, is the application of genomic technologies such as expression profiling, high-throughput gene sequencing, and single-nucleotide polymorphisms (SNPs) to study variations due to multiple genes in drug efficacy, metabolism, and toxicity.[1] The promise of pharmacogenetics lies in individualized therapy with the aim of maximizing drug efficacy while reducing toxicity. A related concept, personalized therapy, is increasingly discussed, but it primarily concerns choosing the right drug for a specific patient's tumor.[2] For drugs with narrow therapeutic indices, such as many anticancer agents, knowledge of a patient's pharmacogenetic susceptibility is key in promoting drug safety.[3]

Compared to other fields, the impact of pharmacogenetics in oncology is greater because chemotherapeutic agents affecting a variety of tissues and tumors are chemically diverse. The metabolism of anticancer drugs is typically very complex, and the therapeutic window is a careful balance between enzyme systems involved in activation and detoxification. Polymorphisms in either system can have profound effects on drug efficacy or toxicity. Tumors also evolve resistance to drugs, either at the target level as shown for imatinib or through enhanced detoxification, as shown for multidrug resistance transporters.

Pharmacogenetics has the potential to lower healthcare costs, streamline drug development, improve drug safety, and reduce disparities between ethnic groups (because of racial differences in expression of gene variants). The NIH now mandates inclusion of minorities in NIH-supported human research,[4] and the higher incidence of mutations (or gene variants) such as those affecting the EGFR receptors in lung cancer patients of East Asian ancestry highlights the importance of understanding these differences.[5] By identifying patients most likely to benefit from a drug, pharmacogenetic technologies may reduce the number needed to treat, resulting in healthcare savings.[6] Addition of pharmacogenetics to post-marketing surveillance, or Phase IV studies, may likewise improve drug safety by identifying patients most susceptible to adverse drug effects.[6]

Translation of pharmacogenomic research has produced diagnostic tests that allow physicians to tailor therapy to specific patients for several drugs. The U.S. FDA now recommends that patients treated with the monoclonal antibody EGF receptor inhibitors cetuximab or panitumumab be tested for K-ras mutations since patients with the wild type gene respond better.[7] Careful selection of patients based on pharmacogenetic profiles is routinely employed to identify patients with variants in methyl thiopurine metabolism for pediatric ALL treatment.[8] Other pharmacogenetic tests that attempt to predict toxicity of specific drugs are available, as listed in Table 6-1. To encourage pharmacogenomics/genetics in new drug development, the FDA published a Guidance for Industry: Pharmacogenomic Data Submission that created a pathway for submitting genomic data during an investigational new drug application.[8] Currently, approximately 10% of labels for drugs approved by the FDA contain pharmacogenomic information, and an estimated one fourth of all outpatients receive drugs with pharmacogenomic label information.[9]

The majority of clinically relevant pharmacogenetic variants occur in drug-metabolizing enzymes, transporters, or targets.[10] Genetic differences cause variation of drug targets at a molecular level (pharmacodynamics) and in differences in drug metabolism and absorption (pharmacokinetics). Examples include drug transporters, such as the P-glycoprotein MDR1, drug-inactivating enzymes, and drug targets such as the B2-adrenergic receptor, and angiotensin-converting enzyme.[11] Extensive work has detailed genetic differences in phase I metabolism (hydrolysis, oxidation/reduction) by enzymes such as cytochrome P450s, and in phase II metabolism (glucuronidation, sulfation, methyl/acetylation).[3] For example, considerable population differences in drug response due to certain cytochrome P450 isoforms led pharmaceutical companies to avoid drug candidates primarily metabolized by highly polymorphic alleles such as *CYP2D6*.[2]

Pharmacogenetic testing has several key advantages over direct monitoring of plasma drug levels. Monitoring plasma drug samples is impractical in most clinical settings and requires close coordination and special laboratory capabilities. Single plasma levels may not predict toxicity if patients are predisposed to slower drug elimination. It can be difficult and expensive to develop assays for numerous drug metabolites. On the other hand, pharmacogenetic testing requires rigorous validation in clinical trials as delivery of suboptimal doses of chemotherapy may preclude effective treatment.[8] "Environmental" conditions such as drug-drug interactions, organ dysfunction, age, or protein binding may introduce variables that change drug disposition and diminish the utility of pharmacogenetic test results. For example, studies of cytochrome P450 2C19 activity in patients with advanced cancer found metabolism to be much slower than predicted by genotype, including one study performed in the absence of renal or hepatic failure.[12,13]

<table>
| TABLE 6.1 | *Public resources for pharmacogenetics* |
</table>

GeneTests (www.genetests.org)

Joint effort between NIH, NCBI, and the University of Washington that offers medical genetics information, peer-reviewed genetic disease descriptions, and lists of genetic testing laboratories organized by state and country

Pharmacogenetics of Anticancer Agents Research Group (www.pharmacogenetics.org)

Consortium of pharmacogeneticists devoted to understanding how genetic variability leads to variability in drug response and to improving clinical translation of such knowledge

Pharmacogenetics Research Network (http://www.nigms.nih.gov/Initiatives/PGRN)

Consortium of 12 centers created by the NIH Roadmap to advance knowledge of the genetic basis for variable drug responses[2]

Pharmacogenetics for Every Nation Initiative (pgeni.unc.edu)

Integrates pharmacogenetics into public health decision making, applying pharmacogenetic testing in 104 countries

Pharmacogenomics Knowledgebase (www.pharmgkb.org)

Public repository of genotype and phenotype information for pharmacogenetics developed by the NIH-funded Pharmacogenetics Research Network.[231] Includes curated literature and detailed descriptions of drug mechanism, pharmacokinetics, and genes responsible for metabolism. Displays information by disease area, drug therapeutic category, gene/SNP, and therapeutic/pharmacokinetic/pharmacodynamic pathways

Pharmacogenetic testing is not a substitute for close clinical monitoring of patients, but can be an additional clinical data point used in formulating a treatment plan or anticipating toxicity, and is especially useful in identifying patients at risk for extreme toxicity or poor response.[8]

For oncologists, pharmacogenetics promises to minimize variations in therapeutic response and drug toxicity. Numerous gene variants that influence the efficacy and toxicity of cancer chemotherapeutics have been identified. Genetic testing of tumor and host is growing in importance as a tool for optimizing clinical trials and clinical practice. In this chapter, we discuss the scientific basis for pharmacogenetics and review the impact of key host variants on toxicity and response to cancer therapeutic agents. A list of public resources for clinicians wishing to incorporate pharmacogenetics into clinical practice is provided in Table 6-2. A list of laboratories offering pharmacogenetic testing (and their Web sites) is provided in Table 6-1.

Impact of Genetic Variation on Cancer Chemotherapy

Human genetic variability is a determinant of anticancer drug efficacy and safety. This variability, which is the basis of the disciplines of pharmacogenetics and pharmacogenomics, encompasses an array of different types of DNA sequence modifications as well as individual differences in gene expression and regulation. In the present overview, we focus on the most common form of variation in genetic sequence, known as SNP. A polymorphism is defined as a "Mendelian or monogenic trait that exists in the population in at least two phenotypes (and presumably at least two genotypes), neither of which is rare—that is, neither of which occurs with a

<table>
| TABLE 6.2 | *Companies offering pharmacogenetic tests in oncology* |
</table>

Drug	Test	Company(ies)[a]
Fluorouracil	DPYD*2A mutation	Arup, Myriad, Specialty
	Fluorouracil drug concentration monitoring	Arup, Myriad
	TS promoter mutations	Myriad
Irinotecan	UGT1A1 full gene sequencing	Mayo
	UGT1A1 gene polymorphism (TA repeat)	Arup, Genzyme, Kimball, Mayo, Quest, Specialty
Mercaptopurine	Mercaptopurine drug level monitoring	Arup
	MTHFR C677T and A1298C mutation	Arup
	TGN levels	Prometheus
	TMPT activity	Arup, Prometheus
	TMPT genotype	Prometheus, Specialty
Methotrexate	Methotrexate levels	Arup
Tamoxifen	CYP2D6	Arup, DNAdirect

[a]Companies: Arup Laboratories (www.aruplab.com); DNAdirect (www.dnadirect.com); Genzyme Genetics (www.genzymegenetics.com); Kimball Genetics (www.kimballgenetics.com); Mayo Medical Laboratories (www.mayomedicallaboratories.com); Myriad Genetics (www.myriad.com); Oncotype Dx by Genomic Health (www.oncotypedx.com); Response Genetics (www.responsegenetics.com); Specialty Laboratories (www.specialtylaboratories.com); Quest Diagnostics (www.questdiagnostics.com/hcp/topics/hem_onc/hem_onc.html?hem_onc). See text for explanation of test abbreviations.

frequency of less than 1% to 2%."[14] Such polymorphisms may include nonsynonymous SNPs, which are within the open reading frame of the gene and may result in significant amino acid substitutions in the encoded protein, affecting protein function or quantity. Other SNPs are characterized as synonymous polymorphisms in the coding region of the DNA, or SNPs in promoter and enhancer regions of a gene that affect transcription and gene regulation, and intronic SNPs, which may lead to splice variants.[1,3,11,15–17] In addition to these SNPs, other sources of variation in DNA sequence include insertions, deletions, and gene duplications, all of which contribute to the complex and multifactorial phenotypes of drug efficacy and safety.

Although virtually all drugs are susceptible to the consequences of genetic variability, the application of pharmacogenetic concepts may be especially important in anticancer chemotherapeutic treatment. Anticancer agents frequently are prodrugs that require enzymatic bioactivation to their cytotoxic active forms, while the active forms of these compounds may also undergo further enzymatic detoxification. In both instances, the involved enzyme systems may exhibit genetic polymorphisms and therefore small but significant changes in anticancer drug metabolism, distribution, transport, or excretion due to modifications such as decreased production of an altered protein (e.g., an enzyme) or increases in the protein amount can lead to interpatient variability in drug effect. Anticancer agents generally have a relatively narrow therapeutic index. In the current treatment strategy, anticancer agents are administered in "standard" doses to patients. This uniform approach to pharmacotherapy ignores interindividual variability in drug metabolism and disposition as part of an individualized drug treatment plan.

Chemotherapeutic drug response is a complex outcome, or phenotype, that is affected by interactions between a network of different genes, including interactions between host and tumor genomes, as most anticancer agents do not selectively target tumor tissue. Genetic polymorphisms in pharmacokinetic pathways may collectively impact drug efficacy and host or tumor toxicity through regulation of drug bioavailability, retention, and efflux and detoxification or metabolism in host or tumor cells. Genetic polymorphisms may further occur in genes that encode drug targets or signal pathways involved in drug response as well as in genes that influence tumor or disease characteristics such as invasiveness and drug resistance. The complexity of variability in human drug response may be additionally affected by differences in the frequencies and types of genetic polymorphisms that are prevalent in ethnically defined populations as well as the specific characteristics of the drugs and disease status, all of which may impact out come. A major aim of pharmacogenetics and pharmacogenomics is to discern which genetic polymorphisms are important in drug response and how knowledge of this variability can be used in the individualization of drug therapy.

Genotypic Tests and Dose Adjustment or Drug Selection in Individual Patients

Once a particular pharmacogenetic syndrome has been identified, pharmacokinetic analysis may be of limited clinical feasibility due to its labor-intensiveness. In addition, observation of changes in

drug concentration alone does not provide an understanding of the pathways responsible for drug metabolism. Therefore, genotypic or phenotypic tests can be more beneficial than pharmacokinetic studies in therapeutic drug monitoring and the individualization of drug therapy. Its potential advantages over pharmacokinetic analysis are summarized below:

- Genotypic and phenotypic tests are less invasive, as they require a single blood, plasma, serum, urine, or tissue sample for assessment of polymorphisms that may affect drug pharmacokinetics and response.
- Genotypic or phenotypic tests can help predict drug response and toxicity. Drug treatment may be altered to prevent potentially lethal toxicity or lack of efficacy due to genetic polymorphisms in genes that influence drug effects.
- The genotypic or phenotypic profile may also be informative in combination treatment with other therapeutic agents.
- The genotypic or phenotypic profile may be applicable to the individual patient's treatment with a drug in the same or a different drug class (e.g., metabolized through the same polymorphic drug-metabolizing enzyme).
- The genotypic or phenotypic test may provide insight into pharmacodynamic variability and the mechanistic basis for variability in drug response or may help in the identification of patients possibly at risk for rapid disease progression or tumor invasiveness.

Research Strategies in Pharmacogenetics

Candidate Gene Approach

The candidate gene approach to pharmacogenetic investigation attempts to link a phenotype with an alteration in a specific gene through hypothesis-based testing. Recognition that specific genes contribute to variation in drug toxicity occurred in the 1950s with three key discoveries[11] (Fig. 6-1). Alving et al.[18] identified a relationship between glucose-6-phosphate dehydrogenase deficiency and hemolysis in patients treated with primaquine. Kalow correlated acetylcholinesterase deficiency and prolonged paralysis from succinylcholine.[19] Evans et al.[20] found that the rate of isoniazid acetylation influenced the development of peripheral neuropathy. Since then, variation in numerous other genes has been shown to affect drug efficacy and toxicity, with a 2009 review reporting 541 genes studied.[21]

Even more potential for discovery exists in the over 1.4 million SNPs in the human genome, and 60,000 SNPs in gene-encoding regions.[22] SNPs are common variations that occur at a given location when two DNA sequences are compared,[23] for example:

AT**G**TA
AT**C**TA

SNPs occur every 100 to 300 bases and can have a variety of effects—they may be silent (synonymous), producing no change in amino acid sequence, or may change a single amino acid (nonsynonymous) that greatly affects protein function. They may introduce a stop codon, which produces a truncated protein.[24] SNPs that occur in the promoter or enhancer regions of a gene may affect RNA expression and protein levels while SNPs in intron-exon boundaries may lead to splice variants. Within the field of oncology, SNPs

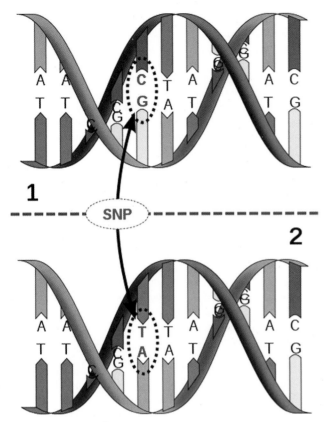

FIGURE 6-1   The DNA sequence for the same allele may differ among individuals by virtue of a change in single base (in this case, a C to T change), creating a variant, or polymorphism, that may or may not have functional significance. (Reprinted with implied consent of copyright holder David Hall from www.wikipedia.org   [http://en.wikipedia.org/wiki/Single_nucleotide_polymorphism]. This file is licensed under the Creative Commons Attribution ShareAlike 3.0 License. Official license.)

have been associated with numerous variations in responsiveness and side effects of chemotherapeutic agents.[10] The C677T polymorphism in 5,10-methylenetetrahydrofolate reductase (MTHFR) slows the activation of leucovorin rescue and in some studies is associated with increased methotrexate toxicity. Glutathione-S-transferase enzymes metabolize drugs through glutathione conjugation. The GSTP1 Ile105Val mutation is associated with lower enzyme activity and increased survival for oxaliplatin/5-fluorouracil (5-FU) regimens (24.9 months for the V105 homozygote versus 13.3 months for the I105 homozygote).[25,26] The *Arg399Gln SNP* in the DNA repair protein XRCC1 is associated with resistance to oxaliplatin/5-FU (discussed below).[10] Lapatinib, a tyrosine kinase inhibitor metabolized by cytochrome P450 enzymes, is associated with diarrhea and rash in patients with the *CYP2C19*2/*2* SNP.[27] In addition to SNP variants, nucleotide insertions, deletions, repeats, and variations in copy number also contribute to genetic diversity.[28] As technologies to identify SNPs improve, more associations will be added.

Family Studies

Cancer chemotherapy drugs are too toxic for the family study approach to assessing patterns of inheritance of drug response used for drugs from other therapeutic classes.[29] Other phenotypic tests such as assessment of the activity of a drug-metabolizing enzyme or

determination of substrate levels in family members can define the pattern of inheritance.

Once a pharmacokinetic or pharmacodynamic alteration has been defined in an individual patient, studies in the family can provide insight into whether the genetic polymorphism is an autosomal or sex-linked trait and whether the pattern of inheritance is dominant, codominant, or recessive. With availability of data from the human genome project and the functional assignment of enzyme activity to a particular gene, it is becoming possible to delineate the inheritance of a specific gene. Techniques that can identify a specific DNA sequence or SNP, such as allele-specific polymerase chain reaction-based (PCR-based) methods, should make this technically straightforward.[30]

Population Studies

Population studies are aimed at the assessment of the frequency of the pharmacogenetic syndrome within the general population as well as frequency differences between populations. As with family studies, population studies can use either phenotypic or genotypic tests. The frequency of individuals with particular phenotypic characteristics can be estimated using the Hardy-Weinberg equation.[31] Population studies to assess the specific phenotype or activity of a particular protein may show unimodal or bimodal patterns of distribution. A unimodal distribution in the activity of a particular enzyme, such as a Gaussian or normal distribution pattern, suggests mutations or genetic alterations that lead to a range of activities in the population studied. In contrast, bimodal distributions may indicate mutations that lead to reduced or greater than normal activity in a subset of the population.[32] The evaluation of particular phenotypes in population studies related to chemotherapeutic drug metabolism may require assessments using a safer probe drug that is metabolized through the same potential polymorphic drug-metabolizing enzyme but without posing a risk of toxicity to the healthy individual participating in the study. Results from a population study comparing cancer patients to healthy volunteers indicated that cancer stage may also influence the phenotype of an important drug-metabolizing enzyme CYP2C19, for which genotype normally predicts phenotype in the healthy population.[13,33] In this study, patients with advanced cancer had the extensive metabolizer genotype; however, 25% of the patients displayed a poor metabolizer phenotype. This discordance between phenotype and genotype and the decreased activity of CYP2C19 observed in terminally ill cancer patients may influence the clinical efficacy and toxicity of therapeutic agents (e.g., cyclophosphamide) and should be investigated with respect to other drug-metabolizing enzymes.[13] The characterization of genes and related phenotypes involved in anticancer drug pharmacokinetic or pharmacodynamic variability or those involved in cancer predisposition may be limited to investigations using individuals with the particular cancer or those already being treated with a particular chemotherapeutic agent.

After an assessment of phenotypic and genotypic markers in the general population, it may be useful to undertake surveys in other populations, including patients affected with specific types of cancer or being treated with a particular chemotherapeutic agent. Such studies may define the frequency of the pharmacogenetic syndrome in the cancer patient population at risk. Other demographic factors, such as race, age, and gender, may influence the risk to specific groups.

The methodologies discussed above have had specific applications in the identification of SNPs in single genes using the candidate gene approach. The genetic polymorphisms in single genes have not thus far explained a large proportion of the individual variability in drug response, mainly because most drug response phenotypes are thought to be determined by the interactions among multiple genes as well as with the environment. Therefore, the candidate gene strategy has limited value for identifying polygenic determinants of variability in drug response. On the other hand, this approach may offer an advantage for testing "specific" biological or pharmacological hypotheses in a given and often limited clinical sample of patients. Genome-wide studies require larger numbers of subjects to achieve statistical power to identify multiple low-penetrance genes, a requirement seldom fulfilled in small heterogeneous patient samples.

Genomic Approaches

Efforts using a candidate gene approach were highly successful in identifying genetic causes for severe drug toxicity such as related to glucose-6-phosphate dehydrogenase deficiency.[34] A genome-wide scanning (GWAS) approach is now increasingly used to look for variants that influence the risk of disease and explain differences in drug effect conferred by variants in metabolic enzymes, drug transporters, and drug targets.[34] Evolving technologies such as microarrays, proteomics, and mouse genetics promise to provide many exciting results that influence clinical practice. Commercial gene chips are available to measure entire classes of genes (i.e., cytochrome P450s) or the entire human genome.[35] In recognition of the emerging role of pharmacogenetics in the clinic, the NIH roadmap sponsored creation of the 12-center Pharmacogenetics Research Network.[2] Pharmacogenomic approaches are hampered by the requirement for large sample sizes to generate statistically significant results and by the high numbers of false-positive findings.[28] For example, recent work using the International HapMap, which has genotyped 3.3 million SNPs, predicted the thiopurine methyltransferase phenotype, although 96 genes in this analysis ranked higher.[36]

> Gene expression arrays of tumor provide an alternative approach to SNP arrays and gene variant analysis for predicting response to drugs. Arrays are primarily of value in predicting the need for, and potential success of treatment. Rather than relying on polymorphisms in a single gene, expression patterns of multiple genes or proteins can be assayed to create a "signature" reflective of a drug's effect. These expression patterns may result from gene variants, but verification of the presence of a variant requires gene sequencing and is usually not done in conjunction with the development of predictive arrays. In contrast to the candidate gene approach, genomic experiments provide an unbiased, hypothesis generating picture of drug effects.[28] Using DNA microarrays on ALL cells, 124 genes were associated with resistance or sensitivity to four chemotherapeutic drugs.[37] A parallel study identified 45 genes differentially expressed in patients resistant to all four drugs.[38] Microarray experiments predict the sensitivity of cancer cells to docetaxel and multidrug regimens and estimate response to treatment.[39-41] Gene signature analysis has also been incorporated into clinical trials of breast cancer patients, and they seemed to predict pathologic complete response.[42]

One of the first pharmacogenomic tests available is the Oncotype DX, which is recommended in the 2007 Update of Recommendations for the Use of Tumor Markers in Breast Cancer from the American Society of Clinical Oncology and the National Comprehensive Cancer Network 2008 Clinical Practice Guidelines in Oncology Breast Cancer.[35,43] Oncotype DX is used to identify which newly diagnosed, node-negative, ER-positive breast cancer patients may benefit from tamoxifen, and may not need adjuvant chemotherapy.[43] The Oncotype DX assay uses RT-PCR to gauge the expression of 21 genes, including those involved in proliferation (Ki67, STK 15, surviving, cyclin B1, MYBL2), invasion (stromelysin 3, cathepsin L2), HER2 (GRB7, HER2), estrogen (ER, PGR, BCL2, SCUBE2), miscellaneous (GSTM1, CD68, BAG1), and five reference genes.[44] RNA extracted from paraffin-embedded tissue is used.[44] Gene expression levels are analyzed by an algorithm that calculates a recurrence score that predicts the likelihood of distant recurrence in tamoxifen-treated patients.[44] The goal of the assay is to identify patients with a good prognosis that may avoid adjuvant chemotherapy.[45]

The use of the Oncotype DX assay in predicting the likelihood of recurrence in women with node-negative ER-positive breast cancer treated with tamoxifen was validated in a trial of 668 patients from the National Surgical Adjuvant and Bowel clinical trial.[44] The recurrence score was used to cluster patients into low-, intermediate-, and high-risk groups. In the patient population studied, 51%, 22%, and 27% of patients fell in the low-, intermediate-, or high-risk groups, respectively, with a 6.8%, 14.3%, and 30.5% chance of distant recurrence at 10 years, respectively.[44] The Oncotype DX assay provided additional information beyond tumor grade as determined by three pathologists.[44] One limitation of the Oncotype DX assay is that results may be influenced by the tumor block selected.[46]

Other genomics based tests include MammaPrint (FDA approved 2007), which uses a 70-gene profile to classify tumors from stage I or II breast cancer patients as low or high risk for recurrence[47] and the Rotterdam Signature, a 76-gene profile that does not overlap with MammaPrint or Oncotype DX. Medicare covers Oncotype DX, which has shown to be cost-effective. If used to classify a hypothetical cohort of 100 patients, Oncotype DX was estimated to result in an increase in quality-adjusted survival by 8.6 years and reduce cost by $202,828.[48] A prospective validation of Oncotype DX is underway in a randomized clinical trial (TAILORx).[49]

In the following section, discussion will be considered for the important SNP variants that influence response to and toxicity of commonly used anticancer drugs. The list of potentially important variants is not all-inclusive; the actual confirmation of an important role for a given variant requires characterization of protein function and large-scale trials, which are often beyond the scope of funding available for such research. Thus, many of the variants of interest have only been assessed through retrospective analysis of toxicity or response patterns in trials not designed for pharmacogenetic study. For most of these variants, understanding of the impact on drug metabolism, transport, or target interaction in human patient populations is incomplete. As will be seen below, genetic variants in drug-metabolizing enzymes are of particular relevance in explaining variable drug responses, especially toxicity. The relationship between polymorphism and toxicity is best established by data demonstrating that the variant affects enzyme activity, that enzyme activity predicts pharmacokinetic behavior, and that drug levels or AUC predict efficacy or toxicity.

Gene Variants and Anticancer Drug Response

Fluorouracil

The phosphorylated form of 5-FU inhibits thymidylate synthase (TS), blocking DNA synthesis and repair.[32] Capecitabine is an oral prodrug that is metabolized to fluorouracil.[50] These agents are used in the treatment of breast and colorectal cancers, in over two million patients a year.[51] Fluorouracil is inactivated by dihydropyridine dehydrogenase (DPD) in the liver, and this enzyme accounts for 80% of removal in cancer patients.[52] Genetic variations in both DPD and TS affect fluorouracil efficacy and toxicity.

Dihydropyridine Dehydrogenase

DPD exhibits a wide interindividual variation in activity of up to 20-fold, and patients with low or negligible DPD activity are unable to efficiently inactivate 5-FU, leading to decreased catabolism, which can produce severe 5-FdUMP–mediated gastrointestinal, hematopoietic, and neurological toxicities.[53–57] An estimated 3% and 0.1% of the population are heterozygous and homozygous, respectively, for inactivating mutations in DPD that involve a splice error leading to an exon deletion.[32] These patients are at increased risk for severe myelosuppression, neurologic, and gastrointestinal side effects due to fluorouracil toxicity.[32] Indeed, decreased DPD activity was detected in 60% of patients with grade 3 to 4 toxicity on fluorouracil.[58] DPD also appears to serve a critical role in tumor response to 5-FU, with low intratumor expression of DPD shown to predict favorable response to this agent and increased survival time in patients with colorectal cancer.[59] Pharmacokinetic studies in patients receiving 5-FU by continuous infusion have demonstrated that plasma 5-FU levels have a circadian variation. This circadian variation was further shown to inversely correlate with the circadian variation in DPD activity from peripheral blood mononuclear cells, suggesting that plasma 5-FU levels are regulated by DPD.[60] There is also considerable variation in DPD activity across different ethnicities.[61]

More than 50 sequence variations in the DPYD gene have been identified, producing multiple complex heterozygote genotypes that are inherited in an autosomal codominant fashion.[62] Analyses of the prevalence of the specific variant alleles have shown that the most common inactivating allele (DPYD*2A), accounting for 25% of patients with toxicity, is characterized by a G to A transition at the invariant GT splice donor site flanking exon 14 of the DPYD gene.[57,63] This mutation leads to truncated mRNA due to skipping of exon 14, which results in a nonfunctional protein.[57,64,65] A second single nucleotide polymorphism associated with DPD deficiency is DPYD*13, which is characterized by a T to G transition at a domain important to enzyme activity.[66]

Familial studies have indicated that DPD deficiency is inherited in an autosomal codominant fashion and that DPD deficiency most likely results from multiple mutations at a single gene locus. For instance, a profoundly deficient patient with heterozygous mutations for both DPYD*13 and DPYD*2A and a spouse with normal DPD activity had two partially deficient offspring (one child being

heterozygous for the DPYD*2A variant allele and one child being heterozygous for the DPYD*13 variant allele).[66] To date, however, the identified DPYD variant alleles do not explain all observed cases of DPD deficiency as many patients with severe 5-FU toxicity have no detected mutations in the DPYD gene.[67]

Previous reports of sequence variations in this gene have not consistently predicted DPD enzyme activity and identified patients at risk for 5-FU–mediated toxicity due to DPD deficiency.[67–70] Less than 50% of patients with severe toxicity from fluorouracil treatment have mutations in the DPYD gene or decreased DPD activity.[71] This suggests that in addition to the investigation of variations in the DPYD gene, further investigations should explore other markers that may act alone or together with DPD to produce 5-FU toxicity.

Several tests are used to assess for DPD deficiency in a research setting, including radioimmunoassay and sequencing, and a ^{13}C-uracil breath test shows great promise for application in the clinic.[51,72] The gold-standard for testing is considered to be measurement of DPD activity in peripheral blood mononuclear cells, with activity levels correlating with heterozygosity for the DPYD*2A allele.[73] In this assay, radiolabeled 5-FU is incubated with patient cells and the rate of catabolite formation is measured by HPLC.[74,75] PCR-based testing is available commercially for the DYPD*2A mutation, which accounts for 52% of patients with complete or severe DPD deficiency and is found in 1% of Caucasians (Table 6-2).[56,76,77] Commercial tests are also available to measure fluorouracil levels in patients receiving continuous infusion (Table 6-2). The use of genetic screening for DPD deficiency should be used cautiously given patients with mutations do not always experience severe toxicity, creating the risk of an unnecessary dose reduction in chemotherapy.[61] For example, a study of 487 patients in France found of 10 patients with a DYPD*2A allele 6 experienced severe toxicity while 4 did not.[78]

Thymidylate Synthase

Like polymorphisms in genes important for drug metabolism, polymorphisms in the genes for drug targets are also important determinants of drug response and disease outcome. TS is the main target of 5-FU. The 5-FU metabolite FdUMP produces a stable complex with TS and a methyl cofactor, leading to inhibition of dTMP synthesis and DNA synthesis.[79] Variability in response to 5-FU has been linked to several TS gene (TYMS) genetic polymorphisms.[80–82]

To date, several polymorphisms in the TYMS gene have been identified. A polymorphism within the 5′-promoter enhancer region (TSER) of the TYMS gene consists of tandem repeats of 28 base pairs ranging from two (TSER*2) to nine (TSER*9) copies.[83] The role of most of these alleles in TS expression is currently unknown; however, patients homozygous for the TSER*3 genotype have increased intratumor TS messenger RNA levels[84] and elevated TS protein levels[85] compared with patients with the homozygous TSER*2 genotype.[84,86,87] Two additional polymorphisms have been identified. The first is a single nucleotide polymorphism within the second repeat of the TSER*3 allele (G→C, 3RG and 3RC alleles). It has been suggested this polymorphism affects the level of TS expression by abolishing a USF1-binding site.[88] The second polymorphism described is a 6–base-pair deletion located in the 3′UTR, 447 base pairs downstream from the stop codon.[89]

The polymorphisms in which there is a double (*TSER*2*) and triple (*TSER*3*) tandem repeat of 28 bp are observed most frequently in Caucasian populations, with higher repeats (*TSER*4*, *TSER*5*, and *TSER*9* alleles) mainly found in African populations.[90] When Asian populations are considered, the homozygous (*TSER*3*) genotype is approximately twice as frequent (67%) as in Caucasians (38%). Using RFLP analysis, the frequency of the *3RC* allele in different ethnic populations was determined to be 56%, 47%, 28%, and 37% for non-Hispanic Whites, Hispanic Whites, African Americans, and Singapore Chinese, respectively.[88] Lastly, the 6–base pair deletion polymorphism displayed frequencies of 41%, 26%, 52%, and 76% in non-Hispanic Whites, Hispanic Whites, African Americans, and Singapore Chinese, respectively.[91]

The efficacy of fluorouracil is reduced in patients with overexpression of TS due to an increased number of tandem repeats in the promoter region.[32,92–96] Patients with metastatic colorectal cancer treated with fluorouracil who are homozygous for three tandem (*TSER*3*) repeats in the TS promoter (increased TS levels) have a median survival of 12 versus 16 months for patients homozygous for two tandem repeats (*TSER*2*).[87] Pullarkat et al.[84] demonstrated that patients homozygous for the *TSER*3* allele had a 3.6-fold higher level of TS mRNA than those homozygous for the *TSER*2* allele. These researchers also found that colorectal cancer patients homozygous for the *TSER*2* genotype had a response rate of 50%, compared with 9% for those homozygous for the *TSER*3* genotype.[84] In another study, colorectal cancer patients homozygous or heterozygous (*TSER*2*/*TSER*3*) for the *TSER*2* allele displayed a higher probability of pathological downstaging (60%) subsequent to neoadjuvant 5-FU–based chemotherapy than patients homozygous for the *TSER*3* allele (22%).[86] The *TSER*3* allele is associated with less grade III or IV toxicity, which was found in 3% of homozygotes for *TSER*3* versus 18% for *TSER*3*/ *TSER*2* versus 43% for *TSER*2* homozygotes.[97]

With respect to the *3RC* variant allele, in a trial with 208 colorectal cancer patients, a 1.3-fold (95% CI, 0.9 to 1.9) increased risk of colorectal cancer was found in patients with the *3RG* allele compared with controls; however, the specific functional significance of this polymorphism is unclear.[98] Another study reported a decreased response to 5-FU in patients homozygous for the variant 6–base-pair deletion located in the 3′UTR (447 base pairs downstream from the stop codon), with an odds ratio of 2.0 for 5-FU–based chemotherapy.[99] Despite strong genetic evidence suggesting an association between TS expression and outcomes, protein levels as measured by immunohistochemistry were not predictive of survival in patients with stage III colon cancer treated with fluorouracil regimens.[100]

Overall, these studies suggest that determination of the *TSER* genotype may be a clinically useful tool in the prediction of response to 5-FU. A commercial test is available for TS promoter mutations (Table 6-2).

Methylenetetrahydrofolate Reductase

MTHFR modulates intracellular folate concentration, and the activity of this enzyme affects the efficacy of antifolate drugs like fluorouracil. Because the active 5-FU metabolite forms a ternary complex with 5,10-methylenetetrahydrofolate and TS, increasing concentrations of 5,10-methylenetetrahydrofolate may augment the efficacy of 5-FU.[101] At least 65 polymorphisms have been identified in the MTHFR gene and surrounding DNA.[102] Two common polymorphisms, *C677T* and *A1298C*, decrease enzyme activity (discussed below). At least 19 studies involving 2,851 patients have examined the relationship between different alleles, with conflicting results. Twelve studies found no effect for the *C677T* or *A1298C* alleles.[103–114] Two studies found that the *A1298C* allele was associated with a shorter survival and the *C677T* allele had no effect,[115,116] while two studies found that the *C677T* allele had a better response rate or lower recurrence.[115,117,118] Two studies found that the *C677T* and *A1298* alleles were associated with worse response to treatment,[119] or shorter survival if found with *TSER*3*.[120] As is the case for MTHFR polymorphisms in methotrexate response and toxicity, there are likely numerous other factors influencing outcome, illustrating the difficulty of applying a candidate gene approach to a complex pathway such as folate metabolism.

Irinotecan

Irinotecan (CPT-11), a synthetic analog of camptothecin, is commonly used in the treatment of several solid tumors, including advanced colorectal cancer. It is converted by carboxylesterase to SN-38, which is a 100- to 1,000-fold more potent topoisomerase I inhibitor.[32] Phase II metabolism in the liver inactivates SN-38 via glucuronidation by UDP glucuronosyltransferase 1A1 (UGT1A1). This enzyme is also involved in bilirubin conjugation, and decreased promoter activity due to variability in the number of promoter TA repeats results in decreased expression and is thought to underlie Gilbert's syndrome.[32] Patients may either be homozygous for six TA repeats, seven TA repeats, or be heterozygous for six and seven repeats.[121] Homozygosity for seven TA repeats is associated with 70% lower protein expression and Gilbert's syndrome.[122,123] In studies of cancer patients treated with irinotecan, the distribution of the wild-type 6/6 genotype is 39% to 49%, the 6/7 genotype 35% to 50%, and the 7/7 genotype (*UGT1A1*28*) 10% to 20%.[121] There is racial variability in the predominance of the 6/6 genotype (76% of Asians versus 46% in Caucasians)[124] and 11% of Caucasians were observed to have the 7/7 genotype versus 0% of Asians.[125] Interestingly, other missense mutations in the coding region of UGT1A1 are thought to be responsible for cases of Gilbert's syndrome observed in Asian populations. Particularly, the most common variant present in Asian populations is the *UGT1A1*6* allele, which has an allelic frequency from 13% to 23%.[126,127]

Patients with decreased UGT1A1 levels due to promoter mutation may also be more likely to experience diarrhea and myelosuppression during irinotecan therapy due to higher SN-38 levels.[32] Diarrhea is thought primarily due to reactivation of SN-38-glucuronide by glucuronidase in the bowel.[121] Four studies involving 351 patients demonstrated that homozygotes for seven TA repeats (n = 34) had a 2.5- to 17-fold greater chance of irinotecan toxicity compared to patients with the normal promoter.[128–131] This led the FDA and Pfizer in 2004 to change irinotecan's package insert to recommend that patients homozygous for the 7/7 (*UGT1A1*28*/*28*) genotype receive a lower initial dose.[132] In 2005, the FDA approved a diagnostic test for the 7/7 genotype.[133]

Subsequent studies linked the 7/7 genotype with neutropenia but not diarrhea,[129,131,134] diarrhea but not neutropenia,[130,135] and some patients with the wild type promoter experienced serious toxicity, further complicating the picture.[132] Neither UGT1A1 polymorphism nor baseline bilirubin level predicted neutropenia in a study of 113 patients.[136] A larger study of 454 patients treated with irinotecan failed to find an association between UGT1A1 7/7 or 6/7 with toxicity, leading the authors to question use of this testing in routine clinical practice.[137] A meta-analysis of nine studies including 821 patients found that the risk of diarrhea in UGT1A1 7/7 homozygotes was not associated with irinotecan dose, but the risk of hematologic toxicity was associated with the 7/7 genotype at higher irinotecan doses.[132] A phase I trial of 59 patients treated with FOLFIRI examining the UGT1A1 genotype identified the maximum tolerated dose in wild-type and heterozygous patients as 370 and 310 mg/m^2, respectively.[138] Another study of 27 patients treated with doxifluridine found a biweekly irinotecan starting dose of 150 mg/m^2 for wild-type patients and 70 mg/m^2 for heterozygotes.[139]

The complexity in associating irinotecan side effects with genotype highlights the effects of variation in patient health, treatment schedules, use of other chemotherapeutic agents, and the influence of other genes on metabolism.[132] For example, severe diarrhea in irinotecan-treated patients has been associated with baseline diarrhea, impaired performance status, higher stage, and primary tumor resection.[140] A recent study of 12 candidate genes in the irinotecan metabolism pathway found the SLC and ABC transporters, which move irinotecan into and out of hepatocytes, respectively, have a significant role in variation seen for neutropenia.[141] Other genes that may modify irinotecan's effect include variations in the carboxylesterases that convert irinotecan into SN-38 and removal via multidrug resistance proteins.[142] Irinotecan may also undergo phase I oxidative metabolism through CYP3A4 and CYP3A5, which leads to inactive metabolites.[143] Other polymorphisms in the UGT1A1 promoter have been reported to cooperatively decrease transcription in combination with the 7/7 variant, resulting in severe toxicity.[144] Mutations may occur in the UGT1A1 protein–coding region that decrease enzyme activity. In addition to UGT1A1, at least five other members of the UGT1 family metabolize SN-38.[121]

Commercial testing for UGT1A1 variants allows selection of irinotecan dose and predicts toxicity (Table 6-2), but the test has not entered common use in clinical practice, as most episodes of severe myelosuppression or diarrhea are managed by dose reduction in subsequent cycles.

Mercaptopurine, Thioguanine, and Azathioprine

The thiopurine group of drugs are used to treat AML and childhood ALL. Mercaptopurine and thioguanine are prodrugs converted by hypoxanthine phosphoribosyl transferase into thioguanine nucleotides (TGNs) that are incorporated into DNA and inhibit purine nucleotide synthesis, triggering cell cycle arrest and apoptosis.[32] S-methylation via the enzyme thiopurine-S-methyltransferase (TPMT) in hematopoietic tissues decreases the intracellular pool of parent drug and decreases formation of the active TGNs.[2] Knowledge of TPMT pharmacogenetics is important in predicting toxicity and efficacy, and tests for variants are employed in routine clinical practice.

TPMT activity in human erythrocytes has a trimodal distribution, with approximately 89% of erythrocytes from a sample of 298 Caucasian blood donors showing high enzyme activity, 11% with intermediate activity, and 0.3% with undetectable activity.[145] There is an inverse relationship between TGN concentration and TPMT activity, with lower TGN levels seen with higher TPMT activity.[146] Children with ALL who had lower levels of TGN had higher levels of TPMT and higher relapse rates.[146] Subsequent genotyping studies showed that children with ALL who were heterozygotes for TPMT with lower activity (thus higher TGN levels) had a 2.9-fold reduction for minimal residual disease,[147] and that TPMT wild-type homozygotes had an increased risk of relapse.[148]

There are at least 24 different TPMT mutations, with 17 associated with reduced activity.[149] Of these, three polymorphisms (TPMT*2, TPMT*3A, and TPMT*3C) account for 90% of observed variation.[149,150] The frequency of TPMT allele distribution varies by ethnicity.[151] Intermediate activity is found in patients heterozygous for one wild type and one variant allele. Approximately 5% of Caucasian patients harbor the TPMT*3A allele, which produces an enzyme rapidly degraded by ubiquitination, leading to higher risk for fatal myelosuppression at standard doses.[2,152]

Additional studies suggest that TPMT heterozygotes are at increased risk of mercaptopurine toxicity compared to wild type, as some studies report higher rates of toxicity[153,154] while others report no difference.[147,155] It is uncertain whether TPMT heterozygotes benefit from dose reduction. It is equally unclear whether ALL patients with low TPMT activity are at increased risk for secondary malignancies after treatment with mercaptopurine. Some studies observed higher rates of secondary malignancies such as myelodysplasia, brain tumors, or AML in patients with low TPMT activity,[156–158] while another study failed to confirm this finding.[159] Whether low TPMT activity underlies a correlation of greater toxicity with higher rates of malignancy from thiopurine treatment has important implications for the growing numbers of patients who take azathioprine chronically for organ transplantation, rheumatoid arthritis, and inflammatory bowel disease.

Discrepancies in these studies could stem, in part, from the influence of other factors on TPMT activity such as promoter polymorphisms and the influence of other pharmacokinetic factors on thiopurine levels.[151] TPMT activity varies in erythrocytes of different age, with older erythrocytes having lower activity, thus biasing measurement if marrow production is impaired by ALL.[160] There is also considerable overlap between TPMT activity levels in patients who are wild-type homozygotes or have one or two mutant alleles, further complicating the predictive power of measuring TPMT activity.[161] Cancer cells may overexpress one or both TPMT alleles resulting in a discrepancy with germ-line genotype or enzyme activity.[162] It has been proposed that heterozygous patients be started on a lower dose of thiopurines with dose escalation if tolerated.[151]

To prevent side effects, treatment protocols at hospitals like St. Jude Children's Research Hospital include testing for TPMT variants, and the FDA updated the labeling of mercaptopurine to include information on TPMT.[8,32] Commercially available tests measure TPMT activity, mercaptopurine levels, and the TPMT gene sequence (Table 6-2). Genotyping TPMT in ALL patients may be cost-effective, with a cost of $2,900 per life-year gained by avoiding 6-MP–induced neutropenia during maintenance therapy.[163]

Methotrexate

Methotrexate inhibits dihydrofolate reductase (DHFR), which blocks DNA synthesis and is a mainstay of childhood leukemia treatment[164] (see Chapter 8 and Fig. 8-2 for pathway). Genetic differences in methotrexate uptake and metabolism along with variations in DHFR have all been identified as possible modulators of methotrexate efficacy.[32] The human reduced folate carrier (RFC1) transports methotrexate into cells, and decreased transport is a mechanism of resistance.[165] Variations in each of the proteins involved in methotrexate transport, metabolism, and target influence the response and toxicity of methotrexate therapy.

Reduced Folate Carrier

The RFC1, also known as the *SLC19A1* gene, transports methotrexate into cells. The RFC gene is located on chromosome 21 and patients with duplication of this chromosome due to Down syndrome or hyperdiploidy are more sensitive to methotrexate.[166,167] At least twelve polymorphisms in the RFC gene or promoter have been described, with the most frequently studied being *SCL19A1* G80A, which reduces the activity of the transporter.[168] Of eight studies involving 890 patients, three showed no difference in toxicity,[169–171] three showed increased risk of hepatotoxicity[172] or GI toxicity,[171,173] one study showed an increased risk of relapse,[174] and one study showed no difference in relapse.[175]

Folypolyglutamate Synthetase

Once methotrexate enters cells it is polyglutamated by the enzyme folypolyglutamate synthetase (FPGS), and this modification increases the potency of inhibition of DHFR, TS, and purine synthetic enzymes, and drug accumulation in cells.[164] At least 34 SNPs have been identified in the *FPGS* gene.[176] Children with B-lineage ALL have better responses to methotrexate treatment compared to patients with T-lineage ALL, and higher FPGS levels in B-lineage cells are thought to account for this increased sensitivity.[177] Polyglutamylation of methotrexate is reversed in part by the lysosomal enzyme γ-glutamyl hydrolase (GGH). A SNP in the substrate-binding domain of GGH is associated with lower enzyme activity and higher concentrations of polyglutamylated methotrexate in ALL patient samples.[178] GGH expression is also influenced by promoter DNA methylation, adding an epigenetic level of regulation.[179]

Methylenetetrahydrofolate Reductase

MTHFR converts 5,10-methylenetetrahydrofolate to 5-methyltetrahydrofolate. At least five polymorphisms have been reported, the most frequently studied being *C677T* and *A1298C*, which decrease enzyme activity level, with *C677T* having lower activity.[168,180,181] The C677T allele is found in 35% of Caucasians and 15% of African-Americans, and 15% of Caucasians are heterozygous for both polymorphisms.[182,183] Attempts to link efficacy or toxicity with the *C677T* or *A1298C* polymorphisms have been unsuccessful. The *C677T* allele has been the subject of 18 studies involving 3,175 patients,[182] with six studies showing no difference in toxicity,[169,170,172,173,184,185] four studies showed an increased risk of bone marrow and liver toxicity or treatment interruption or mucositis and prolonged neutropenia,[171,186–188] one study found a decreased risk of bone marrow and liver toxicity,[189] and another found decreased risk of graft versus host disease.[190] With respect to relapse, three studies of the *C677T* allele found no difference,[175,185,187,191] three studies found a higher risk of relapse,[192–194] and one study found a reduced risk of relapse when found along with the A1298C allele.[195] Seven studies

of 1,409 patients examining the *A1298C* allele found either no difference[173,187,194] or a decrease in toxicity[169,184] or relapse.[193,195]

Dihydrofolate Reductase

DHFR acts to reduce dihydrofolate to tetrahydrofolate, and this enzyme is a primary target of methotrexate. Alterations in DHFR levels or reduced binding to methotrexate is thought to underlie resistance.[196] Promoter polymorphisms that increase transcription of DHFR have been reported to reduce event-free survival in children with ALL.[197,198] A SNP at a micro-RNA–binding site in the *DHFR* 3′ untranslated region was found to decrease micro-RNA binding resulting in overexpression of DHFR and resistance to methotrexate, although a study of 37 patients found no relation to drug toxicity.[199,200]

Tamoxifen

The antiestrogen compound tamoxifen is commonly used for prevention and treatment of breast cancer. The parent compound binds to the cytoplasmic estrogen receptor alpha and inhibits estrogen-mediated stimulation of breast cancer proliferation. Tamoxifen undergoes hydroxylation by CYP2D6 to an active metabolite (4-OH-tamoxifen); a second metabolite, *N*-desmethyltamoxifen, is also hydroxylated by the same enzyme to a second active metabolite, endoxifen (Fig. 35-8), which is the predominant form of the active drug found in plasma. Both hydroxy metabolites have significantly increased (100-fold) potency as inhibitors of ER function, as compared to tamoxifen, and have longer half-lives in plasma (see Chapter 35). *CYP 2D6* exists in multiple polymorphic forms, many of which have reduced (*10, 41*) or absent (*3, *4, *5*) catalytic activity. Patients with reduced 2D6 activity produce much reduced levels of endoxin in plasma.[201] The *4 variant is most common, and it was homozygous in 6% of patients in the initial retrospective analysis that suggested a link between this genotype and recurrence.[202] Other retrospective analyses, such as conducted by Bonanni, failed to reproduce a link between the *4/*4 genotype and breast cancer occurrence in a large prevention trial.[203] These analyses only examined the *4 variant. Other, more comprehensive trials have provided supporting evidence that patients hemizygous or homozygous for alleles with reduced or absent activity have a higher recurrence rate when treated in the adjuvant setting.[202,204] In a retrospective analysis of outcomes of 1,325 postmenopausal patients receiving tamoxifen as adjuvant therapy, recurrence rates were 14.9% for extensive metabolizers, 20.9% for intermediate metabolizers (heterozygous for a variant gene or homozygous for *10 or *41), or 29% for those homozygous for reduced metabolizing alleles.[202] A detailed analysis of 282 patients from Asia and North America, in whom multiple risk alleles were genotyped and pharmacokinetic studies were conducted, found a strong association with the presence of two variant alleles and shorter recurrence-free survival. They also examined alleles of the drug efflux transporter, ABCC2, and found that patients with two variant alleles for *CYP 2D6* and two for *ABCC2* had lower plasma levels of both OH-tamoxifen and endoxifen.[205] However, other studies, summarized by Dezentje,[206] have presented inconclusive or contradictory findings, supporting the position that larger, prospective, and carefully planned studies are needed to quantify the role of *CYP2D6* variants in outcomes of treatment.

Related to pharmacogenomic determinants of tamoxifen is the finding that breast cancer patients taking tamoxifen who use certain serotonin reuptake inhibitors (SSRIs, such as parotexine) have a higher risk of death, perhaps related to the inhibitory effect of the SSRIs on CYP2D6 activity.[207] Again the evidence is conflicting as fluoxetine, a strong enzyme inhibitor, had no effect in the same trial.

Although the FDA has amended the label of tamoxifen to call attention to the apparent increased risk of recurrence in patients with variant alleles of CYP 2D6, and the test is available commercially, it is sporadically used in clinical practice, perhaps due to the lack of agreement among experts regarding the strength of the data.

Other polymorphic genes may influence the outcome of tamoxifen therapy. Two classes of enzyme, the uridinylphosphate-gluconyltransferases (UGT) and the phenol sulfotransferases, degrade the active metabolites. Both exist in polymorphic forms. SULT1A1*2 codes for an Arg to His substitution, resulting in a 10-fold decrease in enzyme activity for individuals homozygous for the variant allele.[208] The variant allele is found in very low (<1%) frequency in both Caucasian and Nigerian subjects and is of uncertain significance in determining the success of therapy. One study found that patients homozygous for the SULT1A1*2 allele had a threefold increased risk of death, a surprising finding for an enzyme that inactivates the functional metabolites.[209]

Regarding UGT polymorphisms, the UGT2B7 (268 Tyr) variant has much reduced ability to glucuronidate and inactive the hydroxy metabolites, but its functional importance in the therapeutic setting is not known.[210]

Anthracyclines

The primary variant implicated in anthracycline pharmacology affects the carbonyl reductase 3 gene (CBR3), which converts doxorubicin to its alcohol metabolite, which has decreased antitumor activity but greater cardiotoxicity (see Chapter 18 for structures). At least six different enzymes are capable of making the two-electron reduction of the parent anthracyclines to their alcohol.

In an analysis of liver enzyme activities, CBR 1, not CBR3, was the most abundant of the carbonyl and aldoketo reductases; expression level varied 70-fold in samples from 80 patients. The variation in activity did not correlate with genetic variants but likely resulted from nongenetic factors.[211] CBR1 D2 diplotype correlated with slower clearance of parent drug and lower levels of the alcohol metabolite, and it is known from in vitro studies to have impaired ability to reduce anthracyclines.[212] No such relationship was found for CBR3 haplotypes or diplotypes and pharmacokinetics.[213]

However, the local effect of the CBR3 enzyme on drug metabolism in the tumor and heart is of interest. The enzyme is present in both tissues. The CBR 3 variant V244 substitutes valine for methionine, has greater activity in converting the parent to its alcohol, and confers an eightfold increase in risk for cardiotoxicity in children who are homozygous for the variant, although the p-value of this retrospective case-control study, compromised by the small sample size, was of borderline significance.[214] The same variant was associated with higher doxorubicinol levels in plasma and higher CBR3 in breast tumor tissue, but its presence was not correlated with breast cancer tumor reduction.[215] In the same study, another CBR 3

variant (11G > A), found with an allelic frequency of 0.48, was associated with higher doxorubicinol levels, greater tumor reduction, and lower CBR3 expression in breast cancer tissue in Singapore patients receiving doxorubicin.[215] Further studies are needed to establish the significance of the CBRs with respect to anthracycline metabolism, antitumor activity, and toxicity, but the relationships suggested by preliminary data are intriguing.

Platinum Compounds

There has been considerable interest in determining the biological and therapeutic impact of variants of proteins that are components of the fundamental DNA repair pathways. Two pathways have attracted particular interest: the nucleotide excision repair group consists of at least nine proteins that excise segments of DNA damaged by oxidation, UV radiation, carcinogens, and bulky adducts produced by alkylation and platination; and base excision repair, a group of proteins that excise damaged bases, fill the gap and relegate the broken strand.

ERCC1

ERCC1 is a component of the NER pathway, and its expression appears to be tightly linked to that of other members of the pathway (XPA, XPB, XPD). A high-frequency SNP at codon 118 of ERCC1 (118C/T) precedes the helix-turn-helix segment of the protein and results in decreased gene expression and lower protein levels[216,217] in 46% of the population. A second polymorphism, C8092A, has a lower frequency (4%) and decreases the message stability.[218] Early studies linked ERCC1 expression to response to platinum-based therapy for ovarian cancer (see Chapter 15).[219,220] In a lung cancer study, the homozygous C8092 genotype had better overall survival of 22.3 months as compared to 13.4 months for the heterozygous C9092/A 8092 or A8092/A8092.[218] No significant effect of the 118C/T SNP was found in the same study. However, Viguier et al.[221] found that the latter SNP predicted for response to oxaliplatin in colon cancer patients, a finding confirmed in other studies of ovarian[222] and colorectal cancer.[26,221]

XPD

XPD SNPs include a lysine to glutamine transition at codon 751, which appears to confer sensitivity to platinating drugs,[223] and a nonsynonymous substitution, Asp312Asn, of uncertain biological significance.[216] Both variants were less effective in repairing benzo(a)pyrene adducts and UV damage.[224,225] The polymorphisms have a high prevalence in the general population (29% and 42%, respectively). The Lys751Gln variant in XPD protein was associated with a lower response to 5-FU-oxaliplatin in 73 patients with metastatic colorectal cancer (10% in homo- or heterozygous variant patients versus 24% in wild-type patients) and a shorter survival, an unexpected finding if XPD variants are less effective in repairing adducts.[223]

XRCC1

The XRCC1 gene participates in base excision repair, an alternative route for excising and replacing damaged bases. Arginine substitution for glutamine at codon 399 displays decreased DNA repair capacity, compared to those with the wild-type gene.[226] In 61 patients with metastatic colorectal cancer receiving 5-FU and oxaliplatin, the majority of responders (8 of 11 or 72%) carried the wild-type alleles (*Arg/Arg*) and three responders were heterozygous at this locus, while only 34% of nonresponders had *Arg/Arg* at this codon.[227] These findings are in conflict with the notion that the *Arg* allele is more competent for DNA repair. In a number of subsequent studies, the variant alleles were associated with improved response and survival in small numbers of patients with colorectal cancer and non–small cell lung cancer.[227] However, in a much larger study of 914 patients with ovarian cancer, treated with carboplatin and paclitaxel, no correlations were observed with response or survival for 27 different variants of DNA repair genes, including *XRCC1: R399Gln* and for *ERCC1: C8092A*.[228] Wang found a correlation of the *Arg/Arg* and *Gln/Arg* genotype with serious (grade 3/4) toxicity in lung cancer patients.[229]

Thus, no consistent associations of specific polymorphisms and response or survival have emerged from these studies. ERCC1 expression appears to be the strongest candidate for influencing platinum-based therapy but the influence of specific SNPs of this gene has not been clearly established. *XRCC1* variants deserve further study. Significant gaps remain in understanding the biological function of the various alleles and their effect on repair of DNA damage inflicted by multiagent chemotherapy regimens.

Cytidine Deaminase (CD)

Cytidine deaminase (CD) detoxifies cytosine arabinoside and gemcitabine to inactive uracil metabolites. The *G208A* allele (designated *3) produces a nonsynonymous substitution of threonine for alanine at *codon 70 of CD*. The allelic frequency in a Japanese population was 0.037. Japanese subjects heterozygous for *3 had a significantly higher (fivefold) AUC of gemcitabine in plasma, as compared to ala/ala subjects, and an increased incidence of grade 3 or higher neutropenia. A homozygous *3 subject had extreme elevation of the plasma AUC and a dramatically lower clearance.[230]

References

1. Evans WE, Relling MV. Pharmacogenomics: translating functional genomics into rational therapeutics. Science 1999;286:487–491.
2. Weinshilboum R, Wang L. Pharmacogenomics: bench to bedside. Nat Rev Drug Discov 2004;3:739–748.
3. Weinshilboum R. Inheritance and drug response. N Engl J Med 2003;348:529–537.
4. Tate SK, Goldstein DB. Will tomorrow's medicines work for everyone? Nat Genet 2004;36:S34–S42.
5. Rosell R, et al. Screening for epidermal growth factor receptor mutations in lung cancer. N Engl J Med 2009;361:958–967.
6. Roses AD. Pharmacogenetics and the practice of medicine. Nature 2000;405:857–865.
7. Dolgin E. FDA narrows drug label usage. Nature 2009;460:1069.
8. Lesko LJ, Woodcock J. Translation of pharmacogenomics and pharmacogenetics: a regulatory perspective. Nat Rev Drug Discov 2004;3:763–769.
9. Frueh FW, et al. Pharmacogenomic biomarker information in drug labels approved by the United States food and drug administration: prevalence of related drug use. Pharmacotherapy 2008;28:992–998.
10. Goldstein DB, Tate SK, Sisodiya SM. Pharmacogenetics goes genomic. Nat Rev Genet 2003;4:937–947.
11. Evans WE, McLeod HL. Pharmacogenomics—drug disposition, drug targets, and side effects. N Engl J Med 2003;348:538–549.
12. Helsby NA, et al. CYP2C19 pharmacogenetics in advanced cancer: compromised function independent of genotype. Br J Cancer 2008;99: 1251–1255.
13. Williams ML, et al. A discordance of the cytochrome P450 2C19 genotype and phenotype in patients with advanced cancer. Br J Clin Pharmacol 2000;49:485–488.
14. Vogel F, Motulsky A. Human Genetics. Problems and Approaches. Berlin: Springer, 1986:498–544.
15. Evans WE, Johnson JA. Pharmacogenomics: the inherited basis for interindividual differences in drug response. Annu Rev Genomics Hum Genet 2001;2:9–39.
16. Meyer UA, Zanger UM. Molecular mechanisms of genetic polymorphisms of drug metabolism. Annu Rev Pharmacol Toxicol 1997;37:269–296.
17. Weinshilboum R, Wang L. Pharmacogenetics: inherited variation in amino acid sequence and altered protein quantity. Clin Pharmacol Ther 2004;75:253–258.
18. Alving AS, Carson PE, Flanagan CL, et al. Enzymatic deficiency in primaquine-sensitive erythrocytes. Science 1956;124:484–485.
19. Kalow W. Human pharmacogenomics: the development of a science. Hum Genomics 2004;1:375–380.
20. Evans DA, Manley KA, Mc KV. Genetic control of isoniazid metabolism in man. Br Med J 1960;2:485–491.
21. Holmes MV, et al. Fulfilling the promise of personalized medicine? Systematic review and field synopsis of pharmacogenetic studies. PLoS One 2009;4:e7960.
22. Sachidanandam R, et al. A map of human genome sequence variation containing 1.42 million single nucleotide polymorphisms. Nature 2001;409: 928–933.
23. Stoneking M. Single nucleotide polymorphisms. From the evolutionary past. Nature 2001;409:821–822.
24. The Wellcome Trust Case Control Consortium. Genome-wide association study of 14,000 cases of seven common diseases and 3,000 shared controls. Nature 2007;447:661–678.
25. Stoehlmacher J, et al. Association between glutathione S-transferase P1, T1, and M1 genetic polymorphism and survival of patients with metastatic colorectal cancer. J Natl Cancer Inst 2002;94:936–942.
26. Stoehlmacher J, et al. A multivariate analysis of genomic polymorphisms: prediction of clinical outcome to 5-FU/oxaliplatin combination chemotherapy in refractory colorectal cancer. Br J Cancer 2004;91:344–354.
27. Roses AD. Pharmacogenetics in drug discovery and development: a translational perspective. Nat Rev Drug Discov 2008;7:807–817.
28. Yong WP, Innocenti F. Translation of pharmacogenetic knowledge into cancer therapeutics. Clin Adv Hematol Oncol 2007;5:698–706.
29. Kalow W. Pharmacoanthropology and the genetics of drug metabolism. In: Kalow W, ed. Pharmacogenetics of Drug Metabolism. New York: Pergamon Press, 1992:865–877.
30. Sasvari-Szekely M, Gerstner A, Ronai Z, et al. Rapid genotyping of factor V Leiden mutation using single-tube bidirectional allele-specific amplification and automated ultrathin-layer agarose gel electrophoresis. Electrophoresis 2000;21:816–821.
31. Lu Z, Diasio R. Polymorphic drug-metabolizing enzymes. In: Schilsky R, Milano G, Ratain M, eds. Principles of Antineoplastic Drug Development and Pharmacology. New York: Dekker, 1996:281–385.
32. Relling MV, Dervieux T. Pharmacogenetics and cancer therapy. Nat Rev Cancer 2000;1:99–108.
33. Chang TK, Yu L, Goldstein JA, et al. Identification of the polymorphically expressed CYP2C19 and the wild-type CYP2C9-ILE359 allele as low-Km catalysts of cyclophosphamide and ifosfamide activation. Pharmacogenetics 1997;7:211–221.
34. Ulrich CM, Robien K, McLeod HL. Cancer pharmacogenetics: polymorphisms, pathways and beyond. Nat Rev Cancer 2003;3:912–920.
35. Huang RS, Ratain MJ. Pharmacogenetics and pharmacogenomics of anticancer agents. CA Cancer J Clin 2009;59:42–55.
36. Jones TS, Yang W, Evans WE, et al. Using HapMap tools in pharmacogenomic discovery: the thiopurine methyltransferase polymorphism. Clin Pharmacol Ther 2007;81:729–734.
37. Holleman A, et al. Gene-expression patterns in drug-resistant acute lymphoblastic leukemia cells and response to treatment. N Engl J Med 2004;351:533–542.
38. Lugthart S, et al. Identification of genes associated with chemotherapy cross-resistance and treatment response in childhood acute lymphoblastic leukemia. Cancer Cell 2005;7:375–386.

39. Potti A, et al. Genomic signatures to guide the use of chemotherapeutics. Nat Med 2006;12:1294–1300.

40. Salter KH, et al. An integrated approach to the prediction of chemotherapeutic response in patients with breast cancer. PLoS One 2008;3:e1908.

41. Acharya CR, et al. Gene expression signatures, clinicopathological features, and individualized therapy in breast cancer. JAMA 2008;299:1574–1587.

42. Bonnefoi H, et al. Validation of gene signatures that predict the response of breast cancer to neoadjuvant chemotherapy: a substudy of the EORTC 10994/BIG 00-01 clinical trial. Lancet Oncol 2007;8:1071–1078.

43. Harris L, et al. American Society of Clinical Oncology 2007 update of recommendations for the use of tumor markers in breast cancer. J Clin Oncol 2007;25:5287–5312.

44. Paik S, et al. A multigene assay to predict recurrence of tamoxifen-treated, node-negative breast cancer. N Engl J Med 2004;351:2817–2826.

45. Bast RC Jr, Hortobagyi GN. Individualized care for patients with cancer—a work in progress. N Engl J Med 2004;351:2865–2867.

46. Geradts J. Molecular prediction of recurrence of breast cancer. N Engl J Med 2005;352:1605–1607; author reply 1605–1607.

47. van de Vijver MJ, et al. A gene-expression signature as a predictor of survival in breast cancer. N Engl J Med 2002;347:1999–2009.

48. Hornberger J, Cosler LE, Lyman GH. Economic analysis of targeting chemotherapy using a 21-gene RT-PCR assay in lymph-node-negative, estrogen-receptor-positive, early-stage breast cancer. Am J Manag Care 2005;11:313–324.

49. Zujewski JA, Kamin L. Trial assessing individualized options for treatment for breast cancer: the TAILORx trial. Future Oncol 2008;4:603–610.

50. Midgley R, Kerr DJ. Capecitabine: have we got the dose right? Nat Clin Pract Oncol 2009;6:17–24.

51. Ezzeldin H, Diasio R. Dihydropyrimidine dehydrogenase deficiency, a pharmacogenetic syndrome associated with potentially life-threatening toxicity following 5-fluorouracil administration. Clin Colorectal Cancer 2004;4:181–189.

52. Heggie GD, Sommadossi JP, Cross DS, et al. Clinical pharmacokinetics of 5-fluorouracil and its metabolites in plasma, urine, and bile. Cancer Res 1987;47:2203–2206.

53. Diasio RB. Clinical implications of dihydropyrimidine dehydrogenase on 5-FU pharmacology. Oncology (Williston Park) 2001;15:21–26; discussion 27.

54. Diasio RB, Beavers TL, Carpenter JT. Familial deficiency of dihydropyrimidine dehydrogenase. Biochemical basis for familial pyrimidinemia and severe 5-fluorouracil-induced toxicity. J Clin Invest 1988;81:47–51.

55. Innocenti F, Ratain MJ. Update on pharmacogenetics in cancer chemotherapy. Eur J Cancer 2002;38:639–644.

56. van Kuilenburg AB, et al. Lethal outcome of a patient with a complete dihydropyrimidine dehydrogenase (DPD) deficiency after administration of 5-fluorouracil: frequency of the common IVS14+1G>A mutation causing DPD deficiency. Clin Cancer Res 2001;7:1149–1153.

57. Wei X, McLeod HL, McMurrough J, et al. Molecular basis of the human dihydropyrimidine dehydrogenase deficiency and 5-fluorouracil toxicity. J Clin Invest 1996;98:610–615.

58. Van Kuilenburg AB, Meinsma R, Zoetekouw L, et al. High prevalence of the IVS14 + 1G>A mutation in the dihydropyrimidine dehydrogenase gene of patients with severe 5-fluorouracil-associated toxicity. Pharmacogenetics 2002;12:555–558.

59. Salonga D, et al. Colorectal tumors responding to 5-fluorouracil have low gene expression levels of dihydropyrimidine dehydrogenase, thymidylate synthase, and thymidine phosphorylase. Clin Cancer Res 2000;6:1322–1327.

60. Harris BE, Song R, Soong SJ, et al. Relationship between dihydropyrimidine dehydrogenase activity and plasma 5-fluorouracil levels with evidence for circadian variation of enzyme activity and plasma drug levels in cancer patients receiving 5-fluorouracil by protracted continuous infusion. Cancer Res 1990;50:197–201.

61. Yen JL, McLeod HL. Should DPD analysis be required prior to prescribing fluoropyrimidines? Eur J Cancer 2007;43:1011–1016.

62. Maekawa K, et al. Genetic variations and haplotype structures of the DPYD gene encoding dihydropyrimidine dehydrogenase in Japanese and their ethnic differences. J Hum Genet 2007;52:804–819.

63. van Kuilenburg AB, De Abreu RA, van Gennip AH. Pharmacogenetic and clinical aspects of dihydropyrimidine dehydrogenase deficiency. Ann Clin Biochem 2003;40:41–45.

64. Johnson MR, et al. Life-threatening toxicity in a dihydropyrimidine dehydrogenase-deficient patient after treatment with topical 5-fluorouracil. Clin Cancer Res 1999;5:2006–2011.

65. van Kuilenburg AB. Dihydropyrimidine dehydrogenase and the efficacy and toxicity of 5-fluorouracil. Eur J Cancer 2004;40:939–950.

66. Johnson MR, Wang K, Diasio RB. Profound dihydropyrimidine dehydrogenase deficiency resulting from a novel compound heterozygote genotype. Clin Cancer Res 2002;8:768–774.

67. Collie-Duguid ES, Etienne MC, Milano G, et al. Known variant DPYD alleles do not explain DPD deficiency in cancer patients. Pharmacogenetics 2000;10:217–223.

68. Fernandez-Salguero PM, et al. Lack of correlation between phenotype and genotype for the polymorphically expressed dihydropyrimidine dehydrogenase in a family of Pakistani origin. Pharmacogenetics 1997;7:161–163.

69. Vreken P, Van Kuilenburg AB, Meinsma R, et al. Dihydropyrimidine dehydrogenase (DPD) deficiency: identification and expression of missense mutations C29R, R886H and R235W. Hum Genet 1997;101:333–338.

70. Mattison LK, et al. Rapid identification of dihydropyrimidine dehydrogenase deficiency by using a novel 2-13C-uracil breath test. Clin Cancer Res 2004;10:2652–2658.

71. Saif MW, Choma A, Salamone SJ, et al. Pharmacokinetically guided dose adjustment of 5-fluorouracil: a rational approach to improving therapeutic outcomes. J Natl Cancer Inst 2009;101:1543–1552.

72. Mattison LK, et al. The uracil breath test in the assessment of dihydropyrimidine dehydrogenase activity: pharmacokinetic relationship between expired 13CO2 and plasma [2−13C]dihydrouracil. Clin Cancer Res 2006;12:549–555.

73. van Kuilenburg AB. Screening for dihydropyrimidine dehydrogenase deficiency: to do or not to do, that's the question. Cancer Invest 2006;24:215–217.

74. Johnson MR, Yan J, Shao L, et al. Semi-automated radioassay for determination of dihydropyrimidine dehydrogenase (DPD) activity. Screening cancer patients for DPD deficiency, a condition associated with 5-fluorouracil toxicity. J Chromatogr B Biomed Sci Appl 1997;696:183–191.

75. Van Kuilenburg AB, Van Lenthe H, Van Gennip AH. Radiochemical assay for determination of dihydropyrimidinase activity using reversed-phase high-performance liquid chromatography. J Chromatogr B Biomed Sci Appl 1999;729:307–314.

76. Raida M, et al. Prevalence of a common point mutation in the dihydropyrimidine dehydrogenase (DPD) gene within the 5′-splice donor site of intron 14 in patients with severe 5-fluorouracil (5-FU)-related toxicity compared with controls. Clin Cancer Res 2001;7:2832–2839.

77. Van Kuilenburg AB, et al. Genotype and phenotype in patients with dihydropyrimidine dehydrogenase deficiency. Hum Genet 1999;104:1–9.

78. Morel A, et al. Clinical relevance of different dihydropyrimidine dehydrogenase gene single nucleotide polymorphisms on 5-fluorouracil tolerance. Mol Cancer Ther 2006;5:2895–2904.

79. Watters JW, McLeod HL. Cancer pharmacogenomics: current and future applications. Biochim Biophys Acta 2003;1603:99–111.

80. Chu E, Ju J, Schmitz J. Antifolate drugs in cancer therapy. In: Jackman A, ed. Anticancer Drug Development Guide. Totowa, NJ: Humana Press, 1999:397–408.

81. Chu E, et al. Autoregulation of human thymidylate synthase messenger RNA translation by thymidylate synthase. Proc Natl Acad Sci U S A 1991;88:8977–8981.

82. Dolnick BJ. Thymidylate synthase and the cell cycle: what should we believe? Cancer J 2000;6:215–216.

83. Copur MS, Chu E. Thymidylate synthase pharmacogenetics in colorectal cancer. Clin Colorectal Cancer 2001;1:179–180.

84. Pullarkat ST, et al. Thymidylate synthase gene polymorphism determines response and toxicity of 5-FU chemotherapy. Pharmacogenomics J 2001;1:65–70.

85. Kawakami K, Omura K, Kanehira E, et al. Polymorphic tandem repeats in the thymidylate synthase gene is associated with its protein expression in human gastrointestinal cancers. Anticancer Res 1999;19:3249–3252.

86. Villafranca E, et al. Polymorphisms of the repeated sequences in the enhancer region of the thymidylate synthase gene promoter may predict downstaging after preoperative chemoradiation in rectal cancer. J Clin Oncol 2001;19:1779–1786.

87. Marsh S, McKay JA, Cassidy J, et al. Polymorphism in the thymidylate synthase promoter enhancer region in colorectal cancer. Int J Oncol 2001; 19:383–386.

88. Mandola MV, et al. A novel single nucleotide polymorphism within the 5′ tandem repeat polymorphism of the thymidylate synthase gene abolishes USF-1 binding and alters transcriptional activity. Cancer Res 2003;63: 2898–2904.

89. Ulrich CM, et al. Searching expressed sequence tag databases: discovery and confirmation of a common polymorphism in the thymidylate synthase gene. Cancer Epidemiol Biomarkers Prev 2000;9:1381–1385.

90. Marsh S, et al. Novel thymidylate synthase enhancer region alleles in African populations. Hum Mutat 2000;16:528.

91. Mandola MV, et al. A 6 bp polymorphism in the thymidylate synthase gene causes message instability and is associated with decreased intratumoral TS mRNA levels. Pharmacogenetics 2004;14:319–327.

92. Aschele C, et al. Immunohistochemical quantitation of thymidylate synthase expression in colorectal cancer metastases predicts for clinical outcome to fluorouracil-based chemotherapy. J Clin Oncol 1999;17:1760–1770.

93. Johnston PG, et al. The role of thymidylate synthase expression in prognosis and outcome of adjuvant chemotherapy in patients with rectal cancer. J Clin Oncol 1994;12:2640–2647.

94. Kornmann M, et al. Thymidylate synthase is a predictor for response and resistance in hepatic artery infusion chemotherapy. Cancer Lett 1997; 118:29–35.

95. Lenz HJ, et al. Thymidylate synthase mRNA level in adenocarcinoma of the stomach: a predictor for primary tumor response and overall survival. J Clin Oncol 1996;14:176–182.

96. Pestalozzi BC, et al. Increased thymidylate synthase protein levels are principally associated with proliferation but not cell cycle phase in asynchronous human cancer cells. Br J Cancer 1995;71:1151–1157.

97. Lecomte T, et al. Thymidylate synthase gene polymorphism predicts toxicity in colorectal cancer patients receiving 5-fluorouracil-based chemotherapy. Clin Cancer Res 2004;10:5880–5888.

98. Stoehlmacher I, Mandola M, Yun J. Alterations of the thymidylate synthase (TS) pathway and colorectal cancer risk: the impact of three TS polymorphisms. Proc Am Assoc Cancer Res 2003;44:597.

99. McLeod H, Sargent D, Marsh, S. Pharmacogenetic analysis of systemic toxicity and response after 5-fluorouracil (5FU)/CPT-11, 5FU/oxaliplatin (oral), or CPT-11/oxal therapy for advanced colorectal cancer. Proc Am Assoc Clin Oncol 2003;22:252.

100. Westra JL, et al. Predictive value of thymidylate synthase and dihydropyrimidine dehydrogenase protein expression on survival in adjuvantly treated stage III colon cancer patients. Ann Oncol 2005;16:1646–1653.

101. De Mattia E, Toffoli G. C677T and A1298C MTHFR polymorphisms, a challenge for antifolate and fluoropyrimidine-based therapy personalisation. Eur J Cancer 2009;45:1333–1351.

102. Martin YN, et al. Human methylenetetrahydrofolate reductase pharmacogenomics: gene resequencing and functional genomics. Pharmacogenet Genomics 2006;16:265–277.

103. Afzal S, et al. MTHFR polymorphisms and 5-FU-based adjuvant chemotherapy in colorectal cancer. Ann Oncol 2009;20:1660–1666.

104. Wisotzkey JD, Toman J, Bell T, et al. MTHFR (C677T) polymorphisms and stage III colon cancer: response to therapy. Mol Diagn 1999;4:95–99.

105. Marcuello E, Altes A, Menoyo A, et al. Methylenetetrahydrofolate reductase gene polymorphisms: genomic predictors of clinical response to fluoropyrimidine-based chemotherapy? Cancer Chemother Pharmacol 2006;57: 835–840.

106. Suh KW, et al. Which gene is a dominant predictor of response during FOLFOX chemotherapy for the treatment of metastatic colorectal cancer, the MTHFR or XRCC1 gene? Ann Surg Oncol 2006;13:1379–1385.

107. Ruzzo A, et al. Pharmacogenetic profiling in patients with advanced colorectal cancer treated with first-line FOLFOX-4 chemotherapy. J Clin Oncol 2007;25:1247–1254.

108. Ruzzo A, et al. Pharmacogenetic profiling in patients with advanced colorectal cancer treated with first-line FOLFIRI chemotherapy. Pharmacogenomics J 2008;8:278–288.

109. Lurje G, et al. Thymidylate synthase haplotype is associated with tumor recurrence in stage II and stage III colon cancer. Pharmacogenet Genomics 2008; 18:161–168.

110. Schwab M, et al. Role of genetic and nongenetic factors for fluorouracil treatment-related severe toxicity: a prospective clinical trial by the German 5-FU Toxicity Study Group. J Clin Oncol 2008;26:2131–2138.

111. Pare L, et al. Influence of thymidylate synthase and methylenetetrahydrofolate reductase gene polymorphisms on the disease-free survival of breast cancer patients receiving adjuvant 5-fluorouracil/methotrexate-based therapy. Anticancer Drugs 2007;18:821–825.

112. Sarbia M, Stahl M, von Weyhern C, et al. The prognostic significance of genetic polymorphisms (methylenetetrahydrofolate reductase C677T, methionine synthase A2756G, thymidilate synthase tandem repeat polymorphism) in multimodally treated oesophageal squamous cell carcinoma. Br J Cancer 2006;94:203–207.

113. Ruzzo A, et al. Pharmacogenetic profiling and clinical outcome of patients with advanced gastric cancer treated with palliative chemotherapy. J Clin Oncol 2006;24:1883–1891.

114. Lee J, et al. Clinical significance of thymidylate synthase and methylenetetrahydrofolate reductase gene polymorphism in Korean patients with gastric cancer. Korean J Gastroenterol 2005;46:32–38.

115. Cohen V, et al. Methylenetetrahydrofolate reductase polymorphism in advanced colorectal cancer: a novel genomic predictor of clinical response to fluoropyrimidine-based chemotherapy. Clin Cancer Res 2003;9: 1611–1615.

116. Zhang W, et al. Association of methylenetetrahydrofolate reductase gene polymorphisms and sex-specific survival in patients with metastatic colon cancer. J Clin Oncol 2007;25:3726–3731.

117. Wu X, et al. Genetic variations in radiation and chemotherapy drug action pathways predict clinical outcomes in esophageal cancer. J Clin Oncol 2006;24:3789–3798.

118. Jakobsen A, Nielsen JN, Gyldenkerne N, et al. Thymidylate synthase and methylenetetrahydrofolate reductase gene polymorphism in normal tissue as predictors of fluorouracil sensitivity. J Clin Oncol 2005;23: 1365–1369.

119. Terrazzino S, et al. A haplotype of the methylenetetrahydrofolate reductase gene predicts poor tumor response in rectal cancer patients receiving preoperative chemoradiation. Pharmacogenet Genomics 2006;16: 817–824.

120. Capitain O, et al. The influence of fluorouracil outcome parameters on tolerance and efficacy in patients with advanced colorectal cancer. Pharmacogenomics J 2008;8:256–267.

121. Schulz C, et al. UGT1A1 gene polymorphism: impact on toxicity and efficacy of irinotecan-based regimens in metastatic colorectal cancer. World J Gastroenterol 2009;15:5058–5066.

122. Bosma PJ, et al. Mechanisms of inherited deficiencies of multiple UDP-glucuronosyltransferase isoforms in two patients with Crigler-Najjar syndrome, type I. FASEB J 1992;6:2859–2863.

123. Monaghan G, Ryan M, Seddon R, et al. Genetic variation in bilirubin UPD-glucuronosyltransferase gene promoter and Gilbert's syndrome. Lancet 1996;347:578–581.

124. Liu JY, Qu K, Sferruzza AD, et al. Distribution of the UGT1A1*28 polymorphism in Caucasian and Asian populations in the US: a genomic analysis of 138 healthy individuals. Anticancer Drugs 2007;18:693–696.

125. Lampe JW, Bigler J, Horner NK, et al. UDP-glucuronosyltransferase (UGT1A1*28 and UGT1A6*2) polymorphisms in Caucasians and Asians: relationships to serum bilirubin concentrations. Pharmacogenetics 1999; 9:341–349.

126. Akaba K, et al. Neonatal hyperbilirubinemia and mutation of the bilirubin uridine diphosphate-glucuronosyltransferase gene: a common missense mutation among Japanese, Koreans and Chinese. Biochem Mol Biol Int 1998;46:21–26.

127. Sato H, Adachi Y, Koiwai O. The genetic basis of Gilbert's syndrome. Lancet 1996;347:557–558.

128. Ando Y, et al. Polymorphisms of UDP-glucuronosyltransferase gene and irinotecan toxicity: a pharmacogenetic analysis. Cancer Res 2000;60: 6921–6926.

129. Innocenti F, et al. Genetic variants in the UDP-glucuronosyltransferase 1A1 gene predict the risk of severe neutropenia of irinotecan. J Clin Oncol 2004;22:1382–1388.

130. Marcuello E, et al. UGT1A1 gene variations and irinotecan treatment in patients with metastatic colorectal cancer. Br J Cancer 2004;91:678–682.

131. Rouits E, et al. Relevance of different UGT1A1 polymorphisms in irinotecan-induced toxicity: a molecular and clinical study of 75 patients. Clin Cancer Res 2004;10:5151–5159.

132. Hoskins JM, Goldberg RM, Qu P, et al. UGT1A1*28 genotype and irinotecan-induced neutropenia: dose matters. J Natl Cancer Inst 2007; 99:1290–1295.

133. Hasegawa Y, et al. Rapid detection of UGT1A1 gene polymorphisms by newly developed Invader assay. Clin Chem 2004;50:1479–1480.

134. Cote JF, et al. UGT1A1 polymorphism can predict hematologic toxicity in patients treated with irinotecan. Clin Cancer Res 2007;13:3269–3275.

135. Massacesi C, et al. Uridine diphosphate glucuronosyl transferase 1A1 promoter polymorphism predicts the risk of gastrointestinal toxicity and fatigue induced by irinotecan-based chemotherapy. Cancer 2006;106: 1007–1016.

136. Parodi L, Pickering E, Cisar LA, et al. Utility of pretreatment bilirubin level and UGT1A1 polymorphisms in multivariate predictive models of neutropenia associated with irinotecan treatment in previously untreated patients with colorectal cancer. Arch Drug Inf 2008;1:97–106.

137. Braun MS, et al. Association of molecular markers with toxicity outcomes in a randomized trial of chemotherapy for advanced colorectal cancer: the FOCUS trial. J Clin Oncol 2009;27:5519–5528.

138. Toffoli G, et al. Genotype-driven phase I study of irinotecan administered in combination with fluorouracil/leucovorin in patients with metastatic colorectal cancer. J Clin Oncol 2010;28:866–871.

139. Hazama S, et al. Phase I study of irinotecan and doxifluridine for metastatic colorectal cancer focusing on the UGT1A1*28 polymorphism. Cancer Sci 2009;101:722–727.

140. Dranitsaris G, Shah A, Spirovski B, et al. Severe diarrhea in patients with advanced-stage colorectal cancer receiving FOLFOX or FOLFIRI chemotherapy: the development of a risk prediction tool. Clin Colorectal Cancer 2007;6:367–373.

141. Innocenti F, et al. Comprehensive pharmacogenetic analysis of irinotecan neutropenia and pharmacokinetics. J Clin Oncol 2009;27:2604–2614.

142. Toffoli G, Cecchin E, Corona G, et al. Pharmacogenetics of irinotecan. Curr Med Chem Anticancer Agents 2003;3:225–237.

143. Santos A, et al. Metabolism of irinotecan (CPT-11) by CYP3A4 and CYP3A5 in humans. Clin Cancer Res 2000;6:2012–2020.

144. Kitagawa C, et al. Genetic polymorphism in the phenobarbital-responsive enhancer module of the UDP-glucuronosyltransferase 1A1 gene and irinotecan toxicity. Pharmacogenet Genomics 2005;15:35–41.

145. Weinshilboum RM, Sladek SL. Mercaptopurine pharmacogenetics: monogenic inheritance of erythrocyte thiopurine methyltransferase activity. Am J Hum Genet 1980;32:651–662.

146. Lennard L, Lilleyman JS, Van Loon J, et al. Genetic variation in response to 6-mercaptopurine for childhood acute lymphoblastic leukaemia. Lancet 1990;336:225–229.

147. Stanulla M, et al. Thiopurine methyltransferase (TPMT) genotype and early treatment response to mercaptopurine in childhood acute lymphoblastic leukemia. JAMA 2005;293:1485–1489.

148. Schmiegelow K, et al. Thiopurine methyltransferase activity is related to the risk of relapse of childhood acute lymphoblastic leukemia: results from the NOPHO ALL-92 study. Leukemia 2009;23:557–564.

149. Schaeffeler E, et al. Highly multiplexed genotyping of thiopurine s-methyltransferase variants using MALD-TOF mass spectrometry: reliable genotyping in different ethnic groups. Clin Chem 2008;54:1637–1647.

150. Schaeffeler E, et al. Comprehensive analysis of thiopurine S-methyltransferase phenotype-genotype correlation in a large population of German-Caucasians and identification of novel TPMT variants. Pharmacogenetics 2004;14:407–417.

151. McLeod HL, Siva C. The thiopurine S-methyltransferase gene locus—implications for clinical pharmacogenomics. Pharmacogenomics 2002;3: 89–98.

152. Tai HL, et al. Enhanced proteasomal degradation of mutant human thiopurine S-methyltransferase (TPMT) in mammalian cells: mechanism for TPMT protein deficiency inherited by TPMT*2, TPMT*3A, TPMT*3B or TPMT*3C. Pharmacogenetics 1999;9:641–650.

153. Evans WE, et al. Preponderance of thiopurine S-methyltransferase deficiency and heterozygosity among patients intolerant to mercaptopurine or azathioprine. J Clin Oncol 2001;19:2293–2301.

154. Relling MV, et al. Mercaptopurine therapy intolerance and heterozygosity at the thiopurine S-methyltransferase gene locus. J Natl Cancer Inst 1999;91:2001–2008.

155. McLeod HL, et al. Analysis of thiopurine methyltransferase variant alleles in childhood acute lymphoblastic leukaemia. Br J Haematol 1999;105: 696–700.

156. Bo J, et al. Possible carcinogenic effect of 6-mercaptopurine on bone marrow stem cells: relation to thiopurine metabolism. Cancer 1999;86: 1080–1086.

157. Relling MV, et al. High incidence of secondary brain tumours after radiotherapy and antimetabolites. Lancet 1999;354:34–39.

158. Schmiegelow K, et al. Methotrexate/6-mercaptopurine maintenance therapy influences the risk of a second malignant neoplasm after childhood acute lymphoblastic leukemia: results from the NOPHO ALL-92 study. Blood 2009;113:6077–6084.

159. Stanulla M, et al. Thiopurine methyltransferase genetics is not a major risk factor for secondary malignant neoplasms after treatment of childhood acute lymphoblastic leukemia on Berlin-Frankfurt-Munster protocols. Blood 2009;114:1314–1318.

160. Lennard L, Chew TS, Lilleyman JS. Human thiopurine methyltransferase activity varies with red blood cell age. Br J Clin Pharmacol 2001;52: 539–546.

161. Fakhoury M, et al. Should TPMT genotype and activity be used to monitor 6-mercaptopurine treatment in children with acute lymphoblastic leukaemia? J Clin Pharm Ther 2007;32:633–639.

162. Marsh S, Van Booven DJ. The increasing complexity of mercaptopurine pharmacogenomics. Clin Pharmacol Ther 2009;85:139–141.

163. van den Akker-van Marle ME, et al. Cost-effectiveness of pharmacogenomics in clinical practice: a case study of thiopurine methyltransferase genotyping in acute lymphoblastic leukemia in Europe. Pharmacogenomics 2006;7:783–792.

164. Gorlick R, et al. Intrinsic and acquired resistance to methotrexate in acute leukemia. N Engl J Med 1996;335:1041–1048.

165. Gorlick R, et al. Defective transport is a common mechanism of acquired methotrexate resistance in acute lymphocytic leukemia and is associated with decreased reduced folate carrier expression. Blood 1997;89: 1013–1018.

166. Belkov VM, et al. Reduced folate carrier expression in acute lymphoblastic leukemia: a mechanism for ploidy but not lineage differences in methotrexate accumulation. Blood 1999;93:1643–1650.

167. Taub JW, Ge Y. Down syndrome, drug metabolism and chromosome 21. Pediatr Blood Cancer 2005;44:33–39.

168. Aplenc R, Lange B. Pharmacogenetic determinants of outcome in acute lymphoblastic leukaemia. Br J Haematol 2004;125:421–434.

169. Huang L, Tissing WJ, de Jonge R, et al. Polymorphisms in folate-related genes: association with side effects of high-dose methotrexate in childhood acute lymphoblastic leukemia. Leukemia 2008;22:1798–1800.

170. Kishi S, et al. Homocysteine, pharmacogenetics, and neurotoxicity in children with leukemia. J Clin Oncol 2003;21:3084–3091.

171. Shimasaki N, et al. Influence of MTHFR and RFC1 polymorphisms on toxicities during maintenance chemotherapy for childhood acute lymphoblastic leukemia or lymphoma. J Pediatr Hematol Oncol 2008;30: 347–352.

172. Imanishi H, et al. Genetic polymorphisms associated with adverse events and elimination of methotrexate in childhood acute lymphoblastic leukemia and malignant lymphoma. J Hum Genet 2007;52:166–171.

173. Kishi S, et al. Ancestry and pharmacogenetics of antileukemic drug toxicity. Blood 2007;109:4151–4157.

174. Laverdiere C, Chiasson S, Costea I, et al. Polymorphism G80A in the reduced folate carrier gene and its relationship to methotrexate plasma levels and outcome of childhood acute lymphoblastic leukemia. Blood 2002;100:3832–3834.

175. Rocha JC, et al. Pharmacogenetics of outcome in children with acute lymphoblastic leukemia. Blood 2005;105:4752–4758.

176. Leil TA, et al. Identification and characterization of genetic variation in the folylpolyglutamate synthase gene. Cancer Res 2007;67: 8772–8782.

177. Galpin AJ, et al. Differences in folylpolyglutamate synthetase and dihydrofolate reductase expression in human B-lineage versus T-lineage leukemic

lymphoblasts: mechanisms for lineage differences in methotrexate polyglutamylation and cytotoxicity. Mol Pharmacol 1997;52:155–163.

178. Cheng Q, et al. A substrate specific functional polymorphism of human gamma-glutamyl hydrolase alters catalytic activity and methotrexate polyglutamate accumulation in acute lymphoblastic leukaemia cells. Pharmacogenetics 2004;14:557–567.

179. Cheng Q, et al. Epigenetic regulation of human gamma-glutamyl hydrolase activity in acute lymphoblastic leukemia cells. Am J Hum Genet 2006;79:264–274.

180. Frosst P, et al. A candidate genetic risk factor for vascular disease: a common mutation in methylenetetrahydrofolate reductase. Nat Genet 1995;10:111–113.

181. Weisberg I, Tran P, Christensen B, et al. A second genetic polymorphism in methylenetetrahydrofolate reductase (MTHFR) associated with decreased enzyme activity. Mol Genet Metab 1998;64:169–172.

182. Schmiegelow K. Advances in individual prediction of methotrexate toxicity: a review. Br J Haematol 2009;146:489–503.

183. Botto LD, Yang Q. 5,10-Methylenetetrahydrofolate reductase gene variants and congenital anomalies: a HuGE review. Am J Epidemiol 2000;151:862–877.

184. Pakakasama S, et al. Genetic polymorphisms of folate metabolic enzymes and toxicities of high dose methotrexate in children with acute lymphoblastic leukemia. Ann Hematol 2007;86:609–611.

185. Seidemann K, et al. MTHFR 677 (C→T) polymorphism is not relevant for prognosis or therapy-associated toxicity in pediatric NHL: results from 484 patients of multicenter trial NHL-BFM 95. Ann Hematol 2006;85:291–300.

186. Chiusolo P, et al. Preponderance of methylenetetrahydrofolate reductase C677T homozygosity among leukemia patients intolerant to methotrexate. Ann Oncol 2002;13:1915–1918.

187. Chiusolo P, et al. MTHFR polymorphisms' influence on outcome and toxicity in acute lymphoblastic leukemia patients. Leuk Res 2007;31:1669–1674.

188. Ulrich CM, et al. Pharmacogenetics of methotrexate: toxicity among marrow transplantation patients varies with the methylenetetrahydrofolate reductase C677T polymorphism. Blood 2001;98:231–234.

189. Costea I, Moghrabi A, Laverdiere C, et al. Folate cycle gene variants and chemotherapy toxicity in pediatric patients with acute lymphoblastic leukemia. Haematologica 2006;91:1113–1116.

190. Robien K, et al. Methylenetetrahydrofolate reductase and thymidylate synthase genotypes and risk of acute graft-versus-host disease following hematopoietic cell transplantation for chronic myelogenous leukemia. Biol Blood Marrow Transplant 2006;12:973–980.

191. Timuragaoglu A, Dizlek S, Uysalgil N, et al. Methylenetetrahydrofolate reductase C677T polymorphism in adult patients with lymphoproliferative disorders and its effect on chemotherapy. Ann Hematol 2006;85:863–868.

192. Krajinovic M, et al. Role of polymorphisms in MTHFR and MTHFD1 genes in the outcome of childhood acute lymphoblastic leukemia. Pharmacogenomics J 2004;4:66–72.

193. Nuckel H, Frey UH, Durig J, et al. Methylenetetrahydrofolate reductase (MTHFR) gene 677C>T and 1298A>C polymorphisms are associated with differential apoptosis of leukemic B cells in vitro and disease progression in chronic lymphocytic leukemia. Leukemia 2004;18:1816–1823.

194. Aplenc R, et al. Methylenetetrahydrofolate reductase polymorphisms and therapy response in pediatric acute lymphoblastic leukemia. Cancer Res 2005;65:2482–2487.

195. Robien K, et al. Methylenetetrahydrofolate reductase genotype affects risk of relapse after hematopoietic cell transplantation for chronic myelogenous leukemia. Clin Cancer Res 2004;10:7592–7598.

196. Saikawa Y, et al. Decreased expression of the human folate receptor mediates transport-defective methotrexate resistance in KB cells. J Biol Chem 1993;268:5293–5301.

197. Dulucq S, et al. DNA variants in the dihydrofolate reductase gene and outcome in childhood ALL. Blood 2008;111:3692–3700.

198. Al-Shakfa F, et al. DNA variants in region for noncoding interfering transcript of dihydrofolate reductase gene and outcome in childhood acute lymphoblastic leukemia. Clin Cancer Res 2009;15:6931–6938.

199. Mishra PJ, et al. A miR-24 microRNA binding-site polymorphism in dihydrofolate reductase gene leads to methotrexate resistance. Proc Natl Acad Sci U S A 2007;104:13513–13518.

200. Goto Y, et al. A novel single-nucleotide polymorphism in the 3′-untranslated region of the human dihydrofolate reductase gene with enhanced expression. Clin Cancer Res 2001;7:1952–1956.

201. Hoskins JM, Carey LA, McLeod HL. CYP2D6 and tamoxifen: DNA matters in breast cancer. Nat Rev Cancer 2009;9:576–586.

202. Schroth W, et al. Association between CYP2D6 polymorphisms and outcomes among women with early stage breast cancer treated with tamoxifen. JAMA 2009;302:1429–1436.

203. Bonanni B, et al. Polymorphism in the CYP2D6 tamoxifen-metabolizing gene influences clinical effect but not hot flashes: data from the Italian Tamoxifen Trial. J Clin Oncol 2006;24:3708–3709; author reply 3709.

204. Brauch H, Murdter TE, Eichelbaum M, et al. Pharmacogenomics of tamoxifen therapy. Clin Chem 2009;55:1770–1782.

205. Kiyotani K, et al. Significant effect of polymorphisms in CYP2D6 and ABCC2 on clinical outcomes of adjuvant tamoxifen therapy for breast cancer patients. J Clin Oncol 2010;28:1287–1293.

206. Dezentje VO, Guchelaar HJ, Nortier JW, et al. Clinical implications of CYP2D6 genotyping in tamoxifen treatment for breast cancer. Clin Cancer Res 2009;15:15–21.

207. Kelly CM, et al. Selective serotonin reuptake inhibitors and breast cancer mortality in women receiving tamoxifen: a population based cohort study. Br Med J 2010;340:c693.

208. Raftogianis RB, Wood TC, Otterness DM, et al. Phenol sulfotransferase pharmacogenetics in humans: association of common SULT1A1 alleles with TS PST phenotype. Biochem Biophys Res Commun 1997;239:298–304.

209. Nowell S, et al. Association between sulfotransferase 1A1 genotype and survival of breast cancer patients receiving tamoxifen therapy. J Natl Cancer Inst 2002;94:1635–1640.

210. Blevins-Primeau AS, et al. Functional significance of UDP-glucuronosyltransferase variants in the metabolism of active tamoxifen metabolites. Cancer Res 2009;69:1892–1900.

211. Kassner N, et al. Carbonyl reductase 1 is a predominant doxorubicin reductase in the human liver. Drug Metab Dispos 2008;36:2113–2120.

212. Bains OS, Karkling MJ, Grigliatti TA, et al. Two nonsynonymous single nucleotide polymorphisms of human carbonyl reductase 1 demonstrate reduced in vitro metabolism of daunorubicin and doxorubicin. Drug Metab Dispos 2009;37:1107–1114.

213. Lal S, et al. CBR1 and CBR3 pharmacogenetics and their influence on doxorubicin disposition in Asian breast cancer patients. Cancer Sci 2008;99:2045–2054.

214. Blanco JG, et al. Genetic polymorphisms in the carbonyl reductase 3 gene CBR3 and the NAD(P)H:quinone oxidoreductase 1 gene NQO1 in patients who developed anthracycline-related congestive heart failure after childhood cancer. Cancer 2008;112:2789–2795.

215. Fan L, et al. Genotype of human carbonyl reductase CBR3 correlates with doxorubicin disposition and toxicity. Pharmacogenet Genomics 2008;18:621–631.

216. Shen MR, Jones IM, Mohrenweiser H. Nonconservative amino acid substitution variants exist at polymorphic frequency in DNA repair genes in healthy humans. Cancer Res 1998;58:604–608.

217. Yu JJ, et al. A nucleotide polymorphism in ERCC1 in human ovarian cancer cell lines and tumor tissues. Mutat Res 1997;382:13–20.

218. Zhou W, et al. Excision repair cross-complementation group 1 polymorphism predicts overall survival in advanced non-small cell lung cancer patients treated with platinum-based chemotherapy. Clin Cancer Res 2004;10:4939–4943.

219. Dabholkar M, Vionnet J, Bostick-Bruton F, et al. Messenger RNA levels of XPAC and ERCC1 in ovarian cancer tissue correlate with response to platinum-based chemotherapy. J Clin Invest 1994;94:703–708.

220. Metzger R, et al. ERCC1 mRNA levels complement thymidylate synthase mRNA levels in predicting response and survival for gastric cancer patients receiving combination cisplatin and fluorouracil chemotherapy. J Clin Oncol 1998;16:309–316.

221. Viguier J, et al. ERCC1 codon 118 polymorphism is a predictive factor for the tumor response to oxaliplatin/5-fluorouracil combination chemotherapy in patients with advanced colorectal cancer. Clin Cancer Res 2005;11:6212–6217.

222. Isla D, et al. Single nucleotide polymorphisms and outcome in docetaxel-cisplatin-treated advanced non-small-cell lung cancer. Ann Oncol 2004;15:1194–1203.

223. Park DJ, et al. A Xeroderma pigmentosum group D gene polymorphism predicts clinical outcome to platinum-based chemotherapy in patients with advanced colorectal cancer. Cancer Res 2001;61:8654–8658.

224. Spitz MR, et al. Modulation of nucleotide excision repair capacity by XPD polymorphisms in lung cancer patients. Cancer Res 2001;61:1354–1357.

225. Qiao Y, et al. Modulation of repair of ultraviolet damage in the host-cell reactivation assay by polymorphic XPC and XPD/ERCC2 genotypes. Carcinogenesis 2002;23:295–299.

226. Hughes HB, Biehl JP, Jones AP, et al. Metabolism of isoniazid in man as related to the occurrence of peripheral neuritis. Am Rev Tuberc 1954;70:266–273.

227. Stoehlmacher J, et al. A polymorphism of the XRCC1 gene predicts for response to platinum based treatment in advanced colorectal cancer. Anticancer Res 2001;21:3075–3079.

228. Marsh S, et al. Pharmacogenetic assessment of toxicity and outcome after platinum plus taxane chemotherapy in ovarian cancer: the Scottish Randomised Trial in Ovarian Cancer. J Clin Oncol 2007;25:4528–4535.

229. Wang Z, et al. XRCC1 polymorphisms and severe toxicity in lung cancer patients treated with cisplatin-based chemotherapy in Chinese population. Lung Cancer 2008;62:99–104.

230. Sugiyama E, et al. Pharmacokinetics of gemcitabine in Japanese cancer patients: the impact of a cytidine deaminase polymorphism. J Clin Oncol 2007;25:32–42.

231. Klein TE, Altman RB. PharmGKB: the pharmacogenetics and pharmacogenomics knowledge base. Pharmacogenomics J 2004;4:1.

Physical Barriers to Drug Delivery

Brendan D. Curti

Our understanding of cancer biology has been transformed over the last 20 years. An illustration of how much our consciousness about oncology has changed can be found by looking at the topics covered in the educational sessions of the annual American Society of Clinical Oncology meetings from 1990 through 2009. In 1989, most sessions were named after cancer diagnoses, such as "Breast Cancer," or "Adult Lymphoma."[1] In 1999, educational sessions were held on angiogenesis, signal transduction, and tumor suppressor genes.[2] In 2009, the focus of the meeting was on using real-time and comprehensive knowledge of genomics, signaling pathways, proteomics, and informatics to understand the biology of tumors from individual patients.[3] Although genetic events and receptor-protein interactions are central to the biology of any cancer, insights about the macroscopic aspects of tumor physiology complement this molecular knowledge. The study of tumor physiology and the interstitial space of tumors, pioneered by Gullino in the 1960s and continued most recently by Jain and colleagues, suggests a new basis for understanding drug delivery problems in tumors.[4–7] Their work has defined tumor nodules in vivo as distinct physiologic entities with unique, biophysical properties compared to normal tissues. These properties cannot be deduced or reproduced by in vitro work because of the complex interaction of growing tumor cells with the new blood vessels they induce and the surrounding normal tissues. The microenvironment of tumor nodules can generate physical barriers to most therapeutic agents. These barriers cannot be ignored when designing new cancer treatments. Therapeutic agents that target tumor vasculature may alter some of these physiological barriers causing "vessel normalization," a term first coined in 1972[8] but now applied to the changes in the tumor vasculature induced by antiangiogenic therapies.[9]

The characteristics of tumor blood vessels and their behavior in the aggregate influence the transport processes used for the delivery of nutrients and therapeutic agents and the disposal of metabolic wastes. These vessels also have a profound secondary effect on the properties of the interstitial space of tumors. The emphasis here will be to provide a general discussion of physiologic spaces, transport variables, and the properties of tumor blood vessels. These basic concepts will be used as a framework for the discussion of intratumoral pharmacokinetics, selected models for the transport of therapeutic agents in tumors, and measurements of the physical barriers to drug delivery.

Transport Compartments and Variables

The vascular space, vascular endothelium, and vessel basement membrane must be traversed before a therapeutic molecule can percolate through the tumor interstitium to reach the cancer. Each of these physiologic spaces contains potential impediments to transport. To understand these impediments, the general mechanisms for transport of any molecule must be understood.

Convection and diffusion are the most important ways that solutes (i.e., nutrients, toxins, and therapeutic agents) are propelled through physiologic spaces. The relative contribution of these variables to transport depends on the size and physical properties of the molecule and the physiologic space it is moving through. In this discussion, transcytosis is not considered as it does not significantly influence cancer drug delivery. Each transport variable is discussed separately, followed by an explanation of how these variables interact and are influenced by the complex behavior of tumor vasculature.

Convection

Convection is defined as the movement of a solute in the direction of solvent flow. This process can be envisioned as water flowing down a pipe. If a solute (e.g., sodium chloride) is dissolved in the water, the salt molecules will travel with the water flow. Convection depends on a series of constants that describe how the solute and solvent move together, multiplied by a pressure gradient.[10]

Convection in tumors has been measured in a number of model systems. Fluorescent photobleaching has been applied to the study of single vessels in granulation tissue and VX2 carcinoma grown in a rabbit ear chamber model.[11] The velocity of the fluid moving through the interstitium of this preparation was comparable in both granulation tissue and tumor, suggesting that convective flux was the same in these model systems. Indirect data, using gravimetric or implanted chamber techniques, indicate a convective flux from the tumor to surrounding normal tissues that is 10 to 1,000 times greater than in normal tissues. These numbers reflect bulk flow and do not define the events occurring at the blood vessel–tumor interface. Data obtained from measurements of arterial and venous hematocrits in tissue-isolated tumors (i.e., tumors on a vascular pedicle with one artery entering the tumor nodule and one vein leaving it) show a marked hemoconcentration from the arterial to venous circulation.[12] In models using Walker 256 and MTW-9 mammary carcinomas, the hematocrit of the tumor efferent veins averaged 1.043 times greater than aortic arterial blood. The authors estimated that 4.5% to 10.2% of the perfusing plasma volume was lost into the tumor interstitium. This implies that plasma left the tumor blood vessels and percolated through the tumor, and it was

by vascular shunting or flow heterogeneity. This also implies that the distribution of therapeutic molecules in tumors is likely to be heterogeneous.

Tumor blood flow can be altered by several factors. Viscosity of blood in tumors has been measured and was found to be greater than normal vessels. Viscosity also varies directly with hematocrit and increases with decreasing blood pressure.[84] The reason that intratumoral blood viscosity is different from that of normal vessels is thought to stem from extravasation of plasma from leaky vessels and changes in the flow characteristics of red blood cells in tumor vessels due to turbulence.

One of the most difficult physiologic barriers to understand and influence is the heterogeneous blood flow in tumors. As described previously, IP can change tumor blood flow, but what accounts for the spatial heterogeneity of blood flow in tumors? Baish et al. devised a network model for a regular mesh of vessels and for a pair of vessels (artery and vein) of equal diameter embedded in a medium with similar characteristics to tumor interstitium. By using a statistical method known as *invasion percolation* and several measures of the heterogeneity of the vessel distribution and path, a network model for the tumor vessels was formulated.[85,86] The model looked at factors coupling vascular, transvascular, and interstitial fluid flow. As the leakiness and compliance of blood vessels were increased, blood flow was diverted away from the center of the tumor. Elevated IP altered the vascular pressure distribution and contributed to the low flow state in the tumor center. This model provides further insight into the difficulties of delivering therapeutic agents, even when tumor blood vessels are highly permeable. A number of clinical trials have been designed to increase vessel leakiness to enhance antibody or biologic response modifier penetration in the tumor.[87,88] These strategies have failed. Based on the physiological models described above, the reason is that increasing vessel leakiness increases IP and decreases blood flow in tumors. The biologics and antibodies tested are large molecules, which can only reach the center of high IP nodules by the slow process of diffusion and not by convection.

Intratumoral Pharmacokinetics in Humans

The increasing sophistication of NMR and PET scanning now permits real-time intratumoral analysis of some chemotherapy drugs in humans. One of the first reports used fluorine 19 (^{19}F)-labeled 5-FU imaged by NMR spectroscopy to estimate the accumulation of drug in metastatic adenocarcinoma deposits in humans.[89] Four out of four patients with 5-FU "trapping" in tumor deposits (time range, 20 to 78 minutes compared to 5 to 15 minutes in blood) had regression in those sites (pelvis, breast, lung, and liver). The three patients who did not show measurable amounts of 5-FU trapping did not have tumor regression. ^{18}F-labeled fluorouracil PET scanning was used to study patients with liver metastases from colorectal carcinoma.[90,91] A variety of 5-FU regimens were used (bolus, infusional, and regional) in these patients. PET scanning was done 120 minutes after drug injection. ^{18}F-labeled fluorouracil trapping was highly variable among patients and at different metastatic sites within the same patient. Patients who achieved higher drug uptake with the tumor were more likely to achieve stable disease or tumor regression and had a significantly longer mean survival.

Another approach was taken by Muller et al.,[92,93] who used microdialysis probes to measure intratumoral and normal tissue uptake of 5-FU and MTX in women with breast cancer. Patients received one of the following regimens: cyclophosphamide (CTX), MTX and 5-FU; or, 5-FU, epirubicin, and CTX. The kinetics of 5-FU clearance were similar in the tumor and subcutaneous tissues. Patients with high intratumoral 5-FU were significantly more likely to respond. Response was not associated with plasma or normal tissue uptake of drug. Similarly, in the patients having MTX measurements, plasma and tumor drug levels were not correlated and a high degree of variability among patients was noted. MTX levels in the tumor did not correlate with response.

Transport Models in Tumors

Therapeutic monoclonal antibodies, or antibodies used in imaging human tumors, have shown that the antibodies will localize to the tumor but are unevenly distributed.[94–96] Common distribution patterns include finding the antibody in the peritumoral area or focally deposited around intratumoral blood vessels. The amount of antibody measured in the tumor is also much less than predicted by in vitro binding experiments. This is illustrated by a study performed by Shockley et al.,[97] who examined a melanoma xenograft model. Melanoma-specific antigen concentrations were 15 to 70 times less than that suggested by a three-compartment kinetic model, which translated into markedly lower antibody concentrations in the tumor 72 hours after injection. Another study compared diphtheria toxin and an immunoconjugate of diphtheria toxin and the human transferrin receptor in a human xenograft tumor model.[98] Although the plasma-to-tissue transport constants were high in the tumors, the amount of immunotoxin that localized in vivo was 530 times less than predicted by in vitro binding affinities. These findings suggest that expression of antigen-binding sites or binding affinity does not predict antibody distribution. Another study used autoradiography to quantify the spatial distribution of diphtheria toxin and a variety of binding and nonbinding diphtheria toxin immunoconjugates.[99] The nonbinding conjugates and unconjugated toxin showed the most homogeneous distribution in RD2 rhabdomyosarcoma xenografts. The reduced penetration of the binding immunoconjugates was attributed to their greater MW and to antigen binding (so-called binding site barrier). The growth rate of RD2 tumor xenografts in vivo was inhibited more effectively by the diphtheria toxin, which penetrated into the tumor, but not by immunoconjugate with lower penetration. In vitro growth retardation by the two agents was similar. The authors concluded that tumor response may be correlated with the spatial distribution of the therapeutic agent.

In the development of monoclonal antibodies, two of the central issues are the binding affinity of the antibody and the distribution of antigen within the tumor. Fujimori et al.[100] developed a spherical tumor nodule model that looked at the distribution of antibodies with varying affinities and different tumor antigen concentrations. Their model also took into account the effective interstitial diffusion coefficient, capillary permeability, initial concentration of the antibody in the serum, and valence of the antibody. This modeling scheme showed that as the number of antibody-antigen binding events increased, the percolation of the antibody through the tumor decreased. This reduced the heterogeneity of antibody distribution and produced a binding site barrier. Direct evidence for the binding site barrier hypothesis was obtained using double-labeled immunohistochemistry and autoradiography.[101] Monoclonal antibody D3 was given to guinea pigs bearing line 10 carcinomas implanted intradermally. A low level of D3 antibody binding to antigen significantly impaired antibody penetration in the tumor. An irrelevant antibody distributed uniformly through the tumor, indicating that other physiologic barriers were not present.

Sung et al.[102] developed a plasma and tissue compartmental model that accounted for interstitial fluid flow and estimated antibody-antigen binding. The model predicted that increasing antibody affinity at low doses of antibody would result in increased tumor uptake. When antigen saturation was approached, binding affinity had a smaller effect. Another implication of this model was that if antigen density could be increased, antibody localization also could be increased. This point was illustrated by an animal model comparing two different melanomas with different surface antigen concentrations grown subcutaneously. The melanoma with the greater antigen density (SK-MEL-2) had greater antibody uptake. Other researchers have concluded that antigen density is of salient importance to antibody distribution in model systems that used antibodies to epidermal growth factor receptors, carcinoembryonic antigen, and cell surface ovarian carcinoma antigens.[103–105]

Another modeling approach incorporated IP as a variable to explain heterogeneous antibody distribution in tumors. In the model described by Baxter et al.,[106] IP opposed the tendency of fluid and macromolecules to leave tumor blood vessels. It also resulted in net convective forces that are directed radially outward from the center of the tumor and are of a magnitude sufficient to counteract the tendency of any molecule present in the area surrounding the tumor nodule to diffuse back into the interior of the tumor. The human IP data reviewed above indicate an IP pressure gradient from the tumor to surrounding tissues exceeding 30 mm Hg in some tumor types, which is a much larger gradient than that explored in this model system, which modeled 5 mm Hg IP gradients. Thus, outward convection in human tumors is likely to be even more significant at impairing antibody targeting. A number of other assumptions were made in this IP-based antibody distribution model, including, that the tumor was uniformly perfused, that IP was spatially dependent, and that the macromolecules modeled were free to move in the tumor interstitium (e.g., no binding-site barrier). With these constraints, the model predicted that smaller molecules such as Fab fragments reached higher concentrations for a given radial position in the tumor than IgG after bolus injections. Continuous infusion of the antibody resulted in higher intratumoral concentrations of both IgG and Fab. The distribution of IgG, Fab2, of Fab predicted by the model was heterogeneous. By modeling IP and not the binding characteristics of the therapeutic agent, it was concluded that tumors would have regions with different concentrations of macromolecules delivered intravenously.

Gene therapy generally requires large vectors for delivery, such as engineered viral particles, measuring 100 to 300 nm in diameter. Particles of this size must traverse transvascular pores in tumor vessels. Hobbs et al.[107] studied this problem in human and murine tumors implanted in dorsal skin-fold chambers or cranial windows. They also tested the influence of hormone-induced tumor regression on transvascular pore size. Pore size was measured between

200 nm and 1.2 µm. Subcutaneous tumor vessels had larger pores than intracranial tumor vessels, but hormone-induced tumor regression diminished the size of transvascular pores in subcutaneous tumors. Thus, the delivery of gene vector therapy or liposome-encapsulated therapeutics may face additional barriers to delivery. The model also illustrates that the physical properties of tumor vessels may differ by site of tumor implantation, even when using the same tumor cell lines.

A mathematical model was developed to characterize the distribution of herpes simplex virus (HSV) in a tumor spheroid after intratumoral administration.[108] The assumption made by many extant clinical trials of oncolytic viral vector vaccines is that intratumoral injection of the vectors will efficiently distribute virus within the injected tumor deposit. The model took into account the binding of virus to tumor cell surface (via the interaction between viral glycoprotein and tumor cell surface heparan sulfate), internalization of the virus and the limits of internalization, viral degradation, the volume of injection, collagen content of the tumor interstitium, and diffusion of virus through tumor interstitium. The size of the tumor spheroid used in the modeling was 0.05 cm, which is considerably smaller than lesions that would be injected in a human clinical trial. The model demonstrated that viral binding and internalization were much more rapid than diffusion. Diffusion coefficients were chosen based on data available in the medical literature and suggest that as collagen content increases, the diffusion of virus decreases. The model suggested that it would take an HSV viral particle 22 minutes to traverse one tumor cell diameter. Due to the rapid internalization of virus, very little diffuses beyond the initial site of injection. By decreasing binding affinity of the virus, spread of the virus by diffusion was enhanced by 1.5-fold. These data parallel the findings of hindered antibody diffusion by a binding site barrier. Decreased binding affinity may enhance diffusion of therapeutic agents but also would be expected to decrease efficacy if the drug has a lower affinity for its target. It is not clear how to balance binding site barriers with target affinity to optimize penetration and efficacy.

The focus of discussion has been on the physiologic forces that influence drug and biologic delivery to tumors. Do these same forces influence the metastatic process (e.g., the delivery of cancer cells to new sites in the body)? As discussed above, cancer cells can form a part of the vascular endothelium of tumors and should allow ready access of tumor cells to the circulation. The physical movement of a cancer cell from the wall of a tumor vessel to the general circulation has not been observed directly, but there is a growing literature quantifying CTC and how this finding influences survival. Immunomagnetic selection of circulating endothelial cells using anti-EpCAM antibodies is the most commonly used technique currently for assessing the number of CTC in a 7.5-mL sample of blood. For instance, Liu et al.[109] have demonstrated that finding five or more CTC in the peripheral of blood of women with metastatic breast cancer during chemotherapy or estrogen receptor modulators correlates with diminished progression-free survival and lower incidence of radiographic responses. Similar data exist for prostate, lung, colon, and ovarian cancers.

Although there are many promoters of angiogenesis, VEGF is the most important mediator in this process. There are different VEGF subtypes, and VEGF-C is also an important driver of lymphangiogenesis. Isaka et al.[110] showed that VEGF-C causes hyperplasia of both normal and peritumoral lymphatics in B16F10 melanomas in a murine model. Evans blue dye and intravital microscopy were used to characterize lymph vessel morphology and function, as viewed through dorsal skin chambers. The newly induced lymph channels were functional but displayed retrograde flow. The same group also measured the number of tumor cells in draining lymph nodes and lymph vessels.[111] They used a VEGF-C-overexpressing B16F10 melanoma cell line. There was a striking 200-fold increase in the number of tumor cells found in draining lymph nodes. Anti-VEGF antibodies suppressed this process. These data support that the aberrant physiology of tumor blood and lymph vessels promote the spread of malignant cells.

Conclusions

The heterogeneity of tumor blood vessels and blood flow, the varied composition of the tumor interstitium, and disturbed convection and diffusion in the interstitial space of tumors all create significant physical barriers to the delivery of therapeutic agents to neoplastic cells in vivo. This vascular chaos creates an extremely hypoxic and acidic milieu around the growing tumor. How could this toxic environment possibly be an advantage to a growing tumor other than its ability to decrease the penetration and effectiveness of anticancer treatments? Wouldn't tumor cells survive and grow even more rapidly if their growth induced an environment with normal oxygen and pH, with a constant supply of energy and other nutrients? In vitro experiments with tumor cell lines strongly support that cancer cells grow best in conditions that favor normal cell growth.

The answer to these questions cannot yet be found in the medical literature. A possible answer comes from the observation that the process of angiogenesis and lymphangiogenesis supports the metastatic process. The cancer is less "concerned" with the survival or size of any solitary nodule but rather strives to assure the spread of the cancer. This is in stark contrast to normal organs which limit their size within narrow constraints, even during conditions of physiologic stress or injury and repair. In geometric terms, one could say that tumor desires to grow to a considerably larger degree than any normal organ and is not significantly limited by nutrient supply or physiologic stress to which it is subjected. This is in concert with the experience of every oncologist that patients almost always die from metastatic disease and rarely from local complications of the cancer.

The vasculature has become an important target in cancer treatment, but no vascular targeting agent has cured a patient with advanced cancer. Observations showing rapid changes in the flow properties of tumor vasculature after VEGF-targeted therapy are an important insight, yet the full potential of this strategy has not been realized. The ability of cancers to survive vascular targeting and spread causing eventual death of the patient underscores the complexity of the angiogenic process and the multiple mechanisms of resistance that cancers employ.

These considerations of tumor vasculature and its influence on drug delivery point out the complex interplay between tumor and the vascular system. The study of individual cancer cells has greatly advanced our understanding of the genetics and regulatory pathways in cancer. Much further work is needed to understand the larger-scale behavior of cancers cells when they are organized into tumors, and how these "cancer organs" influence the vasculature, immune system, and the function of normal organs.

References

1. 1990 Program and Proceedings, American Society of Clinical Oncology Annual Meeting, Washington, DC.
2. 1999 Program and Proceedings, American Society of Clinical Oncology Annual Meeting, Atlanta, GA.
3. 2009 ASCO Annual Meeting Proceedings. J Clin Oncol 2009;27(155): 1s–790s.
4. Gullino PM, Clark SH, Grantham FH. The interstitial fluid of solid tumors. Cancer Res 1964;24:780–794.
5. Gullino PM, Grantham FH. Studies on the exchange of fluids between host and tumor. I. A method for growing "tissue-isolated" tumors in laboratory animals. J Natl Cancer Inst 1961;27:679–693.
6. Jain RK. Delivery of novel therapeutic agents in tumors: physiological barriers and strategies. J Natl Cancer Inst 1989;81:570–576.
7. Jain RK, Tong RT, Munn LL. Effect of vascular normalization by antiangiogenic therapy on interstitial hypertension, peritumor edema, and lymphatic metastasis: insights from a mathematical model. Cancer Res 2007;67:2729–2735.
8. Le Serve AW, Hellmann K. Metastases and the normalization of tumour blood vessels by ICRF 159: a new type of drug action. Br Med J 1972;1:597–601.
9. Winkler F, Kozin SV, Tong RT, et al. Kinetics of vascular normalization by VEGFR2 blockade governs brain tumor response to radiation: role of oxygenation, angiopoietin-1, and matrix metalloproteinases. Cancer Cell 2004;6:553–563.
10. Jain RK. Transport of molecules in the tumor interstitium: a review. Cancer Res 1987;47:3039–3051.
11. Chary SR, Jain RK. Direct measurement of interstitial convection and diffusion of albumin in normal and neoplastic tissues by fluorescence photobleaching. Proc Natl Acad Sci U S A 1989;86:5385–5389.
12. Butler TP, Grantham FH, Gullino PM. Bulk transfer of fluid in the interstitial compartment of mammary tumors. Cancer Res 1975;35:3084–3088.
13. Clauss MA, Jain RK. Interstitial transport of rabbit and sheep antibodies in normal and neoplastic tissues. Cancer Res 1990;50:3487–3492.
14. Padhani AR, Liu G, Koh DM, et al. Diffusion-weighted magnetic resonance imaging as a cancer biomarker: consensus and recommendations. Neoplasia 2009;11:102–125.
15. Charles-Edwards EM, deSouza NM. Diffusion-weighted magnetic resonance imaging and its application to cancer. Cancer Imaging 2006;6:135–143.
16. Kilickesmez O, Bayramoglu S, Inci E, et al. Value of apparent diffusion coefficient measurement for discrimination of focal benign and malignant hepatic masses. J Med Imaging Radiat Oncol 2009;53:50–55.
17. Chauhan VP, Lanning RM, Diop-Frimpong B, et al. Multiscale measurements distinguish cellular and interstitial hindrances to diffusion in vivo. Biophys J 2009;97:330–336.
18. Gullino PM, Grantham FH, Clark SH. The collagen content of transplanted tumors. Cancer Res 1962;22:1031–1037.
19. Gullino PM, Grantham FH, Smith SH. The interstitial water space of tumors. Cancer Res 1965;25:727–731.
20. O'Connor SW, Bale WF. Accessibility of circulating immunoglobulin G to the extravascular compartment of solid rat tumors. Cancer Res 1984;44:3719–3723.
21. Sylven B, Bois I. Protein content and enzymatic assays of interstitial fluid from some normal tissues and transplanted mouse tumors. Cancer Res 1960;20:831–836.
22. Choi HU, Meyer K, Swarm R. Mucopolysaccharide and protein—polysaccharide of a transplantable rat chondrosarcoma. Proc Natl Acad Sci U S A 1971;68:877–879.
23. Thistlethwaite AJ, Leeper DB, Moylan DJ III, et al. pH distribution in human tumors. Int J Radiat Oncol Biol Phys 1985;11:1647–1652.
24. Ashby BS. pH studies in human malignant tumors. Lancet 1966;2:312–315.

25. Newell K, Franchi A, Pouyssegur J, et al. Studies with glycolysis-deficient cells suggest that production of lactic acid is not the only cause of tumor acidity. Proc Natl Acad Sci U S A 1993;90:1127–1131.

26. Vaupel P, Kallinowski F, Okunieff P. Blood flow, oxygen and nutrient supply, and metabolic microenvironment of human tumors: a review. Cancer Res 1989;49:6449–6465.

27. Vaupel P, Schlenger K, Knoop C, et al. Oxygenation of human tumors: evaluation of tissue oxygen distribution in breast cancers by computerized O2 tension measurements. Cancer Res 1991;51:3316–3322.

28. Helmlinger G, Yuan F, Dellian M, et al. Interstitial pH and pO2 gradients in solid tumors in vivo: high-resolution measurements reveal a lack of correlation. Nat Med 1997;3:177–182.

29. Durand RE, LePard NE. Modulation of tumor hypoxia by conventional chemotherapeutic agents. Int J Radiat Oncol Biol Phys 1994;29:481–486.

30. Loeffler DA, Juneau EA, Heppner GH. Natural killer-cell activity under conditions reflective of tumour micro-environment. Intl J Cancer 1991;48:895–899.

31. Loeffler DA, Juneau PL, Masserant S. Influence of tumour physico-chemical conditions on interleukin-2-stimulated lymphocyte proliferation. Br J Cancer 1992;66:619–622.

32. Caldwell CC, Kojima H, Lukashev D, et al. Differential effects of physiologically relevant hypoxic conditions on T lymphocyte development and effector functions. J Immunol 2001;167:6140–6149.

33. Guyton AC. A concept of negative interstitial pressure based on pressures in implanted perforated capsules. Circ Res 1963;12:399–414.

34. Wiig H, Reed RK, Aukland K. Measurement of interstitial fluid pressure: comparison of methods. Ann Biomed Eng 1986;14:139–151.

35. Hargens AR, Mubarak SJ, Owen CA, et al. Interstitial fluid pressure in muscle and compartment syndromes in man. Microvasc Res 1977;14:1–10.

36. McMaster PD. The pressure and interstitial resistance prevailing in the normal and edematous skin of animals and man. J Exp Med 1946;84:473–494.

37. Young JS, Lumsden CE, Stalker AL. The significance of the tissue pressure of normal testicular and of neoplastic (Brown-Pearce carcinoma) tissue in the rabbit. J Pathol Bacteriol 1950;62:313–333.

38. Boucher Y, Kirkwood JM, Opacic D, et al. Interstitial hypertension in superficial metastatic melanomas in humans. Cancer Res 1991;51:6691–6694.

39. Curti BD, Urba WJ, Alvord WG, et al. Interstitial pressure of subcutaneous nodules in melanoma and lymphoma patients: changes during treatment. Cancer Res 1993;53:2204–2207.

40. Gutmann R, Leunig M, Feyh J, et al. Interstitial hypertension in head and neck tumors in patients: correlation with tumor size. Cancer Res 1992;52:1993–1995.

41. Less JR, Posner MC, Boucher Y, et al. Interstitial hypertension in human breast and colorectal tumors. Cancer Res 1992;52:6371–6374.

42. Roh HD, Boucher Y, Kalnicki S, et al. Interstitial hypertension in carcinoma of uterine cervix in patients: possible correlation with tumor oxygenation and radiation response. Cancer Res 1991;51:6695–6698.

43. Boucher Y, Lee I, Jain RK. Lack of general correlation between interstitial fluid pressure and oxygen partial pressure in solid tumors. Microvasc Res 1995;50:175–182.

44. Boucher Y, Jain RK. Microvascular pressure is the principal driving force for interstitial hypertension in solid tumors: implications for vascular collapse. Cancer Res 1992;52:5110–5114.

45. Boucher Y, Leunig M, Jain RK. Tumor angiogenesis and interstitial hypertension. Cancer Res 1996;56:4264–4266.

46. Netti PA, Baxter LT, Boucher Y, et al. Time-dependent behavior of interstitial fluid pressure in solid tumors: implications for drug delivery. Cancer Res 1995;55:5451–5458.

47. Boucher Y, Baxter LT, Jain RK. Interstitial pressure gradients in tissue-isolated and subcutaneous tumors: implications for therapy. Cancer Res 1990;50:4478–4484.

48. Zlotecki RA, Baxter LT, Boucher Y, et al. Pharmacologic modification of tumor blood flow and interstitial fluid pressure in a human tumor xenograft: network analysis and mechanistic interpretation. Microvasc Res 1995;50:429–443.

49. Schwartzentruber DJ. Guidelines for the safe administration of high-dose interleukin-2. J Immunother 2001;24:287–293.

50. Escudier B, Eisen T, Stadler WM, et al. Sorafenib in advanced clear-cell renal-cell carcinoma. N Engl J Med 2007;356:125–134.

51. Motzer RJ, Rini BI, Bukowski RM, et al. Sunitinib in patients with metastatic renal cell carcinoma. JAMA 2006;295:2516–2524.

52. Yang JC, Haworth L, Sherry RM, et al. A randomized trial of bevacizumab, an anti-vascular endothelial growth factor antibody, for metastatic renal cancer. N Engl J Med 2003;349:427–434.

53. Milosevic MF, Fyles AW, Hill RP. The relationship between elevated interstitial fluid pressure and blood flow in tumors: a bioengineering analysis. Int J Radiat Oncol Biol Phys 1999;43:1111–1123.

54. Lee I, Demhartner TJ, Boucher Y, et al. Effect of hemodilution and resuscitation on tumor interstitial fluid pressure, blood flow, and oxygenation. Microvasc Res 1994;48:1–12.

55. Tong RT, Boucher Y, Kozin SV, et al. Vascular normalization by vascular endothelial growth factor receptor 2 blockade induces a pressure gradient across the vasculature and improves drug penetration in tumors. Cancer Res 2004;64:3731–3736.

56. Fukumura D, Gohongi T, Kadambi A, et al. Predominant role of endothelial nitric oxide synthase in vascular endothelial growth factor-induced angiogenesis and vascular permeability. Proc Natl Acad Sci U S A 2001;98:2604–2609.

57. Kashiwagi S, Izumi Y, Gohongi T, et al. NO mediates mural cell recruitment and vessel morphogenesis in murine melanomas and tissue-engineered blood vessels. J Clin Invest 2005;115:1816–1827.

58. Kashiwagi S, Tsukada K, Xu L, et al. Perivascular nitric oxide gradients normalize tumor vasculature. Nat Med 2008;14:255–257.

59. Lahdenranta J, Hagendoorn J, Padera TP, et al. Endothelial nitric oxide synthase mediates lymphangiogenesis and lymphatic metastasis. Cancer Res 2009;69:2801–2808.

60. Willett CG, Duda DG, di Tomaso E, et al. Efficacy, safety, and biomarkers of neoadjuvant bevacizumab, radiation therapy, and fluorouracil in rectal cancer: a multidisciplinary phase II study. J Clin Oncol 2009;27:3020–3026.

61. Willett CG, Boucher Y, di Tomaso E, et al. Direct evidence that the VEGF-specific antibody bevacizumab has antivascular effects in human rectal cancer. Nat Med 2004;10:145–147.

62. Zhu AX, Sahani DV, Duda DG, et al. Efficacy, safety, and potential biomarkers of sunitinib monotherapy in advanced hepatocellular carcinoma: a phase II study. J Clin Oncol 2009;27:3027–3035.

63. Batchelor TT, Sorensen AG, di Tomaso E, et al. AZD2171, a pan-VEGF receptor tyrosine kinase inhibitor, normalizes tumor vasculature and alleviates edema in glioblastoma patients. Cancer Cell 2007;11:83–95.

64. Sorensen AG, Batchelor TT, Zhang WT, et al. A "vascular normalization index" as potential mechanistic biomarker to predict survival after a single dose of cediranib in recurrent glioblastoma patients. Cancer Res 2009;69:5296–5300.

65. Miller AB, Hoogstraten B, Staquet M, et al. Reporting results of cancer treatment. Cancer 1981;47:207–214.

66. Therasse P, Arbuck SG, Eisenhauer EA, et al. New guidelines to evaluate the response to treatment in solid tumors. European Organization for Research and Treatment of Cancer, National Cancer Institute of the United States, National Cancer Institute of Canada. J Natl Cancer Inst 2000;92:205–216.

67. Swabb EA, Wei J, Gullino PM. Diffusion and convection in normal and neoplastic tissues. Cancer Res 1974;34:2814–2822.

68. Jain RK, Baxter LT. Mechanisms of heterogeneous distribution of monoclonal antibodies and other macromolecules in tumors: significance of elevated interstitial pressure. Cancer Res 1988;48:7022–7032.

69. Tunggal JK, Cowan DS, Shaikh H, et al. Penetration of anticancer drugs through solid tissue: a factor that limits the effectiveness of chemotherapy for solid tumors. Clin Cancer Res 1999;5:1583–1586.

70. Kedem O, Katchalsky A. Thermodynamic analysis of the permeability of biological membranes to non-electrolytes. 1958. Biochim Biophys Acta 1989;1000:413–430.

71. Brock TA, Dvorak HF, Senger DR. Tumor-secreted vascular permeability factor increases cytosolic Ca2+ and von Willebrand factor release in human endothelial cells. Am J Pathol 1991;138:213–221.

72. Dvorak HF, Nagy JA, Dvorak JT, et al. Identification and characterization of the blood vessels of solid tumors that are leaky to circulating macromolecules. Am J Pathol 1988;133:95–109.

73. Keck PJ, Hauser SD, Krivi G, et al. Vascular permeability factor, an endothelial cell mitogen related to PDGF. Science 1989;246:1309–1312.

74. Senger DR, Perruzzi CA, Feder J, et al. A highly conserved vascular permeability factor secreted by a variety of human and rodent tumor cell lines. Cancer Res 1986;46:5629–5632.

75. Yeo KT, Wang HH, Nagy JA, et al. Vascular permeability factor (vascular endothelial growth factor) in guinea pig and human tumor and inflammatory effusions. Cancer Res 1993;53:2912–2918.

76. Vaupel P, Kluge M, Ambroz MC. Laser Doppler flowmetry in subepidermal tumours and in normal skin of rats during localized ultrasound hyperthermia. Int J Hyperthermia 1988;4:307–321.

77. Mantyla M, Heikkonen J, Perkkio J. Regional blood flow in human tumours measured with argon, krypton and xenon. Br J Radiol 1988;61: 379–382.

78. Tveit E, Weiss L, Lundstam S, et al. Perfusion characteristics and norepinephrine reactivity of human renal carcinoma. Cancer Res 1987;47:4709–4713.

79. Eskey CJ, Koretsky AP, Domach MM, et al. 2H-nuclear magnetic resonance imaging of tumor blood flow: spatial and temporal heterogeneity in a tissue-isolated mammary adenocarcinoma. Cancer Res 1992;52: 6010–6019.

80. Alexander AA, Nazarian LN, Capuzzi DM Jr, et al. Color Doppler sonographic detection of tumor flow in superficial melanoma metastases: histologic correlation. J Ultrasound Med 1998;17:123–126.

81. Lyng H, Skretting A, Rofstad EK. Blood flow in six human melanoma xenograft lines with different growth characteristics. Cancer Res 1992; 52:584–592.

82. Sevick EM, Jain RK. Geometric resistance to blood flow in solid tumors perfused ex vivo: effects of tumor size and perfusion pressure. Cancer Res 1989;49:3506–3512.

83. Eskey CJ, Wolmark N, McDowell CL, et al. Residence time distributions of various tracers in tumors: implications for drug delivery and blood flow measurement. J Natl Cancer Inst 1994;86:293–299.

84. Sevick EM, Jain RK. Viscous resistance to blood flow in solid tumors: effect of hematocrit on intratumor blood viscosity. Cancer Res 1989;49:3513–3519.

85. Baish JW, Gazit Y, Berk DA, et al. Role of tumor vascular architecture in nutrient and drug delivery: an invasion percolation-based network model. Microvasc Res 1996;51:327–346.

86. Gazit Y, Baish JW, Safabakhsh N, et al. Fractal characteristics of tumor vascular architecture during tumor growth and regression. Microcirculation 1997;4:395–402.

87. LeBerthon B, Khawli LA, Alauddin M, et al. Enhanced tumor uptake of macromolecules induced by a novel vasoactive interleukin 2 immunoconjugate. Cancer Res 1991;51:2694–2698.

88. Schultz KR, Badger CC, Dombi GW, et al. Effect of interleukin-2 on biodistribution of monoclonal antibody in tumor and normal tissues in mice bearing SL-2 thymoma. J Natl Cancer Inst 1992;84:109–113.

89. Presant CA, Wolf W, Albright MJ, et al. Human tumor fluorouracil trapping: clinical correlations of in vivo 19F nuclear magnetic resonance spectroscopy pharmacokinetics. J Clin Oncol 1990;8:1868–1873.

90. Dimitrakopoulou-Strauss A, Strauss LG, Schlag P, et al. Fluorine-18-fluorouracil to predict therapy response in liver metastases from colorectal carcinoma. J Nucl Med 1998;39:1197–1202.

91. Moehler M, Dimitrakopoulou-Strauss A, Gutzler F, et al. 18F-labeled fluorouracil positron emission tomography and the prognoses of colorectal carcinoma patients with metastases to the liver treated with 5-fluorouracil. Cancer 1998;83:245–253.

92. Muller M, Brunner M, Schmid R, et al. Interstitial methotrexate kinetics in primary breast cancer lesions. Cancer Res 1998;58:2982–2985.

93. Muller M, Mader RM, Steiner B, et al. 5-fluorouracil kinetics in the interstitial tumor space: clinical response in breast cancer patients. Cancer Res 1997;57:2598–2601.

94. Begent RH, Pedley RB. Antibody targeted therapy in cancer: comparison of murine and clinical studies. Cancer Treat Rev 1990;17:373–378.

95. Larson SM. Radioimmunology. Imaging and therapy. Cancer 1991;67:1253–1260.

96. Shockley TR, Lin K, Nagy JA, et al. Spatial distribution of tumor-specific monoclonal antibodies in human melanoma xenografts. Cancer Res 1992;52:367–376.

97. Shockley TR, Lin K, Sung C, et al. A quantitative analysis of tumor specific monoclonal antibody uptake by human melanoma xenografts: effects of antibody immunological properties and tumor antigen expression levels. Cancer Res 1992;52:357–366.

98. Sung C, Youle RJ, Dedrick RL. Pharmacokinetic analysis of immunotoxin uptake in solid tumors: role of plasma kinetics, capillary permeability, and binding. Cancer Res 1990;50:7382–7392.

99. Juweid M, Neumann R, Paik C, et al. Micropharmacology of monoclonal antibodies in solid tumors: direct experimental evidence for a binding site barrier. Cancer Res 1992;52:5144–5153.

100. Fujimori K, Covell DG, Fletcher JE, et al. A modeling analysis of monoclonal antibody percolation through tumors: a binding-site barrier. J Nucl Med 1990;31:1191–1198.

101. Sung C, Dedrick RL, Hall WA, et al. The spatial distribution of immunotoxins in solid tumors: assessment by quantitative autoradiography. Cancer Res 1993;53:2092–2099.

102. Sung C, Shockley TR, Morrison PF, et al. Predicted and observed effects of antibody affinity and antigen density on monoclonal antibody uptake in solid tumors. Cancer Res 1992;52:377–384.

103. Boerman O, Massuger L, Makkink K, et al. Comparative in vitro binding characteristics and biodistribution in tumor-bearing athymic mice of anti-ovarian carcinoma monoclonal antibodies. Anticancer Res 1990;10:1289–1295.

104. Goldenberg A, Masui H, Divgi C, et al. Imaging of human tumor xenografts with an indium-111-labeled anti-epidermal growth factor receptor monoclonal antibody. J Natl Cancer Inst 1989;81:1616–1625.

105. Philben VJ, Jakowatz JG, Beatty BG, et al. The effect of tumor CEA content and tumor size on tissue uptake of indium 111-labeled anti-CEA monoclonal antibody. Cancer 1986;57:571–576.

106. Baxter LT, Zhu H, Mackensen DG, et al. Biodistribution of monoclonal antibodies: scale-up from mouse to human using a physiologically based pharmacokinetic model. Cancer Res 1995;55:4611–4622.

107. Hobbs SK, Monsky WL, Yuan F, et al. Regulation of transport pathways in tumor vessels: role of tumor type and microenvironment. Proc Natl Acad Sci U S A 1998;95:4607–4612.

108. Mok W, Stylianopoulos T, Boucher Y, et al. Mathematical modeling of herpes simplex virus distribution in solid tumors: implications for cancer gene therapy. Clin Cancer Res 2009;15:2352–2360.

109. Liu MC, Shields PG, Warren RD, et al. Circulating tumor cells: a useful predictor of treatment efficacy in metastatic breast cancer. J Clin Oncol 2009;27:5153–5159.

110. Isaka N, Padera TP, Hagendoorn J, et al. Peritumor lymphatics induced by vascular endothelial growth factor-C exhibit abnormal function. Cancer Res 2004;64:4400–4404.

111. Hoshida T, Isaka N, Hagendoorn J, et al. Imaging steps of lymphatic metastasis reveals that vascular endothelial growth factor-C increases metastasis by increasing delivery of cancer cells to lymph nodes: therapeutic implications. Cancer Res 2006;66:8065–8075.

Section II
Cytotoxic Agents

Antifolates

Bruce A. Chabner and Carmen J. Allegra

The folate-dependent enzymes represent attractive targets for antitumor chemotherapy because of their critical role in the synthesis of the nucleotide precursors of DNA (Fig. 8-1). In 1948, Farber et al.[1] were the first to show that aminopterin, a 4-amino analog of folic acid, could inhibit the proliferation of leukemic cells and produce remissions in acute leukemia cases. Their findings ushered in the era of antimetabolite chemotherapy and generated great interest in the antifolate class of agents. Since then, antifolate compounds have become extremely valuable in the treatment of hematologic and nonhematologic malignancies as well as nonneoplastic disorders, including rheumatoid arthritis,[2] psoriasis,[3] and bacterial, fungal, and parasitic infections.[4] High-dose regimens have further expanded the role of methotrexate (MTX) and have become the mainstay of therapy for primary central nervous system lymphomas and for prevention of meningeal leukemia,[5] where it has replaced cranial irradiation in children with acute lymphoblastic leukemia (ALL). At this time, the antifolates are one of the best understood and most versatile of all the cancer chemotherapeutic drug classes. The key features of MTX, the most commonly used antifolate, are presented in Table 8-1.

Mechanism of Action

Substitution of an amino group for the hydroxyl at the 4-N position of the pteridine ring critically changes the structure of folate compounds, leading to their enzyme inhibitory and antitumor activities. This change transforms the molecule from a substrate to a tight-binding inhibitor of dihydrofolate reductase (DHFR), a key enzyme in intracellular folate homeostasis. The critical importance of DHFR stems from the fact that folic acid compounds are active as coenzymes only in their fully reduced, tetrahydrofolate, form. Two specific tetrahydrofolates play essential roles as one-carbon carriers in the synthesis of DNA precursors. The cofactor 10-formyltetrahydrofolate provides its one-carbon group for the de novo synthesis of purines in reactions mediated by glycineamide ribonucleotide (GAR) transformylase and aminoimidazole carboxamide ribonucleotide (AICAR) transformylase. A second cofactor, 5,10-methylenetetrahydrofolate (CH_2-FH_4), donates its one-carbon group to the reductive methylation reaction that converts deoxyuridylate (dUMP) to thymidylate (TMP) (Fig. 8-2). In addition to contributing a one-carbon group, CH_2FH_4 is oxidized to dihydrofolate (FH_2), which must then be reduced to tetrahydrofolate by the enzyme DHFR to enable it to rejoin the pool of active reduced-folate cofactors. In actively proliferating tumor cells, inhibition of DHFR by

MTX or other 2,4-diamino antifolates leads to an accumulation of folates in the inactive FH_2 form, with variable depletion of reduced folates.[6–12] Folate depletion, however, does not fully account for the metabolic inhibition associated with antifolate treatment because the critical reduced-folate pools may be relatively preserved even in the presence of cytotoxic concentrations of MTX. Additional factors may contribute to MTX-associated cytotoxicity, including metabolism of the parent compound to polyglutamated derivatives and the accumulation of dihydrofolate polyglutamates (PGs) as a consequence of DHFR inhibition.[6,7,13–15] MTX and dihydrofolate PGs represent potent direct inhibitors of the folate-dependent enzymes of thymidylate and purine biosynthesis.[16–19] Thus, inhibition of DNA biosynthesis by 2,4-diamino folates is a multifactorial process consisting of both partial depletion of reduced-folate substrates and direct inhibition of folate-dependent enzymes. The relative roles of each of these mechanisms in determining antifolate-associated metabolic inhibition may depend on factors specific to various cancer cell lines and tumors.

Chemical Structure

The physiological folate structure, as shown in Figure 8-1, consists of a pteridine ring, which connects via an N-10 bridge to benzoic acid and thence to a terminal glutamic acid. Various heterocyclic compounds with the 2,4-diamino configuration may bind to DHFR and have antifolate activity in microbial organisms and include pyrimidine analogs such as pyrimethamine and trimethoprim[18–25]; the antimicrobial compounds are in general weak inhibitors of the mammalian DHFR. The antifolates with DHFR inhibitory activity conserve the inhibitory 2,4-diamino configuration but have the added structural features of folates; these compounds include classical pteroyl glutamates such as aminopterin and MTX[2]; compounds with an altered pteridine ring, such as those with replacement of the 5- or 8-N position, or both, with a carbon atom (the quinazolines) lipid-soluble derivatives lacking a terminal glutamate (trimetrexate and piritrexim[22,23]); or folate-like compounds with alterations in the N-10 bridge (pralatrexate[24]). Each of these changes alters the pharmacological properties (transport, enzyme binding, and polyglutamation) of the folate inhibitory molecule, as described below. Investigators have designed antifolate analogs directed at targets other than DHFR, such as those folate-dependent enzymes required for the de novo synthesis of purines and thymidylate synthase (TS). Potent TS inhibitors, which utilize physiological pathways for transport and polyglutamation, include raltitrexed (ZD1694,

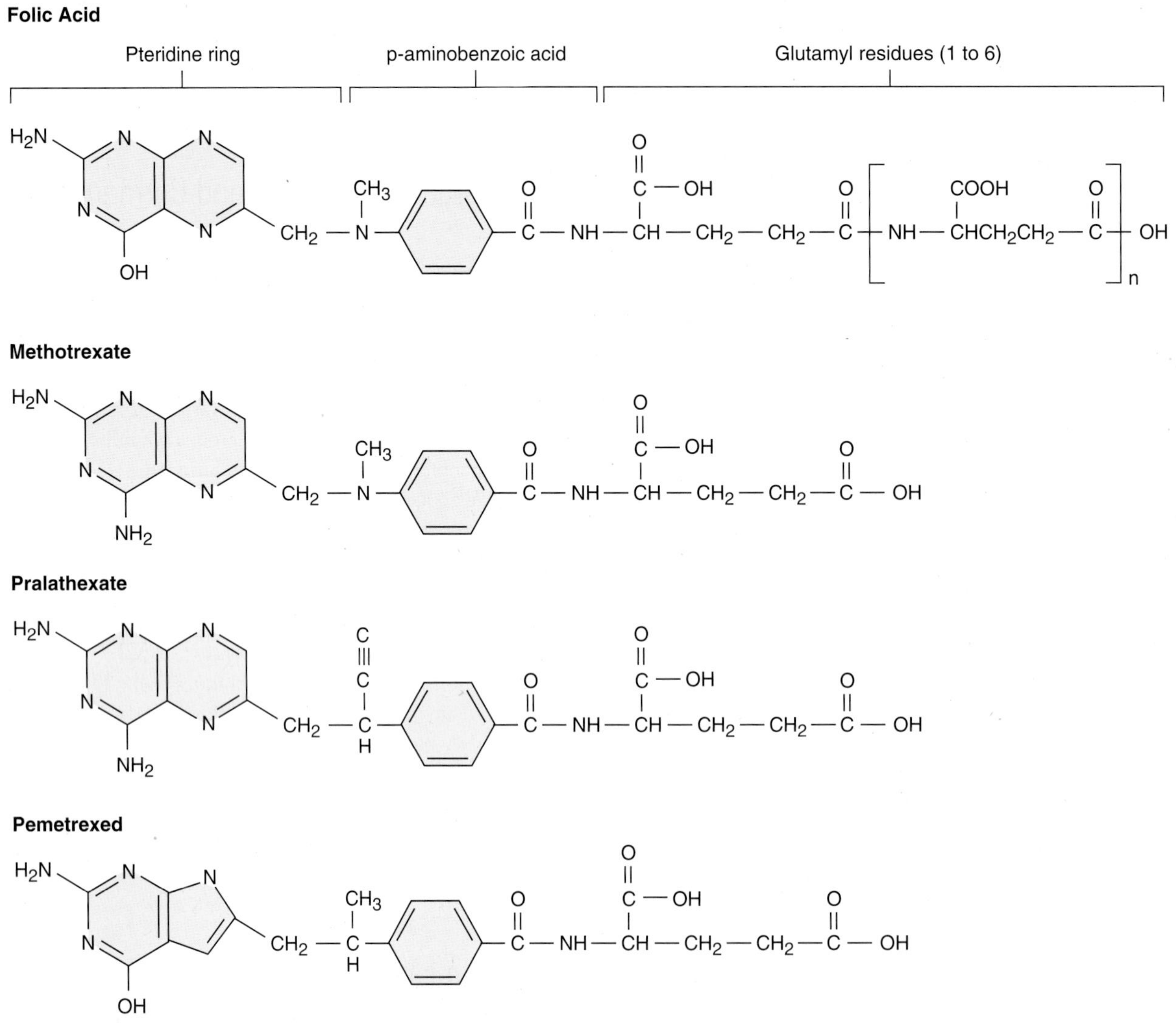

Folic Acid

Methotrexate

Pralathexate

Pemetrexed

FIGURE **8-1**   Structure of folic acid PG, showing its component subgroups (pteroic acid, para-amino benzoic acid, glutamate). Also shown are the analogues methotrexate, pralatrexate, and pemetrexed, which preserve most of the essential features of folates and are readily converted to PGs within cells. MTX and pralatrexate contain the critical 2, 4 diamino configuration that inhibits DHFR. Pemetrexed inhibits TS and GARTF (see text).

Tomudex) and pemetrexed (LY231514, Alimta).[25–28] The antifolates conserve the 2-amino, 4-hydroxy configuration of physiological folates and are weaker inhibitors of DHFR. Pemetrexed is approved for marketing in the United States and elsewhere, based on its activity in mesothelioma and adenocarcinoma of the lung. MTX is considered first in this chapter.

Cellular Pharmacology and Mechanisms of Resistance

In this section, the sequence of events that leads to the cytotoxic action of MTX is considered, beginning with drug movement across the cell membrane, followed by its intracellular metabolism to the PG derivatives, binding to DHFR and other folate-dependent enzymes, effects on intracellular folates, and, finally, inhibition of DNA synthesis.

Transmembrane Transport

Folate influx into mammalian cells proceeds via three distinct transport systems: (a) the reduced-folate carrier (RFC) system, (b) the folate receptor (FR) system (Table 8-2),[29–32] and (c) a pH-sensitive transporter first identified in the intestinal epithelium and found in most tissues and in selected tumor cells[33] (see Table 8-2). The proliferative or kinetic state of tumor cells, as well as the temperature and pH of the extracellular environment, influences the rate of folate and MTX transport. In general, rapidly dividing cells have a greater rate of MTX uptake and a lower rate of drug efflux than cells that are either in the stationary phase or that are slowly growing.[34] The RFC system, with its large transport capacity, transports folic acid inefficiently (K_t [transport coefficient] = 200 μmol/L) and is a primary transport mechanism of the reduced folates and antifolates like MTX (K_t = 0.7 to 6.0 μmol/L), at pharmacologic drug concentrations.[35–37] The RFC system also transports the naturally occurring reduced folates, including the rescue agent

TABLE 8.1 — Key features of methotrexate sodium (MTX)

Mechanism of action	Inhibition of DHFR leads to partial depletion of reduced folates PGs of MTX and dihydrofolate inhibit purine and thymidylate biosynthesis
Metabolism	Converted to PGs in normal and malignant tissues. 7-Hydroxylation in liver
Pharmacokinetics	$t_{1/2}\,\alpha = 2$–3 h; $t_{1/2}\,\beta = 8$–10 h
Elimination	Primarily as intact drug in urine
Drug interactions	Toxicity to normal tissues rescued by leucovorin calcium L-Asparaginase blocks toxicity and antitumor activity Pretreatment with MTX increases 5-fluorouracil and cytosine arabinoside nucleotide formation Nonsteroidal anti-inflammatory agents decrease renal clearance and increase toxicity
Toxicity	Myelosuppression Mucositis, gastrointestinal epithelial denudation Renal tubular obstruction and injury Hepatotoxicity Pneumonitis Hypersensitivity reactions Neurotoxicity
Precaution	Reduce dose in proportion to creatinine clearance Do not administer high-dose MTX to patients with abnormal renal function Monitor plasma concentrations of drug, hydrate patients during high-dose therapy (see Tables 8-3 and 8-4)

$t_{1/2}$, half-life

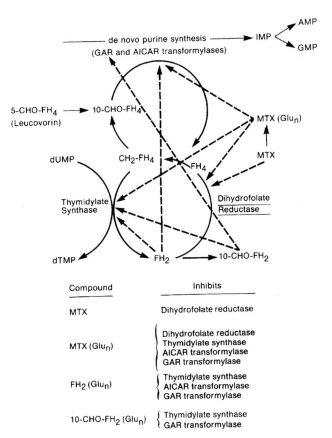

Compound	Inhibits
MTX	Dihydrofolate reductase
MTX (Glu$_n$)	Dihydrofolate reductase Thymidylate synthase AICAR transformylase GAR transformylase
FH$_2$ (Glu$_n$)	Thymidylate synthase AICAR transformylase GAR transformylase
10-CHO-FH$_2$ (Glu$_n$)	Thymidylate synthase GAR transformylase

FIGURE 8-2 Sites of action of methotrexate (MTX), its polyglutamated metabolites (MTX[(Glu$_n$]), and folate byproducts of the inhibition of DHFR, including dihydrofolate (FH$_2$) and 10-formyldihydrofolate (10-CHO-FH$_2$). Also shown are 5,10-methylenetetrahydrofolate (CH$_2$-FH$_4$), the folate cofactor required for thymidylate synthesis and 10-formyltetrahydrofolate (10-CHO-FH$_4$), the required intermediate in the synthesis of purine precursors. AICAR; aminoimidazole carboxamide ribonucleotide; AMP, adenosine monophosphate; dUMP, deoxyuridylate; dTMP, thymidylate; GAR; glycineamide ribonucleotide; GMP, guanosine monophosphate; IMP, inosine monophosphate. (Dashed lines indicate inhibition.) (From DeVita VT, Hellman S, Rosenberg SA, eds. Cancer: Principles and Practice of Oncology. Philadelphia: JB Lippincott, 1989:349–397.)

TABLE 8.2 — Folate transporters and their substrates

Transporter	Folic Acid	Reduced folates	MTX	PMD[a]	PRTX[b]
Reduced folate carrier	+	++++	+++	++++	+++++
Folate receptor	+++	+++ (5-methyl THF)	+	+++	?
Proton-coupled transporter	+++	+++	++	++++	?

Pluses (+) indicate relative affinity.
[a]Pemetrexed.
[b]Pralatrexate.
Source: Mauritz R, Peters GJ, Kathmann I, et al. Dynamics of antifolate transport via the reduced folate carrier and the membrane folate receptor in murine leukemia cells in vitro and in vivo. Cancer Chemother Pharmacol 2008;62:937–948.

5-formyltetrahydrofolate (leucovorin).[30,31,38] The RFC gene resides on the long arm of chromosome 21 and encodes a protein with predicted molecular size of 58 to 68 kD.[39,40] Mutations in the RFC, affecting glutamic acid residue 45 and other sites, have been associated with MTX resistance.[41–43] The proton-coupled transporter may become the predominant folate carrier under relatively acidic conditions, as may be expected in poorly perfused areas of solid tumor masses.[33,44]

A second folate transport mechanism consists of isoforms of the FR, which mediates the internalization of folates via a high-affinity membrane-bound 38-kD glycoprotein. The FR gene family encodes three homologous glycoproteins that share a similar folate-binding site. The α and β FRs are anchored to the plasma membrane by a carboxyl-terminal glycosylphosphatidylinositol tail and transport the reduced folates and MTX at a lower capacity than the RFC system.

The function of the FR-γ is unknown. The FRs are expressed in normal tissues and, at high levels, on the surface of some epithelial tumors such as ovarian cancer.[45,46]

The FR system has a higher affinity for folic acid and the reduced folates (1 nM) than for MTX (5 to 10 nM). In addition, MTX PGs demonstrate a 75-fold increased affinity for FR compared with the monoglutamate form of MTX.[47] The FR is strongly expressed on ovarian cancer cells as the CA-125 antigen and is now the target of experimental monoclonal antibody therapy.[48] Variation in exogenous folate concentrations and normal physiologic conditions, such as pregnancy, can alter the tissue expression of FR. Intracellular levels of homocysteine, which increase under folate-deficient conditions, are a critical modulator of the translational up-regulation of FRs.[49] Under conditions of relative folate deficiency, elevated levels of homocysteine stimulate the interaction between heterogeneous nuclear ribonucleoprotein E1 and an 18–base-pair region in the 5′-untranslated region of the FR mRNA resulting in increased translational efficiency and therefore elevated cellular levels of FR protein. This mechanism of transcriptional regulation through protein binding to its message is operative in DHFR and TS protein synthesis as well.

The FR isoforms (α, β, γ) are independently expressed in mammalian cells and normal human tissues.[50] FR-α is expressed on the apical and luminal surfaces of placenta, chorioid plexus, renal tubules, and alveolar cells and in human epithelial neoplasms (ovarian cancer, papillary serous endometrial cancer, renal cell cancers, and non–small cell lung cancers).[51] In nasopharyngeal KB carcinoma cells, FR-α is up-regulated by folate depletion and down-regulated in folate-replete medium.[29,36] Elwood et al.[52] and others[53,54] have shown that FR-α expression is regulated at a molecular level by promoters upstream from exons 1 and 4 and by differential messenger RNA (mRNA) splicing of 5′ exons. FR-β is expressed in human placenta and nonepithelial tumors. FR-γ, found in hematopoietic and lymphatic cells and tissues, lacks a glycosylphosphatidylinositol membrane anchor and is secreted. Although human FR-α, FR-β, and FR-γ share 70% amino acid sequence homology, they differ in binding affinities for stereoisomers of folates.[55]

The precise mechanism of FR-mediated folate uptake remains controversial[56]; two separate pathways for FR-mediated folate uptake have been reported: (a) the classic receptor-mediated internalization of the ligand-receptor complex through clathrin-coated pits with subsequent formation of secondary lysosomes, and (b) a mechanism of small molecule uptake, termed potocytosis,[57–59] in which receptor complexes accumulate within distinct subdomains of the plasma membrane known as caveolae that internalize to form intracellular vesicles.[60] Once internalization has occurred, acidification within the vesicle causes the folate-receptor complex to dissociate and translocate across the cell membrane. Although questions remain as to the relative importance of the FR and RFC transport systems in the uptake of antifolates during chemotherapy, studies suggest that the RFC system is the more relevant transporter of MTX in most mammalian cells and tumors.[61,62]

The third transporter for folates and analogues, the low-pH, proton-coupled transporter, was first identified in intestinal cells, but is found in many normal tissues as well as tumors, and mediates folate transport into the central nervous system.[63,64] It utilizes an inwardly directed H^+ gradient to move folates and analogues into cells and is lacking in an inherited folate malabsorption disorder.[33,64]

It efficiently transports pemetrexed (K_m = 0.2 to 0.8 μM) but has a lower affinity for MTX and reduced folates.

Role of Transporters in Resistance to MTX

Both in vitro and in vivo experimental systems and limited clinical studies have identified decreased transport as a common mechanism of intrinsic or acquired resistance to MTX. A number of MTX-resistant cell lines with functional defects in the RFC have now been described.[65–68] An MTX-resistant human lymphoblastic CCRF-CEM/MTX cell line maintained in physiologic (micromolar) concentrations of folate (2 nmol/L) lacked the RFC protein and, for this reason, were resistant to MTX.[69] These cells retained the FR, however, and used this transport process to maintain growth even in nanomolar concentrations of folic acid.

A mutated murine RFC (RFC1) with increased affinity for folic acid and decreased affinity for MTX contained an amino acid substitution at glutamic acid residue 45. This region of the RFC is also a cluster site for mutations that occur when cells are placed under selective pressure with antifolates that use RFC1 as the major route of entry into mammalian cells.[70,71] However, none of 121 samples of ALL cells from drug-resistant patients contained a mutation of glutamic acid residue 45.[72]

Other studies provide suggestive but inconclusive evidence for a role of transport deficiency in MTX resistance in both ALL and in solid tumors.[73–78] A sensitive competitive displacement assay using the fluorescent analog of MTX[73] revealed that blast cells from two of four patients in relapse after initial treatment with MTX-based combination chemotherapy demonstrated defective MTX uptake. In two studies of patients with newly diagnosed ALL, low RFC expression at diagnosis correlated with a significantly reduced event-free survival.[74,75] In osteosarcoma treatment, 17 of 26 posttreatment tumor samples (65%) derived from patients with high-grade tumors and with poor response to chemotherapy had decreased RFC expression.[76] Poor response to MTX-based chemotherapy was also observed in tumor samples with low levels of RFC at diagnosis.[77] Thus, impaired transport of MTX may be a common mechanism of intrinsic resistance in osteosarcoma.

Some newer antifolate analogues have improved transport properties. The lipid-soluble nonglutamated antifolates such as trimetrexate and piritrexim, as well as the glutamyl esters of MTX, do not require active cellular transport and demonstrate activity against transport-resistant mutants[79,80] but lack polyglutamation and have minimal activity as antitumor agents. Pralatrexate, the newest addition to the field and now approved for cutaneous T-cell lymphomas, is one of several 10-deaza-aminopterins with a 10-fold or greater efficiency than MTX as a substrate for the reduced folate transporter.[81,82] In contrast to MTX (which has a relatively poor affinity for FR), other antifolate inhibitors (CB3717, raltitrexed, DDATHF, [LY231514], and BW1843U89) rely on the FR for transport.[83,84] Because pemetrexed is efficiently transported by both FR and proton-coupled folate transport systems, it may be less susceptible to the emergence of clinical resistance resulting from alterations in RFC.[85,86]

Low folate conditions may increase the toxicity of antifolates as a consequence of the up-regulations of FR in normal tissues in response to folate starvation.[87] Folate supplementation of patients receiving either pemetrexed or pralatrexate reduces the incidence of severe myelosuppression related to these drugs.[88]

MTX Efflux Mechanisms

Early studies suggested the presence of active efflux mechanisms for MTX and the folates.[89–91] Subsequent experiments have revealed that the multidrug resistance–associated protein family of ATP-binding cassette transporters, particularly MRP-1, MRP-2, and MRP-3 and the breast cancer resistance protein (BCRP), actively extrude MTX in both normal and tumor cells, affecting both drug pharmacokinetics and resistance.[92–95] MRP-2 and BRCP or ABCG2 excrete MTX from liver cells into the bile and efflux drug into the intestinal lumen and urine in mice. Knockout of BCRP produces increased MTX levels in the systemic circulation in mice as a consequence of decreased biliary and urinary excretion.

Experiments in mice suggest that efflux alterations may contribute to MTX resistance. Overexpression of MRP-1 was associated with MTX resistance in murine tumor experiments, and inhibitors of MRP-1 (probenecid) reversed antifolate resistance.[96] Interestingly, others found that loss of MRP-1 expression may expand intracellular folate pools and result in antifolate resistance.[97] BCRP is associated with increased cellular efflux of both MTX and PGs with two or three glutamic acid residues, and its overexpression or mutations may lead to MTX resistance.[98]

Intracellular Transformation

Naturally occurring folates exist within cells in a polyglutamated form (Fig. 8-1). The polyglutamation of folate substrates is directed by folylpolyglutamyl synthetase (FPGS), an enzyme that adds up to eight glutamyl groups in γ peptide linkage. This reaction serves several purposes for folates and antifolates: (a) it facilitates the accumulation of intracellular folates in a selectively retained form, in vast excess of a monoglutamate pool that is freely transportable into and out of cells, (b) it allows selective intracellular retention of these relatively large anionic molecules and thus prolongs intracellular half-life, under conditions of reduced folate availability, and (c) it enhances folate cofactor affinity for folate-dependent enzymes. The MTX PGs are slightly more potent inhibitors of DHFR but significantly more potent antagonists of TS, AICAR transformylase, and GAR transformylase as compared to the parent, MTX-Glu$_1$.[13,14] MTX and the other glutamyl-terminal analogs also undergo polyglutamation in normal liver cells and bone marrow myeloid precursors,[99,100] likely enhancing their toxicity. Polyglutamation occurs in most tumors to varying degrees and likely determines antitumor response.[100–103]

The efficiency of the polyglutamation reaction for various folate substrates and antifolates varies considerably. Pralatrexate is 10-fold more avidly polyglutamated than MTX.[88] The polyglutamation of MTX occurs progressively over several hours of exposure; after 24 hours, 80% or more of intracellular drug exists in the PG form.[101,104–106] Human liver retains MTX PGs for several months after drug administration.[107] Thus, selective retention and depot formation in excess of free monoglutamate, as seen with physiologic folates, characterize MTX PGs as well.

FPGS is a 62-kD magnesium-, adenosine triphosphate-, and potassium-dependent protein.[108–111] The FPGS gene is located on chromosome region 9q34.11 and produces two proteins, the major one having 537-amino acids and a second with 579 amino acids found in mitochondria. The most avid substrate for this enzyme is dihydrofolate (K_m [binding affinity] = 2 μmol/L), with the following folates and analogues in descending order of affinity: tetrahydrofolate (K_m = 6 μmol/L) > 10-formyltetrahydrofolate or 5-methyltetrahydrofolate > aminopterin > leucovorin > MTX. Because of the relatively slow rate of formation of MTX PGs compared with the naturally occurring folate PGs, reductions in FPGS activity or cellular glutamate levels may have little effect on folate PG pools but may critically reduce MTX PG formation and decrease cytotoxicity of MTX and likely other antifolates.

The intracellular content of PG derivatives represents a balance between the activity of two different enzymes: FPGS, which synthesizes PGs, and γ-glutamyl hydrolase (GGH, conjugase),[112] a γ-glutamyl-specific peptidase that removes terminal glutamyl groups and returns MTX PGs to their monoglutamate form.[113]

While the functional importance of GGH in determining response to MTX is not known, the St. Jude group has found a substrate specific polymorphism (C452T) of the enzyme, present in 10% of Caucasian patients, that reduces catalytic activity and allows greater accumulation of MTX PGs in leukemic cells (Fig. 8-3).[114] Yao et al.[115] isolated and cloned the complementary DNA (cDNA) for GGH, which codes for an enzyme of 318 amino acids and has a molecular weight of 36 kD. Although it may be expected that overexpression of hydrolase may result in MTX resistance, particularly with brief drug exposures, such was not the case in several human cell line models in which hydrolase was overexpressed.[116]

MTX PGs exist essentially only within cells and enter or exit cells sparingly in vitro.[102,117] The diglutamate form has an uptake velocity of one-fifteenth that of MTX,[118] whereas higher glutamates have even slower transport rates.[102,117] Thus, MTX PGs are selectively retained in preference to parent drug as extracellular levels of MTX fall.

Cellular activity of FPGS correlates directly with the rate of cell growth[103,119] and inversely with the level of intracellular folates.[119,120] Enhancement of cell proliferation with growth factors such as insulin, dexamethasone, tocopherol, and estrogen in hormone-responsive cells increases polyglutamation, whereas deprivation of essential amino acids[121] results in inhibition of polyglutamation. MTX and L-asparaginase are frequently used in combination for the treatment of acute leukemia. Conversion of MTX to PG forms

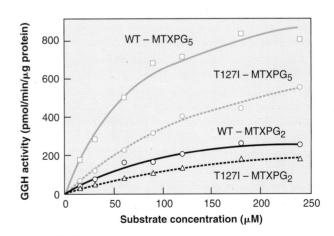

FIGURE 8-3 Catalytic activity of T127I variant gamma-glutamylhydrolase (GGH) on MTX PG substrates, as compared to wild type (WT) enzyme. Enzymes were incubated with MTX PGs with chain length of 2 and 5 glutamyl groups. A 2.7 fold increase in K_m was observed for the variant enzyme. (From Cheng Q, et. al. A substrate specific functional polymorphism of human gamma-glutamyl hydrolase alters catalytic activity and methotrexate polyglutamate accumulation in acute lymphoblastic leukemia cells. Pharmacogenetics 2004;14:557–567.)

can be markedly inhibited by pretreatment with L-asparaginase, presumably through amino acid deprivation with resultant growth arrest.[122] Increasing intracellular folate pools through exposure of cells to high concentrations of leucovorin or 5-methyltetrahydrofolate results in a decrease in MTX polyglutamation.[120] Conversely, the process is enhanced in human hepatoma cells either by incubating cells with MTX in folate-free medium or by first depleting the intracellular folates by "permeabilizing" cell membranes in a folate-free environment.[119]

An important factor in the selective nature of MTX cytotoxicity may derive from modest PG formation in normal tissues relative to that in malignant tissues. Although little metabolism to PGs is observed in normal murine intestinal cells in vivo, most murine leukemias and Ehrlich ascites tumor cells efficiently convert MTX to higher PG forms in tumor-bearing animals.[37,123] Additionally, normal human and murine myeloid progenitor cells form relatively small amounts of MTX PGs compared with leukemic cells.[99,100]

In addition to increasing its retention within cells, polyglutamation of MTX enhances its inhibitory effects on specific folate-dependent enzymes. The pentaglutamates have a slower dissociation rate from DHFR than does MTX[124] and a markedly enhanced inhibitory potency for TS (K_i = 50 nmol/L), AICAR transformylase (K_i = 57 nmol/L), and, to a lesser extent, GAR transformylase (K_i = 2 μmol/L) in the presence of monoglutamated folate substrates.[12] The well-described incomplete depletion of physiologic folate cofactors by MTX suggests that direct enzymatic inhibition by MTX PGs may contribute to MTX cytotoxicity. These effects may also explain the competitive nature of leucovorin rescue and the relatively selective rescue of normal versus malignant tissues, in that rescue may depend on the ability of leucovorin and its derived tetrahydrofolates to compete with MTX PGs at sites other than DHFR.

The ability of antifolate analogs to undergo polyglutamation is one of several properties that influence cytotoxic potency. Aminopterin is a better substrate for FPGS than is MTX and is a more potent cytotoxic agent. A fluorinated MTX analog, PT430, is a weak substrate for FPGS and has little cytotoxic activity.[125] As mentioned previously pemetrexed and particularly pralatrexate are more efficient substrates than MTX. The ability to generate PGs has been correlated with sensitivity to MTX and to other antifolate agents that undergo polyglutamation, including pemetrexed and raltitrexed, and is often defective in drug-resistant human and murine tumor cell lines.[126–130]

Although defective polyglutamation may coexist with other metabolic alterations, examples of pure polyglutamation defects have been described in human leukemia cell lines (CCRF-CEM)[131,132] and in human squamous cancer cell lines derived from head and neck tumors and have been implicated as the specific cause of MTX resistance in human B- and T-cell types of ALL.[132–141]

A decrease in MTX PGs was found in small cell carcinomas resistant in vitro after clinical treatment with MTX.[135] In ALL, the balance of FPGS and GGH activities before treatment predicted PG formation and therapeutic outcome in a small prospective trial.[136] Examples of defective splicing of the folylpolyglutamate mRNA were identified in cell lines selected for MTX resistance, exon 12 skipping was found in bone marrow samples from two ALL patients at diagnosis and one at relapse after MTX therapy.[132] Another study reported a decreased binding affinity (higher K_m) for MTX as a substrate for FPGS in enzyme from blast cells of patients with acute myelogenous leukemia (AML) as opposed to ALL cells. This difference in affinity resulted in a predominance of MTX-Glu$_1$ species in AML cells, and MTX Glu$_{3–5}$ in ALL cells.

Leukemic cells differ greatly in their expression of FPGS (Fig. 8-4). Hyperdiploid status in childhood ALL is a good prognostic feature; cells with hyperdiploid chromosomes show higher levels of synthesis of cytotoxic MTX PGs than cells of diploid, T-cell, TEL-AML1 or E2APBX1 lymphoblasts.[114] Investigators have found a higher concentration of MTX long-chain PGs in B than in T lymphoblasts and an increased level of expression of FPGS mRNA in B-lineage cells.[137,138] These findings suggest that the higher response rates observed in patients with B-cell ALL may result from increased levels of FPGS activity that, in turn, facilitate enhanced intracellular formation of more cytotoxic MTX PGs.

A study involving 52 children with B-cell ALL did not confirm that MTX accumulation and polyglutamation have prognostic significance in patients receiving prolonged oral MTX therapy.[139] This finding supports the notion that, under the conditions of continuous low dose drug exposure, the activity of MTX may not depend on cellular polyglutamation to sustain intracellular levels and antitumor effect. The role of PG formation in solid tumor therapy with MTX has been addressed in very few studies. In specimens from patients with soft tissue sarcoma, 12 of 15 tumors exhibited impaired polyglutamation, although the relationship to clinical response was uncertain.[140,141]

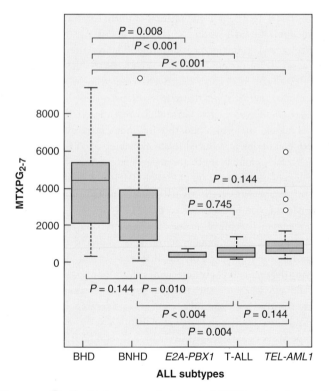

FIGURE 8-4 Methotrexate polyglutamate (MTXPG) content (p moles/ 109 bone marrow ALL cells) of subtypes of ALL following treatment in vivo with 1 g/m² MTX over 24 hours. Hyperdiploid B-cell ALL (BHD), nonhyperdiploid B-cell (BNHD), ALL with E2A-PBX1 fusion, T-cell ALL, and ALL with TEL-AML1 fusion are subsets. One hundred-and-one patients' samples were studied. Medians, quartiles, and ranges excluding outliers are shown, and *P* values from pair-wise comparisons (Wilcoxon rank sum test, adjusted for multiple tests) are given. (From Kager L, et al. Folate pathway gene expression differs in subtypes of acute lymphoblastic leukemia and influences methotrexate pharmacodynamics. J Clin Invest 2005;115:110–117.)

The role of genetic variation in determining function of FPGS is suggested by the finding that two variants (R424C and S457F) slow the rate of PG formation for both folates and MTX and decrease cytotoxicity of MTX when expressed in Aux B1 cells.[142]

In summary, limited experimental and clinical evidence suggests, but does not conclusively prove, a relationship between clinical response and FPGS or GGH activity. The role of genetic variation in contributing to FPGS and GGH activities and PG formation remains to be defined.

Binding to Dihydrofolate Reductase

The physical characteristics of binding of NADPH (reduced form of nicotinamide adenine dinucleotide phosphate [NADP]) and MTX to DHFR of various species have been established by x-ray crystallographic studies, nuclear magnetic resonance spectroscopy, amino-acid sequencing of native and chemically modified enzyme, and site-directed mutagenesis, using enzymes from microbial, chicken, and mammalian sources[143-148]; strong amino acid sequence homology is found at positions involved in substrate cofactor and inhibitor binding.[149] In general, a long hydrophobic pocket binds MTX and is formed in part by the isoleucine-5, alanine-7, aspartate-27, phenylalanine-31 (Phe-31), and phenylalanine-34 (Phe-34), and other amino acid residues. Several particularly important interactions contribute to the binding potency of the 4-amino antifolates: (a) hydrogen bonding of the carbonyl oxygen of isoleucine-5 to the 4-amino group of the inhibitor; (b) a salt bridge between aspartate and the N-1 position of MTX, which is not involved in binding to the physiologic substrates; (c) hydrophobic interactions of the inhibitor with DHFR, particularly with Phe-31 and Phe-34; (d) hydrogen bonding of the 2-amino group to aspartate-27 and to a structurally consistent bound water molecule; and (e) hydrogen binding of the terminal glutamate to an invariant arginine-70 residue. Investigations have identified the importance of the interactions of MTX with Phe-31 and Phe-34 because mutations in these positions result in a 100-fold and 80,000-fold decrease in MTX affinity for the enzyme, respectively.[150] Mutation of arginine-70 results in a decrease in MTX affinity by greater than 22,000-fold but does not alter the binding affinity of trimetrexate, which lacks the terminal glutamate moiety involved in this interaction.[151] Mutations outside the enzyme active site also may result in marked reductions in folate and antifolate affinities.[152] In addition, the physiologic substrate dihydrofolate is bound to the enzyme in an inverted, or "upside down," configuration compared with the inhibitor MTX.[147,153] The reader is referred to more detailed reviews of this subject for consideration of substrate and cofactor binding characteristics and studies of mutated DHFR.[145-148,154-157]

Optimal binding of MTX to DHFR depends on the concentration of NADPH. NADH (reduced form of nicotinamide adenine dinucleotide) may also act as a cosubstrate for DHFR but, unlike NADPH, it does not promote binding of MTX to the enzyme.[158] Thus, the intracellular ratios of NADPH/NADP and NADPH/NADH may play an important role in the selective action of MTX to the extent that the cosubstrate ratios may differ in malignant and in normal tissues.[123,158] In the presence of excess NADPH, the binding affinity of MTX for DHFR has been estimated to lie between 10 and 200 pM,[159,160] although this affinity is significantly affected by pH, salt concentration, and the status of enzyme sulfhydryl groups.

Under conditions of low pH and with a low ratio of inhibitor to enzyme, binding is essentially stoichiometric, that is, one molecule of MTX is bound to one molecule of DHFR.

Binding of MTX to DHFR isolated from parasitic, bacterial, and mammalian sources in the presence of NADPH generates a slowly formed ternary complex. The overall process has been termed slow, tight-binding inhibition and involves an initial rapid but weak enzyme-inhibitor interaction followed by a slow but extremely tight-binding isomerization to the final complex.[145,157,161] The final isomerization step probably involves a conformational change of the enzyme with subsequent binding of the para-aminobenzoyl moiety to the enzyme.[148] Other folate analogs, such as aminopterin, follow the same slow, tight-binding kinetic process, in contrast to the pteridines and pyrimethamine, which behave as classic single step inhibitors of the bacterial enzymes. Trimethoprim is considered to be a classic, albeit weak, inhibitor of mammalian DHFR. Of note, it does not undergo an isomerization process to the ternary complex form.[157]

In the therapeutic setting, and in intact cells, MTX acts as a tight-binding but reversible inhibitor. Under conditions of high concentrations of competitive substrate (dihydrofolate) and at neutral intracellular pH, a considerable excess of free drug is required to fully inhibit the enzyme. As drug concentration falls below 10^{-8} M in tissue culture and at lower concentrations in cell-free systems, enzyme activity resumes, and tritium-labeled MTX bound to intracellular enzyme can be displaced by exposure of cells to unlabeled drug or dihydrofolate,[7,162,163] or reduced folates such as leucovorin and 5-methyltetrahydrofolate,[123] which indicates a slow but definite "off rate" or dissociation of MTX from the enzyme.[123,164] Thus, an excess of free, or unbound, drug is required to maintain total inhibition of DHFR.[165]

MTX PGs have similar potency in their tight-binding inhibition of mammalian DHFR[101,157,166] and possess a slower rate of dissociation from the enzyme than the parent compound. In pulse-chase experiments using intact human breast cancer cells, MTX pentaglutamate was found to have a dissociation half-life of 120 minutes compared with 12 minutes for the parent compound. Cell-free experiments using purified preparations of mammalian enzyme indicate that MTX polyglutamation has a modest effect in enhancing binding and catalytic inhibition (twofold to sixfold) of DHFR.[12,157,160,167] As with MTX, enzyme-bound MTX PGs may also be displaced by reduced folates[123] and high concentrations of dihydrofolate,[168,169] albeit at a slower rate than MTX.

These observations indicate that, in the absence of free drug, a small fraction of intracellular DHFR, either through new synthesis or through dissociation from the inhibitor, becomes available for catalytic activity and is adequate to allow for continued intracellular metabolism. The requirement for excess free drug to inhibit enzyme activity completely is important in understanding the clinical effects and toxicity of this agent and is fundamental to the relationship between pharmacokinetics and pharmacodynamics.

Resistance to MTX as a result of decreased DHFR binding affinity for MTX has been described in murine leukemic cells,[152,170,171] Chinese hamster ovary[172] and lung[173] cells, and murine and hamster lung fibroblast cells.[174,175] These mutant enzymes may have several 1,000-fold reduced binding affinity for MTX and, in general, are less efficient in catalyzing the reduction of dihydrofolate than is wild-type DHFR.

Drug-sensitive Chinese hamster lung cells express two different forms of DHFR encoded by distinct alleles.[176,177] The two species differ in molecular weight and isoelectric point (21,000 versus 20,000 and 6.7 versus 6.5), a difference that results from a single amino acid substitution of asparagine for aspartic acid at position 95. Either allele may be predominantly expressed in various subclones of the parent cell line. This observation raises the possibility that distinct naturally occurring DHFR alleles may exist in a variety of tissues and, to the extent that they may confer differential sensitivity to MTX, this DHFR genetic polymorphism of the host may serve as a mechanism by which cells may become clinically MTX resistant.

DHFR with reduced affinity for MTX may represent a clinically important mechanism of MTX resistance, as this phenomenon was observed in the leukemic cells of 4 of 12 patients with resistant AML.[178] Transfection of MTX-resistant, mutant DHFR has become a tool for creating drug-resistant hematopoietic progenitor cells and several laboratories have developed vectors to efficiently transduce human progenitor cells with the hope that such technology could be used to enable the use of higher, and hopefully more effective, doses of chemotherapeutic agents to treat human maligancies.[179–181]

A common finding in both laboratory and clinical studies of MTX-resistant cells is an increase in the expression of DHFR protein with no associated change in the enzyme's affinity for MTX. Elevations in DHFR may persist for many generations of cell renewal in tumor cells from resistant patients. In resistant murine leukemic cells, the increased DHFR activity results from reduplication of the DHFR gene (Fig. 8-5), a process that occurs by exposing murine and human leukemia and carcinoma cells in culture to stepwise increases in the concentration of MTX.[173,176,182–184] Gene duplication may take the form of a homogeneously staining region (HSR) on chromosomes or nonintegrated pieces of DNA known as double-minute chromosomes (DMs) (Fig. 8-5). Although HSRs appear to confer stable resistance to the cell, double-minute chromosomes are unequally distributed during cell division,[175,183] and in the absence of the continued selective pressure of drug exposure, the cells revert to the original low-DHFR genotype. Evidence exists that gene amplification occurs initially in the form of double-minute chromosomes because this is the predominant abnormality in low-level drug-resistant cells, whereas HSRs occur in highly resistant cells that contain multiple gene copies.[175,183,184] Other investigations suggest the opposite sequence wherein chromosomal breaks result in HSRs, which are then processed to DMs or not, depending on how different cell types handle extra chromosomal sequences.[185] Another mechanism of gene amplification has been identified in an MTX-resistant HeLa 10B3 cell line in which were found submicroscopic extrachromosomal elements (amplisomes) containing amplified DHFR genes. These amplisomes appeared early in the development of MTX resistance and were not found to be integrated into the chromosome, nor were they associated with double-minute chromosomes. Although these amplisomes were lost in the absence of the selective pressure of MTX, they disappeared at a much slower rate than would be predicted from simple dilution of nonreplicating elements.

Although MTX resistance through DHFR gene amplification becomes apparent only after the prolonged selective pressure of drug exposure, highly MTX-resistant cells may be generated by gene amplification within a single cell cycle.[186] Early S-phase cells

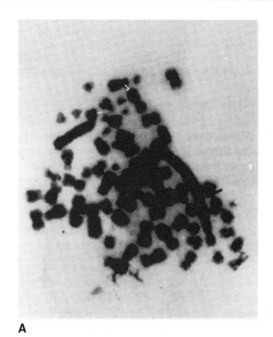

A

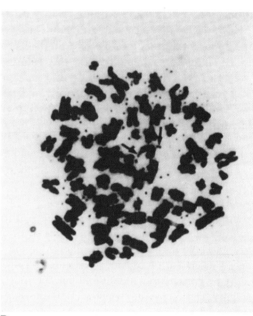

B

FIGURE 8-5 A. Marker chromosomes found in methotrexate (MTX)-resistant breast cancer cells. A human breast cancer cell line, MCF-7, resistant to MTX was isolated by growing cells in gradually increasing drug concentrations. These cells are resistant to drug concentrations more than 200-fold higher than those that kill wild-type cells and contain more than 30-fold increases in DHFR. The *arrow* indicates a marker chromosome with a greatly expanded homogenously staining region. **B.** Metaphase plate of a small cell lung cancer carcinoma cell line taken from a patient with clinical MTX resistance. The prominent double-minute chromosomes (*arrows*) were associated with amplification of the drug target enzyme, DHFR. (From Curt GA, Carney DN, Cowan KH, et al. Unstable methotrexate resistance in human small-cell carcinoma associated with double minute chromosomes. N Engl J Med 1983;308:199–202.)

exposed transiently to agents that block DNA synthesis (e.g., hydroxyurea) may undergo reduplication of multiple genes synthesized during early S phase, including DHFR, after removal of the DNA synthetic inhibitor. This finding has broad implications for

otherwise lethal doses in a 4- to 36-hour infusion, followed by a 24- to 48-hour period of multiple leucovorin doses to terminate the toxic effect of MTX. Several of the more commonly used high-dose regimens and their related pharmacokinetics are presented in Table 8-5. For each regimen, successful rescue by leucovorin depends on the rapid elimination of MTX by the kidneys. Early experience with high-dose regimens, however, indicated that MTX itself may have acute toxic effects on renal function during the period of drug infusion, which can lead to delayed drug clearance, ineffective rescue by leucovorin, and a host of secondary toxicities, including severe myelosuppression, mucositis, and epithelial desquamation.[244] During the early clinical trials of high-dose MTX, a number of toxic deaths were recorded.[289]

Drug-induced renal dysfunction, which is usually manifested as an abrupt rise in serum blood urea nitrogen and creatinine with a corresponding fall in urine output, arises from the precipitation of MTX and possibly its less soluble metabolites, 7-OH-MTX and DAMPA, in acidic urine.[273] A direct toxic effect of antifolates on the renal tubule, however, has been suggested by the observation that aminopterin, an equally soluble compound that is used at one-tenth the dose of MTX, is also associated with renal toxicity; however, a direct nephrotoxic role of MTX has not been substantiated in clinical investigations.[290] The syndrome of MTX-induced renal failure has been reproduced in a monkey model system, in which was demonstrated precipitation of both MTX and 7-OH-MTX in the renal tubules.[273] Both of these compounds have limited solubility under acid pH conditions (Table 8-4). To prevent precipitation, most centers use vigorous hydration (2.5 to 3.5 L of fluid per square meter per 24 hours, beginning 12 hours before MTX infusion and continuing for 24 to 48 hours), with alkalinization of the urine (45 to 50 mEq of sodium bicarbonate per liter of intravenous fluid). The MTX infusion should not begin until urine flow exceeds 100 mL/h and urine pH is 7.0 or higher, and these parameters should be carefully monitored during the course of drug infusion.

With this regimen, the incidence of renal failure and myelosuppression has been markedly reduced. No change in the rate of MTX excretion or alteration of plasma pharmacokinetics results from the intense hydration used in the preparatory regimen previously described[256]; thus, these safety measures should have no deleterious effect on the therapeutic efficacy of the regimen. Despite careful attention to the details of hydration and alkalinization, occasional patients can develop serious or even fatal toxicity.[289] Almost all of these toxic episodes are associated with delayed MTX clearance from plasma and can be predicted by routine monitoring of drug

---

TABLE 8.5   High-dose methotrexate (HD MTX) therapy

Hydration and urinary alkalinization

Administer a total of 2.5–3.5 L/m²/d of IV fluids starting 12 h before and continuing for 24–48 h after administration of MTX drug infusion. Sodium bicarbonate 45–50 mEq/L of IV fluid to keep urine pH > 7.0.

Commonly used drug infusion regimens

MTX dose	Duration (h)	Fluid (L/24 h)	Bicarbonate (mEq/24 h)	Leucovorin calcium rescue	Onset of rescue (h after start of MTX)
1.5–7.5 g/m²	6.0	3/m²	NS	15 mg IV q3h × 3, then 15 mg PO q6h × 7	18
8–12 g/m²	4.0	1.5–2.0/m²	2–3/kg	10 mg PO q6h × 10	20
3.0–7.5 g/m²	0.3	3/m²	288	10 mg/m² IV × 1, then 10 mg/m² PO q6h × 12	24
1 g/m²	24.0	2.4/m²	48/m²	15 mg/m² IV q6h × 2, then 3 mg/m² PO q12h × 3	36
1.0–7.5 g/m²	0.5	3/m²	288	10 mg/m² IV × 1, then 10 mg/m² PO q6h × 11	24

IV, intravenously; NS, not specified; PO, per os.
Adapted from Ackland SP, Schilsky RL. High-dose methotrexate: a critical reappraisal. J Clin Oncol 1987;5:2017–2031.

Suggested Monitoring Points

MTX drug levels above 5×10^{-7} mol/L at 48 h after the start of MTX infusion require continued leucovorin rescue.[a] A general guideline for leucovorin rescue is as follows:

MTX level	Leucovorin dosage
5×10^{-7} mol/L	15 mg/m² q6h × 8
1×10^{-6} mol/L	100 mg/m² q6h × 8
2×10^{-6} mol/L	200 mg/m² q6h × 8

[a] MTX drug levels should be measured every 24 h and the dosage of leucovorin adjusted until the MTX level is $<5 \times 10^{-8}$ mol/L.

concentration in plasma at appropriate times after drug infusion.[291] In an analysis of 790 patients treated with high-dose MTX for osteosarcoma, the incidence of delayed MTX clearance (plasma level >5 uM at 24 hours postinfusion) was 1.6% per cycle of treatment.[292] The specific time for monitoring, and the guidelines for distinguishing between normal and dangerously elevated levels, must be determined for each regimen and for each assay procedure. In general, a time point well into the final phase of drug disappearance, such as 24 or 48 hours after the start of infusion, should be chosen. Ketoprofen and other nonsteroidal anti-inflammatory drugs (NSAIDs) decrease glomerular filtration and MTX excretion and have been associated with severe MTX toxicity.[293] A review of 118 cases of single-agent, high-dose MTX therapy revealed four cases of fatal toxicity associated with the use of NSAIDs. Patients treated with NSAIDs demonstrated a marked prolongation of serum MTX half-life that was postulated to be caused by decreased renal elimination secondary to inhibition of renal prostaglandin synthesis or competitive inhibition of human organic anion transporters (hOATs) responsible for MTX excretion in the kidney.[294,295]

Early detection of elevated concentrations of MTX allows institution of specific clinical measures. Continuous medical supervision is warranted until the severity and duration of myelosuppression can be determined. Leucovorin in increased doses is required and must be continued until plasma MTX concentration falls below 100 nmol/L. Because of the competitive relationship between MTX and leucovorin, the leucovorin dose must be increased in proportion to the plasma concentration of MTX. Small doses of leucovorin are unable to prevent toxicity in patients with markedly elevated drug levels, even when leucovorin is continued beyond 48 hours.[291] As a general rule, a reasonable course is to treat with leucovorin at a dosage of 100 mg/m² every 6 hours for patients with MTX levels of 1 μmol/L and to increase this dosage in proportion to the MTX level above 1 uM up to a maximum of 500 mg/m² leucovorin. Subsequent leucovorin dosage adjustments should be based on repeated plasma MTX levels taken at 24-hour intervals. The results of in vitro studies indicate that leucovorin alone may not be able to rescue patients with plasma MTX concentrations above 10 μmol/L.

The absorption of oral leucovorin is saturable such that the bioavailability of the compound is limited above total doses of 40 mg. The fractional absorption of a 40-mg dose is 0.78, whereas that of 60- and 100-mg doses is 0.62 and 0.42, respectively. For this reason, leucovorin is usually administered intravenously to assure its absorption especially in the presence of high concentrations of MTX in plasma.

Because of the variable effectiveness of leucovorin in preventing toxicity in patients with levels of 10 μmol/L or greater at 48 hours, alternative methods of rescue have been developed. Both intermittent hemodialysis and peritoneal dialysis are ineffective in removing significant quantities of MTX. However, continuous flow hemodialysis has been effective in reducing plasma MTX concentration and preventing toxicity in patients with MTX-induced failure.[297] Clearance of MTX from plasma with continuous flow, high flux hemodialysis approached 0.77 mL/min/kg, very close to the value of 1 mL/min/kg found in patients with normal renal function. Peritoneal dialysis produces clearance rates significantly lower, but one case report describes its successful use in a patient with an intracerebral lymphoma and renal failure receiving HD MTX.[297] The use of charcoal hemoperfusion columns is capable of removing MTX and other antineoplastic drugs from whole blood and has been applied successfully in a few patients; however, platelet adherence to these columns may lead to thrombocytopenia.

A bacterial enzyme, CPDG2, which inactivates MTX by removal of its terminal glutamate, instantly destroys circulating MTX when infused intravenously.[278] One potential disadvantage of CPDG2, however, is its relatively high affinity for natural folates as well as MTX. DeAngelis et al.[298] conducted a pilot study to determine the efficacy of CPDG2 rescue after high-dose MTX in patients with recurrent cerebral lymphoma. All patients had at least a 2-log decline in plasma MTX levels within 5 minutes of CPDG2 administration, whereas CSF MTX concentrations remained elevated for 4 hours after CPDG2. No MTX or CPDG2 toxicity was observed, and anti-CPDG2 activity antibodies were not detected in any patient. The authors concluded that CPDG2 rescue was a safe and effective alternative to leucovorin rescue after high-dose MTX chemotherapy. Additional utility of CPDG2 as a safe and effective means for preventing severe MTX toxicity was demonstrated in several reports of patients with delayed MTX clearance.[299,300] CPDG2 is indicated for patients with persistently high MTX level (above 10 uM) and renal failure, after attempts at drug removal through continuous flow hemodialysis.

In the experimental setting, MTX toxicity can also be blocked by drugs that prevent cell progression into the S phase of the cell cycle. The antagonistic effect of L-asparaginase on MTX toxicity is a representative example; through depletion of the amino acid asparagine[301] blocks progression into S phase and inhibits MTX action. During recovery turn L-asparaginase, leukemic cells may become supersensitive to MTX.

Other Toxicities

Hepatotoxicity

In addition to its inhibitory effects on rapidly dividing tissues, MTX has toxic effects on nondividing tissues not explained by its primary action on DNA synthesis. High-dose MTX commonly causes brief but rapidly reversible hepatic enzyme elevations, but rarely significant long-term damage. In chronic MTX therapy for psoriasis or rheumatoid arthritis, elevated liver enzymes were detected in 13% of patients over the course of a year, but only 4% or less stopped treatment because of liver toxicity. Less than 3% are found to have portal fibrosis on biopsy, and on rare occasions, this lesion may progress to frank cirrhosis.[302] These estimates are much lower than previously thought and may relate to patient selection (particularly elimination of patients with underlying and alternative causes of liver disease); earlier studies estimated that up to 30% of psoriatic patients receiving chronic treatment with MTX develop cirrhosis.[303] Cirrhosis does not always progress with continued antifolate treatment. Of 11 patients with psoriasis who showed cirrhotic changes on liver biopsy and continued to receive treatment, only 3 showed progression on subsequent biopsy and 3 had no pathologic findings on a follow-up biopsy.[303] The use of "pulsed" weekly therapy rather than continuous daily treatment appears to lessen the incidence of MTX-associated hepatotoxicity, and weekly doses of 25 to 30 mg/wk subcutaneously give the optimal therapeutic response.[302,304,305] Several studies suggest that the incidence of hepatic cirrhosis is no different in patients with rheumatoid arthritis treated with MTX pulse therapy than in untreated patients despite long-term therapy (longer than 5 years).[306,307]

Acute elevations of liver enzymes after high-dose MTX administration usually return to normal within 10 days. The frequency and severity of liver enzyme elevations appear to be directly related to the number of MTX doses received.[308] Liver biopsy reveals fatty infiltration but no evidence of hepatocellular necrosis or periportal fibrosis. The late occurrence of cirrhosis in patients treated with high-dose MTX has not been reported.

Pneumonitis

Treatment with MTX is associated with a poorly characterized, self-limited pneumonitis, with fever, cough, and an interstitial pulmonary infiltrate.[309,310] Eosinophilia has not been a consistent finding, either in the peripheral blood or in open lung biopsy specimens. Lung biopsies have revealed a variety of findings, from simple interstitial edema and a mononuclear infiltrate to noncaseating granulomas. The possibility that MTX pneumonitis may not represent a hypersensitivity phenomenon has been raised because of the failure of some patients to react to reinstitution of MTX therapy. However, bronchoalveolar lavage in three patients with presumptive MTX-induced lung damage revealed a predominance of T8 suppressor lymphocytes. In contrast to peripheral lymphocytes obtained from MTX-treated patients with no lung damage, lymphocytes from the study patients elaborated leukocyte inhibitory factor in response to MTX exposure.[311] This study supports an immunologic basis for MTX-related lung damage. The possibility exists, however, that many case reports of "MTX lung" in fact represent unrecognized viral infections or allergic reactions to unsuspected allergens. With the use of long-term weekly low-dose MTX therapy for rheumatoid arthritis, cases of MTX-associated lung damage have been reported.[312,313] A review of 168 patients treated with MTX for rheumatoid arthritis uncovered 9 cases (5%) of probable MTX-associated lung toxicity.[314] Using a retrospective combined-cohort review and abstraction from the medical literature, Kremer et al.[315] characterized the clinical features of MTX-associated lung injury in patients with rheumatoid arthritis. Clinical symptoms of MTX toxicity in the cohort included the subacute development of shortness of breath (93%), cough (82%), and fever (69%); 5 of 27 patients experienced a fatal outcome. The authors concluded that early symptom recognition and the cessation of MTX administration could avoid the serious and sometimes fatal outcome of this MTX-associated toxicity. Corticosteroids have been used in a small number of patients who ultimately recovered,[316] but the utility of this approach has yet to be established. Alarcon et al.[317] found that the strongest predictors of MTX-induced lung injury in rheumatoid arthritis patients included older age, presence of diabetes, rheumatoid pleuropulmonary involvement, presence of hypoalbuminemia, and prior use of disease-modifying antirheumatic drugs.

Induction of EBV related Lymphoproliferative Disorder

Patients on long-term MTX for immunosuppression are prone to develop a *lymphoproliferative disorder* (LPD) related to reactivation of Epstein-Barr Virus (EBV). A spectrum of presentations have been reported, including benign mononucleosis like illness, malignant lymphomas, and vasculitis with lymphoid infiltration of the skin.[318] In some instances, the lymphoid infiltrates regress with discontinuation of the drug, although in frank malignant lymphomas, the tumor progresses in the absence of treatment[318,319] Skin ulcerations independent of LPD have been described as a toxic adverse effect of MTX.

Hypersensitivity

Acute hypersensitivity reaction to MTX occurs rarely.[320,321] Symptoms may range from urticaria and wheezing to acute cardiovascular collapse, which may recur on rechallenge of such patients. Patients receiving bacille Calmette-Guérin or other immune stimulants may be at increased risk. In a few instances, patients had hypersensitivity to folic acid as well.[322] The cross-reactivity to folic acid would not affect the major circulating forms of the vitamin, which are found in a reduced form in tissues and in the systemic circulation. In the authors' limited experienced desensitization in patients with mild initial reactions, using small graded increase in dose dosage with corticosteroids and antihistamines may enable retreatment at full doses of MTX.

Toxic erythema and desquamation of the hands were reported in patients receiving high doses (1.5 g/m^2) of MTX for the treatment of non-Hodgkin's lymphoma.[323] This toxic reaction was associated with severe mucositis and was ameliorated by MTX dose reductions on subsequent treatment.

Reversible oligospermia with testicular failure has been reported in men treated with high-dose MTX.[324] No alterations in follicle-stimulating hormone, luteinizing hormone, estradiol, or progesterone have been observed in women exposed to MTX.

Pharmacokinetics and Toxicity of Methotrexate in the Central Nervous System

Because of its high degree of ionization at physiologic pH, MTX penetrates into the CSF with difficulty. During a constant intravenous drug infusion,[325] the ratio of venous MTX concentration to CSF concentration is approximately 30:1 at equilibrium. Thus, plasma levels in excess of 30 μmol/L would be required to achieve the concentration of 1 μmol/L that is thought to be necessary for killing of leukemic cells. Protocols for prophylaxis against meningeal leukemia and lymphoma using systemic high-dose infusions of MTX have demonstrated that high-dose MTX infusions are a reasonable treatment alternative to intrathecal prophylaxis.[5] Overt meningeal leukemia increases the CSF: plasma ratio and experience supports the use of MTX at a loading dose of 700 mg/m² followed by a 23-hour infusion of 2,800 mg/m², with leucovorin rescue as an excellent treatment alternative for patients with carcinomatous meningitis. This regimen achieves the requisite CSF levels of 1 μmol/L.[326,327] In children with ALL, a diminished CSF: plasma ratio has been found to be a predictor of CNS relapse.[328]

Direct intrathecal injection of MTX has become a standard measure for the treatment and prophylaxis of meningeal malignancy. The readers are referred to a comprehensive review on this topic.[329] Drug injected into the intrathecal space distributes in a total volume of approximately 120 mL for patients over 3 years of age. Thus, a maximal total dose of 12 mg is advised for all patients over 3 years, with lower doses indicated for younger children. Based on pharmacokinetic studies, Bleyer[246] has recommended a dose of 6 mg for age 1 or younger, 8 mg for ages 1 to 2, and 10 mg for ages 2 to 3. The peak CSF concentration achieved by this schedule is approximately 100 μmol/L. Lumbar CSF drug concentrations decline in a biphasic pattern with a terminal half-life of 7 to 16 hours. This terminal phase of disappearance may be considerably prolonged in patients with active meningeal disease and in older-age patients.[329,330] Injection of radiolabeled MTX into the ventricular space of rabbits demonstrated rapid but variable distribution of MTX in the gray matter adjacent to the CSF, which suggests a mechanism for the various syndromes associated with MTX neurotoxicity.[331] MTX is cleared from spinal fluid by bulk resorption of spinal fluid (i.e., "bulk flow"), a process that may be prolonged by increases in intracranial pressure and the administration of acetazolamide. A second component of resorption involves the active transport of this organic anion by the choroid plexus. A prolongation of the terminal half-life is also found in patients who develop drug-related neurotoxicity, although a causal relationship between abnormal pharmacokinetics and neurotoxicity has not been firmly established.

MTX administered into the lumbar space distributes poorly over the cerebral convexities and into the ventricular spaces.[325] The concentration gradient between lumbar and ventricular CSF may exceed 10:1. Although this uneven distribution has no documented role in determining clinical relapse of patients treated for meningeal leukemia, awareness of this potential problem has led to clinical trials using direct intraventricular injection of MTX via an Ommaya reservoir. Bleyer et al.[332] have demonstrated that a concentration × time regimen in which 1 mg MTX was injected into the Ommaya reservoir every 12 hours for 3 days, yielding continuous CSF levels above 0.5 μmol/L, achieved therapeutic results equivalent to those with the conventional intralumbar injection of 12 mg every 4 days. Moreover, this concentration × time regimen was associated with a considerable reduction in neurotoxic side effects, presumably owing to the avoidance of high peak levels of drug associated with higher MTX doses. Glantz et al.[333] reported on the use of high-dose intravenous MTX as the sole treatment for nonleukemic meningeal tumor. Sixteen patients with solid tumor neoplastic meningitis received high-dose intravenous MTX (8 g/m² over 4 hours) with leucovorin rescue. Compared with a reference group of patients receiving standard intrathecal MTX, the high-dose intravenous group exhibited cytotoxic CSF and serum MTX concentrations that were maintained much longer than with intrathecal dosing. In addition, median survival in the high-dose intravenous MTX group was 13.8 versus 2.3 months for the intrathecal reference group ($P = 0.003$).

Three different neurotoxic syndromes have been observed after treatment with intrathecal MTX.[332] The most common and most immediate neurotoxic side effect is an acute chemical arachnoiditis manifested as severe headache, nuchal rigidity, vomiting, fever, and inflammatory cell pleocytosis of the spinal fluid. This constellation of symptoms appears to be a function of the frequency and dose of drug administered and may be ameliorated either by reduction in dose or by a change in therapy to intrathecal cytosine arabinoside. A less acute but more serious neurotoxic syndrome has been observed in approximately 10% of patients treated with intrathecal MTX. This subacute toxicity appears during the 2nd or 3rd week of treatment, usually in adult patients with active meningeal leukemia, and is manifested as motor paralysis of the extremities, cranial nerve palsy, seizures, or coma. Because MTX pharmacokinetics is abnormal in these patients, the suspicion is that this subacute neurotoxicity may be the result of extended exposure to toxic drug concentrations.[329] Finally, a more chronic demyelinating encephalopathy has been observed in children months or years after intrathecal MTX therapy. The primary symptoms of this toxicity are dementia, limb spasticity, and, in more advanced cases, coma. Computerized axial tomography (CT) has revealed ventricular enlargement, white matter changes, cortical thinning, and diffuse intracerebral calcification in children who have received prophylactic intrathecal MTX.[334,335] Most of these patients had also received cranial irradiation (>2,000 rad), and all had received systemic chemotherapy.

Treatment with repeated courses of high-dose intravenous MTX may also result in encephalopathy.[336] In these patients, symptoms of dementia and paresis may develop in the 2nd or 3rd month after treatment and may also be associated with diffuse cortical changes on MRI and CT scans. A second form of cerebral dysfunction associated with high-dose MTX is an acute transient dysfunction, which has been described in 4% to 15% of treated patients.[337–339] The syndrome consists of any combination of paresis, aphasia, behavioral abnormalities, and seizures. The neurologic events occur on an average of 6 days after the MTX dose and in most cases, completely resolve, usually within 48 to 72 hours. Patients may have received any number of MTX doses before the onset of this neurotoxic event, and some patients may have repeat episodes with subsequent MTX doses. In general, CSF and head CT scans are normal, but low-density lesions have been noted in some cases.[340] The electroencephalogram may represent the only abnormal study and shows a diffuse or focal slowing. No clinical evidence exists to support the use of leucovorin, either acutely after intrathecal MTX or over the long-term in patients who develop neurotoxic symptoms. Although leucovorin can enter the CSF, its penetration appears to be poor.[341,342] A comparison of neurologic toxicities was undertaken in a randomized trial involving 49 children with acute leukemia treated with either intrathecal MTX plus radiation or high-dose systemic MTX for central nervous system prophylaxis.[343] Long-term toxicities were similar with either treatment option, and overall decreases in intelligence quotients were found to be clinically significant in 61% of the children. In addition, 58% of the patients treated with systemic therapy had abnormal electroencephalograms and 57% of those treated with intrathecal MTX and radiation experienced somnolence syndrome. Mahoney et al.[344] described the incidence of acute neurotoxicity in 1,304 children with lower risk B-precursor lymphoid leukemia treated as part of the Pediatric Oncology Group trial. After remission induction, patients were randomized into one of three 24-week intensification schedules (intermediate-dose MTX or divided-dose oral MTX with or without intravenous mercaptopurine and extended intrathecal therapy). Overall, acute neurotoxicity occurred in 7.8% (95 of 1,218) of eligible patients, and the authors found that intensification with repeated intravenous MTX and low-dose leucovorin rescue was associated with a higher risk of acute neurotoxicity and leukoencephalopathy, especially in patients who received concomitant triple intrathecal therapy (MTX, dexamethasone, and cytosine arabinoside).

The etiology of the MTX-associated neurotoxicity is unknown. Vascular events in the form of vasospasm or emboli have been proposed to explain these neurologic abnormalities, and studies have suggested alterations in brain glucose metabolism after MTX treatment.[345] Investigators from St. Jude Children's Research Hospital found that the incidence of seizures in children treated for acute leukemia with MTX was related to acute elevations in serum homocysteine levels following MTX treatment.[346] Of interest, these investigators did not find an association between seizures and MTHFR genotype. Long-term exposure of rat cerebellar explants to 1 μmol/L MTX resulted in axonal death 2 weeks after drug exposure and loss of myelin sheaths in 5 weeks, which suggests a direct toxic effect of MTX on axonal cells.[347] DHFR is present in brain tissue, but its biochemical role in the cerebral cortex, the primary site of MTX neurotoxicity, is uncertain.

Cranial radiation appears to increase blood-brain barrier permeability to serum proteins and MTX.[348] Because radiation and MTX are frequently used together, this interaction may be an important mechanism for enhanced toxicity.

Inadvertent overdose of intrathecal MTX generally has a fatal outcome. Immediate lumbar puncture with CSF removal along with ventriculolumbar perfusion has been successfully used to avert catastrophe in such situations.[349]

Clinical Dosage Schedules

A variety of dosage schedules and routes of administration are used clinically, including high-dose therapy with the addition of leucovorin rescue. The selection of an appropriate schedule depends largely on the specific disease being treated, on other antineoplastic agents or radiation to be used in combination regimens, on the patient's tolerance for host toxicity, and on other factors that might alter pharmacokinetics. Parenteral schedules are preferred for induction therapy regimens in which maximal concentrations and duration of exposure are desirable in an effort to achieve complete remission. High-dose MTX regimens and leucovorin rescue offer the advantage of minimal bone marrow toxicity. This regimen, however, can safely be used only in patients with normal renal and hepatic function and under conditions in which no large extracellular accumulations of fluid are present. As emphasized previously, high-dose regimens should be instituted only when plasma monitoring is available to determine the adequacy of drug clearance and the risk of serious toxicity. Furthermore, because leucovorin may rescue tumor cells as well as normal cells, the optimal dose, schedule, and clinical utility of high-dose MTX with leucovorin rescue need to be more carefully defined.

Other Antifolates

Pemetrexed

TS represents a logical target for new drug development using folate analogs. Of the many antifolates synthesized as TS antagonists, pemetrexed (LY231514,), a pyrrolo(2,3-d)pyrimidine-based antifolate analog (see Fig. 8-1), is the most effective. Its key features are shown in Table 8-6. Pemetrexed is readily transported into cells via the RFC and by the proton-coupled carrier described earlier.[350,351] It is avidly metabolized to its PGs, which are more 50-fold more potent inhibitors of TS than corresponding MTX PGs. The multitargeting effect of pemetrexed was seen in studies by Shih et al.,[350] who suggested that, at higher concentrations, pemetrexed and its PGs not only act as TS inhibitors, depleting dTTP pools, but also inhibit other key folate-requiring enzymes, including GARTF, and to a lesser extent DHFR and AICARTF. The combined inhibitory effects of pemetrexed give rise to a cellular level end-product reversal pattern that is different from those of other inhibitors such as MTX and the quinazoline antifolates; at low concentrations, thymidine reverses its toxicity, while at high concentrations, both

TABLE 8.6	Key features of pemetrexed and pralatrexate	
	Pemetrexed	**Pralatrexate**
Mechanism of action	Inhibition of TS, GARTF	Inhibition of DHFR
Metabolism	Minimal	Minimal
Elimination	Renal excretion	Renal excretion
Drug interactions	None	None
Pharmacokinetics (plasma $t_{1/2}$)	4 h	4–8 h
Toxicity	Myelosuppression Pulmonary infiltrates Rash	Myelosuppression
Precautions	Toxicity lessened by pretreatment with folic acid and B-12	

thymidine and purines are required. Pemetrexed has less effect on the folate and purine nucleotide pools as compared to MTX.[352]

Its antitumor efficacy against human tumor cell lines is modulated by external folate concentrations such that reduced folate (RF) supplementation inhibits its effects, while cells adapted to growth in low-folate medium and up-regulating the RF transporter were rescued by leucovorin but not by folic acid, which prefers the FR transporter.[353] Pretreatment with folic acid protects normal tissues from pemetrexed while preserving the antitumor activity in patients. Severe myelosuppression due to pemetrexed correlates with high pretreatment serum concentrations of homocysteine, an indicator of folate deficiency. In other toxic patients, B_{12} deficiency was thought to be responsible for pemetrexed toxicity. Addition of vitamin B_{12} (1 mg intramuscularly) and folic acid (1 mg/d for 2 weeks beginning 2 weeks prior to pemetrexed) resulted in a greatly improved and predictable toxicity profile, without diminishing antitumor efficacy, in patients with mesothelioma treated with pemetrexed.[354,355] The primary toxicities of pemetrexed are myelosuppression, diarrhea, and a rash that responds to corticosteroids. At the doses commonly used, 500 mg/m[2] every 3 weeks, the drug is extremely well tolerated, even for patients who have progressed through multiple other regimens.[356]

Resistance to pemetrexed in the clinical setting is poorly understood but, in experimental systems, has variously been attributed to mutations in FPGS, increased TS activity, or loss of transport, although the role of specific transporters may depend on the relative expression of the RF and proton-coupled systems.[351]

Clinical Pharmacokinetics and Toxicity

Pemetrexed is eliminated primarily by renal excretion as unchanged drug. It has a serum half-life of approximately 4 hours in patients with normal renal function, but the half-life increases markedly in subjects who have a creatinine clearance of 30 mL/min or less.[357] At approved doses, the drug can be given safely to patients with a glomerular filtration rate of at least 40 mL/min. The drug is usually administered as a brief infusion once every 3 weeks. Patients with normal renal function tolerate doses up to 1,000 mg/m^2 in adults and 2,000 mg/m^2 in children, with folate supplementation, and with dose-limiting toxicities of myelosuppression and rash.[358,359] However, there is no proven therapeutic benefit of escalating dose above the approved 500 mg/m^2 every 3 weeks.

Pemetrexed, in combination with cisplatin, has been approved for treatment of mesothelioma. In a randomized phase III investigation of 456 patients with mesothelioma, comparing cisplatin with the combination, patients treated with the doublet enjoyed a significantly improved response rate (41% versus 17%), time to disease progression (5.7 versus 3.9 months), and overall survival (12.1 versus 9.3 months). Pemetrexed is also approved for second-line therapy of non–small cell lung cancer, for which it has a 16% response rate in untreated patients.[356] In a phase III trial of 571 patients randomized patients with advanced and refractory non–small cell lung cancer to either pemetrexed or docetaxel, the drugs produced equivalent efficacy outcomes, but the pemetrexed was associated with a significantly improved toxicity profile.[360] Aside from myelosuppression and intestinal toxicity, pemetrexed causes a rash in 40% of patients. The rash is suppressed by the administration of dexamethasone, 4 mg two times a day, on days 1, 0, and +1.

Pralatrexate

The newest folate analog approved for clinical use, Pralatrexate, (Fig. 8-1), resulted from a series of experiments to develop analogues that had favorable transport properties (see Table 8-2). While its inhibition of DHFR was comparable or slightly less potent than that of MTX, it proved to have 10 fold greater affinity for the RF transporter than MTX and inhibited tumor cell growth at 30- to 40-fold lower extracellular concentrations than MTX; its increased potency is likely related to its more efficient transport and its more avid polyglutamation as compared to MTX. It cured mice with breast and lung cancer xenografts that responded only partially to MTX.[88] Clinical trials demonstrated consistent activity against cutaneous T-cell lymphoma and peripheral T-cell lymphoma, for which it is now approved.[361]

The recommended dose of pralatrexate is 30 mg/m^2/wk for 6 of 7 weeks, the dose-limiting toxicities being stomatitis, rash, thrombocytopenia, and neutropenia. The incidence of stomatitis was reduced by supplementing folic acid (5 mg/d for 3 days prior to, the day of, and the day after pralatrexate) and B12 (1,000 μg orally or 100 μg IM every 8 to 9 weeks). The drug is cleared by excretion in the urine and has a plasma $t_{1/2}$ of 4 to 8 hours, although studies are preliminary.[88] No guidelines are available for modifying dose for renal dysfunction, but it is likely that reductions in proportion to abnormalities in creatine clearance will be necessary.

References

1. Farber S, Diamond LK, Mercer RD, et al. Temporary remission in acute leukemia in children produced by folic acid antagonist 4-amethopteroylglutamic acid (aminopterin). N Engl J Med 1948;238:787.
2. Hoffmeister RT. Methotrexate therapy in rheumatoid arthritis: 15 years' experience. Am J Med 1983;75:69–73.
3. Rees RB, Bennett JH, Maibach HI, et al. Methotrexate for psoriasis. Arch Dermatol 1967;95:2–11.
4. Allegra CJ, Chabner BA, Tuazon CU, et al. Trimetrexate for the treatment of Pneumocystis carinii pneumonia in patients with the acquired immunodeficiency syndrome. N Engl J Med 1987;317:978–985.
5. Pui C-H, Campana D, Pei D, et al. Treating childhood acute lymphoblastic leukemia without cranial irradiation. N Engl J Med 2009;360:2730–2741.
6. Allegra CJ, Fine RL, Drake JC, et al. The effect of methotrexate on intracellular folate pools in human MCF-7 breast cancer cells. Evidence for direct inhibition of purine synthesis. J Biol Chem 1986;261:6478–6485.
7. Matherly LH, Barlowe CK, Phillips VM, et al. The effects of 4-aminoantifolates on 5-formyltetrahydrofolate metabolism in L1210 cells. J Biol Chem 1987;262:710–717.
8. Baram J, Allegra CJ, Fine RL, et al. Effect of methotrexate on intracellular folate pools in purified myeloid precursor cells from normal human bone marrow. J Clin Invest 1987;79:692–697.
9. Kesavan V, Sur P, Doig MT, et al. Effects of methotrexate on folates in Krebs ascites and L1210 murine leukemia cells. Cancer Lett 1986;30:55–59.
10. Bunni M, Doig MT, Donato H, et al. Role of methylenetetrahydrofolate depletion in methotrexate-mediated intracellular thymidylate synthesis inhibition in cultured L1210 cells. Cancer Res 1988;48:3398–3404.
11. Seither RL, Trent DF, Mikulecky DC, et al. Folate-pool interconversions and inhibition of biosynthetic processes after exposure of L1210 leukemia cells to antifolates. Experimental and network thermodynamic analyses of the role of dihydrofolate polyglutamylates in antifolate action in cells. J Biol Chem 1989;264:17016–17023.
12. Priest DG, Bunni M, Sirotnak FM. Relationship of reduced folate changes to inhibition of DNA synthesis induced by methotrexate in L1210 cells in vivo. Cancer Res 1989;49:4204–4209.
13. Allegra CJ, Hoang K, Yeh GC, et al. Evidence for direct inhibition of de novo purine synthesis in human MCF-7 breast cells as a principal mode of metabolic inhibition by methotrexate. J Biol Chem 1987;262:13520–13526.
14. Baram J, Chabner BA, Drake JC, et al. Identification and biochemical properties of 10-formyldihydrofolate, a novel folate found in methotrexate-treated cells. J Biol Chem 1988;263:7105–7111.
15. Kumar P, Kisliuk RL, Gaumont Y, et al. Inhibition of human dihydrofolate reductase by antifolyl polyglutamates. Biochem Pharmacol 1989;38:541–543.
16. Allegra CJ, Chabner BA, Drake JC, et al. Enhanced inhibition of thymidylate synthase by methotrexate polyglutamates. J Biol Chem 1985;260:9720–9726.
17. Allegra CJ, Drake JC, Jolivet J, et al. Inhibition of phosphoribosylaminoimidazolecarboxamide transformylase by methotrexate and dihydrofolic acid polyglutamates. Proc Natl Acad Sci USA 1985;82:4881–4885.
18. Baggott JE, Vaughn WH, Hudson BB. Inhibition of 5-aminoimidazole-4-carboxamide ribotide transformylase, adenosine deaminase and 5'-adenylate deaminase by polyglutamates of methotrexate and oxidized folates and by 5-aminoimidazole-4-carboxamide riboside and ribotide. Biochem J 1986;236:193–200.
19. Chu E, Drake JC, Boarman D, et al. Mechanism of thymidylate synthase inhibition by methotrexate in human neoplastic cell lines and normal human myeloid progenitor cells. J Biol Chem 1990;265:8470–8478.
20. Morrison PF, Allegra CJ. Folate cycle kinetics in human breast cancer cells. J Biol Chem 1989;264:10552–10566.
21. Lyons SD, Sant ME, Christopherson RI. Cytotoxic mechanisms of glutamine antagonists in mouse L1210 leukemia. J Biol Chem 1990;265:11377–11381.
22. O'Dwyer PJ, Shoemaker DD, Plowman J, et al. Trimetrexate: a new antifol entering clinical trials. Invest New Drugs 1985;3:71–75.
23. Sigel CW, Macklin AW, Woolley JL Jr, et al. Preclinical biochemical pharmacology and toxicology of piritrexim, a lipophilic inhibitor of dihydrofolate reductase. J Natl Cancer Inst Monogr 1987;5:111–120.
24. Sirotnak FM, DeGraw JI, Schmid FA, et al. New folate analogs of the 10-deaza-aminopterin series. Further evidence for markedly increased antitumor efficacy compared with methotrexate in ascitic and solid murine tumor models. Cancer Chemother Pharmacol 1984;12:26–30.
25. Kamen BA, Eibl B, Cashmore A, et al. Uptake and efficacy of trimetrexate (TMQ, 2,4-diamino-5-methyl-6-[(3,4,5-trime-thoxyanilino) methyl] quinazoline), a non-classical antifolate in methotrexate-resistant leukemia cells in vitro. Biochem Pharmacol 1984;33:1697–1699.
26. Jones TR, Calvert AH, Jackman AL, et al. A potent anti-tumor quinazoline inhibitor of thymidylate synthetase, biological properties and therapeutic results in mice. Eur J Cancer 1981;17:11–19.

27. Cheng YC, Dutschman GE, Starnes MC, et al. Activity of the new antifolate N10-propargyl-5,8-dideazafolate and its polyglutamates against human dihydrofolate reductase, human thymidylate synthetase, and KB cells containing different levels of dihydrofolate reductase. Cancer Res 1985;45:598–600.

28. Grindey GB, Shih C, Barnett CJ, et al. LY231514, a novel pyrrolopyrimidine antifolate that inhibits thymidylate synthase (TS). Proc Am Assoc Cancer Res Annu Meet 1992;33:411.

29. Antony AC, Kane MA, Portillo RM, et al. Studies of the role of a particulate folate-binding protein in the uptake of 5-methyltetrahydrofolate by cultured human KB cells. J Biol Chem 1985;260:14911–14917.

30. Kamen BA, Capdevila A. Receptor-mediated folate accumulation is regulated by the cellular folate content. Proc Natl Acad Sci USA 1986;83:5983–5987.

31. Fan J, Vitols KS, Huennekens FM. Biotin derivatives of methotrexate and folate. Synthesis and utilization for affinity purification of two membrane-associated folate transporters from L1210 cells. J Biol Chem 1991;266:14862–14865.

32. Brigle KE, Westin EH, Houghton MT, et al. Characterization of two cDNAs encoding folate-binding proteins from L1210 murine leukemia cells. Increased expression associated with a genomic rearrangement. J Biol Chem 1991;266:17243–17249.

33. Zhao R, Qui A, Tsai E, et al. The proton-coupled folate transporter: inpact on pemetrexed Transport and on antifolates activities compared with the reduced folate carrier. Mol Pharmacol 2008;74:854–862.

34. Chello PL, Sirotnak FM, Dorick DM. Alterations in the kinetics of methotrexate transport during growth of L1210 murine leukemia cells in culture. Mol Pharmacol 1980;18:274–280.

35. Knight CB, Elwood PC, Chabner BA. Future directions for antifolate drug development. Adv Enzyme Regul 1989;29:3–12.

36. Kane MA, Portillo RM, Elwood PC, et al. The influence of extracellular folate concentration on methotrexate uptake by human KB cells. Partial characterization of a membrane-associated methotrexate binding protein. J Biol Chem 1986;261:44–49.

37. Price EM, Freisheim JH. Photoaffinity analogues of methotrexate as folate antagonist binding probes. 2. Transport studies, photoaffinity labeling, and identification of the membrane carrier protein for methotrexate from murine L1210 cells. Biochemistry 1987;26:4757–4763.

38. Matherly LH, Czajkowski CA, Angeles SM. Identification of a highly glycosylated methotrexate membrane carrier in K562 human erythroleukemia cells up-regulated for tetrahydrofolate cofactor and methotrexate transport. Cancer Res 1991;51:3420–3426.

39. Moscow JA, Gong M, He R, et al. Isolation of a gene encoding a human reduced folate carrier (RFC1) and analysis of its expression in transport-deficient, methotrexate-resistant human breast cancer cells. Cancer Res 1995;55:3790–3794.

40. Prasad PD, Ramamoorthy S, Leibach FH, et al. Molecular cloning of the human placental folate transporter. Biochem Biophys Res Commun 1995;206:681–687.

41. Zhao R, Gao F, Wang PJ, etal. Role of the amino acid 45 residue in reduced folate carrier function and ion-dependent transport as characterized by site-directed mutagenesis. Mol Pharmacol 2000;57(2):317–323.

42. Zhao R, Wang PJ, Gao F, etal. Residues 45 and 404 in the murine reduced folate carrier may interact to alter carrier binding and mobility. Biochim Biophys Acta 2003;1613(1–2):49–56.

43. Sharina IG, Zhao R, Wang Y, et al. Mutational analysis of the functional role of conserved arginine and lysine residues in transmembrane domains of the murine reduced folate carrier. Mol Pharmacol 2001;59(5):1022–1028.

44. Zhao R, Gao F, Hanscom M, et al. A prominent low-pH methotrexate transport activity in human solid tumors: contribution to the preservation of methotrexate pharmacologic activity in HeLa cells lacking the reduced folate carrier. Clin Cancer Res 2004;10(2):718–727.

45. Campbell IG, Jones TA, Foulkes WD, et al. Folate-binding protein is a marker for ovarian cancer. Cancer Res 1991;51:5329–5338.

46. Coney LR, Tomassetti A, Carayannopoulos L, et al. Cloning of a tumor-associated antigen: MOv18 and MOv19 antibodies recognize a folate-binding protein. Cancer Res 1991;51:6125–6132.

47. Elwood PC, Kane MA, Portillo RM, et al. The isolation, characterization, and comparison of the membrane-associated and soluble folate-binding proteins from human KB cells. J Biol Chem 1986;261:15416–15423.

48. Spannuth WA, Sood AK, Coleman RL. Farletuzumab in epithelial ovarian carcinoma. Expert Opin Biol Ther 2010;10(3):431–437.

49. Shen F, Ross JF, Wang X, et al. Identification of a novel folate receptor, a truncated receptor, and receptor type beta in hematopoietic cells: cDNA cloning, expression, immunoreactivity, and tissue specificity. Biochemistry 1994;33:1209–1215.

50. Roberts SJ, Petropavlovskaja M, Chung KN, et al. Role of individual N-linked glycosylation sites in the function and intracellular transport of the human alpha folate receptor. Arch Biochem Biophys 1998;351:227–235.

51. Allard JE, Risinger JI, Morrison C, et al. Overexpression of folate biinding protein is associated with shortened progression-free survival in uterine adenocarcinomas. Gyn Oncol 2007;107:52–5.

52. Elwood PC, Nachmanoff K, Saikawa Y, et al. The divergent 5' termini of the alpha human folate receptor (hFR) mRNAs originate from two tissue-specific promoters and alternative splicing: characterization of the alpha hFR gene structure. Biochemistry 1997;36:1467–1478.

53. Roberts SJ, Chung KN, Nachmanoff K, et al. Tissue-specific promoters of the alpha human folate receptor gene yield transcripts with divergent 5' leader sequences and different translational efficiencies. Biochem J 1997;326:439–447.

54. Sun XL, Murphy BR, Li QJ, et al. Transduction of folate receptor cDNA into cervical carcinoma cells using recombinant adeno-associated virions delays cell proliferation in vitro and in vivo. J Clin Invest 1995;96:1535–1547.

55. Shen F, Zheng X, Wang J, et al. Identification of amino acid residues that determine the differential ligand specificities of folate receptors alpha and beta. Biochemistry 1997;36:6157–6163.

56. Wu M, Fan J, Gunning W, et al. Clustering of GPI-anchored folate receptor independent of both cross-linking and association with caveolin. J Membr Biol 1997;159:137–147.

57. Anderson RG, Kamen BA, Rothberg KG, et al. Potocytosis: sequestration and transport of small molecules by caveolae. Science 1992;255:410–411.

58. Kamen BA, Smith AK, Anderson RG. The folate receptor works in tandem with a probenecid-sensitive carrier in MA104 cells in vitro. J Clin Invest 1991;87:1442–1449.

59. Chang WJ, Rothberg KG, Kamen BA, et al. Lowering the cholesterol content of MA104 cells inhibits receptor-mediated transport of folate. J Cell Biol 1992;118:63–69.

60. Smart EJ, Mineo C, Anderson RG. Clustered folate receptors deliver 5-methyltetrahydrofolate to cytoplasm of MA104 cells. J Cell Biol 1996;134:1169–1177.

61. Spinella MJ, Brigle KE, Sierra EE, et al. Distinguishing between folate receptor-alpha-mediated transport and reduced folate carrier-mediated transport in L1210 leukemia cells. J Biol Chem 1995;270:7842–7849.

62. Westerhof GR, Rijnboutt S, Schornagel JH, et al. Functional activity of the reduced folate carrier in KB, MA104, and IGROV-I cells expressing folate-binding protein. Cancer Res 1995;55:3795–3802.

63. Zhao R, Min SH, Wang Y, et al. A role for the proton-coupled folate transporter, (PCFT-SLC46A1) in folate receptor-mediated endocytosis. J Biol Chem 2009;284:4567–4274.

64. Zhao R, Min SH, Qui A, et al. The Spectrum of mutations in the PCFT gene, coding for an intestinal folate transporter, that are the basis for hereditary folate malabsorption. Blood 2007;110:1147–1152.

65. Schuetz JD, Matherly LH, Westin EH, et al. Evidence for a functional defect in the translocation of the methotrexate transport carrier in a methotrexate-resistant murine L1210 leukemia cell line. J Biol Chem 1988;263:9840–9847.

66. Assaraf YG, Schimke RT. Identification of methotrexate transport deficiency in mammalian cells using fluoresceinated methotrexate and flow cytometry. Proc Natl Acad Sci USA 1987;84:7154–7158.

67. Rodenhuis S, McGuire JJ, Narayanan R, et al. Development of an assay system for the detection and classification of methotrexate resistance in fresh human leukemic cells. Cancer Res 1986;46:6513–6519.

68. Schuetz JD, Westin EH, Matherly LH, et al. Membrane protein changes in an L1210 leukemia cell line with a translocation defect in the methotrexate-tetrahydrofolate cofactor transport carrier. J Biol Chem 1989;264:16261–16267.

69. Jansen G, Westerhof GR, Kathmann I, et al. Identification of a membrane-associated folate-binding protein in human leukemic CCRF-CEM cells with transport-related methotrexate resistance [published erratum appears in Cancer Res 1995;55(18):4203]. Cancer Res 1989;49:2455–2459.

70. Zhao R, Assaraf YG, Goldman ID. A mutated murine reduced folate carrier (RFC1) with increased affinity for folic acid, decreased affinity for methotrexate, and an obligatory anion requirement for transport function. J Biol Chem 1998;273:19065–19071.

71. Zhao R, Assaraf YG, Goldman ID. A reduced folate carrier mutation produces substrate-dependent alterations in carrier mobility in murine leukemia cells and methotrexate resistance with conservation of growth in 5-formyltetrahydrofolate. J Biol Chem 1998;273:7873–7879.

72. Gifford AJ, Haber M, Witt TL etal. Role of the E45K-reduced folate carrier gene mutation in methotrexate resistance in human leukemia cells. Leukemia 2002;16(12):2379–2387.

73. Trippett T, Schlemmer S, Elisseyeff Y, et al. Defective transport as a mechanism of acquired resistance to methotrexate in patients with acute lymphoblastic leukemia. Blood 1992;80:1158–1162.

74. Levy AS, Sather HN, Steinherz PG etal. Reduced folate carrier and dihydrofolate reductase expression in acucte lymphocytic leukemia may predict outcome: a Children's Cancer Group Study. J Pediatr Hematol Oncol 2003;25(9):688–695.

75. Ge Y, Haska CL, LaFiura K, et al. Prognostic role of the reduced folate carrier, the major membrane transporter for methotrexate, in childhood acute lymphoblastic leukemia: a report from the children's oncology group. Clin Cancer Res 2007;13:451–457.

76. Guo W, Healey JH, Meyers PA, et al. Mechanisms of methotrexate resistance in osteosarcoma. Clin Cancer Res 1999;5:621–627.

77. Ifergan I, Meller I, Issakov J, etal. Reduced folate carrier protein expression in osteosarcoma: implications for the prediction of tumor chemosensitivity. Cancer 2003;98(9):1958–1966.

78. Liu S, Song L, Bevins R, et al. The murine-reduced folate carrier gene can act as a selectable marker and a suicide gene in hematopoietic cells in vivo. Hum Gene Ther 2002;13(14):1777–1782.

79. Taylor IW, Slowiaczek P, Friedlander ML, et al. Selective toxicity of a new lipophilic antifolate, BW301U, for methotrexate-resistant cells with reduced drug uptake. Cancer Res 1985;45:978–982.

80. Mini E, Moroson BA, Franco CT, et al. Cytotoxic effects of folate antagonists against methotrexate-resistant human leukemic lymphoblast CCRF-CEM cell lines. Cancer Res 1985;45:325–330.

81. Sirotnak FM, DeGraw JI. A new analogue of 10-deazaanimopterin with markedly enhanced curative effects against human tumor xenografts in mice. Cancer Chemother Pharmacol 1998;42:313–318.

82. Schmid FA, Sirotnak FM, Otter GM, et al. Combination chemotherapy with a new folate analog: activity of 10-ethyl-10-deaza-aminopterin compared to methotrexate with 5-fluorouracil and alkylating agents against advanced metastatic disease in murine tumor models. Cancer Treat Rep 1987;71:727–732.

83. Jansen G, Schornagel JH, Westerhof GR, et al. Multiple membrane transport systems for the uptake of folate-based thymidylate synthase inhibitors. Cancer Res 1990;50:7544–7548.

84. Westerhof GR, Jansen G, van Emmerik N, et al. Membrane transport of natural folates and antifolate compounds in murine L1210 leukemia cells: role of carrier- and receptor- mediated transport systems. Cancer Res 1991;51:5507–5513.

85. Wang Y, Zhao R, Goldman ID. Decreased expression of the reduced folate carrier and folylpolyglutamate synthetase is the basis for acquired resistance to the pemetrexed antifolate (LY231514) in an L1210 murine leukemia cell line. Biochem Pharmacol 2003;65(7):1163–1170.

86. Zhao R, Hanscom M, Chattopadhyay S, et al. Selective Preservation of pemetrexed pharmacological activity in HeLa cells lacking the reduced folate carrier: association with the presence of a secondary transport pathway. Cancer Res 2004;64(9):3313–3319.

87. Ohe Y, Ichinose Y, Nakagawa K, et al. Efficacy and safety of two doses of pemetrexed supplemented with folic acid and vitamin B$_{12}$ in previously treated patients with non-small cell lung cancer. Clin Cancer Res 2008;14: 4206–4212.

88. Molina JR. Pralatexate, a dihydrofolate reductase inhibitor for the potential treatment of several malignancies. IDrugs 2008;11:508–521.

89. Henderson GB, Zevely EM. Inhibitory effects of probenecid on the individual transport routes which mediate the influx and efflux of methotrexate in L1210 cells. Biochem Pharmacol 1985;34:1725–1729.

90. Henderson GB, Tsuji JM. Methotrexate efflux in L1210 cells. Kinetic and specificity properties of the efflux system sensitive to bromosulfophthalein and its possible identity with a system which mediates the efflux of 3',5'-cyclic AMP. J Biol Chem 1987;262:13571–13578.

91. Henderson GB, Tsuji JM, Kumar HP. Characterization of the individual transport routes that mediate the influx and efflux of methotrexate in CCRF-CEM human lymphoblastic cells. Cancer Res 1986;46:1633–1638.

92. Assaraf YG, Rothem L, Hooijberg JH, et al. Loss of multidrug resistance protein 1 expression and folate efflux activity results i a highly concentrative folate transport in human leukemia cells. J Biol Chem 2003;278(9):6680–6686.

93. Vlaming MLH, Pala Z, van Esch A, et al. Impact of Abcc2 (Mrp2) and Abcc3 (Mrp3) on the in vivo elimination of methotrexate and its main toxic metabolite 7-hydroxymethotrexate. Clin Cancer Res 2008;14:8152–8160.

94. Vlaming MLH, Pala Z, van Esch A, et al. Functionally overlapping roles of Abcg2 (Bcrp1) and Abcc2 (Mrp2) in the elimination of methotrexate and its main toxic metabolite 7-hydroxymethotrexate in vivo. Clin Cancer Res 2009;15:3084–93.

95. Kitamura Y, Hirouchi M, Kusuhara H, et al. Increasing systemic exposure of methotrexate by active efflux mediated by multidrug resistance-associated protein 3 (Mrp3/Abcc3). J Pharmacol Exp Ther 2008;327:465–473.

96. Sirotnak FM, Wendel HG, Bornmann WG, et al. Co-administration of probenecid, an inhibitor of a cMOAT/MRP-like plasma membrane ATPase, greatly enhanced the efficacy of a new 10-deazaaminopterin against human solid tumors in vivo. Clin Cancer Res 2000;6(9):3705–3712.

97. Stark M, Rothem L, Jansen G, et al. Antifolate resistance associated with loss of MRP1 expression and function in Chinese hamster ovary cells with markedly impaired export of folate and cholate. Mol Pharmacol 2003;64(2): 220–227.

98. Chen ZS, Robey RW, Belinsky MG, et al. Transport of methotrexate polyglutamates, and 17 beta-estradiol 17-(beta-D-glucuronide) by ABCG2: effects of acquired mutations as R482 on methotrexate transport. Cancer Res 2003;63(14):4048–4054.

99. Koizumi S, Curt GA, Fine RL, et al. Formation of methotrexate polyglutamates in purified myeloid precursor cells from normal human bone marrow. J Clin Invest 1985;75:1008–1014.

100. Fabre I, Fabre G, Goldman ID. Polyglutamylation, an important element in methotrexate cytotoxicity and selectivity in tumor versus murine granulocytic progenitor cells in vitro. Cancer Res 1984;44:3190–3195.

101. Schilsky RL, Bailey BD, Chabner BA. Methotrexate polyglutamate synthesis by cultured human breast cancer cells. Proc Natl Acad Sci USA 1980;77:2919–2922.

102. Jolivet J, Schilsky RL, Bailey BD, et al. Synthesis, retention, and biological activity of methotrexate polyglutamates in cultured human breast cancer cells. J Clin Invest 1982;70:351–360.

103. Kennedy DG, Van den Berg HW, Clarke R, et al. The effect of the rate of cell proliferation on the synthesis of methotrexate poly-gamma-glutamates in two human breast cancer cell lines. Biochem Pharmacol 1985;34: 3087–3090.

104. Jolivet J, Chabner BA. Intracellular pharmacokinetics of methotrexate polyglutamates in human breast cancer cells. Selective retention and less dissociable binding of 4-NH2- 10-CH3-pteroylglutamate4 and 4-NH2-10-CH3-pteroylglutamate5 to dihydrofolate reductase. J Clin Invest 1983;72:773–778.

105. Winick NJ, Kamen BA, Balis FM, et al. Folate and methotrexate polyglutamate tissue levels in rhesus monkeys following chronic low-dose methotrexate. Cancer Drug Deliv 1987;4:25–31.

106. Shane B. Folylpolyglutamate synthesis and role in the regulation of one-carbon metabolism. Vitam Horm 1989;45:263–335.

107. Gewirtz DA, White JC, Randolph JK, et al. Formation of methotrexate polyglutamates in rat hepatocytes. Cancer Res 1979;39:2914–2918.

108. Clarke L, Waxman DJ. Human liver folylpolyglutamate synthetase: biochemical characterization and interactions with folates and folate antagonists. Arch Biochem Biophys 1987;256:585–596.

109. Cichowicz DJ, Shane B. Mammalian folylpoly-gamma-glutamate synthetase. 1. Purification and general properties of the hog liver enzyme. Biochemistry 1987;26:504–512.

110. Cichowicz DJ, Shane B. Mammalian folylpoly-gamma-glutamate synthetase. 2. Substrate specificity and kinetic properties. Biochemistry 1987;26:513–521.

111. McGuire JJ, Hsieh P, Franco CT, et al. Folylpolyglutamate synthetase inhibition and cytotoxic effects of methotrexate analogs containing 2,omega-diaminoalkanoic acids. Biochem Pharmacol 1986;35:2607–2613.

112. Galivan J, Johnson T, Rhee M, et al. The role of folylpolyglutamate synthetase and gamma-glutamyl hydrolase in altering cellular folyl- and antifolylpolyglutamates. Adv Enzyme Regul 1987;26:147–155.

113. Panetta JC, Wall A, Pui CH, et al. Methotrexate intracellular disposition in acute lymphoblastic leukemia: a mathematical model of gamma-glutamyl hydrolase activity. Clin Cancer Res 2002;8(7):2423–2429.

114. Kager L, Cheok M, Yang W, et al. Folate pathway gene expression differs in subtypes of acute lymphoblastic leukemia and influences methotrexate pharmacodynamics. J Clin Invest 2005;115:110–117.

115. Yao R, Schneider E, Ryan TJ, et al. Human gamma-glutamyl hydrolase: cloning and characterization of the enzyme expressed in vitro. Proc Natl Acad Sci USA 1996;93:10134–10138.

116. Cole PD, Kamen BA, Gorlick R, et al. Effects of overexpression of gamma-glutamyl hydrolase on methotrexate metabolism and resistance. Cancer Res 2001;61(11):4599–4604.

117. Longo GS, Gorlick R, Tong WP, et al. Disparate affinities of antifolates for folylpolyglutamate synthetase from human leukemia cells. Blood 1997;90:1241–1245.

118. Sirotnak FM, Chello PL, Piper JR, et al. Growth inhibitory, transport and biochemical properties of the gamma-glutamyl and gamma-aspartyl peptides of methotrexate in L1210 leukemia cells in vitro. Biochem Pharmacol 1978;27:1821–1825.

119. Galivan J, Nimec Z, Balinska M. Regulation of methotrexate polyglutamate accumulation in vitro: effects of cellular folate content. Biochem Pharmacol 1983;32:3244–3247.

120. Jolivet J, Faucher F, Pinard MF. Influence of intracellular folates on methotrexate metabolism and cytotoxicity. Biochem Pharmacol 1987;36:3310–3312.

121. Jolivet J, Cole DE, Holcenberg JS, et al. Prevention of methotrexate cytotoxicity by asparaginase inhibition of methotrexate polyglutamate formation. Cancer Res 1985;45:217–220.

122. Sur P, Fernandes DJ, Kute TE, et al. L-asparaginase-induced modulation of methotrexate polyglutamylation in murine leukemia L5178Y. Cancer Res 1987;47:1313–1318.

123. Matherly LH, Fry DW, Goldman ID. Role of methotrexate polyglutamylation and cellular energy metabolism in inhibition of methotrexate binding to dihydrofolate reductase by 5-formyltetrahydrofolate in Ehrlich ascites tumor cells in vitro. Cancer Res 1983;43:2694–2699.

124. Allegra CJ, Drake JC, Jolivet J, et al. Inhibition of folate-dependent enzymes by methotrexate polyglutamates. In: Goldman ID, ed. Proceedings of the Second Workshop on Folyl and Antifolyl Polyglutamates. New York: Praeger, 1985:348–359.

125. Galivan J, Inglese J, McGuire JJ, et al. Gamma-fluoromethotrexate: synthesis and biological activity of a potent inhibitor of dihydrofolate reductase with greatly diminished ability to form poly-gamma-glutamates. Proc Natl Acad Sci USA 1985;82:2598–2602.

126. Samuels LL, Moccio DM, Sirotnak FM. Similar differential for total polyglutamylation and cytotoxicity among various folate analogues in human and murine tumor cells in vitro. Cancer Res 1985;45:1488–1495.

127. Matherly LH, Voss MK, Anderson LA, et al. Enhanced polyglutamylation of aminopterin relative to methotrexate in the Ehrlich ascites tumor cell in vitro. Cancer Res 1985;45:1073–1078.

128. Cowan KH, Jolivet J. A methotrexate-resistant human breast cancer cell line with multiple defects, including diminished formation of methotrexate polyglutamates. J Biol Chem 1984;259:10793–10800.

129. Mauritz R, Peters GJ, Priest DG, et al. Multiple mechanisms of resistance to methotrexate and novel antifolates in human CCRF-CEM leukemia cells and their implications for folate homeostasis. Biochem Pharmacol 2002;63(2):105–115.

130. Liani E, Rothem L, Bunni MA, et al. Loss of folylpoly-gamma-glutamate synthetase activity is a dominant mechanism of resistance to polyglutamation-dependent novel antifolates in multiple human leukemia sublines. Int J Cancer 2003;103(5):587–599.

131. Pizzorno G, Mini E, Coronnello M, et al. Impaired polyglutamylation of methotrexate as a cause of resistance in CCRF-CEM cells after short-term, high-dose treatment with this drug. Cancer Res 1988;48:2149–2155.

132. Stark M, Wichman C, Avivi I, Assaraf YG. Aberrant splicing of folylpolglutamate synthetase as a novel mechanism of antifolate resistance in leukemia. Blood 2008;113:4362–4369.

133. Pizzorno G, Chang YM, McGuire JJ, et al. Inherent resistance of human squamous carcinoma cell lines to methotrexate as a result of decreased polyglutamylation of this drug. Cancer Res 1989;49:5275–5280.

134. McCloskey DE, McGuire JJ, Russell CA, et al. Decreased folylpolyglutamate synthetase activity as a mechanism of methotrexate resistance in CCRF-CEM human leukemia sublines. J Biol Chem 1991;266:6181–6187.

135. Curt GA, Jolivet J, Carney DN, et al. Determinants of the sensitivity of human small-cell lung cancer cell lines to methotrexate. J Clin Invest 1985;76:1323–1329.

136. Longo GS, Gorlick R, Tong WP, et al. Gamma-glutamyl hydrolase and folylpolyglutamate synthetase activities predict polyglutamylation of methotrexate in acute leukemias. Oncol Res 1997;9:259–263.

137. Galpin AJ, Schuetz JD, Masson E, et al. Differences in folylpolyglutamate synthetase and dihydrofolate reductase expression in human B-lineage versus T-lineage leukemic lymphoblasts: mechanisms for lineage differences in methotrexate polyglutamylation and cytotoxicity. Mol Pharmacol 1997;52:155–163.

138. Panetta JC, Yanishevski Y, Pui CH, et al. A mathematical model of in vivo methotrexate accumulation in acute lymphoblastic leukemia. Cancer Chemother Pharmacol 2002;50(5):419–428.

139. Mantadakis E, Smith AK, Hynan L etal. Methotrexate polyglutamation may lack prognostic significance in children with B-cell precursor acute lymphoblastic leukemia treated with intensive oral methotrexate. J Pediatr Hematol Oncol 2002;24(8):736–642.

140. Li WW, Lin JT, Tong WP, et al. Mechanisms of natural resistance to antifolates in human soft tissue sarcomas. Cancer Res 1992;52:1434–1438.

141. Li WW, Lin JT, Schweitzer BI, et al. Intrinsic resistance to methotrexate in human soft tissue sarcoma cell lines. Cancer Res 1992;52:3908–3913.

142. Leil TA, Endo C, Adjei AA, et al. Identification and characterization of genetic variation in the folylpolglutamate synthase gene. Cancer Res 2007;67:8772–8782.

143. Matthews DA, Alden RA, Bolin JT, et al. X-ray structural studies of dihydrofolate reductase. In: Kisliuk RL, Brown GM, eds. Chemistry and Biology of Pteridines. New York: Elsevier/North Holland, 1979:465.

144. Matthews DA, Alden RA, Bolin JT, et al. Dihydrofolate reductase: x-ray structure of the binary complex with methotrexate. Science 1977;197:452–455.

145. Appleman JR, Howell EE, Kraut J, et al. Role of aspartate 27 in the binding of methotrexate to dihydrofolate reductase from Escherichia coli. J Biol Chem 1988;263:9187–9198.

146. Taira K, Benkovic SJ. Evaluation of the importance of hydrophobic interactions in drug binding to dihydrofolate reductase. J Med Chem 1988;31:129–137.

147. Oefner C, D'Arcy A, Winkler FK. Crystal structure of human dihydrofolate reductase complexed with folate. Eur J Biochem 1988;174:377–385.

148. Cody V, Ciszak E. Computer graphic modeling in drug design—conformational analysis of antifolate binding to avian dihydrofolate reductase: crystal and molecular structures of 2,4-diamino-5-cyclohexyl-6-methylpyrimidine and 5-cyclohexyl-6-methyluracil. Anticancer Drug Des 1991;6:83–93.

149. Freisheim JH, Kumar AA, Blankenship D. Structure-function relationships of dihydrofolate reductases: sequence homology considerations and active center residues. In: Kislink RL, Brown GM, eds. Chemistry and Biology of Pteridines. New York: Elsevier/North Holland, 1979:419.

150. Schweitzer BI, Srimatkandada S, Gritsman H, et al. Probing the role of two hydrophobic active site residues in the human dihydrofolate reductase by site-directed mutagenesis. J Biol Chem 1989;264:20786–20795.

151. Thompson PD, Freisheim JH. Conversion of arginine to lysine at position 70 of human dihydrofolate reductase: generation of a methotrexate-insensitive mutant enzyme. Biochemistry 1991;30:8124–8130.

152. Dicker AP, Waltham MC, Volkenandt M, et al. Methotrexate resistance in an in vivo mouse tumor due to a non- active-site dihydrofolate reductase mutation. Proc Natl Acad Sci USA 1993;90:11797–11801.

153. Bystroff C, Kraut J. Crystal structure of unliganded Escherichia coli dihydrofolate reductase. Ligand-induced conformational changes and cooperativity in binding. Biochemistry 1991;30:2227–2239.

154. Zhao SC, Banerjee D, Mineishi S, et al. Post-transplant methotrexate administration leads to improved curability of mice bearing a mammary tumor transplanted with marrow transduced with a mutant human dihydrofolate reductase cDNA. Hum Gene Ther 1997;8:903–909.

155. Flasshove M, Banerjee D, Leonard JP, et al. Retroviral transduction of human CD34+ umbilical cord blood progenitor cells with a mutated dihydrofolate reductase cDNA. Hum Gene Ther 1998;9:63–71.

156. Mareya SM, Sorrentino BP, Blakley RL. Protection of CCRF-CEM human lymphoid cells from antifolates by retroviral gene transfer of variants of murine dihydrofolate reductase. Cancer Gene Ther 1998;5:225–235.

157. Appleman JR, Prendergast N, Delcamp TJ, et al. Kinetics of the formation and isomerization of methotrexate complexes of recombinant human dihydrofolate reductase. J Biol Chem 1988;263:10304–10313.

158. Kamen BA, Whyte-Bauer W, Bertino JR. A mechanism of resistance to methotrexate. NADPH but not NADH stimulation of methotrexate binding to dihydrofolate reductase. Biochem Pharmacol 1983;32:1837–1841.

159. Jackson RC, Hart LI, Harrap KR. Intrinsic resistance to methotrexate of cultured mammalian cells in relation to the inhibition kinetics of their dihydrofolate reductases. Cancer Res 1976;36:1991–1997.

160. Kumar P, Kisliuk RL, Gaumont Y, et al. Interaction of polyglutamyl derivatives of methotrexate, 10-deazaaminopterin, and dihydrofolate with dihydrofolate reductase. Cancer Res 1986;46:5020–5023.

161. Blakley RL, Cocco L. Role of isomerization of initial complexes in the binding of inhibitors to dihydrofolate reductase. Biochemistry 1985;24:4772–4777.

162. White JC. Reversal of methotrexate binding to dihydrofolate reductase by dihydrofolate. Studies with pure enzyme and computer modeling using network thermodynamics. J Biol Chem 1979;254:10889–10895.

163. Allegra CJ, Boarman D. Interaction of methotrexate polyglutamates and dihydrofolate during leucovorin rescue in a human breast cancer cell line (MCF-7). Cancer Res 1990; 50:3574–3578.

164. Cohen M, Bender RA, Donehower R, et al. Reversibility of high-affinity binding of methotrexate in L1210 murine leukemia cells. Cancer Res 1978;38:2866–2870.

165. White JC, Loftfield S, Goldman ID. The mechanism of action of methotrexate. III. Requirement of free intracellular methotrexate for maximal suppression of (14C)formate incorporation into nucleic acids and protein. Mol Pharmacol 1975;11:287–297.

166. Galivan J. Evidence for the cytotoxic activity of polyglutamate derivatives of methotrexate. Mol Pharmacol 1980;17:105–110.

167. Drake JC, Allegra CJ, Baram J, et al. Effects on dihydrofolate reductase of methotrexate metabolites and intracellular folates formed following methotrexate exposure of human breast cancer cells. Biochem Pharmacol 1987;36:2416–2418.

168. Boarman DM, Baram J, Allegra CJ. Mechanism of leucovorin reversal of methotrexate cytotoxicity in human MCF-7 breast cancer cells. Biochem Pharmacol 1990;40:2651–2660.

169. Kruger-McDermott C, Balinska M, Galivan J. Dihydrofolate-mediated reversal of methotrexate toxicity to hepatoma cells in vitro. Cancer Lett 1986;30:79–84.

170. Goldie JH, Dedhar S, Krystal G. Properties of a methotrexate-insensitive variant of dihydrofolate reductase derived from methotrexate-resistant L5178Y cells. J Biol Chem 1981;256:11629–11635.

171. McIvor RS, Simonsen CC. Isolation and characterization of a variant dihydrofolate reductase cDNA from methotrexate- resistant murine L5178Y cells. Nucleic Acids Res 1990;18:7025–7032.

172. Flintoff WF, Essani K. Methotrexate-resistant Chinese hamster ovary cells contain a dihydrofolate reductase with an altered affinity for methotrexate. Biochemistry 1980;19:4321–4327.

173. Melera PW, Davide JP, Hession CA, et al. Phenotypic expression in Escherichia coli and nucleotide sequence of two Chinese hamster lung cell cDNAs encoding different dihydrofolate reductases. Mol Cell Biol 1984;4:38–48.

174. Melera PW, Lewis JA, Biedler JL, et al. Antifolate-resistant Chinese hamster cells. Evidence for dihydrofolate reductase gene amplification among independently derived sublines overproducing different dihydrofolate reductases. J Biol Chem 1980;255:7024–7028.

175. Haber DA, Schimke RT. Unstable amplification of an altered dihydrofolate reductase gene associated with double- minute chromosomes. Cell 1981;26:355–362.

176. Cowan KH, Goldsmith ME, Levine RM, et al. Dihydrofolate reductase gene amplification and possible rearrangement in estrogen-responsive methotrexate-resistant human breast cancer cells. J Biol Chem 1982;257:15079–15086.

177. Melera PW, Davide JP, Oen H. Antifolate-resistant Chinese hamster cells. Molecular basis for the biochemical and structural heterogeneity among dihydrofolate reductases produced by drug-sensitive and drug-resistant cell lines. J Biol Chem 1988;263:1978–1990.

178. Dedhar S, Hartley D, Fitz-Gibbons D, et al. Heterogeneity in the specific activity and methotrexate sensitivity of dihydrofolate reductase from blast cells of acute myelogenous leukemia patients. J Clin Oncol 1985;3:1545–1552.

179. Takebe N, Nakahara S, Zhao SC, et al. Comparison of methotrexate resistance conferred by a mutated dihydrofolate reductase cDNA in two different retroviral vectors. Cancer Gene Ther 2000;7(6):910–919.

180. Meisel R, Bardenheuer W, Strehblow C, et al. Efficient protection from methotrexate toxicity and selection of transduced human hematopoietic cells following gene transfer of dihydrofolate reductase mutants. Exp Hematol 2003;31(12):1215–1222.

181. Bertino, JR. Transfer of drug resistance genes into hematopoietic stem cells for marrow protection. The Oncologist 2009;13:1036–1042.

182. Hamlin JL, Biedler JL. Replication pattern of a large homogenously staining chromosome region in antifolate-resistant Chinese hamster cell lines. J Cell Physiol 1981;107:101–114.

183. Brown PC, Beverley SM, Schimke RT. Relationship of amplified dihydrofolate reductase genes to double minute chromosomes in unstably resistant mouse fibroblast cell lines. Mol Cell Biol 1981;1:1077–1083.

184. Meltzer PS, Cheng YC, Trent JM. Analysis of dihydrofolate reductase gene amplification in a methotrexate-resistant human tumor cell line. Cancer Genet Cytogenet 1985;17:289–300.

185. Singer MJ, Mesner LD, Friedman CL, et al. Amplification of the human dihydrofolate reductase gene via double minutes is initiated by chromosome breaks. Proc Natl Acad Sci USA 2000;97(14):7921–7926.

186. Hoy CA, Rice GC, Kovacs M, et al. Over-replication of DNA in S phase Chinese hamster ovary cells after DNA synthesis inhibition. J Biol Chem 1987;262:11927–11934.

187. Fanin R, Banerjee D, Volkenandt M, et al. Mutations leading to antifolate resistance in Chinese hamster ovary cells after exposure to the alkylating agent ethylmethanesulfonate. Mol Pharmacol 1993;44:13–21.

188. Sharma RC, Schimke RT. Enhancement of the frequency of methotrexate resistance by gamma-radiation in Chinese hamster ovary and mouse 3T6 cells. Cancer Res 1989;49:3861–3866.

189. Barsoum J, Varshavsky A. Mitogenic hormones and tumor promoters greatly increase the incidence of colony-forming cells bearing amplified dihydrofolate reductase genes. Proc Natl Acad Sci USA 1983;80:5330–5334.

190. Newman EM, Lu Y, Kashani-Sabet M, et al. Mechanisms of cross-resistance to methotrexate and 5-fluorouracil in an A2780 human ovarian carcinoma cell subline resistant to cisplatin. Biochem Pharmacol 1988;37:443–447.

191. Rice GC, Ling V, Schimke RT. Frequencies of independent and simultaneous selection of Chinese hamster cells for methotrexate and doxorubicin (Adriamycin) resistance. Proc Natl Acad Sci USA 1987;84:9261–9264.

192. Schuetz JD, Gorse KM, Goldman ID, et al. Transient inhibition of DNA synthesis by 5-fluorodeoxyuridine leads to overexpression of dihydrofolate reductase with increased frequency of methotrexate resistance. J Biol Chem 1988;263:7708–7712.

193. Wright JA, Smith HS, Watt FM, et al. DNA amplification is rare in normal human cells. Proc Natl Acad Sci USA 1990;87:1791–1795.

194. Al-Shakfa F, Dulucq S, Brukner I, et al. DNA variants in region for noncoding interfering transcript of dihydrofolate reductase gene and outcome in childhood acute lymphoblastic leukemia. Clin Cancer Res 2009;15:OF1–OF8.

195. Mishra PJ, Humeniuk R, Mishra PJ, et al. An miR-24 microRNA binding-site polymorphism in dihydrofolate reductase gene leads to methotrexate resisance. PNAS 2007;104:13513–13518.

196. Sowers R, Toguchida J, Qin J etal. MRNA expression levels of E2F transcription factors correlate with dihydrofolate reductase, reduced folate carrier, and thymidylate synthase mRNA expression in osteosarcoma. Mol Cancer Ther 2003;2(6):535–541.

197. Cowan KH, Goldsmith ME, Ricciardone MD, et al. Regulation of dihydrofolate reductase in human breast cancer cells and in mutant hamster cells transfected with a human dihydrofolate reductase minigene. Mol Pharmacol 1986;30:69–76.

198. Chu E, Takimoto CH, Voeller D, et al. Specific binding of human dihydrofolate reductase protein to dihydrofolate reductase messenger RNA in vitro. Biochemistry 1993;32:4756–4760.

199. Ercikan-Abali EA, Banerjee D, Waltham MC, et al. Dihydrofolate reductase protein inhibits its own translation by binding to dihydrofolate reductase mRNA sequences within the coding region. Biochemistry 1997;36:12317–12322.

200. Curt GA, Carney DN, Cowan KH, et al. Unstable methotrexate resistance in human small-cell carcinoma associated with double minute chromosomes. N Engl J Med 1983;308:199–202.

201. Curt GA, Jolivet J, Bailey BD, et al. Synthesis and retention of methotrexate polyglutamates by human small cell lung cancer. Biochem Pharmacol 1984;33:1682–1685.

202. Seither RL, Rape TJ, Goldman ID. Further studies on the pharmacologic effects of the 7-hydroxy catabolite of methotrexate in the L1210 murine leukemia cell. Biochem Pharmacol 1989;38:815–822.

203. Rhee MS, Balinska M, Bunni M, et al. Role of substrate depletion in the inhibition of thymidylate biosynthesis by the dihydrofolate reductase inhibitor trimetrexate in cultured hepatoma cells. Cancer Res 1990;50:3979–3984.

204. Rhee MS, Coward JK, Galivan J. Depletion of 5,10-methylenetetrahydrofolate and 10-formyltetrahydrofolate by methotrexate in cultured hepatoma cells. Mol Pharmacol 1992;42:909–916.

205. Trent DF, Seither RL, Goldman ID. Compartmentation of intracellular folates. Failure to interconvert tetrahydrofolate cofactors to dihydrofolate in mitochondria of L1210 leukemia cells treated with trimetrexate [published erratum appears in Biochem Pharmacol 1991;42(12):2405]. Biochem Pharmacol 1991;42:1015–1019.

206. Li JC, Kaminskas E. Accumulation of DNA strand breaks and methotrexate cytotoxicity. Proc Natl Acad Sci USA 1984;81:5694–5698.

207. Hori T, Ayusawa D, Shimizu K, et al. Chromosome breakage induced by thymidylate stress in thymidylate synthase-negative mutants of mouse FM3A cells. Cancer Res 1984;44:703–709.

208. Borchers AH, Kennedy KA, Straw JA. Inhibition of DNA excision repair by methotrexate in Chinese hamster ovary cells following exposure to ultraviolet irradiation or ethylmethanesulfonate. Cancer Res 1990;50:1786–1789.

209. Goulian M, Bleile B, Tseng BY. Methotrexate-induced misincorporation of uracil into DNA. Proc Natl Acad Sci USA 1980;77:1956–1960.

210. Grafstrom RH, Tseng BY, Goulian M. The incorporation of uracil into animal cell DNA in vitro. Cell 1978;15:131–140.

211. Curtin NJ, Harris AL, Aherne GW. Mechanism of cell death following thymidylate synthase inhibition: 2'-deoxyuridine-5'-triphosphate accumulation, DNA damage, and growth inhibition following exposure to CB3717 and dipyridamole. Cancer Res 1991;51:2346–2352.

212. Beck WR, Wright GE, Nusbaum NJ, et al. Enhancement of methotrexate cytotoxicity by uracil analogues that inhibit deoxyuridine triphosphate nucleotidohydrolase (dUTPase) activity. Adv Exp Med Biol 1986;195:97–104.

213. Goker E, Waltham M, Kheradpour A, et al. Amplification of the dihydrofolate reductase gene is a mechanism of acquired resistance to methotrexate in patients with acute lymphoblastic leukemia and is correlated with p53 gene mutations. Blood 1995;86:677–684.

214. Li WW, Fan J, Hochhauser D, et al. Overexpression of p21waf1 leads to increased inhibition of E2F-1 phosphorylation and sensitivity to anticancer drugs in retinoblastoma-negative human sarcoma cells. Cancer Res 1997;57:2193–2199.

215. Pinedo HM, Zaharko DS, Bull J, et al. The relative contribution of drug concentration and duration of exposure to mouse bone marrow toxicity during continuous methotrexate infusion. Cancer Res 1977;37:445–450.

216. Cherry LM, Hsu TC. Restitution of chromatid and isochromatid breaks induced in the G2 phase by actinomycin D. Environ Mutagen 1982;4:259–265.

217. Pinedo HM, Zaharko DS, Bull JM, et al. The reversal of methotrexate cytotoxicity to mouse bone marrow cells by leucovorin and nucleosides. Cancer Res 1976;36:4418–4424.

218. Howell SB, Mansfield SJ, Taetle R. Thymidine and hypoxanthine requirements of normal and malignant human cells for protection against methotrexate cytotoxicity. Cancer Res 1981;41:945–950.

219. Howell SB, Ensminger WD, Krishan A, et al. Thymidine rescue of high-dose methotrexate in humans. Cancer Res 1978;38:325–330.

220. Rustum YM. High-pressure liquid chromatography. I. Quantitative separation of purine and pyrimidine nucleosides and bases. Anal Biochem 1978;90:289–299.

221. Willson JK, Fischer PH, Remick SC, et al. Methotrexate and dipyridamole combination chemotherapy based upon inhibition of nucleoside salvage in humans. Cancer Res 1989;49:1866–1870.

222. Novelli A, Mini E, Liuffi M, et al. Clinical data on rescue of high-dose methotrexate with N5-methyltetrahydrofolate in human solid tumors. In: Periti P, ed. High-Dose Methotrexate Pharmacology, Toxicology and Chemotherapy. Firenze: Giuntina, 1978:299.

223. Matherly LH, Barlowe CK, Goldman ID. Antifolate polyglutamylation and competitive drug displacement at dihydrofolate reductase as important elements in leucovorin rescue in L1210 cells. Cancer Res 1986;46:588–593.

224. Bernard S, Etienne MC, Fischel JL, et al. Critical factors for the reversal of methotrexate cytotoxicity by folinic acid. Br J Cancer 1991;63:303–307.

225. Browman GP, Goodyear MD, Levine MN, et al. Modulation of the antitumor effect of methotrexate by low-dose leucovorin in squamous cell head and neck cancer: a randomized placebo-controlled clinical trial. J Clin Oncol 1990;8:203–208.

226. Pesce MA, Bodourian SH. Evaluation of a fluorescence polarization immunoassay procedure for quantitation of methotrexate. Ther Drug Monit 1986;8:115–121.

227. Donehower RC, Hande KR, Drake JC, et al. Presence of 2,4-diamino-N10-methylpteroic acid after high-dose methotrexate. Clin Pharmacol Ther 1979;26:63–72.

228. Oellerich M, Engelhardt P, Schaadt M, et al. Determination of methotrexate in serum by a rapid, fully mechanized enzyme immunoassay (EMIT). J Clin Chem Clin Biochem 1980;18:169–174.

229. Allegra CJ, Drake JC, Bell BA, et al. Measuring levels of methotrexate [letter]. N Engl J Med 1985;313:184.

230. So N, Chandra DP, Alexander IS, et al. Determination of serum methotrexate and 7-hydroxymethotrexate concentrations. Method evaluation showing advantages of high-performance liquid chromatography. J Chromatogr 1985;337:81–90.

231. Stout M, Ravindranath Y, Kauffman R. High-performance liquid chromatographic assay for methotrexate utilizing a cold acetonitrile purification and separation of plasma or cerebrospinal fluid. J Chromatogr 1985;342:424–430.

232. Palmisano F, Cataldi TR, Zambonin PG. Determination of the antineoplastic agent methotrexate in body fluids by high-performance liquid chromatography with electrochemical detection. J Chromatogr 1985;344:249–258.

233. Slordal L, Prytz PS, Pettersen I, et al. Methotrexate measurements in plasma: comparison of enzyme multiplied immunoassay technique, TDx fluorescence polarization immunoassay, and high pressure liquid chromatography. Ther Drug Monit 1986;8:368–372.

234. Zaharko DS, Dedrick RL, Bischoff KB, et al. Methotrexate tissue distribution: prediction by a mathematical model. J Natl Cancer Inst 1971;46:775–784.

235. Chungi VS, Bourne DW, Dittert LW. Drug absorption VIII: kinetics of GI absorption of methotrexate. J Pharm Sci 1978;67:560–561.

236. Stuart JF, Calman KC, Watters J, et al. Bioavailability of methotrexate: implications for clinical use. Cancer Chemother Pharmacol 1979;3:239–241.

237. Balis FM, Savitch JL, Bleyer WA. Pharmacokinetics of oral methotrexate in children. Cancer Res 1983;43:2342–2345.

238. Balis FM, Holcenberg JS, Poplack DG, et al. Pharmacokinetics and pharmacodynamics of oral methotrexate and mercaptopurine in children with lower risk acute lymphoblastic leukemia: a joint children's cancer group and pediatric oncology branch study. Blood 1998;92:3569–3577.

239. Steele WH, Lawrence JR, Stuart JF, et al. The protein binding of methotrexate by the serum of normal subjects. Eur J Clin Pharmacol 1979;15:363–366.

240. Liegler DG, Henderson ES, Hahn MA, et al. The effect of organic acids on renal clearance of methotrexate in man. Clin Pharmacol Ther 1969;10:849–857.

241. Wan SH, Huffman DH, Azarnoff DL, et al. Effect of route of administration and effusions on methotrexate pharmacokinetics. Cancer Res 1974;4: 3487–3491.

242. Chabner BA, Stoller RG, Hande K, et al. Methotrexate disposition in humans: case studies in ovarian cancer and following high-dose infusion. Drug Metab Rev 1978;8:107–117.

243. Torres IJ, Litterst CL, Guarino AM. Transport of model compounds across the peritoneal membrane in the rat. Pharmacology 1978;17:330–340.

244. Fossa SD, Heilo A, Bormer O. Unexpectedly high serum methotrexate levels in cystectomized bladder cancer patients with an ileal conduit treated with intermediate doses of the drug. J Urol 1990;143:498–501.

245. Kristenson L, Weismann K, Hutters L. Renal function and the rate of disappearance of methotrexate from serum. Eur J Clin Pharmacol 1975;8: 439–444.

246. Bleyer WA. The clinical pharmacology of methotrexate: new applications of an old drug. Cancer 1978;41:36–51.

247. Howell SB, Tamerius RK. Achievement of long duration methotrexate exposure with concurrent low dose thymidine protection: influence of methotrexate pharmacokinetics. Eur J Cancer 1980;16:1427–1432.

248. Evans WE, Crom WR, Stewart CF, et al. Methotrexate systemic clearance influences probability of relapse in children with standard-risk acute lymphocytic leukaemia. Lancet 1984;1:359–362.

249. Evans WE, Crom WR, Abromowitch M, et al. Clinical pharmacodynamics of high-dose methotrexate in acute lymphocytic leukemia. Identification of a relation between concentration and effect. N Engl J Med 1986;314: 471–477.

250. Borsi JD, Moe PJ. Systemic clearance of methotrexate in the prognosis of acute lymphoblastic leukemia in children. Cancer 1987;60:3020–3024.

251. Pearson AD, Amineddine HA, Yule M, et al. The influence of serum methotrexate concentrations and drug dosage on outcome in childhood acute lymphoblastic leukaemia [see comments]. Br J Cancer 1991;64:169–173.

252. Colom H, Farre R, Soy Dolors, et al. Population pharmacokinetics of high-dose methotrexate after intravenous administration in pediatric patients with osteosarcoma. Ther Drug Monit 2009;31:76–85.

253. Calvert AH, Bondy PK, Harrap KR. Some observations on the human pharmacology of methotrexate. Cancer Treat Rep 1977;61:1647–1656.

254. Monjanel S, Rigault JP, Cano JP, et al. High-dose methotrexate: preliminary evaluation of a pharmacokinetic approach. Cancer Chemother Pharmacol 1979;3:189–196.

255. Sasaki K, Tanaka J, Fujimoto T. Theoretically required urinary flow during high-dose methotrexate infusion. Cancer Chemother Pharmacol 1984;13:9–13.

256. Romolo JL, Goldberg NH, Hande KR, et al. Effect of hydration on plasma-methotrexate levels. Cancer Treat Rep 1977;61:1393–1396.

257. Huang KC, Wenczak BA, Liu YK. Renal tubular transport of methotrexate in the rhesus monkey and dog. Cancer Res 1979;39:4843–4848.

258. Iven H, Brasch H. Influence of the antibiotics piperacillin, doxycycline, and tobramycin on the pharmacokinetics of methotrexate in rabbits. Cancer Chemother Pharmacol 1986;17:218–222.

259. Iven H, Brasch H. The effects of antibiotics and uricosuric drugs on the renal elimination of methotrexate and 7-hydroxymethotrexate in rabbits. Cancer Chemother Pharmacol 1988;21:337–342.

260. Iven H, Brasch H. Cephalosporins increase the renal clearance of methotrexate and 7-hydroxymethotrexate in rabbits. Cancer Chemother Pharmacol 1990;26:139–143.

261. Titier K, Lagrange F, Pehourcq F, et al. Pharmacokinetic interaction between high-dose methotrexate and oxacillin. Ther Drug Monit 2002;24(4): 570–572.

262. Dalle JH, Auvrignon A, Vassal G, et al. Interaction between methotrexate and ciprofloxacin. J Pediatr Hematol Oncol 2002;4(4):321–322.

263. Kerr IG, Jolivet J, Collins JM, et al. Test dose for predicting high-dose methotrexate infusions. Clin Pharmacol Ther 1983;33:44–51.

264. Favre R, Monjanel S, Alfonsi M, et al. High-dose methotrexate: a clinical and pharmacokinetic evaluation. Treatment of advanced squamous cell carcinoma of the head and neck using a prospective mathematical model and pharmacokinetic surveillance. Cancer Chemother Pharmacol 1982;9: 156–160.

265. Strum WB, Liem HH. Hepatic uptake, intracellular protein binding and biliary excretion of amethopterin. Biochem Pharmacol 1977;26:1235–1240.

266. Jacobs SA, Derr CJ, Johns DG. Accumulation of methotrexate diglutamate in human liver during methotrexate therapy. Biochem Pharmacol 1977;26:2310–2313.

267. Said HM, Hollander D. Inhibitory effect of bile salts on the enterohepatic circulation of methotrexate in the unanesthetized rat: inhibition of methotrexate intestinal absorption. Cancer Chemother Pharmacol 1986;16: 121–124.

268. Lerne PR, Creaven PJ, Allen LM, et al. Kinetic model for the disposition and metabolism of moderate and high-dose methotrexate in man. Cancer Chemother Rep 1975;59:811–817.

269. Shen DD, Azarnoff DL. Clinical pharmacokinetics of methotrexate. Clin Pharmacokinet 1978;3:1–13.

270. Steinberg SE, Campbell CL, Bleyer WA, et al. Enterohepatic circulation of methotrexate in rats in vivo. Cancer Res 1982;42:1279–1282.

271. Breithaupt H, Kuenzlen E. Pharmacokinetics of methotrexate and 7-hydroxymethotrexate following infusions of high-dose methotrexate. Cancer Treat Rep 1982;66:1733–1741.

272. Erttmann R, Landbeck G. Effect of oral cholestyramine on the elimination of high-dose methotrexate. J Cancer Res Clin Oncol 1985;110:48–50.

273. Jacobs SA, Stoller RG, Chabner BA, et al. 7-Hydroxymethotrexate as a urinary metabolite in human subjects and rhesus monkeys receiving high dose methotrexate. J Clin Invest 1976;57:534–538.

274. Bremnes RM, Slordal L, Wist E, et al. Formation and elimination of 7-hydroxymethotrexate in the rat in vivo after methotrexate administration. Cancer Res 1989;49:2460–2464.

275. Sholar PW, Baram J, Seither R, et al. Inhibition of folate-dependent enzymes by 7-OH-methotrexate. Biochem Pharmacol 1988;37:3531–3534.

276. Clendeninn NJ, Drake JC, Allegra CJ, et al. Methotrexate polyglutamates have a greater affinity and more rapid on-rate for purified human dihydrofolate reductase than MTX. Proc Am Assoc Cancer Res 1985:232.

277. McCullough JL, Chabner BA, Bertino JR. Purification and properties of carboxypeptidase G1. J Biol Chem 1971;246:7207–7213.

278. Abelson HT, Ensminger W, Rosowsky A, et al. Comparative effects of citrovorum factor and carboxypeptidase G1 on cerebrospinal fluid-methotrexate pharmacokinetics. Cancer Treat Rep 1978;62:1549–1552.

279. Chabner BA, Young RC. Threshold methotrexate concentration for in vivo inhibition of DNA synthesis in normal and tumorous target tissues. J Clin Invest 1973;52:1804–1811.

280. Sirotnak FM, Moccio DM. Pharmacokinetic basis for differences in methotrexate sensitivity of normal proliferative tissues in the mouse. Cancer Res 1980;40:1230–1234.

281. Toffoli G, Russo A, Innocenti F, et al. Effect of methylenetetrahydrofolate reductase C677T polymorphism on toxicity and homocysteine plasma level after chronic methotrexate treatment of ovarian cancer patients. Int J Cancer 2003;103(3):294–299.

282. Chiusolo P, Reddiconto G, Casorelli I, et al. Preponderance of methylenethtrahydrofolate reductase C677T homozygosity among leukemia patients intolerant to methotrexate. Ann Oncol 2002;13(12):1915–1918.

283. Ulrich CM, Yasui Y, Storb R, et al. Pharmacogenetics of methotrexate: toxicity among marrow transplantation patients varies with the methylenetetrahydrofolate reductase C677T polymorphism. Blood 2001;98(1): 231–234.

284. Urano W, Taniguchi A, Yamanaka H, et al. Polymorphisms in the methylenetetrahydrofolate reductase gene were associated with both the efficacy and the toxicity of methotrexate used for the treatment of rheumatoid arthritis, as evidenced by single locus haplotype analysis. Pharmacogenetics 2002;12(3):183–190.

285. Van Ede AE, Laan RF, Blom HJ, et al. The C677T mutation in the methylenetetrahydrofolate reductase gene: a genetic risk factor for methotrexate-related elevation of liver enzymes in rheumatoid arthritis patients. Arthritis Rheum 2001;44(11):2525–2530.

286. Schmiegelow K. Advances in individual prediction of methotrexate toxicity: a review. Br J Haematol 2009;146:489–503.

287. Shimasaki N, Mori T, Samejima H, et al. Effects of methylenetetrahydrofolate reductase and reduced folate carrier 1 polymorphisms on high-dose methyotrexate-induced toxicities in children with acute lymphoblastic leukemia or lymphoma. Pediatr Hematol Oncol 2006;64–68.

288. Ackland SP, Schilsky RL. High-dose methotrexate: a critical reappraisal. J Clin Oncol 1987;5:2017–2031.

289. Von Hoff DD, Penta JS, Helman LJ, et al. Incidence of drug-related deaths secondary to high-dose methotrexate and citrovorum factor administration. Cancer Treat Rep 1977;61:745–748.

290. Hempel L, Misselwitz J, Fleck C, etal. Influence of high-dose methotrexate therapy on glomerular and tubular kidney function. Med Pediatr Oncol 2003;40(6):348–354.

291. Stoller RG, Hande KR, Jacobs SA, et al. Use of plasma pharmacokinetics to predict and prevent methotrexate toxicity. N Engl J Med 1977;297:630–634.

292. Bacci G, Ferrari S, Longhi A, et al. Delayed methotrexate clearance in osteosarcoma patients treated with multiagent regimens of neoadjuvant chemotherapy. Oncol Rep 2003;10(4):851–857.

293. Thyss A, Milano G, Kubar J, et al. Clinical and pharmacokinetic evidence of a life-threatening interaction between methotrexate and ketoprofen. Lancet 1986;1:256–258.

294. Takeda M, Khamdang S, Narikawa S, et al. Characterization of methotrexate transport and its drug interactions with human organic anion transporters. J Pharmacol Exp Ther 2002;302(2):666–671.

295. Nozaki Y, Kusuhara H, Endou H, et al. Quantitative evaluation of the drug-drug interactions between methotrexate and nonsteroidal anti-inflammatory drugs in the renal uptake process based on the contribution of organic anion transporters and reduced folate carrier. J Pharmacol Exp Ther 2004;309(1):226–234.

296. Wall SM, Johansen MJ, Molony DA, et al. Effective clearance of methotrexate using high-flux hemodialysis membranes. Am J Kidney Dis 1996;28:846–854.

297. Murashima M, Adamski J, Milone MC, et al. Methotrexate clearance by high-flux hemodialysis and peritoneal dialysis: A case report. Am J Kidney Dis 2009;53:871–874.

298. DeAngelis LM, Tong WP, Lin S, et al. Carboxypeptidase G2 rescue after high-dose methotrexate. J Clin Oncol 1996;14:2145–2149.

299. Mohty M, Peyriere H, Guinet C, et al. Carboxypeptidase G2 rescue in delayed methotrexate elimination in renal failure. Leuk Lymphoma 2000;37(3–4):441–443.

300. Schwartz S, Borner K, Müller K, et al. Glucarpidase (Carboxypeptidase G2) Intervention in adult and elderly cancer patients with renal dysfunction and delayed methotrexate elimination after high-dose methotrexate therapy. The Oncol 2007;12:1299–1308.

301. Yap BS, McCredie KB, Benjamin RS, et al. Refractory acute leukaemia in adults treated with sequential colaspase and high-dose methotrexate. BMJ 1978;2:791–793.

302. Salliot C, van der Heijde D. Long-term safety of methotrexate monotherapy in patients with rheumatoid arthritis: a systematic literature research. Ann Rheum Dis 2009;68:1100–1104.

303. Zachariae H, Kragballe K, Sogaard H. Methotrexate induced liver cirrhosis. Studies including serial liver biopsies during continued treatment. Br J Dermatol 1980;102:407–412.

304. Dahl MG, Gregory MM, Scheuer PJ. Methotrexate hepatotoxicity in psoriasis—comparison of different dose regimens. BMJ 1972;1:654–656.

305. Podurgiel BJ, McGill DB, Ludwig J, et al. Liver injury associated with methotrexate therapy for psoriasis. Mayo Clin Proc 1973;48:787–792.

306. Willkens RF, Clegg DO, Ward JR, et al. Liver biopsies in patients on low-dose pulse methotrexate for the treatment of rheumatoid arthritis [abstract]. In: Sixteenth International Congress on Rheumatology. Sydney, Australia: 1985:88.

307. Mackenzie AH. Hepatotoxicity of prolonged methotrexate therapy for rheumatoid arthritis. Cleve Clin Q 1985;52:129–135.

308. Weber BL, Tanyer G, Poplack DG, et al. Transient acute hepatotoxicity of high-dose methotrexate therapy during childhood. J Natl Cancer Inst Monogr 1987;5:207–212.

309. Clarysse AM, Cathey WJ, Cartwright GE, et al. Pulmonary disease complicating intermittent therapy with methotrexate. JAMA 1969;209:1861–1868.

310. Sostman HD, Matthay RA, Putman CE, et al. Methotrexate-induced pneumonitis. Medicine (Baltimore)1976;55:371–388.

311. Akoun GM, Mayaud CM, Touboul JL, et al. Use of bronchoalveolar lavage in the evaluation of methotrexate lung disease. Thorax 1987;42:652–655.

312. Kremer JM, Phelps CT. Long-term prospective study of the use of methotrexate in the treatment of rheumatoid arthritis. Update after a mean of 90 months. Arthritis Rheum 1992;35:138–145.

313. Searles G, McKendry RJ. Methotrexate pneumonitis in rheumatoid arthritis: potential risk factors. Four case reports and a review of the literature. J Rheumatol 1987;14:1164–1171.

314. Carson CW, Cannon GW, Egger MJ, et al. Pulmonary disease during the treatment of rheumatoid arthritis with low dose pulse methotrexate. Semin Arthritis Rheum 1987;16:186–195.

315. Kremer JM, Alarcon GS, Weinblatt ME, et al. Clinical, laboratory, radiographic, and histopathologic features of methotrexate-associated lung injury in patients with rheumatoid arthritis: a multicenter study with literature review [see comments]. Arthritis Rheum 1997;40:1829–1837.

316. Hargreaves MR, Mowat AG, Benson MK. Acute pneumonitis associated with low dose methotrexate treatment for rheumatoid arthritis: report of five cases and review of published reports. Thorax 1992;47:628–633.

317. Alarcon GS, Kremer JM, Macaluso M, et al. Risk factors for methotrexate-induced lung injury in patients with rheumatoid arthritis. A multicenter, case-control study. Methotrexate Lung Study Group. Ann Intern Med 1997;127:356–364.

318. Shimura C, Satoh T, Takayama K, et al. Methotrexate-related lymphoproliferative disorder with extensive vascular involvement in a patient with rheumatoid arthritis. J Am Acad Dermatol 2009;61:126–129.

319. Clarke LE, Junkins-Hopkins J, Seykora JT, et al. Methotrexate-associated lymphoproliferative disorder in a patient with rheymatoid arthritis presenting in the skin. J Am Acad Dermatol 2007;56:686–690.

320. Goldberg NH, Romolo JL, Austin EH, et al. Anaphylactoid type reactions in two patients receiving high dose intravenous methotrexate. Cancer 1978;41:52–55.

321. Nishitani N, Adachi A, Fukumoto T, et al. Folic acid-induced anaphylaxis showing cross-reactivity wtih methotrexate: a case report and review of the literature. Internat J Dermatol 2009;48:522–524.

322. Ozguven AA, Uysal K, Gunes D, et al. Delayed renal excretion of methotrexate after a severe anaphylactic reaction to methotrexate in a child with osteosarcoma. J Pediatr Hematol Oncol 2009;31:289–291.

323. Doyle LA, Berg C, Bottino G, et al. Erythema and desquamation after high-dose methotrexate. Ann Intern Med 1983;98:611–612.

324. Shamberger RC, Rosenberg SA, Seipp CA, et al. Effects of high-dose methotrexate and vincristine on ovarian and testicular functions in patients undergoing postoperative adjuvant treatment of osteosarcoma. Cancer Treat Rep 1981;65:739–746.

325. Shapiro WR, Young DF, Mehta BM. Methotrexate: distribution in cerebrospinal fluid after intravenous, ventricular and lumbar injections. N Engl J Med 1975;293:161–166.

326. Tatef ML, Margolin KA, Doroshow JH, et al. Pharmacokinetics and toxicity of high-dose intravenous methotrexate in the treatment of leptomeningeal carcinomatosis. Cancer Chemother Pharmacol 2000;46(1):19–26.

327. Bleyer WA, Drake JC, Chabner BA. Neurotoxicity and elevated cerebrospinal-fluid methotrexate concentration in meningeal leukemia. N Engl J Med 1973;289:770–773.

328. Morse M, Savitch J, Balis F, et al. Altered central nervous system pharmacology of methotrexate in childhood leukemia: another sign of meningeal relapse. J Clin Oncol 1985;3:19–24.

329. Blaney SM, Balis FM, Poplack DG. Current pharmacological treatment approaches to central nervous system leukaemia. Drugs 1991;41:702–716.

330. Ettinger LJ, Chervinsky DS, Freeman AI, et al. Pharmacokinetics of methotrexate following intravenous and intraventricular administration in acute lymphocytic leukemia and non-Hodgkin's lymphoma. Cancer 1982;50:1676–1682.

331. Grossman SA, Reinhard CS, Loats HL. The intracerebral penetration of intraventricularly administered methotrexate: a quantitative autoradiographic study. J Neurooncol 1989;7:319–328.

332. Bleyer WA, Poplack DG, Simon RM. "Concentration × time" methotrexate via a subcutaneous reservoir: a less toxic regimen for intraventricular chemotherapy of central nervous system neoplasms. Blood 1978;51:835–842.

333. Glantz MJ, Cole BF, Recht L, et al. High-dose intravenous methotrexate for patients with nonleukemic leptomeningeal cancer: is intrathecal chemotherapy necessary? J Clin Oncol 1998;16:1561–1567.

334. Peylan-Ramu N, Poplack DG, Blei CL, et al. Computer assisted tomography in methotrexate encephalopathy. J Comput Assist Tomogr 1977;1:216–221.

335. Paakko E, Vainionpaa L, Lanning M, et al. White matter changes in children treated for acute lymphoblastic leukemia. Cancer 1992;70:2728–2733.

336. Shapiro WR, Allen JC, Horten BC. Chronic methotrexate toxicity to the central nervous system. Clin Bull 1980;10:49–52.

337. Jaffe N, Takaue Y, Anzai T, et al. Transient neurologic disturbances induced by high-dose methotrexate treatment. Cancer 1985;56:1356–1360.

338. Fritsch G, Urban C. Transient encephalopathy during the late course of treatment with high-dose methotrexate. Cancer 1984;53:1849–1851.

339. Walker RW, Allen JC, Rosen G, et al. Transient cerebral dysfunction secondary to high-dose methotrexate. J Clin Oncol 1986;4:1845–1850.

340. Kubo M, Azuma E, Arai S, et al. Transient encephalopathy following a single exposure of high-dose methotrexate in a child with acute lymphoblastic leukemia. Pediatr Hematol Oncol 1992;9:157–165.

341. Allen J, Rosen G, Juergens H, et al. The inability of oral leucovorin to elevate CSF 5-methyl-tetrahydrofolate following high dose intravenous methotrexate therapy. J Neurooncol 1983;1:39–44.

342. Mehta BM, Glass JP, Shapiro WR. Serum and cerebrospinal fluid distribution of 5-methyltetrahydrofolate after intravenous calcium leucovorin and intra-Ommaya methotrexate administration in patients with meningeal carcinomatosis. Cancer Res 1983;43:435–438.

343. Ochs J, Mulhern R, Fairclough D, et al. Comparison of neuropsychologic functioning and clinical indicators of neurotoxicity in long-term survivors of childhood leukemia given cranial radiation or parenteral methotrexate: a prospective study. J Clin Oncol 1991;9:145–151.

344. Mahoney DH Jr, Shuster JJ, Nitschke R, et al. Acute neurotoxicity in children with B-precursor acute lymphoid leukemia: an association with intermediate-dose intravenous methotrexate and intrathecal triple therapy—a Pediatric Oncology Group study. J Clin Oncol 1998;16:1712–1722.

345. Phillips PC, Dhawan V, Strother SC, et al. Reduced cerebral glucose metabolism and increased brain capillary permeability following high-dose methotrexate chemotherapy: a positron emission tomographic study. Ann Neurol 1987;21:59–63.

346. Kishi S, Griener J, Cheng C, et al. Homocysteine, pharmacogenetics, and neurotoxicity in children with leukemia. J Clin Oncol 2003;21(16):3084–3091.

347. Gilbert MR, Harding BL, Grossman SA. Methotrexate neurotoxicity: in vitro studies using cerebellar explants from rats. Cancer Res 1989;49:2502–2505.

348. Livrea P, Trojano M, Simone IL, et al. Acute changes in blood-CSF barrier permselectivity to serum proteins after intrathecal methotrexate and CNS irradiation. J Neurol 1985;231:336–339.

349. Spiegel RJ, Cooper PR, Blum RH, et al. Treatment of massive intrathecal methotrexate overdose by ventriculolumbar perfusion. N Engl J Med 1984;311:386–388.

350. Shih C, Chen VJ, Gossett LS, et al. LY231514, a pyrrolo[2,3-d]pyrimidine-based antifolate that inhibits multiple folate-requiring enzymes. Cancer Res 1997;57:1116–1123.

351. Chattopadhyay S, Moran RD, Goldman ID. Pemetrexed: biochemical and cellular pharmacology, mechanisms and clinical applications. Mol Cancer Ther 2007;6:404–417.

352. Shih C, Habeck LL, Mendelsohn LG, et al. Multiple folate enzyme inhibition: mechanism of a novel pyrrolopyrimidine-based antifolate LY231514 (MTA). Adv Enzyme Regul 1998;38:135–152.

353. Worzalla JF, Shih C, Schultz RM. Role of folic acid in modulating the toxicity and efficacy of the multitargeted antifolate, LY231514. Anticancer Res 1998;18:3235–3239.

354. Scagliotti GV, Shin DM, Kindler HL, et al. Phase II study of pemetrexed with and without folic acid and vitamin B12 as front-line therapy in malignant pleural mesothelioma. J Clin Oncol 2003;21(8):1556–1561.

355. Vogelzang NJ, Rusthoven JJ, Symanowski J, et al. Phase III study of pemetrexed in combination with cisplatin versus cisplatin alone in patients with malignant pleural mesothelioma. J Clin Oncol 2003;21(14):2636–2644.

356. Clarke SJ, Abatt R, Goedhals L, et al. Phase II trial of pemetrexed disodium (Alimta, LY231514) in chemotherapy-naive patients with advanced non-small-cell lung cancer. Ann Oncol 2002;13(5):737–741.

357. Mita AC, Sweeney CJ, Baker SD, et al. Phase I and pharmacokinetic study of pemetrexed administered every 3 weeks to advance cancer patients with normal and impaired renal function. J Clin Oncol 2006;24:552–562.

358. Takimoto CH, Hammond-Thelin LA, Latz JE, et al. Phase I and pharmacokinetic study of pemetrexed with high-dose folic acid supplementation of multivitamin supplementation in patients with locally advanced or metastatic cancer. Clin Cancer Res 2007;13:2675–2683.

359. Malempati S, Nicholson HS, Reid JM, et al. Phase I trial and pharmacokinetic study of pemetrexed in children with refractory solid tumors: The children's oncology group. J Clin Oncol 2007;25:1505–1511.

360. Hanna N, Shepherd FA, Fossella FV, et al. Randomized phase III trial of pemetrexed versus docetaxel in patients with non-small-cell lung cancer previously treated with chemotherapy. J Clin Oncol 2004;22(9):1589–1597.

361. O'Connor OA, Horwitz S, Hamlin P, et al. Phase II-I-II study of two different doses and schedules of pralatrexate, a high-affinity substrate for the reduced folate carrier, in patients with relapsed or refractory lymphoma reveals marked activity in T-Cell malignancies. J Clin Oncol 2009;27:4357–4364.

5-Fluoropyrimidines

Jean L. Grem, Bruce A. Chabner, David P. Ryan, and Raymond C. Wadlow

The 5-fluorinated pyrimidines were rationally synthesized by Heidelberger et al.[1] on the basis of the observation that rat hepatomas incorporate radiolabeled uracil in nucleic acids more avidly than nonmalignant tissues, a finding that suggested differences in the enzymatic pathways for uracil metabolism. Fluorouracil (5-FU) has become particularly important in the treatment of gastrointestinal (GI) adenocarcinomas, squamous cell carcinomas arising in the head and neck, and many other solid tumors of epithelial derivation. Enhancement of 5-FU activity by leucovorin (LV) and synergistic interaction of fluoropyrimidines with other antitumor agents and with irradiation have further broadened its spectrum of use and effectiveness.

Structure and Cellular Pharmacology

The chemical structures of the initial 5-fluoropyrimidines in clinical use in the United States are shown in Figure 9-1. The simplest derivative, 5-FU (molecular weight [MW] = 130), has the slightly bulkier fluorine atom substituted at the carbon-5 position of the pyrimidine ring in place of hydrogen. The key features of 5-FU are outlined in Table 9-1. Activation to the nucleotide level is essential to antitumor activity. The ribonucleoside derivative 5-fluorouridine (FUrd) has been used exclusively in preclinical studies. The deoxyribonucleoside derivative 5-fluoro-2'-deoxyuridine (FdUrd, MW = 246) is commercially available (floxuridine, FUDR) but only employed for hepatic arterial infusion.

Transport

5-FU shares the same facilitated-transport system as uracil, adenine, and hypoxanthine. In human erythrocytes, 5-FU and uracil exhibited similar saturable (K [binding affinity] ~4 mmol/L; V_{max} 500 pmol/s/5 μL cells) and nonsaturable (rate constant approximately 80 pmol/s/5 μL cells) components of influx. The system is neither temperature dependent nor energy dependent.[2,3] 5-FU permeation is pH dependent and reaches a steady status in 3 to 5 minutes. Ionization of the hydroxyl group attached to the fourth carbon (pK [ionization constant of acid] = 8.0) markedly depresses its transmembrane passage. 5-FU entry into erythrocytes via nonfacilitated diffusion and a facilitated nucleobase transport system clearly differs from entry mechanisms used by pyrimidine nucleosides.[3]

FdUrd is a deoxynucleoside. There are at least four major nucleoside transport (NT) systems in mammalian cells that vary in substrate specificity, sodium dependence, and sensitivity to nitrobenzylthioinosine.[4] Two basic classes of human NT systems are present: equilibrative (bidirectional) and concentrative (sodium dependent, unidirectional). Human equilibrative nucleoside transport (ENT-1) and concentrative nucleoside transport (CNT-1) systems are selective for pyrimidines; the former is present in most cell types, including cancer cells, and the latter is present in liver, kidney, intestine, choroid plexus, and some tumor cells. In Ehrlich ascites cells, intracellular FdUrd reaches equilibrium with extracellular drug within 15 seconds.[5] Total intracellular drug continues to accumulate thereafter from rate-limiting phosphorylation to form fluorodeoxyuridylate (5-fluoro-2'-deoxyuridine-5'monophosphate, FdUMP) and other nucleotides.

Metabolic Activation

Activation of 5-FU to the ribonucleotide level may occur through one of two pathways, as outlined in Figure 9-2[6-15]: direct transfer of a ribose phosphate to 5-FU from 5-phosphoribosyl-1-pyrophosphate (PRPP) as catalyzed by orotic acid phosphoribosyl transferase (OPRTase); and the addition of a ribose moiety by uridine (Urd) phosphorylase followed by phosphorylation by Urd kinase. Sequential action of uridine/cytidine monophosphate (UMP/CMP) kinase and pyrimidine diphosphate kinase results in the formation of fluorouridine diphosphate (FUDP) and fluorouridine triphosphate (FUTP); the latter is incorporated into RNA by the action of RNA polymerase.

The pathway catalyzed by OPRTase may be of primary importance for 5-FU activation in healthy tissues because its inhibition by a nucleotide metabolite of allopurinol diminishes toxicity to bone marrow and GI mucosa,[7,12,14] but it is also the dominant route of 5-FU activation in many murine leukemias.[6] Other cancer cell lines appear to activate the drug by the action of Urd phosphorylase and Urd kinase.[7-11,14] Although one activation pathway may appear to predominate in a given cancer cell under certain conditions, both pathways are often available.

In the presence of a 2'-deoxyribose-1-phosphate (dR-1-P) donor, 5-FU is converted to FdUrd by a third activation pathway involving thymidine (dThd) phosphorylase.[15,16] dThd kinase then forms FdUMP, a potent inhibitor of thymidylate synthase (TS). FdUMP can be also be formed by ribonucleotide reductase-mediated conversion of FUDP to fluorodeoxyuridine diphosphate (FdUDP), followed by dephosphorylation to FdUMP. FdUMP and FdUDP are substrates for dThd monophosphate and diphosphate kinases, respectively, resulting in the formation of fluorodeoxyuridine triphosphate (FdUTP). FdUTP can be incorporated into DNA by DNA polymerase.

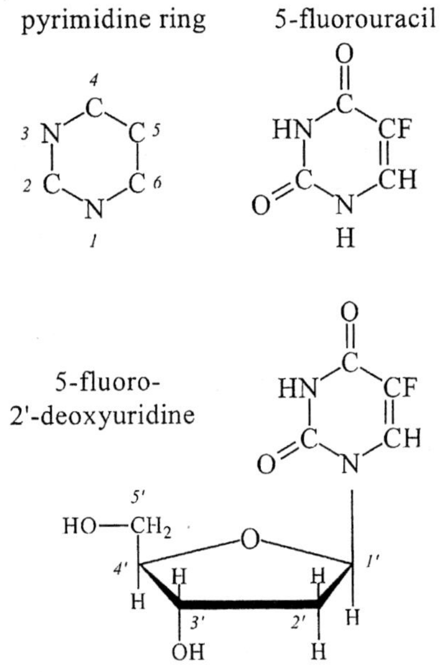

pyrimidine ring   5-fluorouracil

5-fluoro-
2'-deoxyuridine

FIGURE **9-1**   Structures of pyrimidine ring, 5-FU, and FdUrd.

Physiologic Urd metabolites are largely present in vivo as nucleotide sugars that are necessary for the glycosylation of proteins and lipids. 5-FU nucleotide sugars, such as FUDP-glucose, FUDP-hexose, FUDP-N-acetylglucosamine, and FdUDP-N-acetylglucosamine, have been detected in mammalian cells.[17] The extent to which 5-FU nucleotide sugars are incorporated into proteins and lipids and any possible metabolic consequences are unclear.

Catabolic enzymes also play important roles in nucleoside metabolism. Acid and alkaline phosphatases nonspecifically remove phosphate groups to convert nucleotides to nucleosides. 5'-Nucleotidases also remove a phosphate group from the nucleotide. Nucleosidases break the glycosyl linkage to release a free base. Pyrophosphatases remove two phosphate groups from the 5'-position of the nucleotide, with release of a monophosphate. The pyrimidine phosphorylases catalyze the reversible conversion from pyrimidine base to nucleoside and back. FdUrd serves as a substrate for both Urd and dThd phosphorylases in a tissue-dependent manner, yielding 5-FU.[15,16] dThd phosphorylase is homologous to platelet-derived endothelial growth factor, a cytokine involved in angiogenesis.

TABLE
9.1   *Key features of 5-FU*

Mechanism of action	Incorporation of FdUMP into RNA interferes with RNA processing and function. FdUMP inhibits TS, depletes dThd nucleotides. Incorporation of fluorouridine and Urd nucleotides into DNA triggers DNA repair and strand breaks, apoptosis.
Metabolism	Converted to active nucleotides by multiple pathways intracellularly. DPD catalyzes the initial, rate-limiting step in 5-FU catabolism and clearance.
Pharmacokinetics	Plasma $t_{1/2}$ 8–14 min after IV bolus. Saturable catabolism leads to nonlinear pharmacokinetics: total-body clearance decreases with increasing doses; clearance is faster with infusional schedules. Volume of distribution slightly exceeds extracellular fluid space.
Elimination	90% eliminated by metabolism (catabolism/anabolism). <10% unchanged drug excreted by kidneys after infusion or bolus.
Drug interactions	Pharmacological inhibitors of DPD: see Tables 9-7 and 9-8. Cimetidine (but not ranitidine) may decrease the clearance of 5-FU. Interferon-α may decrease 5-FU clearance in a dose- and schedule-dependent manner. LV increases intracellular folates, enhances ternary TS complex with 5-FU Oxaliplatin down-regulates expression of TS
Toxicity	GI epithelial ulceration Myelosuppression Dermatologic: rash, palmar-plantar dysesthesia Conjunctival irritation, keratitis Neurotoxicity (cognitive dysfunction and cerebellar ataxia) Cardiac (coronary spasm) Biliary sclerosis (after hepatic arterial infusion)
Precautions	Nonlinear pharmacokinetics: difficulty in predicting plasma concentrations and toxicity at high doses. Patients with deficiency of DPD may have life-threatening or fatal toxicity if treated with 5-fluoropyrimidines. Patients receiving sorivudine should not receive concurrent 5-fluoropyrimidines (4-wk washout period recommended). Older, female, and poor-performance–status patients have greater risk of toxicity. Closely monitor prothrombin time and INR in patients receiving concurrent warfarin DPD.

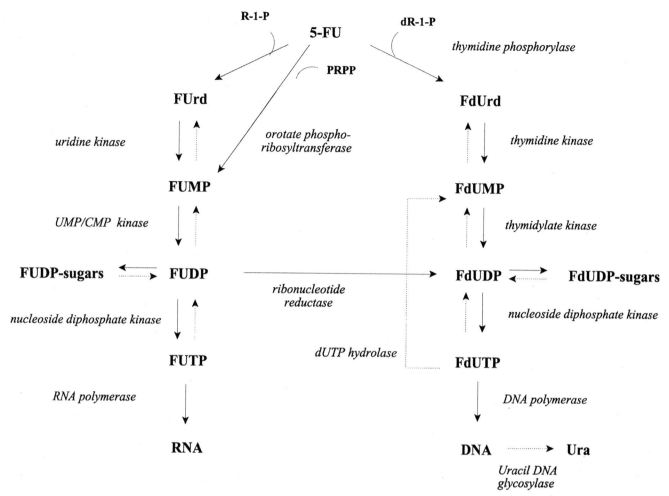

FIGURE 9-2 Intracellular activation of 5-FU, 5-fluorouracil; dUTP, deoxyuridine triphosphate; FdUDP, fluorodeoxyuridine diphosphate; FdUMP, fluorodeoxyuridylate; FdUrd, 5-fluoro-2'-deoxyuridine; FdUTP, fluorodeoxyuridine triphosphate; FUDP, fluorouridine diphosphate; FUMP, fluorouridine monophosphate; FUrd, 5-fluorouridine triphosphate; PPRP, phosphoribosyl phosphate.

Mechanism of Action

Inhibition of Thymidylate Synthase

At least two primary mechanisms of action appear capable of causing cell injury: inhibition of TS and incorporation into RNA. FdUMP binds tightly to TS and prevents formation of thymidylate (thymidine 5'-monophosphate, dTMP), the essential precursor of thymidine 5'-triphosphate (dTTP), which is required for DNA synthesis and repair. The functional TS enzyme comprises a dimer of two identical subunits, each of MW ~30 kDa (bacterial) or ~36 kDa (human). Each subunit has a nucleotide-binding site and two distinct folate-binding sites, one for 5,10-methylenetetrahydrofolate (5,10-CH$_2$ FH$_4$) monoglutamate or polyglutamate, and one for dihydrofolate polyglutamates. FdUMP competes with the natural substrate 2'-deoxyuridine monophosphate (dUMP) for the TS catalytic site.[20,21] During methylation of dUMP, transfer of the folate methyl group to dUMP occurs by elimination of hydrogen attached to the pyrimidine carbon-5 position (Fig. 9-3). This elimination cannot occur with the more tightly bound fluorine atom of FdUMP, and the enzyme is trapped in a slowly reversible ternary complex with FdUMP and folate (Fig. 9-4). The "thymineless state" that ensues is toxic to actively dividing cells. Toxicity can be cir-

cumvented by salvage of dThd in cells that contain dThd kinase. The circulating concentrations of dThd in humans are not thought to be sufficient (approximately 0.1 μmol/L) to afford protection.[22] The plasma levels of dThd are approximately tenfold higher in rodents, which complicates preclinical evaluation of the antitumor activity of various TS inhibitors.

A reduced-folate cofactor is required for tight binding of the inhibitor to TS. The natural cofactor for the TS reaction, 5,10-CH$_2$ FH$_4$, in its monoglutamate and polyglutamate forms, binds through its methylene group to the carbon-5 position of FdUMP. The polyglutamates of 5,10-CH$_2$ FH$_4$ are much more effective in stabilizing the FdUMP-TS-folate ternary complex.[23] Other naturally occurring folates promote FdUMP binding to the enzyme but form a more readily dissociable complex. Polyglutamated forms of dihydrofolic acid (FH$_2$) promote extremely tight binding of FdUMP to the enzyme.[24] FH$_2$ accumulates in cells exposed to methotrexate (MTX). Although MTX is a relatively weak inhibitor of TS in cell-free experiments, MTX polyglutamates are more potent inhibitors.[24] MTX polyglutamates decrease the rate of ternary complex formation among FdUMP, folate cofactor, and TS. The ability of MTX polyglutamates to inhibit ternary-complex formation is influenced by the glutamation state of the reduced-folate cofactor and is substantially reduced in the presence of 5,10-CH$_2$ FH$_4$

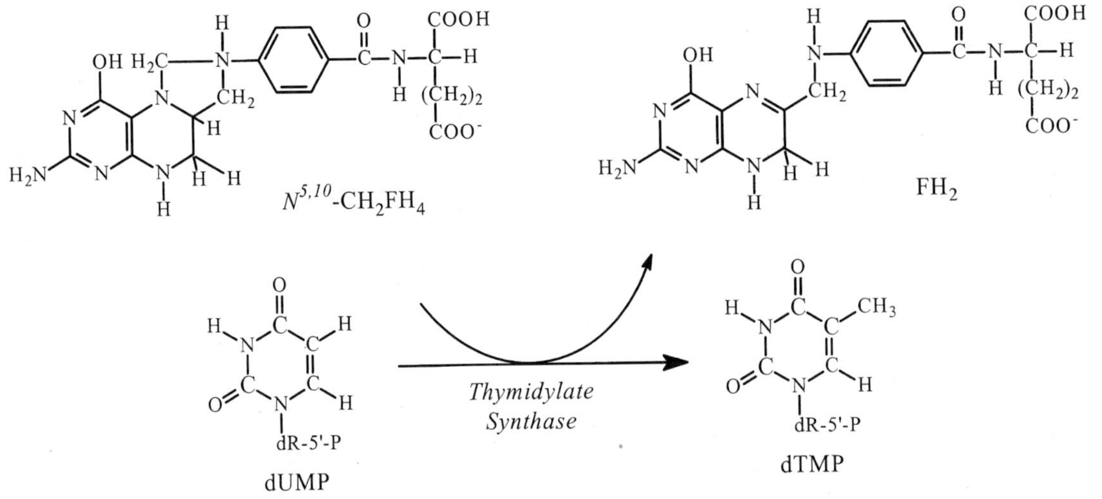

FIGURE **9-3**   Thymidylate synthase reaction, with cofactor 5,10 methylene tetrahydrofolate, converting deoxyuridylate (dUMP) to deoxythymidylate (dTMP).

pentaglutamate.[24] Similarly, in tissue culture, MTX-induced depletion of intracellular reduced folates causes a marked reduction in the rate of formation of ternary complex.[25]

FdUMP binds avidly to the mammalian enzyme, with a dissociation half-life ($t_{1/2}$) of 6.2 hours.[26] Elucidation of the crystal structure of TS has permitted a complex kinetic and thermodynamic description of ternary complex formation.[27,28] The interaction proceeds by an ordered mechanism with initial nucleotide binding followed by 5,10-CH$_2$ FH$_4$ binding to form a rapidly reversible noncovalent ternary complex (Fig. 9-4). Enzyme-catalyzed conversions result in the formation of a covalent bond between carbon-5 of FdUMP and the one-carbon unit of the cofactor. The overall dissociation constant of 5,10-CH$_2$ FH$_4$ from the covalent complex is approximately 1×10^{-11} mol/L.

Despite the high specificity and potency of TS inhibition by FdUMP and the well-established lethality of dTMP and dTTP depletion, inhibition of TS may not be the sole cause of 5-FU toxicity. If 5-FU toxicity results from dTTP depletion, then dThd should

reverse the toxic effects. Examples of complete protection from 5-FU cytotoxicity by dThd have been reported, but dThd shows variable effectiveness in rescuing cells exposed to 5-FU.[29] Experimental evidence from in vitro and in vivo studies supports the concept that, depending on the target cell, drug concentration, and modulating factors, 5-FU toxicity may be partially independent of its effect on TS. Coadministration of 5-FU and dThd prevents the early inhibition of DNA synthesis but markedly increases 5-FU toxicity to healthy tissues in the whole animal, increases the antitumor effect of 5-FU against various animal tumors, and increases [³H]FUrd incorporation into RNA.[30] Pharmacologic measures that increase FUTP formation and its RNA incorporation also increase its toxicity.

RNA-Directed Effects

5-FU is extensively incorporated into nuclear and cytoplasmic RNA fractions, which may result in alterations in RNA processing

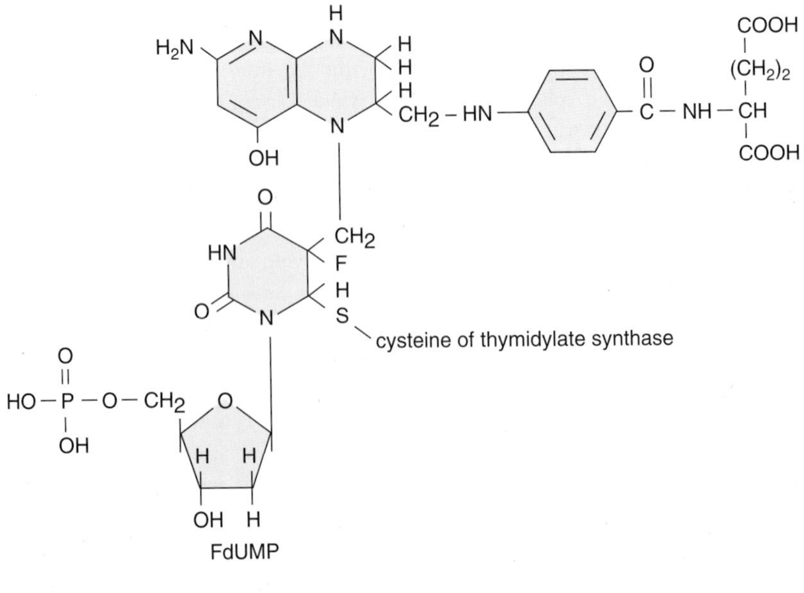

FIGURE **9-4** • Interaction of fluorodeoxyuridylate (FdUMP) with thymidylate synthase and N$^{5-10}$ CH$_2$ FH$_4$ to form an essentially irreversible complex.

and function, such as inhibiting the processing of initial pre-rRNA transcripts to the cytoplasmic rRNA species in a dose- and time-dependent manner.[31–34]

Net RNA synthesis may be inhibited during and after fluoropyrimidine exposure in a concentration- and time-dependent fashion. In some cancer cell lines, a highly significant relationship exists between 5-FU incorporation into total cellular RNA and the loss of clonogenic survival.[35] 5-FU is incorporated into all species of RNA; substantial amounts of [3H] 5-FU accumulate in low-MW (4S) RNA at lethal drug concentrations.[33] Although the analog replaces only a small percentage of uracil residues in RNA, the incorporated 5-FU residues appear to be stable and to persist in RNA for many days after drug administration.[36]

5-FU exposure affects mRNA processing and translation. Polyadenylation of mRNA and methylation of tRNA are inhibited at relatively low concentrations of 5-FU,[37,38] and altered metabolism of specific proteins such as dihydrofolate reductase (DHFR) precursor mRNA has been reported.[39] Incorporation of 5-FU into RNA may affect quantitative and qualitative aspects of protein synthesis.[40,41]

In vitro-transcribed TS mRNA with 100% substitution of 5-FU has an altered secondary structure but no differences in the translational efficiency.[40] Hundred percent substitution of uracil residues in human-TS complementary DNA (cDNA) with either FUTP or 5-bromouridine 5′-triphosphate (BrUTP) only inhibited the translational rate in the presence of BrUTP-substituted cDNA.[41] The stability of the transcribed mRNA in a cell-free system is *increased* by threefold and tenfold with FUTP and BrUTP, respectively.

Changes in the structure, levels, and function of small nuclear RNAs (snRNA) and small nuclear ribonuclear proteins (snRNP) result from 5-FU treatment.[42,65] The substitution of FUTP for uridine triphosphate (UTP) in a cell-free system (84% replacement of uracil residues by 5-FU) leads to pH-dependent missplicing of [32P]-labeled human β-globin precursor mRNA; pH values favoring 5-FU ionization promote missplicing.[43]

Further, 5-FU substitution greatly increases the pH and temperature sensitivity of the process. Partial ionization of 5-FU residues at physiologic pH (pK 5-FU = 7.8 versus pK uracil = 10.1) may therefore destabilize the active conformation of RNA.[44]

Another potential locus of 5-FU action is inhibition of enzymes involved in posttranscriptional modification of RNA particularly the formation of methylated uracil bases that have profound effects on splicing.[45a,b–47] Although 5-FU-associated cytotoxicity in cancer cells exposed in the presence of sufficient concentrations of dThd to circumvent TS inhibition is presumed to result from RNA-directed effects of 5-FU, it is paradoxical that significant incorporation of 5-FU into RNA may occur in some cancer cell lines in the absence of toxicity. The factors that influence whether 5-FU–RNA incorporation results in cytotoxicity are not clear. The rate of RNA incorporation and the species into which the fluoropyrimidine is incorporated may be more important determinants of cytotoxicity than the total amount incorporated. 5-FU and FUrd may be channeled into different ribonucleotide compartments and, ultimately, into distinct classes of RNA.[48]

In summary, the changes that result in altered pre-RNA processing and mRNA metabolism are not uniform for all RNA species after 5-FU exposure. Effects on precursor and mature rRNA, precursor and mature mRNA, tRNA, and snRNA species suggest inhibition of processing; incorporated 5-FU residues also inhibit enzymes involved in posttranscriptional modification of uracil. Many of the RNA-directed effects of 5-FU undoubtedly occur as a consequence of its fraudulent incorporation into various RNA species. The changes in certain key mRNAs resulting from 5-FU exposure may be relevant to its cytotoxicity. 5-FU-mediated interference with the production of enzymes involved in DNA repair may have cytotoxic consequences, such as 5-FU-mediated inhibition of ERCC-1 mRNA expression in cisplatin-resistant cancer cells.[49]

DNA-Directed Mechanisms of Potential Toxicity

The biochemical consequences of TS inhibition and the potential effects on DNA integrity have been extensively studied, but their relationship to cytotoxicity is incompletely understood. Inhibition of TS results in depletion of dTMP and dTTP, thus leading to inhibition of DNA synthesis and interference with DNA repair. Accumulation of dUMP occurs behind the blockade of TS, and further metabolism to the deoxyuridine triphosphate (dUTP) level may occur.[50] Inhibition of TS is accompanied by elevated concentrations of deoxyuridine in the extracellular media in cell culture models and in plasma of rodents; monitoring changes in plasma deoxyuridine levels may, therefore, serve as an indirect reflection of TS inhibition.

FdUTP and dUTP are substrates for DNA polymerase, and their incorporation into DNA is a possible mechanism of cytotoxicity.[51–54] 5-FU cytotoxicity in some models correlates with the level of 5-FU-DNA.[52,53] Two mechanisms prevent incorporation of FdUTP and dUTP into DNA. The enzyme dUTP pyrophosphatase or dUTP hydrolase catalyses the hydrolysis of FdUTP to FdUMP and inorganic pyrophosphate.[55,56] The DNA repair enzyme uracil-DNA-glycosylase hydrolyzes the 5-FU-deoxyribose glycosyl bond of the FdUMP residues in DNA, thereby creating an apyrimidinic site.[57] The base deoxyribose 5′-monophosphate is subsequently removed from the DNA backbone by an AP (apurinic/apyrimidinic) endonuclease, creating a single-strand break, which is subsequently repaired. With dThd triphosphate depletion, however, the efficiency of the repair process is substantially weakened. Uracil-DNA-glycosylase is a cell cycle–dependent enzyme with maximal levels of activity at the G1 and S interface, such that excision of the fraudulent bases occurs before DNA replication. The activity of uracil-DNA-glycosylase inversely correlates with the level of FdUrd incorporation into DNA in human lymphoblastic cells. Because the affinity of human uracil-DNA-glycosylase is much lower for 5-FU than for uracil, 5-FU is removed more slowly from DNA by this mechanism.[57] FdUTP itself inhibits the activity of uracil-DNA-glycosylase.[58] Accumulation of deoxyadenosine triphosphate (dATP) accompanies TS inhibition.[59] The combined effects of deoxyribonucleotide imbalance (high dATP, low dTTP, high dUTP) and misincorporation of FdUTP into DNA may have deleterious consequences affecting DNA synthesis, the integrity of nascent DNA, and induction of apoptosis.

A variety of DNA-directed effects have been described.[60–64] 5-FU treatment inhibits DNA elongation and decreases the average DNA chain length.[60] DNA strand breaks accumulate in 5-FU-treated cells and correlate with excision of [3H]5-FU from DNA. 5-FU and FdUrd result in single- and double-stranded DNA breaks in HCT-8 cells in a concentration- and time-dependent fashion, a process that is enhanced by LV and limited by dThd.[61] FdUrd exposure may result in the formation of large (1 to 5 Mb) DNA fragments as a result of double-strand DNA breaks; the time course and extent of DNA megabase fragmentation correlate with loss of clonogenicity in HT29 cells.[62] The pattern of DNA fragmentation is distinct from that associated with γ radiation, which produces random breaks. The pattern of high-MW DNA damage differs in SW620 cells, which are equally sensitive as HT29 cells to FdUrd-induced inhibition of TS, but require higher drug concentrations and longer exposures to achieve a comparable degree of DNA fragmentation and cytotoxicity. Resistance to 5-FU appears to be related to the higher activity of dUTPase and failure to accumulate dUTP of SW620 cells.[63] Simple dThd starvation of a TS-deficient murine cell line produces much smaller DNA fragments, 50 to 200 kb in length.[64]

Inhibition of protein synthesis by cycloheximide within 8 hours of FdUrd exposure dramatically reduces DNA double-strand breakage and lethality in murine FM3A cells, suggesting that FdUrd exposure triggers the synthesis of an endonuclease capable of inducing DNA strand breaks.[60] Factors that regulate recognition of DNA damage and apoptosis contribute to 5-FU lethality. The oncogene *p53* plays a pivotal role in the regulation of cell-cycle progression and apoptosis and influences the sensitivity of murine embryonic fibroblasts to 5-FU.[65] Transfection and expression of the *bcl-2* oncogene in a human-lymphoma cell line render it resistant to FdUrd. TS inhibition, dTTP depletion, and induction of single-strand breaks in nascent DNA are similar in vector control cells and *bcl-2*-expressing cells.[66] In vector control cells, induction of double-stranded DNA fragmentation in parental DNA coincides with onset of apoptosis. The contribution of DNA damage to cell lethality varies among different malignant lines, and DNA fragmentation does not appear to contribute to 5-FU-mediated cytotoxicity in some cancer cell lines.[67]

In summary, TS inhibition, as seen in "pure" form with FdUrd treatment in the absence of dThd salvage, and 5-FU incorporation into RNA are capable of producing lethal effects on cells. DNA damage also contributes to cytotoxicity and can occur in the absence of detectable FdUTP incorporation into DNA. The combined effects of deoxyribonucleotide imbalance (high dATP, low dTTP, high dUTP) and misincorporation of FdUTP and dUTP into DNA result in deleterious consequences affecting DNA synthesis and the integrity of nascent DNA. The pattern and extent of DNA damage induced by fluoropyrimidines in human colorectal cancer cells vary and may be affected by the activity of enzymes involved in DNA repair and by downstream pathways that are required to implement cellular destruction.

> It is now recognized that the genotoxic stress resulting from TS inhibition activates programmed cell-death pathways, resulting in induction of parental DNA fragmentation. Depending on the cell line in question, two different patterns of parental DNA damage may be noted: internucleosomal DNA laddering, the hallmark of classical apoptosis, and high-MW DNA fragmentation with segments ranging from approximately 50 kb to 1 to 3 Mb. Differences in the type and activity of endonucleases and DNA-degradative enzymes triggered in a given cell line most likely explain these disparate patterns of parental DNA fragmentation. In "apoptosis-competent" cancer cell lines, such as HL60 promyelocytic leukemia cells, genotoxic stress results in rapid (within hours) induction

of programmed cell death, with classic DNA laddering. In contrast, many cancer cell lines derived from epithelial tumors, including colon cancer, appear to undergo delayed programmed cell death. This phenomenon may reflect a "postmitotic" cell death, in which one or more rounds of mitosis are needed before cell death occurs.[68] In such cell lines, the duration of the genotoxic insult may determine whether induction of cytostasis or programmed cell death occurs. One possible explanation for delayed apoptosis is that originally sublethal damage to genes, essential for cell survival, may ultimately lead to cell death with subsequent rounds of DNA replication.

Factors operating downstream from TS clearly influence the cellular response to genotoxic stress, such as overexpression of the cellular oncoproteins *bcl-2* and mutant *p53*. Disruption of the signal pathways that sense genotoxic stress or lead to induction of programmed cell death, or both, may render a cancer cell inherently resistant to 5-FU. In some cancer cell lines, thymineless death may be mediated by Fas and Fas-ligand interactions.[69] Cancer cell lines insensitive to Fas-mediated apoptosis are insensitive to 5-FU, suggesting that modulation of their expression may influence sensitivity to 5-FU.[70] As previously mentioned, base excision repair (BER) plays an essential role in removing incorporated 5-FU and uracil residues from DNA, resulting in single-strand DNA breaks. BER recognizes the mispairing of 5-FU with guanine in DNA and excises the fluoropyrimidine. Because BER involves multiple proteins, deficiencies in one of the components, such as uracil DNA glycosylase, XRCC1 or DNA polymerase-β, may reduce the toxic effects of TS inhibitors.[71] Abrogation of uracil DNA glycosylase activity affords protection from cytotoxicity in selected cell lines[72,73] but not others.[73]

Microsatellite instability (MSI) is a manifestation of genomic instability in human cancers that have a decreased overall ability to faithfully replicate DNA and is a surrogate phenotypic marker of underlying functional inactivation of the human DNA mismatch repair (MMR) genes.[74] In vitro studies suggest that MMR recognizes DNA breaks resulting from 5-FU incorporated into DNA and signals cell cycle (G2M) arrest. Functional loss of a MMR gene results from inactivation of both alleles via some combination of coding region mutations, loss of heterozygosity, and/or promoter methylation, which leads to gene silencing. In vitro studies suggest that MMR-proficient cells are more sensitive to 5-FU or FdUrd than MMR-deficient cells.[75,76] The loss of MMR proficiency leads to fluoropyrimidine resistance in some cell lines, but not others,[77] perhaps because of differences in cell lines and conditions of drug concentration and duration of exposure in vitro. The MSI phenotype has been associated with a better prognosis in stage-for-stage matched tumors in primary colorectal cancer,[78] but data are conflicting as to whether MSI status influences benefit from 5-FU-based adjuvant therapy. The MSI phenotype has been associated with a better prognosis in stage for stage-matched tumors in primary colorectal cancer. While there is conflicting evidence for the predictive effect of the MSI phenotype in stage 3 and 4 patients, there is an emerging consensus that stage 2 patients with an MSI high phenotype do not gain any benefit from adjuvant 5-FU therapy and may actually be harmed by 5-FU treatment through undetermined mechanisms.[392] An ongoing prospective trial in stage 2 colon cancer patients will help clarify this issue.

Relative Importance of RNA- Versus DNA-Directed Effects

The relative contributions of DNA- and RNA-directed mechanisms to the cytotoxicity of 5-FU are influenced by the specific patterns of intracellular drug metabolism, which vary among different healthy and tumor tissues. 5-FU concentration and duration of exposure play pivotal roles in determining the basis of cytotoxicity. The improved response rates observed with LV modulation of bolus 5-FU therapy, the correlation between high TS expression in tumor tissue and insensitivity to 5-FU-based therapy, and the clinical activity of the antifolate-based TS inhibitors provide strong evidence that TS is the most important therapeutic target. In some models, RNA-directed effects have been predominant, particularly with prolonged duration of exposure, and are not necessarily cell-cycle dependent, whereas DNA-directed effects have been important during short-term exposure of cells in S phase. However, this generalization does not hold for all experiments with selected tumor cell lines.[79]

In two human colon carcinoma cell lines, the determinants of cytotoxicity with prolonged (120-hour) exposure to 5-FU at pharmacologically relevant concentrations (0.1 to 1.0 μmol/L) suggested that DNA-directed effects (inhibition of TS and induction of single-strand breaks in nascent DNA) and the gradual and stable accumulation of 5-FU into RNA both contribute to 5-FU toxicity.[80] Thus, the primary mechanism of 5-FU cytotoxicity varies among cancer cell lines and can change within a given cell line by alterations in schedule or the circumstances of drug exposure (the presence or absence of potential modulators of toxicity). More than one mechanism of action may be operative, and each may contribute to cytotoxicity.

Determinants of Sensitivity to Fluoropyrimidines

Because of the complexity of fluoropyrimidine metabolism and the multiple sites of biochemical action, multiple factors may be associated with responsiveness to this class of antimetabolites (Table 9-2). Deletion of or diminished activity of the various activating enzymes may result in resistance to 5-FU.[81–83] Conversely, elevated levels of certain activating enzymes have been associated with increased fluoropyrimidine sensitivity. Clones derived from murine leukemia selected for stable resistance to either 5-FU, FUrd, or FdUrd are each deficient in one enzyme involved in pyrimidine metabolism: decreased OPRT was associated with 5-FU resistance, whereas FdUrd and FUrd resistance were associated with deletion of dThd and Urd kinase, respectively.[84,85] Clones retained sensitivity to alternate fluoropyrimidines; thus, resistance to 5-FU may not preclude sensitivity to FdUrd, or vice versa.

In addition to the importance of these activating enzymes, the availability of ribose-1-phosphate, dR-1-P, and PRPP may influence activation and response.[84,85] Guanine nucleotides augment 5-FU activation to the ribonucleotide and deoxyribonucleotide levels by serving as a source of ribose-1-phosphate and dR-1-P.

The formation of 5-fluoropyrimidine nucleotides within target cells and the size of the competitive physiologic pools of UTP and dTTP also influence 5-FU cytotoxicity.[86,87] The extent of 5-FU incorporation into RNA depends on FUTP formation and the size of the competing pool of UTP. Strategies that increase FUTP

TABLE

9.2 *Determinants of sensitivity to 5-FU*

Extent of 5-FU anabolism to FdUMP and triphosphate nucleotides
    Activity of anabolic enzymes
    Availability of (deoxy)ribose-1-phosphate donors and
        phosphoribosyl phosphate
Activity of catabolic pathways
    Alkaline and acid phosphatases
    Dihydropyrimidine dehydrogenase
Thymidylate synthase
    Baseline activity of TS
    Intracellular reduced-folate content
    Polyglutamation of folate cofactor
    Concentration of competitive dUMP
    Upregulation of TS protein expression or TS amplification or
        mutation
Extent of fluorouridine triphosphate incorporation into RNA
    Concentration of competing normal substrates (UTP)
Extent of dUTP and FdUTP incorporation into DNA
    Ability to increase pools of dUTP (dUTP hydrolase activity)
    Uracil-DNA-glycosylase activity
Extent and type of DNA damage
    Single-strand breaks
    Double-strand breaks
    Newly synthesized DNA versus parental DNA
    DNA repair
Cellular response to genotoxic stress
    Cytostasis and repair of DNA versus cell death
    Intact programmed cell death signaling pathways
    Duration of genotoxic stress

FdUrd, 5-fluoro-2′-deoxyuridine; FUrd, 5-fluoro-uridine; dUMP, deoxyuridine monophosphate; FdUMP, 5-fluoro-2′deorguridine monophosphate; TS, thymidylate synthase; 5-FU, 5-flurouracil; dUTP, deoxyuridine triphosphate; FdUTP, dUTP deoxyuridine triphosphate; UTP, uridine triphosphate.

formation generally increase incorporation of FUTP into RNA and enhance 5-FU toxicity. Modulators including 6-methylmercaptopurine riboside (MMPR), N-phosphonoacetyl-L-aspartic acid (PALA), pyrazofurin, MTX, and dThd may increase FUTP formation by virtue of inhibiting de novo purine or pyrimidine synthesis, thereby increasing PPRP levels. Through feedback inhibition, expansion of dTTP pools decreases FdUMP formation by two means: blocking phosphorylation of FdUrd by dThd kinase and inhibiting the reduction of FUDP to FdUDP. In contrast, expansion of UTP or cytidine triphosphate (CTP) pools inhibits formation of fluorouridine monophosphate (FUMP) by Urd kinase. Changes in nucleotide pool size have been implicated in 5-FU resistant murine S49 lymphoma sublines that increased CTP synthase activity, increased CTP pools, and decreased UTP pools.[88]

Because RNA- and DNA-directed effects of 5-FU may differ in importance among different malignant cell lines, any single manipulation of 5-FU metabolism may produce conflicting results if different tumor models are compared. The development and application of sensitive assays that permit reliable measurement of FUTP, 5-FU-RNA levels, and TS inhibition in patient samples will help elucidate clinical determinants of sensitivity to fluorinated pyrimidines given by various schedules. In one study, RNA and DNA incorporation in tumor biopsy specimens taken 2, 24, or 48 hours from patients receiving bolus 5-FU (500 mg/m^2) were measured using gas chromatography/mass spectrometry (GC/MS) after complete degradation of isolated RNA and DNA to bases. Maximal incorporation occurred 24 hours after 5-FU administration: 1.0 pmol/mg RNA ($n = 59$) and 127 pmol/mg DNA ($n = 46$). Incorporation into RNA, but not DNA, significantly correlated with intratumoral 5-FU levels. The extent of TS inhibition, but not RNA or DNA incorporation, correlated with response to 5-FU therapy.[89] Results of such studies in clinical samples from patients receiving various infusional schedules of 5-FU are needed for a fuller understanding of determinants of response.

Determinants of Thymidylate Synthase Inhibition

The ability of FdUMP to inhibit TS is influenced by several variables, including the concentration of enzyme, the amount of FdUMP formed and its rate of breakdown, the levels of the competing healthy substrate (dUMP) and 5,10-CH$_2$ FH$_4$ cofactor, and the latter's extent of polyglutamation. The degree and persistence of TS inhibition are a crucial determinant of cytotoxicity. Blockade of TS can lead to a gradual expansion of the intracellular dUMP pool; resumption of DNA synthesis is a function of three factors: the rate of decrease of intracellular FdUMP, the rate of increase in dUMP, which competes with FdUMP for newly synthesized TS and for enzyme that has dissociated from the ternary complex, and the rate of synthesis of new TS.

FdUMP accumulates rapidly in both responsive L1210 leukemia and resistant Walker 256 carcinoma, but more rapid recovery of DNA synthesis in the insensitive line correlates with accelerated decline in intracellular free FdUMP concentrations.[86] The basis for resistance in some cells may be explained by the rate of nucleotide inactivation rather than slower formation of the active product.

Determination of TS content in tumor tissue may help to clarify the relationship between pretreatment TS levels and prognosis, response, or both, to 5-FU therapy. Biochemical assays permit measurement of dUMP, TS, the ternary complex, and free FdUMP in tissue samples.[87,90,91] Their application to clinical tumor samples is limited by the need for relatively large quantities of tissue (at least 50 mg) as well as fresh or frozen tumor tissue. In one study, biopsies of liver metastases were obtained 20 to 240 minutes after 500 mg/m^2 5-FU among 21 patients undergoing elective surgery, and maximal TS inhibition occurred within 90 minutes and averaged 70% to 80% in tumor tissue.[92] Large variations in TS binding and catalytic activity were noted in primary colon tumors, but the overall enzyme levels were significantly higher than in adjacent healthy colonic tissue.[93]

Measurement of TS gene expression provides an alternative to directly assaying intracellular TS enzyme. Overexpression to TS in tumor biopsies correlates with insensitivity to 5-FU-based regimens.[94,95]

Monoclonal antibodies have been developed that are capable of detecting human TS in immunoprecipitation and enzyme-linked immunosorbent assays (ELISA) and by immunoblot analysis. A number of studies have reported a strong relationship between TS expression in clinical specimens and prognosis; a systematic review of such studies in colorectal cancer has found great variability in methodology, clinical regimens, and combinations of drugs employed and concluded that high TS expression had the most consistent correlation with decreased survival in patients with metastatic disease,[96] although defective mismatch repair was also implicated in an improved over-all prognosis but a poorer response to 5-FU.[97]

Quantitative and qualitative changes in TS have been identified in cells with innate or acquired resistance to fluoropyrimidines. Amplification of the TS gene, with corresponding elevation of enzyme content, has been found in lines resistant to 5-FU or FdUrd.[98–100] Resistant cell lines may have an altered TS protein with either decreased binding affinity for FdUMP or decreased affinity for 5,10-CH$_2$ FH$_4$.[101–104] Adequate reduced-folate pools are required to form and maintain a stable ternary complex. Administration of exogenous reduced folates enhances the cytotoxicity of 5-FU and FdUrd in preclinical models, and clinical administration of LV is used to elevate the reduced-folate content in the cancer cell.[105,106] Tumor cells transport LV intracellularly and convert the folates to more potent and stable polyglutamates. Deficiency of the low-affinity, high-capacity folate transport system (impaired membrane transport) or reduced folylpolyglutamate synthetase activity (impaired polyglutamation) would likely impair the ability of LV to expand the reduced-folate pools, although their mechanisms of resistance have not been found in experiments to date.

In summary, to inhibit TS, 5-FU must enter the tumor and then be metabolized to FdUMP. Additional factors influence the ability of FdUMP to inhibit TS, including enzyme concentration, mutations affecting TS binding, and cofactor concentration. The tumor cell must enter the vulnerable synthetic phase of the cell cycle during drug exposure. A final factor, the ratio of endogenous dUMP to FdUMP pools can affect the duration of TS inhibition.

Regulation of Thymidylate Synthase

TS is required for DNA replication; its activity is higher in rapidly proliferating cells than in noncycling cells. When nonproliferating cells are synchronized and stimulated to enter the synthetic phase of the cell cycle, TS content may increase up to 20-fold.[107] In proliferating cancer cells, TS activity varies by fourfold to eightfold from resting to synthetic phase.[108] Increased expression of the TS gene at the G1-S boundary is controlled by both transcriptional and posttranscriptional regulation.[109,110] Elements in the promoter region of the human TS gene are regulated by the transcription factor LSF, which is in turn controlled by the astrocyte elevated gene-1 (AEG-1) AEG-1, when overexpressed in hepatocyte Uular carcinoma cells, up-regulates TS and dihydropyrimidine dehydrogenase (DPD), and confers resistance to 5-FU.[110]

In both experimental and clinical[111,112] observations,[113] 5-FU exposure may be accompanied by an acute increase in TS content, which may in turn permit recovery of enzymatic activity, and the magnitude of the increase is influenced by drug concentration and time of exposure. In NCI-H630 colon cancer cells, TS content increases up to 5.5-fold during 5-FU exposure and is regulated at the translational level.[114]

TS protein binds to specific regions in its corresponding TS-mRNA, which contributes to the regulation of TS-mRNA translation.[115,116] Antisense oligodeoxynucleotides targeted at the AUG translational start site of TS-mRNA inhibit translation in rabbit reticulocyte lysate; transfection of KB31 nasopharyngeal cancer cells with a plasmid construct containing the TS antisense fragment decreases the expression of TS protein and enhances the sensitivity to FdUrd by eightfold.[117] Reduced-folate content also influences TS expression. TS (TS-C1) with reduced affinity for its folate cofactor has normal clonogenic growth in the presence of high folate levels, suggesting folate responsiveness of the TS-C1 mutant.[118] Exposure of TS-C1 cells to 20 μmol/L LV stimulated de novo dTMP synthesis, whereas TS activity was lost by 24 hours after LV removal.[118]

Importance of Schedule of Administration in Preclinical Models

Drug concentration and duration of exposure in vitro are important determinants of response to 5-FU.[29,36,119–121] High drug concentrations (above 100 μmol/L) are generally required for cytotoxicity if the duration of exposure is brief (<6 hours), whereas prolonged exposure (>72 hours) to concentrations between 1 and 10 μmol/L effectively kills many tumors in culture. Schedules designed to provide extended exposure are currently preferred in current clinical regimens, usually in combination with LV.

> Other molecular pathways undoubtedly modulate fluoropyrimidine toxicity. Loss of protein expression of pRB (the retinoblastoma protein which controls cell cycle entry and proliferation rates) correlates with sensitivity to FU and to MTX in mouse embryo fibroblasts and in selected breast and colon cancer cell lines,[122] and the same correlation was found for pRB expression in tumor samples from breast cancer patients treated with adjuvant cyclophosphamide, 5-FU, and MTX. However, the number of patients with tumors lacking pRB immunostaining was very small (<5%). The authors hypothesize that the lack of cell cycle control allowed cells to proceed through DNA synthesis while accumulating DNA damage due to drug treatment.
>
> FU treatment activates the MAP kinase pathway and the downstream Egr1 transcription factor, and thereby stimulates production of thrombospondin-1, an antiangiogenic cytokine. This finding leads to speculation that fluoropyrimidines may synergize with inhibitors of the vascular endothelial growth factor (VEGF) pathway,[123] as has been observed clinically with bevicizumab.

Clinical Pharmacology of 5-Fluorouracil

The pharmacokinetics of 5-FU are important because of the choices of routes and schedules of administration available for this drug. Regional approaches permit selective exposure of specific tumor-bearing sites to high local concentrations of drug. Pharmacokinetic studies have played an important role in assessing these alternative schedules and routes of administration.

Clinical Pharmacology Assay Methods

5-FU has been assayed in biologic fluids using high-performance liquid chromatography (HPLC) and GC-MS. In general, an initial deproteination step is performed by chemical or filtration techniques. HPLC methods using ultraviolet detection of 5-FU are typically associated with limits of detection in the range of 0.2 to 1.0 μmol/L. Column or valve-switching techniques and the use of microbore-HPLC columns can further improve the limits of detection. Radio immuno assays of 5-FU, with high specificity and sensitivity, have also been developed.

The nucleoside metabolites of 5-FU can be separated from parent drug on reversed-phase and ion-exchange columns, whereas separation of the nucleotide metabolites is obtained with either anion-exchange or reversed-phase ion-pairing methods. Preclinical studies describing intracellular metabolism generally typically use radiolabeled 5-FU; HPLC with inline liquid scintillation detection is used to quantify the metabolites.

Derivatization of 5-FU is required for GC-MS. MS generally provides much greater sensitivity than that achievable with HPLC, with limits of detection as low as 0.5 ng/mL (4 nmol/L) for a 1-mL plasma sample.[124,125] Recent advances in fluorine-19 magnetic resonance imaging (MRI) have permitted monitoring of the pharmacokinetics and cellular pharmacology of 5-FU, thus allowing noninvasive determination of 5-FU content in tissues.[126]

5-FU is unstable in whole blood and plasma at room temperature, and catabolism is much more rapid in whole blood than in plasma.[127] Blood samples should be placed on ice immediately; plasma should be quickly isolated. 5-FU is stable in plasma at 4°C for up to 24 hours and is stable for prolonged periods when stored at −20°C.

Absorption and Distribution

Bioavailability of 5-FU by the oral route is highly variable. Less than 75% of a dose reaches the systemic circulation.[128] When administered by intravenous bolus or infusion, 5-FU readily penetrates the extracellular space, cerebrospinal fluid (CSF), and extracellular "third-spaces" such as effusions. The volume of distribution (V_d) ranges from 13 to 18 L (8 to 11 L/m^2) after intravenous bolus doses of 370 to 720 mg/m^2, which slightly exceeds extracellular fluid space.[124,129]

Plasma Pharmacokinetics

The pharmacokinetic profile of 5-FU varies according to dose and schedule of administration. After intravenous bolus injection of 370 to 720 mg/m^2, peak plasma concentrations (C_p) of 5-FU vary widely and primarily lie in the range of 300 to 1,000 μmol/L (Table 9-3).[124,129–131] Rapid metabolic elimination accounts for a primary $t_{1/2}$ of 8 to 14 minutes; 5-FU C_p fall below 1 μmol/L within 2 hours.

The most sensitive assays detect triexponential elimination of intravenous bolus 5-FU with $t_{1/2}$ values of 2, 12, and 124 minutes.[132] A prolonged third elimination phase of 5-FU was noted by GC-MS after bolus administration with a $t_{1/2}$ of 5 hours: 5-FU plasma concentration ranged from 36 to 136 nmol/L 4 to 8 hours after intravenous bolus doses of 500 to 720 mg/m^2 and may reflect tissue release.[124]

The clearance of 5-FU is much faster with continuous infusion (CI) (Table 9-4) than with bolus administration and increases as the dose rate decreases (Fig. 9-5).[125,128,133–138] As the duration of 5-FU infusion increases, the tolerated daily dose decreases.

TABLE

9.3   *Pharmacokinetics of 5-FU given by intravenous bolus*

Investigators	Dose (mg/m^2)	No.	Half-life (min)	Clearance (mL/min/m^2)	Plasma concentration (µmol/L)	AUC per dose (µmol/min/L)
Grem et al.[129]	370	16	8.1 ± 0.4	862 ± 24	C_0: 332 ± 27 15 min: 82 ± 6 60 min: 4 ± 1	3,761 ± 286
Macmillan et al.[152]	400	8	11.4 ± 1.5	744 ± 145	5 min: 469 ± 85 20 min: 100 ± 20 60 min: 13 ± 6	9,885 ± 1,569
Heggie et al.[130]	500	10	12.9 ± 7.3	594 ± 7.3	5 min: 420 ± 102 20 min: 114 ± 52 60 min: 10 ± 11	7,125 ± 2,371
van Gröeningen et al.[124]	500	15	9.8 ± 2.4	558	Not stated	7,338 ± 1,708
	600	18		404		12,000 ± 2,446
	720	7	14.4 ± 2.5	349		16,200 ± 2,446
Grem et al.[131]	425	11	9.8 ± 0.5 (all doses)	743 ± 81	C_0: 378 ± 46	4,401 ± 363
	490	13		713 ± 28	393 ± 24	5,304 ± 227

AUC, area under the concentration time curve; C_0, estimated initial concentration.
Note: If either AUC or clearance was not provided, it was calculated from the following equation: intravenous dose/AUC = clearance. The MW of 5-FU = 130.1.

TABLE

9.4   *Pharmacokinetics of 5-FU given by continuous intravenous infusion*

Investigators	Duration of infusion	Daily dose (mg/m^2)	No.	C_{ss} (µmol/L)	Clearance (mL/min/m^2)
Grem et al.[136]	Protracted	64–200	24	0.30 ± 0.04 (0.14–1.04)	3,050 ± 330
Anderson et al.[125]	Protracted	176–300	3	0.32 (0.05–0.57)	Not provided
Harris et al.[135]	Protracted	300	7	0.13 ± 0.01	Not provided
Yoshida et al.[134]	Protracted	190–600	19	1.15 ± 0.15 (0.08–2.40)	2,033
Petit et al.[137]	120 h	450–966	7	2.6 ± 0.2	Not provided
Fleming et al.[138]	120 h	1,000	57	2.1	2,523 ± 684
Fraile et al.[128]	96 h	1,000–1,100	6	24–48 h, 1.3 ± 0.1 72–96 h, 1.8 ± 0.3	Not provided
Benz et al.[133]	24 h	1,500	7	4 (1.94–5.63)	2,118 (1,235–3,471)
Erlichman et al.[139]	120 h	1,250	15	3.4 ± 0.4	2,410
		1,500	6	5.1 ± 1.0	1,790
		1,750	14	6.4 ± 0.9	1,990
		2,000	25	7.2 ± 0.7	1,910
		2,250	17	7.5 ± 1.0	2,000
Remick et al.[140]	72 h	1,655	6	5.4 ± 0.3	1,750 ± 105
		2,875	8	13.9 ± 0.5	1,117 ± 37
Grem et al.[141]	72 h	1,150–1,525	19	3.4 ± 0.5	3,011 ± 356
		1,750	31	5.0 ± 0.5	2,671 ± 563
		2,000	53	6.5 ± 0.9	2,651 ± 324
		2,300	14	8.8 ± 1.3	2,116 ± 572
		2,645	10	10.0 ± 2.1	2,247 ± 443

C_{ss}, plasma concentration at steady state.
Note: Plasma clearance converted from milliliter per minute assuming an average body surface area of 1.7 m^2 and from milliliter per kilogram assuming a conversion factor of 37 from kg to m^2.

biliary sclerosis, and is believed to result from diminished vascular perfusion via small vessel injury for the gallbladder and upper bile duct but may also be due to nonvascular events. In more severely affected patients, cholangiograms reveal characteristic radiographic changes: narrowing of the common hepatic duct and the lobar ducts, varying degrees of intrahepatic ductal stricture, and sparing of the common bile duct. Liver biopsy reveals canalicular cholestasis and focal pericholangitis. The hepatocytes appear normal, although reactive changes (hyperplasia, intracellular bile staining, and small clusters of neutrophils in association with aggregates of Kupffer's cells) are present. Some patients require cholecystectomy for acalculous cholecystitis; at surgery, the gallbladder appears shrunken, hypovascular, and densely fibrotic. The onset of biliary sclerosis can be delayed by decreasing the initial dose (median time to toxicity at 0.2 or 0.3 mg/kg/d is three or five cycles). Although FdUrd may be reinstituted at a lower dose after normalization of liver enzymes, most patients became progressively intolerant. The clinical picture may not improve after interruption of therapy.

Patients receiving HAI FdUrd should have careful monitoring of the liver enzymes; therapy should be interrupted if elevations of alkaline phosphatase or transaminases occur. Imaging studies should rule out tumor progression. A randomized trial comparing HAI of FdUrd (0.3 mg/kg/d for 14 of 28 days) with or without dexamethasone (20 mg total) showed the incidence of patients experiencing a more than a twofold increase in bilirubin decreased from 30% to 9%.[227] The incidence of biliary sclerosis, 12%, seemed to be higher when low-dose LV was given concurrently with HAI FdUrd.[228] In a subsequent phase 2 study in which dexamethasone, 20 mg total dose, was added to FdUrd (0.30 mg/kg/d) and LV (15 mg/m^2/d) as a 14-day HAI, the incidence of biliary sclerosis was only 3%.[229]

Catheter-related complications include arterial thrombosis, hemorrhage or infection at the arterial puncture site, and slippage of the catheter into the arterial supply of the duodenum or stomach, with necrosis of the intestinal epithelium, hemorrhage, and perforation. The occurrence of epigastric pain or vomiting should alert the clinician to promptly reassess the catheter position. In some patients, HAI may be impossible because of difficulties in catheter placement, thrombosis of the portal vein, or variations in vascular anatomy.

Age and Gender as Prognostic Factors for 5-Fluorouracil Clinical Toxicity

A number of clinical studies have reported significantly greater clinical toxicity in female and older patients treated with 5-FU-based therapy.[230–235] The Meta-Analysis Group in Cancer, using individual data from six randomized trials comparing infusional with bolus 5-FU, found that female patients, older patients, and those with poorer performance had a significantly higher risk of diarrhea, mucositis, nausea, and vomiting.[233] HFS was 2.6-fold more common in patients receiving infusional 5-FU versus bolus drug (34% versus 13%, $P < 0.0001$); female patients and older patients also had a higher risk of HFS. Grade 3 to 4 hematologic toxicity, mainly neutropenia, was sevenfold more common with bolus 5-FU therapy (31% versus 4%, $P < 0.0001$); poor performance status was a significant prognostic factor for serious hematologic toxicity.

Folprecht et al. evaluated pooled data from 19 randomized studies for patients with metastatic colorectal cancer receiving 5-FU.[393]

There was no difference in efficacy in the metastatic setting between patients younger or older than 70. While toxicity data were not available, 60 day mortality was similar between patients over or younger than 70. Sargent et al. performed a pooled analysis of seven randomized trials evaluating the role of adjuvant 5-FU.[394] Patients over the age of 70 experienced the same magnitude of benefit from adjuvant 5-FU. Older patients treated with 5-FU and levamisole had an increased incidence of leucopenia; whereas this association was of borderline statistical significance for patients treated with 5-FU and LV. Older patients did not experience significantly more diarrhea and mucositis.

The possible influence of age and gender on 5-FU clearance and DPD activity (in PBMCs or liver tissue) has yielded inconsistent results in different studies.[236–238] Even in trials that report a difference according to gender, there is considerable overlap in the values between men and women, and the correlation between either age and gender and 5-FU clearance or DPD activity has not been evident. Age-related physiologic changes in the liver, perhaps involving organ mass and function, and alterations in regional blood flow might account for the reduced elimination of metabolized drugs, such as 5-FU, in the older population.[239]

Because of the reports of increased clinical toxicity, it seems prudent to closely monitor blood counts and symptoms in older and female patients during 5-FU-based therapy with appropriate dose adjustments according to toxicity. The dose of 5-FU should not be lowered a priori in elderly subsets.

Randomized Trials Comparing Various Fluoropyrimidine Routes and Schedules

A series of meta-analyses has been performed by the Advanced Colorectal Cancer Meta-Analysis Group (Table 9-5).[240–244] They concluded CI yields superior response rate as compared to intravenous bolus 5-FU (22% versus 11%) when given as a single agent; HFS is significantly more common with CI (34% versus 13%); diarrhea and hematologic toxicity are much less frequent (4% versus 31%).[242] HAI of 5-FU or FdUrd consistently produced higher response rates in patients with liver metastases compared with systemic infusion of 5-FU or FdUrd,[243] although evidence for improved survival is inconclusive. LV enhanced response rates of single agent bolus 5-FU (13.6% versus 22.5%).[244]

Modulation of Fluoropyrimidines

The multiple enzymatic steps in the activation and catabolism of 5-FU offered opportunities for enhancing cytotoxicity or decreasing host toxicity by combining 5-FU with second agents that affect its metabolism. Many such combinations have reached the stage of clinical trial, but with the exception of LV enhancement, only the empirical combinations of 5-FU with cisplatin and with other independently active neoplastic agents have become standard elements of patient care. Other mechanism-driven trials have failed.

The combinations explored for host protection are summarized in Table 9-6. Allopurinol, and its active metabolite, oxypurinol, inhibit orotidylate decarboxylase[7,9] expanding the pool of orotidylate, an inhibitor of OPRT. Animal experiments indicated that host tissues, including bone marrow preferentially activated 5-FU by this pathway. However, the hypothesis that allopurinol would protect host but not tumor was not borne out in clinical trials.[200] Urd

TABLE

9.5   *Meta-analyses comparing routes and schedules of 5-fluoropyrimidine therapy*

Reference	Comparison	No. of patients	% Responding (*P* value)	Median survival (months) (*P* value)
240	Bolus 5-FU	578	11.1	11
	Bolus 5-FU + LV	803	22.5 ($<1 \times 10$) –7	11.5
241	5-FU	570	10	9.1
	5-FU + MTX	608	19 (<0.0001)	10.7 (0.024)
242	Bolus 5-FU	551	13.6	11.3
	CI 5-FU	552	22.5 (0.0002)	12.1 (0.04)
243	IV 5-FU or FdUrd or supportive care	655 (391 got 5-FU or FdUrd)	14	11 (12 mo + chemotherapy)
	HAI FdUrd	654	41 ($<1 \times 10$) – 10	16 (0.0009 versus all controls) (0.14 versus + IV chemotherapy)

expands cellular pools of dUTP and UTP, decreases 5-FU incorporation into nucleic acids, and seems to provide selective rescue of bone marrow or intestinal epithelium in mouse tumor models.[245] However, it proved difficult to achieve adequate Urd levels in humans, and the nucleoside provided only partial protection.[246]

Pharmacokinetic studies reveal diurnal fluctuation in plasma drug concentrations in patients receiving CI of 5-FU. The underlying metabolic events responsible for these fluctuations were never clarified, but drug levels peaked at 4 A.M. and reached a trough at 4 P.M. By infusing drug at variable rates through out the day, it was

TABLE

9.6   *Modulation of 5-FU toxicity to host and tumor*

Modulator	Putative mechanism	Evidence for positive effect in clinical trials (see text)
Sparing of host toxicity		
Allopurinol	Oxypurinol ribonucleotide inhibits orotate decarboxylase; buildup of orotate inhibits 5-FU activation by OPRTase	Uncertain results
Uridine	Urd nucleotides prevent 5-FU nucleotide incorporation into DNA and RNA	Impossible to reach required drug concentrations of Urd. Rescue of host tissue unpredictable
Chronomodulation of 5-FU infusion	Compensate for chronological variability in 5-FU clearance rates from plasma	Difficult to reproduce exact clinical control of infusion rates. Higher doses of 5-FU well tolerated
Increasing tumor toxicity		
Methotrexate	Given before 5-FU, MTX inhibits purine biosynthesis and elevates cellular pools of PRPP, increasing 5-FU activation.	Mixed results. Timing MTX pretreatment uncertain and may differ for different tumors. Inconvenient. Combination rarely used.
Leucovorin	Given before or with 5-FU, LV expands pool of required folate cofactor for ternary complex with 5-FdUMP and TS.	Consistent benefit seen in clinical trials with 5-FU/LV, although toxicity enhanced. Benefit of LV with capecitabine unproven.
PALA (*N*-(phospho-L-aspartic acid)	PALA blocks de novo pyrimidine synthesis, decreased pools of dUTP, UTP that compete with 5-FU nucleotides for incorporation into nucleic acids. Also increases PRPP availability for 5-FU activation.	Randomized trials show no benefit.
Platinum analogues	5-FU decreases dTTP pools, inhibits DNA repair. Oxaliplatin down-regulates TS expression.	Multiple positive combination trials in aerodigestive cancer.
Irradiation	5-FU decreases dTTP pools, inhibits DNA repair.	Multiple positive combination trials in aerodigestive cancer.

possible to even out peaks and troughs of drug concentration and minimize toxicity in animals and humans. However, randomized trials of 5-FU/LV, comparing chronomodified versus continuous dosing, failed to confirm earlier positive results[248] and interest has waned in chronomodification.

Enhancement of Antitumor Effects

Other research efforts have explored ways of enhancing cytotoxicity of 5-FU (Table 9-6). The antifolate and fluoropyrimidine pathways have multiple points of intersection (Fig. 9-7). The antifolate polyglutamates and dihydrofolate polyglutamates directly inhibit TS and could have additive inhibitory effects on the 5-FdMP target (see Chapter 8). MTX polyglutamates inhibit two steps in de novo purine biosynthesis, and thereby expands the pool of PRPP available for 5-FU activation.[249] The opposite sequence, 5-FU before MTX, produces unfavorable interaction as 5-FU inhibits TS, blocks the generation of oxidized folates by this reaction, preserves the cellular pool of reduced folates, and negates the impact of inhibition of dihydrofolate reductase by MTX.[250] The benefits of sequencing MTX before 5-FU were readily demonstrated in cell culture and in selected mouse models, but clinical trials results exploring multiple different sequences and regimens yielded conflicting evidence of benefit.[251,252] In clinical practice, such as with the CMF (cyclophosphamide, methotrexate, and 5-FU) regimen in breast cancer, the drugs are given simultaneously for reasons of convenience.

Leucovorin Modulation

The most successful approach to enhancing 5-FU antitumor activity resulted from tissue culture and animal experiments showing that LV (5-formyl tetrahydrofolate) could enhance 5-FU killing.[253–257] LV is a readily transportable and stable, but inactive precursor of the active cofactors, 5 to 10 methylene tetrahydrofolate (5 to 10 CH_2 FH_4), used in thymidylate synthesis, and 10-formyl FH_4, used in purine synthesis. Optimal concentrations of LV for forming the tight ternary complex of F-dUMP with TS are 1 µM or greater in plasma, and need to be maintained throughout the period of 5-FU exposure.[258,259] The optimal conditions for LV administration, before or during 5-FU, may vary among cell lines and in clinical treatment,[260–267] pretreatment for 4 to 18 hours with LV allowing an optimal buildup of folate polyglutamates, while longer exposures of drug likely requiring lower concentrations of continuous LV.[259]

LV is available through chemical synthesis, the clinical material consisting of equal amounts of the R- (or D-) and S- (or L-) isomers. The active or S-isomer must be converted to the active 5 to 10 CH_2 FH_4 in a multistep process. There appears to be no advantage to using the active isomer, as opposed to the racemic mixture.[268,269] Methylene FH_4 reductase, a key enzyme in the sequence, occurs in polymorphic forms, and it may limit the effectiveness of LV.[168] Tumor cells with impaired ability to transport and polyglutamate folates (see Chapter 8) will also become insensitive to LV modulation of 5-FU.[266]

Various combinations of 5-FU and LV are used in clinical regimens. With intravenous bolus doses of 50 mg LV, plasma concentrations of reduced folate remain above 1 µM for 1 hour, while 500 mg LV intravenously yields plasma levels of 5 to 10 CH_2 FH_4, the active cofactor, or greater than 2 µM. With a 2-hour infusion of 500 mg LV, peak levels of reduced folate exceed 40 µM.[270–273] Oral absorption of LV, as with other folates, is saturable, and therefore, this route is less reliable for 5-FU enhancement.

Randomized trials have supported the benefit of LV in enhancing response rates, but there is no obvious survival advantage.[274] LV has become a standard component of most 5-FU regimens, although it is not used with capecitabine, as evidence for enhancement of capecitabine, either improved response or survival rates, is lacking.

Thymidine Enhancement of 5-FU

Thymidine attracted interest as a tool for enhancing 5-FU incorporation into RNA, while at the same time circumventing the effects of 5-FdUMP on TS and preventing fluoropyrimidine incorporation into DNA.[30,275–277] The previous edition of this book described the relevant experiments in detail. However, the promise of dThd rescue in tissue culture and in mice was not borne out in clinical trials, in which massive doses of dThd (up to 8 g/d, by infusion) produced severe bone marrow and epithelial toxicity and diarrhea due to markedly delayed 5-FU clearance.[174,277,278] Further attempts to develop this combination have been abandoned.

5-FU and Inhibitors of de Novo Pyrimidine Synthesis

Efforts to enhance 5-FU antitumor activity led to experimental and clinical trials with inhibitors of pyrimidine synthesis. The trials were based on the concept that these inhibitors would elevate intracellular pools of PRPP and decrease the competitive pools of UTP and dUMP that mitigate fluoropyrimidine effects on RNA, DNA, and TS.

PALA (N-phosphono-acetyl-L-aspartic acid), an extremely tight binding and effective inhibitor of the second step in de novo pyrimidine biosynthesis,[279] enhanced 5-FU incorporation into RNA,

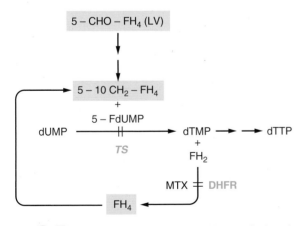

FIGURE 9-7 Interaction of folate and thymidylate synthesis pathways. 5-FdUMP and 5 to 10 CH_2 FH_4 (5 to 10 methylene tetrahydrofolate) form a ternary complex with thymidylate synthase (TS), blocking formation of thymidylate (dTMP) and inhibiting DNA synthesis. Exogenous folate, in the form of LV (5-formyl tetrahydrofolate, 5-CHO FH_4), is converted in a multistep reaction to 5 to 10 CH_2 FH_4 and expands the cellular pool of the required cofactor. Dihydrofolate (FH_2) generated in any residual TS catalytic activity must be recycled to tetrahydrofolate reductase, which is inhibited by MTX. Complete inhibition of TS negates the generation of FH_2 and renders MTX ineffective.

increased TS inhibition, and augmented cytotoxicity in preclinical studies. However, despite metabolic evidence of effective inhibition of pyrimidine biosynthesis in humans, PALA with 5-FU failed to produce a clear benefit, as compared to 5-FU alone, in randomized clinical trials.[184]

5-FU and Inhibitors of Nucleoside Transport

Multiple concentrative or equilabrative transporters share responsibility for the influx of nucleosides for RNA and DNA synthesis. While the understanding of the specific role of any one of these transporters in human tumors is incomplete, investigators have explored the concept that inhibiting NT might enhance the activity of 5-FU. One such transport inhibitor is dipyridamiole, which did enhance 5-FU toxicity against selected cell lines.[280] However, in clinical experiments, the target plasma levels of dipyridamole (50 nM) could not be maintained, 5-FU clearance was accelerated, and the combination proved to be no better than 5-FU alone.[148,281]

5-FU in Combination with Other Cytotoxics and Irradiation

In clinical practice, 5-FU is rarely used as a single agent. In most regimens, it is combined with LV and with other cytotoxic agents, particularly cisplatin or oxaliplatin, cyclophosphamide, and, in breast cancer treatment, with MTX and anthracyclines. In general, these combinations of drugs are more successful than single-agent therapy, and there is empirical experimental and clinical evidence to support specific drug combinations.

Of greatest importance are the combinations of 5-FU and cisplatin with irradiation in head and neck cancer, cervical cancer, endometrial cancer, and anal cancer. Preclinical studies have demonstrated that 5-FU enhances the cytotoxicity of cisplatin,[282–285] probably by either its depletion of thymidylate nucleotides. The effect of dTTP depletion is to inhibit repair of radiation induced DNA strand breaks.

The combination of 5-FU/LV and oxaliplatin (FOLFOX) has become standard and highly effective for both adjuvant therapy of colorectal cancer and for metastatic disease.[287,288] Oxaliplatin differs from cisplatin in its lack of dependence on mismatch repair for recognition of DNA breaks and apoptosis, and its cytotoxic mechanism and repair of its adducts differ in other respect from cisplatin (see Chapter 15). One noteworthy feature of oxaliplatin is its downregulation of TS in certain colon cancer cell lines.[286]

5-FULV is commonly combined with irinotecan in an alternative regimen for colon cancer. Irinotecan (FOLFIRI) exerts its tumor killing effects when it creates single-strand DNA breaks, which are converted to lethal double-strand breaks during active replication. In experimental systems, the combination is most effective when irinotecan precedes 5-FU/L, as irinotecan cytotoxicity is inhibited when DNA synthesis is blocked by earlier 5-FU.[289,290] In clinical practice, sequencing of drug administration is inconvenient and not demonstrably more effective. Unlike the FOLFOX regimen where the interaction of 5-FU and oxaliplatin is synergistic, the combination of 5-FU and irinotecan in regimens such as FOLFIRI is generally considered to be additive in terms of efficacy.

Interaction with Radiation

Early in its clinical development, 5-FU was found to sensitize cells to irradiation.[291] Continuous 5-FU exposure of cells for a period longer than cell doubling time during irradiation produces the greatest cell kill,[292] a finding confirmed by the superior results of continuous drug infusion in rectal cancer trials.[293] Thus, in clinical practice, 5-FU is often administered by continuous intravenous infusion with daily or twice daily irradiation for tumors of the aerodigestive tracts.[294] The mechanism underlying the synergy of fluoropyrimidines and irradiation is not well understood but likely results from inhibition of DNA repair due to dTTP depletion or incorporation of 5-FU nucleotide into DNA.[295] The actual efficacy of 5-FU with irradiation may result from the drug's systemic effects rather than enhancement of irradiation locally.

The concept of radiation sensitization of 5-FU has been challenged in recent years on the basis of clinical data in patients with rectal cancer. While there is ample data demonstrating that the use of 5-FU improves the response rate against tumors, there is little data demonstrating improved local control. Patients with T3 or node positive rectal cancer had improved survival with chemoradiation compared with radiation therapy alone.[395] Subsequently, the Intergroup compared the effectiveness of CI 5-FU versus bolus 5-FU during radiation in patients with T3 or node positive rectal cancer.[396] All patients received systemic 5-FU before and after the radiation. CI 5-FU was associated with an improved overall survival, but local control was similar in both arms. While this study was interpreted at the time of publication of proof of radiation sensitization, future authors have questioned this conclusion because local control was similar and perhaps CI was a more effective way of delivering 5-FU against micrometastatic disease. Subsequently, EORTC 22,921 randomized patients with clinical T3 rectal cancer preoperatively to either chemoradiation with 5-FU or radiation therapy alone.[397] There was no difference in clinical outcome. Bujko et al. randomized patients with clinical T3 rectal cancer to preoperative chemoradiation with 5-FU versus short course radiation therapy alone and there was no difference in local or systemic control of disease.[398] Despite these results, the concept of radiation sensitization with the use of 5-FU continues in multiple tumor types.

Orally Bioavailable 5′-Fluoropyrimidines

Table 9-7 summarizes oral preparations of 5-FU or 5-FU prodrugs. The structures of selected oral 5-FU-prodrugs are shown in Figure 9-8. Key features of capecitabine are displayed in Table 9-8.

Ftorafur and UFT

Ftorafur [1-(2-tetrahydrofuranyl)-5-FU, tegafur; MW = 200], a furan nucleoside prodrug, was the first successful orally administered analogue of 5-FU. It is slowly metabolized to 5-FU by two major metabolic pathways (Fig. 9-9). One pathway is mediated by microsomal cytochrome P-450 oxidation at the 5′-carbon of the tetrahydrofuran moiety, resulting in the formation of a labile intermediate (5′-hydroxyftorafur) that spontaneously cleaves to produce

136. Grem JL, McAtee N, Balis F, et al. A phase II study of continuous infusion 5-fluorouracil and leucovorin with weekly cisplatin in metastatic colorectal carcinoma. Cancer 1993;72:663–668.

137. Petit E, Milano G, Levi F, et al. Circadian rhythm-varying plasma concentration of 5-fluorouracil during a five-day continuous venous infusion at a constant rate in cancer patients. Cancer Res 1988;48:1676–1680.

138. Fleming RF, Milano G, Thyss A, et al. Correlation between dihydropyrimidine dehydrogenase activity in peripheral mononuclear cells and systemic clearance of fluorouracil in cancer patients. Cancer Res 1982;52:2899–2902.

139. Erlichman C, Fine S, Elhakim T. Plasma pharmacokinetics of 5-FU given by continuous infusion with allopurinol. Cancer Treat Rep 1986;70:903–904.

140. Remick SC, Grem JL, Fischer PH, et al. Phase I trial of 5-fluorouracil and dipyridamole administered by 72-hour concurrent continuous infusion. Cancer Res 1990;50:2667–2672.

141. Grem JL, McAtee N, Steinberg SM, et al. A phase I study of continuous infusion 5-fluorouracil plus calcium leucovorin in combination with n-(phosphonacetyl)-L-aspartate in metastatic gastrointestinal adenocarcinoma. Cancer Res 1993;53:4828–4836.

142. Ensminger WD, Rosowsky A, Raso VO, et al. A clinical pharmacological evaluation of hepatic arterial infusion of 5-fluoro-2′-deoxyuridine and 5-fluorouracil. Cancer Res 1978;38:3784–3792.

143. Collins JM, Dedrick RL, King FG, et al. Nonlinear pharmacokinetic models for 5-fluorouracil in man: intravenous and intraperitoneal routes. Clin Pharmacol Ther 1980;28:235–246.

144. Wagner JG, Gyves JW, Stetson PL, et al. Steady-state nonlinear pharmacokinetics of 5-fluorouracil during hepatic arterial and intravenous infusions in cancer patients. Cancer Res 1986;46:1499–1506.

145. Thyss A, Milano G, Renee N, et al. Clinical pharmacokinetic study of 5-FU in continuous 5-day infusions for head and neck cancer. Cancer Chemother Pharmacol 1986;16:64–66.

146. Trump DL, Egorin MJ, Forrest A, et al. Pharmacokinetic and pharmacodynamic analysis of fluorouracil during 72-hour continuous infusion with and without dipyridamole. J Clin Oncol 1991;9:2027–2035.

147. Fety R, Rolland F, Barberi-Heyob M. Clinical impact of pharmacokinetically-guided dose adaptation of 5-fluorouracil: results from a multicentric randomized trial in patients with locally advanced head and neck carcinomas. Clin Cancer Res 1998;4:2039–2045.

148. Santini J, Milano G, Thyss A, et al. 5-FU therapeutic monitoring with dose adjustment leads to an improved therapeutic index in head and neck cancer. Br J Cancer 1989;59:287–290.

149. Saif MW, Choma A, Salamone SJ, Chu E. Pharmacokinetically guided dose adjustment of 5-fluorouracil: a rational approach to improving therapeutic outcomes. Yonsei Med J 2009;50(6):796–802.

150. Di Paolo A, Lencioni M, Amatori F, et al. 5-Fluorouracil pharmacokinetics predics disease-free survival in patients administered adjuvant chemotherapy for colorectal cancer. Clin Cancer Res 2008;14:2749–2755.

151. Walko CM, McLoed HL. Will we ever be ready for blood level-guided therapy? J Clin Oncol 2008;26:2078–2079.

152. MacMillan WE, Wolberg WH, Welling PG. Pharmacokinetics of fluorouracil in humans. Cancer Res 1978;38:3479–3482.

153. Creaven PJ, Rustum YM, Petrelli NJ, et al. Phase I and pharmacokinetic evaluation of floxuridine/leucovorin given on the Roswell Park weekly regimen. Cancer Chemother Pharmacol 1994;34:261–265.

154. Sigurdson ER, Ridge JA, Kemeny N. Tumor and liver drug uptake following hepatic artery and portal vein infusion. J Clin Oncol 1987;5:1836–1840.

155. Speyer JL, Collins JM, Dedrick RL, et al. Phase I and pharmacologic studies of 5-fluorouracil administered intraperitoneally. Cancer Res 1980;40:567–572.

156. Sugarbaker PH, Gianola FJ, Speyer JC, et al. Prospective, randomized trial of intravenous versus intraperitoneal 5-fluorouracil in patients with advanced primary colon or rectal cancer. Surgery 1985;98:414–422.

157. Schilsky RL, Choi KE, Grayhack J, et al. Phase I clinical and pharmacologic study of intraperitoneal cisplatin and fluorouracil in patients with advanced intra-abdominal cancer. J Clin Oncol 1990;8:2054–2061.

158. Grem JL, Harold N, Shapiro J, et al. A phase I and pharmacokinetic trial of weekly oral 5-fluorouracil given with eniluracil and low-dose leucovorin. J Clin Oncol 2000;18:3952–3963.

159. Lu Z, Zhang R, Diasio RB. Purification and characterization of dihydropyrimidine dehydrogenase from human liver. J Biol Chem 1992;267:17102–17109.

160. Naguib FN, El Kouni MH, Cha S. Enzymes of uracil catabolism in normal and neoplastic tissues. Cancer Res 1985;45:5405–5412.

161. Ansfield FJ, Ramirez G, Davis HL, et al. Further clinical studies with intra-hepatic arterial infusion with 5-fluorouracil. Cancer 1975;36:2413–2417.

162. Zhang R, Soong S-J, Liu T, et al. Pharmacokinetics and tissue distribution of 2-fluoro-β-alanine in rats: potential relevance to toxicity pattern of 5-fluorouracil. Drug Metab Dispos 1992;20:113–119.

163. Dobritzsch D, Schneider G, Schnackerz KD, et al. Crystal structure of dihydropyrimidine dehydrogenase, a major determinant of the pharmacokinetics of the anti-cancer drug 5-fluorouracil. EMBO J 2001;20(4):650–660.

164. Etienne MC, Lagrange JL, Dassonville O, et al. Population study of dihydropyrimidine dehydrogenase in cancer patients. J Clin Oncol 1994;12:2248–2253.

165. Lu A, Zhang R, Diasio RB. Dihydropyrimidine dehydrogenase activity in human peripheral blood mononuclear cells and liver: population characteristics, newly identified deficient patients, and clinical implication in 5-fluorouracil chemotherapy. Cancer Res 1993;53:5433–5438.

166. Milano G, Etienne MC, Pierrefite V, et al. Dihydropyrimidine dehydrogenase deficiency and fluorouracil-related toxicity. Br J Cancer 1999;79:627–630.

167. Loganayagam A, Arenas-Hernandez M, Fairbanks L, et al. The contribution of deleterious DPYD gene sequence variants to fluoropyrimidine toxicity in British cancer patients. Cancer Chemother Pharmacol 2010;65(2):403–406.

168. Ezzeldin HH, Diasio RB. Predicting fluorouracil toxicity: Can we finally do it? J Clin Oncol 2008;26:2080–2082.

169. Yokota H, Fernandez-Salguero P, Furuya H, et al. cDNA cloning and chromosome mapping of human dihydropyrimidine dehydrogenase, an enzyme associated with 5-fluorouracil toxicity and congenital thymine uraciluria. J Biol Chem 1994;269:23192–23196.

170. Takai S, Fernandez-Salguero P, Kimura S, et al. Assignment of the human dihydropyrimidine dehydrogenase gene (DPYD) to chromosome region 1p22 by fluorescence in situ hybridization. Genomics 1994;24:613–614.

171. Johnson MR, Diasio RB, Albin N, et al. Structural organization of the human dihydropyrimidine dehydrogenase gene. Cancer Res 1997;57:1660–1663.

172. Ridge SA, Sludden J, Wei X, et al. Dihydropyrimidine dehydrogenase pharmacogenetics in patients with colorectal cancer. Br J Cancer 1998;77:497–500.

173. Fernandez-Salguero PM, Gonzalez FJ, Idle JR, et al. Lack of correlation between phenotype and genotype for the polymorphically expressed dihydropyrimidine dehydrogenase in a family of Pakistani origin. Pharmacogenetics 1997;7:161–163.

174. Au JL-S, Rustum YM, Ledesma EJ, et al. Clinical pharmacological studies of concurrent infusion of 5-fluorouracil and thymidine in treatment of colorectal carcinomas. Cancer Res 1982;42:2930–2937.

175. Harvey VJ, Slevin ML, Dilloway MR, et al. The influence of cimetidine on the pharmacokinetics of 5-fluorouracil. Br J Clin Pharmacol 1984;18:421–430.

176. Diasio RB. Sorivudine and 5-fluorouracil; a clinically significant drug-drug interaction due to inhibition of dihydropyrimidine dehydrogenase. Br J Clin Pharmacol 1998;46:1–4.

177. Poon MA, O'Connell MJ, Moertel CG, et al. Biochemical modulation of fluorouracil: evidence of significant improvement of survival and quality of life in patients with advanced colorectal carcinoma. J Clin Oncol 1989;7:1407–1418.

178. Petrelli N, Douglass HD, Herrera L, et al. The modulation of fluorouracil with leucovorin in metastatic colorectal carcinoma: a prospective randomized phase III trial. J Clin Oncol 1991;7:1419–1426.

179. Seifert P, Baker L, Reed ML, et al. Comparison of continuously infused 5-fluorouracil with bolus injection in treatment of patients with colorectal adenocarcinoma. Cancer 1975;36:123–128.

180. Rougier P, Paillot B, LaPlanche A, et al. 5-Fluorouracil (5-FU) continuous intravenous infusion compared with bolus administration. Final results of a randomised trial in metastatic colorectal cancer. Eur J Cancer 1997;33:1789–1793.

181. Sullivan RD, Young CW, Miller E, et al. The clinical effects of the continuous administration of fluorinated pyrimidines (5-fluorouracil and 5-fluoro-2′-deoxyuridine). Cancer Chemother Rep 1960;8:77–83.

182. Leichman CG, Fleming TR, Muggia FM, et al. Phase II study of fluorouracil and its modulation in advanced colorectal cancer: a Southwest Oncology Group study. J Clin Oncol 1995;13:1303–1311.

183. Kohne CH, Schoffski P, Wilke H, et al. Effective biomodulation by leucovorin of high-dose infusion fluorouracil given as a weekly 24-hour infusion: results of a randomized trial in patients with advanced colorectal cancer. J Clin Oncol 1998;16:418–426.

184. O'Dwyer PJ, Manola J, Valone FH, et al. Fluorouracil modulation in colorectal cancer: lack of improvement with N-phosphonoacetyl-l-aspartic acid or oral leucovorin or interferon, but enhanced therapeutic index with weekly 24-hour infusion schedule—an Eastern Cooperative Oncology Group/Cancer and Leukemia Group B Study. J Clin Oncol 2001;19:2413–2421.

185. Aranda E, Diaz-Rubio E, Cervantes A, et al. Randomized trial comparing monthly low-dose leucovorin and fluorouracil bolus with weekly high-dose 48-hour continuous-infusion fluorouracil for advanced colorectal cancer: a Spanish Cooperative Group for Gastrointestinal Tumor Therapy (TTD) study. Ann Oncol 1998;9:727–731.

186. Lokich JJ, Ahlgren JD, Gullo JJ, et al. A prospective randomized comparison of continuous infusion fluorouracil with a conventional bolus schedule in metastatic colorectal carcinoma: a Mid-Atlantic Oncology Program Study. J Clin Oncol 1989;7:425–432.

187. de Gramont A, Bosset JF, Milan C, et al. Randomized trial comparing monthly low-dose leucovorin and fluorouracil bolus with bimonthly high-dose leucovorin and fluorouracil bolus plus continuous infusion for advanced colorectal cancer: a French intergroup study. J Clin Oncol 1997;15:808–815.

188. Beerblock K, Rinaldi Y, Andre T, et al. Bimonthly high dose leucovorin and 5-fluorouracil 48-hour continuous infusion in patients with advanced colorectal carcinoma. Groupe d'Etude et de Recherche sur les Cancers de l'Ovaire et Digestifs (GERCOD). Cancer 1997;79:1100–1105.

189. Ansfield F, Ramirez G, Skibba JL, et al. Intrahepatic arterial infusion with 5-fluorouracil. Cancer 1971;28:1147–1151.

190. Kerr DJ, Ledermann JA, McArdle CS, et al. Phase I clinical and pharmacokinetic study of leucovorin and infusional hepatic arterial fluorouracil. J Clin Oncol 1995;13:2968–2972.

191. Sullivan RD, Miller E. The clinical effects of prolonged intravenous infusion of 5-fluoro-2′-deoxyuridine. Cancer Res 1965;25:1025–1030.

192. Kemeny N, Daly J, Reichman B, et al. Intrahepatic or systemic infusion of fluorodeoxyuridine in patients with liver metastases from colorectal carcinoma. Ann Intern Med 1987;107:459–465.

193. Hohn D, Stagg R, Friedman M, et al. A randomized trial of continuous intravenous versus hepatic intraarterial floxuridine in patients with colorectal cancer metastatic to the liver: the Northern California Oncology Group trial. J Clin Oncol 1989;7:1646–1654.

194. Anderson N, Lokich J, Bern M, et al. A phase I clinical trial of combined fluoropyrimidines with leucovorin in a 14-day infusion. Demonstration of biochemical modulation. Cancer 1989;63:233–237.

195. Martin JK, O'Connell MJ, Wieand HS, et al. Intra-arterial floxuridine vs systemic fluorouracil for hepatic metastases from colorectal cancer. Arch Surg 1990;125:1022–1027.

196. Creaven PJ, Rustum YM, Petrelli NJ, et al. Phase I and pharmacokinetic evaluation of floxuridine/leucovorin given on the Roswell Park weekly regimen. Cancer Chemother Pharmacol 1994;34:261–265.

197. Vokes EE, Raschko JW, Vogelzang NJ, et al. Five day infusion of fluorodeoxyuridine with high-dose oral leucovorin: a phase I study. Cancer Chemother Pharmacol 1991;28:69–73.

198. Kelvin FM, Gramm HF, Gluck WL, et al. Radiologic manifestations of small-bowel toxicity due to floxuridine therapy. AJR Am J Roentgenol 1986;146:39–43.

199. Benson AB III, Ajana JA, Catalano RB, et al. Recommended guidelines for the treatment of cancer treatment-induced diarrhea. J Clin Oncol 2004;22:2918–2926.

289. Loprinzi CL, Cianflone SG, Dose AM, et al. A controlled evaluation of an allopurinol mouthwash as prophylaxis against 5-fluorouracil induced stomatitis. Cancer 1990;65:1879–1882.

201. Yen-Revollo JL, Goldberg RM, McLeod HL. Can inhibiting dihydropyrimidine dehydrogenase limit hand-foot syndrome caused by fluoropyrimidines? Clin Cancer Res 2008;14:8–13.

202. DeSpain JD. Dermatologic toxicity of chemotherapy. Semin Oncol 1992;19:501–507.

203. Vukelja SJ, Bonner MW, McCollough M, et al. Unusual serpentine hyperpigmentation associated with 5-fluorouracil. Case report and review of

cutaneous manifestations associated with systemic 5-fluorouracil. J Am Acad Dermatol 1991;25:905–908.

204. Pujol RM, Rocamora V, Lopez-Pousa A, et al. Persistent supravenous erythematous eruption. A rare local complication of intravenous 5-fluorouracil therapy. J Am Acad Dermatol 1998;39:839–842.

205. Riehl JL, Brown WJ. Acute cerebellar syndrome secondary to 5-fluorouracil therapy. Neurology 1964;14:961–967.

206. Moertel CG, Reitemeier RJ, Bolton CF, et al. Cerebellar ataxia associated with fluorinated pyrimidine therapy. Cancer Chemother Rep 1964;41:15–18.

207. Lynch HT, Droszcz CP, Albano WA, et al. "Organic brain syndrome" secondary to 5-fluorouracil toxicity. Dis Colon Rectum 1981;24:130–131.

208. Moore DH, Fowler WC Jr, Crumpler LS. 5-Fluorouracil neurotoxicity. Gynecol Oncol 1990;36:152–154.

209. Tuxen MK, Hansen SW. Neurotoxicity secondary to antineoplastic drugs. Cancer Treat Rev 1994;20:191–214.

210. Bygrave HA, Geh JI, Jani Y, et al. Neurological complications of 5-fluorouracil chemotherapy. Case report and review of the literature. Clin Oncol 1998;10:334–336.

211. Diasio RB, Beavers TL, Carpenter T. Familial deficiency of dihydropyrimidine dehydrogenase: biochemical basis for familial pyrimidinemia and severe 5-fluorouracil-induced toxicity. J Clin Invest 1998;81:47–51.

212. Harris BE, Carpenter JT, Diasio RB. Severe 5-fluorouracil toxicity secondary to dihydropyrimidine dehydrogenase deficiency. Cancer Res 1991;68:499–501.

213. Takimoto CH, Lu Z-H, Zhang R, et al. Severe neurotoxicity following 5-fluorouracil-based chemotherapy in a patient with dihydropyrimidine dehydrogenase deficiency. Clin Cancer Res 1996;2:477–481.

214. Hook CC, Kimmel DW, Kvols LK, et al. Multifocal inflammatory leukoencephalopathy with 5-fluorouracil and levamisole. Ann Neurol 1992;31:262–267.

215. Davis ST, Joyner SS, Baccanari DP, et al. 5-Ethynyluracil (776C85). Protection from 5-fluorouracil-induced neurotoxicity in dogs. Biochem Pharmacol 1994;48:233–236.

216. Tsavaris N, Kosmas C, Vadiaka M, et al. Cardiotoxicity following different doses and schedules of 5fluorouracil administration for malignancy—a survey of 427 patients. Med Sci Monit 2002;8:151–157.

217. Jones RL, Ewer MS. Cardiac and cardiovascular toxicity of nonanthracycline anticancer drugs. Expert Rev Anticancer Ther 2006;6:1249–1269.

218. Meyer CC, Calis KA, Burke LB, et al. Symptomatic cardiotoxicity associated with 5-fluorouracil. Pharmacotherapy 1997;17:729–736.

219. Grandi AM, Pinotti G, Morandi E, et al. Noninvasive evaluation of cardiotoxicity of 5-fluorouracil and low doses of folinic acid. A one-year follow-up study. Ann Oncol 1997;8:705–708.

220. Wang WS, Hsieh RK, Chiou TJ, et al. Toxic cardiogenic shock in a patient receiving weekly 24-hr infusion of high-dose 5-fluorouracil and leucovorin. Jpn J Clin Oncol 1998;28:551–554.

221. Mosseri M, Fingert HJ, Varticovski L, et al. In vitro evidence that myocardial ischemia resulting from 5-fluorouracil chemotherapy is due to protein kinase C-mediated vasoconstriction of vascular smooth muscle. Cancer Res 1993;53:3028–3033.

222. al-Tweigeri T, Nabholtz JM, Mackey JR. Ocular toxicity and cancer chemotherapy. A review. Cancer 1996;78:1359–1373.

223. Eiseman AS, Flanagan JC, Brooks AB, et al. Ocular surface, ocular adnexal, and lacrimal complications associated with the use of systemic 5-fluorouracil. Ophthal Plast Reconstr Surg 2003;19:216–224.

224. Loprinzi CL, Wender DB, Veeder MH, et al. Inhibition of 5-fluorouracil-induced ocular irritation by ocular ice packs. Cancer 1994;74:945–948.

225. Boyle FM, Smith RC, Levi JA. Continuous hepatic artery infusion of 5-fluorouracil for metastatic colorectal cancer localised to the liver. Aust N Z J Med 1993;23:32–34.

226. Hohn DC, Rayner AA, Economou JS, et al. Toxicities and complications of implanted pump hepatic arterial and intravenous floxuridine infusion. Cancer 1986;57:465–470.

227. Kemeny N, Seiter K, Niedzwiecki D, et al. A randomized trial of intrahepatic infusion of fluorodeoxyuridine with dexamethasone versus fluorodeoxyuridine alone in the treatment of metastatic colorectal cancer. Cancer 1992;69:327–334.

228. Kemeny N, Seiter K, Conti JA, et al. Hepatic arterial floxuridine and leucovorin for unresectable liver metastases from colorectal carcinoma. New dose schedules and survival update. Cancer 1994;73:1134–1142.

229. Kemeny N, Conti JA, Cohen A, et al. Phase II study of hepatic arterial floxuridine, leucovorin, and dexamethasone for unresectable liver metastases from colorectal carcinoma. J Clin Oncol 1994;12:2288–2295.

230. Stein BN, Petrelli NJ, Douglass HO, et al. Age and sex are independent predictors of 5-fluorouracil toxicity. Cancer 1995;75:11–17.

231. Zalcberg J, Kerr D, Seymour L, et al. Haematological and non-haematological toxicity after 5-fluorouracil and leucovorin in patients with advanced colorectal cancer is significantly associated with gender, increasing age and cycle number. Tomudex International Study Group. Eur J Cancer 1998;34:1871–1875.

232. Tepper JE, O'Connell MJ, Petroni GR, et al. Adjuvant post-operative fluorouracil-modulated chemotherapy combined with pelvic radiation therapy for rectal cancer. Initial results of intergroup 0114. J Clin Oncol 1997;15:2030–2039.

233. Meta-Analysis Group in Cancer. Toxicity of fluorouracil in patients with advanced colorectal cancer. Effect of administration schedule and prognostic factors. J Clin Oncol 1988;16:3537–3541.

234. Sloan JA, Goldberg RM, Sargent DJ, et al. Women experience greater toxicity with fluorouracil-based chemotherapy for colorectal cancer J Clin Oncol 2002;20:1491–1498.

235. Popescu RA, Norman A, Ross PJ, et al. Adjuvant or palliative chemotherapy for colorectal cancer in patients 70 years or older. J Clin Oncol 1999;17:2412–2418.

236. Port RE, Daniel B, Ding RW, et al. Relative importance of dose, body surface area, sex and age for 5-fluorouracil clearance. Oncology 1991;48:277–281.

237. Milano G, Etienne MC, Cassuto-Viguier E, et al. Influence of sex and age on fluorouracil clearance. J Clin Oncol 1992;10:1171–1175.

238. Etienne MC, Chatelut E, Pivot X, et al. Co-variables influencing 5-fluorouracil clearance during continuous venous infusion. A NONMEM analysis. Eur J Cancer 1998;34:92–97.

239. Wildiers H, Highley MS, de Bruijn EA, et al. Pharmacology of anticancer drugs in the elderly population. Clin Pharmacokinet 2003;42:1213–1242.

240. The Advanced Colorectal Cancer Meta-Analysis Project. Modulation of fluorouracil by leucovorin in patients with advanced colorectal cancer. Evidence in terms of response rate. J Clin Oncol 1992;10:896–903.

241. The Advanced Colorectal Cancer Meta-Analysis Project. Meta-analysis of randomized trials testing the biochemical modulation of fluorouracil by methotrexate in metastatic colorectal cancer. J Clin Oncol 1994;12:960–969.

242. Meta-Analysis Group in Cancer. Efficacy of intravenous continuous infusion of fluorouracil compared with bolus administration in advanced colorectal cancer. J Clin Oncol 1998;16:301–308.

243. Meta-Analysis Group in Cancer. Reappraisal of hepatic arterial infusion in the treatment of nonresectable liver metastases from colorectal cancer. J Natl Cancer Inst 1996;88:252–258.

244. Thirion P, Piedbois P, Buyse M, et al. Alpha-interferon does not increase the efficacy of 5-fluorouracil in advanced colorectal cancer. Br J Cancer 2001;84:611–620.

245. Peters GJ, van Dijk J, Laurensse E, et al. In vitro biochemical and in vivo biological studies of the uridine "rescue" of 5-fluorouracil. Br J Cancer 1988;57:259–265.

246. van Groeningen CJ, Peters GJ, Nadal JC, et al. Clinical and pharmacological study of orally administered uridine. J Natl Cancer Inst 1991;83:437–441.

247. Levi F, Zidani R, Misset JL. Randomised multicentre trial of chronotherapy with oxaliplatin, fluorouracil, and folinic acid in metastatic colorectal cancer. International organization for cancer chronotherapy. Lancet 1997;350:681–686.

248. Giacchetti S, Bjarnason G, Garufi C, et al. First line infusion of5-fluorouracil, leucovorin and oxaliplatin for metastatic colorectal cancer: 4-day chronomodulated (FFL4–10) versus 2-day FOLFOX2. A multicenter randomized Phase III trial of the Chronotherapy Group of the European Organization for Research and Treatment of Cancer (EORTC 05963). Proc Am Soc Clin Oncol 2004;22(14 Suppl): abstr 3526.

249. Donehower RC, Allegra JC, Lippman ME, et al. Combined effects of methotrexate and 5-fluoropyrimidines on human breast cancer cells in serum-free tissue culture. Eur J Cancer 1980;16:655–661.

250. Bertino JR, Sawicki WL, Linquist CA, et al. Schedule-dependent antitumor effects of methotrexate and 5-fluorouracil. Cancer Res 1977;37:327–328.

251. Kemeny N, Ahmed T, Michaelson R, et al. Activity of sequential low-dose methotrexate and fluorouracil in advanced colorectal carcinoma. Attempt at correlation with tissue and blood levels of phosphoribosylpyrophosphate. J Clin Oncol 1984;2:311–315.

252. Marsh JC, Bertino JR, Katz KH, et al. The influence of drug interval on the effect of methotrexate and fluorouracil in the treatment of advanced colorectal cancer. J Clin Oncol 1991;9:371–380.

253. Houghton JA, Maroda SJ, Phillips JO, et al. Biochemical determinants of responsiveness to 5-fluorouracil and its derivatives in xenografts of human colorectal adenocarcinomas in mice. Cancer Res 1981;41:144–149.

254. Houghton JA, Torrance PM, Radparvar S, et al. Binding of 5-fluorodeoxyuridylate to thymidylate synthase in human colon adenocarcinoma xenografts. Eur J Cancer Clin Oncol 1986;22:505–510.

255. Spears CP, Gustavsson BG, Fiosing R. Folinic acid modulation of fluorouracil. Tissue kinetics of bolus administration. Invest New Drugs 1989;7:27–36.

256. Evans RM, Laskin JD, Hakala MT. Effects of excess folates and deoxyinosine on the activity and site of action of 5-fluorouracil. Cancer Res 1981;41:3288–3295.

257. Yin M-B, Zakrzewski SF, Hakala MT. Relationship of cellular folate cofactor pools to the activity of 5-fluorouracil. Mol Pharmacol 1983;23:190–197.

258. Cao S, Frank C, Rustum YM. Role of fluoropyrimidine Schedule and (6R,S) leucovorin dose in a preclinical animal model of colorectal carcinoma. J Natl Cancer Inst 1996;88:430–436.

259. Drake JC, Voeller DM, Allegra CJ, et al. The effect of dose and interval between 5-fluorouracil and leucovorin on the formation of thymidylate synthase ternary complex in human cancer cells. Br J Cancer 1995;71:1145–1150.

260. Keyomarsi K, Moran R. Folinic acid augmentation of the effects of fluoropyrimidines on murine and human leukemic cells. Cancer Res 1986;46:5229–5235.

261. Matherly LH, Czaijkowski CA, Muench SP, et al. Role for cytosolic folate binding proteins in compartmentation of endogenous tetrahydrofolates and the formyltetrahydrofolate-mediated enhancement of 5-fluoro-2′-deoxyuridine antitumor activity in vitro. Cancer Res 1990;50:3262–3269.

262. Nadal JC, van Groeningen CJ, Pinedo HM, et al. In vivo potentiation of 5-fluorouracil by leucovorin in murine colon carcinoma. Biomed Pharmacother 1988;42:387–393.

263. Radparvar S, Houghton PJ, Houghton JA. Effect of polyglutamylation of 5,10-methylenetetrahydrofolate on the binding of 5-fluoro-2-deoxyuridylate to thymidylate synthase purified from a human colon adenocarcinoma xenograft. Biochem Pharmacol 1989;38:335–342.

264. Wright JE, Dreyfuss A, El-Magharbel I, et al. Selective expansion of 5,10-methylenetetrahydrofolate pools and modulation of 5-fluorouracil antitumor activity by leucovorin in vivo. Cancer Res 1989;49:2592–2596.

265. Carlsson G, Gustavsson BG, Spears CP, et al. 5-Fluorouracil plus leucovorin as adjuvant treatment of an experimental liver tumor in rats. Anticancer Res 1990;10:813–816.

266. Houghton JA, Williams LG, Cheshire PJ, et al. Influence of dose of [6RS]-leucovorin on reduced folate pools and 5-fluorouracil-mediated thymidylate synthase inhibition in human colon adenocarcinoma xenografts. Cancer Res 1990;50:3940–3946.

267. Houghton JA, Williams WG, deGraaf SS, et al. Comparison of the conversion of 5-formyltetrahydrofolate and 5-methyltetrahydrofolate to 5,10-methylenetetrahydrofolates and tetrahydrofolates in human colon tumors. Cancer Commun 1989;1:167–174.

268. Bertrand R, Jolivet J. Lack of interference by the unnatural isomer of 5-formyltetrahydrofolate with the effects of the natural isomer in leucovorin preparations. J Natl Cancer Inst 1989;81:1175–1178.

269. Straw JA, Szapary D, Wynn WT. Pharmacokinetics of the diastereoisomers of leucovorin after intravenous and oral administration to normal subjects. Cancer Res 1984;44:3114–3119.

270. Machover D, Goldschmidt E, Chollet P, et al. Treatment of advanced colorectal and gastric adenocarcinomas with 5-fluorouracil and high-dose folinic acid. J Clin Oncol 1986;4:685–696.

271. Trave F, Rustum YM, Petrelli NJ, et al. Plasma and tumor tissue pharmacology of high dose intravenous leucovorin calcium in combination with fluorouracil in patients with advanced colorectal carcinoma. J Clin Oncol 1988;6:1181–1188.

272. Newman EA, Straw JA, Doroshow JH. Pharmacokinetics of diastereoisomers of (6R,S)-folinic acid (leucovorin) in humans during constant high-dose intravenous infusion. Cancer Res 1989;49:5755–5760.

273. Priest DG, Schmitz JC, Bunni MA, et al. Pharmacokinetics of leucovorin metabolites in human plasma as a function of dose administered orally and intravenously. J Natl Cancer Inst 1991;83:1806–1812.

274. The Advanced Colorectal Cancer Meta-Analysis Project. Modulation of fluorouracil by leucovorin in patients with advanced colorectal cancer. Evidence in terms of response rate. J Clin Oncol 1992;10:896–903.

275. Santelli G, Valeriote F. In vivo enhancement of 5-fluorouracil cytotoxicity to AKR leukemia cells by thymidine in mice. J Natl Cancer Inst 1978; 61:843–847.

276. Carrico CK, Glazer RI. Augmentation by thymidine of the incorporation and distribution of 5-fluorouracil into ribosomal RNA. Biochem Biophys Res Commun 1979;87:664–670.

277. O'Dwyer PJ, King SA, Hoth DF, et al. Role of thymidine in biochemical modulation. A review. Cancer Res 1987;47:3911–3919.

278. Vogel SJ, Presant CA, Ratkin FA, et al. Phase I study of thymidine plus 5-fluorouracil infusions in advanced colorectal carcinoma. Cancer Treat Rep 1979;63:1–5.

279. Grem JL, King SA, O'Dwyer PJ, et al. Biochemistry and clinical activity of n-(phosphonacetyl)-l-aspartate. A review. Cancer Res 1988;48:4441–4454.

280. Grem JL, Fischer PH. Augmentation of 5-fluorouracil cytotoxicity in human colon cancer cells by dipyridamole. Cancer Res 1985;45:2967–2972.

281. Köhne C-H, Hiddemann W, Schüller J, et al. Failure of orally administered dipyridamole to enhance the antineoplastic activity of fluorouracil in combination with leucovorin in patients with advanced colorectal cancer. A prospective randomized trial. J Clin Oncol 1995;13:1201–1208.

282. Scanlon KJ, Newman EM, Lu Y, et al. Biochemical basis for cisplatin and 5-fluorouracil synergism in human ovarian carcinoma cells. Proc Natl Acad Sci U S A 1986;83:8923–8925.

283. Pratesi G, Gianni L, Manzotti C, et al. Sequence dependence of the antitumor and toxic effects of 5-fluorouracil and cis-diamminedichloroplatinum combination on primary colon tumors in mice. Cancer Chemother Pharmacol 1988;20:237–241.

284. Esaki T, Nakano S, Tatsumoto T, et al. Inhibition by 5-fluorouracil of cis-diamminedichloroplatinum(II)-induced DNA interstrand cross-link removal in a HST-1 human squamous carcinoma cell line. Cancer Res 1992;52:6501–6506.

285. Johnston PG, Geoffroy F, Drake J, et al. The cellular interaction of 5-fluorouracil and cisplatin in a human colon carcinoma cell line. Eur J Cancer 1996;32A:2148–2154.

286. Yeh K-H, Cheng A-L, Wan J-P, et al. Down-regulation of thymidylate synthase expression and its steady-state mRNA by oxaliplatin in colon cancer cells. Anticancer Drugs 2004;15:371–376.

287. de Gramont A, Figer A, Seymour M, et al. Leucovorin and fluorouracil with or without oxaliplatin as first-line treatment in advanced colorectal cancer. J Clin Oncol 2000;18:2938–2947.

288. Andre T, Boni C, Mounedji-Boudiaf L, et al. Oxaliplatin, fluorouracil, and leucovorin as adjuvant treatment for colon cancer. N Engl J Med 2004;350:2343–2351.

289. Mans DR, Grivicich I, Peters GJ, et al. Sequence-dependent growth inhibition and DNA damage formation by the irinotecan-5-fluorouracil combination in human colon carcinoma cell lines. Eur J Cancer 1999;35:1851–1861.

290. Azrak RG, Cao S, Slocum HK, et al. Therapeutic synergy between irinotecan and 5-fluorouracil against human tumor xenografts. Clin Cancer Res 2004;10:1121–1129.

291. Heidelberger C, Griesvach L, Montag BJ, et al. Studies on fluorinated pyrimidines. II. Effects on transplanted tumors. Cancer Res 1958;18:305–317.

292. Ishikawa T, Tanaka Y, Ishitsuka H, et al. Comparative antitumor activity of 5-fluorouracil and 5′-deoxyfluorouridine in combination with radiation therapy in mice bearing colon 26 adenocarcinoma. Cancer Res 1989;80:583–591.

293. Cooper JS, Guo MD, Herskovic A, et al. Chemoradiotherapy of locally advanced esophageal cancer. Long-term follow-up of a prospective randomized trial (RTOG 85-01). Radiation Therapy Oncology Group. JAMA 1999;281:1623–1627.

294. O'Connell MJ, Martenson JA, Wieand HS, et al. Improving adjuvant therapy for rectal cancer by combining protracted infusion fluorouracil with radiation therapy after curative surgery. N Engl J Med 1994;33:502–507.

295. Shewach DS, Lawrence TS. Antimetabolite radiosensitizers. J Clin Oncol 2007;25:4043–4050.

296. El Sayed YM, Sadee W. Metabolic activation of ftorafur. the microsomal oxidative pathway. Biochem Pharmacol 1982;31:3006–3008.

297. Komatsu T, Yamazaki H, Shimada N, et al. Involvement of microsomal cytochrome P450 and cytosolic thymidine phosphorylase in 5-fluorouracil formation from tegafur in human liver. Clin Cancer Res 2001;7:675–681.

298. Antilla MI, Sotaniemi EA, Kaiaralcoma MI, et al. Pharmacokinetics of ftorafur after intravenous and oral administration. Cancer Chemother Pharmacol 1983;10:150–153.

299. Benvenuto J, Lu K, Hall SW, et al. Metabolism of 1-(tetrahydro-2-furanyl)-5-fluorouracil (ftorafur). Cancer Res 1978;38:3867–3870.

300. Ansfield FJ, Kallas GJ, Singson JP. Phase I–II studies of oral tegafur (ftorafur). J Clin Oncol 1983;1:107–110.

301. Kajanti MJ, Pyrhönen SO, Maiche AG. Oral tegafur in the treatment of metastatic breast cancer. A phase II study. Eur J Cancer 1993;29A:863–866.

302. Palmeri S, Gebbia V, Russo A, et al. Oral tegafur in the treatment of gastrointestinal tract cancers. A phase II study. Br J Cancer 1990;61:475–478.

303. Ota K, Taguchi T, Kimura K. Report on nationwide pooled data and cohort investigation in UFT phase II study. Cancer Chemother Pharmacol 1988;22:333–338.

304. Sulkes A, Benner SE, Canetta RM. Uracil-ftorafur. An oral fluoropyrimidine active in colorectal cancer. J Clin Oncol 1998;16:3461–3475.

305. Carmichael J, Tadeusz P, Radstone D, et al. Randomized comparative study of tegafur/uracil and oral leucovorin versus parenteral fluorouracil and leucovorin in patients with previously untreated metastatic colorectal cancer. J Clin Oncol 2002;20:3617–3627.

306. Douillard J-Y, Hoff PM, Skillings JR, et al. Multicenter phase III study of uracil/tegafur and oral leucovorin versus fluorouracil and leucovorin in patients with previously untreated metastatic colorectal cancer. J Clin Oncol 2002;20:3605–3616.

307. Lembersky BC, Wieand HS, Petrelli NJ, et al. Oral uracil and tegafur plus leucovorin compared with intravenous fluorouracil and leucovorin in stage II and III carcinoma of the colon: results from National Surgical Adjuvant Breast and Bowel Project Protocol C-06. J Clin Oncol 2006;24:2059–2064.

308. Noguchi S, Koyama H, Uchino J, et al. Postoperative adjuvant therapy with tamoxifen, tegafur plus uracil, or both in women with node-negative breast cancer: a pooled analysis of six randomized controlled trials. J Clin Oncol 2005;23:2172–2184.

309. Dooley M, Goa KL. Capecitabine. Drugs 1999;58(1):69–76.

310. O'Shaughnessy J, Miles D, Vukelja S, et al. Superior survival with capecitabine plus docetaxel combination therapy in anthracycline-pretreated patients with advanced breast cancer: phase III trial results. J Clin Oncol 2002;20:2812–2823.

311. Geyer CE, Forster J, Lindquist D, et al. Lapatinib plus capecitabine for HER2-positive advanced breast cancer. N Engl J Med 2006;355:2733–2743.

312. Cassidy J, Clarke S, Díaz-Rubio E, et al. Randomized phase III study of capecitabine plus oxaliplatin compared with fluorouracil/folinic acid plus oxaliplatin as first-line therapy for metastatic colorectal cancer. J Clin Oncol 2008;26:2006–2012.

313. Tabata T, Katoh M, Tokudome S, et al. Identification of the cytosolic carboxylesterase catalyzing the 5′-deoxy-5-fluorocytidine formation from capecitabine in human liver. Drug Metab Dispos 2004;32:1103–1110.

314. Budman DR, Meropol NJ, Reigner B, et al. Preliminary studies of a novel oral fluoropyrimidine carbamate. Capecitabine. J Clin Oncol 1998;16:1795–1802.

315. Mackean M, Planting A, Twelves C, et al. Phase I and pharmacologic study of intermittent twice-daily oral therapy with capecitabine in patients with advanced and/or metastatic cancer. J Clin Oncol 1998;16:2977–2985.

316. Miwa M, Ura M, Nishida M, et al. Design of a novel oral fluoropyrimidine carbamate, capecitabine, which generates 5-fluorouracil selectively in tumours by enzymes concentrated in human liver and cancer tissue. Eur J Cancer 1998;34:1274–1281.

317. Ishikawa T, Utoh M, Sawada N, et al. Tumor selective delivery of 5-fluorouracil by capecitabine, a new oral fluoropyrimidine carbamate, in human cancer xenografts. Biochem Pharmacol 1998;55:1091–1097.

318. Ishikawa T, Sekiguchi F, Fukase Y, et al. Positive correlation between the efficacy of capecitabine and doxifluridine and the ratio of thymidine phosphorylase to dihydropyrimidine dehydrogenase activities in tumors in human cancer xenografts. Cancer Res 1998;58:685–690.

319. Schuller J, Cassidy J, Dumont E, et al. Preferential activation of capecitabine in tumor following oral administration to colorectal cancer patients. Cancer Chemother Pharmacol 2000;45:291–297.

320. Reigner B, Blesch K, Weidekamm E. Clinical pharmacokinetics of capecitabine. Clin Pharmacokinet 2001;40:85–104.

321. Reigner B, Verweij J, Dirix L, et al. Effect of food on the pharmacokinetics of capecitabine and its metabolites following oral administration in cancer patients. Clin Cancer Res 1998;4:941–948.

322. Twelves C, Glynne-Jones R, Cassidy J, et al. Effect of hepatic dysfunction due to liver metastases on the pharmacokinetics of capecitabine and its metabolites. Clin Cancer Res 1999;5:1696–1702.

323. Poole C, Gardiner J, Twelves C, et al. Effect of renal impairment on the pharmacokinetics and tolerability of capecitabine (Xeloda) in cancer patients. Cancer Chemother Pharmacol 2002;49:225–234.

324. Walkhorm B, Fraunfelder FT. Severe ocular irritation and corneal deposits associated with capecitabine use. New Engl J Med 2004;343:740–741.

325. Couch LS, Groteluschen DL, Stewart JA, et al. Capecitabine-related neurotoxicity presenting as trismus. Clin Colorectal Cancer 2003;3:121–123.

326. Hoff PM, Ansari R, Batist G, et al. Comparison of oral capecitabine versus intravenous fluorouracil plus leucovorin as first-line treatment in 605 patients with metastatic colorectal cancer: results of a randomized phase III study. J Clin Oncol 2001;19:2282–2292.

327. Van Cutsem E, Twelves C, Cassidy J, et al. Oral capecitabine compared with intravenous fluorouracil plus leucovorin in patients with metastatic colorectal cancer: results of a large phase III study. J Clin Oncol 2001;19:4097–4106.

328. Milano G, Etienne-Grimaldi MC, Mari M, et al. Candidate mechanisms for capecitabine-related hand-foot syndrome. Br J Clin Pharmacol 2008;66:88–95.

329. Yen-Revollo JL, Goldberg RM, McLeod HL. Can inhibiting dihydropyrimidine dehydrogenase limit hand-foot syndrome caused by fluoropyrimidines? Clin Cancer Res 2008;14:8–13.

330. Saif MW, Diasio R. Is capecitabine safe in patients with gastrointestinal cancer and dihydropyrimidine dehydrogenase deficiency? Clin Colorectal Cancer 2006;5:359–362.

331. Midgley R, Kerr DJ, Capecitabine: have we got the dose right? Nat Clin Pract Oncol 2009;6:17–24.

332. Hennessy BT, Gauthier AM, Michaud LB, et al. Lower dose capecitabine has a more favorable therapeutic index in metastatic breast cancer: retrospective analysis of patients treated at M. D. Anderson Cancer Center and a review of capecitabine toxicity in the literature. Ann Oncol 2005;16:1289–1296.

333. Twelves C, Wong A, Nowacki MP, et al. Capecitabine as adjuvant treatment for stage III colon cancer. N Engl J Med 2005;352(26):2696–2704.

334. Largillier R, Etienne-Grimaldi MC, Formento JL, et al. Pharmacogenetics of capecitabine in advanced breast cancer patients. Clin Cancer Res 2006;12:5496–5502.

335. Sharma R, Hoskins JM, Rivory LP, et al. Thymidylate synthase and methylenetetrahydrofolate reductase gene polymorphisms and toxicity to capecitabine in advanced colorectal cancer patients. Clin Cancer Res 2008;14:817–825.

336. Jensen SA, Sorensen JB. Risk factors and prevention of cardiotoxicity induced by 5-fluorouracil or capecitabine. Cancer Chemother Pharmacol 2006;58:487–493.

337. Ng M, Cunningham D, Norman AR. The frequency and pattern of cardiotoxicity observed with capecitabine used in conjunction with oxaliplatin in patients treated for advanced colorectal cancer (CRC). Eur J Cancer 2005;41:1542–1546.

338. Van Cutsem E, Hoff PM, Blum JL, et al. Incidence of cardiotoxicity with the oral fluoropyrimidine capecitabine is typical of that reported with 5-fluorouracil. Ann Oncol 2002;13:484–485.

339. Farina A, Malafronte C, Valsecchi MA, et al. Capecitabine-induced cardiotoxicity: when to suspect? How to manage? A case report. J Cardiovasc Med (Hagerstown) 2009;10:722–726.

340. Goldsmith YB, Roistacher N, Baum MS. Capecitabine-induced coronary vasospasm. J Clin Oncol 2008;26:3802–3804.

341. Hoff PM, Pazdur R, Lassere Y, et al. Phase II study of capecitabine in patients with fluorouracil-resistant metastatic colorectal carcinoma. J Clin Oncol 2004;22:2078–2083.

342. Lee JJ, Kim TM, Yu SJ, et al. Single-agent capecitabine in patients with metastatic colorectal cancer refractory to 5-fluorouracil/leucovorin chemotherapy. Jpn J Clin Oncol 2004;34:400–404.

343. Cunningham D, Starling N, Rao S, et al. Capecitabine and oxaliplatin for advanced esophagogastric cancer. N Engl J Med 2008;358:36–46.

344. Overman MJ, Varadhachary GR, Kopetz S, et al. Phase II study of capecitabine and oxaliplatin for advanced adenocarcinoma of the small bowel and ampulla of Vater. J Clin Oncol 2009;27:2598–2603.

345. Herrmann R, Bodoky G, Ruhstaller T, et al. Gemcitabine plus capecitabine compared with gemcitabine alone in advanced pancreatic cancer: a randomized, multicenter, phase III trial of the Swiss Group for Clinical Cancer Research and the Central European Cooperative Oncology Group. J Clin Oncol 2007;25(16):2212–2217.

346. Bartsch R, Wenzel C, Altorjai G, et al. Capecitabine and trastuzumab in heavily pretreated metastatic breast cancer. J Clin Oncol 2007;25:3853–3858.

347. Cameron D, Casey M, Press M, et al. A phase III randomized comparison of lapatinib plus capecitabine versus capecitabine alone in women with advanced breast cancer that has progressed on trastuzumab: updated efficacy and biomarker analyses. Breast Cancer Res Treat 2008;112:533–543.

348. Saltz LB, Clarke S, Díaz-Rubio E, et al. Bevacizumab in combination with oxaliplatin-based chemotherapy as first-line therapy in metastatic colorectal cancer: a randomized phase III study. J Clin Oncol 2008;26:2013–2019.

349. Souglakos J, Kalykaki A, Vamvakas L, et al. Phase II trial of capecitabine and oxaliplatin (CAPOX) plus cetuximab in patients with metastatic colorectal cancer who progressed after oxaliplatin-based chemotherapy. Ann Oncol 2007;18:305–310.

350. Arkenau HT, Arnold D, Cassidy J, et al. Efficacy of oxaliplatin plus capecitabine or infusional fluorouracil/leucovorin in patients with metastatic colorectal cancer: a pooled analysis of randomized trials. J Clin Oncol 2008;26:5910–5917.

351. Fuchs CS, Marshall J, Barrueco J. Randomized, controlled trial of irinotecan plus infusional, bolus, or oral fluoropyrimidines in first-line treatment of metastatic colorectal cancer: results from the BICC-C Study. J Clin Oncol 2007;25:4779–4786.

352. Puglisi F, Cardellino GG, Crivellari D, et al. Thymidine phosphorylase expression is associated with time to progression in patients receiving low-dose, docetaxel-modulated capecitabine for metastatic breast cancer. Ann Oncol 2008;19:1541–1546.

353. Uchida K, Danenberg PV, Danenberg KD, et al. Thymidylate synthase, dihydropyrimidine dehydrogenase, ERCC1, and thymidine phosphorylase gene expression in primary and metastatic gastrointestinal adenocarcinoma tissue in patients treated on a phase I trial of oxaliplatin and capecitabine. BMC Cancer 2008;8:386.

354. Mori K, Hasegawa M, Nishida M, et al. Expression levels of thymidine phosphorylase and dihydropyrimidine dehydrogenase in various human tumor tissues. Int J Oncol 2000;17:33–38.

355. Honda J, Sasa M, Moriya T, et al. Thymidine phosphorylase and dihydropyrimidine dehydrogenase are predictive factors of therapeutic efficacy of capecitabine monotherapy for breast cancer-preliminary results. J Med Invest 2008;55:54–60.

356. Endo M, Shinbori N, Fukase Y, et al. Induction of thymidine phosphorylase expression and enhancement of efficacy of capecitabine or 5′-deoxy-5-fluorouridine by cyclophosphamide in mammary tumor models. Int J Cancer 1999;83:127–134.

357. Blanquicett C, Gillespie GY, Nabors LB, et al. Induction of thymidine phosphorylase in both irradiated and shielded, contralateral human U87MG glioma xenografts: implications for a dual modality treatment using capecitabine and irradiation. Mol Cancer Ther 2002;1:1139–1145.

358. Xiao YS, Tang ZY, Fan J, et al. Interferon-alpha 2a up-regulated thymidine phosphorylase and enhanced antitumor effect of capecitabine on hepatocellular carcinoma in nude mice. J Cancer Res Clin Oncol 2004;130: 546–550.

359. Magne N, Fischel JL, Dubreuil A, et al. ZD1839 (Iressa) modifies the activity of key enzymes linked to fluoropyrimidine activity: rational basis for a new combination therapy with capecitabine. Clin Cancer Res 2003;9:4735–4742.

360. Bazarbashi S, El-Bassiouni M, Abdelsalam M, et al. A modern regimen of pre-operative concurrent chemo-radiation therapy in locally advanced rectal cancer. J Surg Oncol 2008;98:167–174.

361. Craven I, Crellin A, Cooper R, et al. Preoperative radiotherapy combined with 5 days per week capecitabine chemotherapy in locally advanced rectal cancer. Br J Cancer 2007;97:1333–1337.

362. De Paoli A, Chiara S, Luppi G, et al. Capecitabine in combination with preoperative radiation therapy in locally advanced, resectable, rectal cancer: a multicentric phase II study. Ann Oncol 2006;17:246–251.

363. Desai SP, El-Rayes BF, Ben-Josef E, et al. A phase II study of preoperative capecitabine and radiation therapy in patients with rectal cancer. Am J Clin Oncol 2007;30:340–345.

364. Dunst J, Debus J, Rudat V, et al. Neoadjuvant capecitabine combined with standard radiotherapy in patients with locally advanced rectal cancer: mature results of a phase II trial. Strahlenther Onkol 2008;184:450–456.

365. Dupuis O, Vie B, Lledo G, et al. Preoperative treatment combining capecitabine with radiation therapy in rectal cancer: a GERCOR Phase II Study. Oncology 2007;73:169–176.

366. Kim JC, Kim TW, Kim JH, et al. Preoperative concurrent radiotherapy with capecitabine before total mesorectal excision in locally advanced rectal cancer. Int J Radiat Oncol Biol Phys 2005;63:346–353.

367. Kim JS, Kim JS, Cho MJ, et al. Preoperative chemoradiation using oral capecitabine in locally advanced rectal cancer. Int J Radiat Oncol Biol Phys 2002;54:403–408.

368. Kim JS, Kim JS, Cho MJ, et al. Comparison of the efficacy of oral capecitabine versus bolus 5-FU in preoperative radiotherapy of locally advanced rectal cancer. J Korean Med Sci 2006;21:52–57.

369. Krishnan S, Janjan NA, Skibber JM, et al. Phase II study of capecitabine (Xeloda) and concomitant boost radiotherapy in patients with locally advanced rectal cancer. Int J Radiat Oncol Biol Phys 2006;66:762–771.

370. Porter DJ, Chestnut WG, Merrill BM, et al. Mechanism-based inactivation of dihydropyrimidine dehydrogenase by 5-ethynyluracil. J Biol Chem 1992;267:5236–5242.

371. Spector T, Harrington JA, Porter DJ. 5-Ethynyluracil (776C85). Inactivation of dihydropyrimidine dehydrogenase in vivo. Biochem Pharmacol 1993;46:2243–2248.

372. Baccanari DP, Davis ST, Knick VC, et al. 5-Ethynyluracil (776C85). A potent modulator of the pharmacokinetics and antitumor efficacy of 5-fluorouracil. Proc Natl Acad Sci U S A 1993;90:11064–11068.

373. Cao S, Rustum YM, Spector T. 5-Ethynyluracil (776C85). Modulation of 5-fluorouracil efficacy and therapeutic index in rats bearing advanced colorectal carcinoma. Cancer Res 1994;54:1507–1510.

374. Spector T, Cao S, Rustum YM, et al. Attenuation of the antitumor activity of 5-fluorouracil by (R)-5-fluoro-5,6-dihydrouracil. Cancer Res 1995;55:1239–1241.

375. Davis ST, Joyner SS, Baccanari DP, et al. 5-Ethynyluracil (776C85). Protection from 5-fluorouracil-induced neurotoxicity in dogs. Biochem Pharmacol 1994;48:233–236.

376. Mani S, Hochster H, Beck T, et al. Multicenter phase II study to evaluate a 28-day regimen of oral fluorouracil plus eniluracil in the treatment of patients with previously untreated metastatic colorectal cancer. J Clin Oncol 2000;18:2894–2901.

377. Smith IE, Johnston SR, O'Brien ME, et al. Low-dose oral fluorouracil with eniluracil as first-line chemotherapy against advanced breast cancer: a phase II study. J Clin Oncol 2000;18:2378–2384.

378. Schilsky RL, Levin J, West WH, et al. Randomized, open-label, phase III study of a 28-day oral regimen of eniluracil plus fluorouracil versus intravenous fluorouracil plus leucovorin as first-line therapy in patients with metastatic/advanced colorectal cancer. J Clin Oncol 2002;20:1519–1526.

379. Schilsky RL, Hohneker J, Ratain MJ, et al. Phase I clinical and pharmacologic study of eniluracil plus fluorouracil in patients with advanced cancer. J Clin Oncol 1998;16:1450.

380. Fujii S, Fukushima M, Shimamoto Y, et al. Antitumor activity of BOF-A2, a new 5-fluorouracil derivative. Jpn J Cancer Res 1989;80:173–181.

381. Schöfski P. The modulated oral fluoropyrimidine prodrug S-1, and its use in gastrointestinal cancer and other solid tumors. Anticancer Drugs 2004;15:85–106.

382. Sakamoto J, Kodaira S, Hamada C, et al. An individual patient data meta-analysis of long supported adjuvant chemotherapy with oral carmofur in patients with curatively resected colorectal cancer. Oncol Rep 2001;8:697–703.

383. Rich TA, Shepard RC, Mosley ST. Four decades of continuing innovation with fluorouracil: current and future approaches to fluorouracil chemoradiation therapy. J Clin Oncol 2004;22:2214–2232.

384. Fujita K, Nakayama H, Yamamoto W, et al. Pharmacokinetics of 5-flourouracil in elderly Japanese patients with cancer treated with S-1 (a combination of Tegafure and dihydropyrimidine dehydrogenase inhibitor 5-chloro-2,4-dihydropyridine). Drug Metab Dispos 2009;37(7):1375–1377.

385. Sakuramoto S, Sasako M, Yamaguchi T, et al. Adjuvant chemotherapy for gastric cancer with S-1, an oral fluoropyrimidine. N Engl J Med 2007;357:1810–1820.

386. Koizumi W, Narahara H, Hara T, et al. S-1 plus cisplatin versus S-1 alone for first-line treatment of advanced gastric cancer (SPIRITS trial): a phase III trial. Lancet Oncol 2008;9:215–221.

387. Brickell K, Porter D, Thompson P. Phenytoin toxicity due to fluoropyrimidines (5FU/capecitabine): three case reports. Br J Cancer 2003;89:615–616.

388. Shah HR, Ledbetter L, Diasio R, et al. A retrospective study of coagulation abnormalities in patients receiving concomitant capecitabine and warfarin. Clin Colorectal Cancer 2006;5:354–358.

389. Masci G, Magagnoli M, Zucali PA, et al. Minidose warfarin prophylaxis for catheter-associated thrombosis in cancer patients: can it be safely associated with fluorouracil-based chemotherapy? J Clin Oncol 2003;21: 736–739.

390. Camidge R, Reigner B, Cassidy J, et al. Significant effect of capecitabine on the pharmacokinetics and pharmacodynamics of warfarin in patients with cancer. J Clin Oncol 2005;23:4719–4725.

391. Gunes A, Coskun U, Boruban C, et al. Inhibitory effect of 5-fluorouracil on cytochrome P450 2C9 activity in cancer patients. Basic Clin Pharmacol Toxicol 2006;98:197–200.

392. Popat S, Hubner R, Houlston RS. Systematic review of microsatellite instability and colorectal cancer prognosis. J Clin Oncol 2005;23:609–618.

393. Folprecht G, Cunningham D, Ross P, et al. Efficacy of 5-fluorouracil-based chemotherapy in elderly patients with metastatic colorectal cancer: a pooled analysis of clinical trials. Ann Oncol 2004;15:1330–1338.

394. Sargent DJ, Goldberg RM, Jacobson SD, et al. A pooled analysis of adjuvant chemotherapy for resected colon cancer in elderly patients. N Engl J Med 2001;345:1091–1097.

395. Krook JE, Moertel CG, Gunderson LL, et al. Effective surgical adjuvant therapy for high-risk rectal carcinoma. N Engl J Med 1991;310:737–743.

396. Mayer RJ, Davis RB, Schiffer CA, et al. Intensive postremission chemotherapy in adults with acute myeloid leukemia. Cancer and Leukemia Group B. N Engl J Med 1994;331:896–903.

397. Bosset JF, Collette L, Calais G, et al. Chemotherapy with preoperative radiotherapy in rectal cancer. N Engl J Med 2006;355(11):1114–1123.

398. Bujko K, Nowacki MP, Nasierowska-Guttmejer A, et al. Long-term results of a randomized trial comparing preoperative short-course radiotherapy with preoperative conventionally fractionated chemoradiation for rectal cancer. Br J Surg 2006;93:1215–1223.

Cytidine Analogues

Bruce A. Chabner and Jacob Glass

Nucleoside analogs have earned an important place in the treatment of acute leukemia. Through modification of the base or sugar component, chemists have been able to create molecules that mimic the physiological counterparts but potently inhibit aspects of DNA synthesis or function. Among these analogues are the arabinose nucleosides, a unique class of antimetabolites isolated from the sponge *Cryptothethya crypta*[1] but now produced synthetically.[2] They differ from the physiologic deoxyribonucleosides in the presence of a $2'$-OH group in the *cis* configuration relative to the *N*-glycosyl bond between cytosine and the arabinose sugar (Fig. 10-1). Several arabinose nucleosides, including cytosine arabinoside (ara-C, cytarabine), 2-fluoro-ara-adenosine monophosphate, and nelarabine, a guanine analogue, have been important agents for treating hematological cancers.

Cytosine Arabinoside

Ara-C is one of the most effective agents in the treatment of acute myelogenous leukemia (AML)[3] and is incorporated into virtually all standard induction regimens for this disease, generally in combination with an anthracycline (daunorubicin hydrochloride or idarubicin hydrochloride). Ara-C is also a component of consolidation and maintenance regimens in AML after remission is attained.[4] High-dose ara-C confers particular benefit in AML patients with certain cytogenetic abnormalities related to the core binding factor that regulates hematopoiesis (t8:21, inv 16, del 16, t16:16).[5] Ara-C is also active against other hematologic malignancies, including Burkitt's lymphoma,[6] acute lymphocytic leukemia,[7] and chronic myelogenous leukemia[8] but has little value as a single agent against solid tumors. This limited spectrum of activity has been attributed to the lack of metabolic activation of this agent in solid tumors and its selective action against rapidly dividing cells. The essential features of ara-C pharmacology are described in Table 10-1.

Mechanism of Action

Ara-C acts as an analogue of deoxycytidine (CdR) and has multiple effects on DNA synthesis. Ara-C undergoes phosphorylation to form arabinosylcytosine triphosphate (ara-CTP), which competitively inhibits DNA polymerase α in opposition to the normal substrate deoxycytidine $5'$-triphosphate (dCTP).[9] This competitive inhibition has been demonstrated with crude DNA polymerase from calf thymus[9] and with purified enzyme from human leukemic cells[10] and from murine tumors.[11] Ara-CTP has an affinity for human leukemia cell DNA polymerase α in the range of 1×10^{-6} mol/L and com-

petes with dCTP. In intact cells, its effects are antagonized by the addition of CdR, the precursor of dCTP.[12] Ara-CTP inhibits DNA polymerase β with lesser potency.[13] The effects of ara-C on DNA polymerase activity extend not only to semiconservative DNA replication but also to DNA repair. Repair of ultraviolet light damage to DNA, a function of polymerase α, is blocked more potently than the repair of photon-induced or γ radiation-induced strand breaks,[14] which are repaired by a different polymerase. In addition to its inhibition of DNA synthesis, however, it becomes incorporated into DNA, a feature that correlates closely with cytotoxicity[15,16] (Fig. 10-2). In fact, a preponderance of evidence suggests that this is the major cytotoxic lesion in ara-C–treated cells. Drugs that prevent ara-C incorporation into DNA, such as aphidicolin, block its cytotoxicity.[17] In cell culture experiments, a linear relationship exists between picomoles of ara-C incorporated into DNA and the log of cell survival for a wide range of drug concentrations and durations of exposure. Thus, drug toxicity is a direct function of incorporation into DNA, and the latter varies directly with drug concentration and duration of exposure.[18] Once incorporated into DNA, ara-C is excised slowly,[19] and the incorporated ara-C inhibits template function and chain elongation.[17,20,21] In experiments with purified enzyme and calf thymus DNA, the consecutive incorporation of two ara-C or two arabinosyl-5-azacytidine (ara-5–aza-C) residues effectively stops chain elongation.[10] At high concentrations of ara-C, one finds a greater than expected proportion of ara-C residues at the $3'$-terminus, a finding that implies potent chain termination.[19] These observations support the hypothesis that ara-C incorporation into DNA is a prerequisite for drug action and is responsible for cytotoxicity.

Ara-C also causes an unusual reiteration of DNA segments.[22] Human lymphocytes exposed to ara-C in culture synthesize small reduplicated segments of DNA, which results in multiple copies of limited portions of DNA. These reduplicated segments increase the possibility of recombination, crossover, and gene amplification; gaps and breaks are observed in karyotype preparations after ara-C treatment. The same mechanism, reiteration of DNA synthesis after its inhibition by an antimetabolite, may explain the high frequency of gene reduplication induced by methotrexate, 5-fluorouracil, and hydroxyurea (see relevant chapters). In summary, although ara-C has multiple effects on DNA synthesis, the most important antitumor mechanism seems to be its incorporation into DNA.

Other biochemical actions of ara-C have been described, including a relatively weak inhibition of ribonucleotide reductase[23] and formation of arabinosylcytosine diphosphate (ara-CDP)-choline. The latter functions as an analog of cytidine $5'$-diphosphocholine

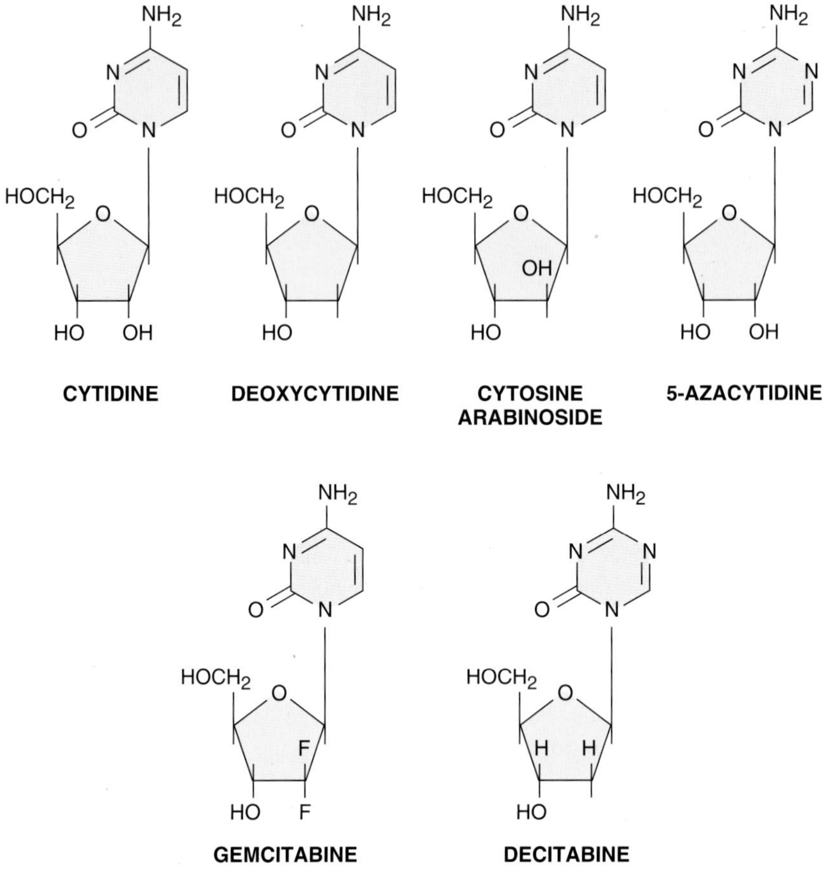

FIGURE **10-1**   Structure of cytidine analogs.

TABLE

10.1   *Key features of ara-C pharmacology*

Factor	Result
Mechanism of action	Inhibits DNA polymerase α, is incorporated into DNA, and terminates DNA chain elongation
Metabolism	Activated to triphosphate in tumor cells. Degraded to inactive ara-U by deamination
	Converted to ara-CDP choline derivative
Pharmacokinetics	Plasma: $t_{1/2}\alpha$ 7–20 min, $t_{1/2}\beta$ 2 h; CSF: $t_{1/2}$ 2 h
Elimination	Deamination in liver, plasma, and peripheral tissues—100%
Drug interactions	Methotrexate increases ara-CTP formation
	THU, 3-deazauridine inhibit deamination
	Fludarabine phosphate increases ara-CTP formation
	Ara-C blocks DNA repair, enhances activity of alkylating agents
Toxicity	Myelosuppression
	Gastrointestinal epithelial ulceration
	Intrahepatic cholestasis, pancreatitis
	Cerebellar and cerebral dysfunction (high dose)
	Conjunctivitis (high dose)
	Hidradenitis
	Noncardiogenic pulmonary edema
Precautions	High incidence of cerebral-cerebellar toxicity with high-dose ara-C in the elderly, especially in those with compromised renal function

ara-CDP, arabinosylcytosine diphosphate; ara-CTP, arabinosylcytosine triphosphate; ara-U, uracil arabinoside; CSF, cerebrospinal fluid; $t_{1/2}$, half-life; THU, tetrahydrouridine; ara-C, cytosine arabinoside.

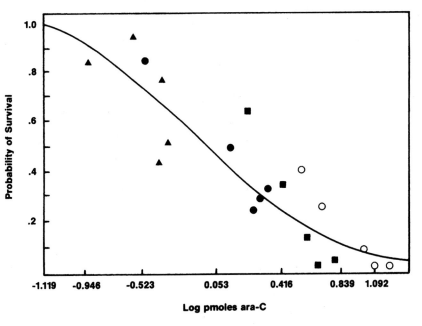

Figure **10-2** Relationship between AML blast clonogenic survival and incorporation of tritium-labeled ara-C into DNA at ara-C concentrations of 10^{-7} mol/L (▲), 10^{-6} mol/L (●), 10^{-5} mol/L (■), and 10^{-4} mol/L (○) during periods of 1, 3, 6, 12, and 24 hours. (From Kufe DW, Spriggs DR. Biochemical and cellular pharmacology of cytosine arabinoside. Semin Oncol 1985;12:34.)

(CDP-choline) and inhibits synthesis of membrane glycoproteins and glycolipids.[24] Ara-C also has the interesting property of promoting differentiation of leukemic cells in tissue culture, an effect that is accompanied by decreased c-*myc* oncogene expression.[25] These changes in morphology and oncogene expression occur at concentrations above the threshold for cytotoxicity and may simply represent terminal injury of cells. After exposure to ara-C, both normal and malignant cells undergo apoptosis in experimental models.[26]

The mechanism by which ara-C induces apoptosis is uncertain. It may be triggered by p53 in response to DNA breaks (see above) and by futile attempts to excise incorporated ara-C nucleotides. Ara-C stimulates the formation of ceramide, a potent inducer of apoptosis.[27] Ara-C induces production of diacylglycerol, which activates protein kinase C (PKC), a response that opposes apoptosis in hematopoietic cells. The lethal actions of ara-C may depend, at least partially, on its relative effects on the PKC and ceramide pathways.

Cells exposed to ara-C display marked alterations in transcription factors. Ara-C induces AP-1 (a dimer of jun-fos or jun-jun proteins) and NF-kB, and induction has been temporally associated with apoptosis.[28,29] PKC inhibitors promote ara-C–induced apoptosis despite their antagonizing c-*jun* up-regulation, calling into question the involvement of c-*jun* expression in apoptosis secondary to ara-C.[30] Ara-C induces pRb phosphatase activity, another possible mechanism responsible for p53-independent G_1 arrest and apoptosis.[31] The resulting hypophosphorylated pRb binds to and inactivates the E2F transcription factor, which inhibits the transcription of genes responsible for cell-cycle progression.[32]

Cellular Pharmacology and Metabolism

Ara-C penetrates cells by a carrier-mediated process shared by physiologic nucleosides.[33] Several different classes of transporters for nucleosides have been identified in mammalian cells; the most extensively characterized in human tumors is hENT1, the equilibrative transporter, identified by its binding to nitrobenzylthioinosine (NBMPR). The number of transport sites on the cell membrane is greater in AML cells than in acute lymphocytic leukemia cells and can be enumerated by incubation of cells with NBMPR.[34] The hENT1 transporter is highly upregulated in biphenotypic leukemia associated with the 11q23 MLL gene (4:11) translocation.[35] Uptake occurs rapidly. A steady-state level of intracellular drug is achieved within 90 seconds at 37°C.[36,37] Studies of Wiley et al.[33] and others[34,37] suggest that the NBMPR transporter plays a limiting role in the action of this agent in that the formation of the ultimate toxic metabolite ara-CTP is strongly correlated with the number of transporter sites on leukemic cells (Fig. 10-3). A single point

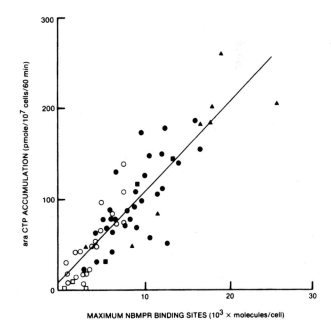

Figure **10-3** Correlation between accumulation of ara-CTP and nucleoside transport capacity measured by the maximal number of NBMPR binding sites on leukemic cells ($r = 0.87$; $P < 0.0001$). Ara-CTP accumulation was measured after incubation of cells with 1 μmol/L of tritium-labeled ara-C for 60 minutes. ●, acute myelogenous leukemia; ○, non-T-cell acute lymphoblastic leukemia; ▲, T-cell leukemia/lymphoma, lymphoblastic leukemia; ■, acute undifferentiated leukemia; ϒ, chronic lymphocytic leukemia. (From Wiley JS, Taupin J, Jamieson GP, et al. Cytosine arabinoside transport and metabolism in acute leukemias and T-cell lymphoblastic lymphoma. J Clin Invest 1985;75:632.)

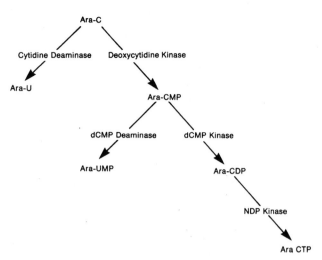

FIGURE **10-4**   Metabolism of ara-C by tumor cells. The conversion of ara-UMP to a triphosphate has not been demonstrated in mammalian cells. Ara-CMP, arabinosylcytosine monophosphate; ara-CDP, arabinosylcytosine diphosphate; ara-CTP, arabinosylcytosine triphosphate; ara-U, uracil arabinoside; dCMP, deoxycytidine monophosphate; NDP, nucleoside diphosphate.

mutation in the hENT1 carrier confers resistance in leukemic cell lines in vitro.[36] At drug concentrations above 10 μmol/L, the transport process becomes saturated, and further entry takes place by passive diffusion.[37] hENT1 is strongly inhibited by various receptor tyrosine kinase inhibitors, an interaction that could limit ara-C use with targeted drugs.[38]

As shown in Figure 10-4, ara-C must be converted to its active form, ara-CTP, through the sequential action of three enzymes: (a) CdR kinase, (b) deoxycytidine monophosphate (dCMP) kinase, and (c) nucleoside diphosphate (NDP) kinase. Ara-C is subject to degradation by cytidine deaminase, forming the inactive product uracil arabinoside (ara-U); arabinosylcytosine monophosphate (ara-CMP) is likewise degraded by a second enzyme, dCMP deaminase, to the

inactive arabinosyluracil monophosphate (ara-UMP). Each of these enzymes, with the exception of NDP kinase, has been examined in detail because of its possible relevance to ara-C resistance.

The first activating enzyme, CdR kinase, is found in lowest concentration (Table 10-2) and is believed to be rate limiting in the process of ara-CTP formation. The enzyme is a 30.5-kDa protein that phosphorylates ara-C and many pyrimidine and purine nucleosides and their analogs. The gene coding for CdR kinase and a mutated version found in ara-C resistant cells have been cloned.[39,40] The rate-limiting role of CdR kinase in ara-C activation is illustrated by transfection of malignant cell lines with retroviral vectors containing CdR kinase cDNA, a maneuver that substantially increases the susceptibility of cells to ara-C, gemcitabine, and purine analogues.[41] Ara-C cytotoxicity increases when intracerebral gliomas in rats are transduced with CdR kinase.[42]

CdR kinase activity is highest during the S phase of the cell cycle.[43] The K_m, or affinity constant, for ara-C is 20 μmol/L, compared with the higher affinity or 7.8 μmol/L for the physiologic substrate CdR.[44] This enzyme is strongly inhibited by dCTP but weakly inhibited by ara-CTP. This lack of "feedback" inhibition allows accumulation of the ara-C nucleotide to higher concentrations. PKC-α, the activity of which is increased after ara-C exposure, has been implicated in phosphorylation and activation of CdR kinase. This observation raises the possibility that ara-C at high doses may potentiate its own metabolism by induction of the PKC activator, diacylglycerol.[45]

The second activating enzyme, dCMP kinase,[46] is found in several hundred-fold higher concentration than CdR kinase. Its affinity for ara-CMP is low (K_m = 680 μmol/L) but greater than the affinity for the competitive physiologic substrate dCMP. Because of its relatively poor affinity for ara-CMP, this enzyme could become rate limiting at low ara-CMP concentrations. The third activating enzyme, the diphosphate kinase, appears not to be rate limiting because it is present in very high concentration and the intracellular pool of ara-CDP is only a fraction of the ara-CTP pool.[47]

TABLE
10.2   *Kinetic parameters of enzymes that metabolize ara-C*

Enzyme	Substrate	K_m (mol/L)	Activity in AML cells (nmol/h/mg protein at 37°C)
CdR kinase	Ara-C	2.6×10^{-5}	15.4 ± 16
	CdR	7.8×10^{-6}	
dCMP kinase	Ara-CMP	6.8×10^{-4}	$1,990 \pm 1,500$
	dCMP	1.9×10^{-3}	
dCDP kinase	Ara-CDP	?	Not known
	Other NDPs	?	
CR deaminase	Ara-C	8.8×10^{-5}	372 ± 614
	CdR	1.1×10^{-5}	
dCMP deaminase	Ara-CMP	Ara-CMP has higher K_m than dCMP; exact K_m not determined	1,250 (five patients)
	dCMP		

AML, acute myelogenous leukemia; Ara-C, cytosine arabinoside; ara-CDP, arabinosylcytosine diphosphate; ara-CMP, arabinosylcytosine monophosphate; CdR, deoxycytidine; CR, cytidine; dCDP, deoxycytidine diphosphate; dCMP, deoxycytosine monophosphate; NDPs, nucleoside diphosphates.

Opposing the activation pathway are two deaminases found in high concentration in some tumor cells as well as in normal tissues. Cytidine deaminase is widely distributed in mammalian tissues, including intestinal mucosa, liver, and granulocytes.[48] It is found in granulocyte precursors and in leukemic myeloblasts in lower concentrations than in mature granulocytes, but even in these immature cells, the deaminase level exceeds the activity of CdR kinase, the initial activating enzyme.[44,48] The second degradative enzyme, dCMP deaminase (Fig. 10-4), regulates the flow of physiologic nucleotides from the dCMP pool into the deoxyuridine monophosphate (dUMP) pool from which point dUMP is ultimately converted to deoxythymidine 5′-phosphate (dTMP) by thymidylate synthase.[49] The enzyme dCMP deaminase is strongly activated by intracellular dCTP (K_m = 0.2 μmol/L) and strongly inhibited by deoxythymidine triphosphate in concentrations of 0.2 μmol/L or greater. Ara-CTP weakly activates this enzyme (K_m = 40 μmol/L[50] and, thus, would not promote degradation of its own precursor nucleotide, ara-CMP. The affinity of dCMP deaminase for ara-CMP is somewhat higher than the affinity of dCMP kinase for the same substrate, but the activity of these competitive enzymes depends greatly on their degree of activation or inhibition by regulatory triphosphates (dCTP), and dCMP deaminase concentration in leukemic myeloblasts is slightly less than that of dCMP kinase (Table 10-2).

The balance between activating and degrading enzymes, thus, is crucial in determining the quantity of drug converted to the active intermediate, ara-CTP. This enzymatic balance varies greatly among cell types.[44] CdR kinase activity is higher and cytidine deaminase activity lower in lymphoid leukemia than in acute myeloblastic leukemia. Enzyme activities vary also with cell maturity; deaminase increases dramatically with maturation of granulocyte precursors, whereas kinase activity decreases correspondingly.[48] Thus, admixture of normal granulocyte precursors with leukemic cells in human bone marrow samples complicates the interpretation of enzyme measurements unless normal and leukemic cells are separated. In general, cytidine deaminase (D) activity greatly exceeds kinase (K). The kinase:deaminase ratio averages 0.03 in human AML, whereas the enzyme activities are approximately equal in acute lymphoblastic leukemia and Burkitt's lymphoma. Thus, the biochemical setting seems to favor drug activation by lymphoblastic leukemia cells if these initial enzymes play a rate-limiting role.

In fact, this may not be the case. Chou et al.[47] found that human AML cells formed 12.8 ng of ara-CTP per 10^6 cells after 45 minutes of incubation with 1×10^{-5} mol/L ara-C. Acute lymphoblastic leukemia cells formed less ara-CTP, 6.3 ng/10^6 cells, and as expected, the more mature chronic myelocytic and chronic lymphocytic leukemia cells formed lesser amounts of ara-CTP (4.7 to 5.2 ng/10^6 cells). The likelihood is that other factors, such as transport across the cell membrane and regulatory effects of intracellular nucleoside triphosphate concentrations, may limit ara-CTP formation.

In addition to its activation to ara-CTP, ara-C is converted intracellularly to ara-CDP-choline,[51] an analog of the physiologic CDP-choline lipid precursor. However, ara-C does not inhibit incorporation of choline into phospholipids of normal or transformed hamster embryo fibroblasts.[24] Ara-CMP does inhibit the transfer of galactose, N-acetylglucosamine, and sialic acid to cell surface glycoproteins. Further, high concentrations (approaching 1 mM) of ara-CTP inhibit the synthesis of cytidine monophosphate (CMP)–acetylneuraminic acid, an essential substrate in sialylation of glycoproteins.[52] Thus, ara-C treatment could alter membrane structure, antigenicity, and function.

Biochemical Determinants of Cytosine Arabinoside Resistance

The foregoing consideration of ara-C metabolism and transport makes it clear that a number of factors could affect ara-C response. Not surprisingly, many of these factors have been implicated in various preclinical models of ara-C resistance. The most frequent abnormality found in resistant leukemic cells recovered from mice treated with ara-C has been decreased activity of CdR kinase.[53] In cultured cells exposed to a mutagen and then to low concentrations of ara-C, some single-step mutants developed high-level resistance to ara-C through loss of activity of CdR kinase, whereas other resistant clones exhibited markedly expanded dCTP pools, presumably through increased cytidine-5′-triphosphate (CTP) synthetase activity or through deficiency of dCMP deaminase.[54,55] As mentioned previously, specific mutations and deletions in the gene coding for CdR kinase derived from resistant cells have been described.[39,40]

The role of cytidine deaminase in experimental models of resistance is less clear. Retrovirus-mediated transfer of the cytidine deaminase cDNA into 3T3 murine fibroblast cells significantly increases drug resistance to ara-C and other analogs such as 5-aza-2′-CdR and gemcitabine. This phenotype of increased cytidine deaminase activity and drug resistance is reversed by the cytidine deaminase inhibitor tetrahydrouridine (THU).[56] Other genes, including proto-oncogenes, may affect ara-C response. Transfection of rodent fibroblasts and human mammary HBL 100 cells with c-H-ras conferred resistance to ara-C, an event attributed to decreased activity of CdR kinase.[57] On the other hand, N-ras or K-ras mutations strongly correlated with increased ara-C sensitivity in the screening of human tumor cell lines from the National Cancer Institute's in vitro drug screen.[58] Ras mutations are found in 20% of AML cases, and these patients appear to derive greatest benefit from high-dose ara-C regimens.[59] Although various molecular lesions have been implicated as causing ara-C resistance in animals, their relevance to resistance in human leukemia is less certain. Clinical studies have described specific biochemical changes in drug-resistant cells from patients with leukemia, including deletion of CdR kinase,[60] increased cytidine deaminase,[61] a decreased number of nucleoside transport sites,[62] and increased dCTP pools.[63] Other clinical investigators have not been able to correlate resistance with either CdR kinase or cytidine deaminase or their ratio.[64,65] All studies have shown extreme variability in enzyme levels among patients with leukemia. Thus, no agreement exists as to the specific changes responsible for resistance in human leukemia.

Although specific biochemical lesions associated with resistance in humans are unclear, the current understanding of ara-C action suggests that the ultimate formation of ara-CTP and the duration of its persistence in leukemic cells determine response.[47,66] Chou et al.[47] found greater ara-CTP formation in leukemic cells of responders when these cells were incubated in vitro with ara-C, but even this correlation was not confirmed in other studies.[67–69]

Preisler et al.[70] found that the duration of remission induced by ara-C–containing regimens was strongly correlated with the ability of cells to retain ara-CTP in vitro after removal of ara-C from the medium. Attempts to monitor ara-CTP formation in leukemic cells taken from patients during therapy have not disclosed useful correlations of ara-CTP levels or intracellular persistence with response.[69,71] Ara-CTP has an intracellular half-life of about 3 to 4 hours. Again, considerable variability has been observed in the rates of formation of ara-CTP, and this rate does not correlate well with plasma ara-C pharmacokinetics in individual patients (Fig. 10-5).

The cellular response to ara-C–mediated DNA damage also governs whether the genotoxic insult results in cell death. Ara-C incorporation into DNA stalls the replication fork for cells in active DNA synthesis, activating ATR and Chk 1, checkpoint kinases that block cell cycle progression and allow for removal of ara-C from DNA. Absence of either of these checkpoints sensitizes cells to apoptosis. Levels of expression of apoptotic proteins influence response. Overexpression of the antiapoptotic proteins Bcl-2 and Bcl-X$_L$ in leukemic blasts causes in vitro resistance to ara-C–mediated apoptosis.[72] The intracellular metabolism of ara-C and its initial effects on DNA are not modified by Bcl-2 expression, which suggests that Bcl-2 primarily regulates the more distal steps in the ara-C–induced cell death pathway. Although the precise mechanism by which these proteins prevent ara-C–induced cytotoxicity remains to be elucidated, Bcl-2 and Bcl-X$_L$ have been shown to antagonize ara-C–mediated cell death by caspase activation.[72] The fact that antisense oligonucleotides directed against Bcl-2 increase the susceptibility of leukemic blasts to ara-C–induced apoptosis in vitro,[73] and that patients whose blasts express high levels of Bcl-2 respond poorly to ara-C–containing regimens,[74] further suggests the pivotal role of Bcl-2 in ara-C resistance.

Phosphorylation of apoptotic or DNA damage response factors may also determine the outcome of ara-C exposure. Phosphorylation of Bcl-2 is required for its antiapoptotic function, and a functional role for PKC-α in Bcl-2 phosphorylation and suppression of apoptosis has been postulated,[75] although this observation has not been confirmed by others.[76] Attempts at pharmacological inhibition of PKC-α activity have increased ara-CTP formation but had variable effects on cytotoxicity in culture, possibly due to their simultaneous activation of BcL-2.[76] Altered phosphorylation of transcription factors also influences the cellular response to ara-C toxic insult. Ara-C–induced activation of PKC and mitogen-activated protein kinase (MAPK) increases c-*jun* expression and phosphorylation,[27,77] and hyperphosphorylation of the AP-1 transcription factor has been associated with ara-C resistance in human myeloid leukemic cell lines in vitro.[78]

Clinical studies of determinants of ara-C response are complicated by the fact that ara-C is almost always given in combination with an anthracycline or an anthraquinone. Thus, a complete response or long remission duration does not necessarily imply sensitivity to ara-C. A lack of response does imply resistance to both agents in the combination, except for the not-infrequent cases in which failure can be attributed to infection or inability to administer full dosages of drug. With these limitations, the duration of complete response is probably the most appropriate and most important single yardstick of drug sensitivity because it reflects the fractional cell kill during induction therapy, but no single factor has emerged as a determinant of remission duration.

Cell Kinetics and Cytosine Arabinoside Cytotoxicity

In addition to biochemical factors that determine response, cell kinetic properties exert an important influence on the results of ara-C treatment. As an inhibitor of DNA synthesis, ara-C has its greatest cytotoxic effects during the S phase of the cell cycle perhaps because of the requirement for its incorporation into DNA and the greater activity of anabolic enzymes during S phase. The duration of exposure of cells to ara-C is directly correlated with cell kill because the longer exposure period allows ara-C to be incorporated into the DNA of a greater percentage of cells as they pass through S phase. The cytotoxic action of ara-C is not only cell-cycle phase–dependent but is influenced by the rate of DNA synthesis. That is, cell kill in tissue culture is greatest if cells are exposed during periods of maximal rates of DNA synthesis, as in the recovery period after exposure to a cytotoxic agent. In experimental situations, it has been possible to schedule sequential doses of ara-C to coincide with the peak in recovery of DNA synthesis and thus to improve the therapeutic results.[79]

In humans, the influence of tumor cell kinetics on response is unclear. Although earlier studies showed that the complete remission rate seems to be *higher* in patients who have a high percentage of cells in S phase,[80] remissions are *longer* in patients with leukemias that have long cell-cycle time.[81]

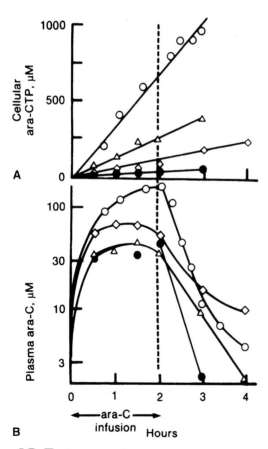

FIGURE 10-5 Pharmacokinetics of ara-CTP in leukemia cells and of ara-C in plasma. Blood samples were drawn at the indicated times during and after infusion of ara-C, 3 g/m², to patients with acute leukemia in relapse. Symbols for each analysis are the same for individual patients. (From Plunkett W, Liliemark JO, Estey E, et al. Saturation of ara-CTP accumulation during high-dose ara-C therapy: pharmacologic rationale for intermediate-dose ara-C. Semin Oncol 1987;14[2 (Suppl 1)]:159.)

Clinical Pharmacology—Assay Methods

The preferred method for assay of ara-C and its primary metabolite ara-U is high-pressure liquid chromatography, which has the requisite specificity and adequate (0.1 μmol/L) sensitivity.[82] An alternative method using gas chromatography–mass spectrometry combines high specificity with greater sensitivity (4 nmol/L) but requires derivatization of samples and thus prolonged performance time.[83] Because of the presence of cytidine deaminase in plasma, the deaminase inhibitor THU must be added to plasma samples immediately after blood samples are obtained.

Pharmacokinetics

The important factors that determine ara-C pharmacokinetics are its high aqueous solubility and its susceptibility to deamination in liver, plasma, granulocytes, and gastrointestinal tract. Ara-C is amenable to use by multiple schedules and routes of administration and has shown clinical activity in dosages ranging from 3 mg/m² twice weekly to 3 g/m² every 12 hours for 6 days. Remarkably, over this wide dosage range, its pharmacokinetics remains quite constant and predictable.

Distribution

As a nucleoside, ara-C is transported across cell membranes by a nucleoside transporter and distributes rapidly into total-body water.[84] It then crosses into the central nervous system (CNS) with surprising facility for a water-soluble compound and reaches steady-state levels at 20% to 40% of those found simultaneously in plasma during constant intravenous infusion. At conventional doses of ara-C (100 mg/m² by 24-hour infusion), spinal fluid levels reach 0.2 μmol/L, which is probably above the cytotoxic threshold for leukemic cells. High doses of ara-C yield proportionately higher ara-C levels in the spinal fluid.[85]

Plasma Pharmacokinetics

The pharmacokinetics of ara-C are characterized by rapid disappearance from plasma owing to deamination, with some variability seen among individual patients.[83] Peak plasma concentrations reach 10 μmol/L after bolus doses of 100 mg/m² and are proportionately higher (up to 150 μmol/L) for doses up to 3 g/m² given over a 1- or 2-hour infusion[86] (Fig. 10-6). Thereafter, the plasma concentration of ara-C declines, with a half-life of 7 to 20 minutes. A second phase of drug disappearance has been detected after high-dose ara-C infusion, with a terminal half-life of 30 to 150 minutes, but the drug concentration during this second phase has cytotoxic potential only in patients treated with high-dose ara-C.[87,88] Seventy to eighty percent of a given dose is excreted in the urine as ara-U,[87] which, within minutes of drug injection, becomes the predominant compound found in plasma. Ara-U has a longer half-life in plasma (3.2 to 5.8 hours) than does ara-C and may enhance the activation of ara-C through feedback inhibition of ara-C deamination in leukemic cells.[87] The steady-state level of ara-C in plasma achieved by constant intravenous infusion remains proportional to dose for dose rates up to 2 g/m²/d. At this dosage, steady-state plasma levels approximate 5 μmol/L. Above this rate of infusion, the deamination reaction is saturated and ara-C plasma levels rise unpredictably, which leads to severe toxicity in some patients.[88] To accelerate the achievement of a steady-state concentration, one may give a

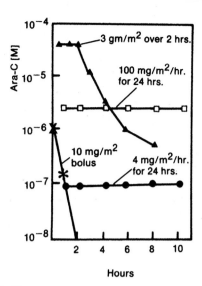

FIGURE 10-6 Ara-C pharmacokinetics in plasma after doses of 3 g/m² given over 2 hours, 100 mg/m²/h by continuous infusion for 24 hours, 4 mg/m²/h (a conventional antileukemic dose) by continuous intravenous infusion, and 10 mg/m² subcutaneously or intravenously as a bolus.

bolus dose of three times the hourly infusion rate before infusion.[89] Equivalent drug exposure (area under the curve [AUC]) is achieved by subcutaneous or intravenous infusion of ara-C, although one study has reported higher ara-CTP concentrations in leukemia cells after subcutaneous administration.[90]

Owing to the presence of high concentrations of cytidine deaminase in the gastrointestinal mucosa and liver, orally administered ara-C provides much lower plasma levels than does direct intravenous administration. Threefold to tenfold higher doses must be given in animals to achieve a biologic effect equivalent to that produced by intravenous drug. The oral route, therefore, is not routinely used in humans.

Ara-C may also be administered by intraperitoneal infusion for treatment of ovarian cancer.[91] After instillation of 100 μmol/L of drug, ara-C levels fall in the peritoneal cavity with a half-life of approximately 2 hours. Simultaneous plasma levels are 100- to 1,000-fold lower, presumably because of deamination of ara-C in liver before it reaches the systemic circulation. In 21-day continuous infusion, patients tolerated up to 100 μmol/L intraperitoneal concentrations but developed peritonitis at higher concentrations.[92]

Cerebrospinal Fluid Pharmacokinetics

After intravenous administration of 100 mg/m² of ara-C, parent drug levels reach 0.1 to 0.3 μmol/L in the cerebrospinal fluid (CSF). Thereafter, levels decline with a half-life of 2 hours. Proportionately higher CSF levels are reached by intravenous high-dose ara-C regimens; for example, a 3 g/m² infusion intravenously over 1 hour yields peak CSF concentrations of 4 μmol/L,[86] whereas the same dose over 24 hours yields peak CSF ara-C concentrations of 1 μmol/L.[88]

Ara-C is effective when administered intrathecally for the treatment of metastatic neoplasms. A number of dosing schedules for giving intrathecal ara-C have been recommended, but twice weekly or weekly schedules of administration are the most often used. The dose of ara-C ranges from 30 to 50 mg/m². The dose is generally adjusted in pediatric patients according to age (15 mg for children below 1 year of age, 20 mg for children between 1 and 2 years, 30 mg for children between 2 and 3 years, and 40 mg for children older than 3 years). The clinical pharmacology of ara-C in the CSF following intrathecal administration differs considerably from that seen in the plasma following a parenteral dose. Systematically administered ara-C is rapidly eliminated by biotransformation to the inactive metabolite ara-U. In contrast, little conversion of ara-C to ara-U takes place in the CSF following an intrathecal injection. The ratio of ara-U to ara-C is only 0.08, a finding that is consistent with the very low levels of cytidine deaminase present in the brain and CSF. Following an intraventricular administration of 30 mg of ara-C, peak levels exceed 1 to 2 mM, and levels decline slowly, with the terminal half-life of approximately 3.4 hours.[93] Concentrations above the threshold for cytotoxicity (0.1 μg/mL, or 0.4 μmol/L) are maintained in the CSF for 24 to 48 hours. The CSF clearance is 0.42 mL/min, which is similar to the CSF bulk flow rate. This finding suggests that drug elimination occurs primarily by this route. Plasma levels following intrathecal administration of 30 mg/m² of ara-C are less than 1 μmol/L, which illustrates again the advantage of intracavitary therapy with a drug that is rapidly cleared in the systemic circulation.

Depocytarabine (DTC 101) is a depot formulation in which ara-C is encapsulated in microscopic Gelfoam particles (DepoFoam) for sustained release into the CSF so that the need for repeated lumbar punctures is avoided. The encapsulation of ara-C in DepoFoam results in a 55-fold increase in CSF half-life after intraventricular administration in rats, from 2.7 to 148 hours. Cytotoxic concentrations of free ara-C (>0.4 μmol/L) in CSF are maintained for more than 1 month following a single intrathecal dose administration of 2 mg of DTC 101 in rhesus monkeys. A phase I trial of DTC 101 given intraventricularly has been performed in patients with leptomeningeal metastasis. Free ara-C CSF concentration decreased biexponentially. After a dose of 50 mg of DTC, ara-C concentrations were maintained above the cytotoxic threshold for 12 ± 3 days. The maximum tolerated dosage was 75 mg administered every 3 weeks, and the dose-limiting toxicity was headache and arachnoiditis.[94] A randomized study involving patients with lymphomatous meningitis demonstrated a possible prolongation of time to neurologic progression in patients treated with 50 mg of DTC 101 every 2 weeks compared with patients treated with standard intrathecal ara-C.[95] DTC appears to give equivalent results to standard intrathecal methotrexate, given every 4 days, for treatment of carcinomatous meningitis.[96]

Alternate Schedules of Administration

Although ara-C is used most commonly in regimens of 100 to 200 mg/m²/d for 7 days, other high-dose and low-dose schedules have been used in treating leukemia. The more effective of these newer regimens have been high-dose schemes, usually 2 to 3 g/m² every 12 hours for six doses.[97] High-dose ara-C is used primarily in the consolidation phase for acute myelocytic leukemia.[4] The rationale for the higher-dose regimen initially rested on the assumption that ara-C phosphorylation is the rate-limiting intracellular step in the drug's activation and could be promoted by raising intracellular concentrations to the K_m of CdR kinase for ara-C, or approximately 20 μmol/L. Above this level, further increases in ara-C do not lead to increased ara-CTP because the phosphorylation pathways enzymes become saturated.[98]

Others have examined the clinical activity of low-dose ara-C, particularly in older patients with myelodysplastic syndromes.[99] These regimens have used dosages in the range of 3 to 20 mg/m²/d for up to 3 weeks, with the expectation that low doses would produce less toxicity and promote leukemic cell differentiation (or apoptosis). The persistence of chromosomal markers for the leukemic cell line in remission granulocytes has been documented, findings that support induction of differentiation.[100] In general, although the low-dose regimens produce less toxicity, myelosuppression often supervenes and less than 20% of patients achieve meaningful improvement in blood counts.

Toxicity

The primary determinants of ara-C toxicity are drug concentration and duration of exposure. Because ara-C is cell cycle phase specific, the duration of cell exposure to the drug is critical in determining the fraction of cells killed.[101] In humans, single-bolus doses of ara-C as large as 4.2 g/m² are well tolerated because of the rapid inactivation of the parent compound and the brief period of exposure, whereas constant infusion of drug for 48 hours using total doses of 1 g/m² produces severe myelosuppression.[102]

Myelosuppression and gastrointestinal epithelial injury are the primary toxic side effects of ara-C. With the conventional 5- to 7-day courses of treatment, the period of maximal toxicity begins during the first week of treatment and lasts 14 to 21 days. The primary targets of ara-C are platelet production and granulopoiesis, although anemia also occurs. Little acute effect is seen on the lymphocyte count, although a depression of cell-mediated immunity is found in patients receiving ara-C.[103] Megaloblastic changes consistent with suppression of DNA synthesis are observed in both the white and red cell precursors.[104]

Gastrointestinal symptoms, including nausea, vomiting, and diarrhea, are frequent during the period of drug administration but subside quickly after treatment. Severe gastrointestinal lesions occur in patients treated with ara-C as part of complex chemotherapy regimens, and the specific contribution of ara-C is difficult to ascertain in these cases. All parts of the gastrointestinal tract are affected. Oral mucositis may be severe and prolonged in patients receiving more than 5 days of continuous treatment. Clinical symptoms of diarrhea, ileus, and abdominal pain may be accompanied by gastrointestinal bleeding, electrolyte abnormalities, and protein-losing enteropathy. Radiologic evidence of dilatation of the terminal ileum, termed typhlitis, may be associated with progressive abdominal pain and bowel perforation. Pathologic findings include denudation of the epithelial surface and loss of crypt cell mitotic activity. Reversible intrahepatic cholestasis with jaundice occurs frequently in patients receiving ara-C for induction therapy but requires a discontinuation of therapy in fewer than 25% of patients.[105] It is manifested primarily as an increase in hepatic enzymes in the serum, together with mild jaundice, and rapidly reverses with discontinuation of treatment. Ara-C has been implicated as the cause of pancreatitis in a small number of patients.[106]

Toxicity of High-Dose Cytosine Arabinoside

High-dose ara-C significantly increases the incidence and severity of bone marrow and gastrointestinal toxic effects.[4] Hospitalization for fever and neutropenia is required in 71% of the treatment courses in patients receiving 3 g/m^2 per 12 hours given on alternative days for six doses, and platelet transfusions are required in 86%.[4] Treatment-related deaths, primarily the result of infection, occur in 5% of the patients treated with this schedule. In addition, high-dose ara-C produces pulmonary toxicity, including noncardiogenic pulmonary edema, in approximately 10% of patients, and a surprisingly high incidence of *Streptococcus viridans* pneumonia is seen, especially in pediatric populations.[107] The pulmonary edema syndrome presents 1 to 2 weeks after drug administration with fever, dyspnea, and pulmonary infiltrates and is fatal in 10% to 20% of patients with this complicatoin.[108]

Cholestatic jaundice and elevation of serum glutamic-oxaloacetic transaminase, serum glutamic-pyruvic transaminase, and alkaline phosphatase, with underlying cholestasis and passive congestion on liver biopsy, are also frequently observed with the high-dose regimen.[109] These changes, however, are generally clinically unimportant and reversible. A more dangerous toxicity involving cerebral and cerebellar dysfunction occurs in 10% of patients receiving 3 g/m^2 for 6 doses[4] and in two thirds of patients receiving 4.5 g/m^2 for 12 doses.[110] Age over 40 years, abnormal alkaline phosphatase activity in serum, and compromised renal function[111] are risk factors associated with an increased susceptibility to CNS toxicity, which is manifested as slurred speech, unsteady gait, dementia, and coma.[110] Thirty-seven percent of patients with two or more of these risk factors treated with high-dose ara-C develop CNS toxicity in 37% of the cases, whereas the incidence is less than 1% when fewer than two of these criteria are present.[111] Symptoms of neurologic toxicity resolve within several days in approximately 20% of patients and gradually recede over several weeks in approximately 40%; however, a permanent disability is present in the remaining 40%, and occasionally patients have died of CNS toxicity.[4] Progressive brainstem dysfunction[112] and an ascending peripheral neuropathy[113] also have been reported after high-dose ara-C.

Other bothersome toxicities complicate high-dose Ara-C. Conjunctivitis, responsive to topical steroids, also has been a frequent side effect of high-dose ara-C.[114] Rarely, skin rash and even anaphylaxis have been noted.[115] Neutrophilic eccrine hydradenitis, an unusual febrile cutaneous reaction manifested as plaques or nodules during the second week after chemotherapy, is being reported with increasing frequency after high-dose ara-C.[116] Finally, sporadic reports of cardiac toxicity have implicated ara-C, generally at high dosages. Findings have included arrhythmias, pericarditis, and congestive heart failure. None of these reports provide conclusive evidence for a cause-and-effect relationship.[117]

Toxicity of Intrathecal Cytosine Arabinoside

Ara-C given intrathecally is infrequently associated with fever and seizures occurring within 24 hours of administration, and arachnoiditis occurring within 4 to 7 days.[118] Rarely, ara-C causes a progressive brainstem toxicity that may be fatal.[119] Intrathecal ara-C should be used with caution in patients who are receiving systemic high-dose methotrexate and in those who have previously experienced methotrexate neurotoxicity.

Although ara-C causes chromosomal breaks in cultured cells and in the bone marrow of patients receiving therapy, it is not an established carcinogen in humans. The drug is teratogenic in animals.[120]

Drug Interactions

Ara-C has synergistic antitumor activity with a number of other antitumor agents in animal tumor models. These other agents include alkylating agents (cyclophosphamide,[121] cisplatin,[122] purine analogs, methotrexate,[123] and etoposide).[124] The basis for ara-C potentiation of alkylating agents and cisplatin is thought to be inhibition of repair of DNA-alkylator adducts. The hypothesis is consistent with the finding that ara-C exposure preceding cisplatin is synergistic—perhaps allowing for inhibition of repair[125]—whereas ara-C after cisplatin is not.[122]

THU, a potent inhibitor of cytidine deaminase ($K_i = 3 \times 10^{-8}$ mol/L), enhances ara-CTP formation in acute myelocytic leukemia cells in vitro but not in chronic lymphocytic leukemia cells, which lack deaminase activity.[126] THU enhances the growth-inhibitory effects of sublethal concentrations of ara-C in experiments with the sarcoma 180 cell line, which contains high amounts of cytidine deaminase.[127] Initial clinical evaluation of the combination indicates that THU in intravenous doses of 50 mg/m^2 markedly prolongs the plasma half-life of ara-C from 10 to 120 minutes and causes a corresponding enhancement of toxicity to bone marrow.[128] In combination with THU, the tolerable dosage of ara-C is reduced 30-fold to 0.1 mg/kg/d for 5 days. Whether the combination has greater therapeutic effects and a better therapeutic ratio than ara-C alone is unclear.

Inhibitors of ribonucleotide reductase such as hydroxyurea[129] and fludarabine[130] decrease dCTP pools and increase ara-CTP formation several fold. A decrease in dCTP should have several beneficial effects on ara-C activity. CdR kinase, the enzyme that converts ara-C to ara-CMP, is inhibited by dCTP, whereas dCMP deaminase, which would convert ara-CMP to the inactive ara-UMP, is activated by dCTP; a decrease in dCTP pools should thus increase ara-CTP formation. Second, because ara-CTP and dCTP compete for the same active site on DNA polymerase, a decrease in dCTP pools should lead to a relative increase in the amount of ara-C incorporated into DNA. The favorable effects of fludarabine on ara-CTP concentration have not led to improvement of clinical therapy outcome in patients with AML,[131] perhaps due to their additive toxicity.

Ara-C is commonly used in combination with daunorubicin or etoposide for the treatment of AML. In experimental systems, minute (0.01 μmol/L) concentrations of ara-C cause an increase in levels of topoisomerase II, enhance the rate of protein-associated DNA strand breaks induced by etoposide, and increase etoposide cytotoxicity.[132]

Considerable interest has focused on the use of ara-C in combination with hematopoietic growth factors (HGFs). The theoretical gain of this combination would be that administration of HGFs before the administration of a cell-cycle–specific drug, such as ara-C, would recruit leukemia cells into the susceptible S phase of the cell cycle, which would thereby enhance cytotoxicity.[133] Randomized clinical trials have shown no advantage in response rate or survival in patients with acute myelocytic leukemia treated with HGFs in combination with ara-C compared with patients treated with ara-C alone.[134]

Aza-Cytidine Analogs

5-Aza-analogs of cytidine have become important therapeutic agents and tools for investigating epigenetic modification of DNA.

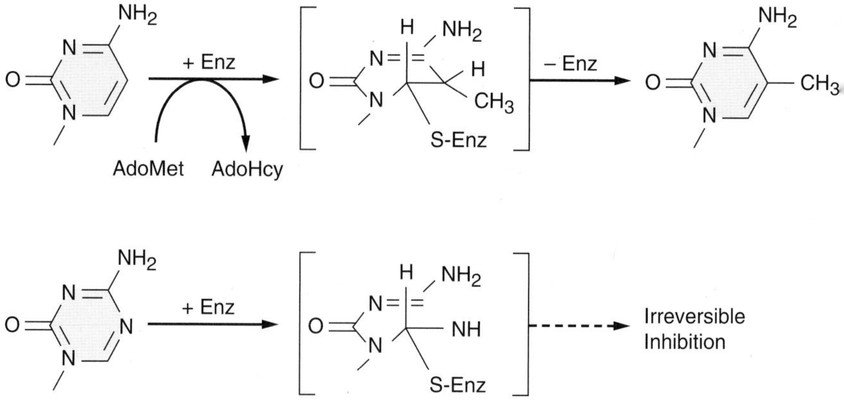

Figure 10-7 Formation of a dihydropyrimidine intermediate during methylation of a target DNA containing (a) CdR, or (b) 5-azacytidine nucleotide in a CpG sequence. DNA methyltransferase forms a covalent bond with the 5-N of the aza-nucleotide. (Adapted from Christman JK. 5-Azacytidine and 5-aza-2′-deoxycytidine as inhibitors of DNA methylation: mechanistic studies and their implications for cancer therapy. Oncogene 2002;21:5483–5495.)

Although first discovered and tested as a treatment for AML, 5-azacytidine and more recently, 2-deoxy-5-azacytidine (decitabine) have become standard agents for management of myeolodysplasia, a preleukemic syndrome characterized by defective maturation of cells of the myeloid series, but affecting all bone marrow hematopoietic lineages. They normalize bone marrow morphology in up to 10% of patients and reduce red blood cell and platelet transfusion requirements in more than one third of such patients; 5-azacytidine treatment leads to an increase in survival of MDS patients as compared to best supportive care.[135]

Both drugs are incorporated into DNA and inhibit DNA methylation (Fig. 10-7), thereby modifying gene expression and promoting differentiation of both normal and malignant cells in experimental systems inhibitors of DNA methylation.[136] 5-Azacytidine has greater incorporation into RNA precursors, a property that may modify and contribute to its antitumor activity. Decitabine, which is exclusively incorporated into DNA, is a more effective inducer of erythroid differentiation than its related analog 5-azacytidine, with less acute cell toxicity. Decitabine is more potent as an antileukemic agent than ara-C when the two drugs were compared in vitro on a panel of human leukemia cell lines of different phenotypes[137] and in animal models of leukemia.[138] Both azacytidine analogues continue to be investigational agents in various types of leukemia, but their primary use is for treatment of myelodysplasia.[139,140]

5-Azacytidine

The success of ara-C as an antileukemic agent encouraged the search for other cytidine analogs, particularly those that would not require activation by CdR kinase (the enzyme deleted in many ara-C–resistant tumors). It was logical to consider ribonucleosides with structural changes in the basic pyrimidine ring because these would likely be activated by uridine-cytidine kinase, an entirely separate enzyme. 5-azacytidine, an analog of cytidine, was synthesized by Sorm and colleagues in 1963[141] and later isolated as a product of fungal cultures.[142] The compound was found to be toxic to both bacterial and mammalian cells. In clinical trials, however, its most important cytostatic action was exerted against myeloid leukemias and myelodysplasia (MDS).[143] Other actions of 5-azacytidine attracted the interest among biologists and clinicians, particularly its ability to inhibit DNA cytosine methylation and, as a consequence, to promote expression of "suppressed" genes. For example, the drug promotes the synthesis of fetal hemoglobin by red cell precursors in sickle cell anemia, an effect believed to be mediated by hypomethylation of the γ-globin gene.[144] 5-Azacytidine has been widely used for DNA demethylation in molecular biology studies, but its value as a treatment for hemoglobinopathies has been limited by its bone marrow toxicity and by concerns about carcinogenesis. The important features of the pharmacokinetics and clinical effects of 5-azacytidine are summarized in Table 10-3.

Structure and Mechanism of Action

The biochemistry and pharmacology of 5-azacytidine[145] derive from it close structural similarity to cytidine, with the caveat of

TABLE
10.3 *Key features of 5-azacytidine (aza) and decitabine (DAC) pharmacology*

Factor	Result
Mechanism of action	AZA incorporated into DNA and RNA; DAC incorporated into DNA. Primary effect of both is to inhibit DNA methylation
Metabolism	Both drugs are activated to a deoxytriphosphate. Uridine-cytidine kinase activates aza; CdR kinase activates DAC.
	Both drugs are degraded to inactive metabolites by cytidine deaminase
Pharmacokinetics and elimination	AZA: $t_{1/2}$ 20–40 min
Drug interactions	THU inhibits deamination, increases toxicity
Toxicity	Myelosuppression
	Nausea, vomiting after bolus dose
	Hepatocellular dysfunction (AZA, high dose)
	Muscle tenderness, weakness (AZA, high dose)
	Lethargy, confusion, coma (AZA, high dose)
Precautions	Hepatic failure may occur in patients with underlying liver dysfunction (AZA)
	Use with caution in patients with altered mental status

the nitrogen at the 5 position of the heterocyclic ring (Fig. 10-1). This substitution renders the ring chemically unstable and leads to spontaneous decomposition of the compound in neutral or alkaline solution, with a half-life of approximately 4 hours. The product of this ring opening, N-formylamidinoribofuranosylguanylurea, may recyclyze to form the parent compound but is also spontaneously decomposed to ribofuranosylurea.[146] This chemical instability is important in the drug's use in two ways: (a) the subsequent spontaneous decomposition of the ring may contribute to its cytotoxicity, once incorporated into DNA or RNA, and (b) the clinical formulation must be administered within several hours of its dissolution in dextrose and water or saline. In buffered solutions such as Ringer's lactate and at acidic pH, the agent is considerably more stable, with a half-life of 65 hours at 25°C and 94 hours at 20°C.[147]

5-Azacytidine has multiple molecular and biological effects that may contribute to its antitumor activity. As a triphosphate, it competes with CTP for incorporation into RNA,[148] the primary event that leads to a number of different effects on RNA processing and function.[149] These effects include an inhibition of the formation of ribosomal 28 S and 18 S RNA from higher molecular-weight species,[149,150] defective methylation[151] and acceptor function of transfer RNA,[152] disassembly of polyribosomes,[153] and a marked inhibition of protein synthesis.[154]

Other effects of 5-azacytidine, however, are likely more relevant to its antitumor activity. This analog is incorporated into DNA,[155] although to a lesser extent than into RNA. 5-A zacytidine incorporation into DNA leads to inhibition of DNA methylation of daughter cells following replication of DNA. The mechanism of inhibition of DNA methyltransferase is shown in Figure 10-7.[146] In both normal and malignant cells, the methylation of cytosine residues in regulatory sequences of DNA inactivates transcription of a broad set of

genes, depending on the cell type studied.[156] Transferase inhibition prevents methylation of daughter strands of DNA following replication and allows reactivation of these silenced genes. Inhibition of DNA methyltransferase by the 5-azacytidine analogues occurs through formation of a covalent bond between the azacytidine base at N-5 and a prolylcysteine dipeptide group on the enzyme,[139,146] an interaction that leads to proteosomal degradation of the complex.

It has been well established that unusually dense clusters of the CpG dinucleotide, sequence known as CpG islands, are found in a hypomethylated state in normal tissue but acquire methylation in various solid and hematologic malignancies,[157] a finding that likely reflects a broader pattern of epigenetic dysregulation. The consequence of CpG methylation is a silencing of gene expression through methylation of a regulatory region associated with that gene. Methylation of at least one tumor suppressor gene promoter in a given tumor is a relatively common occurrence,[158] and reversal of tumor suppressor methylation can result in gene reactivation.[159] The treatment of cells with 5-azacytidine leads to enhanced expression of a broad variety of genes, depending on the cell type studied.[156,160] The relative contribution of DNA methylation inhibition to the clinical antineoplastic effects of 5-azacytidine has yet to be fully elucidated; however, recent studies indicate synergy of methylation blockers and HDAC inhibitors,[161] indicating the importance of epigenetic regulation as a target for cancer treatment.

Cellular Pharmacology

The analog 5-azacytidine readily enters mammalian cells by an equilibrative nucleoside transporter.[162] It is then converted to a monophosphate by uridine-cytidine kinase (Fig. 10-8), which is found in low concentration in human acute myelocytic leukemia cells,[163] has low

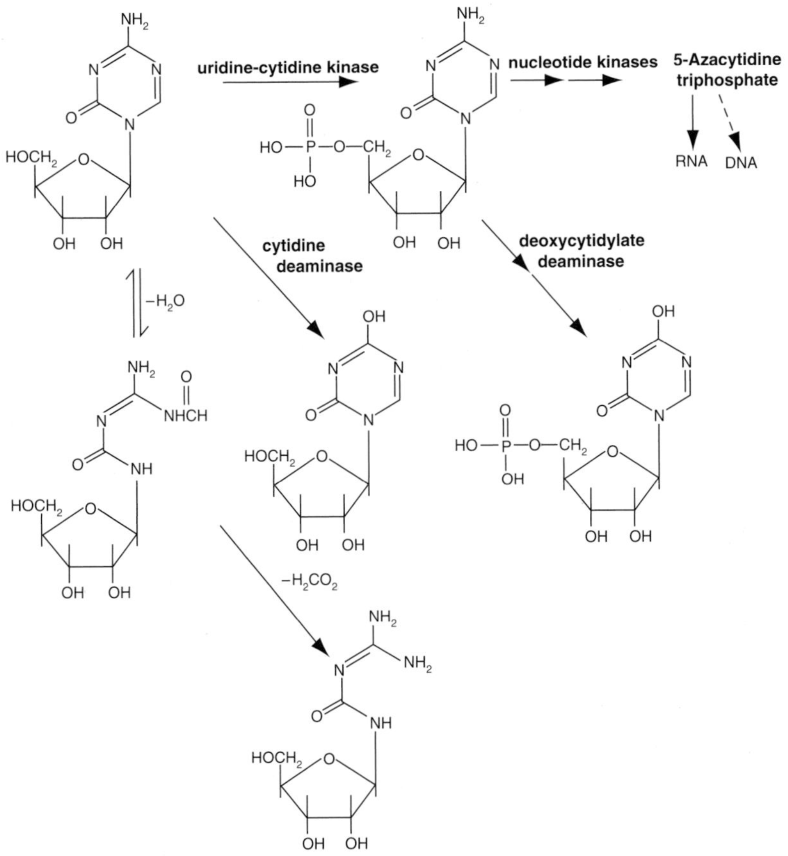

FIGURE 10-8 Metabolic pathway of 5-azacytidine metabolism.

affinity for 5-azacytidine ($K_m = 0.2$ to 11 mmol/L),[163] and probably represents the rate-limiting step in 5-azacytidine activation. Either uridine[164] or cytidine is capable of preventing 5-azacytidine toxicity in the whole animal and in tissue culture by competitively inhibiting its phosphorylation. Deletion of uridine-cytidine kinase has been observed in cells resistant to 5-azacytidine.[165] Cytidine deaminase, found in 10- to 30-fold higher concentration than uridine-cytidine kinase in leukemic cells, degrades 5-azacytidine to 5-azauridine. The role of this enzyme in resistance to 5-azacytidine has not been defined.

Further activation of 5-azacytidine monophosphate (5-aza-CMP) to a triphosphate probably occurs by the enzyme dCMP kinase and nucleoside NDP kinase. One hour after exposure of cells to the radiolabeled drug, 60% to 70% of acid-soluble radioactivity in cells was identified as 5-azacytidine triphosphate.[166]

Both drug concentration and duration of exposure are important determinants of 5-azacytidine cytotoxicity in tissue culture, a finding consistent with a preferential action on rapidly dividing cells. In tissue culture experiments, it has greatest lethality for cells in the S phase of the cell cycle and relatively little effect against nondividing cells.[167]

The differentiating action of 5-azacytidine has not been attributed to expression of specific genes as its effects are global.[156,160,167–174] Through its inhibition of DNA methylation, it induces the synthesis of various proteins, including hepatic enzymes (tyrosine aminotransferase),[167] metallothionein,[168] β- and γ-globin, histocompatibility proteins,[169] and T-cell surface markers.[170] It can reactivate repressed genes coding for thymidine kinase,[171] hypoxanthine-guanine phosphoribosyl transferase,[172] or DNA repair.[173] Probably through its effects on DNA methylation, 5-azacytidine is able to increase the immunogenicity of tumor cells and induce senescence in cell lines.[174] The drug has mutagenic and teratogenic effects,[175,176] but it is not known to be carcinogenic in humans.

Decitabine

Decitabine follows a somewhat different path of activation to a triphosphate. Like ara-C, its first phosphorylation is accomplished by CdR kinase, an enzyme lost in drug-resistant cell lines. Thereafter, it follows the same activation pathway as ara-C. Its clearance depends on deamination.

Assay Methods

5-Azacytidine is assayed by high-performance liquid chromatography with tandem mass spectrometry,[177,178] which has the requisite sensitivity and specificity for clinical studies.

Clinical pharmacology and pharmacokinetics of 5-azacytidine initial studies using drug labeled with radioactive carbon (^{14}C)[179,180] provided an incomplete understanding of drug disposition because of the drug's extensive metabolism and chemical decomposition. After subcutaneous injection, [^{14}C]5-azacytidine rapidly distributes into a volume approximately equal to or greater than total-body water (0.58 to 1.15 L/kg) with little plasma protein binding. Isolated measurements of radioactivity in the CSF indicate poor penetration of drug, with a CSF:plasma ratio of less than 0.1.

For treatment of MDS, the drug is given subcutaneously, 75 mg/m^2/d for 7 days in a 28-day cycle. After either subcutaneous (89% bioavailability) or intravenous bolus administration of 75 mg/m^2, the drug reaches a C_{max} of approximately 2 to 10 μM, and has an AUC of 4 μmol·h/mL. Its volume of distribution is

approximately 75 L.[177,181] It undergoes rapid deamination, with a clearance from plasma of 146 to 167 L/h and a plasma half-life of 20 to 40 minutes. An unquantified fraction undergoes renal excretion, and the package insert advises discontinuing treatment until serum creatinine or BUN returns to normal and then using a 50% reduction in dose. A longer $t_{1/2}$ of 1.2 hours was reported in an adolescent patient with renal failure, who received a subcutaneous dose of 45 mg/m^2.[181]

The identity of metabolites is unclear in humans.[182] 5-Azacytidine is known to undergo spontaneous ring opening in vitro, generating metabolites previously described in this chapter, and is also susceptible to deamination by cytidine deaminase,[183] an enzyme found in high concentrations in liver, granulocytes, and intestinal epithelium and in lower concentration in plasma. A number of metabolic products have been identified in the urine of dogs, including 5-azacytosine, 5-azauracil, and ring cleavage products.[143] The last-named product may result from decomposition of the parent compound or of its deamination product, 5-azauridine.

Toxicity

In patients with AML, a number of schedules of administration have been used for 5-azacytidine,[184] including single weekly intravenous doses of up to 750 mg/m^2, daily doses of 150 to 200 mg/m^2 for 5 to 10 consecutive days, and continuous infusion of similar daily doses for up to 5 days. With each of these schedules, the primary toxicity was leukopenia, although nausea and vomiting were prominent symptoms after bolus administration, which has led some investigators to favor continuous intravenous infusion,[182] a schedule also supported by cell kinetic considerations. The continuous infusion of 5-azacytidine requires fresh preparation of drug at frequent intervals, usually every 3 to 4 hours, because of the chemical instability of the agent. The response rate to 5-azacytidine in previously treated patients with acute myelocytic leukemia varied from 17% to 36% and was the same for the bolus and continuous-infusion schedules.

In patients with MDS, a lower dose of 75 mg/m^2/d for 7 days repeated every 28 days yields a best response after the fifth cycle of therapy.[143] Maximal dosages, used in AML, produce profound leukopenia and somewhat lesser thrombocytopenia. Hepatotoxicity also has been observed, particularly in patients with preexisting hepatic dysfunction.[185] The lower doses in MDS cause an initial decrease in peripheral blood counts, with a subsequent rise with onset of response.

In treating AML with higher doses of 5-azacytidine, occasional patients have developed hepatic enzyme elevations and hyperbilirubinemia.[185] A syndrome of neuromuscular toxicity was observed in patients receiving 200 mg/m^2/d by intravenous bolus injection. Neurotoxicity has been reported only sporadically by other investigators using this agent.[186] Several less worrisome acute toxic reactions have been associated with 5-azacytidine, including transient fever, a pruritic skin rash, and, rarely, hypotension during or immediately after bolus intravenous administration.

5-Azacytidine was approved for treatment of patients with MDS in 2004, based on the results of a randomized phase III trial comparing the drug to best supportive care. Thirty-five percent of patients achieved either a clear improvement in blood counts or decreased transfusion requirements, the transfusion benefits lasting a median of more than 330 days.[143] In an overview of published trials on 5-azacytidine in MDS, 6% achieved a complete response in bone marrow and peripheral blood.[187]

Decitabine was approved by the FDA for treatment of myelodysplasia using a regimen of 15 mg/m² intravenously every 3 hours for 3 days. Subsequent trials established the equal efficacy of a more convenient outpatient regimen of 20 mg/m²/d for 5 days per month, given intravenously.[140] Its toxicity profile is the same (most prominently myelosuppression and gastrointestinal symptoms), although neutropenia may prevent its use beyond a limited number of cycles of therapy.

Gemcitabine

Gemcitabine (2,2-difluorodeoxycytidine, dFdC) is the most important cytidine analog to enter clinical trials since ara-C (Fig. 10-1). It has become a standard first-line therapy for patients with pancreatic cancer, and it is also used for non–small cell lung cancer, ovarian cancer, and transitional cell cancer of the bladder.[189–191] The drug was selected for development on the basis of its impressive activity against murine solid tumors and human xenografts in nude mice.[192] In tissue culture, it is generally more potent than ara-C; the 50% inhibition concentration values for human leukemic cells range from 3 to 10 nM for 48-hour exposure compared with 26 to 52 nM for ara-C.[193] Although its metabolism to triphosphate status and its effects on DNA in general mimic those of ara-C, differences are found in kinetics of inhibition and additional sites of action of the newer compound, and clearly its spectrum of clinical activity is different.

Cellular Pharmacology, Metabolism, and Mechanism of Action

Gemcitabine retains many of the characteristics of ara-C. Its key features are shown in Table 10-4. Influx of gemcitabine through the cell membrane occurs via the hENT equilibrative nucleoside transporter. A concentrative transporter may also participate in its uptake.[194] CdR kinase phosphorylates gemcitabine intracellularly to produce difluorodeoxycytidine monophosphate (dFdCMP), from which point it is converted to its diphosphate and triphosphate difluorodeoxycytidine (dFdCDP, dFdCTP) (Fig. 10-9).[195] Its affinity for CdR kinase is threefold lower than the affinity of the natural substrate, CdR, whereas it has a 50% lower affinity for cytidine deaminase than CdR.[196] Cytidine deaminase conversion of gemcitabine to difluorodeoxyuridine (dFdU) represents the main catabolic pathway and is responsible for its brief 15 minute half-life in the systemic circulation.[197] To a lesser extent, pyrimidine nucleoside phosphorylase clears gemcitabine by cleaving the pyrimidine base from the furanose ring.

As with ara-C, in vitro studies of gemcitabine suggest potent inhibition of DNA synthesis as a major component of its mechanism of action,[192,195,198] but kinetic studies indicate that the killing effects of gemcitabine are not confined to the S phase of the cell cycle, and the drug is as effective against confluent cells as it is against cells in log-phase growth.[199] The cytotoxic activity may be a result of several actions on DNA synthesis: dFdCTP competes with dCTP as a weak inhibitor of DNA polymerase[198]; dFdCDP is a potent inhibitor of ribonucleotide reductase, which results in depletion of deoxyribonucleotide pools necessary for DNA synthesis.[200] The mechanism of inhibition of RNR proceeds via formation of a tight complex between the difluoro sugar of gemcitabine, six catalytic alpha subunits of RNR, and ATP[201] (Fig. 10-10). dFdCTP is a substrate for incorporation into DNA and, after the incorporation of one more nucleotide, leads to DNA strand termination.[202] This "extra" nucleotide may be important in hiding the dFdCMP from DNA repair enzymes because incorporation of gemcitabine into DNA appears to be resistant to DNA repair.[203] Incorporation of dFdCTP into

TABLE 10.4	Key features of gemcitabine
Factor	**Result**
Mechanism of Action	Incorporation into DNA terminates chain elongation
	Inhibits ribonucleotide reductase
	Inhibits DNA repair
"Metabolism"	Converted to a triphosphate
	Deaminated to inactive 2'-2' di fluorouridine
Pharmacokinetics	Plasma $t_{1/2}$ 8 min
Elimination	Deamination in liver, plasma, and peripheral tissues
	Reduce doses in patients with elevated serum bilirubin
Drug Interactions	Radiosensitizer
	Sensitizes cells to platinum-induced DNA damage
Toxicity	Myelosuppression
	Gastrointestinal epithelial ulceration
	Flu-like symptoms
	Abnormal liver function tests
	Microangiopathic anemia-uremia
	Pulmonary infiltrates

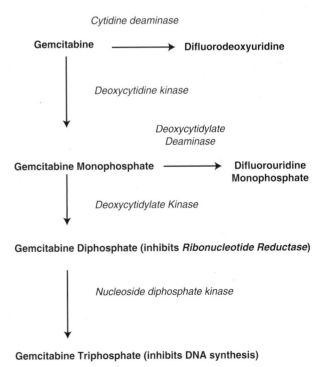

FIGURE 10-9 Key steps in gemcitabine activation and degradation.

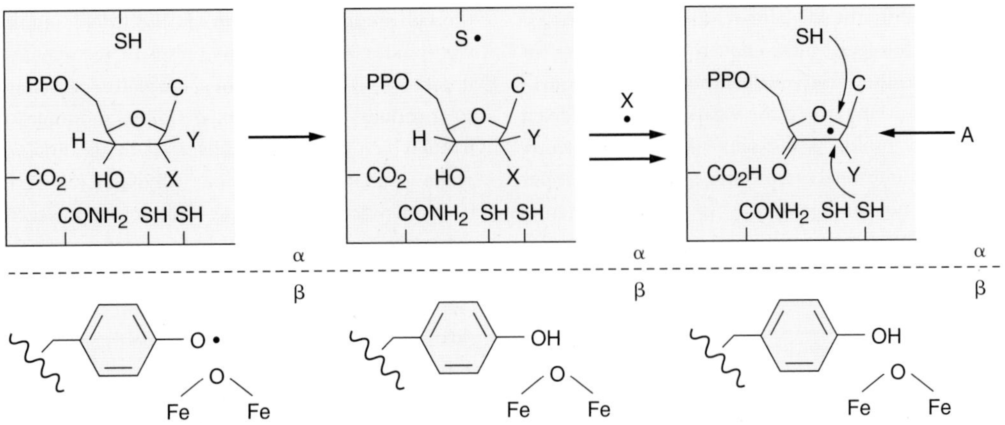

FIGURE 10-10 Sequential steps in reduction of NDP by ribonucleotide reductase. A tyrosyl diferric oxide radical transfers an electron to a sulfhydryl group in the alpha subunit of the enzyme, and the thylyl radical reduces the 2′ carbon of the ribose. α and β depict the subunit faces of RNR. X represents the 2′-OH group. (Adapted from Wang J, Lohman GJS, Stubbe J. Enhanced subunit interactions with gemcitabine-5′-diphosphate inhibit ribonucleotide reductase. PNAS 2007;104:14323–14329.)

DNA, as facilitated by RNR inhibition, is the critical event leading to apoptosis.[204]

Several important differences exist between ara-C and gemcitabine (Fig. 10-11). First, dFdCTP has a biphasic elimination from leukemic cells with α half-life ($t_{1/2}\alpha$) of 3.9 hours and β half-life ($t_{1/2\beta}$) of 16 hours, whereas ara-CTP has a monophasic elimination with $t_{1/2} = 0.7$ to 3.5 hours.[205] Also, dFdCDP is a much stronger inhibitor of ribonucleotide reductase (50% inhibition concentration of 4 µmol/L), and exposure to the drug blocks incorporation of labeled cytidine into the competitive cellular pool of dCTP.[200] Further, dFdC causes a decrease in all intracellular deoxynucleotide triphosphates, consistent with inhibition of ribonucleotide reductase. The ribonucleotide reductase inhibition is likely an important contributor to its potent radiosensitization and, by reducing competitive dCTP pools, enhances its incorporation into DNA. Some cell lines selected for resistance to other inhibitors of this enzyme, such as hydroxyurea and deoxyadenosine, do not show cross-resistance to dFdC, likely because their mechanisms of inhibiting RNR differ,[201] and the mutant forms of RNR generated by the other inhibitors remain sensitive to gemcitabine.[205] Resistance

to gemcitabine has been demonstrated through overexpression of ribonucleotide reductase.[206] Ribonucleotide reductase inhibition may potentiate other sites of gemcitabine action.[207] For example, deamination of dFdCMP by dCMP deaminase requires activation by dCTP. As dCTP pools become depleted by the effect of gemcitabine on ribonucleotide reductase, less deamination of gemcitabine monophosphate occurs and intracellular accumulation of gemcitabine metabolites increases. Furthermore, high intracellular concentration of dFdCTP appears to inhibit dCMP deaminase directly.[197]

The activity of dFdCTP on DNA repair mechanisms increases the cytotoxicity of other chemotherapeutic agents, particularly platinum compounds. Cisplatin works by creating interstrand and intrastrand cross-links. A mechanism of resistance may be removal of these cross-links by nucleotide excision repair (NER). Preclinical studies of tumor cell lines show that cisplatin-DNA adducts are enhanced in the presence of gemcitabine.[208] In cisplatin-resistant tumor cell lines, which have increased expression of NER, the addition of gemcitabine inhibited the repair of cisplatin-induced DNA lesions and increased cytotoxic.[208] Combined gemcitabine

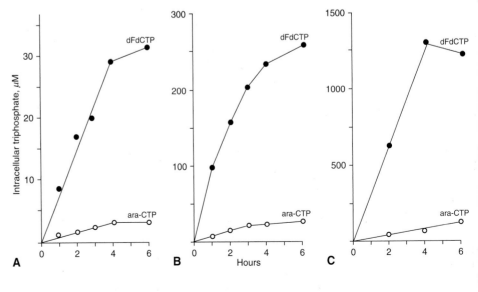

FIGURE 10-11 Accumulation of difluorodeoxycytidine triphosphate (dFdCTP) and ara-CTP as a function of time after incubation of cells with either dFdCTP or ara-C at drug concentrations of 1 µmol/L (**A**), 10 µmol/L (**B**), and 100 µmol/L (**C**). (Adapted from Heinemann V, Hertel LW, Grindey GB, et al. Comparison of the cellular pharmacokinetics and toxicity of 2′,2′-difluorodeoxycytidine and 1-beta-ᴅ-arabinofuranosylcytosine. Cancer Res 1988;48:4024–4031.)

and cisplatin are standard agents in the treatment of non–small cell lung cancer and transitional cell carcinoma of the bladder.

Mechanisms of Resistance

Resistance to gemcitabine is not fully understood. In vitro studies have suggested several possible mechanisms. Gemcitabine resistance has been correlated with tumor levels of CdR kinase.[209] Induction of cytidine deaminase[210] and high concentrations of heat-shock protein have also conferred gemcitabine resistance to cells.[211] Preclinical studies have also demonstrated that increased expression of ribonucleotide reductase may be associated with gemcitabine resistance.[212] Lastly, inhibition of nucleoside transporters can prevent the influx of gemcitabine through the cell membrane and the absence of transporters has been associated with reduced survival in patients with pancreatic cancer.[213,214]

Pharmacokinetics

In animals, gemcitabine pharmacokinetics is largely determined by deamination.[215] In mice and dogs, the predominant elimination product is dFdU. In cell lines and in cells taken from patients during treatment, maximal accumulation of dFdCTP occurs when plasma (or tissue culture) drug concentrations are in the range of 10 to 20 μmol/L, a level achieved during 3-hour infusions of 300 mg/m^2.[216]

Abbruzzese et al.[217] performed a phase I study of gemcitabine given weekly as a 30-minute infusion on days 1, 8, and 15, followed by a 1-week rest in patients with refractory solid tumors. The maximum tolerated dose (MTD) was 1,000 mg/m^2/wk. The dose-limiting toxicity was myelosuppression characterized by thrombocytopenia with relative sparing of granulocytes. Pharmacokinetic analysis showed a $t_{1/2}$ of 8 minutes for the parent compound and a biphasic elimination of dFdU, with $t_{1/2\alpha}$ = 27 minutes and $t_{1/2\beta}$ = 14 hours. No relationship was found between degree of myelosuppression and any of the pharmacokinetic parameters. The AUC of plasma dFdC was proportional to the dose over a range of 10 to 1,000 mg/m^2/wk. Clearance was dose independent but varied widely among individuals (39 to 1,239 L/h/m^2 at a dose of 1,000 mg/m^2).

A higher gemcitabine dose of 2,200 mg/m^2 administered over 30 minutes on days 1, 8, and 15 can be safely given to less heavily treated or chemonaïve patients.[218] The question remains unanswered as to whether cells generate higher concentration of the active metabolite as the dose rate increases. In the case of ara-C, the ability of peripheral blood mononuclear cells to accumulate ara-CTP saturates at ara-C concentrations of >10 μmol/L.[219] A similar series of studies with gemcitabine have demonstrated that activation of gemcitabine by CdR kinase to dFdCTP is saturated at infusion rates of approximately 10 mg/m^2/min.[215,220,221] This "dose-rate infusion" produced steady-state dFdC levels of 15 to 20 μmol/L in plasma. Based on a phase I study using constant dose-rate infusion of gemcitabine on days 1, 8, and 15 every 28 days was carried out in patients with metastatic solid tumors.[222] Although the first-cycle MTD was estimated to be 2,250 mg/m^2 over 225 minutes, the recommended phase II dose of gemcitabine administered as a dose-rate infusion is 1,500 mg/m^2 over 150 minutes because of the occurrence of cumulative neutropenia and thrombocytopenia at higher doses. In a proof-of-concept study, Tempero et al.[223] performed a randomized phase II study of constant dose-rate infusion at 10 mg/m^2/min

for 150 minutes versus dose-intense infusion of 2,200 mg/m^2 over 30 minutes in patients with advanced pancreatic cancer. Constant dose-rate infusion resulted in a twofold increase in intracellular gemcitabine triphosphate in peripheral blood mononuclear cells compared with the standard 30-minute infusion. However, no improvement in therapeutic outcome was seen.[224]

Gemcitabine has been studied in children, and the MTD of gemcitabine given as a 30-minute infusion weekly for 3 of 4 weeks is 1,200 mg/m^2. Myelosuppression is the dose-limiting toxicity, and pharmacokinetics in pediatric patients is similar to the adult population.[225]

Toxicity

The dose-limiting toxicity of gemcitabine is invariably hematologic, and the toxicity profile differs according to schedule. In general, the longer-duration infusions lead to greater myelosuppression. The MTD for a daily × 5 schedule every 21 days is 12 mg/m^2/d or 60 mg/m^2/cycle.[226] The MTD for twice-weekly doses of gemcitabine administered for 3 weeks with a 1-week rest period depends on the time of infusion. When the drug is administered over 5 minutes, the MTD is 150 mg/m^2, and when it is administered as a 30-minute infusion, the MTD is 75 mg/m^2.[227] For a 24-hour infusion given weekly in 3 of 4 weeks, the MTD is 180 mg/m^2 per dose.[228]

The weekly dose schedule is the standard regimen and is implemented as a 30-minute infusion for 3 of 4 weeks. The MTD for chemonaïve patients is 2,200 mg/m^2/wk, and the MTD for pretreated patients is 800 to 1,000 mg/m^2/wk.[216,217] A dose of 1,000 mg/m^2/wk, for 3 to 4 weeks, given over 30 minutes, is recommended for treatment of pancreatic cancer and other solid tumors, and in other tumor types, it is often given in combination with cis- or carboplatin. The safety of gemcitabine has been evaluated in a database including 22 studies using the once-weekly treatment regimen.[229] Nine hundred seventy-nine patients received at least one dose of gemcitabine and were evaluable for toxicity. World Health Organization (WHO) grade 3 and 4 neutropenia occurred in 19.3% and 6% of patients, respectively. WHO grade 3 and 4 thrombocytopenia occurred in 4.1% and 1.1% of patients, respectively. Clinically significant consequences of hematologic toxicity were uncommon: only 1.1% of patients experienced WHO grade 3 infection and 0.7% of patients required platelet transfusions. Among nonhematologic toxicities, flu-like symptoms including fever, headache, back pain, and myalgias occur in approximately 45% of patients. The duration of these symptoms was short, and <1% of patients discontinued therapy because of flu-like symptoms. Asthenia is also common, occurring in 42% of patients. A transient, mild elevation in liver function test results (WHO grade 1 or 2 elevations in alanine aminotransferase) was detected in 41% of cycles.

Although severe nonhematologic reactions are rare, several specific syndromes complicating gemcitabine therapy have emerged from its expanding clinical experience.[230–235] Thrombotic microangiopathy as manifested by hemolytic-uremic syndrome or thrombotic thrombocytopenic purpura has been reported as a complication of gemcitabine therapy,[230–232] and a review of the manufacturer's database estimated an overall incidence rate of 0.015%.[229] However, a large single institution review demonstrated 9 cases of gemcitabine-associated microangiopathy among a total of 2,586 cases of microangiopathy for an estimated incidence of 0.31%.[232] Patients who are treated for prolonged periods (i.e., longer than 1 year) may be at higher risk for developing hemolytic-uremic syndrome or thrombotic microangiopathy.

Severe pulmonary toxicity as manifested by acute respiratory distress syndrome, capillary leak syndrome, or interstitial pneumonitis has been reported in patients treated with gemcitabine.[233-235] A review of the Lilly world-wide database identified 91 patients with serious pulmonary toxicity for an estimated incidence of less than 0.1%.[234] Caution is warranted when combining gemcitabine with drugs known to cause pulmonary dysfunction, such as bleomycin. A study substituting gemcitabine for etoposide in the BEACOPP regimen in Hodgkin's lymphoma led to severe pulmonary toxicity, possibly as a result of interaction with bleomycin.[235]

A multicenter study evaluated the role of gemcitabine in patients with hepatic or renal dysfunction.[236] Patients with elevated bilirubin experienced increased toxicity and should receive reduced doses, whereas, patients with elevated transaminases did not experience increased toxicity. Patients with elevated creatinine appeared to be more sensitive to gemcitabine but did not require dose reductions.

Radiation Sensitization

Because of its inhibition of ribonucleotide reductase and DNA polymerase, gemcitabine has strong radiosensitizing effects. Preclinical studies of gemcitabine have shown potent radiosensitization in human colon, pancreatic, head and neck, and cervical cancer cell lines.[237,238] These effects parallel the intracellular depletion of deoxyadenosine triphosphate and are most prominent when gemcitabine is administered before radiation therapy. Interestingly, the radiosensitization effect had no correlation with dFdCMP incorporation into DNA, which suggests that the inhibition of ribonucleotide reductase is the key mechanism of action. In vitro studies suggest that maximal enhancement of radiation sensitization occurs when gemcitabine is administered before radiation, and in vivo studies suggest that this effect is most pronounced when the time interval is 24 to 60 hours.[237,239,240] Gemcitabine radiosensitization is most evident in mismatch repair-deficient cells,[241] and correlates with mismatch incorporation of deoxynucleotides into DNA.[242]

Despite the radiosensitization seen in preclinical studies, the initial phase I and II studies of gemcitabine and radiation therapy have not demonstrated markedly improved clinical activity and are associated primarily with increased toxicity. In a phase I trial of twice-weekly gemcitabine and concurrent radiation in patients with advanced pancreatic cancer, the MTD was 40 mg/m[2] administered over 30 minutes on Monday and Thursday of each week.[243] The dose-limiting toxicities were grade 3 neutropenia, thrombocytopenia, nausea, and vomiting. This regimen was subsequently evaluated in phase II study for patients with locally advanced pancreatic cancer, and the median survival was 7.9 months.[244] When given once weekly with radiation at gemcitabine doses of 300 to 500 mg/m[2] to patients with locally advanced pancreatic cancer, the drug caused severe toxicity and no improvement in survival when results were compared with historical controls using fluoropyrimidines with external beam radiation therapy.[245] An attempt to combine weekly gemcitabine with fluorouracil and external beam radiation therapy in patients with locally advanced pancreatic cancer was stopped

when five of the first seven patients experienced dose-limiting toxicities at gemcitabine doses of 100 and 50 mg/m[2].[246]

The inability to deliver full-dose gemcitabine concurrent with radiation has been demonstrated in other tumor types as well. A phase II study of gemcitabine administered weekly with concurrent external beam radiation therapy in patients with unresectable head and neck cancer required dose de-escalation from 300 to 50 mg/m[2]/wk as the result of a high rate of mucosa-related toxicity.[247] A phase I study of weekly gemcitabine with concurrent radiotherapy in patients with locally advanced lung cancer established a maximally tolerated dose of 300 mg/m[2].[248] Dose-limiting toxicities included grade 3 esophagitis and grade 3 pneumonitis. There is little interest at this time in continuing studies of the combination of gemcitabine and irradiation.

References

1. Bergmann W, Feeney R. Contributions to the study of marine products: XXXII. The nucleosides of sponges. J Org Chem 1951;16:981.
2. Roberts WK, Dekker CA. A convenient synthesis of arabinosylcytosine (cytosine arabinoside). J Org Chem 1967;32:84.
3. Ellison RR, Holland JF, Weil M, et al. Arabinosyl cytosine: a useful agent in the treatment of acute leukemia in adults. Blood 1968;32:507.
4. Mayer RJ, Davis RB, Schiffer CA, et al. Intensive chemotherapy in adults with acute myeloid leukemia. N Engl J Med 1994;331:896.
5. Bloomfield CD, Lawrence D, Byrd JC, et al. Frequency of prolonged remission duration after high-dose cytarabine by cytogenetic subtype. Cancer Res 1998;58:4173.
6. Cadman E, Farber L, Berd D, et al. Combination therapy for diffuse lymphocytic lymphoma that includes antimetabolites. Cancer Treat Rep 1977;61:1109.
7. Bryan JH, Henderson ES, Leventhal BG. Cytosine arabinoside and 6-thioguanine in refractory acute lymphocytic leukemia. Cancer 1974;33:539.
8. Guilhot F, Chastang C, Michallet M, et al. Interferon alfa-2b combined with cytarabine versus interferon alone in chronic myelogenous leukemia. N Engl J Med 1997;337:223.
9. Furth JJ, Cohen SS. Inhibition of mammalian DNA polymerase by the 5′-triphosphate of 9-β-D-arabinofuranosylcytosine and the triphosphate of 9-β-D-arabinofuranosyladenine. Cancer Res 1968;28:2061.
10. Townsend AJ, Cheng YC. Sequence-specific effects of ara-5-aza-CTP and ara-CTP on DNA synthesis by purified human DNA polymerases in vitro: visualization of chain elongation on a defined template. Mol Pharmacol 1987;32:330.
11. Graham FL, Whitmore GF. Studies in mouse L-cells on the incorporation of 1-β-D-arabinofuranosylcytosine into DNA and on inhibition of DNA polymerase by 1-β-D-arabinofuranosylcytosine-5′-triphosphate. Cancer Res 1970;30:2636.
12. Chu MY, Fischer GA. A proposed mechanism of action of 1-β-D-arabinofuranosylcytosine as an inhibitor of the growth of leukemic cells. Biochem Pharmacol 1962;11:423.
13. Yoshida S, Yamada M, Masaki S. Inhibition of DNA polymerase-α and -β of calf thymus by 1-β-D-arabinofuranosylcytosine-5′-triphosphate. Biochim Biophys Acta 1977;477:144.
14. Fram RJ, Kufe DW. Inhibition of DNA excision repair and the repair of x-ray-induced DNA damage by cytosine arabinoside and hydroxyurea. Pharmacol Ther 1985;31:165.
15. Kufe WE, Major PP, Egan EM, et al. Correlation of cytotoxicity with incorporation of araC into DNA. J Biol Chem 1980;255:8997.
16. Fram RJ, Egan EM, Kufe DW. Accumulation of leukemic cell DNA strand breaks with adriamycin and cytosine arabinoside. Leuk Res 1983;7:243.
17. Kufe DW, Munroe D, Herrick D, et al. Effects of 1-β-D-arabinofuranosylcytosine incorporation on eukaryotic DNA template function. Mol Pharmacol 1984;26:128.
18. Kufe DW, Spriggs DR. Biochemical and cellular pharmacology of cytosine arabinoside. Semin Oncol 1985;12:34.

19. Major P, Egan E, Herrick D, et al. The effect of araC incorporation on DNA synthesis. Biochem Pharmacol 1982;31:2937.

20. Mikita T, Beardsley GP. Functional consequences of the arabinosylcytosine structural lesion in DNA. Biochemistry 1988;27:4698.

21. Ross DD, Cuddy DP, Cohen N, et al. Mechanistic implications of alterations in HL-60 cell nascent DNA after exposure to 1-β-D-arabinofuranosylcytosine. Cancer Chemother Pharmacol 1992;31:61.

22. Woodcock DM, Fox RM, Cooper IA. Evidence for a new mechanism of cytotoxicity of 1-β-D-arabinofuranosylcytosine. Cancer Res 1979;39:418.

23. Moore EC, Cohen SS. Effects of arabinonucleotides on ribonucleotide reduction by an enzyme system from rat tumor. J Biol Chem 1967;242:2116.

24. Hawtrey AO, Scott-Burden T, Robertson G. Inhibition of glycoprotein and glycolipid synthesis in hamster embryo cells by cytosine arabinoside and hydroxyurea. Nature 1974;252:58.

25. Bianchi Scarra GL, Romani M, Civiello DA, et al. Terminal erythroid differentiation in the K-562 cell line by 1-β-D-arabinofuranosylcytosine: accompaniment by c-myc messenger RNA decrease. Cancer Res 1986;46:6327.

26. Gunji H, Kharbanda S, Kufe D. Induction of internucleosomal DNA fragmentation in human myeloid leukemia cells by 1-β-D-arabinofuranosylcytosine. Cancer Res 1991;51:741.

27. Strum JC, Small GW, Pauig SB, et al. 1-β-D-arabinofuranosylcytosine stimulates ceramide and diglyceride formation in HL-60 cells. J Biol Chem 1994;269:15493.

28. Kharbanda S, Datta R, Kufe D. Regulation of c-jun gene expression in HL-60 leukemia cells by 1-β-D-arabinofuranosylcytosine. Potential involvement of a protein kinase C dependent mechanism. Biochemistry 1991;30:7947.

29. Brach MA, Kharbanda SM, Herrmann F, et al. Activation of the transcription factor kB in human KG-1 myeloid leukemia cells treated with 1-β-D-arabinofuranosylcytosine. Mol Pharmacol 1992;41:60.

30. Bullock G, Ray S, Reed J, et al. Evidence against a direct role for the induction of c-jun expression in the mediation of drug-induced apoptosis in human acute leukemia cells. Clin Cancer Res 1995;1:559.

31. Dou QP, An B, Will P. Induction of a retinoblastoma phosphatase activity by anticancer drugs accompanies p53-independent G_1 arrest and apoptosis. Proc Natl Acad Sci U S A 1995;92:9019.

32. Ikeda M, Jakoi L, Nevins J. A unique role for the Rb protein in controlling E2F accumulation during cell growth and differentiation. Proc Natl Acad Sci U S A 1996;93:3215.

33. Wiley JS, Jones SP, Sawyer WH, et al. Cytosine arabinoside influx and nucleoside transport sites in acute leukemia. J Clin Invest 1982;69:479.

34. Belt JA, Noel DL. Isolation and characterization of a mutant of L1210 murine leukemia deficient in nitrobenzylthioinosine-insensitive nucleoside transport. J Biol Chem 1988;263:13819.

35. Pui CH, Relling MV, Downing JR. Acute lymphoblastic leukemia. N Engl J Med 2004;350:1535–1548.

36. Cai J, Damaraju VL, Groulx N, et al. Two distinct molecular mechanisms underlying cytarabine resistance in human leukemic cells. Cancer Res 2008;68:2349–2357.

37. White JC, Rathmell JP, Capizzi RL. Membrane transport influences the rate of accumulation of cytosine arabinoside in human leukemia cells. J Clin Invest 1987;79:380.

38. Damaraju VL, Damarjus S, Young JD, et al. Nucleoside anticancer drugs: The role of nucleoside transporters in resistance to cancer chemotherapy. Oncogene 2003;22:7524.

39. Owens JK, Shewach DS, Ullman B, et al. Resistance to 1-β-D-arabinofuranosylcytosine in human T lymphoblasts mediated by mutations within the deoxycytidine kinase gene. Cancer Res 1992;52:2389.

40. Cai J, Damaraju VL, Groulx N, et al. Two distinct molecular mechanisms underlying cytarabine resistance in human leukemic cells. Cancer Res 2008;68:2349–2357.

41. Hapke DM, Stegmann APA, Mitchell BS. Retroviral transfer of deoxycytidine kinase into tumor cell lines enhances nucleoside toxicity. Cancer Res 1996;56:2343.

42. Manome Y, Wen PY, Dong Y, et al. Viral vector transduction of the human deoxycytidine kinase cDNA sensitizes glioma cells to the cytotoxic effects of cytosine arabinoside in vitro and in vivo. Nat Med 1996;2:567.

43. Gandhi V, Plunkett W. Cell cycle-specific metabolism of arabinosyl nucleosides in K562 human leukemia cells. Cancer Chemother Pharmacol 1992;31:11.

44. Coleman CN, Stoller RG, Drake JC, et al. Deoxycytidine kinase: properties of the enzyme from human leukemic granulocytes. Blood 1975;46:791.

45. Wang L, Kucera GL. Deoxycytidine kinase is phosphorylated in vitro by protein kinase Cα. Biochim Biophys Acta 1994;1224:161.

46. Hande KR, Chabner BA. Pyrimidine nucleoside monophosphate kinase from human leukemic blast cells. Cancer Res 1978;38:579.

47. Chou T-C, Arlin Z, Clarkson BD, et al. Metabolism of 1-β-D-arabinofuranosylcytosine in human leukemic cells. Cancer Res 1977;37:3561.

48. Chabner B, Johns D, Coleman C, et al. Purification and properties of cytidine deaminase from normal and leukemic granulocytes. J Clin Invest 1974;53:922.

49. Jackson RC. The regulation of thymidylate biosynthesis in Novikoff hepatoma cells and the effects of amethopterin, 5-fluorodeoxyuridine, and 3-deazauridine. J Biol Chem 1978;253:7440.

50. Ellims P, Kao AH, Chabner BA. Deoxycytidylate deaminase: purification and kinetic properties of the enzyme isolated from human spleen. J Biol Chem 1981;256:6335.

51. Lauzon GJ, Paran JH, Paterson ARP. Formation of 1-β-D-arabinofuranosylcytosine diphosphate choline in cultured human leukemic RPMI 6410 cells. Cancer Res 1978;38:1723.

52. Myers-Robfogel MW, Spatato AC. 1-β-D-Arabinofuranosylcytosine nucleotide inhibition of sialic acid metabolism in WI-38 cells. Cancer Res 1980;40:1940.

53. Chu MY, Fischer GA. Comparative studies of leukemic cells sensitive and resistant to cytosine arabinoside. Biochem Pharmacol 1965;14:333.

54. De Saint Vincent BR, Dechamps M, Buttin G. The modulation of the thymidine triphosphate pool of Chinese hamster cells by dCMP deaminase and UDP reductase. J Biol Chem 1980;255:162.

55. De Saint Vincent BR, Buttin G. Studies on 1-β-D-arabinofuranosyl cytosine-resistant mutants of Chinese hamster fibroblasts: IV. Altered regulation of CTP synthetase generates arabinosylcytosine and thymidine resistance. Biochim Biophys Acta 1980;610:352.

56. Eliopoulos N, Cournoyer D, Momparler RL. Drug resistance to 5-aza-2′-deoxycytidine, 2′,2′-difluorodeoxycytidine, and cytosine arabinoside conferred by retroviral-mediated transfer of human cytidine deaminase cDNA into murine cells. Cancer Chemother Pharmacol 1998;42:373.

57. Riva C, Khyari SE, Rustum Y, et al. Resistance to cytosine arabinoside in cells transfected with activated Ha-ras oncogene. Anticancer Res 1995;15:1297.

58. Koo H, Monks A, Mikheev A, et al. Enhanced sensitivity to 1-β-D-arabinofuranosylcytosine and topoisomerase II inhibitors in tumor cell lines harboring activated ras oncogenes. Cancer Res 1996;56:5211.

59. Neubauer A, Maharry K, Mrózek K, et al. Patients with acute myeloid leukemia and RAS mutations benefit most from postremission high-dose cytarabine: a Cancer and Leukemia Group B study. J Clin Oncol 2008;26:4603.

60. Tattersall MNH, Ganeshaguru K, Hoffbrand AV. Mechanisms of resistance of human acute leukaemia cells to cytosine arabinoside. Br J Haematol 1974;27:39.

61. Steuart CD, Burke PJ. Cytidine deaminase and the development of resistance to arabinosylcytosine. Nature New Biol 1971;233:109.

62. White JC, Rathmell JP, Capizzi RL. Membrane transport influences the rate of accumulation of cytosine arabinoside in human leukemia cells. J Clin Invest 1987;79:380.

63. Chiba P, Tihan T, Szekeres T, et al. Concordant changes of pyrimidine metabolism in blasts of two cases of acute myeloid leukemia after repeated treatment with araC in vivo. Leukemia 1990;4:761.

64. Chang P, Wiernik PH, Reich SD, et al. Prediction of response to cytosine arabinoside and daunorubicin in acute nonlymphocytic leukemia. In: Mandelli F, ed. Therapy of Acute Leukemias: Proceedings of the Second International Symposium, Rome, 1977. Rome: Lombardo Editore, 1979:148.

65. Smyth JF, Robins AB, Leese CL. The metabolism of cytosine arabinoside as a predictive test for clinical response to the drug in acute myeloid leukaemia. Eur J Cancer 1976;12:567.

66. Estey E, Plunkett W, Dixon D, et al. Variables predicting response to high dose cytosine arabinoside therapy in patients with refractory acute leukemia. Leukemia 1987;1:580.

67. Ross DD, Thompson BW, Joneckis CC, et al. Metabolism of araC by blast cells from patients with ANLL. Blood 1986;68:76.

68. Rustum YM, Riva C, Preisler HD. Pharmacokinetic parameters of 1-β-D-arabinofuranosylcytosine and their relationship to intracellular metabolism

of araC, toxicity, and response of patients with acute nonlymphocytic leukemia treated with conventional and high-dose araC. Semin Oncol 1987;14:141.

69. Estey EH, Keating MJ, McCredie KB, et al. Cellular ara-CTP pharmacokinetics, response, and karyotype in newly diagnosed acute myelogenous leukemia. Leukemia 1990;4:95.

70. Preisler HD, Rustum Y, Priore RL. Relationship between leukemic cell retention of cytosine arabinoside triphosphate and the duration of remission in patients with acute non-lymphocytic leukemia. Eur J Cancer Clin Oncol 1985;21:23.

71. Plunkett W, Iacoboni S, Keating MJ. Cellular pharmacology and optimal therapeutic concentrations of 1-β-D-arabinofuranosylcytosine 5′-triphosphate in leukemic blasts during treatment of refractory leukemia with high-dose 1-β-D-arabinofuranosylcytosine. Scand J Haematol 1986;34:51.

72. Ibrado AM, Uang Y, Fang G, et al. Overexpression of Bcl-2 or Bcl-xL inhibits araC-induced CPP32/Yama protease activity and apoptosis of human acute myelogenous leukemia HL-60 cells. Cancer Res 1996;56:4743.

73. Keith FJ, Bradbury DA, Zhu Y, et al. Inhibition of bcl-2 with antisense oligonucleotides induces apoptosis and increases the sensitivity of AML blasts to araC. Leukemia 1995;9:131.

74. Campos L, Rouault J, Sabido O, et al. High expression of bcl-2 protein in acute myeloid leukemia cells is associated with poor response to chemotherapy. Blood 1993;81:3091.

75. Ruvolo PR, Deng X, Carr BK, et al. A functional role for mitochondrial protein kinase Cα Bcl2 phosphorylation and suppression of apoptosis. J Biol Chem 1998;273:25436.

76. Wang S, Vrana JA, Bartimole TM, et al. Agents that down-regulate or inhibit protein kinase C circumvent resistance to 1-β-D-arabinofuranosylcytosine–induced apoptosis in human leukemia cells that overexpress Bcl-2. Mol Pharmacol 1997;52:1000.

77. Kharbanda S, Emoto Y, Kisaki H, et al. 1-β-D-arabinofuranosylcytosine activates serine/threonine protein kinases and c-jun gene expression in phorbol ester-resistant myeloid leukemia cells. Mol Pharmacol 1994;46:67.

78. Kolla SS, Studzinski GP. Constitutive DNA binding of the low mobility forms of the AP-1 and SP-1 transcription factors in HL60 cells resistant to 1-β-D-arabinofuranosylcytosine. Cancer Res 1994;54:1418.

79. Young RC, Schein PS. Enhanced antitumor effect of cytosine arabinoside given in a schedule dictated by kinetic studies in vivo. Biochem Pharmacol 1973;22:277.

80. Preisler HD, Azarnia N, Raza A, et al. Relationship between percent of marrow cells in S phase and the outcome of remission induction therapy for acute nonlymphocytic leukemia. Br J Haematol 1984;56:399.

81. Raza A, Preisler HD, Day R, et al. Direct relationship between remission duration in acute myeloid leukemia and cell cycle kinetics: a leukemia intergroup study. Blood 1990;76:2191.

82. Sinkule JA, Evans WE. High-performance liquid chromatographic assay for cytosine arabinoside, uracil arabinoside, and some related nucleosides. J Chromatogr 1983;274:87.

83. Harris AL, Potter C, Bunch C, et al. Pharmacokinetics of cytosine arabinoside in patients with acute myeloid leukaemia. Br J Clin Pharmacol 1979;8:219.

84. Van Prooijen R, van der Kleijn E, Haanen C. Pharmacokinetics of cytosine arabinoside in acute leukemia. Clin Pharmacol Ther 1977;21:744.

85. Slevin ML, Piall EM, Aherne GW, et al. Effect of dose and schedule on pharmacokinetics of high-dose cytosine arabinoside in plasma and cerebrospinal fluid. J Clin Oncol 1983;1:546.

86. Early AP, Preisler HD, Slocum H, et al. A pilot study of high-dose of 1-β-D-arabinofuranosylcytosine for acute leukemia and refractory-lymphoma: clinical response and pharmacology. Cancer Res 1982;42:1587.

87. Capizzi RL, Yang JL, Ching E, et al. Alterations of the pharmacokinetics of high-dose araC by its metabolite, high araU in patients with acute leukemia. J Clin Oncol 1983;1:763.

88. Donehower RC, Karp JE, Burke PJ. Pharmacology and toxicity of high-dose cytarabine by 72-hour continuous infusion. Cancer Treat Rep 1986;70:1059.

89. Wau SH, Huffman DH, Azarnoff DL, et al. Pharmacokinetics of 1-β-D-arabinofuranosylcytosine in humans. Cancer Res 1974;34:392.

90. Liliemark JO, Paul CY, Gahrton CG, et al. Pharmacokinetics of 1-β-D-arabinofuranosylcytosine 5′-triphosphate in leukemic cells after intravenous and subcutaneous administration of 1-β-D-arabinofuranosylcytosine. Cancer Res 1985;45:2373.

91. Markman M. The intracavitary administration of cytarabine to patients with nonhematopoietic malignancies: pharmacologic rationale and results of clinical trials. Semin Oncol 1985;12(Suppl 3):177.

92. Kirmani S, Zimm S, Cleary SM, et al. Extremely prolonged continuous intraperitoneal infusion of cytosine arabinoside. Cancer Chemother Pharmacol 1990;25:454.

93. Ho DHW, Frei E III. Clinical pharmacology of 1-β-D-arabinofuranosylcytosine. Clin Pharmacol Ther 1971;12:944.

94. Chamberlain MC, Khatibi S, Kim JC, et al. Treatment of leptomeningeal metastasis with intraventricular administration of Depot cytarabine (DTC 101). Arch Neurol 1993;50:261.

95. Howell SB, Glantz MJ, LaFollette S, et al. A controlled trial of Depocyt™ for the treatment of lymphomatous meningitis [abstract 34]. Proc Am Soc Clin Oncol 1999;18:11a.

96. Cole BF, Glantz MJ, Jaeckle KA, et al. Quality-of-life-adjusted survival comparison of sustained-release cytosine arabinoside versus intrathecal methotrexate for treatment of solid tumor neoplastic meningitis. Cancer 2003;97:3053.

97. Capizzi RL, Powell BL, Cooper MR, et al. Dose-related pharmacologic effects of high-dose araC and its use in combination with asparaginase for the treatment of patients with acute nonlymphocytic leukemia. Scand J Haematol 1986;34(Suppl 44):17.

98. Plunkett W, Iacoboni S, Estey E, et al. Pharmacologically directed araC therapy for refractory leukemia. Semin Oncol 1985;12(Suppl 3):20.

99. Wisch JS, Griffin JD, Kufe DN. Response of preleukemic syndromes to continuous infusion of low-dose cytarabine. N Engl J Med 1983;309:1599.

100. Tilly H, Bastard C, Bizet M, et al. Low-dose cytarabine: persistence of a clonal abnormality during complete remission of acute nonlymphocytic leukemia. N Engl J Med 1986;314:246.

101. Raijmakers R, DeWitte T, Linssen P, et al. The relation of exposure time and drug concentration in their effect on cloning efficiency after incubation of human bone marrow with cytosine arabinoside. Br J Haematol 1986;62:447.

102. Frei E III, Bickers JN, Hewlett JS, et al. Dose schedule and antitumor studies of arabinosyl cytosine (NSC 63878). Cancer Res 1969;29:1325.

103. Mitchell MS, Wade ME, DeConti RC, et al. Immunosuppressive effects of cytosine arabinoside and methotrexate in man. Ann Intern Med 1969;70:535.

104. Talley RW, Vaitkevicius VK. Megaloblastosis produced by a cytosine antagonist, 1-β-D-arabinofuranosyl cytosine. Blood 1963;21:352.

105. Slavin RE, Dias MA, Saral R. Cytosine arabinoside-induced gastrointestinal toxic alterations in sequential chemotherapeutic protocols. Cancer 1978;42:1747.

106. Altman A, Dinndorf P, Quinn JJ. Acute pancreatitis in association with cytosine arabinoside therapy. Cancer 1982;49:1384.

107. Weisman SJ, Scoopo FJ, Johnson GM, et al. Septicemia in pediatric oncology patients: the significance of viridans streptococcal infections. J Clin Oncol 1990;8:453.

108. Forghieri F, Luppi M, Morselli M, et al. Cytarabine-related lung infiltrates on high resolution computerized tomography: a possible complication with benign outcome in leukemic patients. Haematologica 2007;92:e85.

109. George CB, Mansour RP, Redmond J, et al. Hepatic dysfunction and jaundice following high-dose cytosine arabinoside. Cancer 1984;54:2360.

110. Herzig RH, Hines JD, Herzig GP, et al. Cerebellar toxicity with high-dose cytosine arabinoside. J Clin Oncol 1987;5:927.

111. Rubin EH, Anderson JW, Berg DT, et al. Risk factors for high-dose cytarabine neurotoxicity: an analysis of a cancer and leukemia group B trial in patients with acute myeloid leukemia. J Clin Oncol 1992;10:948.

112. Shaw PJ, Procopis PG, Menser MA, et al. Bulbar and pseudobulbar palsy complicating therapy with high-dose cytosine arabinoside in children with leukemia. Med Pediatr Oncol 1991;19:122.

113. Paul M, Joshua D, Rahme N, et al. Fatal peripheral neuropathy associated with axonal degeneration after high-dose cytosine arabinoside in acute leukemia. Br J Haematol 1991;79:521.

114. Castleberry RP, Crist WM, Holbrook T, et al. The cytosine arabinoside syndrome. Med Pediatr Oncol 1981;9:257.

115. Rassiga AL, Schwartz HJ, Forman WB, et al. Cytarabine-induced anaphylaxis: demonstration of antibody and successful desensitization. Arch Intern Med 1980;140:425.

116. Flynn TC, Harris TJ, Murphy GF, et al. Neutrophilic eccrine hidradenitis: a distinctive rash associated with cytarabine therapy and acute leukemia. J Am Acad Dermatol 1984;11:584.

117. Reykdal S, Sham R, Kouides P. Cytarabine-induced pericarditis: a case report and review of the literature of the cardio-pulmonary complications of cytarabine. Leuk Res 1995;19:141.

118. Eden OB, Goldie W, Wood T, et al. Seizures following intrathecal cytosine arabinoside in young children with acute lymphoblastic leukemia. Cancer 1978;42:53.

119. Kleinschmidt-DeMasters BK, Yeh M. "Locked-in syndrome" after intrathecal cytosine arabinoside therapy for malignant immunoblastic lymphoma. Cancer 1992;70:2504.

120. Dixon RL, Adamson RH. Antitumor activity and pharmacologic disposition of cytosine arabinoside (NSC 63878). Cancer Chemother Rep 1965;48:11.

121. Schabel FM Jr. In vivo leukemic cell kill kinetics and curability in experimental systems. In: The Proliferation and Spread of Neoplastic Cells. Baltimore, MD: Williams & Wilkins, 1968:379.

122. Kern DH, Morgan CR, Hildebrand-Zanki SU. In vitro pharmacodynamics of 1-β-D-arabinofuranosylcytosine: synergy of antitumor activity with cis-diamminedichloroplatinum(II). Cancer Res 1988;48:117.

123. Burchenal JH, Dollinger MR. Cytosine arabinoside in combination with 6-mercaptopurine, methotrexate, or fluorouracil in L1210 mouse leukemia. Cancer Chemother Rep 1967;51:435.

124. Chresta CM, Hicks R, Hartley JA, et al. Potentiation of etoposide-induced cytotoxicity and DNA damage in CCRF-CEM cells by pretreatment with non-cytotoxic concentrations of arabinosyl cytosine. Cancer Chemother Pharmacol 1992;31:139.

125. Swinnen LJ, Barnes DM, Fisher SG, et al. 1-β-D-Arabinofuranosyl-cytosine and hydroxyurea: production of cytotoxic synergy with cis-diamminedichloroplatinum(II) and modifications in platinum-induced DNA interstrand crosslinking. Cancer Res 1989;49:1383.

126. Ho DHW, Carter CJ, Brown NS, et al. Effects of tetrahydrouridine on the uptake and metabolism of 1-β-D-arabinofuranosylcytosine in human normal and leukemic cells. Cancer Res 1980;40:2441.

127. Chabner BA, Hande KR, Drake JC. AraC metabolism: implications for drug resistance and drug interactions. Bull Cancer 1979;66:89.

128. Wong PP, Currie VE, Mackey RW, et al. Phase I evaluation of tetra-hydrouridine combined with cytosine arabinoside. Cancer Treat Rep 1979;63:1245.

129. Rauscher F III, Cadman E. Biochemical and cytokinetic modulation of L1210 and HL-60 cells by hydroxyurea and effect on 1-1-β-D-arabino-furanosylcytosine metabolism and cytotoxicity. Cancer Res 1983;43:2688.

130. Kemena A, Gandhi V, Shewach DS, et al. Inhibition of fludarabine metabolism by arabinosylcytosine during therapy. Cancer Chemother Pharmacol 1992;31:193.

131. Gandhi V, Estey E, Du M, et al. Minimum dose of fludarabine for the maximal modulation of 1-β-D-arabinofuranosylcytosinetriphosphate in human leukemia blasts during therapy. Clin Cancer Res 1997;3:1539.

132. Bakic M, Chan D, Andersson BS, et al. Effect of 1-β-D-arabinofuranosylcy-tosine on nuclear topoisomerase II activity and on the DNA cleavage and cytotoxicity produced by 4'-(9-acridinylamino)methanesulfon-m-anisidide and etoposide in m-AMSA-sensitive and -resistant human leukemia cells. Biochem Pharmacol 1987;36:4067.

133. Karp JE, Burke PJ, Donehower RC. Effects of rhGM-CSF on intracellular araC pharmacology in vitro in acute myelocytic leukemia: comparability with drug-induced humoral stimulatory activity. Leukemia 1990;4:553.

134. Stone RM, Berg DT, George SL, et al. Granulocyte-macrophage colony-stimulating factor after initial chemotherapy for elderly patients with primary acute myelogenous leukemia. N Engl J Med 1995;332(25):1671–1677.

135. Stone RM. How I treat patients with myelodysplastic syndromes. Blood 2009;113:6296–6303.

136. Christman JK. 5-Azacytidine and 5-aza-2'-deoxycytidine as inhibitors of DNA methylation: mechanistic studies and their implications for cancer therapy. Oncogene 2002;21:5483–5495.

137. Momparler RL, Onetto-Pothier N, Momparler LF. Comparison of the anti-leukemic activity of cytosine arabinoside and 5-aza-2'-deoxycytidine against human leukemic cells of different phenotype. Leuk Res 1990;14:755.

138. Richel DJ, Colly LP, Lurvink E, et al. Comparison of the anti-leukemic activity of 5-aza-2'-deoxycytidine and arabinofuranosyl-cytosine arabino-side in rats with myelocytic leukemia. Br J Cancer 1988;58:730.

139. Issa J-P, Kantarjian HM. Targeting DNA methylation. Clin Cancer Res 2009;15:3938.

140. Steensma DP, Baer MR, Slack JL, et al. Multicenter study of decitabine administered daily for 5 days every 4 weeks to adults with myelodysplastic syndromes: the alternative dosing for outpatient treatment (ADOPT) trial. J Clin Oncol 2009;27:3842.

141. Sorm F, Piskala A, Cihak A, et al. 5-Azacytidine, a new highly effective cancerostatic. Experientia 1964;20:202.

142. Hanka LJ, Evans JS, Mason DJ, et al. Microbiological production of 5-azacy-tidine: 1. Production and biological activity. Antimicrob Agents Chemother 1966;6:619.

143. Silverman LR, Demakos EP, Peterson BL, et al. Randomized controlled trial of azacitidine in patients with the myelodysplastic syndrome: a study of the cancer and leukemia group B. J Clin Oncol 2002;20:2429–2440.

144. Galanello R, Stamatoyannopoulos G, Papayannopoulou T. Mechanism of Hb F stimulation by S-stage compounds: in vitro studies with bone marrow cells exposed to 5-azacytidine, araC, or hydroxyurea. J Clin Invest 1988;81:1209.

145. Glover AB, Leyland-Jones B. Biochemistry of azacytidine: a review. Cancer Treat Rep 1987;71:959.

146. Beisler J. Isolation, characterization, and properties of a labile hydro-lysis product of the antitumor nucleoside, 5-azacytidine. J Med Chem 1978;21:204.

147. Notari RE, De Young JL. Kinetics and mechanisms of degradation of the antileukemic agent 5-azacytidine in aqueous solutions. J Pharm Sci 1975;64:1148.

148. Vesely J, Cihak A. 5-Azacytidine: mechanism of action and biological effects in mammalian cells. Pharmacol Ther 1978;2:813.

149. Glazer RI, Peale AL, Beisler JA, et al. The effects of 5-azacytidine and dihydro-5-azacytidine on nucleic ribosomal RNA and poly(A) RNA synthesis in L1210 cells in vitro. Mol Pharmacol 1980;17:111.

150. Weiss JW, Pitot HC. Inhibition of ribosomal precursor RNA maturation by 5-azacytidine and 8-azaguanine in Novikoff hepatoma cells. Arch Biochem Biophys 1974;165:588.

151. Lee T, Karon MR. Inhibition of protein synthesis in 5-azacytidine-treated HeLa cells. Biochem Pharmacol 1976;25:1737.

152. Kalousek F, Raska K, Jurovik M, et al. Effect of 5-azacytidine on the acceptor activity of sRNA. Coll Czech Chem Commun 1966;31:1421.

153. Cihak A, Vesela H, Sorm F. Thymidine kinase and polyribosomal distribution in regenerating rat liver following 5-azacytidine. Biochim Biophys Acta 1968;166:277.

154. Cihak A, Vesely J. Prolongation of the lag period preceding the enhancement of thymidine and thymidylate kinase activity in regenerating rat liver by 5-azacytidine. Biochem Pharmacol 1972;21:3257.

155. Plagemann PGW, Behrens M, Abraham D. Metabolism and cytotoxicity of 5-azacytidine in cultured Novikoff rat hepatoma and P388 mouse leukemia cells and their enhancement by preincubation with pyrazofurin. Cancer Res 1978;38:2458.

156. Jones PA, Taylor SM, Wilson V. DNA modification, differentiation, and transformation. J Exp Zool 1983;228:287.

157. Issa JP. CpG island methylator phenotype in cancer. Nat Rev Cancer 2004;4:988.

158. Yang B, House MG, Guo M, et al. Promoter methylation profiles of tumor suppressor genes in intrahepatic and extrahepatic cholangiocarcinoma. Mod Pathol 2005;18:412.

159. Daskalakis M, Nguyen TT, Nguyen C, et al. Demethylation of a hyperm-ethylated P15/INK4B gene in patients with myelodysplastic syndrome by 5-Aza-2'-deoxycytidine (decitabine) treatment. Blood 2002;100:2957.

160. Barletta JM, Rainier S, Feinberg AP. Reversal of loss of imprinting in tumor cells by 5-aza-2'-deoxycytidine. Cancer Res 1997;57:48.

161. Cameron EE, Bachman KE, Myohanen S, et al. Synergy of demethylation and histone deacetylase inhibition in the re-expression of genes silenced in cancer. Nat Genet 1999;21:103.

162. Streisemann C, Lyko F. Modes of action of the DNA methyltransferase inhibitors azacytidine and decitabine. Int J Cancer 2008;123:8–13.

163. Drake JC, Stoller RG, Chabner BA. Characteristics of the enzyme uridine-cytidine kinase isolated from a cultured human cell line. Biochem Pharmacol 1977;26:64.

164. Vadlamudi S, Padarathsingh M, Bonmassar E, et al. Reduction of antileukemic and immunosuppressive activities of 5-azacytidine in mice by concurrent treatment with uridine. Proc Soc Exp Biol Med 1970;133:1232.

165. Vesely J, Cihak A, Sorm F. Biochemical mechanisms of drug resistance: IV. Development of resistance to 5-azacytidine and simultaneous depression of pyrimidine metabolism in leukemic mice. Int J Cancer 1967;2:639.

166. Adams RL, Burdon RH. DNA methylation in eukaryotes. Crit Rev Biochem 1992;13:349.

167. Cihak A, Lamar C, Pitot HC. Studies on the mechanism of the stimulation of tyrosine aminotransferase activity in vivo by pyrimidine analogs: the role of enzyme synthesis and degradation. Arch Biochem Biophys 1973; 156:176.

168. Stallings RL, Crawford BD, Tobey RA, et al. 5-Azacytidine-induced conversion to cadmium resistance correlated with early S phase replication of inactive metallothionein genes in synchronized CHO cells. Somat Cell Mol Genet 1986;12:423.

169. Bonal FJ, Pareja E, Martin J, et al. Repression of class I H-2K, H-2D antigens or GR9 methylcholanthrene-induced tumour cell clones is related to the level of DNA methylation. J Immunogenet 1986;13:179.

170. Richardson B, Kahl L, Lovett EJ, et al. Effect of an inhibitor of DNA methylation on T cells: I. 5-Azacytidine induces T4 expression on T8+ T cells. J Immunol 1986;137:35.

171. Liteplo RG, Alvarez E, Frost P, et al. Induction of thymidine kinase activity in a spontaneously enzyme-deficient murine tumor cell line by exposure in vivo to the DNA-hypomethylating agent 5-aza-2′-deoxycytidine: implications for mechanisms of tumor progression. Cancer Res 1985;45:5294.

172. Jones PA, Taylor SM, Mohandas T, et al. Cell cycle-specific reactivation of an inactive X-chromosome locus by 5-azadeoxycytidine. Proc Natl Acad Sci U S A 1982;79:1215.

173. Jeggo PA, Holliday R. Azacytidine-induced reactivation of a DNA repair gene in Chinese hamster ovary cells. Mol Cell Biol 1986;6:2944.

174. Holliday R. Strong effects of 5-azacytidine on the in vitro lifespan of human diploid fibroblasts. Exp Cell Res 1986;166:543.

175. Karon M, Benedict W. Chromatid breakage: differential effect of inhibitors of DNA synthesis during G_2 phase. Science 1972;178:62.

176. Seifertova M, Vesely J, Cihak A. Enhanced mortality in offspring of male mice treated with 5-azacytidine prior to mating: morphological changes in testes. Neoplasma 1976;23:53.

177. Zhao M, Rudek MA, He P, et al. Quantification of 5-azacytidine in plasma by electrospray tandem mass spectrometry coupled with high-performance liquid chromatography. J Chromatogr B Analyt Technol Biomed Life Sci 2004;813:81.

178. Marcucci G, Silvermann L, Eller M, et al. Bioavailability of azacitidine subcutaneous versus intravenous in patients with the myelodysplastic syndromes. J Clin Pharmacol 2005;45:597.

179. Chan KK, Staroscik JA, Sadee W. Synthesis of 5-azacytidine-6-³C and -6-¹⁴C. J Med Chem 1977;20:598.

180. Troetel WM, Weiss AJ, Stambaugh JE, et al. Absorption, distribution, and excretion of 5-azacytidine (NSC-102816) in man. Cancer Chemother Rep 1972;56:405.

181. Tsao CF, Dalal J, Peters C, et al. Azacitidine pharmacokinetics in an adolescent patient with renal compromise. J Pediatr Hematol Oncol 2007;29:330.

182. Israili ZH, Vogler WR, Mingioli ES, et al. The disposition and pharmacokinetics in humans of 5-azacytidine administered intravenously as a bolus or by continuous infusion. Cancer Res 1976;36:1453.

183. Chabner BA, Drake JC, Johns DC. Deamination of 5-azacytidine by a human leukemia cell cytidine deaminase. Biochem Pharmacol 1973;22:2763.

184. Vogler WR, Miller DS, Keller JW. 5-Azacytidine (NSC-102816): a new drug for the treatment of myeloblastic leukemia. Blood 1976;48:331.

185. Bellet RE, Mastrangelo MJ, Engstrom PF, et al. Hepatotoxicity of 5-azacytidine (NSC-102816): a clinical and pathologic study. Neoplasma 1973;20:303.

186. Levi J, Wiernik P. A comparative clinical trial of 5-azacytidine and guanazole in previously treated adults with acute nonlymphocytic leukemia. Cancer 1976;38:36.

187. Kaminskas E, Farrell AT, Wang YC, et al. FDA Drug approval summary: azacytidine (5 azacytidine, Vidaza™) for injectable suspension. Oncologist 2005;10:176–182.

188. Wijermans P, Lubbert M, Verhoef G, et al. Low-dose 5-aza-2′-deoxycytidine, a DNA hypomethylating agent, for the treatment of high-risk myelodysplastic syndrome: a multicenter phase II study in elderly patients. J Clin Oncol 2000;18:956–962.

189. Burris HA III, Moore MJ, Andersen J, et al. Improvements in survival and clinical benefit with gemcitabine as first-line therapy for patients with advanced pancreas cancer: a randomized trial. J Clin Oncol 1997;15:2403.

190. von der Maase H, Hansen SW, Robert JT, et al. Gemcitabine and cisplatin versus methotrexate, vinblastine, doxorubicin, and cisplatin in advanced or metastatic bladder cancer: results of a large, randomized, multinational, multicenter phase III study. J Clin Oncol 2000;18:3068–3077.

191. Schiller JH, Harrington D, Belani CP, et al. Comparison of four chemotherapy regimens for advanced non-small cell lung cancer. N Engl J Med 2002;346:92–98.

192. Hertel LW, Boder GB, Kroin JS, et al. Evaluation of the antitumor activity of gemcitabine (2′,2′-difluoro-2′-deoxycytidine). Cancer Res 1990;50:4417.

193. Bouffard DY, Laliberte J, Momparler RL. Comparison of antineoplastic activity of 2-2-difluoro-2-deoxycytidine and cytosine arabinoside against human myeloid and lymphoid leukemic cells. Anticancer Drugs 1991;2:49.

194. Mackey JR, Mani RS, Selner M, et al. Functional nucleoside transporters are required for gemcitabine influx and manifestation of toxicity in cancer cell lines. Cancer Res 1998;58:4349.

195. Heinemann V, Hertel LW, Grindey GB, et al. Comparison of the cellular pharmacokinetics and toxicity of 2′,2′-difluorodeoxycytidine and 1-beta-D-arabinofuranosylcytosine. Cancer Res 1988;48:4024.

196. Bouffard DY, Laliberte J, Momparler RL. Kinetic studies on 2′,2′-difluorodeoxycytidine (gemcitabine) with purified human deoxycytidine kinase and cytidine deaminase. Biochem Pharmacol 1993;45:1857.

197. Heinemann V, Xu YZ, Chubb S, et al. Cellular elimination of 2′,2′-difluorodeoxycytidine 5′-triphosphate: a mechanism of self-potentiation. Cancer Res 1992;52:533.

198. Gandhi V, Plunkett W. Modulatory activity of 2′,2′-difluorodeoxycytidine on the phosphorylation and cytotoxicity of arabinosyl nucleosides. Cancer Res 1990;50:3675.

199. Rockwell S, Grindey GB. Effect of 2′,2′-difluorodeoxycytidine on the viability and radiosensitivity of EMT6 cells in vitro. Oncol Res 1992; 4:151.

200. Heinemann V, Xu YZ, Chubb S, et al. Inhibition of ribonucleotide reduction in CCRF-CEM cells by 2′,2′-difluorodeoxycytidine. Mol Pharmacol 1990;38:567.

201. Wang J, Lohman GJS, Stubbe J. Enhanced subunit interactions with gemcitabine-5′-diphosphate inhibit ribonucleotide reductase. PNAS 2007;104:14323–14329.

202. Huang P, Chubb S, Hertel LW, et al. Action of 2′,2′-difluorodeoxycytidine on DNA synthesis. Cancer Res 1991;51:6110.

203. Gandhi V, Legha J, Chen F, et al. Excision of 2′,2′-difluorodeoxycytidine (gemcitabine) monophosphate residues from DNA. Cancer Res 1996;56:4453.

204. Huang P, Plunkett W. Fludarabine- and gemcitabine-induced apoptosis: incorporation of analogs into DNA is a critical event. Cancer Chemother Pharmacol 1995;36:181.

205. Cory AH, Hertel LW, Kroin JS, et al. Effects of 2′,2′-difluorodeoxycytidine (gemcitabine) on wild type and variant mouse leukemia L1210 cells. Oncol Res 1993;5:59.

206. Goan YG, Zhou B, Hu E, et al. Overexpression of ribonucleotide reductase as a mechanism of resistance to 2′,2′-difluorodeoxycytidine in human KB cancer line. Cancer Res 1999;59:4204.

207. Van Moorsel CJ, Pinedo HM, Veerman G, et al. Mechanisms of synergism between cisplatin and gemcitabine in ovarian and non-small-cell cancer cell lines. Br J Cancer 1999;80:981.

208. Lang LY, Li L, Jiang H, et al. Expression of ERCC1 Antisense RNA abrogates gemcitabine-mediated cytotoxic synergism with cisplatin in human colon tumor cells defective in mismatch repair but proficient in nucleotide excision repair. Clin Cancer Res 2000;6:773.

if they are homozygous for a variant TMPT gene and 65% if they are heterozygous.[28]

Several studies,[29,30] but not all,[16] have suggested that children with high TPMT activity are at greater risk of disease relapse as a result of decreased drug activation. In a large Scandinavian study in children with ALL, the risk of relapse following therapy was 18% for patients with wild type TPMT versus 6% for patients heterozygous or deficient in TMPT activity ($P = 0.03$).[31] Despite a lower probability of relapse, patients with low TPMT activity did not have superior survival ($P = 0.08$), perhaps due to an increased rate of drug toxicity including the development of secondary malignancies.

While screening for TMPT variants with decreased enzymatic activity identifies individuals at risk for mercaptopurine toxicity, the association is not perfect. Toxicity still occurs in individuals with wild-type TMPT. Individuals heterozygous for TPMT*2, *3A and *3C can have a wide range of TPMT activity. Mercaptopurine metabolism is not dependent on a single gene (Fig. 11-2). Inosine triphosphate pyrophosphatase (ITPA) catalyzes the hydrolysis of inosine triphosphate (ITP) to inosine monophosphate which protects cells from the accumulation of potentially harmful nucleotides. A polymorphism in the ITPA gene occurring in roughly 10% of individuals results in a 25% decrease in enzyme activity in heterozygous individuals.[32] ITPA inactivates the potentially toxic thioinosine triphosphate metabolite from patients receiving mercaptopurine or azathioprine (Fig. 11-2). In children with ALL who have had their mercaptopurine dose adjusted based on TMPT phenotype, the ITPA mutant allele has been associated with an increase incidence of febrile neutropenia[33] and myelosuppression.[34] However, an association of ITPA polymorphism with drug toxicity has not been seen in all studies.[32]

6-Thioguanine

6-TG is available as 40-mg tablets for oral use. An intravenous preparation is investigational. As with 6-MP, the absorption of 6-TG in humans is variable and incomplete (mean bioavailability is 30%; range: 14% to 46%).[35] Peak plasma levels of 0.03 to 5 μM occur 2 to 4 hours after ingestion; the median drug half-life is 90 minutes but with wide variability reported.[36] Intravenously administered 6-TG has been evaluated. Clearance of drug (600 to 1,000 mL/min/m^2) appears to be dose dependent, suggesting saturation of clearance at doses over 10 mg/m^2/h.[37] Plasma concentrations of 4 to 10 μM can be achieved.

The catabolism of 6-TG differs from that of 6-MP. Thioguanine is not a substrate for xanthine oxidase. Thioguanine is converted to 6-thioinosine (an inactive metabolite) by the action of the enzyme, guanase. Because thioguanine inactivation does not depend on the action of xanthine oxidase, allopurinol will not block the detoxification of thioguanine. In humans, methylation of thioguanine, via TPMT, is more extensive than methylation of 6-MP. The product of methylation, 2-amino-6-methylthiopurine, is substantially less active and less toxic than thioguanine.

Azathioprine

Azathioprine is a prodrug of mercaptopurine. About 90% of an administered dose of azathioprine is non-enzymatically converted to 6-MP by sulfhydryl-containing compounds such as glutathione or cysteine. The metabolic pathways following conversion to mercaptopurine are identical to those just described for 6-MP.[38] In transplant patients taking 2 mg/kg/d azathioprine, peak 6-MP plasma concentrations ($T_{max} < 2$ hours) are low (75 ng/mL) and plasma drug half-life is short (1.9 hours).[39] Plasma 6-MP concentrations exceed those of azathioprine within an hour of drug administration. Loss of renal function does not alter the plasma kinetics of either azathioprine or 6-MP. 6-MP was not detected in significant quantities in breast milk of women taking azathioprine and plasma concentrations of thiopurine metabolites were not found in infants breast-fed by women taking azathioprine.[40]

Toxicity

6-Mercaptopurine

The dose-limiting toxicity of 6-MP is myelosuppression, occurring 1 to 4 weeks following the onset of therapy and reversible when the drug is discontinued. Platelets, granulocytes, and erythrocytes are all affected. Weekly monitoring of blood counts during the first 2 months of therapy is recommended. Myelosuppression following 6-MP therapy is related to TPMT phenotype. Most patients (65%) with excessive toxicity following 6-MP or azathioprine administration have TMPT deficiency or heterozygosity.[41]

6-MP is an immunosuppressant. Immunity to infectious agents or vaccines is subnormal in patients receiving 6-MP. Gastrointestinal mucositis and stomatitis are modest. Approximately one quarter of treated patients experienced nausea, vomiting, and anorexia. Gastrointestinal side effects appear to be more common in adults than in children. Pancreatitis is seen in 3% of patients with long-term therapy, with rash, fever, or joints pains seen in 2%.[41] Three types of hepatotoxicity can bee seen with thiopurine therapy.[42] A small percentage of patients have transient, asymptomatic elevation in transaminases, which return to normal with follow-up and do not require dose alterations. Thiopurines may induce a several cholestatic jaundice that may not regress. Thiopurine therapy should be discontinued in this situation. Thiopurines may cause endothelial cell injury with raised portal pressures (VOD or veno-occlusive disease). The development of hepatotoxicity, in contrast to myelosuppression, is not associated with TPMT polymorphisms[43] but is correlated with the dose of 6-MP given and with the formation of methylated metabolites of 6-MP (but not with 6-TG nucleotide formation).[44]

At very high doses (>1,000 mg/m^2), the limited solubility of 6-MP can cause precipitation of drug in the renal tubules with hematuria and crystalluria.[45] Thioguanine therapy does not appear to markedly increase a patient's rates of developing a second malignancy.[46] However, an increased risk of myelodysplastic syndrome or AML was found in children treated with mercaptopurine for ALL who had reduced TMPT activity.[47]

Thioguanine

As with 6-MP, the primary toxicity of 6-TG is myelosuppression.[48] Blood counts should be frequently monitored because there may be a delayed effect during oral drug administration. Higher doses result in mucositis. Thioguanine produces gastrointestinal toxicities similar to 6-MP but less frequently. Jaundice and hepatic VOD have been reported more frequently (11% incidence) with 6-TG than with mercaptopurine or azathioprine.[49,50] At present, 6-TG should be used only as second-line thiopurine therapy. There is suggestive data that VOD may be caused by the formation of methylmercaptopurine nucletides.[51]

Azathioprine

Adverse effects from azathioprine are similar to those seen with 6-MP. These effects include leukopenia, diarrhea, nausea, abnormal liver function tests, and skin rashes. Frequent monitoring of the complete blood count is warranted throughout therapy (weekly during the first 8 weeks of therapy). Molecular testing for TMPT may be a cost-effective way of identifying the 10% of the population at high risk for toxicity.[32]

A hypersensitivity reaction, generally characterized by fever, chills, severe nausea, diarrhea, hypertension, and hepatic dysfunction, has been reported.[52] The mechanism for the hypersensitivity reaction is unclear. Chronic azathioprine therapy results in a 3% per patient-year incidence of myelotoxicity (1% severe). The cumulative risk of infectious complications among azathioprine myelosuppressed patients is 6.5%.[53] Patients homozygous and heterozygous for mutant TPMT are at high risk for toxicity and dose modification.[54]

Use and Drug Interactions

6-MP is a standard component of maintenance therapy for ALL. It has little role in therapy of solid tumors or remission induction in myeloid leukemias. 6-MP is also used to treat inflammatory bowel disease. 6-TG should be used only rarely as second- or third-line therapy for leukemias and lymphomas given its greater incidence of hepatic toxicity. Azathioprine is used as an immunosuppressant in preventing rejection of organ transplants and in the therapy of illnesses believed autoimmune in character (such as lupus, rheumatoid arthritis, and ulcerative colitis). Thiopurines are considered the standard of care for the treatment of Crohn's disease.

As previously mentioned, allopurinol inhibits the catabolism of 6-MP and increases its bioavailability.[17] Oral doses of 6-MP and azathioprine should be reduced by at least 75% in patients also receiving allopurinol. Combined use of standard dose azathioprine (or 6-MP) with allopurinol will result in life-threatening toxicity.[55] Methotrexate causes a modest increase in 6-MP bioavailability but not to an extent significant enough to warrant dosage reduction.[15] Methotrexate increases 6-MP plasma concentrations slightly but antagonizes thiopurine metabolite disposition in leukemia blasts resulting in lower thioguanine nucleotide incorporation.[56] Olsalazine, mesalazine, and sulfasalazine are inhibitors of TPMT and can increase the toxicity of mercaptopurine or azathioprine.[57] Other agents including furosemide and various nonsteroidal anti-inflammatory agents can inhibit TPMT in vitro but the clinical importance of this finding remains unclear.

Adenosine Analogs

Adenosine analogs with documented clinical utility are fludarabine, pentostatin, cladribine (2′-chlorodeoxyadenosine), and clofarabine (Fig. 11-3). Key pharmacologic features of the adenosine analogs are listed in Tables 11-4 to 11-7. Adenosine arabinoside is cytotoxic in vitro but in man is quickly inactivated by the enzyme adenosine deaminase (ADA). Substitution of a halogen (fluorine in fludarabine or chlorine in cladribine) at the two position of deoxyadenosine produces molecules which are resistant to the action of ADA.

Fludarabine (Fludara)

Fludarabine (or 9-β-D-arabinofuranosyl-2-fluoroadenine monophosphate) is a monophosphate analog of adenosine arabinoside (Fig. 11-3). The monophosphate moiety results in aqueous solubility allowing intravenous administration.[58] Key features of fludarabine are summarized in Table 11-4.

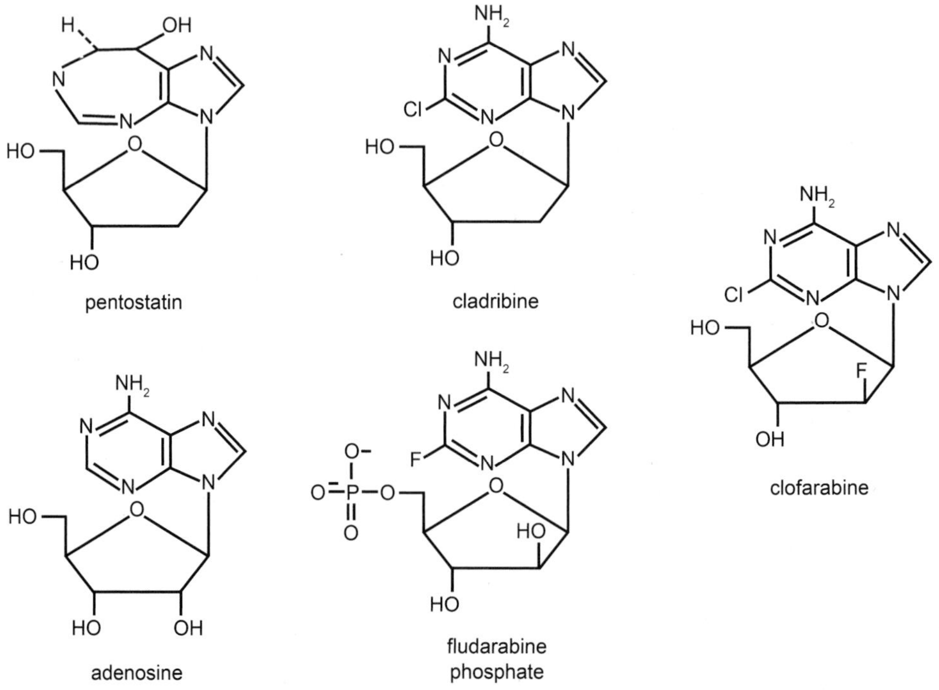

FIGURE **11-3** • Chemical structure of adenosine analogs.

TABLE **11.5**	*Key features of pentostatin*
Factor	**Result**
Mechanism of action	1. Inhibits ADA with subsequent accumulation of dATP pools, which inhibit ribonucleotide reductase and DNA methylation 2. Inhibition of DNA replication and repair by dATP
Metabolism	Minimal
Pharmacokinetics	Clearance rate of 8 mL/min/m², which decreases with decreasing creatinine clearance
Elimination	Majority of drug is excreted unchanged in the urine.
Drug interactions	Increased risk of pulmonary toxicity when continued with fludarabine
Toxicity	1. Well tolerated at low doses 2. At higher doses; nausea, immunosuppression, nephrotoxicity and CNS disturbances
Precautions	Dose reductions for patients with renal failure

mechanisms are relevant to proliferating cells. The mechanism of action of pentostatin on nonproliferating cells is unclear.

Pentostatin enters cells via the nucleoside transport system[88] with a rate of cellular uptake that parallels that of other nucleosides. Pentostatin exerts tight-binding inhibition of ADA.[86] Pentostatin was originally postulated to be more effective in T-cell lymphocytic tumors with high ADA levels. However, pentostatin has subsequently shown activity in both T- and B-cell lymphocytic neoplasms. The antineoplastic activity appears to depend, to a certain extent, on the intracellular ADA concentration of the neoplasm. In indolent lymphoid neoplasms in which cellular ADA levels are lower, ADA can be inhibited at pentostatin concentrations, which are low and produce minimal systemic side effects.[89]

Clinical Pharmacology

Pentostatin is reasonably stable at neutral pH; however, care must be taken if the drug is extensively diluted with 5% dextrose in water as pentostatin's stability is compromised at pH $\leq$ 5.[90] Pentostatin has a large volume of distribution with little protein binding.[91] The terminal elimination half-life averages 6 hours.[92,93] Plasma levels of pentostatin 1 hour after administration exceed the ADA inhibitory concentration by approximately 10⁶, supporting the recommendation for an intermittent infusion schedule. Only a small amount of pentostatin is metabolized; 40% to 80% of the drug is excreted in urine unchanged within 24 hours.[92,93] In patients with impaired renal function (creatinine clearance < 60 mL/min), drug half-life is prolonged (~18 hours). Dose reductions are suggested for patients with renal function impairment. Patients with a creatinine

clearance greater than 60 mL/min should receive a dose of 4 mg/m² every 14 days, patients with Cl_{cr} of 41 to 60 mL/min should receive 3 mg/m² every 2 weeks, and patients with a Cl_{cr} of 20 to 40 mL/min should receive a 2 mg/m² dose every 14 days.[94] Pentostatin is not orally bioavailable. Pentostatin crosses the blood-brain barrier with CSF concentrations 10% to 13% of serum drug concentrations.[95]

Toxicity

At commonly used doses (4 mg/m² every 2 weeks), pentostatin toxicity is modest and therapy is usually well tolerated.[96] In a large intergroup trial of 313 patients, grade 3 to 4 toxicity was uncommon.[97] Twenty-two percent of patients treated at 4 mg/m² every 2 weeks develop grade 3 to 4 neutropenia. Nausea and vomiting (>grade 3) occur in 11% of patients. The most common nonmyelosuppressive drug toxicity is nausea (11% of patients at standard doses). Nausea and vomiting may be delayed (12 to 72 hours after administration). Mild-to-moderate lethargy (3% incidence), rash, and reactivation of herpes zoster have been reported. Toxicity from higher doses of pentostatin ($\geq$10 mg/m²/d) includes immunosuppression, conjunctivitis, renal impairment, hepatic enzyme elevation, and central nervous system disturbances.[95] Renal toxicity seen in early trials is minimized with the use of lower drug doses and adequate hydration. Nephrotoxicity occurs 10 to 20 days after drug administration. Cardiac complications in older patients have been described but appear to be uncommon.[98] Patients with poor performance status or impaired renal function have a higher incidence of life-threatening toxicity. An increased risk of opportunistic infections is seen.[99] Initial concerns regarding an increased risk of second malignancies following use of pentostatin have not been confirmed.[100]

Clinical Use

Pentostatin, delivered in low doses, produces responses in over 90% of patients with hairy-cell leukemia with estimated disease-free survival at 5 and 10 years in over 85% and 65%, respectively.[100] Pentostatin has also been shown to produce responses in a number of other closely related disorders, including B-cell CLL, Waldenstrom's macroglobulinemia, refractory multiple myeloma, and adult T-cell lymphomas.[101] Pentostatin's immunosuppressive effects have been used to treat graft versus host disease developing after stem cell transplantation.[102]

Cladribine or 2-Chlorodeoxyadenosine (Leustatin)

Cladribine or 2-chlorodeoxyadenosine is a purine nucleoside analog with antineoplastic activity against low-grade lymphoproliferative diseases, childhood leukemias, and multiple sclerosis. Its important pharmacologic features are noted in Table 11-6.

Mechanism of Action

Cladribine (2-CdA) (Fig. 11-3) is a prodrug that requires intracellular phosphorylation for activation.[64] The 5'-triphosphate metabolite (2-chloro-2'-deoxyadenosine 5-triphosphate [2-CdATP]) accumulates in cells rich in deoxycytidine kinase[103] (Fig. 11-5). 2-CdATP is incorporated into DNA, producing DNA strand breaks and inhibition of DNA synthesis.[104] Cladribine, incorporated into DNA promoter sequences, acts as a transcription antagonist.[105] High

<table>
<tr><td colspan="2">TABLE
11.6 *Key features of cladribine
(2-chlorodeoxyadenosine)*</td></tr>
</table>

Factor	Result
Mechanism of action	1. Incorporated into DNA as a false nucleotide resulting in DNA stand breaks 2. Inhibits DNA polymerase 3. Inhibits ribonucleotide reductase
Metabolism	Activation to 2-CdATP within cells
Pharmacokinetics	1. Significant variability in cladribine plasma AUC 2. 40%–50% oral bioavailability 3. 50% urinary excretion
Drug interactions	Increase toxicity of cytarabine Rash when used with allopurinol
Toxicity	1. Myelosuppression 2. Fever 3. Immunosuppression with resulting infection complications 4. Rash

intracellular concentrations of 2-CdATP also inhibit DNA polymerases[106] and ribonucleotide reductase,[61] causing an imbalance in deoxyribonucleotide triphosphate pools with subsequent impairment of DNA synthesis and repair.

The mechanism for triggering apoptosis in nondividing cells by 2-CdATP is not clear. Cysteine proteases, referred to as caspases, are activated by cladribine.[107] 2-CdATP interacts with cytochrome C and protease activating factor-1 (PAF-1) to initiate the caspase cascade leading to DNA degradation, even in the absence of cell division.[108] Cladribine resistance can result from deficiency in deoxycytidine kinase[109] (the initial enzyme in the activation pathway) and p53 mutations.[110]

Clinical Pharmacology

Liquid chromatography is used to determine plasma concentrations of cladribine and its primary metabolite, 2-chlorodeoxyadenosine.[111] Cladribine is a prodrug. It is activated within the cell to cladribine nucleotides. Cladribine nucleotides are retained in leukemic cells with an intracellular half-life of 9 to 30 hours. Intracellular concentrations are 100-fold higher than plasma concentrations.[112] The AUC for active intracellular cladribine nucleotide is similar for continuous infusion and intermittent dosing. The long intracellular nucleotide half-life supports the use of intermittent drug administration.[113] Unfortunately, no correlations have been found between the plasma AUC of cladribine or intracellular cladribine concentrations and the response to treatment.[114]

Following a 2-hour infusion of 0.12 mg/kg cladribine, peak serum concentrations of roughly 100 nM are achieved.[113] A linear dose-concentration relationship is present up to doses of 2.5 mg/m²/h. Cladribine clearance rates of 664 to 978 mL/h/kg have been reported with significant interpatient variability (±50%). The drug is weakly bound to plasma protein (20%). Renal clearance accounts for 50% of total drug clearance, with 20% to 30% of drug excreted as unchanged cladribine within the first 24 hours.[113,115] Little information is available regarding dose adjustments for renal or hepatic insufficiency. However, given the high renal drug clearance, caution should be taken in using cladribine in patients with renal failure. Chloroadenine is the major metabolite formed. Renal excretion of chloroadenine accounts for clearance of 3% of administered cladribine.[113]

Bioavailability of subcutaneously administered cladribine is excellent (100%).[116] An oral preparation has been evaluated with bioavailability of 40% to 50%. Increased metabolism to chloroadenine is seen following oral administration suggesting a first-pass effect.[111,116] Significant patient-to-patient variability (±28%) exists in the AUC achieved following administration of drug by any method.[113,115] Oral drug is not yet FDA approved. FDA approval is for intravenous drug administration, but several studies suggest that the subcutaneous administration of 3.4 mg/m²/d for 7 days is equivalent to intravenous administration of 0.1 mg/kg/d for 7 days.[117] A single subcutaneous dose of 0.25 mg/kg was found ineffective.[118] Cladribine penetrates the blood-brain barrier, and CSF concentrations are 25% of plasma cladribine concentrations.[118]

Toxicity

The primary toxicity using a standard dosage of 0.7 mg/kg/cycle of cladribine (usually as a continuous 7-day infusion at 0.1 mg/m²/d) is myelosuppression.[119] Nausea, alopecia, hepatic and renal toxicity rarely occur at this dose. Fever (temperature > 100°F) is seen in two thirds of patients treated with cladribine, mostly during the period of neutropenia but may occur without neutropenia. Only

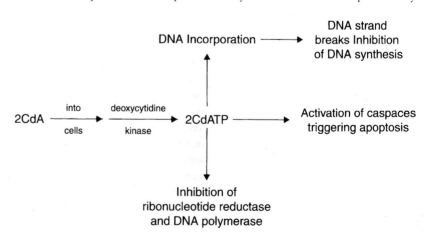

Figure **11–5** Activation of cladribine (2-chorodeoxyadenosine or 2 CdA).

10% to 15% of febrile patients will have documented infections. Myelosuppression and immunosuppression with development of opportunistic infections are the major adverse events.[99] Grade 3 to 4 neutropenia and lymphopenia occur in half of treated patients. Neutrophil counts decrease 1 to 2 weeks after starting therapy and persist for 3 to 4 weeks.[120] Twenty percent of patients develop grade 3 to 4 thrombocytopenia. Infections occur in 15% to 40% of patients, often opportunistic infections, such as *Candida* or *Aspergillus*.[121] Betticher et al.[121] have found that reducing the dose of 2CdA from 0.7 to 0.5 mg/kg/cycle decreases the grade 3 myelosuppression rate (33% to 8%) and the infection rate (30% to 7%) without a change in response rate. A weekly schedule of 0.12 mg/kg CdA has been evaluated.[122] Response rates and toxicities were not different from a daily × 5 schedule given for 1 week. Toxicities other than myelosuppression and infections are rare but have been reported. Following high dose 2-CdA (five to ten times the recommended therapeutic dose), renal failure, and motor weakness has been described. Autoimmune hemolytic anemia, eosinophilia, nausea, and fatigue have been reported.

Clinical Use and Drug Interactions

Cladribine's spectrum of activity is similar to that of other adenosine analogs. It has become the treatment of choice for patients with hairy cell leukemia due to the high remission rate and long-term survival of patient treated with cladribine.[123] Patients with CLL, low-grade non-Hodgkin's lymphomas, cutaneous T-cell lymphoma, Waldenstrom's macroglobulinemia, mantle cell lymphoma, mastocytosis, and blast-phase chronic myelogenous leukemia have responded to cladribine therapy.[124,125] A drug-drug interaction between cladribine and cytarabine has been reported. Pretreatment of patients with cladribine increases the intracellular accumulation of ara-CTP, the active metabolite of cytarabine, by 40%.[126] An increased frequency of drug rash has been noted when cladribine and allopurinol have been used concomitantly.[127]

Clofarabine (Clolar)

Clorfarabine was synthesized in a search for new 2-halo-2′-halo-deoxyarabinofuranosyl adenine analogs with potentially better activity than fludarabine or cladribine.[128] Clofarabine (Fig. 11-3) retains the 2-chloroadenine aglycone of cladribine making it resistant to inactivation by ADA. It also has a fluorine at the 2′ position of the carbohydrate in the arabinosyl configuration, which is thought essential to the DNA activity of the compound. The substitution of the fluorine at the C-2′ position decreases phosphorolytic cleavage by purine nucleoside phosphorylase (PNP) to one third that of fludarabine and cladribine.[129] The key features of clofarabine are summarized in Table 11-7.

Mechanism of Action

Following cellular uptake, clofarabine must be converted to the 5′ triphosphate metabolite, in a manner similar to fludarabine and cladribine (Figs. 11-4 and 11-5). Clofarabine is a better substrate for deoxycytidine kinase than either fludarabine or cladribine.[129] The triphosphate form of clofarabine inhibits DNA synthesis and repair. Clofarabine triphosphate is incorporated into DNA, inhibits

TABLE 11-7	Key features of clofarabine
Factor	Result
Mechanism of action	1. Triphosphate metabolites are incorporated into DNA, inhibiting DNA primer extension. 2. Inhibits ribonucleotide reductase lowering deoxynucleotide pools needed for DNA synthesis
Metabolism	Activation to triphosphate metabolite within cells
Pharmacokinetics	50%–60% renal excretion
Drug interactions	Increases toxicity of cytarabine
Toxicity	1. Myelosuppression 2. Infections 3. Elevated liver function tests 4. Rash

ribonucleotide reductase, inhibits DNA polymerases, depletes intracellular deoxynucleotides, and inhibits elongation of DNA strands.[130,131] Clofarabine and fludarabine are superior to cladribine as inhibitors of DNA polymerases. Clofarabine can induce cellular apoptosis via induction of mitochondrial damage, an effect not seen with fludarabine.[132]

Clinical Pharmacology

Clofarabine has been most commonly administered at doses of 2 to 40 mg/m² for 5 days. The recommended dose for patients with acute myeloid leukemia has been 40 mg/m² for 5 days.[133] Lower doses (2 to 4 mg/m²/d for 5 days) have been used in patients with chronic leukemia or solid tumors.[134] Plasma concentrations of roughly 1.5 μM can be achieved with significant patient-to-patient variability.[134,135] Plasma concentrations appear to be dose proportional.[135] Clofarabine's plasma half-life is about 5 hours, with 50% to 60% of the drug excreted in the urine unchanged. No data are currently available to make recommendations for dosing in patients with renal or hepatic insufficiency. Intracellular clofarabine triphosphate concentrations are similar to those achieved with cladribine and fludarabine with an intracellular half-life of over 24 hours.[134]

Toxicity

The primary toxicity with clofarabine, as with fludarabine and cladribine, is myelosuppression resulting in an increased risk of infectious complications.[134,135] Reversible hepatic transaminase elevation is noted in up to 15% to 25% of patients.[136] Other side effects include nausea, fatigue, edema, and skin rash. In children, febrile neutropenia, anorexia, hypotension, and nausea have been the most commonly reported toxicities.[137]

Clinical Use and Drug Interactions

Clofarabine was approved by the FDA in 2004 for the treatment of pediatric patients with relapsed or refractory ALL following the use of at least two prior therapies. Clofarabine has produced occasional responses in adults with AML and myelodysplastic syndrome.[136] Clofarabine increases the intracellular concentrations of cytosine arabinoside, potentiating ara-C cytotoxicity. The combination of clofarabine and cytarabine, compared to clofarabine alone, improves the response rate in the treatment of AML with similar toxicity.[138]

Nelarabine

Nelarabine, like clofarabine, is a purine analog recently approved (2005) by the FDA. It is indicated for treatment of patients with T-cell acute leukemia (T-ALL) and T-cell lymphoblastic lymphoma (T-LBL) who have not responded to or have relapsed after at least two chemotherapy regimens. The key pharmacologic features of nelarabine are listed in Table 11-8.

Mechanism of Action

T cells are particularly sensitive to deoxyguanosine, which becomes phosphorylated within the cell leading to inhibition of DNA synthesis.[139] Deoxyguanosine, however, is not a useful drug as it has a very short half-life in plasma due to rapid deamination by PNP present in red blood cells. 9-β-D arabinofuranosylguanine (ara-G), an analog of deoxyguanine, is resistant to deamination by PNP but is poorly soluble. Nelarabine (Fig 11-1) is a soluble prodrug of ara-G, which is demethylated by ADA to ara-G. Ara-G then accumulates in cells with higher concentrations in T than in B lymphocytes.[140] Ara-G is phosphorylated to ara-GTP via deoxycytidine kinase and dGuo kinase. Ara-GTP is incorporated into DNA where it terminates DNA elongation, leading to inhibition of DNA synthesis and cell death.[141] Ara-GTP also impairs ribonucleotide reductase, leading to impaired DNA synthesis. A positive relationship between accumulation of ara-GTP

within leukemic cells and the development of a complete or partial response to nelarabine therapy has been demonstrated.[142]

Clinical Pharmacology

Following intravenous administration, nelarabine is converted to ara-G by demethoxylation by ADA. By the end of a 1-hour infusion, 94% of nelarabine is converted to ara-G.[143] The half-life of nelarabine is short (30 minutes). The half-life of ara-G is 3 hours with a mean plasma concentration of 115 µmol/L following an infusion of 1,500 mg/m^2 nelarabine.[144] Pediatric patients appear to have an increased clearance rate of ara-G with a resulting shorter plasma half-life (2 hours).[143] Small quantities of nalarabine (5%) and ara-G (23%) are excreted unchanged in the urine. At present, no dose modifications are recommended for patients with renal insufficiency. Most nalarabine is converted to ara-G, which is subsequently hydrolyzed to guanine, which is in turn converted to xanthine and uric acid. Neither nalarabine nor ara-G is significantly protein bound or have and effect on cytochrome P450 (CYP) enzymes.

Intracellular accumulation of ara-GTP has been measured.[145] A median ara-GTP C_{max} of 150 µmol/L is found in T-ALL cells (more than double the concentration found in other cell lineages). The intracellular elimination half-life of ara-GTP varies from 10 to 24 hours. The concomitant use of fludarabine prior to the administration of nelarabine increases intracellular concentrations of ara-GTP by 10%, possibly by upregulating deoxycytidine and deoxyguanosine kinase concentrations.[146]

Toxicity

In Phase I and II trials, the dose-limiting toxicity of nalarabine has been central nervous system (seizures, encephalopathy, obtundation) and peripheral neurotoxicity.[147] The recommended dose of nalarabine in adults is 1,500 mg/m^2 given over 2 hours on days 1, 3, and 5 every 3 weeks and in children is 650 mg/m^2 given over 1 hour for 5 consecutive days every 3 weeks. The most common adverse events are malaise, fever, headache, somnolence, nausea, peripheral neuropathy, and myelosuppression.[144,148] Grade 3 or 4 neurologic events occur in 10% to 15% of patients. As would be expected, in treated leukemic patients, hematologic events are universally noted.

Clinical Use and Drug Interactions

Nalarabine has been approved for treatment of patients with T-ALL and T-LBL who have not responded to or have relapsed after at least two prior chemotherapy regimens. Response rates in patients with relapsed/refractory T-cell malignancies are low and of short duration. The response rate of nalarabine in this population is 23% in pediatric patients and 31% in adults.[140] Some of these patients have proceeded on to stem cell transplantation. The median survival for adult relapsed T-ALL/LBL patients treated with nalarabine is 20 weeks with 25% alive at 1 year. Results to date are based on Phase I and II trials in a small number of patients.

Allopurinol

Allopurinol has no antineoplastic activity. However, it is frequently used in patients with leukemia and lymphoma to prevent hyperuricemia and uric acid nephropathy. The key features of allopurinol are summarized in Table 11-9.

TABLE

11.8 *Key features of nalarabine*

Factor	Result
Mechanism of action	1. Triphosphate metabolites are incorporated into DNA inhibiting DNA primer extension. 2. Inhibits ribonucleotide reductase lowering deoxynucleotide pools needed for DNA synthesis
Metabolism	Activation to guanosine triphosphate metabolite within cells
Pharmacokinetics	Hydrolyzed to guanine (metabolic conversion)
Drug interactions	Increased intracellular drug concentrations when used with fludarabine
Toxicity	1. Neurotoxicity (somnolence, neuropathy, encephalopathy) 2. Myelosuppression 3. Fatigue 4. Nausea and vomiting.

TABLE **11.9**	*Key features of allopurinol*

Factor	Result
Mechanism of action	1. Limits conversion of xanthine and hypoxanthine to uric acid by inhibiting xanthine oxidase 2. Causes feedback inhibition of de novo purine synthesis
Metabolism	Rapid metabolic conversion to oxipurinol, which is the active metabolite
Pharmacokinetics	Allopurinol $t_{1/2}$: 0.7–1.6 h Oxipurinol $t_{1/2}$: 14–28 h
Elimination	Allopurinol: metabolism to oxipurinol Oxipurinol: renal excretion
Drug interactions	1. Prolongs half-life of \ and azathioprine by decreasing rate of metabolic elimination 2. May impair hepatic microsomal enzyme function
Toxicity	1. Rash 2. Hypersensitivity syndrome (TEN, renal failure, liver, hepatic failure) 3. Rare: xanthine nephropathy
Precautions	1. Reduce doses of 6-MP or azathioprine. 2. Reduce allopurinol doses for renal insufficiency. 3. Stop drug for rash.

Mechanism of Action

Allopurinol (4-hydroxypyrazolo [3,4-d] pyrimidine) and its major metabolic product oxipurinol are analogs of hypoxanthine and xanthine, respectively. Allopurinol binds to xanthine oxidase and undergoes internal conversion to oxipurinol, simultaneously reducing and inhibiting xanthine oxidase (Fig 11-6).[149] Allopurinol reduces serum uric acid concentrations not only by inhibiting xanthine oxidase but also by decreasing the rate of de novo purine biosynthesis. Administration of allopurinol to patients with primary gout causes an increase in serum xanthine and hypoxanthine concentrations.[128] Increased conversion of hypoxanthine to inosinic acid and subsequently to adenylic and guanylic acid occurs (Fig. 11-7). Adenylic and guanylic acid are allosteric inhibitors of 5′ phosphoribosyl-1-pyrophosphate (PRPP) aminotransferase, the critical enzyme involved in de novo purine synthesis. Total purine excretion (xanthine plus hypoxanthine plus uric acid) decreases by 30% to 40% after initiation of allopurinol therapy.[150] The effect of allopurinol on de novo purine synthesis is important in the treatment of gout but has negligible benefit in treatment of the tumor lysis syndrome (TLS) where the release of purines from already present DNA occurs.

Clinical Pharmacology

Allopurinol is available in 100- and 300-mg tablets and as an intravenous preparation.[151] Allopurinol is well absorbed orally (50% to 80% bioavailability).[152] The plasma half-life of allopurinol is short (30 to 100 minutes) with rapid conversion of allopurinol to oxipurinol.[153] Most of an administered dose of allopurinol is metabolized to oxipurinol within 1 hour. In patients with normal renal function, steady-state oxipurinol plasma concentrations are 15 mg/L (100 μM) at an allopurinol dose of 300 mg/d. This is in excess of the concentration needed to inhibit xanthine oxidase (25 μM). Oxipurinol clearance and drug half-life are closely tied to creatinine clearance.[154] Patients with renal failure have delayed oxipurinol excretion and require a dose reduction to prevent drug accumulation. Older patients (>70 years) have reduced oxipurinol clearance related to an age-dependent decline in renal function.[155]

Toxicity

Allopurinol therapy is well tolerated in most patients and produces few side effects. Skin rash is seen in 2% of patients taking allopurinol.[156] Gastrointestinal intolerance, fever, and alopecia are rare complications of allopurinol therapy. A severe, potentially life-threatening hypersensitivity syndrome resulting from allopurinol

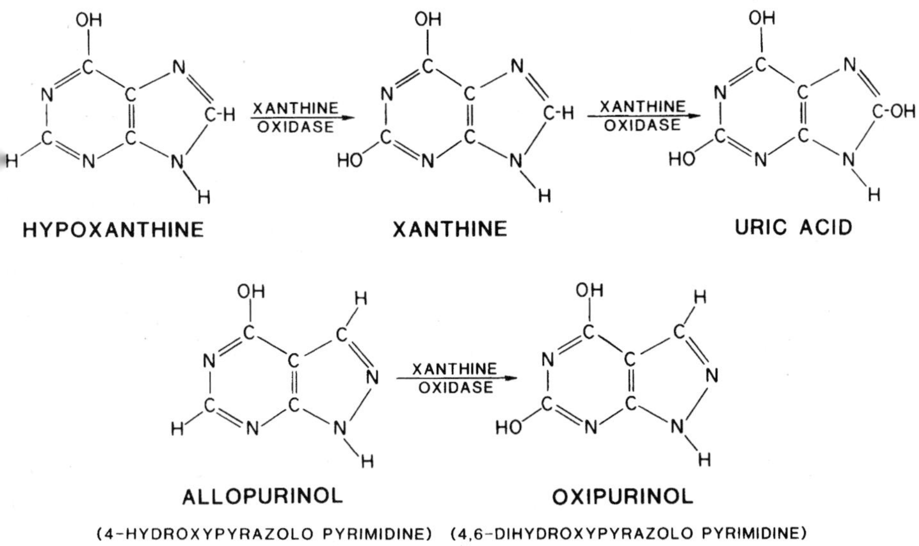

HYPOXANTHINE → (XANTHINE OXIDASE) → **XANTHINE** → (XANTHINE OXIDASE) → **URIC ACID**

ALLOPURINOL → (XANTHINE OXIDASE) → **OXIPURINOL**

(4-HYDROXYPYRAZOLO PYRIMIDINE) (4,6-DIHYDROXYPYRAZOLO PYRIMIDINE)

FIGURE **11-6** Metabolic pathway for the conversion of hypoxanthine and xanthine to uric acid and of allopurinol to oxipurinol.

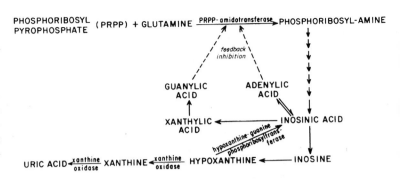

FIGURE **11-7**   Feedback inhibition of de novo purine biosynthesis. Inhibition of xanthine oxidase by allopurinol causes an increase in serum hypoxanthine concentrations which in turn causes increased concentrations of inosinic, xanthylic, adenylic, and guanylic acids. Guanylic and adenylic acids are inhibitors of phosphoribosylpyrophosphate aminotransferase (PRPP-aminotransferase).

use has been reported.[154,157] Patients usually have fever (87% of reported cases), eosinophilia (73%), and skin rash (92%) including toxic epidermal neurolysis, renal dysfunction, and hepatic failure (68%). Death has been reported in 20% of published cases. This hypersensitivity syndrome usually appears 2 to 4 weeks after the initiation of 300 to 400 mg/d allopurinol. Over 80% of patients developing this syndrome have underlying renal failure when allopurinol therapy is started. Steady-state concentrations of oxipurinol are elevated in this situation and may play a role in the development of the toxicity syndrome. Allopurinol has been found to cause a short-term reduction in blood pressure.[158] Xanthine nephropathy is a rare complication of allopurinol therapy in cancer patients.[159] Even though xanthine precipitation is a potential complication of allopurinol therapy in patients who have massive tumor lysis, allopurinol treatment is beneficial to such patients. Allopurinol enables patients to excrete a larger total purine load. Because the solubility of a single purine, such as xanthine, hypoxanthine, or uric acid, is independent of the others, dividing the purine load among these three purines by the use of allopurinol will increase the total amount of purine that can be excreted in the urine.

Clinical Uses and Drug Interactions

In the treatment of primary gout, allopurinol produces a fall in serum uric acid concentration and a decrease in urinary uric acid excretion 1 or 2 days following initiation of therapy and produces a maximal reduction in serum urate levels within 4 to 14 days. In patients who do not respond to 300 mg of allopurinol per day, dosages of 600 to 1,000 mg/d are usually effective in lowering serum uric acid concentrations.

With rapid tumor lysis following cancer treatment, there is a sudden rise in serum uric acid caused by cell destruction with release of purines from degraded DNA. The rapid release of uric acid can result in renal failure because of the precipitation of urate crystals in the distal renal tubules where concentration and acidification are maximal. The development of hyperuricemia after treatment of many leukemias and lymphomas is so common that hydration and allopurinol therapy are recommended before chemotherapy for these diseases is begun. Doses of 300 to 400 mg/m^2/d should be given for 2 to 3 days, with subsequent doses reduced to 300 to 400 mg/d. These doses prevent marked increases in uric acid excretion after chemotherapy,[160,161] although clinically significant tumor lysis is still seen in 5% of patients with high-grade lymphomas and laboratory evidence of lysis in 40%. Xanthine oxidase catalyzes the conversion of both azathioprine and 6-MP to the inactive metabolite, 6-thiouric acid. Oral doses of 6-MP or azathioprine

should be reduced by at least 65% to 75% when allopurinol is concomitantly used. White blood cell counts should be monitored frequently. Even with azathioprine dose reductions of 67%, myelosuppression is seen in over one third of patients also treated with allopurinol.[162]

RASBURICASE (Elitek)

Rasburicase is an enzyme and not a purine analog. However, like allopurinol (a purine analog), rasburicase is used to prevent hyperuricemia and renal failure occurring with the TLS. TLS is characterized by metabolic abnormalities occurring with massive, rapid release of intracellular components into the blood following rapid lysis of malignant cells.[160,161] The primarily intracellular products released are nucleic acids, potassium, and phosphorus. The purines in DNA are degraded to xanthine and hypoxanthine and finally to uric acid (Fig. 11-6). Uric acid is poorly soluble and may precipitate in the renal tubule, where concentration and acidification are maximal, leading to renal failure. Rasburicase has been recommended as part of standard therapy for prevention of TLS in patients with ALL, Burkitt's lymphoma, lymphoblastic lymphoma, and selected patient with non-Hodgkin's lymphoma.[160] Key pharmacologic features of rasburicase are summarized in Table 11-10.

TABLE **11.10**	*Key features of rasburicase*
Factor	Result
Mechanism of action	Converts poorly soluble uric acid to the more soluble allantoin
Metabolism	Protein degradation
Pharmacokinetics	Half-life: 16–21 h
	Distribution thought limited to vascular space
Elimination	Peptide hydrolysis
Drug interactions	None known to date
Toxicity	1. Allergic reaction
	2. Hemolytic anemia and methemaglobinuria

Mechanism of Action

Uric acid is the end product of purine catabolism in man and is poorly soluble in water and urine. Most mammals have the ability to make an enzyme, urate oxidase which converts uric acid to allantoin, which is five to ten times more soluble than uric acid. In humans, there is a nonsense mutation in the coding region of the gene so that no enzyme is formed.[163] When rapid DNA breakdown occurs, purines in the DNA are broken down to uric acid which precipitates in the renal tubule when concentrations exceed solubility. Prevention of uric acid formation can avoid renal failure in such patients.

A nonrecombinant form of urate oxidase has been used for over two decades to treat and prevent hyperuricemia resulting from chemotherapy induces TLC.[163] This nonrecombinant urate oxidase was found effective in lowering serum urate but was associated with a 4.5% rate of hypersensitivity reactions. Rasburicase is a recombinant form of urate oxidase that converts uric acid to allantoin. Rasburicase is formed from a cDNA clone of urate oxidase obtained from *Aspergillus flavus* and expressed in the yeast strain *Saccharomyces cerevisae*. Rasburicase differs from the nonrecombinant product in that the amino acid sequence is preserved during the purification process so that the enzymes has a greater purity and specificity.[164]

Clinical Pharmacology

Rasburicase distribution is thought to be limited to the vascular space.[165] Following the administration of 0.15 or 0.2 mg/kg rasburicase, plasma concentrations of 2.8 to 3.8 µg/L are achieved,[166] with no evidence of accumulation after multiple daily doses. Rasburicase has a long plasma half-life (16 to 21 hours). The clearance of rasburicase is thought to be similar to that of other proteins, peptide hydrolysis. Rasburicase is not expected to interact with drugs metabolized by cytochrome P450 enzymes. Dose adjustments for renal insufficiency are not required.[165]

Toxicity

Rasburicase is generally well tolerated. The most frequently reported toxicities are those of the chemotherapy given with rasburicase. The conversion of uric acid to allantoin by rasburicase results in the formation of hydrogen peroxide as a by-product. Patients with glucose-6-phosphate dehydrogenase deficiency or inherited anemias are at risk of hemolysis due to the formation of hydrogen peroxide. Hemolytic anemia and methemoglobinemia are seen in fewer than 1% of patients.[167] Hypersensitivity reactions occur in 3% to 6% of patients.[165,168] Other reported side effects include fever (5%), skin rash (2%), respiratory distress (3%), and elevations in liver function test (3%). No deaths have been attributed to rasburicase. Discontinuation of treatment due to adverse events occurs in fewer than 1% of patients.[165,166,167]

Clinical Use and Drug Interactions

Rasburicase has been shown to be very effective in lowering serum uric acid concentrations. Within 4 hours of receiving 0.15 mg/kg rasburicase, serum uric acid concentrations fall significantly.[169,170] With hydration and allopurinol therapy alone, serum uric acid concentration declines 12% within 24 hours while there is an 85% to 95% reduction in uric acid concentrations when rasburicase is added to treatment. An improvement in patient survival or improved preservation of renal function has not been yet been demonstrated in leukemia or lymphoma patients pretreated with rasburicase to prevent TLS. However, in a review of 245 patients, only 10 (4%) of patients at risk for TLS required dialysis for hyperphosphemia, azotemia, or both when treated with allopurinol plus rasburicase.[171] In adults, all patients who received rasburicase for greater than 3 days have normal plasma uric acid values following chemotherapy.[170] Rasburicase has been approved for the treatment and prevention of chemotherapy-induced hyperuricemia at a dose of 0.15 to 0.2 mg/kg/d for 5 days. Because the cost of a 5 day treatment is high ($11,000 to $15,000 in adults[163]), a single dose of rasburicase has been evaluated in preliminary studies[172] and may be as effective as a multiple dose regimen.

No drug interactions with rasburicase have been identified.[165]

References

1. Burchenal JH, Murphy ML, Ellison RR, et al. Clinical evaluation of a new antimetabolite, 6-mercaptopurine, in the treatment of leukemia and allied diseases. Blood 1953;8:965–999.
2. Sahasranaman S, Howard, D, Roy S. Clinical pharmacology and pharmacogentics of thiopurines. Eur J Clin Pharmacol 2008;64:753–767.
3. Tidd DM, Patterson ARP. Distinction between inhibition of purine nucleotide synthesis and the delayed cytotoxic reaction of 6-mercaptopurine. Cancer Res 1974;34:733–737.
4. Sommerville L, Krynetski E, Krynetskaia N, et al. Structure and dynamics of thioguanine-modified duplex DNA. J Biol Chem 2003;278:1005–1011.
5. Swann PF, Waters TR, Moulton DC, et al. Role of postreplicative DNA mismatch repair in the cytotoxic action of thioguanine. Science 1996;273:1109–1011.
6. Dervieux T, Blanco JG, Krynetcki EY, et al. Differing contribution of thiopurine methyltransferase to mercaptopurine versus thioguanine effects in human leukemic cells. Cancer Res 2001;61:5810–5816.
7. Fairchild CR, Maybaum J, Kennedy KA. Concurrent unilateral chromatic damage and DNA strand breakage in response to 6-thioguanine treatment. Biochem Pharmacol 1986;35:3533–3541.
8. Pan BF, Nelson JA. Characterization of the DNA damage in 6-thioguanine treated cells. Biochem Pharmacol 1990;40:1063–1069.
9. Erb N, Harms DO, Janka-Schaab G. Pharmacokinetics and metabolism of thiopurines in children with ALL receiving 6-thioguanine versus 6-mercaptopurine. Cancer Chemother Pharmacol 1998;42:266–272.
10. Tiede I, Fritz G, Stand S, et al. C28-dependent RAC activation is the molecular target of azathioprine in primary human CD4 T lymphocytes. J Clin Invest 2003;111:1133–1145.
11. Lavi L, Holcenberg JS. A rapid sensitive high performance liquid chromatography assay for 6-mercaptopurine metabolites in red blood cells. Anal Biochem 1985;144:514–521.
12. Zimm S, Collins JM, Riccardi R, et al. Variable bioavailability of oral mercaptopurine. Is maintenance chemotherapy in ALL being optimally delivered? N Eng J Med 1983;308:1005–1009.
13. Arndt CAS, Balis FM, McCully CL, et al. Bioavailability of low-dose vs high-dose 6-mercaptopurine. Clin Pharmacol Ther 1988;43:588–591.
14. Jacqz-Aigrain E, Nafa S, Medard Y, et al. Pharmacokinetics and distribution of 6-mercaptopurine administered intravenously in children with lymphoblastic leukemia. Eur J Clin Pharmacol 1997;53:71–74.
15. Balis FM, Holcenberg JS, Zimm S, et al. The effect of methotrexate on the bioavailability of oral 6-mercaptopurine. Clin Pharmacol Ther 1987;41:384–387.
16. Balis FM, Holcenberg JS, Poplack DG, et al. Pharmacokinetics and pharmacodynamics of oral methotrexate and mercaptopurine in children with lower risk ALL; a joint Children's Cancer Group and Pediatric Oncology Branch study. Blood 1998;92:3569–3577.
17. Zimm S, Collins JM, O'Neill D, et al. Chemotherapy: inhibition of first-pass metabolism in cancer interaction of 6-mercaptopurine and allopurinol. Clin Pharmacol Ther 1983;34:810–817.

18. Zimm S, Ettinger LJ, Holcenberg JS, et al. Phase I and clinical pharmacological study of mercaptopurine administered as a prolonged intravenous infusion. Cancer Res 1985;45:1869–1873.

19. Lafolie P, Hayder S, Bjork O, et al. Intraindividual variation in 6-mercaptopurine pharmacokinetics during oral maintenance therapy of children with ALL. Eur J Clin Pharmacol 1991;40:599–601.

20. Burton NK, Barnett MJ, Aherne GW, et al. The affect of food on the oral administration of 6-mercaptopurine. Cancer Chemother Pharmacol 1986; 18:90–91.

21. Burton NK, Aherne GW. The effect of cotrimoxazole on the absorption of orally administered 6-mercaptopurine in the rat. Cancer Chemother Pharmacol 1986;16:81–84.

22. Weinshilboum RM. Methyltransferase pharmacogenetics. Pharmacol Ther 1989;43:77–90.

23. Schaeffeler E, Fisher C, Brockmeirer D, et al. Comprehensive analysis of thiopurine S-methyltransferase phenotype-genotype correlation in a large population of German-Caucasians, and identification of novel TMPT variants. Pharmacogenetics. 2004;14:407–414.

24. Tai HL, Krynetski EY, Schueta EG, et al. Enhanced proteolysis of thiopurine S-methyltransferase (TMPT) encoded by mutant alleles in humans (TPMT*3a, TPMT*2) mechanisms for the genetic polymorphism of TMPT activity. Proc Natl Acad Sci 1997;94:6444–6449.

25. Coulthard SA, Howell C, Robson J, et al. The relationship between thiopurine methyltransferase activity and genotype in blasts from patients with acute leukemia. Blood 1998;92:2856–2862.

26. Yates CR, Krynetski EY, Loennechen T, et al. Molecular diagnosis of thiopurine 5-methylltransferase deficiency: genetic basis for azathioprine and mercaptopurine intolerance. Ann Intern Med 1997;126:608–614.

27. Gate Pharmaceuticals. Purinethol (mercaptopurine) prescribing information. http://www.gatepharma.com/Purinethol/PI.pdf; 2007.

28. McLeod HL, Siva C. The thiopurine S-methyltransferase gene locus—implication for clinical pharmacogeneomics. Pharmacogenomics 2002;3:89–98.

29. Koren G, Ferrazini G, Sulh H, et al. Systemic exposures to mercaptopurine as a prognostic factor in acute lymphocytic leukemia. N Engl J Med 1990;323:17–21.

30. Lennard L, Lilleyman JS, Van Loon JA, et al. Genetic variation in response to 6-mercaptopurine for childhood acute lymphoblastic leukemia. Lancet 1991;336:225–229.

31. Schmiegelow K, Forestier E, Kristinsson J, et al. Thiopurine methyltransferase activity is related to the risk of relapse of childhood acute lymphoblastic leukemia. Leukemia 2009;23:557–564.

32. Marsh S, Van Booven DJ. The increasing complexity of mercaptopurine pharmacogenetics. Clin Pharmacol Ther 2009;85:139–141.

33. Stoco G, Cheok MH, Crews KR, et al. Genetic polymorphism of inosine triphosphate pyrophosphatase is a determinant of mercaptopurine metabolism and toxicity during treatment of acute lymphoblastic leukemia. Clin Pharmacol Ther 2009;85:164–171.

34. Hawwa AF, Millership, JS, Collier PS, et al. Pharmacogenomic studies of the anticancer and immunosuppressive thiopurines mercaptopurine and azathioprine. Br J Clin Pharm 2008;66:517–528.

35. LePage GA, Whitecar JP. Pharmacology of 6-thioguanine in man. Cancer Res 1971;31:1627–1631.

36. Brox LW, Birkett L, Belch A. Clinical pharmacology of oral thioguanine in acute myelogenous leukemia. Cancer Chemother Pharmacol 1981;6:35–638.

37. Kitchen BJ, Balis FM, Poplack DG, et al. A pediatric Phase I trial and pharmacokinetic study of thioguanine administered by continuous i.v. infusion. Clin Cancer Res 1997;3:713–717.

38. Liliemark J, Petterson B, Lafolie P, et al. Determination of plasma azathioprine and 6-mercaprine in patients with rheumatoid arthritis treated with oral azathioprine. Ther Drug Monit 1990;12:339–343.

39. Chan CLC, Erdmen GR, Gruber SA, et al. Azathioprine metabolism: Pharmacokinetics of 6-mercaptopurine, 6-thiouric acid and 6-thioguanine nucleotides in renal transplant patients. J Clin Pharm 1990;30:358–363.

40. Sau A, Clark S, Bass J, et al. Azathiprine and breastfeeding: is it safe? BJOG 2007;114:498–501.

41. Evans WE, Hon YY, Bomgaars L, et al. Preponderance of thiopurine S-methyltransferase deficiency and heterozygosity among patients intolerant to mercaptopurine or azathioprine. J Clin Oncol 2001;19:2293–2301.

42. Gisbert JP, Gonzalez-Lama Y, Mate J. Thiopurine-induced liver injury in patients with inflammatory bowel disease: a systemic review. Am J Gastroenterol 2007;102:1518–1527.

43. Gearry RB, Barclay ML, Burt MJ, et al. Thiopurine 5-methltransferase (TPMT) gene type does not predict adverse drug reactions to thiopurine drugs in patients with inflammatory bowel disease. Alimentary Pharmacol Ther 2003;18:395–400.

44. Nygaard U, Toft N, Schmiegelow K. Methylated metabolites of 6-mercaptopurine are associated with hepatotoxicity. Clin Pharmacol Ther 2004;75:274–281.

45. Duttera MJ, Caralla RL, Gallelli JF. Hematuria and crystalluria after high-dose 6-mercaptopurine administration. N Eng J Med 1972;287:292–294.

46. Lewis JD, Bikker WB, Brensinger C, et al. Inflammatory bowel disease is not associated with an increased risk of lymphoma. Gastroenterology 2001;121:1080–1087.

47. Schmiegelow K, Al-Modhwahi I, Andersen MK, et al. Methotrexate/6-mercaptopurine maintenance therapy influences the risk of a second malignant neoplasm after childhood acute lymphoblastic leukemia: results from the NOPHO ALL-92 study. Blood 2009:113:6077–6084.

48. Kovach JS, Rubin J, Creagan ET, et al. Phase I trial of parenteral 6-thioguanine given on 5 consecutive days. Cancer Res 1986;46:5959–5962.

49. Vora A, Mitchell CD, Lennard L, et al. Toxicity and efficacy of 6-thiguanine versus 6-mercaptopurine in childhood acute lymphoblastic leukemia: a randomized trial. Lancet 2006;368:1339–1348.

50. Almer SH, Hjortswang H, Hindorf U. 6-Thioguanine therapy in Crohn's disease—observational data in Swedish patients. Dig Liver Dis 2009;41:194–200.

51. Gardiner SJ, Gearry RB, Burt MJ, et al. Severe hepatotoxicity with high-methylmercaptopurine nucleotide concentrations after thiopurine dose escalation due to low 6-thioguanine nucleotides. Eur J Gastroenterol Hepatol 2008;20:1238–1242.

52. Fields CK, Robinson JW, Roy TM, et al. Hypersensitivity reaction to azathioprine. South Med J 1998;91:471–474.

53. Gisbert JP, Gomolion F. Thiopurine-induced myelotoxicity in patients with inflammatory bowel disease: a review. Am J Gastroenterol 2008:103:1783–1800.

54. Black AJ, McLeod HL, Capell HA, et al. Thiopurine methyltransferase genotype predicts therapy-limiting severe toxicity from azathioprine. Ann Intern Med 1998;129:716–718.

55. Kennedy DT, Hayney MS, Lake KD. Azathioprine and allopurinol: the price of an avoidable drug interaction. Ann Pharmacothera 1996;30:951–954.

56. Dervieux T, Hancock ML, Pui CH, et al. Antagonism by methotrexate on mercaptopurine disposition in lymphoblastic during upfront treatment of acute lymphoblastic leukemia. Clin Pharmacol Ther 2003;73:506–516.

57. Lowry PW, Franklin CL, Weaver AL, et al. Leucopenia resulting from a drug interaction between azathioprine or 6-mercaptopurine and mesalamine, sulphasalazine or balsalazide. Gut 2001;49:656–662.

58. Adkins JC, Peters DH, Markham A. Fludarabine. An update of its pharmacology and use in the treatment of haematological malignancies. Drugs 1997;53:1005–1037.

59. Danhauser L, Plunkett W, Keating M, et al. 9-B-D-arabinofuranosyl-2-fluoroadenine 5′-monophosphate pharmacokinetics in plasma and tumor cells of patients with relapsed leukemia and lymphoma. Cancer Chemother Pharmacol 1986;18:145–152.

60. Molina-Arcas M, Bellosillo B, Casado FJ, et al. Fludarabine uptake mechanisms in B-cell chronic lymphocytic leukemia. Blood 2003;101:2328–2334.

61. Gandhi V, Plunkett W. Cellular and clinical pharmacology of fludarabine. Clin Pharmacokinet 2002;41:93–103.

62. Kamiya K, Huang P, Plunkett W. Inhibition of the 3′→5′ exonucleases of human DNA polymerase epsilon by fludarabine-terminated DNA. J Biol Chem 1996;271:19428–19435.

63. Plunkett W, Begleiter A, Liliemark O, et al. Why do drugs work in CLL? Leuk Lymphoma 1996;22(Suppl 2):1–11.

64. Pettitt A. Mechanism of action of purine analogs in chronic lymphocytic leukemia. Br J Hematol 2003;121:692–702.

65. Sandoval A, Consoli U, Plunkett W. Fludarabine-mediated inhibition of nucleotide excision repair induces apoptosis in quiescent human lymphocytes. Clin Cancer Res 1996;2:1731–1741.

66. Danhauser L, Plunkett W, Liliemark J, et al. Comparison between the plasma and intracellular pharmacology of 1-(-D-arabinofuranosyl-2-fluoro-adenine 5'-monophosphate in patients with relapsed leukemia. Leukemia 1987;1:638–643.

67. Gandhi V, Estey E, Du M, et al. Maximum dose of fludarabine for maximal modulation of arabinosyl-cytosine triphosphate in human leukemic blast cells during therapy. Clin Cancer Res 1997;3:1539–1545.

68. Lichtman SM, Etcubanas E, Budman D, et al. The pharmacokinetics and pharmacodynamics of fludarabine phosphate in patients with renal impairment: a perspective dose adjustment study. Cancer Invest 2002;20:904–913.

69. Aronoff GR, Bennett WM, Berns JS, et al. Drug Prescribing in Renal Failure: Dosing Guidelines for Adults and Children. 5th ed. Philadelphia: American College of Physicians, 2007.

70. Posker GL, Figgitt DP. Oral fludarabine. Drugs 2003;63:2317–2323.

71. Oscier D, Orchard JA, Culligan D, et al. The bioavailability of oral fludarabine phosphate is unaffected by food. Hematol J 2001;2:316–321.

72. Hagenbeck A, Eghbali H, Monfardini S, et al. Phase III intergroup study of fludarabine phosphate compared with cyclophosphamide, vincristine and prednisone chemotherapy in newly diagnosed patients with stage III and IV low-grade malignant non-Hodgkin's lymphoma. J Clin Oncol 2006;24:1590–1596.

73. Byrd JC, Peterson BL, Morrison VA, et al. Randomized Phase II study of fludarabine with concurrent versus sequential treatment with rituximab in symptomatic untreated patients with B-cell chronic lymphocytic leukemia: results from the CALGB 9712. Blood 2003;101:6–14.

74. Frank DA, Mahajan S, Ritz J. Fludarabine-induced immunosuppression is associated with inhibitor of STAT 1 signaling. Nat Med 1999;5:444–447.

75. Keating MJ, O'Brien S, Lerner S, et al. Long-term follow-up of patients with chronic lymphocytic leukemia (CLL) receiving fludarabine regimens as initial therapy. Blood 1998;92:1165–1171.

76. Anaissie EJ, Kontoyiannis DP, O'Brien S, et al. Infections in patients with chronic lymphocytic leukemia treated with fludarabine. Ann Intern Med 1998;129:559–566.

77. Mortell RE, Peterson BL, Cohen HJ, et al. Analysis of age, estimated creatinine clearance and pretreatment hematologic parameters as predictors of fludarabine toxicity in patients treated for chronic lymphocytic leukemia. Chemother Pharmacol 2002;50:37–45.

78. Weiss RB, Freiman J, Kweder SL, et al. Hemolytic anemia after fludarabine therapy for chronic lymphocytic leukemia. J Clin Oncol 1998;16:1885–1889.

79. Cheson BD, Frame JN, Vena D, et al. Tumor lysis syndrome: an uncommon complication of fludarabine therapy of chronic lymphocytic leukemia. J Clin Oncol 1998;16:2313–2320.

80. Cheson BD, Vena DA, Foss FM, et al. Neurotoxicity of purine analogs: a review. J Clin Oncol 1994;12:2216–2228.

81. Helman DL, Byrd JL, Alex NC, et al. Fludarabine-related pulmonary toxicity: a distinct clinical entity in chronic lymphoproliferative syndromes. Chest 2002;127:785–790.

82. Ogawa Y, Hotta T, Watanabe K, et al. Phase I and pharmacokinetic study of oral fludarabine phosphate in relapsed indolent B-cell non-Hodgkin's lymphoma. Ann Oncol 2006;17:330–333.

82. Tam CS, O'Brien S, Wierda W, et al. Long-term results of the fludarabine, cyclophosphamide, and rituximab regimen as initial therapy of chronic lymphocytic leukemia. Blood 2008;112:975–980.

83. Bonin M, Pursche S, Bergeman T, et al. F-ara A pharmacokinetics during reduced intensity conditioning therapy with fludarabine and busulfan. Bone Marrow Transplant 2007;39:201–206.

85. Gandhi V, Huang P, Chapman AJ, et al. Incorporation of fludarabine and 1-beta-D-arabinofuranosylcytosine 5'-triphosphates by DNA polymerase alpha: affinity, interaction and consequences. Clin Cancer Res 1997;3:1347–1355.

86. Agarwal RP. Inhibitors of adenosine deaminase. Pharmacol Ther 1982;17:399–429.

87. O'Dwyer PJ, Wagner B, Leyland-Jones B, et al. 2'-Deoxycoformycin (Pentostatin) for lymphoid malignancies. Ann Intern Med 1988;108:733–743.

88. Wiley JS, Smith CL, Jamieson GP. Transport of 2'deoxycoformycin in human leukemic and lymphoma cells. Biochem Pharmacol 1991;42:708–710.

89. Johnston JB, Glazer RI, Pugh L, et al. The treatment of hairy-cell leukemia with 2'-deoxycoformycin. Br J Haematol 1986;63: 525–534.

90. Al-Razzak KA, Benedetti AE, Waugh WN, et al. Chemical stability of pentostatin (NSC-218321), a cytotoxic and immunosuppressant agent. Pharmaceutical Res 1990;7:452–460.

91. Kane BJ, Kuhn JG, Roush MK. Pentostatin: an adenosine deaminase inhibitor for the treatment of hairy cell leukemia. Ann Pharmacother 1992;26:939–946.

92. Smyth JF, Paine RM, Jackman AL, et al. The clinical pharmacology of the adenosine deaminase inhibitor 2'deoxycorformycin. Cancer Chemother Pharmacol 1980;5:93–101.

93. Major PP, Hgarwal RP, Kufe DW. Clinical pharmacology of deoxycoformycin. Blood 1981;58:91–96.

94. Lathia C, Fleming G, Mayer M, et al. Pentostatin pharmacokinetics and dosing recommendations in patients with mild renal impairment. Cancer Chemother Pharmacol 2002;50:121–126.

95. Major PP, Agarwal RP, Kufe DW. Deoxycoformycin: neurological toxicity. Cancer Chemother Pharmacol 1981;5:193–196.

96. Margolis J, Grever MR. Pentostatin; nipent: a review of potential toxicity and its management. Sem Oncol 2000;27(Suppl)5:9–14.

97. Grever M, Kopecky K, Foucar MK, et al. Randomized comparison of pentostatin versus interferon alfa 2A in previously untreated patients with hairy cell leukemia: an intergroup study. J Clin Oncol 1995;13:974–982.

98. Grem JL, King SA, Chun HG, et al. Cardiac complications observed in elderly patients following 2'deoxycoformycin therapy. Am J Hematol 1991;38:245–247.

99. Samonis G, Kontoyiannis DP. Infectious complications of purine analog therapy. Current Opin Infect Disease 2001;14:409–413.

100. Flinn IW, Kopecky KJ, Foucar MK, et al. Long-term follow-up of remission duration mortality and second malignancy in hairy cell leukemia patients treated with pentostatin. Blood 2000;96:2981–2986.

101. Ho AD, Hensel M. Pentostatin for the treatment of indolent lymphoproliferative disorders. Sem Hematol 2006:43S:S2–S10.

102. Jacobson DA, Chen AR, Zahurak M, et al. Phase II study of pentostatin in patients with corticosteroid-refractory chronic graft-versus-host disease. J Clin Oncol 2007;25:4255–4261.

103. Kawasaki H, Carrera CJ, Piro LO, et al. Relationship of deoxycytidine kinase and cytoplasmic 5' nucleotidase to the chemotherapeutic efficacy of 2-chlorodeoxyadenosine. Blood 1993;81:597–601.

104. Seto S, Carrera CJ, Kubota M, et al. Mechanism of deoxyadenosine and 2-chlorodeoxyadenosine toxicity to non-dividing human lymphocytes. J Clin Invest 1985;75:377–383.

105. Hartman WR, Hantosh P. The antileukemic drug 2-chlorodeoxyadenosine: an intrinsic transcription antagonist. Mol Pharmacol 2004;65:227–234.

106. Hentosh P, Kools R, Blakley RL. Incorporation of 2-halogen-2'- deoxyadenosine 5-triphosphosphates into DNA during replication by human polymerases alpha and beta. J Biol Chem 1990;265:4033–4040.

107. Ceruti S, Beltrami E, Matarrese P, et al. A key role for caspase-2 and caspase-3 in apoptosis induced by 2'chloro-2-deoxyadenosine (cladribine) and 2-chloro adenosine in human astrocytoma cells. Mol Pharmacol 2003;63:1437–1447.

108. Leoni LM, Chao Q, Cottam HB, et al. Induction of an apoptotic program in cell free extracts by 2-chloro-2'deoxyadenosine 5' triphosphate and cytochrome C. Proc Natl Acad Sci USA 1998;95:9567–9571.

109. Mansson E, Spaskoukoskaja T, Sallstrom J, et al. Molecular and biochemical mechanisms of fludarabine and cladribine resistance in a human promyelocytic cell line. Cancer Res 1999;59:5956–5963.

110. Galnarini CM, Voorzanger N, Faletten N, et al. Influence of P53 and P21 (WAFI) expression on sensitivity of cancer cells to cladribine. Biochem Pharmacol 2003:65:121–129.

111. Lindemalm S, Lilemark J, Julinsson G, et al. Cytotoxicity and pharmacokinetic of cladribine metabolite 2-chloroadenine in patients with leukemia. Cancer Lett 2004;210:171–177.

112. Liliemark J, Juliusson G. Cellular pharmacokinetics of 2-chloro-2'-deoxyadenosine nucleotides: comparison of intermittent and continuous intravenous infusion and subcutaneous and oral administration in leukemia patients. Clin Cancer Res 1995;1:385–390.

113. Liliemark J. The clinical pharmacokinetics of cladribine. Clin Pharmacokinet 1997;32:120–131.

114. Albertioni F, Lindemalm S, Reichelova V, et al. Pharmacokinetics of cladribine and its 5'monophosphate and 5' triphosphate in leukemic cells

of patients with chronic lymphocytic leukemia. Clin Cancer Res 1998;4: 653–658.

115. Kearns CM, Blakley RL, Santana VM, et al. Pharmacokinetics of cladribine (2-chlorodeoxyadenosine) in children with acute leukemia. Cancer Res 1994;54:1235–1239.

116. Lilliemark J, Albertioni F, Hansen M, et al. On the bioavailability of oral and subcutaneous 2-chloro2′-deoxyadenosine in humans: alternative routes of administration. J Clin Oncol 1992;10:1514–1518.

117. Zenhausern R, vonRohr A, Rufiback K, et al. Low dose 2-chlordeoxy-adenosine given as a single subcutaneous injection in patients with hairy cell leukemia: a multicentre trial SAKK 32/95. Leuk Lymph 2009;50: 133–136.

118. Juliusson G, Lilemark J. Purine analogs: rationale for development, mechanisms of action and pharmacokinetics in hairy cell leukemia. Hematol Oncol Clin N Am 2006;20:1087–1097.

119. Piro LD, Carrera CJ, Carson DA, et al. Lasting remission in hairy-cell leukemia induced by a single infusion of 2-chlorodeoxyadenosine. N Engl J Med 1990;322:1117–1121.

120. Cheson BD. Infectious and immunosuppressive complications of purine analog therapy. J Clin Oncol 1995;13:2431–2448.

121. Betticher DC, von Rohr A, Ratschiller D, et al. Fewer infections, but maintained antitumor activity with lower-dose vs standard-dose cladribine in pretreated low-grade non-Hodgkin's lymphoma. J Clin Oncol 1998;16:850–858.

122. Robak T, Jamroziak K, Gore-Tybor J, et al. Cladribine in a weekly versus daily schedule for untreated hairy cell leukemia: final report from the Polish Adult Leukemia Group (PALG) of a prospective, randomized, multicenter trial. Blood 2007;109:3672–3675.

123. Chadha P, Rademaker AW, Mendiratta P, et al. Treatment of hairy cell leukemia with 2-cholordeoxyadenosine (2-CdA): long-term follow-up of the Northwestern experience. Blood 2005;106:241–246.

124. Piro LD. 2-Chlorodeoxyadenosine treatment of lymphoid malignancies. Blood 1992;79:843–845.

125. Inwards DJ, Fishkin PA, Hillman DW, et al. Long-term results of treatment of patients with mantle cell lymphoma with cladribine (2-CdA) alone or 2-CdA and rituximab in the North Central Cancer Treatment Group. Cancer 2008;113:108–116.

126. Crews KR, Gandhi V, Srivostava DK, et al. Interim comparison of a continuous infusion versus a short daily infusion of cytarabine given in combination with cladribine for pediatric acute myeloid leukemia. J Clin Oncol 2002;20:4217–4224.

127. Chubar Y, Bennett M. Cutaneous reactions in hairy cell leukemia treated with 2-chlorodeoxyadenosine and allopurinol. Br J Hematol 2003;122: 768–770.

128. Montgomery JA, Shortnay-Fowler AT, Clayton SD, et al. Synthesis and biologic activity of 2′ fluoro 2 halo derivative of 9 beta D arabinosuronaosyladenine. J Med Chem 1992;35:397–401.

129. Parker WB, Shaddix SC, Rose LM, et al. Comparison of the mechanisms of 2-choro-9-(2-deoxy-2-fluoro-β-D-arabinofuranosyl) adenine, of 2-chloro-9 (2-deoxy-2-fluoroβ-D ribofuranosyl adenine and of 2-cholor (2-deoxy-2,2difluoro-β-D-arabinosyl adenine in CEM cells. Mol Pharmacol 1999;55:515–520.

130. Parker WB, Shaddix SC, Chang CH, et al. Effects of 2-cholor-9-(2 deoxy-2-fluoro-β-D arabinofuranosyl) adenine on K562 cellular metabolism and the inhibition of human ribonucletide reductase and DNA polymerases by its 5′-triphosphate. Cancer Res 1991;51:2386–2394.

131. Xie KC. Plunkett W. Deoxynucleotide pool depletion and sustained inhibition of ribonucletide reductase and DNA synthesis after treatment of human lymphoblastoid cells with 2-chlor-(2-deoxy-fluoro-β-D-arabinofuranosyl) adenine. Cancer Res 1996;56:3030–3037.

132. Gemini D, Adachi S, Chao Q, et al. Deoxyadenosine analogs induce programmed cell death in chronic lymphocytes by damaging the DNA and by directly affecting the mitochondria. Blood 2000;96:3537–3543.

133. Cooper T, Kantarjian H, Plunkett W, et al. Clofarabine in adult acute leukemias: clinical success and pharmacokinetics. Nucleosides Nucleotides Nucleic Acids 2004;23:1417–1423.

134. Gandhi V, Plunkett W, Bonate PL, et al. Clinical and pharmacokinetic study of clofarabine in chronic lymphocytic leukemia: strategy for treatment. Clin Cancer Res 2006;12:4011–4017.

135. Kantajarian H, Gandhi V, Kozuch P, et al. Phase I clinical and pharmacologic study of clofarabine in patients with solid tumors and hematologic cancers. J Clin Oncol 2003;21:1167–1173.

136. Kantarjian H, Jehe S, Gandhi V, et al. Clofarabine: past present and future. Leuk Lymph 207;48:1922–1930.

137. Jeha S, Gaynon P, Razzouk B, et al. Phase II study of clofarabine in pediatric patients with refractory or relapsed acute lymphoblastic leukemia. J Clin Oncol 2006;24:1917–1923.

138. Faderk S, Ravandi F, Huang X, et al. A randomized study of clofarabine versus clofarabine plus low-dose cytarabine as front-line therapy for patients aged 60 years and older with acute myeloid leukemia and high risk myelodysplasia. Blood 2008;112:1638–1645.

139. Cohen A, Lee JW, Gelfand EW. Sensitivity of deoxyguanosine and arabinosyl guanine for T-leukemic cells. Blood 1983;61:660–666.

140. DeAngelo DJ. Nalarabine for the treatment of patients with relapsed or refractory T-cell acute lymphoblastic leukemia or lymphoblastic lymphoma. Hematol Oncol Clin N Am 2009;23:1121–1135.

141. Rodriguez CO, Strellrecht CM, Gandhi V. Mechanisms for T-cell selective cytotoxicity of arabinosylguanine. Blood 2003;102:1842–1848.

142. Gandhi V, Tam C, Jewel RC, et al. Phase I trial of nelarabine in indolent leukemias. J Clin Oncol 2008;26:1098–1105.

143. Kisor DF, Plunkett W, Kurtzberg J, et al. Pharmacokinetics of nelarabine and 9-β-D-arabinofuranosyl guanine in pediatric and adult patients during a phase I study of nelarabine for the treatment of refractory hematologic malignancies. J Clin Oncol 2000;18:995–1003.

144. Sanford M, Lyseng-Williamson A. Nelarabine. Drugs 2008;68:439–447.

145. Buie LW, Epstein SS, Lindley CM. Nelarabine: a novel purine antimetabolite antineoplastic agent. Clin Ther 2007;29:1887–1899.

146. Gandhi V, Plunkett W, Weller S, et al. Evaluation of the combination of nalarabine and fludarabine in leukemias: clinical response, pharmacokinetics and pharmacodynamics in leukemia cells. J Clin Oncol 2001;19: 2142–2152.

147. Kurtzberg J, Ernst TJ, Keating MJ, et al. Phase I study of 506U78 administer on a consecutive 5-day schedule in children and adults with refractory malignancies. J Clin Oncol 2000;18:995–1003.

148. DeAngelo DJ, Yu D, Johnson JL, et al. Nelarabine induces complete remissions in adults with relapsed or refractory T-linage acute lymphoblastic leukemia or lymphoblastic lymphoma: a Cancer and Leukemia Group B study. Blood 2007;109:5136–5142.

149. Spector T. Inhibition of urate production by allopurinol. Biochem Pharmacol 1977;26:355–358.

150. Fox IH, Wyngaarden JB, Kelley WN. Depletion of erythrocyte phosphoribosylpyrophosphate in man; a newly observed effect of allopurinol. N Engl J Med 1970;283:1177–1182.

151. Smalley RV, Guaspari A, Haase-Statz S, et al. Allopurinol: intravenous use for prevention of hyperuricemia. J Clin Oncol 2000;18:1758–1763.

152. Guerra P, Frias J, Ruiz B, et al. Bioequivalence of allopurinol and its metabolite oxipurinol in two tablet formulations. Pharm Ther 2001;26:113–119.

153. Hande KR, Reed E, Chabner BA. Allopurinol kinetics. Clin Pharmacol Ther 1978;23:598–605.

154. Hande KR, Noone RM, Stone WJ. Severe allopurinol toxicity; description and guidelines for prevention in patients with renal insufficiency. Am J Med 1984;76:47–56.

155. Turnheim K, Krivanek P, Oberbauer R. Pharmacokinetics and pharmacodynamics of allopurinol in elderly and young subjects. Br J Clin Pharmacol 1999;48:501–509.

156. Boston Collaborative Drug Surveillance Program. Excess of ampicillin rash associated with allopurinol or hyperuricemia. N Engl J Med 1972;286: 505–507.

157. Plum HJ, van Deuren M, Wetzels JFM. The allopurinol hypersensitivity syndrome. Neth J Med 1998;52:107–110.

158. Feig DI, Soletsky B, Johnson RJ. Effect of allopurinol on blood pressure in adolescents with newly diagnosed essential hypertension. JAMA 2009;300:924–932.

159. Green ML, Fujimoto WY, Seegmiller JE. Urinary xanthine stones—a rare complication of allopurinol therapy. N Engl J Med 1969;280:426–427.

160. Coffier B, Altman A, Pui CH, et al. Guidelines for the management of pediatric and adult tumor lysis syndrome: an evidence based review. J Clin Oncol 2008;26:2767–2778.

161. Hande KR, Garrow GC. Acute tumor lysis syndrome in patients with high-grade non-Hodgkin's lymphoma. Am J Med 1993;94:133–139.

162. Cummins D, Sekar M, Halil O, et al. Myelosuppression associated with azathioprine-allopurinol interaction after heart and lung transplantation. Transplantation 1996;61:1661–1662.

163. Yim BT, Sims-McCallum RP, Chong PH. Rasburicase for the treatment and prevention of hyperuricemia. Ann Pharmacother 2003;37:1047–1054.

164. LePlatois P, Le Douarin B, Loison G. High level production of a personal enzyme: *Aspergillus flavus* uricase accumulates intracellularly and is active in *Saccharomyces cerevisiae*. Gene 1992;122:139–145.

165. Oldfield V, Perry CM. Rasburicase: a review of its use in the management of anticancer therapy-induced hyperuricemia. Drugs 2006;66:529–545.

166. Pui CH, Mahmoud HH, Wiley JM, et al. Recombinant urate oxidase for the prophylaxis or treatment of hyperuricemia in patients with leukemia or lymphoma. J Clin Oncol 2001;19:697–704.

167. Jeha S, Kantarjarian H, Irwin D, et al. Efficacy and safety of rasburicase, a recombinant urate oxidase (Elitek) in the management of malignancy-associated hyperuricemia in pediatric and adult patients: final results of a multicenter compassionate use trial. Leukemia 2005;19:34–38.

168. Ishizawa K, Ogura M, Hamaguchi M, et al. Safety and efficacy of rasburicase in a Japanese phase II study. Can Sci 2009;200:357–362.

169. Goldman SC, Holcenberg JS, Finklestein JZ, et al. A randomized comparison between rasburicase and allopurinol in children with lymphoma or leukemia at high risk of tumor lysis. Blood 2001;97:2998–3003.

170. Coffier B, Monnier N, Bologna S, et al. Efficacy and safety of rasburicase, (recombinant urate oxidase) for the prevention and treatment of hyperuricemia during induction chemotherapy of aggressive non-Hodgkin's lymphoma: results of the GRAAL1 study. J Clin Oncol 2003;21:4402–4406.

171. Pui CH, Jeha S, Irvin D, et al. Recombinant urate oxidase (rasburicase) in the prevention and treatment of malignancy-associated hyperuricemia in pediatric and adult patients: results of a compassionate-use trial. Leukemia 2001;15:1505–1509.

172. Compara M, Shord SS, Haaf CM. Single-dose rasburicase for tumor lysis syndrome in adults: weight based approach. J Clin Pharm Ther 2009;34:207–213.

Hydroxyurea

Bruce A. Chabner

Hydroxyurea (HU), one of the simplest of the anticancer drugs, plays a supportive role in the treatment of myeloproliferative disease because of its ability to suppress proliferation of myeloid, erythroid, and platelet precursors, but its value is limited by its inability to induce bone marrow remission and the equally rapid reversibility of its myelosuppressive effect. However, it has other notable clinical properties, including its induction of β-globin synthesis in patients with sickle cell anemia and thalassemia. It has been an invaluable probe for the laboratory study of its intracellular target, ribonucleotide reductase (RR), the rate-limiting step in the de novo synthesis of deoxyribonucleotide triphosphates (dNTPs). Other actions, including the generation of nitroxyl radicals and radiosensitizing effects, have potential clinical applications. The key features of this drug are shown in Table 12-1.

HU (Fig. 12-1) was originally synthesized in Germany in 1860,[1] and it was found to have inhibitory effects on granulocyte production.[2] It displayed antileukemic properties in the National Cancer Institute's screening system,[3] entered clinical trials in the 1960s, and was soon recognized as a potent myelosuppressive agent with a novel mechanism of action and few side effects, properties that have earned it a limited but constant role in cancer chemotherapy. Other inhibitors of RR have since been evaluated in the clinic, including compounds of the thiosemicarbazone series[4] and guanazole,[5] but they have no special therapeutic advantage and greater toxicity. The principal use of HU at present is in controlling lineage proliferation; it provides excellent control of myeloproliferative disorders.[6-8]

Once a primary agent with interferon-α in first-line therapy against chronic myelogenous leukemia (CML),[8] it has been largely replaced by the targeted agent, imatinib mesylate, and is now used primarily for acute control of white cell count at presentation or during blastic transformation. In polycythemia vera (PV), it effectively prevents thrombosis resulting from elevated hematocrit and high platelet count,[6] and it similarly lessens the incidence of thrombosis in patients with essential thrombocythemia (ET) and platelet counts above 1.5 million.[7] Because both PV and ET are chronic, slowly progressive diseases, there is concern that HU may increase the risk of leukemic conversion, a risk that has not been substantiated thus far.[9,10] In younger patients with PV, who have the prospect of long-term treatment, prophylactic phlebotomy is the favored treatment, and in patients with ET, anagrelide and interferon-α are alternatives to HU. Newer drugs that attack the mutation in Jak-2 kinase have entered clinical trial for PV and ET and may displace HU in the future.

A major current use of HU is in the prevention of complications of sickle cell anemia. In patients with sickle cell anemia, HU increases the production of fetal hemoglobin, ameliorates symptoms, and reduces the incidence of painful crisis and hospitalization.[11,12] In vitro incubation of HU with erythroid progenitors induces fetal hemoglobin β-globin production.[13] Whether the induction of fetal hemoglobin represents a response to inhibition of DNA synthesis in red cell progenitors or a specific alteration of γ-globin gene transcription is uncertain.[13] Nitroxy radicals produced by decomposition of HU may directly stimulate γ-globin gene transcription through the Sar 1a promoter.[14,15] The increase in fetal hemoglobin promotes the solubility of hemoglobin and prevents the downward spiral of intravascular red cell sickling that leads to painful crisis. Convincing evidence now exists that induction of fetal hemoglobin is not the only, and perhaps not the major, contributor to the drug's efficacy. The benefit from HU may be partly related to its ability to suppress the neutrophil count and its effects on white and red cell adhesion to vessel walls.[16] A marked decrease in the endothelial adhesion of a patient's blood cells, coincident with a down-regulation of L-selectin on the red cell and white cell surfaces, is observed after 2 weeks of HU therapy, before fetal hemoglobin levels rise. There is a strong inverse correlation between neutrophil count and crisis rate. In terms of clinical efficacy, a randomized, double-blind study has demonstrated that long-term treatment with HU decreases the incidence of painful crisis by 44% in adult patients with sickle cell disease.[17] HU treatment the frequency of acute chest syndrome and hospitalization and the need for blood transfusion. These results establish HU as the first clinically acceptable drug shown to decrease crises in sickle cell disease. HU appears to be as effective in children with sickle cell disease[18] and in patients with sickle cell–β-thalassemia and sickle cell–hemoglobin C disease.[19]

Mechanism of Action and Cellular Pharmacology

The primary site of cytotoxic action for HU is inhibition of the RR enzyme system. This highly regulated enzyme system is responsible for the conversion of ribonucleotide diphosphates to the deoxyribonucleotide form, which can subsequently be used in either de novo DNA synthesis or DNA repair.[20] HU inhibits RR in vitro,[21] and the extent of inhibition of DNA synthesis observed in HU-treated cells correlates closely with the size of the decreased deoxyribonucleotide pools.[22] This enzyme has an important role as a rate-limiting reaction in the regulation of DNA synthesis. In human and other mammalian cells, this unique enzyme consists of two different subunits, usually referred to as M-1 and M-2.[23] Protein M-1 is a dimer with a molecular weight of 170 kD and contains the binding site

TABLE

12.1   *Key features of hydroxyurea*

Mechanism of action	Inhibitor of RR by inactivation of the tyrosyl free radical on the M-2 subunit.
	Regulation of gene expression.
Pharmacokinetics	Nonlinear at high doses.
	Bioavailability of essentially 100%.
	Elimination half-life of 3.5–4.5 h.
	Rapid distribution to tissues and extracellular fluid compartments.
Elimination/metabolism	Renal excretion predominates, although interpatient variability is significant.
	Several enzyme systems capable of metabolism of HU exist, but the extent of metabolism in humans is not known.
Drug interactions	Increases metabolism of AraC to active metabolite and the incorporation of arabinosylcytosine triphosphate into DNA.
	Enhances the effects of other antimetabolites.
	Increases the phosphorylation of antiviral nucleosides and favors their incorporation into viral DNA.
	Enhances effects of ionizing radiation.
Toxicity	Myelosuppression with white blood cells affected to a greater extent than platelets or red blood cells.
	Gastrointestinal effects (nausea, vomiting, changes in bowel habits, ulceration).
	Dermatologic effects (pigmentation, leg ulcers, erythema, rash, atrophy, squamous carcinoma of the skin).
	Renal effects, rare.
	Hepatic effects, occasionally severe.
	Neurologic effects, rare.
	Acute interstitial lung disease, rare.
Precautions	Decrease dosage in renal failure until patient tolerance is demonstrated.
	When given with concomitant radiotherapy, anticipate increased tissue reaction.
	Use with caution when combined with AraC or other antimetabolites.
	Use with caution in pregnant or lactating women.

for the diphosphate substrates as well as the allosteric nucleotide triphosphate regulatory sites.[24] Although considerable variability exists among enzymes from various tissue sources, the general regulatory effects are summarized in Table 12-2. The reduction of all substrates is inhibited and the enzyme complex dissociates in the presence of deoxyadenosine triphosphate.[25] Protein M-1 is present at a relatively constant level throughout the cell cycle, except in cells in G_0 or those that have undergone terminal differentiation, in which it is markedly decreased.[26] The gene coding for the M-1 protein can be mapped to chromosome 11.[26]

Protein M-2 is the catalytic subunit of the enzyme and exists as a dimer with a molecular weight of 88 kD. This unique protein contains stoichiometric amounts of iron and a stable organic free radical localized to a tyrosine residue. The fully conserved tyrosyl radical is essential to enzyme activity and is localized in proximity to and stabilized by the binuclear nonheme iron complex.[27] The cellular concentration of M-2 protein is variable throughout the cell cycle; it peaks in S phase, which suggests that functional enzyme activity depends on the concentration of M-2 protein.[28] The M-2 subunit sequences have been mapped to chromosome 2 in human

cells and seem to be in the same amplification unit as the gene for ornithine decarboxylase.

HU enters cells by passive diffusion. The inhibition of RR occurs as a result of the drug's chelation of iron and its inactivation of the tyrosyl free radical on the M-2 subunit, with disruption of the enzyme's iron-binding center.[29] The fact that this inhibition can be partially reversed in vitro by ferrous iron and that cytotoxicity can be enhanced by iron-chelating agents[30] emphasizes the importance

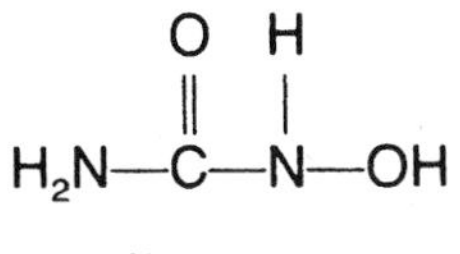

TABLE

12.2   *Regulatory effects of nucleotides triphosphate on ribonucleotide reductase*

Substrate	Activators	Inhibitors
CDP	ATP	dATP, dGTP
UDP		dUTP, dTTP, dATP
ADP	dGTP, GTP	dATP, dTTP
GDP	dTTP	dATP, dGTP

ADP, adenosine diphosphate; ATP, adenosine triphosphate; CDP, cytidine diphosphate; dATP, deoxyadenosine triphosphate; dGTP, deoxyguanosine triphosphate; dTTP, deoxythymidine triphosphate; dUTP, deoxyuridine triphosphate; GDP, guanosine diphosphate; GTP, guanosine triphosphate; UDP, uridine diphosphate.

$$H_2N-\overset{\overset{\displaystyle O}{\|}}{C}-\overset{\overset{\displaystyle H}{|}}{N}-OH$$

FIGURE **12-1**   Structure of hydroxyurea.

of the nonheme iron cofactor in this process. HU selectively kills cells in S phase, and within an S-phase population of cells, those that are most rapidly synthesizing DNA are most sensitive.[31] The cytotoxic effects of HU correlate with dose or concentration achieved, as well as with duration of drug exposure.[32] Following HU exposure, cells progress normally through the cell cycle until they reach the G_1-S interface. Rather than being prevented from entering S phase, as was once thought, cells enter S phase at a normal rate but are accumulated there as a result of the inhibition of DNA synthesis.[33] Cells undergo apoptosis in a process mediated by both *p53* and non-*p53* pathways.

HU may be transformed in vivo to nitric oxide (NO), which is also a RR inhibitor.[34] The possibility, therefore, exists that the RR inhibition observed after HU exposure may be both direct through chelation of iron and indirect and mediated through the NO metabolite. Indeed, HU-borne NO may be the intermediate effector in other actions of the drug, such as its induction of fetal hemoglobin.[14]

Several of the enzymes involved in DNA polymerization and DNA precursor synthesis are assembled in a replitase complex during S phase of the cell cycle to channel metabolites to enzymes sequentially during the synthetic process.[35] Replitase contains DNA polymerases, thymidine kinase, dihydrofolate reductase, nucleoside-5′ phosphate kinase, thymidylate synthase, and RR. Cross-inhibition is a phenomenon observed with enzymes of the replitase complex, in which inhibition of one enzyme in the complex leads to inhibition of a second, unrelated enzyme. This occurs only in intact cells and only in S phase. Evidence suggests that this is the result of a direct allosteric, structural interaction from a remote site within the complex because disruptions of deoxyribonucleotide pools do not explain the findings.[36] HU appears to inhibit DNA polymerases, thymidylate synthase, and thymidine kinase by this mechanism under certain conditions.

A potentially important HU action is acceleration of the loss of extrachromosomally amplified genes that are present in double-minute chromosomes.[37] Acentric extrachromosomal elements are common in the gene amplification process. Exposure to HU at clinically achievable concentrations leads to enhanced loss of both amplified oncogenes and drug-resistance genes.[38]

Mechanisms of Cellular Resistance

The principal mechanism by which cells achieve resistance to HU is elevation in cellular RR activity.[39] Transfection of the human M-2 gene into drug-sensitive KB cells confers resistance by increasing the enzyme activity.[40] Transfection of the M-1 gene does not decrease sensitivity to HU, although transfected cells resist dNTP inhibition of RR activity, probably because of an alteration of the function of effector binding sites. Several different molecular mechanisms can contribute to the increased RR activity in HU-resistant cells. A number of cell lines have amplifications of the gene coding for M-2 protein accompanied by an elevation in M-2 messenger RNA and M-2 protein levels.[41] It also seems that posttranscriptional modifications, such as an increase in initiation factor 4E, can occur during drug selection, which results in an increased translational efficiency. An increase in M-2 protein biosynthetic rate can then occur with no further increase in messenger RNA levels.[42]

In most studies, HU resistance has been associated with a parallel decrease in sensitivity to other RR inhibitors and often to other antimetabolites.[43] Interestingly, some inhibitors of the M-2 subunit, including 3-aminopyridine-2-carboxaldehyde thiosemicarbazone, or 3-AP, retain their antitumor effect in HU-resistant cell lines.[4] In addition, some of these cell lines with increased RR activity display an increased sensitivity to other cytotoxics, particularly, analogs such as 6-thioguanine (via increased conversion to the deoxynucleotide and enhancement of its incorporation into DNA)[44] or gemcitabine (via increased drug uptake by the cells).[45]

Drug Interactions

HU enhances the cytotoxicity of both purine and pyrimidine analogues by reducing the competitive pools of physiologic triphosphates. It causes a significant increase in formation of arabinosylcytosine triphosphate and AraC incorporation into DNA[46] in HU-treated cells and has similar enhancing effect on the antipurines, fludarabine and cladribine. However, clinical trials have not established the synergy of HU in combination with AraC or other antimetabolites in clinical practice.

The major clinical interest in HU in the treatment of solid tumors has been in combination with 5-fluorouracil. Synergy has been demonstrated in experimental tumor models, presumably based on the ability of HU to lower cellular pools of deoxyuridine monophosphate, the competitive substrate for inhibition of thymidylate synthase by 5-fluorodeoxyuridylate.[47] A number of clinical trials of this combination have been performed, but its role remains uncertain.

HU has been evaluated in both clinical and laboratory studies in combination with chemotherapy agents that produce DNA damage, such as alkylating agents, cisplatin, and inhibitors of topoisomerase II.[47] Although synergy has been observed in preclinical testing, the clinical role for such combinations remains speculative. Synchronization in the G_1-S phase drives cells to a condition of increased sensitivity to radiation. By depleting deoxynucleotide pools, HU inhibits DNA repair that follows radiation damage. It has been used as a radiosensitizer in cervical cancer and head and neck cancer, and, experimentally, as a modulator of anti-HIV nucleoside analogues.[48]

Clinical Pharmacology

HU is generally administered orally (an intravenous formulation is also available, but rarely used), and doses are titrated in response to changes in peripheral white blood cell counts. Doses range from 80 mg/kg, given to acute lower leukemic cell counts, to 15 mg/kg/d, the starting dose for patients with sickle cell anemia. In each case, the doses are adjusted to achieve the desired degree of myelosuppression. For sickle cell patients, a neutrophil count of 2,000 cells/mm³ is the target. Neutrophil counts respond rapidly to discontinuation of drug, the period of myelosuppression lasting 2 weeks or less. Although significant interpatient variability is observed, peak concentrations of 0.1 to 2.0 mmol/L are achieved 1.0 to 1.5 hours after doses of 15 to 80 mg/kg.[49] Oral bioavailability is excellent (80% to 100%), and comparable areas under the C × T curve in plasma are seen after oral and intravenous dosing[49,50] (Table 12-3). After

The explanation for the differential effects of the various vinca alkaloids on normal tissues and tumors is not clear. VCR, the most potent of the analogs in humans and the most neurotoxic, has the greatest affinity for tubulin.[51,89] In contrast, VFL's lower affinity for tubulin binding, as well as its greater potential intracellular sequestration, may contribute to its reduced incidence of peripheral neuropathy.[51] Peripheral neurotoxicity, possibly due to drug-induced microtubule loss, steroid hindrance of MAPs, and/or altered microtubule dynamics in axonal processes, is a common adverse effect of first-generation vinca alkaloids.[90] Although the vinca alkaloids may demonstrate similar potencies against preparations of tubulin derived from any given tissue, the differential sensitivities of various tissues to the vinca alkaloids are likely due to several factors.[59,69,87,90–96] One possible factor is tubulin isotype composition, which is highly variable amongst tissues. Intracellular drug accumulation and tubulin binding vary according to tubulin isotype composition.[18,19,97] Neurons are enriched in α-β-tubulin classes II and III, and the relatively high drug binding affinities for these isotypes may explain, in part, why the vinca alkaloids produce neurotoxicity.[88,89,97] The variable potencies of the vinca alkaloids with regard to the induction of tubulin spirals also appear to relate to their relative neurotoxic potencies.[88,89,97] In addition, the differences in the type and concentration of MAPs and posttranslational tubulin modifications between various tissues, which may influence drug interactions with tubulin, as well as differences in the cellular permeability and retention of the various vinca alkaloids, may affect the formation and stability of complexes formed between the vinca alkaloids and tubulin.[27,59,86,89,91,92,98–100] For example, the higher cellular retention of VCR compared with VBL in cultured leukemia cells may explain why VCR is more potent than VBL after brief treatment periods, whereas these effects of the vinca alkaloids differ to a lesser degree with more prolonged exposure times.[91,96,100–103] Additionally, the vinca alkaloids directly inhibit palmitoylation of tubulin, and tubulin palmitoylation may relate to drug sensitivity.[104] The intracellular concentration of GTP concentrations may also influence the type of interactions between the vinca alkaloids and tubulin, and variable vinca alkaloid retention among tumors may relate to GTP hydrolysis.[101–103] Other factors that may explain why various tissues are differentially sensitive to the vinca alkaloid include differences in cellular pharmacology and pharmacokinetics, which is discussed in the next section.

Cellular Pharmacology

Although the vinca alkaloids are rapidly taken up into cells and accumulate intracellularly, steady-state intracellular/extracellular concentration ratios range from 5- to 500-fold depending on the cell type.[91,93,99,103,105] In murine leukemia cells, the intracellular concentrations of VCR are 5- to 20-fold higher than the extracellular concentrations, and this ratio has been reported to range from 150- to 500-fold for other vinca alkaloids in both human and murine leukemia cell lines.[96,105,106] In isolated human hepatocytes, VRL is more rapidly taken up and metabolized than other vinca alkaloids.[96,105–108] Although the vinca alkaloids are retained in cells for long periods and thus may have protracted cellular effects, there are marked differences in cellular retention amongst agents in this class.[109–114] Overall, the most important determinant of drug accumulation and retention is lipophilicity, although a number of other

factors undoubtedly play a role.[105,106] Drug uptake and retention also appear to be determined by tissue-specific and drug-specific factors, as illustrated by studies indicating that the accumulation and retention of VRL in neurons are less than other vinca alkaloids (see the section on "Mechanistic and Functional Differences" under "Vinca Alkaloids").[57,102] Recent studies using cellulose-purified tubulin from porcine brain have demonstrated the following pattern of binding affinities: VCR > VBL > VRL > VFL, which mirrors the relative potential of the vinca alkaloids to induce tubulin spirals.[51,98] As discussed in the last section, the differential tissue uptake of the vinca alkaloid appears to be related to the tissue composition of tubulin isotypes, each possessing different binding characteristics, uptake kinetics, efflux pumps, and intracellular reservoirs for drug accumulation. Although the binding affinity for tubulin appears to be less for VFL than for the other vinca alkaloids, its intracellular accumulation has been demonstrated to be higher than for VBL, VCR, and VRL, which may be due to the sequestration of VFL in, as of yet, undefined intracellular compartments and its slower release over time.[51,75,98]

Temperature-independent, nonsaturable mechanisms, analogous to simple diffusion, seem to account for most transport, and temperature-dependent saturable processes are less important.[27,30,74,93,105,106] Although both drug concentration and treatment duration are important determinants of drug accumulation and cytotoxicity, the duration of exposure above a critical threshold concentration is perhaps the most important determinant of vinca alkaloid cytotoxicity.[96,107] Cytotoxicity is directly related to the extracellular concentration of drug when the duration of treatment is kept constant; for prolonged exposure to VCR, the concentration yielding 50% inhibition ranges from 1 to 5 nmol/L.[107]

Mechanisms of Resistance

Resistance to the vinca alkaloids develops rapidly in vitro with continuous exposure to these agents. Two types of mechanisms of resistance to the vinca alkaloids have been well characterized. The first mechanism is pleiotropic or multidrug resistance (MDR), which can be either innate (primary) or acquired. Although a large number of proteins mediate MDR, the best-characterized ones are the ATP-binding cassette (ABC) transporters, which transport a variety of substrates across cellular compartments and are encoded by a large transporter gene family.[108] These intracellular and extracellular membrane-spanning proteins transport endobiotics and xenobiotics across membranes and confer resistance to the vinca alkaloids, taxanes, and other structurally bulky, natural product chemotherapeutic agents in vitro. The most extensively studied ABC transporters with respect to conferring resistance to the vinca alkaloids are the permeability glycoprotein (Pgp), or the *MDR1* encoded gene product MDR1 (ABC Subfamily B1; ABCB1), and the multidrug resistance protein (MRP) (ABC Subfamily C2; ABCB1).[108–118]

MDR1 is a 170-kDa Pgp energy-dependent transmembrane transport pump that regulates the efflux of a large range of amphipathic hydrophobic substances, resulting in decreased drug accumulation. Pgp forms a channel in the membrane through which drugs are transported, and drug resistance is proportional to the amount of Pgp. Pgp is constitutively overexpressed by various normal tissues, including renal tubular epithelium, colonic mucosa, adrenal medulla, and other epithelial tissues. The efflux protein is also commonly overexpressed by several human cancers, particularly those derived from tissues in which it is constitutively expressed (e.g., kidney and colon cancers). In the clinical setting, Pgp overexpression has been documented following treatment of patients with a variety of malignancies including lymphoma, leukemia, and multiple myeloma.

MDR1 confers varying degrees of cross-resistance to other structurally bulky natural products, such as the taxanes, anthracyclines, epipodophyllotoxins, actinomycin D (dactinomycin), and colchicine.[119–124] These cells may have homogeneously stained chromosomal regions or double-minute chromosomes, which indicates the presence of an amplified gene that codes for Pgp.[110,111] The specific Pgp associated with resistance to the vinca alkaloids shows slight antigenic amino acid sequence differences and a different peptide map after digestion than does Pgp from cells selected for resistance to colchicine or paclitaxel.[116,122] In fact, two forms of the protein are produced by a single clone of VCR-resistant cells, and these forms undergo posttranslational modifications, particularly N-glycosylation and phosphorylation, which results in further structural diversity. This diversity may explain the greater degree of resistance for the specific agent used to induce resistance compared with other MDR substrates, and it also may explain the variable patterns of resistance among cells with the MDR phenotype. The composition of membrane gangliosides in cancer cells resistant to the vinca alkaloids has also been shown to differ from that of wild-type cells.[111] Although VFL is a substrate for Pgp, Pgp overexpression appears to be less involved in conferring resistance to VFL compared with other vinca alkaloids in various types of Pgp-overexpressing human cancers.[118,125] The clinical ramifications of this resistance mechanism are not known, but VCR resistance, as assessed ex vivo, correlates with Pgp overexpression, particularly in childhood acute lymphoblastic leukemia (ALL).[112]

Resistance to the vinca alkaloids is also conferred by MRP1, which is a 190-kDa membrane-spanning protein that shares 15% amino acid homology with MDR1.[116–128] The expression of MRP1, a member of the ABC protein family distantly related to Pgp, is found in many types of cancer and has been implicated as being responsible for the MDR phenotype in cancers of the lung, colon, breast, bladder, and prostate, as well as leukemia.[116–128] Transient increase in MRP1 expression also correlates with resistance to MDR substrate drugs in cell lines transfected with *MRP1*.[123,126] Amplification of *MRP1* has been identified in several laboratory-derived cancer cell lines with elevated levels of MRP1 protein, as well as increased energy-dependent drug efflux.[116–118,128] MRP1 has been shown to transport glutathione conjugates of several types of compounds, including alkylating agents, as well as etoposide and doxorubicin, but it only confers resistance to the latter agents. The MRP1 profile also encompasses resistance to methotrexate but confers a low level of resistance, if any, to the taxanes and colchicine.[112,113,116,118,126–128] Also, MRP1 and other ABC transporters do not confer a significant resistance to VFL.[118,125,129] Expression of MRP in transfected or selected cell lines is principally localized to the plasma membrane and endoplasmic reticulum, suggesting that MRP1 mediates resistance by affecting drug sequestration and/or vesicular transport.[118,127] Several other ABC transporters have also been characterized in vitro, including several that enhance cellular resistance to the vinca alkaloids; how-

ever, their roles in conferring inherent or acquired resistance to the vinca alkaloids in the clinic are even less clear than those of MDR1 and MRP1.

Another important feature of MDR1 and MRP in vitro is that drug resistance may be reversed, in part, after treatment with various agents that have distinctly different structural and functional characteristics, such as the calcium-channel blockers, calmodulin inhibitors, detergents, progestational and antiestrogenic agents, antibiotics, antihypertensives, antiarrhythmics, antimalarials, and immunosuppressives.[130–132] These agents bind directly to Pgp, thereby blocking the efflux of the cytotoxic drugs and increasing intracellular drug concentrations. Therefore, the role of MDR modulators has been a source of great contemporary interest, but the interpretation of clinical studies of resistance modulation has been confounded by the fact that MDR modulators, particularly MDR1 reversal agents, also enhance drug uptake in normal cells, decrease biliary elimination and drug clearance, and lead to enhanced toxicity.[130–132] Overall, strategies aimed at reversing resistance to the vinca alkaloids in the clinic with pharmacologic modulators of both MDR1 and MRP1 have been disappointing, most likely due to the fact that many other proteins besides MDR1 and MRP1 occur in association with the MDR phenotype.[92] Nevertheless, by characterizing the genetics and role of the ABC transporters in normal organ function and in the disposition of chemotherapeutic agents, there is a great deal to learn about how genetic polymorphisms in these proteins impact pharmacokinetics and drug toxicity.

The second well-characterized mechanism of vinca alkaloid resistance relates to tubulin isotypes. Mammalian cells have six α- and seven β-tubulin isotypes, whose expression may influence microtubule dynamics. Structural alterations in α- or β-tubulin due to either genetic mutations and consequential amino acid substitutions or posttranslational modifications, particularly phosphorylation and acetylation, have been identified in cancer cells with acquired resistance to the vinca alkaloids.[18,19,57,69,117,118,133–142] These alterations result in α- and β-tubulins that confer hyperstability to microtubule polymers and are collaterally sensitive to the taxanes and similar tubulin-stabilizing natural products (see "Mechanisms of Resistance" under "Taxanes"). Although the means by which tubulin alterations confer resistance to the vinca alkaloids are not entirely clear, this phenomenon is not apparently due to decreased binding affinity of the altered tubulins for drug.[138–141] Instead, alterations in α- and β-tubulins promote resistance to agents that inhibit microtubule assembly by increasing microtubule stability, perhaps by promoting longitudinal interdimer and intradimer interactions and/or lateral interactions between protofilaments.[142]

Decreased expression of class III β-tubulin, which increases the rate of microtubule assembly, in contrast to overexpression of class III β-tubulin, which is associated with rapid disassembly, is associated vinca alkaloid resistance in vitro.[117,118,137,142–147] Additionally, knockdown of either class II or IVb β-tubulin with siRNA hypersensitizes lung cancer cell lines to the effects of the vinca alkaloids, with the effects more pronounced following knockdown of class IVb β tubulin.[118,137,147] A high level of class III β-tubulin expression also appears to independently predict a poor response and reduced survival in patients with non–small cell lung and breast cancer, following treatment with VRL or the taxanes.[117,118,147–150] These data suggest that class III β-tubulin may alter the dynamic

TABLE

13.3 Key features of the taxanes and epothilones

	Paclitaxel	Docetaxel	PBPPI	Ixabepilone
Mechanism of action	Low concentrations inhibit microtubule dynamics (dynamic instability and treadmilling). High concentrations inhibit depolymerization of tubulin.			
Standard dosage (mg/m²)	175 over 3 h every 3 wk; 135–175 over 24 h every 3 wk; 80 over 1 h weekly	60–100 over 1 h every 3 wk (75 is the most common dose used); 36 over 1 h weekly	260 over 30 min every 3 wk; 100–150 over 30 min weekly	40 (3-h infusion) every 3 wk; should be capped at 2.2 mg/m² for body surface areas exceeding this value.
Principal toxicity	Neutropenia	Neutropenia	Neutropenia	Neutropenia
Other toxicities	Alopecia, peripheral neuropathy, HSR, anemia, thrombocytopenia, myalgia, arthralgia, asthenia	Alopecia, peripheral neuropathy, HSR (mild-moderate), anemia, thrombocytopenia, myalgia, arthralgia, fluid retention, skin and rash toxicity	Alopecia, peripheral neuropathy, anemia, thrombocytopenia, hypersensitivity (mild-moderate)	Peripheral neuropathy, skin, HSRs, anemia, thrombocytopenia
Premedication	Corticosteroids, H_1- and H_2-histamine antagonists before each treatment to prevent HSR (see "Administration")	Corticosteroids with each treatment to prevent fluid retention; H_1-histamine antagonists recommended to HSRs (see "Administration")	None indicated (see "Administration")	H_1- and H_2-histamine antagonists before each treatment to prevent HSR. For patients who experience an HSR, corticosteroids, in addition to pretreatment with H_1-histamine and H_2-histamine antagonists, are recommended. (see "Administration")
Pharmacokinetic behavior	Triexponential; Saturable elimination and distribution; pseudononlinearity due to vehicle	Triexponential; Dose proportional to 115 mg/m²	Biexponential; Dose proportional	Multiexponential; Dose proportional
C_{peak} (µmol/L)	3.37 (100 mg/m² 1-h infusion weekly); 4.30 (175 mg/m² 3-h infusion every 3 wk)	1.9 (36 mg/m² 1-h infusion weekly); 2.3 (75 mg/m² 1-h infusion every 3 wk)		
Plasma half-life (terminal phase) (h)	10–20	10–20	~27	~52
Clearance (L/h)	20–25 (3-h schedule)	~36	~15	36–40
Vd_{ss} (L/m²)	99 (3-h schedule)	67		
Protein binding	>95%; albumin and α_1–acid glycoprotein	>80%–95%; α_1–acid glycoprotein, albumin, and lipoproteins		
Primary route of elimination	Hepatic metabolism and biliary elimination	Hepatic metabolism and biliary elimination	Hepatic metabolism and biliary elimination	Hepatic metabolism and biliary elimination
Precautions	Patients with abnormal liver function should be treated with caution. See section on dosage and schedule for specific dosing guidelines.			

HSR, hypersensitivity reaction; PBPPI, protein-bound paclitaxel particles for injection.

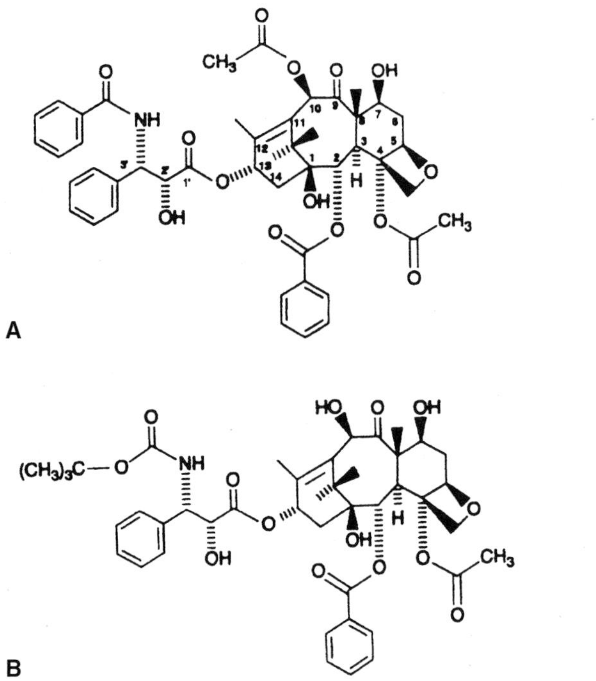

A

B

FIGURE **13-5** Structures of the taxanes: paclitaxel (**A**) and docetaxel (**B**).

(Cremophor EL).[298,319] The role of PBPPI is currently being evaluated in non–small cell, prostate, and other cancers.

Structures

The structures of paclitaxel, docetaxel, and their precursor 10-deacetylbaccatin III are shown in Figure 13-5. The taxanes are complex alkaloid esters, consisting of a 15-member taxane ring system linked to an unusual four-member oxetane ring at positions C-4 and C-5.[320,321] The taxane rings of both paclitaxel and docetaxel, but not 10-deacetylbaccatin III, are linked to an ester at the C-13 position. Structure-function studies suggest that taxane analogs without this ester linkage interact minimally with mammalian tubulin, although they still stabilize microtubules of the amoeba *Physarum polycephalum*. Furthermore, the moieties at the C-2′ and C-3′ positions are essential for the unique antimicrotubule action of the taxanes. Acetyl substitution at C-2′ results in a substantial loss of activity. The structures of paclitaxel and docetaxel differ in substitutions at the C-10 taxane ring position and on the ester side chain attached at C-13, which renders docetaxel slightly more water soluble and more potent than paclitaxel. Neither the acetyl group at C-10 nor the phenyl group at C-5′ is required for in vitro activity, and the structures of paclitaxel and docetaxel differ in linkages at these positions.[321]

Mechanism of Action

The taxanes bind poorly to soluble tubulin, but, instead, bind directly and with high affinity to polymerized tubulin along the length of the microtubule.[292–296] The binding sites are distinct from those of exchangeable GTP, colchicine, podophyllotoxin, and the vinca alkaloids, and the taxanes do not inhibit the binding of these agents to their respective sites. Photoaffinity studies have indicated that paclitaxel principally binds to the N-terminal 1 to 31 amino acids and residues 217 to 233 of the β-tubulin subunit,

and the paclitaxel pharmacophore has been characterized.[322–324] X-ray crystallographic models of the β-tubulin N-terminus indicate that His 227 and Asp 224 are critical to binding the C-2 benzoyl side chain of paclitaxel, and modeling data also indicate that both paclitaxel and docetaxel bind to the interior surface of the microtubule lumen (i.e., shows binding of the taxanes).[14,324–326] Other antimicrotubule natural products with similar mechanisms of action, such as the epothilones and eleutherobins, appear to occupy the same binding sites, although they have an altered core and side chain.[324–326] Paclitaxel binds reversibly to microtubules reassembled in vitro with high affinity (K_d, 10 nmol), whereas the binding affinity for docetaxel, which is slightly more water soluble, is approximately 1.9-fold higher.[2,3,4,14,296,327,328] It has been reported that tubulin assembly induced by docetaxel also proceeds with a critical protein concentration that is 2.1-fold lower than that of paclitaxel.[327] However, these differences, along with the higher potency of docetaxel, do not necessarily mean that docetaxel has a higher therapeutic index as greater potency may also portend more severe toxicity at identical drug concentrations in vivo. Furthermore, both preclinical and clinical studies have been inconsistent about whether the taxanes are completely cross-resistant, possibly because these studies used dose schedules and clinical formulations that are not equivalent.[329–332]

In contrast to the vinca alkaloids, the taxanes disrupt microtubule dynamics by reducing the critical tubulin concentration required for microtubule assembly and promoting both the nucleation and elongation phases of the polymerization reaction, which, in essence, stabilizes the microtubule against depolymerization and enhances polymerization.[2–5,40,72,292–296,333–340] Nevertheless, the vinca alkaloids and taxanes seem to produce similar disruptive effects on the mitotic spindle apparatus and the mitotic process. Binding of the taxanes to their binding site on the inside of the microtubule stabilizes and actually strengthens the microtubule and enhances tubulin polymerization. It induces a conformation change in tubulin, that, by an unknown mechanism, increases tubulin affinity for neighboring tubulin molecules.[2] In essence, these actions profoundly alter the tubulin dissociation rate constants at each end of the microtubule without affecting the association rate constants, thereby suppressing both treadmilling and dynamic instability. There is one paclitaxel binding site on each tubulin molecule of the microtubule, and the ability of paclitaxel to enhance polymerization is associated with nearly 1:1 stoichiometric binding of paclitaxel to tubulin in microtubules. At submicromolar concentrations that are readily achieved in the clinic, binding is stoichiometric and tubulin polymerization is enhanced. However, substoichiometric concentrations suppress microtubule dynamics without increasing the amount of polymerized tubulin.[333,334] The taxanes induce tubulin self-assembly into microtubules in the cold and in the absence of exogenous GTP and MAPs, which are normally required for these processes.[292,294–296,333–340] Furthermore, taxane-treated microtubules are extraordinarily stable, resisting depolymerization in response to cold, calcium, dilution, and depolymerizing agents. This stability impedes dynamic processes, which result in continuous remodeling and reorganization of the microtubule network, essential processes for vital cellular functions in both mitosis and interphase.

The stoichiometry of taxane binding to microtubules in vitro greatly influences the nature of the perturbations of these agents on tubulin dynamics. Both stoichiometric and substoichiometric drug binding inhibit the proliferation of cells, principally by inducing a sustained mitotic block at the metaphase/anaphase boundary. At low concentrations (10 to 50 nmol/L), the binding of small numbers of paclitaxel molecules to microtubules reduces the rate and extent of microtubule shortening at their assembly (plus) ends.[2,3,30,38,334] At higher concentrations (10 to 100 nmol/L), paclitaxel preferentially suppresses tubulin dynamics and induces a modest increase in microtubule length at the plus ends with negligible effect on dynamics at the minus ends. At paclitaxel concentrations ranging from 100 to 1,000 nmol/L, which are readily achieved in cancer patients, growing and shortening rates are suppressed to the same extent, and microtubules remain in a state of attenuation. At very high concentrations (1 to 20 μmol/L), which are likely achieved intracellularly following administration of standard doses due to the high tubulin affinity for the taxanes in almost all tissues, the binding of paclitaxel to microtubules is saturated at a stoichiometry of 1 mole drug/mole tubulin, and the mass of microtubule polymer increases sharply as tubulin is recruited into the microtubules.[333] In HeLa cells, mitosis is half-maximally blocked at 8 nmol/L paclitaxel, whereas polymer mass is half-maximally increased at 80 nmol/L, and there is no increase in microtubule polymer mass below 10 nmol/L.[72] The taxanes inhibit tubulin dissociation at both microtubule ends, but the ends remain free for tubulin addition.[338] The taxanes also inhibit microtubule treadmilling.[2,3] Most studies with docetaxel indicate that it suppresses tubulin dynamics similar to paclitaxel, but the structural aspects of abnormal microtubules induced by paclitaxel and docetaxel may differ. In one report, for example, paclitaxel induced the formation of microtubules with predominantly 12 protofilaments, whereas 13 protofilaments are usually evident in docetaxel-induced microtubules.[327]

As with the vinca alkaloids, the suppression of spindle-microtubule dynamics by the taxanes prevents the dividing cell from progressing from metaphase into anaphase and the cells eventually undergo apoptosis. At low concentrations (<10 nmol/L), mitosis is blocked with no concomitant increase in microtubule mass. The alterations in spindle organization induced by the taxanes resemble those induced by the vinca alkaloids, suggesting that mitotic arrest is the end result of perturbations in microtubule dynamics, irrespective of whether the agent results in microtubule depolymerization or polymerization. At higher concentrations (>100 nmol/L), microtubule mass is increased, mitosis is blocked, and large and dense spindle asters containing prominent bundles of stabilized microtubules are formed. With increasing taxane concentrations, the spindles become monopolar and the chromosomes condense, but do not congress.[30,295] Even substoichiometric taxane concentrations, which are sufficient to induce mitotic arrest without increasing microtubule mass, may induce apoptosis (see the sections on "Drug Resistance" and "Taxanes").[72,341–352]

The taxanes, as well as other antimicrotubule agents that perturb mitosis, are associated with presence of abnormal spindles with uncongressed chromosomes (i.e., failure to line up at the equator), a morphology that is highly predictive of suppression of microtubule dynamics in interphase cells and suppression of centromere dynamics in mitotic cells. Suppression of dynamics has at least two downstream effects on the spindle: it prevents the mitotic spindle from assembling normally, and it reduces the tension at the kinetochores of the chromosomes. The downstream effects of prolonged mitotic arrest are frequent multinucleated cells and/or apoptosis. In addition, the taxanes and other microtubule stabilizing drugs

often induce mitotic cells with multiple spindle poles.[3,336] The precise mechanism by which these drugs cause multipolar spindles is unclear. The taxanes induce disassociation of centrosomal components and it is conceivable that individual centrosomal components may be able to nucleate additional asters in the absence of bonafide centrioles.[3,353]

Perturbations of the mitotic processes and the induction of mitotic arrest by the taxanes trigger several fates for cells that exit mitosis, including cell-cycle progression, cell-cycle arrest and apoptosis, but the precise means by which these fates are governed are not well understood (see the sections on "Mechanism of Action" under "Vinca Alkaloids").[352–355] Nevertheless, the tumor suppressor gene p53 appears to be involved as there is substantial evidence that p53 restrains cell-cycle progression following exit from a prolonged mitotic block. Microtubule disruption induces p53 and inhibitors of cyclin-dependent kinases (CDK; e.g., p21/Waf-1) and modulates several protein kinases.[26,72,341–350] As a consequence, cells are arrested in G_2/M, after which time they may either undergo apoptosis or traverse through G_2/M and divide.[356] Several potential mechanisms may link mitotic arrest induced by the taxanes to the initiating events in the intrinsic pathway of apoptosis. These include the activation of the proapoptotic molecules Bax and Bad, as well as the inactivation of the antiapoptotic regulators Bcl-2 and Bcl$_{xL}$.[357–359] Taxane-induced mitochondrial stress triggering apoptosis occurs through activation of both Jun N-terminal kinase (JNK) and p38 pathways, and various kinases have been implicated in the phosphorylation of Bcl-2 induced by the taxanes and other antimicrotubule agents, including JNK and its proapoptotic effector Bim, c-Raf, extracellular signal-regulated kinase (ERK) 1 and 2, CDK-1, cAMP-dependent protein kinase A, and protein kinase C.[26,358] Phosphorylation (inactivation) of Bcl-2 family members (Bad, BCL-2) and phosphorylation of proapoptotic molecules (activation) stimulate the intrinsic pathway of apoptosis and a wide range of effector caspases.[356,358,360–362] Paclitaxel has also been shown to bind directly to Bcl-2, but Bcl-2 phosphorylation does not appear to play a preeminent role in inducing apoptosis in all types of cancer.[364,365] Furthermore, caspase-independent mechanisms of mitotic death have been described.[366]

The taxanes also disrupt interphase microtubules and inhibit DNA synthesis by an unknown mechanism in nonproliferating cells.[28,368] In nonproliferating cells, the taxanes induce the formation of microtubule bundles, which resemble hoops and ribbons, in interphase cells.[367] Paclitaxel induces the expression of tumor necrosis factor-α (TNF-α), as well as transcription factors and enzymes that mediate proliferation, apoptosis, and inflammation.[344,350,359,364,368,369] The taxanes enhance the effects of ionizing radiation in vitro at clinically achievable concentrations (<50 nmol/L) and in vivo, perhaps by inhibition of cell-cycle progression in the G_2 phase, the most radiosensitive phase of the cell cycle.[369–373] The taxanes and other microtubule-stabilizing agents also disrupt endothelial cells and inhibit angiogenesis at concentrations below those that induce cytotoxicity.[374–378] Interestingly, paclitaxel concentrations as low as 0.1 to 5 nmol/L disrupt microtubule dynamics in endothelial cells, which appear to be less sensitive than tumor cells to the effects of paclitaxel at higher concentrations (100 nmol/L).[377]

The taxanes induce many other cellular effects that may or may not relate to their disruptive effects on microtubule dynamics. Although they principally block cell-cycle traverse in mitosis, the taxanes block G_0 to S phase transition in both normal and malignant cells.[28,367,379,380] Their potential to disrupt tubulin in the cell membrane and/or interphase cytoskeleton, as well as microtubules involved in growth factor signaling, may account for this nonmitotic action.[29,379–381]

The taxanes also inhibit specific functions in nonmalignant tissues, which may be mediated through their disruptive effects on microtubule dynamics.[29] For example, paclitaxel inhibits relevant morphologic and biochemical processes in human neutrophils, including chemotaxis, migration, spreading, polarization, hydrogen peroxide generation, and killing of phagocytozed microorganisms.[29] In addition, paclitaxel antagonizes the effects of microtubule-disrupting drugs on lymphocyte function and cAMP metabolism and inhibits the proliferation of stimulated human lymphocytes.[29] Paclitaxel mimics the effects of endotoxic bacterial lipopolysaccharide on macrophages, which results in a rapid decrement in TNF-α receptors and TNF-α release.[368,381,382] The agent also induces expression of TNF-α, but these activities independent of paclitaxel's disruptive effects on microtubule assembly, which raises the issue of the role of cytokines in the antitumor activities of the taxanes.[368] Additionally, paclitaxel inhibits chorioretinal fibroblast proliferation and contractility in an in vitro model of proliferative vitreoretinopathy, and blocks neointimal smooth muscle cell proliferation after angioplasty in a rat model.[382,383] Cardiac arterial stents coated with paclitaxel received regulatory approval in the United States and elsewhere in 2003 because the coated stents significantly decreased the incidence of restenosis due to fibroblast proliferation and intimal hyperplasia.[384] Finally, paclitaxel inhibits secretory functions in many specialized cells, such as insulin secretion in isolated rat islets of Langerhans, protein secretion in rat hepatocytes, and the nicotinic receptor-stimulated release of catecholamines from chromaffin cells of the adrenal medulla.[29]

PPBPI likely affects malignant and nonmalignant tissues in a manner similar to paclitaxel in conventional formulations. However, the binding of paclitaxel to albumin may result in increased accumulation of paclitaxel molecules in tumor tissue by two mechanisms albumin-specific glycoprotein 60-mediated endothelial cell transcytosis of paclitaxel-bound albumin, and accumulation in the area of tumor by albumin binding to a receptor-like protein, secreted protein acidic and rich in cysteine (SPARC).[385–390] These factors may result in more rapid systemic distribution and clearance of paclitaxel than polyoxyethylated castor oil formulations.[389,390] SPARC up-regulation in tumors may be a poor prognostic factor in several types of malignancies. It has been hypothesized that SPARC-albumin interaction facilitates the accumulation of albumin in the tumor and increases the effectiveness of PPBPI.[385–390]

Mechanisms of Resistance

The MDR phenotype, which is mediated by several members of the ABC transporter family and confers cross-resistance to a wide range of xenobiotics is the best characterized mechanism of resistance to the taxanes (see the section on "Mechanisms of Resistance," under "Vinca Alkaloids"). The most important ABC transporters with respect to conferring taxane resistance is Pgp or the *MDR1* encoded gene product MDR1 (ABC Subfamily B1; ABCB1) and MDR2 (ABC Subfamily ABCB4).[116,344,391] In contrast to the vinca alkaloids, ABCC1 (MRP1) and ABCC2 (MRP2) confer a lower level of resistance to the taxanes.[392,393] The clinical relevance of MRP overexpression, identified in several hematologic and solid malignancies and associated with poor prognosis, still remains to be fully elucidated. Low-level taxane resistance also appears to be conferred by the bile salt export protein (BSEP, also known as ABCC11).[113,116] Early clinical observations of the antitumor profile of the taxanes, particularly in women with breast cancer who respond to the taxanes following the development of progressive disease while receiving treatment with the anthracyclines, suggest that cross-resistance to the taxanes and anthracycline is incomplete, but the role of MDR as a major cause of anthracycline resistance in this setting is not clear. Similar to the vinca alkaloids, taxane resistance associated with the MDR phenotype can be reversed by many classes of drugs, including the calcium channel blockers, tamoxifen, cyclosporine A, and antiarrhythmic agents.[113,116,344,394,395] In fact, plasma concentrations of the principal component of the vehicles used to formulate paclitaxel and docetaxel, polyoxyethylated castor oil (Cremophor EL) and polysorbate-80 (Tween 80), respectively, can also reverse taxane resistance.[396,397] However, the plasma concentrations of polyoxyethylated castor oil achieved with paclitaxel on clinically relevant dose schedules are sufficient to reverse MDR, whereas sufficient modulatory concentrations of polysorbate-80 are not achieved with docetaxel. Strategies aimed at reversing taxane resistance with various transporter substrates in the clinic have resulted in low impact at best; however, the interpretation of these results is confounded by the effects of these agents, particularly those that are MDR substrates, on taxane clearance and toxicity.[344,394,395,397,398] Nevertheless, MDR modulators, including verapamil, cyclosporine A, VX-710, the nonimmunomodulatory cyclosporine analogue PSC 833, and other agents that do not affect taxane pharmacokinetics and toxicity, do not appear to significantly enhance antitumor activity.[113,344,395,398]

Alterations in cytoskeletal components, tubulin-binding sites, or microtubule dynamics have also been implicated in drug resistance to the taxanes. Several taxane-resistant mutant cell lines have structurally altered α-tubulin and β-tubulin proteins and an impaired ability to polymerize into microtubules (see the section on "Mechanisms of Resistance," under "Vinca Alkaloids").[16,139–141,344,399–403] Mutants with "hypostable" microtubules exhibit collateral sensitivity to the vinca alkaloids. Paclitaxel-resistant Chinese hamster ovary cells with mutated β-tubulin alleles that encode the putative taxane binding sites, specifically, leucine moieties at positions 215, 217, and 228 mutated to histidine, arginine, or phenylalanine, have been described.[404,405] Low-level expression was associated with resistance, whereas high-level expression of any of these mutations was linked to impairment of assembly, cell-cycle arrest, and failure to proliferate.[405] Some clinical reports suggest that β-tubulin mutations in non–small cell lung cancer may underlie taxane resistance, but others have found no such relationship in breast and ovarian cancers.[26,406,407] Most β-tubulin gene mutations involve the β-tubulin class III genes but other mutations like β-tubulin gene mutations, particularly class I gene mutations, have been observed. A loss of wild-type γ-actin, with concomitant expression of mutant isoforms identified in human ALL cells and more recently in tumor samples from ALL patients at relapse, enhances selection for resistance to both tubulin-depolymerizing and tubulin-polymerizing agents.[408]

A number of cancers grown in vitro and sampled from patients resistant to tubulin-binding agents, including the taxanes, have alterations in tubulin content, tubulin isotype profiles, and tubulin polymerization dynamics.[344,401–403,409–411] Significantly higher levels of class I, III, and IVa isotypes of β-tubulin have been associated with taxane resistance in both preclinical and clinical studies.[26,136,147,148,344,402,403,411] The most common tubulin isotype aberration that relates to taxane resistance is higher intratumoral levels of the β-III tubulin isotype, which is a typically expressed in low levels. High cellular levels of β-III tubulin increase the dynamic instability of microtubules and impede microtubule assembly, whereas low levels are associated with rapid microtubule assembly.[147–149,402,403,411] High expression of the β-III tubulin isotype has been demonstrated in tumor biopsies sampled from patients with a wide range of taxane-resistant malignancies, most prominently non–small cell and breast cancers, as well as cell lines, with acquired drug resistance.[147–149,344,412–415] High levels of class III β-tubulin RNA levels have also been reported in non–small cell lung cancers of patients who did not respond to taxane-based treatment.[410,416] Further proof that β-III tubulin levels relate to taxane resistance is provided by experiments that demonstrate that antisense oligonucleotides to β-tubulin class III RNA, as well as silencing of β-III tubulin expression, decrease protein expression and increase drug sensitivity in taxane-resistant cells.[26,147,417] Tubulin gene amplifications and isotype switching have also been reported in taxane-resistant cell lines.[105,344,356–359,365]

Aberrant proliferative signaling may contribute to taxane resistance by raising the cell's threshold for apoptosis. For example, insulin-like growth factor I protects responsive breast cancer cell lines from anthracyclines and taxanes, possibly by activating the phosphoinositide 3-kinase (PI3K) pathway and inducing phosphorylation (inactivation) of antiapoptotic factors.[418,421] Mesothelin, a secreted protein expressed in some cancers, can also inhibit paclitaxel-induced cell death by modulating PI3K signaling in the regulation of Bcl-2 family expression.[418,419] Higher levels of phosphorylated Akt have also conferred paclitaxel resistance.[420] Other mediators that may influence the cell's threshold for drug-induced apoptosis include p53, HER-2, auora kinase, survivin, and BRAC1.[421] The centromere-associated serine/threonine kinase, aurora kinase, which is involved in centrosome separation, bipolar spindle formation, and chromosomal kinetochore attachment to the mitotic spindle, overrides the mitotic assembly checkpoint and induces taxane resistance.[11–13,26] In addition, the overexpression of survivin, a member of the inhibitor of apoptosis family of proteins, inhibits caspase activity and apoptosis induced by antimicrotubule agents.[26] The disruption of the tumor-suppressor gene BRAC1, which is implicated in maintaining genomic stability through DNA repair, appears to play a role in conferring resistance to paclitaxel and the inducible expression of BRAC1 may enhance paclitaxel-induced apoptosis.[26] Recently, overexpression of NAC-1, a transcription factor and member of the BTB/POZ gene family, has been shown to relate to recurrent ovarian cancer and paclitaxel resistance.[422] Finally, overexpression of p21, a downstream effector of p53, impedes cell cycle traverse in G_2, thereby blocking progression into the more drug-vulnerable mitotic phase and decreasing taxane sensitivity.[423,424]

MAPs have been implicated in mechanisms of resistance to apoptosis induced by the taxanes and other antimicrotubule agents: MAP4, which is negatively regulated by wild-type p53, increases sensitivity to paclitaxel.[152,153] The MAP stathmin modulates taxane resistance (see the section on "Mechanisms of Resistance," under "Vinca Alkaloids").[425]

Transfection of cells with HER-2, a member of the epidermal growth factor receptor, which is amplified and overexpressed in approximately 30% of breast cancers, confers taxane resistance, and high expression of HER-2 in vitro is associated with taxane resistance.[426,427] Consistent with these observations, down-regulation of HER-2 by the anti–HER-2 antibody trastuzumab sensitizes breast cancer cells to the taxanes, and the treatment of women with HER-2-overexpressing breast cancer with trastuzumab combined with paclitaxel increases survival compared to paclitaxel alone.[306] Nevertheless, the presence of HER-2 amplifications in breast cancer does not adversely influence response to paclitaxel-containing chemotherapy in the clinic.[428,429] In a study evaluating the addition of paclitaxel following adjuvant treatment with doxorubicin plus cyclophosphamide in women with lymph node–positive breast cancer, the presence of HER-2 expression or amplification, or both, did not adversely influence the benefits conferred by adding paclitaxel, regardless of estrogen receptor status, whereas women with HER-2–negative disease derived little benefit, if any from paclitaxel.[428]

Clinical Pharmacology

Analytical Assays

The earliest analytical assays used to measure paclitaxel concentrations in biologic samples were biochemical assays that exploited the ability of paclitaxel to induce tubulin to form cold-resistant polymers that hydrolyze GTP at 0°C; however, such assays lacked requisite sensitivity (0.1 µmol/L) to measure low plasma concentrations achieved in clinical trials and were too cumbersome for monitoring large numbers of clinical samples.[430] Immunologic assays, including indirect competitive inhibition enzyme immunoassays and ELISAs, that were developed for detecting taxanes in plant extracts were highly sensitive (0.3 nmol/L) and amenable to high-throughput procedures, but the degree of cross-reactivity of the antibodies to the taxanes, their metabolites, and other moieties are not known.[431] The earliest chromatographic separation methods, including HPLC with ultraviolet detection, had variable extraction efficiencies, suboptimal lower limits of sensitivity (≥50 nmol/L), and other unfavorable assay performance characteristics. More sensitive HPLC assays, particularly those using tandem mass spectroscopy and solid phase extraction, can detect paclitaxel and docetaxel concentrations in the low nanomolar to picomolar range in minute quantities of plasma (0.05 mL) and several are capable of simultaneously measuring metabolites.[397,432,433] Further improvement in sensitivity and specificity for determining taxane concentrations in human plasma can also be achieved by using ultraperformance liquid chromatography–tandem mass spectrometry.[434]

Pharmacokinetics

The oral bioavailability of both paclitaxel and docetaxel is poor, owing in part to the constitutive overexpression of Pgp and other ABC transporters by enterocytes and/or first-pass metabolism in the liver and/or intestines. Nevertheless, biologically relevant plasma concentrations can be achieved if the taxanes are administered orally with oral modulators of ABC transporters and/or cytochrome P450 mixed-function oxidases such as cyclosporine, but oral administration of taxanes is generally associated with high intraindividual variability in pharmacokinetics, as well as clinical effects.[397,435] Rapid drug distribution and avid binding in all tissues except for central nervous system result in large volumes of distribution, high clearance rates, short distribution $t_{1/2}$ values, and long terminal $t_{1/2}$ values.

Paclitaxel

The pharmacokinetics of paclitaxel on both long and short administration schedules have been characterized (Table 13-3). In early studies that principally evaluated prolonged (6- and 24-hour) schedules, substantial interpatient variability was noted, and nonlinear, dose-dependent behavior was not observed.[398,442,443] In these studies, drug disposition was characterized as biphasic, with values for α- and β-$t_{1/2}$ values averaging 20 minutes and 6 hours, respectively. However, subsequent studies of shorter administration schedules, especially a 3-hour infusion, indicate that the pharmacokinetic behavior of paclitaxel is nonlinear.[397,436–439] Nonlinearity occurs with all administration schedules, but it is more apparent with shorter infusions which result in higher plasma paclitaxel concentrations that are more likely to saturate both drug elimination and tissue distribution processes. Both saturable distribution and elimination may be, in part, responsible for paclitaxel's nonlinear behavior. Tissue distribution becomes saturated at lower drug concentrations (achieved with paclitaxel doses <175 mg/m² over 3 hours) compared with elimination processes that are effectively saturated at higher concentrations (achieved with paclitaxel doses >175 mg/m² over 3 hours). The use of shorter infusion schedules also results in higher plasma concentrations of paclitaxel's polyoxyethylated castor oil vehicle, which may be responsible for an appearance of nonlinearity (or pseudononlinearity).[440,441] A true nonlinear profile may have several important clinical implications, particularly regarding dose modifications at doses associated with nonlinearity because dose escalation may result in a disproportionate increase in drug exposure and hence toxicity, whereas dose reduction may result in a disproportionate decrease in drug exposure, thereby decreasing antitumor activity. Shorter paclitaxel infusion schedules are also associated with reduced clearance and higher concentrations of the polyoxyethylated castor oil vehicle, which may simulate nonlinearity (pseudononlinearity) by binding paclitaxel and reducing clearance. These effects, as well as reduced exposure to unbound paclitaxel, may explain the lower incidence of hematologic toxicity and higher incidence of HSRs with shorter infusions.[441,442]

The volume of distribution of paclitaxel is much larger than that of total body water, which is likely the result of extensive drug distribution and binding to plasma proteins and other tissue elements, particularly tubulin. Estimates of the magnitude of protein binding reach as high as 98% with equilibrium dialysis and ultracentrifugation.[397,443] Protein binding is readily reversible.[397] At clinically relevant concentrations (0.1 to 0.6 µmol/L), protein binding is concentration independent, which may be attributable to nonspecific hydrophobic binding. Despite extensive binding to plasma proteins, paclitaxel is readily eliminated from the plasma compartment, a finding that suggests lower-affinity, reversible binding. Albumin and α_1–acid glycoprotein contribute equally to the binding, with a minor contribution from lipoproteins.[444,445] None of the drugs that are commonly administered with paclitaxel, including ranitidine, dexamethasone, diphenhydramine, doxorubicin, 5-fluorouracil, and cisplatin, substantially alter protein binding.[397,444] Drug binding to platelets is extensive and saturable, whereas binding to red

blood cells is insignificant.[398,449,450] Animal distribution studies with radiolabeled paclitaxel indicate extensive drug uptake and retention by virtually all tissues, except "tumor sanctuary sites" such as the central nervous system and testes.[446] However, paclitaxel appears to have affinity for distribution to specific tissue types. Kidney, lung, spleen, and third-space fluid collections, including ascitic and pleural fluid, have been found to have the high concentrations; however, the highest drug concentrations have been demonstrated to be in liver and tumor tissues.[397,443]

In addition, clearance relates to body surface area, providing a rationale for dosing based on this measurement.[447] In humans, peak plasma concentrations achieved with 3- to 96-hour infusions (>0.05 to 10 µmol/L) and drug concentrations in third-space fluid collections, such as ascites (>0.1 µmol/L), are capable of inducing significant biologic effects in vitro, but drug penetration into the unperturbed central nervous system is negligible.[397,436–439,441,442,447]

Paclitaxel disposition occurs predominantly by cytochrome P450 mixed function oxidase metabolism in the liver followed by the excretion of both parent drug and metabolites into the bile.[397,436,438,443,448–455] Ninety-eight percent of radioactivity is recovered from feces collected for 6 days after rats are treated with radiolabeled paclitaxel, and approximately 71% of an administered dose of paclitaxel is excreted in the feces over 5 days as either parent compound or metabolites in humans, with 6α-hydroxypaclitaxel being the largest component and accounting for 26% of the dose. Only 5% is unchanged paclitaxel. Renal clearance of paclitaxel and metabolites is minimal, accounting for 14% of the administered dose.[397] In humans, the cytochrome P450 mixed-function oxidases CYP2C8 and CYP3A4 are responsible for the bulk of drug disposition. All human paclitaxel metabolites that have been identified are hydroxylated derivatives with intact side chains at taxane ring positions C-2 and C-13, whereas low concentrations of baccatin III, which lacks the side chain at position C-13, are found in rat bile.[449,454] The principal metabolites in human plasma and bile include 6α-hydroxypaclitaxel, a product of CYP2C8; p-hydroxyphenyl-C3′-paclitaxel, a product of CYP3A4; and a dihydroxymetabolite (6α- and C3′-dihydroxypaclitaxel). The metabolites are much less active than paclitaxel in cell culture, but several are as active as paclitaxel in stabilizing microtubules against disassembly in a cell-free system.[455] All three retain some cytotoxicity against human bone marrow cells ex vivo.[455] One possible explanation for this discrepancy is that the cell does not take up these hydroxylated metabolites, which are more polar than paclitaxel.

There is considerable interindividual variability in the qualitative and quantitative aspects of taxane metabolism, which can be attributed to pharmacogenetic differences in P450 metabolism and concurrent medications that variably alter metabolism.[397,436,438,440,443,449–452,456–458] Genetic polymorphisms, often related to ethnicity, can affect CYP2C8 and CYP3A4, as well as CYP3A5 that has overlapping activities with CYP3A4. However, only CYP2C8 polymorphisms have clinical implications. Study data regarding the clinical role of CYP2C8 polymorphisms are discrepant.[443,456,457,459–462] Furthermore, genetic polymorphisms, also related to race and ethnicity, have been found in the Pgp transporter MDR1, as well as MRP1 and MRP2, all of which can affect transport of products of metabolism and parent drugs.[443,457] In fact, both neutropenia and neurotoxicity, as well as antitumor activity, have been related to ABCB1 polymorphisms.[456,463] However, little is known about the relationships between Pgp polymorphisms and specific changes in paclitaxel metabolism.

Pharmacokinetic parameters indicative of drug exposure have been related to the principal toxicities of paclitaxel, the most important of which is the relationship between the severity of neutropenia and the duration of drug exposure above biologically relevant plasma concentrations ranging from 0.05 to 0.1 μmol/L.[397,436–439,453,464] However, a prospective analysis of pharmacokinetic determinants of outcome in patients with advanced non–small cell lung cancer treated with cisplatin combined with paclitaxel at either 135 or 250 mg/m^2 over 24 hours showed that the magnitude of the steady-state plasma paclitaxel concentration correlated poorly with antitumor activity, disease-free survival, and overall survival.[465] In randomized trials evaluating the effects of paclitaxel dose on outcome in patients with advanced ovarian, non–small cell lung, breast, and head and neck cancer, doses above 175 mg/m^2 resulted in neither increased progression-free nor overall survival.

Docetaxel

The pharmacokinetics of docetaxel on a 1-hour schedule are linear at doses of 115 mg/m^2 or less and optimally fit a three-compartment model.[297,466–472] Terminal $t_{1/2}$ values ranging from 11.1 to 18.5 hours have been reported. In one population study, plasma concentration data optimally fit a three-compartment model, and the following pharmacokinetic parameters were generated: $t_{1/2\gamma}$ of 12.4 hours, clearance of 1 L/h/m^2, and steady-state volume of distribution of 74 L/m^2.[469,470,472] The most important determinants of docetaxel clearance were the body surface area, hepatic function, age, and plasma α_1–acid glycoprotein and albumin concentrations. As with paclitaxel, plasma protein binding is high (>85% to 95%), and binding is primarily to α_1–acid glycoprotein, albumin, and lipoproteins.[297,466–472] Higher free fraction values relate to low α_1–acid glycoprotein concentrations and may confer greater toxicity. As with paclitaxel, docetaxel is widely distributed and avidly bound in all tissues except tumor sanctuary sites.[470,472,473] In both dogs and mice treated with radiolabeled drug, fecal excretion accounts for 70% to 80% of total radioactivity, whereas urinary excretion accounts for 10% or less.[470,471] In mice and dogs, tissue [^{14}C]docetaxel rapidly distributes into tissues from plasma with an apparent $t_{1/2}$ of 10 minutes.[470] Immediately after treatment, tissue uptake of radioactivity is highest in the liver, bile, and intestines, a finding that is consistent with substantial hepatobiliary extraction and excretion. High levels of radioactivity are also found in the stomach, which indicates the possibility of gastric secretion, as well as in the spleen, bone marrow, myocardium, skeletal muscles, and pancreas, but not the central nervous system.

The hepatic cytochrome P450 mixed-function oxidase isoenzyme CYP3A, the activity of which, in adults, is represented by the combined activities of CYP3A4, CYP3A5, CYP3A7, and CYP3A43 is responsible for the bulk of docetaxel metabolism.[470,472,474–476] However, CYP3A4 and CYP3A5, to a lesser extent, confer the highest relative contributions to overall CYP3A activity and are primarily involved in biotransformation that, in contrast to paclitaxel, principally affects the C-13 side chain and not the taxane ring.[474–476] CYP2B, and CYP1A also appear to play major roles in biotransformation. The main metabolic pathway consists of oxidation of the tertiary butyl group on the side chain at the C-13 position of the taxane ring, as well as cyclization of the side chain. All metabolites

maintain their 10-deacetylbaccatin III or 7-epi isomer structural backbones. These metabolites seem to be much less active than docetaxel.

The main pharmacokinetic determinants of toxicity, particularly neutropenia, are total drug exposure and the time in which plasma levels exceed biologically relevant concentrations.[472,474–476] A population pharmacodynamic analysis of determinants of outcome in phase 2 trials of docetaxel in patients with metastatic breast cancer has revealed that the most important positive determinants of objective response and progression-free survival are low pretreatment plasma concentration of α_1–acid glycoprotein, number of prior chemotherapeutic regimens, and number of disease sites, whereas both drug exposure and the pretreatment plasma concentration of α_1–acid glycoprotein were strong positive determinants of time to progression in patients with advanced lung cancer.[467,468] Conversely, the pretreatment plasma level of α_{1r}–acid glycoprotein was negatively, albeit significantly, related to the probability of experiencing both severe neutropenia and febrile neutropenia. The concentration of α_1–acid glycoproteins is a principal determinant of interindividual variability in docetaxel clearance.[397,467,468]

Similar to the situation with paclitaxel, various polymorphisms in P450 mixed function oxidases and ABC1 transporter proteins have been associated with variable pharmacokinetics, toxicities, and antitumor responses in patients receiving docetaxel.[456–463,476–483] Most clinically relevant cytochrome P450 isoform polymorphisms appear to involve CYP3A4 and CYP3A5.[456–463,476–483] Interestingly, a pilot study suggested that CYP1B1*3, which is associated with genotype-dependent estrogen metabolism, may be an important marker for estimating docetaxel efficacy in patients with prostate cancer.[479,482] Polymorphisms associated with ABCB1 have been linked to treatment efficacy and the development of neutropenia and neurotoxicity in patients with castrate-resistant prostate cancer and other malignancies.[477,479,480,482,483]

Protein-Bound Paclitaxel Particles for Injection

Following the administration of PBPPI doses ranging from 80 to 360 mg/m^2, paclitaxel pharmacokinetics were dose proportional and plasma concentration data fit a two-compartment model. At the recommended dose of 260 mg/m^2, total clearance averages 15 L/h/m^2 and the mean volume of distribution and terminal half-life values are approximately 632 L/m^2 and 27 hours, respectively.[386,387] Approximately 89% to 98% of paclitaxel is protein bound in vitro studies of PBPPI. In a report of the comparative pharmacokinetics of paclitaxel formulated as either PBPPI or polyoxyethylated castor oil in both rats and humans, the volume of distribution at steady state and clearance for paclitaxel formulated as PBPPI were significantly greater than those for paclitaxel formulated with polyoxyethylated castor oil in rats.[484,485] Fecal excretion was the main elimination pathway with both formulations. Consistent with the preclinical data, paclitaxel clearance and volume of distribution were significantly higher for PBPPI than for the polyoxyethylated castor oil formulation in humans (21.13 versus 14.76 L/h/m^2 [$P = 0.048$] and 663.8 versus 433.4 L/m^2 [$P = 0.040$]), respectively.[485] The greater clearance of paclitaxel following administration of PBPPI has been hypothesized to be due to the binding of paclitaxel to albumin in PPBPI, which results in increased accumulation of paclitaxel molecules in tumor and normal tissue via SPARC.[389,390] In another report of a randomized cross-over pharmacokinetic study of PBPPI (260 mg/m² over 30 minutes) and paclitaxel formulated in polyoxyethylated castor oil (175 mg/m² over 3 hours), the exposure to unbound paclitaxel was significantly higher following PBPPI administration due to a higher free fraction of paclitaxel in PBPPI, which might in part explain the differences in clinical antitumor activity noted between the formulations.[486]

After a 30-minute infusion of 260 mg/m² doses of PBPPI, the mean values for cumulative urinary recovery of unchanged drug (4%) indicate extensive nonrenal clearance. PBPPI paclitaxel has a metabolic profile similar to paclitaxel in polyoxyethylated castor oil formulations.[386,387,484,485] Fecal and urinary excretion accounts for approximately 20% and 4% of the total dose of PBPPI administered, respectively, and less than 1% of the total administered dose is excreted in urine as the metabolites 6α-hydroxypaclitaxel and 3′-p-hydroxypaclitaxel. Fecal excretion approximates 20% of the total dose administered. In vitro studies with human liver microsomes and tissue slices revealed identical CYP2C8- and CYP3A4-induced hydroxylated metabolites as with polyoxyethylated castor oil formulations.

> In a study that examined plasma pharmacokinetics and partitioning of radiolabeled paclitaxel from PBPPI and a polyoxyethylated paclitaxel formulation into red blood cells and tumor tissue for 24 hours following tail vein injection of 20 mg/kg paclitaxel in a MX-1 human breast cancer xenograft model, the distribution of PBPPI was rapid and extensive, as shown by a fivefold larger volume of distribution and much lower peak plasma concentrations and area under the concentration time curve values compared with a polyoxyethylated castor oil formulation.[386] For PBPPI, there was a significantly lower plasma/blood ratio of paclitaxel across all time points and paclitaxel distributed more effectively into tumors. Tumor AUC values of paclitaxel were 1.6-fold higher, on average, with PBPPI and terminal half-life values for paclitaxel significantly longer than from the polyoxyethylated castor oil formulation (17.1 versus 4.0 hours). The prolonged half-life of paclitaxel following administration of PBPPI could be attributed to sequestration in red blood cells that release paclitaxel as plasma levels decrease.

Drug Interactions

Both sequence-dependent pharmacokinetic and toxicologic interactions between paclitaxel and several other chemotherapy agents have been noted, but the number of clinically significant drug-drug interactions has been surprisingly low in light of the importance of cytochrome P450 metabolism in drug disposition.[397,487] Sequence-dependent effects between paclitaxel, especially on protracted infusion schedules, and other chemotherapeutics have been observed. The sequence of cisplatin followed by paclitaxel (24-hour schedule) induces more profound neutropenia than the reverse sequence, which is explained by a 33% reduction in the clearance of paclitaxel after cisplatin.[397,488,489] The least toxic sequence—paclitaxel before cisplatin—was demonstrated to induced more cytotoxicity in vitro; therefore, this drug sequence was selected for clinical development for patients with ovarian and non–small cell lung cancer. As expected, however, sequence dependence does not appear to be a clinically relevant phenomenon on shorter schedules. Treatment with paclitaxel on either a 3- or 24-hour schedule followed

by carboplatin results in equivalent neutropenia and less thrombocytopenia as compared with carboplatin as a single agent, which is not explained by pharmacokinetic interactions.[397,490–492] Although sequence dependence has not been noted with combinations of carboplatin and paclitaxel, which induce less thrombocytopenia than comparable single-agent doses of carboplatin, other paclitaxel-based chemotherapy combinations, most notably those involving the anthracyclines, are associated with this phenomena.[397,490–492] Both neutropenia and mucositis are more severe when paclitaxel on a 24-hour schedule is administered before doxorubicin, compared with the reverse sequence, which is most likely caused by an approximately 32% reduction in the clearance rates of both doxorubicin and doxorubicinol when doxorubicin is administered after paclitaxel.[493,494] Hematologic toxicity has also been more profound with the sequence of cyclophosphamide before paclitaxel (24-hour schedule) than the reverse sequence.[495] Sequence-dependent cytotoxic effects have been reported when the taxanes are combined with 5-fluorouracil, etoposide, cytosine arabinoside, fludarabine, flavopyridol, and other antineoplastic agents in vitro.[397,496]

Although neither sequence-dependent pharmacologic interactions nor acute toxicologic interactions occur between doxorubicin and paclitaxel on a shorter (3-hour) schedule, combined treatment with paclitaxel (3-hour schedule) and doxorubicin as a bolus infusion leads to a higher incidence of cardiotoxicity than would have been expected from an equivalent cumulative doxorubicin dose given without paclitaxel (see the sections on "Cardiac," "Toxicity," "Paclitaxel," and "Taxanes").[493,494,497] The precise etiology for these interactions is unclear. Experimental data indicate that paclitaxel enhances the metabolism of doxorubicin to cardiotoxic metabolites, such as doxorubicinol, in cardiomyocytes.[494,497] Docetaxel does not influence doxorubicin pharmacokinetics, but there are experimental data suggesting that, as with paclitaxel, docetaxel can enhance the metabolism of doxorubicin to toxic species in cardiac tissue.[494,496] Similar decrements in the clearance of epirubicin and its metabolites have been noted in studies of paclitaxel combined with epirubicin, but cardiotoxicity has not been enhanced.[498] Competition for the hepatic or biliary Pgp transport of the anthracyclines with paclitaxel or its polyoxyethylated castor oil vehicle (or both) is an alternate explanation. Enhancement of cardiotoxicity has not been noted with docetaxel, which is not formulated in polyoxyethylated castor oil, but in polysorbate-80.

The taxanes induce thymidine phosphorylase activity, which may increase the metabolic activation of the oral fluoropyrimidine prodrug capecitabine.[499]

Drug interactions may also result from the effects of other classes of drugs. Various inducers of cytochrome P450 mixed-function oxidases, such as the anticonvulsants phenytoin and phenobarbital, accelerate the metabolism of both paclitaxel and docetaxel in human microsomes in vitro and in both children and adults who are concurrently receiving treatment with these anticonvulsants, as manifested by rapid drug clearance and tolerance of high drug doses.[397,449–452,460,474,475,487,500–503] Preclinical evidence suggests that docetaxel has markedly reduced propensity to cause drug interactions related to hepatic CYP3A4 induction.[503] Conversely, many types of agents that inhibit cytochrome P450 mixed-function oxidases, such as orphenadrine, erythromycin, cimetidine, testosterone, ketoconazole, fluconazole, midazolam, polyoxyethylated castor oil, and corticosteroids, interfere with the metabolism of paclitaxel and docetaxel in human microsomes in vitro; however, the clinical relevance of these findings is not known.[397,449–452,474,475,487,500–503] With regard to potential interactions between ketoconazole and the taxanes, inconsistent conclusions have been reached although docetaxel exposure increased in a high proportion of patients receiving concurrent ketoconazole.[504] Besides the potent inhibitors of CYP3A listed previously, other well-established inhibitors and inducers of CYP3A, including grapefruit juice and herbal products (e.g., St. John's wort and Echinacea), may potentially induce pharmacokinetic interactions with the taxanes. Although there has been concern that H_2-receptor antagonists with variable cytochrome P450 inhibitory activities used as components of premedication regimens may affect taxane clearance and hence toxicity, neither toxicologic nor pharmacologic differences between the agents were noted in a randomized clinical trial.[505–507] A review of early clinical trial results with docetaxel has not demonstrated significant alterations in docetaxel clearance by corticosteroids. In addition, interactions between warfarin and the taxanes leading to advancement of anticoagulation may result from effects on protein binding.[506]

It has been a concern that H_2-histamine antagonist premedication may be a potential source of drug interactions. Use of these agents with the taxanes may produce variable pharmacologic and toxicologic effects because these agents differentially inhibit cytochrome P450 metabolism, with cimetidine being the most potent inhibitor. However, H_2 histamine antagonists do not appear to alter the metabolism and pharmacologic disposition of the taxanes in animal and in vitro studies.[505,507,508] In addition, the results of a clinical trial in which patients were randomized to receive either cimetidine or famotidine premedication before their first course of paclitaxel and then crossed over to the alternate premedication during their second course have failed to show significant toxicologic and pharmacologic differences between these H_2 histamine antagonists.[505]

The incidence of congestive heart failure has also been higher in breast cancer patients treated with the combination of trastuzumab and paclitaxel than with paclitaxel alone, but the explanation for this observation is not known.[509]

Although there has been less clinical experience with PBPPI compared to paclitaxel in polyoxyethylated castor oil, preclinical studies indicate that the prospects for drug interactions are likely to be similar. In vitro, the presence of cimetidine, ranitidine, dexamethasone did not affect the protein binding of paclitaxel in PBPPI. Although paclitaxel metabolism is inhibited by many agents, including ketoconazole, verapamil, diazepam, quinidine, dexamethasone, cyclosporin, teniposide, etoposide, and VCR, the concentrations used in these studies exceeded those found in vivo following normal therapeutic doses. Testosterone, 17α-ethinyl estradiol, retinoic acid, and quercetin, a specific inhibitor of CYP2C8, also inhibited the formation of the principal metabolite, 6α-hydroxypaclitaxel, in vitro. Similar to paclitaxel in polyoxyethylated castor oil, paclitaxel pharmacokinetics following PBPPI administration may be altered as a result of interactions with compounds that are substrates, inducers, or inhibitors of CYP2C8 and/or CYP3A4.

Administration, Dose, and Schedule

Paclitaxel

Effective premedication regimens have decreased the incidence of major adverse reactions and have led to evaluations of paclitaxel in a broad range of schedules. Although the paclitaxel dose-schedule consisting of 135 mg/m^2 over 24 hours was initially approved for patients with refractory and recurrent ovarian cancer, regulatory approval was subsequently obtained for paclitaxel, 175 mg/m^2 on a 3-hour schedule in ovarian and other malignancies. In patients with advanced breast and ovarian cancers, the cumulative body of randomized study results indicates that both schedules are equivalent, particularly with regard to event-free and overall survival. However, objective response rates have occasionally been higher with the 24-hour infusion.

Based on in vitro studies, which indicated that the duration of exposure above a biologically relevant threshold is one of the most important determinants of cytotoxicity, more protracted infusion schedules were evaluated.[292,510] Although intriguing results were initially obtained with a 96-hour infusion schedule in patients with advanced breast cancer and non-Hodgkin's lymphoma, there is no clear evidence that protracted schedules are superior to shorter schedules with regard to efficacy, and certain toxicities, particularly myelosuppression and mucositis, appear to more somewhat greater.[510–515] The lack of clearly superior results with protracted schedules in vivo is likely due to the extensive and rapid distribution of the taxanes to peripheral tissues and, more importantly, the avid and protracted tissue binding of these agents, whereas the agents are washed out from cells in tissue culture after short-term exposure. There has also been considerable interest in intermittent schedules, particularly those in which paclitaxel is administered as a 1-hour infusion weekly, which results in substantially less myelosuppression than every 3-week schedules.[301,307–309,510,516–518] Furthermore, in some studies, weekly paclitaxel has yielded superior response rates compared with every 3-week schedules, particularly in the adjuvant and advanced breast cancer settings.[301,307–309,510,516–518] However, no consistent evidence indicates that weekly treatment results in robust activity in tumors unresponsive to the every 3-week schedules. The weekly schedule may be advantageous for patients who are at high risk of developing severe myelosuppression.

Paclitaxel is generally administered every 3 weeks at a dose of 175 mg/m^2 over 3 hours. The alternative dose-schedule of 135 to 175 mg/m^2 over 24 hours every 3 weeks is used less commonly. Several phase 3 studies in patients with advanced lung, head and neck, ovarian, and breast cancers have consistently failed to show that paclitaxel doses greater than 135 to 175 mg/m^2 on a 24-hour schedule or greater than 175 mg/m^2 on a 3-hour schedule confer superior efficacy.[292,519,520] The following doses have been recommended on less conventional schedules: 200 mg/m^2 over 1 hour as either a single dose or three divided doses every 3 weeks; 140 mg/m^2 over 96 hours every 3 weeks; and 80 to 100 mg/m^2 weekly. The most common schedules evaluated in patients with AIDS-associated Kaposi's sarcoma are paclitaxel, 135 mg/m^2 over 3 or 24 hours every 3 weeks, and 100 mg/m^2 every 2 weeks.[310]

Following intracavitary administration, paclitaxel concentrations in the peritoneal and pleural cavities are several orders of magnitude greater than plasma concentrations, which remain biologically relevant, and the results of a single randomized trial indicate that the administration of intraperitoneal paclitaxel in conjunction with carboplatin and paclitaxel administered intravenously confers a survival advantage in previously untreated women with optimally debulked advanced ovarian cancer.[521,522]

The following premedication is recommended to prevent major HSRs: dexamethasone, 20 mg orally or intravenously, 12 and 6 hours before treatment; an H_1-receptor antagonist (such as diphenhydramine, 50 mg intravenously) 30 minutes before treatment; and an H_2-receptor antagonist (such as cimetidine, 300 mg; famotidine, 20 mg; or ranitidine, 150 mg intravenously) 30 minutes before treatment. A single dose of a corticosteroid (dexamethasone, 20 mg intravenously) administered 30 minutes before treatment also appears to confer effective prophylaxis of major HSRs; however, the relative merits of this schedule compared to the more traditional schedule are not known.[523,524] Other schedules, including oral premedication with corticosteroids and antihistamines immediately prior to treatment, may be effective.[525]

Contact of paclitaxel with plasticized polyvinyl chloride equipment or devices must be avoided because of the risk of patient exposures to plasticizers that may be leached from polyvinyl chloride infusion bags or sets. Paclitaxel solutions should be diluted and stored in glass or polypropylene bottles or suitable plastic bags (polypropylene or polyolefin) and administered through polyethylene-lined administration sets that include an in-line filter with a microporous membrane not greater than 0.22 μm.

The extensive involvement of hepatic metabolism and biliary excretion in the disposition of paclitaxel has led to examination of the need for dose modifications related to hepatic dysfunction. Although formal recommendations have not been accepted, patients with moderate-to-severe elevations in serum concentrations of hepatocellular enzymes or bilirubin (or both) are more likely to develop severe toxicity than patients without hepatic dysfunction.[526–528] Therefore, it is prudent to reduce paclitaxel doses by at least 50% in patients with abnormal serum bilirubin or significant (five to ten times or greater) elevations in hepatic transaminases. Renal clearance contributes minimally to overall clearance (5% to 10%), and based on such information and anecdotal data, patients with severe renal dysfunction would not be expected to require dose modification.[529] Nevertheless, it should be noted that paclitaxel clearance was reduced by 34% in rats following a 5/6 partial nephrectomy.[443] Based on the pharmacologic behavior, particularly the wide distributive properties of the taxanes, dose modifications are not required solely for peripheral edema and third-space fluid collections.

Docetaxel

Docetaxel is most commonly administered at a dose of 75 mg/m² over 1 hour every 3 weeks, but regulatory approval was granted in the United States for a dose range of 60 to 100 mg/m² over 1 hour in patients with breast and non–small cell lung cancers, respectively; much less data are available for patients treated at 60 mg/m².[297,530] The most common dose schedule of docetaxel used as a single-agent and in combination regimens is 75 mg/m² over 1 hour, which seems to be more reasonable and so far starting dose, than 100 mg/m² particularly in heavily pretreated patients.[530]

Like paclitaxel, docetaxel is also administered on a chronic weekly schedule. Although a clear advantage of chronic weekly drug administration over the conventional schedule in terms of antitumor activity has not been noted, the weekly schedule actually appears less effective in adjuvant breast cancer therapy, hematologic toxicity is much less than with conventional dose schedules.[307]

However, weekly administration schedules have been associated with a higher incidence of cumulative asthenia and neurotoxicity, particularly with docetaxel doses exceeding 36 mg/m²/wk.[517]

Despite the use of a polysorbate 80 formulation instead of polyoxyethylated castor oil, which is used to formulate paclitaxel, an unacceptably high rate of major HSRs and profound fluid retention in patients who did not receive premedication has led to the several effective premedication regimens, the most popular of which is dexamethasone, 8 mg orally twice daily for 3 or 5 days starting 1 or 2 days, respectively, before docetaxel, with or without both H_1-receptor and H_2-receptor antagonists given 30 minutes before docetaxel.[297,531,532]

In a retrospective review of docetaxel pharmacokinetics and toxicity in patients without hyperbilirubinemia, clearance was reduced by approximately 25% in patients with elevations in serum concentrations of both hepatic transaminases (1.5-fold or greater) and alkaline phosphatase (2.5-fold or greater), regardless of whether the elevations are the result of hepatic metastases.[467,468,526] Therefore, dose reductions by at least 25% are recommended for such patients. However, greater dose reductions (50% or greater) may be required in patients who have moderate or severe hepatic excretory dysfunction (hyperbilirubinemia).[526] As with paclitaxel, there is no rationale for dose modification solely for renal deficiency or third-space fluid accumulation (see the sections on "Administration, Dose, and Schedule," and "Paclitaxel"). Also similar to the case with paclitaxel, glass bottles or polypropylene or polyolefin plastic products should be used for preparation and storage, and docetaxel should be administered through polyethylene-lined administration sets.

Protein-Bound Paclitaxel Particles for Injection

The recommended dosage schedule for PBPPI for the treatment of patients with metastatic breast cancer is 260 mg/m² as a 30-minutes IV infusion. However, notable activity has been observed with PBPPI doses of 100 to 150 mg/m² as a 30-minutes IV infusion weekly for three out of every 4 weeks following failure of previous taxane treatment.[388] No premedication to prevent HSRs or edema is indicated prior to administration. The use of PVC-free containers and administration sets, as well as in-line filters, is not necessary.

The most appropriate doses for patients with hepatic insufficiency (bilirubin ≥ 1.5 mg/dL) and renal insufficiency are not known. However, similar to the case with other taxanes, renal disposition is negligible. It is recommended that patients who experience severe neutropenia (neutrophil < 500/μL for at least 7 days) or severe sensory neuropathy during PBPPI treatment should have the dosage reduced to 220 mg/m² for subsequent courses. Additional dose reduction should be made to 180 mg/m² for further episodes of severe neutropenia and/or sensory neuropathy. In cases of severe sensory neuropathy, it is recommended that treatment be discontinued until resolution to mild or moderate manifestations followed by a dose reduction for all subsequent courses.

Toxicity

Despite having similar structural features, the toxicity spectra of paclitaxel and docetaxel do not completely overlap. Myelosuppression, primarily neutropenia, is the principal toxicity of both agents, but the types and frequencies of several nonhematologic side effects are different.

Paclitaxel

Hematologic

Neutropenia is the principal toxicity of paclitaxel. The onset is usually on days 8 to 10, and recovery is generally complete by days 15 to 21 on every 3-week dosing regimens. A critical pharmacologic determinant of the severity of neutropenia is the duration that plasma drug concentrations are maintained above biologically relevant levels (0.05 to 0.1 μmol/L), which may explain why neutropenia is more severe with more protracted infusions (see the sections on "Pharmacokinetics," and "Paclitaxel").[436,438,453] Which some dosing schedules may be preferred in specific clinical settings (see the sections on "Administration, Dose, and Schedule," and "Paclitaxel"),[307,517,518] the main clinical determinant of the severity of neutropenia is the extent of prior myelotoxic therapy.

Neutropenia is noncumulative, and the duration of severe neutropenia, even in heavily pretreated patients, is usually brief. At paclitaxel doses exceeding 175 mg/m^2 on a 24-hour schedule and 225 mg/m^2 on a 3-hour schedule, nadir neutrophil counts are typically less than 500/μL for fewer than 5 days in most courses, even in untreated patients. Even patients who have received extensive prior therapy can usually tolerate paclitaxel doses of 175 to 200 mg/m^2 over 3 or 24 hours. More frequent administration schedules, particularly weekly treatment schedules with doses of 80 to 100 mg/m^2, are associated with less severe neutropenia. Platelets and red blood cell production is less affected by taxanes, except in heavily pretreated patients.

Hypersensitivity

The incidence of major HSRs in early trials was approximately 30% but declined to 1% to 3% following development of effective prophylaxis.[292,532-535] Major HSRs, which are characterized by dyspnea with bronchospasm, urticaria, hypotension, chest, abdominal and backpain, usually occur within the first 10 minutes after the first (and less frequently after the second) treatment and resolve completely after stopping treatment. They occasionally occur after pretreatment with antihistamines, fluids, and vasopressors. Patients who have major reactions have been rechallenged successfully after receiving high doses of corticosteroids, but this approach has not always been successful.[535-538] Rechallenge appears to be most successful in patients who experience severe hypersensitivity manifestations within minutes of starting treatment, if the infusion is immediately discontinued, and if treatment resumes within approximately 30 minutes, which is likely the result of profound and persistent depletion of histamines and other mediators at the time of rechallenge.[535-538] Although the incidence of minor HSRs, such as isolated flushing and rash, is about 40%, major reactions do not generally occur after minor HSRs. Based on the resemblance of the HSRs to those caused by radiocontrast dyes, they are probably caused by an immunologically mediated release of histamine or other vasoactive substances, owing to the taxane moiety or, more likely, its polyoxyethylated castor oil vehicle, possibly with complement activation.[535,539] The vehicle is the suspected culprit because it induces histamine release and similar manifestations in dogs, and when other drugs are formulated in it (cyclosporine A and vitamin K with the vehicle induce similar reactions). The rates of major HSRs are low on both 3- and 24-hour schedules when patients are premedicated with various regimens of corticosteroids and both H$_1$-receptor and H$_2$-receptor antagonists 2.1% for the 3 hour schedule, versus 1.0% for the 24 hour schedule.[534]

Peripheral Neurotoxicity

Paclitaxel induces a peripheral neuropathy characterized by sensory symptoms, such as numbness in a symmetric glove-and-stocking distribution.[228,229,245,246,292,533,540-542] The most common findings on neurologic examination loss are of sensation and deep tendon reflexes. Neurophysiologic studies support a primary disruption of neuronal microtubules, resulting in axonal degeneration and demyelination neuronopathy is particularly severe at higher doses or when combined with other neurotoxic agents.[228,229,245,246,292,533,540-542] Severe neurotoxicity is uncommon when paclitaxel is given alone at doses below 200 mg/m^2 on a 3- or 24-hour schedule every 3 weeks or below 100 mg/m^2 on a continuous weekly schedule, but almost all "low-risk" patients experience mild or moderate effects. Patients with preexisting neuropathy caused other neurotoxic agents, diabetes mellitus, congenital conditions, or alcoholism, even when manifestations are subclinical, are more prone to paclitaxel-induced neuropathy. Symptoms may begin as soon as 24 to 72 hours after treatment with higher doses ($\geq$250 mg/m^2) but usually occur only after multiple courses at 135 to 250 mg/m^2 every 3 weeks. Neurotoxicity is generally more pronounced when paclitaxel is administered on short infusion schedules, indicating that peak plasma concentration may be a principal pharmacologic determinant. The combination of paclitaxel on a 3-hour schedule and cisplatin is particularly neurotoxic, and while paclitaxel and carboplatin produce less neurotoxicity. Motor and autonomic dysfunction may occur, especially at high doses and in patients with preexisting neuropathies caused by diabetes mellitus and alcoholism. There have been inconsistent reports of glutamate reducing the severity of peripheral neuropathy from high doses of paclitaxel.[270,246,543,544] While anecdotal reports, experimental models, and/or insufficiently powered randomized trials have suggested that the sulfhydryl group scavenger drugs, pyridoxine, or anticonvulsants reduce the neurotoxic effects of paclitaxel, convincing evidence is lacking that any specific measure is effective at preventing or reversing neurotoxicity.[228,229,245,246,292,533,540-544] Transient myalgia and arthralgia of uncertain etiology, usually noted 24 to 48 hours after therapy and apparently dose-related, are also common, and a myopathy has been described in patients receiving high doses with cisplatin.[228,533,540,541,545] Corticosteroids, specifically prednisone 10 mg twice daily for 5 days beginning 24 hours after treatment, may be effective at reducing myalgia and arthralgia.[533,545] Optic nerve disturbances, manifested by scintillating scotoma, and vocal cord paralysis, have also been reported.[546,547] Acute encephalopathy, which can progress to coma and death, has been reported after high doses (600 mg/m^2 or greater).[548] A transient acute encephalopathy has also been observed, rarely, within several hours following paclitaxel in patients who received prior cranial irradiation.[549]

Cardiac

Paclitaxel treatment has been associated with cardiac rhythm disturbances, most of which were discovered using cardiac monitoring.

Their clinical relevance is not known.[532,533,550–552] The most common disturbance, transient, asymptomatic bradycardia, was noted in 29% of patients in one trial in which patients underwent cardiac monitoring, and, in the absence of hemodynamic effects, is not an indication for discontinuing paclitaxel.[5] More important bradyarrhythmias, such as Mobitz type I (Wenckebach's syndrome), Mobitz type II, and third-degree heart block, have been noted, but the incidence in a large National Cancer Institute database was only 0.1%.[552] Most episodes have been asymptomatic and almost all documented events involved patients in early trials in which continuous cardiac monitor was routinely performed, indicating that the incidence of heart block is likely underreported. However, these bradyarrhythmias are likely true adverse effects of paclitaxel as related taxanes affect cardiac automaticity and conduction, and similar arrhythmias have occurred in humans and animals after ingesting various species of yew plants.[552]

Myocardial infarction, cardiac ischemia, atrial arrhythmias, and ventricular tachycardia have been noted, but the causal relationship between paclitaxel and these events is uncertain. There is also no evidence that chronic, long-term treatment with paclitaxel causes progressive cardiac dysfunction. Routine cardiac monitoring during paclitaxel therapy is not necessary but is advisable for patients who may not be able to tolerate bradyarrhythmias, such as those with atrioventricular conduction disturbances or ventricular dysfunction. Although patients with a wide range of cardiac abnormalities and cardiac histories were broadly and empirically restricted from participating in early clinical trials, paclitaxel treatment was well tolerated in a small series of patients with gynecologic cancer and with major cardiac risk factors.[550,552] However, repetitive treatment of patients with the combined regimen of paclitaxel on a 3-hour schedule and doxorubicin as a brief infusion is associated with a higher frequency of congestive cardiotoxicity than would be expected to occur with the same cumulative doxorubicin dose given without paclitaxel (see the sections on "Drug Interactions" and "Taxanes").[464,494,497] In one study of previously untreated women with advanced breast cancer who were treated with escalating doses of paclitaxel as a 3-hour infusion and doxorubicin, 60 mg/m^2 to a cumulative dose of 480 mg/m^2, (a dose that would be predicted to result in a less than 5% incidence of congestive cardiotoxicity in patients treated with doxorubicin alone) the incidence of congestive cardiotoxicity was approximately 25%.[464] However, the incidence of cardiotoxicity was less than 5% when similar patients received identical schedules of paclitaxel and doxorubicin, but the cumulative doxorubicin dose did not exceed 360 mg/m^2. Both experimental and early clinical results suggest that dexrazoxane reduces the cardiotoxicity of the doxorubicin and paclitaxel combination.[553,554] The incidence of congestive heart failure was also significantly higher in patients treated with the combination of trastuzumab and paclitaxel than paclitaxel alone; therefore, careful monitoring of cardiac function in patients receiving this combination is warranted.[509]

Miscellaneous

Drug-related gastrointestinal effects, such as vomiting and diarrhea, are uncommon. Higher paclitaxel doses or protracted (96-hour) infusional administration may cause mucositis.[515,548,555] Rare cases of neutropenic enterocolitis and gastrointestinal necrosis have been noted, particularly in patients given high doses of paclitaxel in combination with doxorubicin or cyclophosphamide.[555–557] Severe hepatotoxicity and pancreatitis have also been noted rarely.[557,558] Acute bilateral pneumonitis has been reported in fewer than 1% of patients treated on a 3-hour schedule in one series, and both interstitial and parenchymal pulmonary toxicity have been reported, but clinically significant pulmonary effects are uncommon.[559,560] In contrast to the vinca alkaloids, the agent is not a potent vesicant but extravasations of large volumes can cause moderate soft-tissue injury. Inflammation at the injection site and along the course of an injected vein may occur. Paclitaxel also induces reversible alopecia of the scalp in a dose-related fashion, and loss of all facial and body hair may result in heavily pretreated patients. Nail disorders have been reported, particularly in patients treated on weekly schedules.[561] Recall reactions in previously irradiated sites have also been noted.

Docetaxel

Hematologic

Following treatment with docetaxel administered over 1 hour every 3 weeks, the onset of neutropenia, the principal toxicity of docetaxel, is usually noted by day 8 and complete resolution typically occurs by days 15 to 21.[297,532,562] At a dose of 100 mg/m^2 administered over 1 hour, neutrophil counts are commonly below 500/μL and the incidence of neutropenic complications is high.[297,530] Although severe neutropenia at 75 mg/m^2 is common, the duration of severe neutropenia and incidence of complications are lower than after the higher dose. As with paclitaxel, neutropenia is significantly less when lower doses are administered on a weekly schedule (see the sections on "Administration, Dose, and Schedule" and "Docetaxel"). The most important determinant of neutropenia is the extent of prior treatment. Significant thrombocytopenia and anemia are uncommon with docetaxel alone.

Hypersensitivity

Despite not being formulated in polyoxyethylated castor oil, HSRs have been reported in approximately 31% of patients receiving docetaxel without premedication in early phase 2 studies.[297,562,563] As with paclitaxel, major reactions characterized by dyspnea, bronchospasm, and hypotension typically occur during the first two courses and within minutes after the start of treatment. Signs and symptoms generally resolve within 15 minutes after cessation of treatment, and docetaxel is usually able to be reinstituted without sequelae, occasionally after treatment with an H$_1$-receptor antagonist. Fortunately, however, most events are minor and rarely result in discontinuation of treatment.[297,532] Both the incidence and severity of HSRs appear to be reduced by premedication with corticosteroids and H$_1$-receptor and H$_2$-receptor antagonists, but the corticosteroid premedication regimen is principally administered to prevent fluid retention (see the sections on "Administration, Dose, and Schedule" and "Docetaxel"). As with paclitaxel, patients who experience major reactions have been retreated successfully after the resolution of symptoms and after treatment with corticosteroids and H$_1$-receptor antagonists. Furthermore, there are several anecdotal reports of patients treated successfully with docetaxel following severe HSRs as the result of taking paclitaxel, but it is not known whether these reactions would have occurred if the patients had been retreated with paclitaxel.[532,562,563]

Fluid Retention

Docetaxel induces a unique fluid retention syndrome characterized by edema, weight gain, and third-space fluid collection.[297,517,531,532,564] Fluid retention is cumulative and unrelated to hypoalbuminemia or cardiac, renal, or hepatic dysfunction. Instead, increased capillary permeability appears to be responsible.[564] Capillary filtration studies in patients who were not receiving corticosteroid premedication have revealed a two-stage process, with progressive congestion of the interstitial space by proteins and water starting between the second and fourth course, followed by insufficient lymphatic drainage.[564] In early studies in which premedication was not used, fluid retention was not usually significant at cumulative docetaxel doses below 400 mg/m², however, the incidence and severity of fluid retention increased sharply at cumulative doses of 400 mg/m² or greater and often resulted in the delay or termination of treatment. Premedication with corticosteroids with or without H_1-receptor and H_2-receptor antagonists reduces the overall incidence of fluid retention and increases the number of courses and cumulative docetaxel dose before the onset of this toxicity (see the sections on "Administration, Dose, and Schedule" and "Docetaxel").[531,562] Fluid retention typically resolves slowly after docetaxel is stopped, but complete resolution occurs several months after treatment in patients with severe toxicity. Aggressive and early treatment with diuretics usually manages fluid retention.[531,532,564] The incidence of fluid retention decreases in studies of lower doses (60 to 75 mg/m²) of docetaxel during each course, but this may be simply the result of lower overall cumulative doses, and the effects of lower doses on antitumor activity are unknown.

Dermatologic

Skin toxicity may occur in as many as 50% to 75% of patients; however, corticosteroid premedication may reduce the incidence.[297,517,532,562,565,566] An erythematous pruritic maculopapular rash affects the forearms, hands, or feet. Other cutaneous effects include desquamation of the hands and feet, which may respond to pyridoxine or cooling, and onychodystrophy characterized by brown discoloration, ridging, onycholysis, soreness, brittleness and loss of the nail plate.[517,532,565–568] Skin and nail changes are most prominent in patients treated with high cumulative doses over long periods, particularly on weekly administration schedules.[517]

Neurotoxicity

Docetaxel produces neurotoxicity, which is qualitatively similar to that of paclitaxel.[297,540,578] Patients typically complain of paresthesia and numbness, but peripheral motor effects may also occur. Both neurosensory and neuromuscular effects are generally less frequent and less severe with docetaxel as compared with paclitaxel, and docetaxel can be considered as a substitute in high-risk patients with underlying neuropathy.[297,532,569,570] Nevertheless, mild-to-moderate peripheral neurotoxicity occurs in approximately 40% of untreated patients, and patients who had received prior cisplatin are particularly susceptible, with the incidence approaching 74% in one trial.[297,516,517,532,562] Severe toxicity has been unusual after repetitive treatment with docetaxel doses less than 100 mg/m², except in patients with antecedent neurotoxicity and relevant disorders, such as alcohol abuse and diabetes mellitus. Similar to the taxanes, various medications, including glutamate and neuroactive steroids like progesterone and dihydroprogesterone, confer protection against the neurotoxic effects of docetaxel in preclinical models but robust clinical evidence has not yet been documented.[246,270,543,544,571] Transient arthralgia and myalgia are occasionally noted within days after treatment. Malaise or asthenia has been prominent complaint in patients who have been treated with large cumulative doses, particularly when docetaxel is administered on a continuous weekly schedule.[297,517,532,562]

Miscellaneous

Stomatitis is more common with docetaxel than paclitaxel, but still infrequent. Significant nausea, vomiting, and diarrhea are also infrequently rare. Empiric use of antiemetic premedication does not appear to be warranted. Mild-to-moderate conjunctivitis, which is responsive to topical corticosteroids, and canalicular stenosis causing excessive lacrimation may also occur, particularly with weekly schedules.[572] Similar to paclitaxel, docetaxel is not a potent vesicant and infusion site reactions are uncommon. Other rare events reported that may or may not be drug-related included arrhythmias, confusion, erythema multiforme, neutropenic enterocolitis, hepatitis, ileus, interstitial pneumonia, seizures, pulmonary fibrosis, hepatitis, radiation recall, and visual disturbances.[517] Cardiovascular manifestations, such as angina, arrhythmia, conduction disturbances, congestive heart failure, hypertension, and hypotension, have been noted rarely following treatment, and these events have not been linked convincingly to docetaxel.

Protein-Bound Paclitaxel Particles for Injection

The toxicity profile of PBPPI is similar to that of paclitaxel, with neutropenia as the principal dose-limiting toxicity.[319,332,385–389] Most other paclitaxel-related toxicities have also been observed with PBPPI. The rate of HSRs, particularly major reactions, appears less with PBPPI than that of paclitaxel formulated in polyoxyethylated castor oil. No premedication regimen to prevent HSRs is recommended. In a pivotal phase 3 trial in which the previously treated breast cancer were randomized to treatment with either 260 mg/m² PBPI administered over 30 minutes or 175 mg/m² paclitaxel in polyoxyethylated castor over 3 hours, the frequencies of severe adverse events were similar.[319] PBPPI caused a greater degree of neutrophils less than 500/μL (9% versus 22%), and more severe sensory neuropathic symptoms (10% versus 2%), severe arthralgia/myalgia (8% versus 2%), and asthenia (8% versus 3%). Additional toxicities, most of which are noted with other taxane formulations, include increased lacrimation, conjunctivitis, radiation recall, Stevens-Johnson syndrome, toxic epidermal necrolysis, photosensitivity reactions, and palmar-plantar erythrodysesthesia in patients previously treated with capecitabine.

Other Natural Products That Enhance Tubulin Polymerization

The success of the taxanes has led to the identification of other natural products that enhance tubulin polymerization and may confer a therapeutic advantage over the taxanes. These include the epothilones isolated from myxobacterium *Sorangium cellulosum*, discodermolide (isolated from the Caribbean sponge *Discodermia dissoluta*), eleutherobin (isolated from the soft coral *Eleutherobia* sp), the tac-calonolides (isolated from *Tacca chantrieri*), peloruside A (isolated from the New Zealand marine sponge *Mycale hentscheli*), lauli-malide (isolated from the marine sponge *Cacospongia mycofijiensis*), and the sarcodictyins (isolated from the Mediterranean stoloniferan coral *Sarcodictyon roseum*). Some of these agents (epothilones, dis-codermolide, eleutherobins, and the sarcodictyins) bind to micro-tubules at or near the taxane-binding site, which has resulted in the identification of a common pharmacophore that may enable the development of hybrid chemical constructs with more desir-able pharmaceutical and clinical characteristics.[2–7,298,573–575] Others, such as laulimalide, appear to bind to unique sites on microtubules. Despite competition for a similar binding site, discodermolide and paclitaxel have demonstrated synergistic cytotoxicity in vitro, suggesting that their tubulin-binding sites and microtubule effects may not be identical.[576] Severe pulmonary toxicity was observed in early clinical studies of a completely synthetic discodermolide (XAA296).[577]

Epothilones

Many of the aforementioned compounds are either poor substrates or lack substrate affinity for Pgp and/or other ABC transporters but retain various degrees of activity against taxane-resistant cells in vitro. Although the clinical implications of these characteristics are not entirely clear, the epothilones have relevant activity in patients who have been previously treated with taxanes, some of whom are clearly taxane resistant. Of the nontaxane tubulin-polymerizing

agents, the epothilones are the furthest along in development, and one epothilone, ixabepilone, a semisynthetic analog of epothilone B, with a chemically modified lactam substitution for the naturally existing lactone, has received regulatory approval in the United States and elsewhere in combination with capecitabine for the treat-ment of patients with metastatic or locally advanced breast cancer resistant to anthracyclines and taxanes or for patients whose cancer is taxane resistant and for whom further anthracycline therapy is not indicated.[578–580] Ixabepilone is also indicated as monotherapy for treating patients with metastatic or locally advanced breast can-cer that is resistant or refractory to anthracyclines, taxanes, and capecitabine.[578–580] Additionally, both ixabepilone and epothilone B (patupilone) have moderate antitumor activity in patients with non–small cell lung and prostate cancer.[589–593] Moderate- to low-level activity has also been reported in patients with malignancies in which the taxanes do not possess relevant efficacy, including pancreatic, gastric, hepatobiliary, renal, urothelial, and colorectal cancers.[580–584] Epothilone D (KOS-862) and its analogs possess anti-cancer activity in patients with breast and ovarian cancers.[580–584]

Structure

The epothilones A and B are 16-member polyketide macrolides with nearly identical structures, except that epothilone B has an additional methyl group at the C-12 position (Fig. 13-6). The lac-tam analogue of epothilone B, ixabepilone (aza-epothilone B), was designed to enhance metabolic stability in the presence of plasma esterases. The antitumor activities of epothilones A and B led to

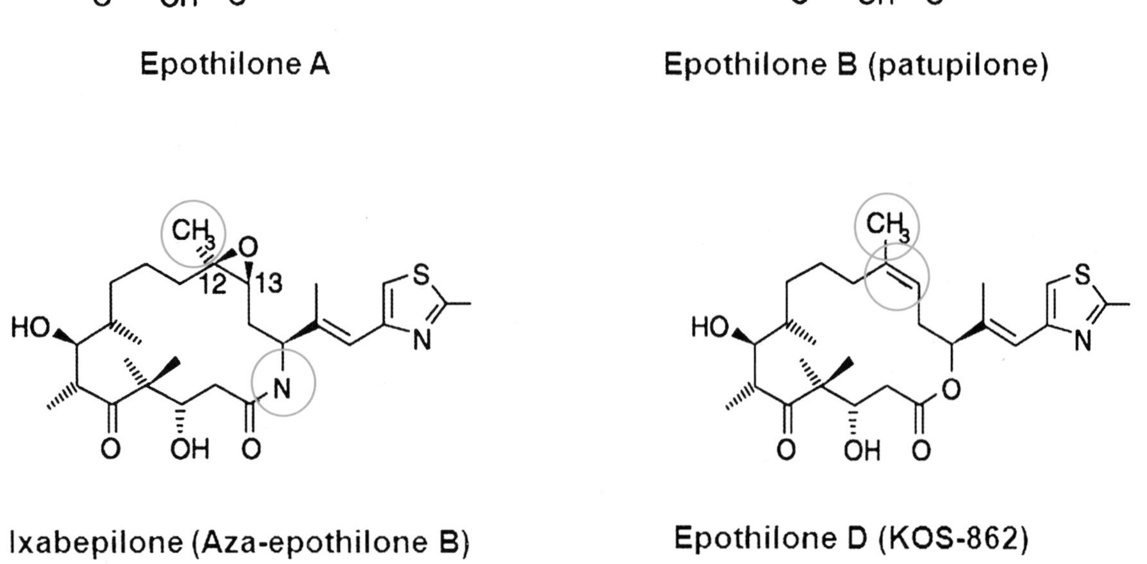

Epothilone A

Epothilone B (patupilone)

Ixabepilone (Aza-epothilone B)

Epothilone D (KOS-862)

FIGURE **13-6**   Structures of the epothilones: epothilone A, B, and D, and ixabepilone.

further modifications of the macrolactone ring (deletion of the epoxide moiety) that resulted in deoxyepothilone B (epothilone D; KOS-862) and the related KOS-1584, which appear to possess similar anticancer activities as epothilones A and B.

Mechanism of Action

Both epitholones A and B competitively inhibit binding of paclitaxel to tubulin polymers in vitro, suggesting that the binding sites of the epothilones and taxanes overlap and the epothilones and taxanes possess a common pharmacophore for microtubule binding.[324,582–586] However, the epothilones may occupy additional binding sites on tubulin and have chemical structural differences that enable them to evade MDR.[587–592]

Both epothilones A and B promote tubulin polymerization in vitro with kinetics similar to paclitaxel, but epothilone B appears to be a more potent than both epothilone A and paclitaxel.[582–585] Similar to the taxanes, the epothilones also induce tubulin polymerization in the absence of GTP and/or MAPs, which results in microtubules that are long, rigid, and resistant to destabilization by cold, temperature, and calcium.[573,582–585,589] Additionally, microtubule bundling may also occur. The antitumor activity of the epothilones directly relates to their ability to arrest cells in the G_2/M phase of the cell cycle.[352,591–593] Following mitotic arrest, epothilone-treated cells undergo p53- and BAX-dependent apoptosis.[582,587] At low concentrations, epothilone B does not induce mitotic arrest but transforms proliferating cells into large anueploid cells, which undergo apoptotic cell death in the G_1 phase of the cell cycle. Thus, protracted mitotic arrest may not be essential for epothilone-induced cytotoxicity, not unlike the effects of concentrations of the taxanes. In an in vitro study, the epothilones demonstrated greater activity against transformed prostate epithelial cells with mutant p53 compared to wild-type p53.[594] After treatment of cancer cells with epothilone A or B at low, albeit equipotent, concentrations, centrosome/spindle pole integrity is strongly affected by epothilone B but not greatly affected by epothilone A.[595]

Mechanisms of Resistance

A critical difference between the epothilones, taxanes, and vinca alkaloids is that overexpression of the ABC transporters Pgp and MRP1 minimally affects the cytotoxicity of the epothilones, which possess low-level or no substrate affinity for these proteins.[582–586,590,591] Epothilones A and B have strong antiproliferative activity in paclitaxel-resistant human cancer cells with high expression of Pgp (ABCB1), and tumor samples obtained from patients with ixabepilone-responsive malignancies show significant expression of both MDR1 and MRP1 mRNA, further suggesting that these proteins may not confer resistance to ixabepilone in the clinic.[582,591]

Although tumor resistance to certain microtubule inhibitors, including the taxanes, may relate to βIII-tubulin overexpression, this phenomenon does not seem to affect sensitivity to the epothilones. Ixabepilone also suppresses the dynamic instability of purified α/βIII-microtubules, whereas paclitaxel is less potent in suppressing the growth rate and catastrophe frequency of purified α/βIII-microtubules.[587] In addition, ixabepilone has exhibited substantially greater potency than both the taxanes and vinca alkaloids against a wide variety of cell lines and xenografts, as well as

activity against taxane- and vinca alkaloid-resistant cancer models, in which taxane-resistance is putatively due to overexpression of βIII-tubulin.[582,587,591]

In preclinical systems, cancer cells with point mutations involving βI and various other β-tubulins at sites that are critical for microtubule stabilization are resistant to the epothilones.[596,597] Additional mechanisms of epothilone resistance, such as α-tubulin mutations, altered expression of tubulin isotypes, altered MAP structure and function, and may be operative in conferring resistance to the epothilones but their clinical significance is not known.[582–585,591,597] Additionally, MRP-7 (ABCC10) appears to confer resistance to epothilone B, other natural products, and nucleoside analogues that are not substrates for Pgp.[598]

Ixabepilone: Clinical Pharmacology

In cancer patients, ixabepilone exhibits dose-proportional pharmacokinetics in the dose range of 15 to 57 mg/m^2 (Table 13-3).[582–584,599] Following administration of a single 40 mg/m^2 dose, C_{max} and terminal phase $t_{1/2}$ values average 252 ng/mL and 52 hours, respectively. Similar to the taxanes and vinca alkaloids, ixabepilone's volume of distribution at steady state is large, with mean values exceeding 1,000 L, reflecting rapid tissue distribution and extensive tissue binding.[599] Human serum protein binding has ranged from 67% to 77% in vitro.

The principal mode of systemic disposition of ixabepilone is hepatic metabolism.[582–584] Following intravenous administration of radiolabeled ixabepilone, 86% of the dose is eliminated within 7 days, with fecal and urinary elimination accounting for 65% and 21% of the dose, respectively. Little parent compound is excreted (1.6% and 5.6% of the dose in feces and urine, respectively). The principal metabolic pathway is oxidative metabolism via CYP3A4.

More than 30 inactive metabolites are excreted into human urine and feces, but no single metabolite accounts for more than 6% of the administered dose.

Drug Interactions

In vitro studies using human liver microsomes have demonstrated that clinically relevant concentrations of ixabepilone do not affect the activities of CYP3A4, CYP1A2, CYP2A6, CYP2B6, CYP2C8, CYP2C9, CYP2C19, or CYP2D6 and therefore would likely not affect the pharmacokinetics and metabolism of drugs that are substrates of these enzymes.[582–584,599] However, coadministration of ixabepilone with ketoconazole, a potent CYP3A4 inhibitor, increases ixabepilone AUC values by 79%, on average, compared to ixabepilone treatment alone. Therefore, strong inhibitors of CYP3A4 should be used judiciously in the context of ixabepilone treatment. With regard to ketoconazole and similar agents, if alternative treatment cannot be administered, a dose adjustment should be considered. Since the effect of mild or moderate CYP3A4 inhibitors (e.g., erythromycin, fluconazole, or verapamil) on exposure to ixabepilone has not been studied, caution should also be exercised when administering such agents in patients receiving ixabepilone and such patients should be carefully monitored for toxicity. Potent inducers of CYP3A4, such as dexamethasone, phenytoin, carbamazepine, rifampin, rifampicin, rifabutin, and phenobarbital, may also decrease ixabepilone concentrations and lead to subtherapeutic levels. Therefore, agents with low CYP3A4 induction potential should be considered for coadministration with ixabepilone.

In studies involving cancer patients who received ixabepilone (40 mg/m^2) in combination with capecitabine ($1,000 \text{ mg/m}^2$), the effects of ixabepilone on the exposure to capecitabine and metabolites, and vice versa, were modest and not clinically relevant.

Toxicity

Neurotoxicity

Peripheral neurotoxicity is the most common serious toxicity observed with ixabepilone as both monotherapy and combined with capecitabine.[578–602] Symptoms include a burning sensation, hyperesthesia, hypoesthesia, paresthesia, discomfort, and neuropathic pain. Sixty-three to sixty-seven percent of breast cancer patients who had previously received a taxane develop peripheral neurotoxicity after treatment with ixabepilone alone or in combination with capecitabine; however, severe (grades 3 and 4) toxicity was noted in 14% on monotherapy and 23% with capecitabine, respectively. In heavily pretreated patients, the onset of neuropathy occurs during the first three cycles and the most serious manifestations are experienced after four cycles. In clinical trials, peripheral neuropathy has been managed using dose reduction, treatment delay, and treatment discontinuation (see the sections on "Administration, Dose, and Schedule" and "Ixabepilone"). Following treatment discontinuation and/or dose reduction, manifestations usually resolve in 4 to 6 weeks, as compared to neuropathy due to the taxanes and vinca alkaloids, which resolves more slowly and incompletely. Patients who have hepatic insufficiency and/or diabetes mellitus are at an increased risk of developing severe neuropathy (see the sections on "Administration, Dose, and Schedule" and "Ixabepilone"). Although the presence of grade 1 neuropathy and prior therapy with neurotoxic chemotherapy do not predict for the development of neuropathy, it should be noted that patients with neuropathy of at least moderate severity were excluded from early clinical trials.

Myelosuppression

Dose-dependent myelosuppression, principally neutropenia, is common following ixabepilone treatment.[578–600] Similar to the taxanes, effects on platelets and red blood cells are less common. Grade 4 neutropenia (<500 cells/μL) has occurred in 36% of patients treated with ixabepilone in combination with capecitabine and in 23% of patients treated with monotherapy; however, febrile neutropenia and infection with neutropenia have been much less common, occurring in 5% or fewer patients on monotherapy or with capecitabine. Myelosuppression does not generally worsen with successive treatment, suggesting that ixabepilone does not significantly affect hematopoietic progenitor cells.

Dose reduction is recommended for patients experiencing severe neutropenia, and dose modification is recommended for patients with moderate hepatic dysfunction (see below).

Hypersensitivity

Since ixabepilone is formulated in polyoxyethylated castor oil, severe HSRs, largely secondary to this diluent, do occur.[578–600] Manifestations of HSRs include flushing, rash, dyspnea, and bronchospasm. For this reason, it is recommended that all patients receive premedication with H_1- and H_2-histamine antagonists approximately 1 hour before treatment (see the sections on "Administration, Dose, and Schedule" and "Ixabepilone"). In the case of severe HSRs, treatment should be stopped and aggressive supportive treatment (e.g., epinephrine, corticosteroids) should be started. In clinical studies, approximately 1% of patients have experienced severe reactions despite various premedication regimens. There have been reports of successful retreatment of patients who had experienced prior reactions after addition of a corticosteroid to H_1- and H_2-histamine antagonists, and extension of the infusion time.

Miscellaneous

Patients treated with ixabepilone have developed cognitive dysfunction, lethargy, and discoordination in the peritreatment period, possibly due to the effects of ethanol in the diluent. Myalgia and arthralgia in the peritreatment period have also been noted. Various cardiac disturbances, including myocardial infarction, supraventricular arrhythmia, left ventricular dysfunction, angina pectoris, atrial flutter, cardiomyopathy, and myocardial ischemia, have also been observed, but these events have not been directly attributed to ixabepilone.

Ileus, colitis, impaired gastric emptying, esophagitis, dysphagia, gastritis, gastrointestinal hemorrhage, hepatic insufficiency, erythema multiforme, various rashes, muscle spasm, and trismus have all been reported as uncommon side effects. Similar to the taxanes, nail disorders, including oncycholyis and subungual hemorrhagic bullaes in the fingernails, may occur and appear to relate to the duration of treatment.[602]

Administration, Dose, and Schedule

The recommended dosage of ixabepilone is 40 mg/m^2 intravenously over 3 hours every 3 weeks.[578–582] Doses for patients with body surface areas greater than 2.2 m^2 should be calculated based on 2.2 m^2 since this method was used to characterize dose-toxicity relationships. Although a range of intermittent dosing schedules have been evaluated, the preponderance of efficacy data relates to the 3-hour infusion every-3-week dosing schedule.

Ixabepilone is intended for intravenous use only after constitution with the supplied diluent, which is a nonpyrogenic solution of 52.8% (w/v) purified polyoxyethylated castor oil and 39.8% (w/v) dehydrated alcohol, USP, and after further dilution with Lactated Ringers Injection, USP. To minimize the chance of occurrence of major HSRs, all patients should be premedicated approximately 1 hour before treatment with both an H_1-histamine antagonist, such as diphenhydramine 50 mg orally or equivalent, and an H_2-histamine antagonist (e.g., ranitidine 150 to 300 mg orally or equivalent). For patients who experience an HSR, premedication with corticosteroids (e.g., dexamethasone 20 mg intravenously, 30 minutes before infusion or orally, 60 minutes before infusion) in addition to pretreatment with H_1-histamine and H_2-histamine antagonists is recommended.

Dose modification and/or treatment delay are recommended for patients who develop clinically relevant grades of neuropathy and/or myelosuppression.

Dose reduction by 20% is recommended for patients who develop neuropathic manifestations of grade 2 severity lasting at

Patients are generally treated for 30 to 90 days before assessment of therapeutic benefit. Chronic oral therapy can be maintained for months or even years. Abbreviated 1-, 3-, and 5-day courses of oral estramustine phosphate have been proposed for use in combination with the taxanes and other chemotherapeutics. Such schedules appear to reduce the gastrointestinal toxicity associated with chronic oral administration.[672,673] In studies with docetaxel using this abbreviated schedule, the recommended dose of estramustine is 280 mg three times daily ($\approx$600 mg/m^2/d) for 5 days.

References

1. Gelfand VI, Bershadsky AD. Microtubule dynamics: mechanism, regulation, and function. Annu Rev Cell Biol 1991;7:93–116.

2. Jordan MA, Wilson L. Microtubules as a target for anticancer drugs. Nat Rev Cancer 2004;4:253–265.

3. Jordan MA, Kamath K. How do microtubule-targeted drugs work? An overview. Curr Cancer Drug Targets 2007;7:730–742.

4. Kavallaris M, Verrills NM, Hill BT. Anticancer therapy with novel tubulin-interacting drugs. Drug Resist Updates 2001;4:392–401.

5. Correia JJ, Lobert S. Physiochemical aspects of tubulin-interacting antimitotic drugs. Curr Pharm Des 2001;7:1213–1228.

6. Gascoigne KA, Taylor SS. How do anti-mitotic drugs kill cancer cells. J Cell Sci 2009;122:2579–2585.

7. Pellegrini F, Budman DR. Review: tubulin function, action of antitubulin drugs, and new drug development. Cancer Invest 2005;23:264–273.

8. Jackson JR, Patrick DR, Dar MM, et al. Targeted antimitotic therapies: can we improve on tubulin agents? Nat Rev Cancer 2007;7:107–117.

9. Schwartz EL. Antivascular actions of microtubule-binding drugs. Clin Cancer Res. 2009;15:2594–2601.

10. Huszar D, Theoclitou ME, Skolnik J, et al. Kinesin motor proteins as targets for cancer therapy. Cancer Metastasis Rev 2009;28:197–208.

11. Gautschi O, Heighway J, Mack PC, et al. Aurora kinases as anticancer drug targets. Clin Cancer Res 2008;14:1639–1648.

12. Pérez de Castro I, de Cárcer G, Montoya G, et al. Emerging cancer therapeutic opportunities by inhibiting mitotic kinases. Curr Opin Pharmacol 2008;8:375–383.

13. Taylor S, Peters JM. Polo and Aurora kinases: lessons derived from chemical biology. Curr Opin Cell Biol 2008;20:77–84.

14. Li H, DeRosier DJ, Nicholson WV, Nogales E, et al. Downing KH Microtubule structure at 8 Å resolution. Structure 2002;10:1317–1328.

15. Nogales E, Whittaker M, Milligan RA, et al. High-resolution model of the microtubule. Cell 1999;96:78–88.

16. Luduena RF. Multiple forms of tubulin: different gene products and covalent modifications. Int Rev Cytol 1998;178:207–275.

17. Zheng Y, Jung MK, Oakley BR. Gamma-tubulin is present in Drosophila melanogaster and Homo sapiens and is associated with the centrosome. Cell 1991;65:817–823.

18. Raff EC. The role of multiple tubulin isoforms in cellular microtubule function. In: Hyams JF, Lloyd CD, eds. Microtubules. New York: Wiley-Liss, 1993:89–104.

19. Khan A, Luduena F. Different effects of vinblastine on the polymerization of isotypicallly purified tubulins from bovine brain. Invest New Drugs 2003;21:3–13.

20. Olmsted JB. Microtubule-associated proteins. Annu Rev Cell Biol 1986;2:421–457.

21. Hammond JW, Cai D, Verhey KJ. Tubulin modifications and their cellular functions. Curr Opin Cell Biol 2008;20:71–76.

22. Wilson L, Panda D, Jordan MA. Modulation of microtubule dynamics by drugs: a paradigm for the actions of cellular regulators. Cell Struct Funct 1999; 24:329–335.

23. Verhey KJ, Gaertig J. The tubulin code. Cell Cycle 2007;6:2152–2160.

24. Schulze E, Asai DJ, Bulinski JC, et al. Post-translational modification and microtubule stability. J Cell Biol 1987;105:2167–2177.

25. Vale RD. Microtubule motors: many new models off the assembly line. Trends Biochem Sci 1992;17:300–304.

26. Bhalla KN. Microtubule-targeted anticancer agents and apoptosis. Oncogene 2003;22:9075–9086.

27. Beck WT. Alkaloids. In: Fox BW, Fox M, eds. Antitumor Drug Resistance. Berlin: Springer-Verlag, 1984;589–656.

28. Crossin KL, Carney DH. Microtubule stabilization by Taxol inhibits initiation of DNA synthesis by thrombin and epidermal growth factor. Cell 1981;27:341–350.

29. Rowinsky EK, Donehower RC. The clinical pharmacology and use of antimicrotubule agents in cancer chemotherapeutics. Pharmacol Ther 1992;52:35–84.

30. Wilson L, Jordan MA. Pharmacological probes of microtubule function. In: Hyams JF, Lloyd CD, eds. Microtubules. New York: Wiley-Liss, 1994: 59–83.

31. Carlier M-F. Role of nucleotide hydrolysis in the polymerization of actin and tubulin. Cell Biophys 1998;12:105–117.

32. Farrell KW, Jordan MA, Miller HP, et al. Phase dynamics at microtubule ends: the coexistence of microtubule length changes and treadmilling. J Cell Biol 1987;104:1035–1046.

33. Mandelkow E-M, Mandelkow E. Microtubule oscillations. Cell Motil Cytoskeleton 1992;22:235–244.

34. Mitchison TJ. Localization of exchangeable GTP binding site at the plus end of microtubules. Science 1993;261:1044–1047.

35. Margolis RL, Wilson L. Microtubule treadmilling: what goes around comes around. Bioessays 1998;20:830–836.

36. Erickson HP, O'Brien ET. Microtubule dynamic instability and GTP hydrolysis. Annu Rev Biophys Biomol Struct 1992;21:145–166.

37. Mitchison T, Kirschner M. Dynamic instability of microtubule growth. Nature 1984;312:237–242.

38. Wilson L, Jordan MA. Microtubule dynamics: taking aim at a moving target. Chem Biol 1995;2:569–573.

39. Zhai Y, Kronebusch PJ, Simon PM, et al. Microtubule dynamics at the G2/M transition: abrupt breakdown of cytoplasmic microtubules at nuclear envelope breakdown and implications for spindle morphogenesis. J Cell Biol 1996;135:201–214.

40. Yvon A-M, Wadsworth P, Jordan MA. Taxol suppresses dynamics of individual microtubules in living human tumor cells. Mol Biol Cell 1999;10:947–959.

41. Johnson IS, Armstrong JG, Gorman M, et al. The vinca alkaloids: a new class of oncolytic agents. Cancer Res 1963;23:1390–1427.

42. Johnson IS. Historical background of vinca alkaloid research and areas of future interest. Cancer Chemother Rep 1968;52:455–461.

43. Dancey J, Steward WP. The role of vindesine in oncology—recommendations after 10 years' experience. Anticancer Drugs 1995;6:625–636.

44. Joel S. The comparative clinical pharmacology of vincristine and vindesine: does vindesine offer any advantage in clinical use? Cancer Treat Rev 1996;21:513–525.

45. Gridelli C, De Vivo R. Vinorelbine in the treatment of non-small cell lung cancer. Curr Med Chem 2002;9:879–891.

46. Domenech GH, Vogel CL. A review of vinorelbine in the treatment of breast cancer. Clin Breast Cancer 2001;2:113–128.

47. Budman DR. Vinorelbine (Navelbine): a third-generation vinca alkaloid. Cancer Invest 1997;15:475–490.

48. Curran MP, Plosker GL. Vinorelbine: a review of its use in elderly patients with advanced non-small cell lung cancer. Drugs Aging 2002;19: 695–721.

49. Rowinsky EK, Noe DA, Lucas VS, et al. A phase I, pharmacokinetic and absolute bioavailability study of oral vinorelbine (Navelbine) in solid tumor patients. J Clin Oncol 1994;12:1754–1763.

50. Yun-San Yip A, Yuen-Yuen Ong E, Chow LW. Vinflunine: clinical perspectives of an emerging anticancer agent. Expert Opin Investig Drugs 2008;17: 583–591.

51. Jordan MA, Horwitz SB, Lobert S, et al. Exploring the mechanisms of action of the novel microtubule inhibitor vinflunine. Semin Oncol 2008;35(3 Suppl 3):S6–S12.

52. Bellmunt J, Delgado FM, George C. Clinical activity of vinflunine in transitional cell carcinoma of the urothelium and other solid tumors. Semin Oncol 2008;35(3 Suppl 3):S34–S43.

53. Bennouna J, Delord JP, Campone M, et al. Vinflunine: a new microtubule inhibitor agent. Clin Cancer Res 2008;14:1625–1632.

54. Kruczynski A, Barret JM, Etiévant C, et al. Antimitotic and tubulin-interacting properties of vinflunine, a novel fluorinated Vinca alkaloid. Biochem Pharmacol 1998;55:635–648.

55. van den Bent MJ. Anaplastic oligodendroglioma and oligoastrocytoma. Neurol Clin 2007;25:1089–1109.

56. Shvidel L, Sigler E, Shtalrid M, et al. Vincristine-loaded platelet infusion for treatment of refractory autoimmune hemolytic anemia and chronic immune thrombocytopenia: rethinking old cures. Am J Hematol 2006;81:423–425.

57. Toso RJ, Jordan MA, Farrell KW, et al. Kinetic stabilization of the microtubule dynamic instability in vitro by vinblastine. Biochemistry 1993;32:185–193.

58. Himes RH, Kersey RN, Heller-Bettinger I, et al. Action of the vinca alkaloids, vincristine and vinblastine, and desacetyl vinblastine amide on microtubules in vitro. Cancer Res 1976;36:3798–3802.

59. Tucker RW, Owellen RJ, Harris SB. Correlation of cytotoxicity and mitotic spindle dissolution by vinblastine in mammalian cells. Cancer Res 1977;37:4346–4351.

60. White JG. Effect of colchicine and vinca alkaloids on human platelets: I. influence on platelet microtubules and contractile function. Am J Pathol 1968;53:281–91.

61. Bruchovsky N, Owen AA, Becker AJ, et al. Effects of vinblastine on the proliferative capacity of L cells and their progress through the division cycle. Cancer Res 1965;25:1232–1237.

62. Schrek R, Stefani SS. Inhibition by ionophore A23187 of the cytotoxicity of vincristine, colchicine and x-rays to leukemic lymphocytes. Oncology 1976;33:132–135.

63. Johnson SA, Harper P, Hortobagyi GN, et al. Vinorelbine: an overview. Cancer Treat Rev 1996;22:127–142.

64. Jordan MA, Thrower D, Wilson L. Mechanism of inhibition of cell proliferation by the vinca alkaloids. Cancer Res 1991;51:2212–2222.

65. Himes RH. Interactions of the catharanthus (vinca) alkaloids with tubulin and microtubules. Pharmacol Ther 1991;51:256–267.

66. Jordan MA, Margolis RL, Himes RH, et al. Identification of a distinct class of vinblastine binding sites on microtubules. J Mol Biol 1986;187:61–73.

67. Jordan MA, Wilson L. Kinetic analysis of tubulin exchange at microtubule ends at low vinblastine concentrations. Biochemistry 1990;29:2730–2739.

68. Singer WD, Jordan MA, Wilson L, et al. Binding of vinblastine to stabilized microtubules. Mol Pharmacol 1989;36:366–370.

69. Donoso JA, Haskins KM, Himes R. Effect of microtubule proteins on the interaction of vincristine and microtubules and tubulin. Cancer Res 1979;39:1604–1610.

70. Palmer CG, Livengood D, Warren AK, et al. The action of the vincaleukoblastine on mitosis in vitro. Experl Cell Res 1960;20:198–201.

71. Devred F, Tsvetkov PO, Barbier P, et al. Stathmin/Op18 is a novel mediator of vinblastine activity. FEBS Lett 2008;582:2484–2488.

72. Jordan MA, Wendell KL, Gardiner S, et al. Mitotic block induced in HeLa cells by low concentrations of paclitaxel (Taxol) results in abnormal mitotic exit and apoptotic cell death. Cancer Res 1996;56:816–825.

73. Fan S, Cherney B, Reinhold W, et al. Disruption of p53 function in immortalized human cells does not affect survival or apoptosis after taxol or vincristine treatment. Clin Cancer Res 1998;4:1047–1054.

74. Blagosklonny MV, Robey R, Bates S, et al. Pretreatment with DNA-damaging agents permits selective killing of checkpoint-deficient cells by microtubule-active drugs. J Clin Invest 2000;105:533–539.

75. Ngan VK, Bellman K, Hill BT, et al. Mechanism of mitotic block and inhibition of cell proliferation by the semisynthetic vinca alkaloids vinorelbine and its newer derivative vinflunine. Mol Pharmacol 2001;60:225–232.

76. Jordan MA, Thrower D, Wilson L. Effects of vinblastine, podophyllotoxin and nocodazole on mitotic spindles. Implications for the role of microtubule dynamics in mitosis. J Cell Sci 1992;102:401–416.

77. Upreti M, Lyle CS, Skaug B, et al. Vinblastine-induced apoptosis is mediated by discrete alterations in subcellular location, oligomeric structure, and activation status of specific Bcl-2 family members. J Biol Chem 2006;281:15941–15950.

78. Du L, Lyle CS, Chambers TC. Characterization of vinblastine-induced Bcl-xL and Bcl-2 phosphorylation: evidence for a novel protein kinase and a coordinated phosphorylation/dephosphorylation cycle associated with apoptosis induction. Oncogene 2005;24:107–117.

79. Wilson L, Miller HP, Farrell KW, et al. Taxol stabilization of microtubules in vitro: dynamics of tubulin addition and loss at opposite microtubule ends. Biochemistry 1985;24:5254–5262.

80. Vacca A, Iurlaro M, Ribatti D, et al. Antiangiogenesis is produced by nontoxic doses of vinblastine. Blood 1999;94:4143–4155.

81. Braguer D, Barret JM, McDaid H, et al. Antitumor activity of vinflunine: effector pathways and potential for synergies. Semin Oncol 2008;35 (3 Suppl 3):S13–S21.

82. Meissner M, Pinter A, Michailidou D, et al. Microtubule-targeted drugs inhibit VEGF receptor-2 expression by both transcriptional and post-transcriptional mechanisms. J Invest Dermatol 2008;128:2084–2091.

83. Pasquier E, André N, Braguer D. Targeting microtubules to inhibit angiogenesis and disrupt tumour vasculature: implications for cancer treatment. Curr Cancer Drug Targets. 2007;7:566–581.

84. Simoens C, Lardon F, Pauwels B, et al. Comparative study of the radiosensitizing and cell cycle effects of vinflunine and vinorelbine, in vitro. BMC Cancer 2008;8:65.

85. Fukuoka K, Arioka H, Iwamoto Y, et al. Mechanism of vinorelbine-induced radiosensitization of human small cell lung cancer cells. Cancer Chemother Pharmacol 2002;49:385–390.

86. Ngan V, Bellman K, Hill B, et al. Novel actions of the antitumor drugs vinflunine and vinorelbine on microtubules. Mol Pharmacol 2001;60:225–232.

87. Jordan MA, Himes RH, Wilson L. Comparison of the effects of vinblastine, vincristine, vindesine, and vinepidine on microtubule dynamics and cell proliferation in vitro. Cancer Res 1985;45:2741–2747.

88. Lobert S, Correia JJ. Energetics of vinca alkaloid interactions with tubulin. Methods Enzymol 2000;323:77–103.

89. Lobert S, Vulevic B, Correria JJ. Interaction of vinca alkaloids with tubulin: a comparison of vinblastine, vincristine, and vinorelbine. Biochemistry 1996;35:6806–6814.

90. Sahenk Z, Barohn R, New P, Mendell JR. Taxol neuropathy. Electrodiagnostic and sural nerve biopsy findings. Arch Neurol 1994;51:726–729.

91. Bowman LC, Houghton JA, Houghton PJ. Formation and stability of vincristine-tubulin complex in kidney cytosols. Role of GTP and GTP hydrolysis. Biochem Pharmacol 1988;37:1251–1257.

92. Ferguson PJ, Cass CE. Differential cellular retention of vincristine and vinblastine by cultured human promyelocytic leukemia HL-60/C-1 cells: the basis of differential toxicity. Cancer Res 1985;45:5480–5488.

93. Bleyer WA, Frisby SA, Oliverio VT. Uptake and binding of vincristine by murine leukemia cells. Biochem Pharmacol 1975;24:633–639.

94. Rahmani R, Zhou XJ, Placidi M, et al. In vivo and in vitro pharmacokinetics and metabolism of vinca alkaloids in rat. I. Vindesine (4-deacetyl-vinblastine 3-carboxyamide). Eur J Drug Metab Pharmacokinet 1990;15:49–55.

95. Zhou XJ, Martin M, Placidi M, et al. In vivo and in vitro pharmacokinetics and metabolism of vinca alkaloids: II. Vinblastine and vincristine. Eur J Drug Metab Pharmacokinet 1990;15:323–332.

96. Ferguson PJ, Phillips JR, Steiner M, et al. Differential activity of vincristine and vinblastine against cultured cells. Cancer Res 1984;44:3307–3312.

97. Sullivan KF. Structure and utilization of tubulin isotypes. Annu Rev Cell Biol 1988;4:687–716.

98. Lobert S, Puozzo C. Pharmacokinetics, metabolites, and preclinical safety of vinflunine. Semin Oncol 2008;35(3 Suppl 3):S28–S33.

99. Bowman LC, Houghton JA, Houghton PJ. GTP influences the binding of vincristine in human tumor cytosols. Biochem Biophys Res Commun 1986;135:695–700.

100. Gout PW, Noble RL, Bruchovsky N, et al. Vinblastine and vincristine growth-inhibitory effects correlate with their retention by cultured Nb2 node lymphoma cells. Int J Cancer 1984;34:245–248.

101. Houghton JA, Williams LG, Houghton PJ. Stability of vincristine complexes in cytosols derived from xenografts of human rhabdomyosarcoma and normal tissues of the mouse. Cancer Res 1985;45:3761–3767.

102. Fellous A, Ohayon R, Vacassin T, et al. Biochemical effects of Navelbine on tubulin and associated proteins. Semin Oncol 1989;16(2 Suppl 4):9–14.

103. Lengfeld AM, Dietrich J, Schultze-Maurer B. Accumulation and release of vinblastine and vincristine in HeLa cells: light microscopic, cinematographic, and biochemical study. Cancer Res 1982;42:3798–3805.

104. Caron JM, Herwood M. Vinblastine, a chemotherapeutic drug, inhibits palmitoylation of tubulin in human leukemic lymphocytes. Chemotherapy 2007;53:51–58.

105. Zhou XJ, Placidi M, Rahmani R. Uptake and metabolism of vinca alkaloids by freshly isolated human hepatocytes in suspension. Anticancer Res 1994;14:1017–1022.

106. Rahmani R, Zhou XJ. Pharmacokinetics and metabolism of vinca alkaloids. In: Workman P, Graham M, eds. Pharmacokinetics and Cancer Chemotherapy: Cancer Surveys. Plainview: Cold Spring Harbor Laboratory Press, 1993:269–285.

107. Jackson DV, Bender RA. Cytotoxic thresholds of vincristine in a murine and human leukemia cell line in vitro. Cancer Res 1979;39:4346–4349.

108. Inaba M, Fujikura R, Sakurai Y. Active efflux common to vincristine and daunorubicin in vincristine-resistant P388 leukemia. Biochem Pharmacol 1981;30:1863–1865.

109. Greenberger LM, Williams SS, Horwitz SB. Biosynthesis of heterogeneous forms of multidrug resistance associated glycoproteins. J Biol Chem 1987;262:13685–13689.

110. Choi K, Chen C, Kriegler M, et al. An altered pattern of cross-resistance in multidrug-resistant human cells results from spontaneous mutations in the mdr1 (P-glycoprotein) gene. Cell 1988;53:519–529.

111. Peterson RHF, Meyers MB, Spengler BA. Alterations of plasma membrane glycopeptides and gangliosides of Chinese hamster cells accompanying development of resistance to daunorubicin and vincristine. Cancer Res 1983;43:222–228.

112. Pieters R, Hongo T, Loonen AH, et al. Different types of non-P-glycoprotein mediated multiple drug resistance in children with relapsed acute lymphoblastic leukaemia. Br J Cancer 1992;65:691–697.

113. Cornwell MM, Tsuruo T, Gottesman MM, et al. ATP-binding properties of P-glycoprotein from multidrug-resistant KB cells. FASEB J 1987;1:51–54.

114. Fojo AT, Ueda K, Slamon DJ, et al. Expression of a multidrug-resistance gene in human tumors and tissues. Proc Natl Acad Sci USA 1987;84:265–269.

115. Beck WT, Mueller TJ, Tanzer LR. Altered cell surface membrane glycoproteins in Vinca alkaloid-resistant human leukemic lymphoblasts. Cancer Res 1979;39:2070–2076.

116. Lockhart AC, Tirona RG, Kim RB. Pharmacogenetics of ATP-binding cassatte transporters in cancer and chemotherapy. Mol Ther 2003;2:685–698.

117. Fojo T, Menefee M. Mechanisms of multidrug resistance: the potential role of microtubule-stabilizing agents. Ann Oncol 2007;18 Suppl 5:3–8.

118. Kavallaris M, Annereau JP, Barret JM. Potential mechanisms of resistance to microtubule inhibitors. Semin Oncol 2008;35(3 Suppl 3):S22–S27.

119. Nooter K, Westerman AM, Flens MJ, et al. Expression of the multidrug resistance-associated protein (MRP) in human tissues and adult solid cancers. Clin Cancer Res 1995;1:1301–1310.

120. Beck WT, Cirtain MC, Lefko JL. Energy-dependent reduced drug binding as a mechanism of Vinca alkaloid resistance in human leukemia lymphoblasts. Mol Pharmacol 1983;24:485–492.

121. Bender RA, Kornreich WD, Wodinsky I. Correlates of vincristine resistance in four murine tumor cell lines. Cancer Lett 1982;15:335–341.

122. Safa AR, Glover CJ, Meyers MB, et al. Vinblastine photoaffinity labeling of a high molecular weight surface membrane glycoprotein specific for multidrug-resistant cells. J Biol Chem 1986;261:6137–6140.

123. Grant CE, Validmarsson G, Hipfner R, et al. Overexpression of multidrug resistance associated protein (MRP) increases resistance to natural product drugs. Cancer Res 1994;54:357–361.

124. Scheper RJ, Broxterman HJ, Scheffer GL. Overexpression of a Mr 110000 vesicular protein in non-P-glycoprotein-mediated multidrug resistance. Cancer Res 1993;53:1475–1479.

125. Etiévant C, Barret J-M, Kruczynski A, et al. Vinflunine (20′,20′-difluoro-3′,4′-dihydrovinorelbine), a novel Vinca alkaloid, which participates in P-glycoprotein (Pgp)-mediated multidrug resistance in vivo and in vitro. Invest New Drugs 1998;16:3–17.

126. Kruh GD, Gaughan KT, Godwin A, et al. Expression pattern of MRP in human tissues and adult solid tumor cell lines. J Natl Cancer Inst 1995;87:1256–1258.

127. Hifpner DR, Deeley RG, Cole SP. Structural, mechanistic, and clinical aspects of MRP1. Biochim Biopsy Acta 1999;1461:359–366.

128. Zaman GJ, Flens JM, van Leusden MR, et al. The human multidrug resistance-protein MRP is a plasma membrane drug-efflux pump. Proc Natl Acad Sci USA 1994;91:8822–8826.

129. Etiévant C, Kruczynski A, Barret J-M, et al. Markedly diminished drug resistance-inducing properties of vinflunine (20′,20′-difluoro-3′,4′-dihydrovinorelbine) relative to vinorelbine, identified in murine and human tumour cells in vivo and in vitro. Cancer Chemother Pharmacol 2001;48:62–70.

130. Betrand Y, Capdeville R, Balduck N, et al. Cyclosporin A used to reverse drug resistance increases vincristine neurotoxicity. Am J Hematol 1992;40:158–159.

131. Pinkerton CR. Multidrug resistance reversal in childhood malignancies: potential for a real step forward? Eur J Cancer 1996;32A:641–645.

132. List AF, Kopecky KJ, Willman CL, et al. Benefit of cyclosporine modulation of drug resistance in patients with poor-risk acute myeloid leukemia: a Southwest Oncology Group Study. Blood 2004;98:3212–3220.

133. Amos LA, Baker TS. The three dimension structure of tubulin protofilaments. Nature 1979;279:607–612.

134. Rai SS, Wolff J. Localization of critical histidyl residues required for vinblastine-induced tubulin polymerization and for microtubule assembly. J Biol Chem 1998;273:31131–31137.

135. Orr GA, Verdier-Pinard P, McDaid H, et al. Mechanisms of Taxol resistance related to microtubules. Oncogene 2003;22:7280–7295.

136. Hari M, Wang Y, Veeraraghavan S, et al. Mutations in α- and β-tubulin that stabilize microtubules and confer resistance to colcemid and vinblastine. Mol Cancer Ther 2003;2:597–605.

137. Gan PP, Kavallaris M. Tubulin-targeted drug action: functional significance of class II and class IVb beta-tubulin in vinca alkaloid sensitivity. Cancer Res 2008;68:9817–9824.

138. Minotti AM, Barlow SB, Cabral F. Resistance to antimitotic drugs in Chinese hamster ovary cells correlates with changes in the level of polymerized tubulin. J Biol Chem 1991;266:3987–3994.

139. Cabral FR, Barlow SB. Resistance to the antimitotic agents as genetic probes of microtubule structure and function. Pharmacol Ther 1991;52:159–171.

140. Cabral FR, Barlow SB. Mechanisms by which mammalian cells acquire resistance to drugs that affect microtubule assembly. FASEB J 1989;3:1593–1599.

141. Cabral FR, Brady RC, Schiber MJ. A mechanism of cellular resistance to drugs that interfere with microtubule assembly. Ann N Y Acad Sci 1986;466:748.

142. Hari M, Wang Y, Veeraraghavan S. Mutations in alpha- and beta-tubulin that stabilize microtubules and confer resistance to colcemid and vinblastine. Mol Cancer Ther 2003;2:597–605.

143. Ranganathan S, Dexter DW, Benetatos CA, et al. Cloning and sequencing of human βIII-tubulin cDNA: induction of betaIII isotype in human prostate carcinoma cells by acute exposure to antimicrotubule agents. Biochim Biophys Acta 1998;1395:237–245.

144. Banerjee A, Roach MC, Trcka P, et al. Increased microtubule assembly in bovine brain tubulin lacking the type III isotype of β-tubulin. J Biol Chem 1990;265:1794–1799.

145. Kavallaris M, Kuo DYS, Burkhart CA, et al. Taxol-resistant ovarian tumors are associated with altered expression of specific beta-tubulin isotypes. J Clin Invest 1997;100:1282–1293.

146. Kavallaris M, Tait AS, Walsh BJ, et al. Multiple microtubule alterations are associated with vinca alkaloid resistance in human leukemia cells. Cancer Res 2001;61:5803–5809.

147. Gan P, Pasquier E, Kavallaris M. Class III β-tubulin mediates sensitivity to chemotherapeutic drugs in non-small cell lung cancer. Cancer Res 2007;67:9356–9363.

148. Sève P, Mackey J, Isaac S, et al. Class III beta-tubulin expression in tumor cells predicts response and outcome in patients with non-small cell lung cancer receiving paclitaxel. Mol Cancer Ther 2005;4:2001–2007.

149. Sève P, Isaac S, Trédan O, et al. Expression of class III β-tubulin is predictive of patient outcome in patients with non-small cell lung cancer receiving vinorelbine-based chemotherapy. Clin Cancer Res 2005;11:5481–5486.

150. Bernard-Marty C, Treilleux I, Dumontet C, et al. Microtubule-associated parameters as predictive markers of docetaxel activity in advanced breast cancer patients: results of a pilot study. Clin Breast Cancer 2002;3:341–345.

151. Arai K, Matsumoto Y, Nagashima Y, Yagasaki K. Regulation of class II beta-tubulin expression by tumor suppressor p53 protein in mouse melanoma cells in response to Vinca alkaloid. Mol Cancer Res 2006;4:247–255.

152. Murphy M, Hinmann A, Levine AJ. Wild-type p53 negatively regulates the expression of a microtubule-associated protein. Genes Dev 1996;10: 2971–2980.

153. Zhang CC, Yang JM, White E, et al. The role of MAP4 expression in the sensitivity to paclitaxel and resistance to vinca alkaloids in p53 mutant cells. Oncogene 1998;16:1617–1624.

154. Kruczynski A, Etiévant C, Perrin D, et al. Characterization of cell death induced by vinflunine, the most recent vinca alkaloid in clinical development. Br J Cancer 2002;86:143–150.

155. Upreti M, Galitovskaya EN, Chu R, et al. Identification of the major phosphorylation site in Bcl-xL induced by microtubule inhibitors and analysis of its functional significance. J Biol Chem 2008;283:35517–35525.

156. Sethi VS, Thimmaiah KN. Structural studies of the degradation products of vincristine dihydrogen sulfate. Cancer Res 1985;45:4386–4389.

157. Castle MC, Margileth DA, Oliverio VT. Distribution and excretion of [3H] vincristine in the rat and the dog. Cancer Res 1976;36:3684–3689.

158. Bender RA, Castle MC, Margileth DA, et al. The pharmacokinetics of [3H]-vincristine in man. Clin Pharmacol Ther 1977;22:430–435.

159. Culp HW, Daniels WD, McMahon RE. Disposition and tissue levels of [3H]-vindesine in rats. Cancer Res 1977;37:3053–3056.

160. Owellen RJ, Hartke CA, Hains FO. Pharmacokinetics and metabolism of vinblastine in humans. Cancer Res 1977;37:2597–2602.

161. Owellen RJ, Root MA, Hains FO. Pharmacokinetic of vindesine and vincristine in humans. Cancer Res 1977;37:2603–2607.

162. Jackson DV, Castle MC, Bender RA. Biliary excretion of vincristine. Clin Pharmacol Ther 1978;24:101–107.

163. Ramirez J, Ogan K, Ratain MJ. Determination of vinca alkaloids in human plasma by liquid chromatography/atmospheric pressure chemical ionization mass spectrometry. Cancer Chemother Pharmacol 1997;39:286–290.

164. Van Tellingen O, Beijnen JH, Nooyen WJ. Analytical methods for the determination of vinca alkaloids in biological specimens: a survey of the literature. J Pharm Biomed Anal 1991;9:1077–1082.

165. Ylinen M, Suhonen P, Naaranlahti T, et al. Gas chromatographic-mass spectrometric analysis of major indole alkaloids of Catharanthus roseus. J Chromatogr 1990;505:429–434.

166. Rahmani R, Bruno R, Iliadis A, et al. Clinical pharmacokinetics of the antitumor drug Navelbine (5'-noranhydrovinblastine). Cancer Res 1987; 47:5796–5799.

167. Nelson RL, Dyke RW, Root MA. Comparative pharmacokinetics of vindesine, vincristine, and vinblastine in patients with cancer. Cancer Treat Rev 1980;7(Suppl):17–24.

168. Rahmani R, Zhou XJ. Pharmacokinetics and metabolism of vinca alkaloids. Cancer Surv 1993;17:269–281.

169. Levêque D, Jehl F. Molecular pharmacokinetics of catharanthus (vinca) alkaloids. J Clin Pharmacol 2007;47:579–588.

170. Rahmani R, Zhou XJ. Pharmacokinetics and metabolism of vinca alkaloids. In: Workman P, Graham M, eds. Pharmacokinetics and Cancer Chemotherapy: Cancer Surveys. Plainview: Cold Spring Harbar Laboratory Press, 1993:269–282.

171. Gidding CE, Kellie SJ, Kamps WA, et al. Vincristine revisited. Crit Rev Oncol Hematol 1999;29:267–287.

172. Sethi VS, Jackson DV, White CT, et al. Pharmacokinetics of vincristine sulfate in adult cancer patients. Cancer Res 1981;41:3551–3555.

173. Jackson DV Jr. The periwinkle alkaloids. In: Lokich JJ, ed. Cancer Chemotherapy by Infusion. Chicago: Precept Press, 1990:155–185.

174. Owellen RJ, Donigian DW. 3H-Vincristine: preparation and preliminary pharmacology. J Med Chem 1972;15:894–898.

175. Jackson DV, Sethi VS, Spurr CL, et al. Pharmacokinetics of vincristine in the cerebrospinal fluid of humans. Cancer Res 1981;41:1466–1468.

176. Jehl F, Quoix E, Leveque D, et al. Pharmacokinetic and preliminary metabolic fate of Navelbine in humans as determined by high performance liquid chromatography. Cancer Res 1991;51:2073–2076.

177. Sethi VS, Castle MC, Surratt P, et al. Isolation and partial characterization of human urinary metabolites of vincristine sulfate. Proc Am Assoc Cancer Res 1981;22:173.

178. Villikka K, Kivistš KT, Mäenpää H, et al. Cytochrome P450-inducing antiepileptics increase the clearance of vincristine in patients with brain tumors. Clin Pharmacol Ther 1999;66:589–593.

179. Gillies J, Hung KA, Fitzsimons E, et al. Severe vincristine toxicity in combination with itraconazole. Clin Lab Haematol 1998;20:123–124.

180. Yao D, Ding S, Burchell B, et al. Detoxication of vinca alkaloids by human P450 CYP3A4-mediated metabolism: implications for the development of drug resistance. J Pharmacol Exp Ther 2000;294:387–395.

181. Tobe SW, Siu LL, Jamal SA, et al. Vinblastine and erythromycin: an unrecognized serious drug interaction. Cancer Chemother Pharmacol 1996;39:176–177.

182. Sathiapalan RK, El-Soth H. Enhanced vincristine neurotoxicity from drug interactions: case report and review of literature. Pediatr Hematol Oncol 2001;18:543–546.

183. Eiden C, Palenzuela G, Hillaire-Buys D, et al. Posaconazole-increased vincristine neurotoxicity in a child: a case report. J Pediatr Hematol Oncol 2009;31:292–295.

184. Yano R, Tani D, Watanabe K, et al. Evaluation of potential interaction between vinorelbine and clarithromycin. Ann Pharmacother 2009;43: 453–458.

185. Renbarger JL, McCammack KC, Rouse CE, et al. Effect of race on vincristine-associated neurotoxicity in pediatric acute lymphoblastic leukemia patients. Pediatr Blood Cancer 2008;50:769–771.

186. Ribrag V, Koscielny S, Casasnovas O, et al. Pharmacogenetic study in Hodgkin's lymphoma reveals the impact of UGT1A1 polymorphisms on patient prognosis. Blood 2009;113:3307–3313.

187. Pan JH, Han JX, Wu JM, et al. CYP450 polymorphisms predict clinic outcomes to vinorelbine-based chemotherapy in patients with non-small-cell lung cancer. Acta Oncol 2007;46:361–366.

188. Lönnerholm G, Frost BM, Abrahamsson J, et al. Vincristine pharmacokinetics is related to clinical outcome in children with standard risk acute lymphoblastic leukemia. Br J Haematol 2008;142:616–621.

189. Steele WH, King DJ, Barber HE, et al. Protein binding of prednisone and vinblastine in the serum of normal subjects and subjects with Hodgkin's disease. Eur J Clin Pharmacol 1983;24:683–687.

190. Hebden HF, Hadfield JR, Beer CT. The binding of vinblastine by platelets in the rat. Cancer Res 1970;30:1417–1424.

191. Creasey WA, Scott AI, Wei CC, et al. Pharmacological studies with vinblastine in the dog. Cancer Res 1975;35:1116–1120.

192. Zhou-Pan XR, Seree E, Zhou XJ, et al. Involvement of human liver cytochrome P450 3A in vinblastine metabolism: drug interactions. Cancer Res 1993;53:5121–5126.

193. Ohnuma T, Norton L, Andrejczuk A, et al. Pharmacokinetics of vindesine given as an intravenous bolus and 24-hour infusion in humans. Cancer Res 1985;45:464–469.

194. Nelson RL, Dyke RW, Root MA. Clinical pharmacokinetics of vindesine. Cancer Chemother Pharmacol 1979;2:243–246.

195. Rahmani R, Martin M, Favre R, et al. Clinical pharmacokinetics of vindesine: repeated treatments by intravenous bolus injections. Eur J Cancer Clin Oncol 1984;20:1409–1417.

196. Rahmani R, Kleisbauer JP, Cano JP, et al. Clinical pharmacokinetics of vindesine infusion. Cancer Treat Rep 1985;69:839–844.

197. Jackson DV Jr, Sethi VS, Long TR, et al. Pharmacokinetics of vindesine bolus and infusion. Cancer Chemother Pharmacol 1994;13:114–119.

198. Hande K, Gay J, Gober J, et al. Toxicity and pharmacology of bolus vindesine injection and prolonged vindesine infusion. Cancer Treat Rev 1980;7(Suppl 1):25–30.

199. Zhou XJ, Zhou-Pan XR, Gauthier T, et al. Human liver microsomal cytochrome P450 3A isoenzymes mediated vindesine biotransformation: metabolic drug interactions. Biomed Pharmacol 1993;4:853–861.

200. Levêque D, Jehl F. Clinical pharmacokinetics of vinorelbine. Clin Pharmacokinet 1996;31:184–197.

201. Urien S, Bree F, Breillout F, et al. Vinorelbine high-affinity binding to human platelets and lymphocytes: distribution in human blood. Cancer Chemother Pharmacol 1993;32:231–234.

202. Levêque D, Quoiz E, Dumont P, et al. Pulmonary distribution of vinorelbine in patients with non-small lung cancer. Cancer Chemother Pharmacol 1993;33:176–178.

203. Rahmani R, Gueritte F, Martin M, et al. Comparative pharmacokinetics of antitumor vinca alkaloids: intravenous bolus injections of Navelbine and related alkaloids to cancer patients and rats. Cancer Chemother Pharmacol 1986;16:223–228.

204. Levêque D, Merle-Melet M, Bresler L, et al. Biliary elimination and pharmacokinetics of vinorelbine in micropigs. Cancer Chemother Pharmacol 1993;32:487–490.

205. Krikorian A, Rahmani R, Bromet M, et al. Pharmacokinetics and metabolism of Navelbine. Semin Oncol 1989;16(Suppl 4):21–25.

206. Sorio R, Robieux I, Galligioni E, et al. Pharmacokinetics and tolerance of vinorelbine in elderly patients with metastatic breast cancer. Eur J Cancer 1997;33:301–303.

207. Robieux I, Sorio R, Borsatti E, et al. Pharmacokinetics of vinorelbine in patients with liver metastases. Clin Pharmacol Ther 1996;59:32–40.

208. de Graeve J, van Heugen JC, Zorza G, et al. Metabolism pathway of vinorelbine (Navelbine) in human: characterisation of the metabolites by HPLC-MS/MS. J Pharm Biomed Anal 2008;47:47–58.

209. Bugat R, Variol P, Roche H, et al. The effects of food on the pharmacokinetic profile of oral vinorelbine. Cancer Chemother Pharmacol 2002;50:285–290.

210. Zhou XJ, Zhou-Pan XR, Favre R, et al. Relative bioavailability of two oral formulations of Navelbine in cancer patients. Biopharm Drug Dispos 1994;15:577–586.

211. Johnson P, Geldart T, Fumoleau P, et al. Phase I study of vinflunine administered as a 10-minute infusion on days 1 and 8 every 3 weeks. Invest New Drugs 2006;24:223–231.

212. Bennouna J, Fumoleau P, Armand JP, et al. Phase I and pharmacokinetic study of the new vinca alkaloid vinflunine administered as a 10-min infusion every 3 weeks in patients with advanced solid tumors. Ann Oncol 2003;14:630–637.

213. Zhao X-P, Liu X-Q, Wang Y-S, et al. Pharmacokinetics, tissue distribution and excretion of vinflunine. Eur J Drug Metab Pharmacokinet 2006;31:59–64.

214. Zhao X-P, Zhong J, Liu X-Q, et al. CYP3A4 mediated in vitro metabolism of vinflunine in human liver microsomes. Acta Pharmacol Sin 2007;28:118–124.

215. Bender RA, Bleyer WA, Frisby SA. Alteration of methotrexate uptake in human leukemia cells by other agents. Cancer Res 1975;35:1305–1308.

216. Zager RF, Frisby SA, Oliverio VT. The effects of antibiotics and cancer chemotherapeutic agents on the cellular transport and antitumor activity of methotrexate in L1210 murine leukemia. Cancer Res 1973;33:1670–1676.

217. Chan JD. Pharmacokinetic drug interactions of vinca alkaloids. Summary of case reports. Pharmacotherapy 1998;18:1304–1307.

218. Bender RA, Nichols AP, Norton L, et al. Lack of therapeutic synergism of vincristine and methotrexate in L1210 murine leukemia in vivo. Cancer Treat Rep 1978;62:997–1003.

219. Yalowich JC. Effect of microtubule inhibition on etoposide accumulation and DNA damage in human K562 cells in vitro. Cancer Res 1987;47:1010–1015.

220. Chatterjee K, Zhang J, Tao R, et al. Vincristine attenuates doxorubicin cardiotoxicity. Biochem Biophys Res Commun 2008;373:555–560.

221. Bollini R, Riva R, Albani R, et al. Decreased phenytoin levels during antineoplastic therapy: a case report. Epilepsia 1983;24:75.

222. Jarosinski PF, Moscow JA, Alexander MS, et al. Altered phenytoin clearance during intensive chemotherapy for acute lymphoblastic leukemia. J Pediatr 1988;112:996–999.

223. Porter CC, Carver AE, Albano EA. Vincristine induced peripheral neuropathy potentiated by voriconazole in a patient with previously undiagnosed CMT1X. Pediatr Blood Cancer 2009;52:298–300.

224. Tobe SW, Siu LL, Jamal SA, et al. Vinblastine and erythromycin: an unrecognized serious drug interaction. Cancer Chemother Pharmacol 1995;35:188–190.

225. Rajaonarison JF, Lacarelle B, Catalin J, et al. Effect of anticancer drugs on the glucuronidation of 3′-azido-3′-deoxythymidine in human liver microsomes. Drug Metab Dispos 1993;21:823–829.

226. Sathiapalan RK, El-Soth H. Enhanced vincristine neurotoxicity from drug interactions: case report and review of literature. Pediatr Hematol Oncol 2001;18:543–546.

227. Sulkes A, Collins JM. Reappraisal of some dosage adjustment guidelines. Cancer Treat Rep 1987;71:229–233.

228. Quasthoff S, Hartung HP. Chemotherapy-induced peripheral neuropathy. J Neurol 2002;249:9–17.

229. Peltier AC, Russell JW. Recent advances in drug-induced neuropathies. Curr Opin Neurol 2002;15:633–638.

230. Costa G, Hreshchyshyn MM, Holland JF. Initial clinical studies with vincristine. Cancer Chemother Rep 1962;24:39–44.

231. Holland JF, Scharlau C, Gailani S, et al. Vincristine treatment of advanced cancer: a cooperative study of 392 cases. Cancer Res 1973;33:1258–1264.

232. Desai ZR, Van den Berg HW, Bridges JM, et al. Can severe vincristine neurotoxicity be prevented? Cancer Chemother Pharmacol 1982;8:211–214.

233. Van den Berg HW, Desai ZR, Wilson R, et al. The pharmacokinetics of vincristine in man: reduced drug clearance associated with raised serum alkaline phosphatase and dose-limiting elimination. Cancer Chemother Pharmacol 1982;8:215–219.

234. Slyter H, Liwnicz B, Herrick MK, et al. Fatal myeloencephalopathy caused by intrathecal vincristine. Neurology 1980;30:867–871.

235. Dyke RW. Treatment of inadvertent intrathecal administration of vincristine. N Engl J Med 1989;321:1270–1271.

236. Jackson DV Jr, Richards F, Spurr CL, et al. Hepatic intra-arterial infusions of vincristine. Cancer Chemother Pharmacol 1984;13:120–122.

237. Kinzel PE, Dorr RT. Anticancer drug renal toxicity and elimination: dosing guidelines for altered renal function. Cancer Treat Rev 1995;21:33–64.

238. Falkson G, Van Dyk JJ, Falkson FC. Oral vinblastine sulfate (NSC 49842) in malignant disease. S Afr Cancer Bull 1968;2:78–83.

239. Zeffren J, Yagoda A, Kelsen D, et al. Phase I-II trial of 5-day continuous infusion of vinblastine sulfate. Anticancer Res 1984;4:411–413.

240. Cvitkovic E, Izzo J. The current and future place of vinorelbine in cancer therapy. Drugs 1992;44(Suppl 4):36–45.

241. Paule B, Saliba F, Gil-Delgado M-A, et al. Phase I and pharmacokinetic (PK) dose-adjusted study of IV vinflunine (VFL) in cancer patients with liver dysfunction (LD) pharmacokinetic results. Proc Am Soc Clin Oncol 2007;15(18S):102S.

242. Legha SS. Vincristine neurotoxicity. Pathophysiology and management. Med Toxicol 1986;1:421–427.

243. Bradley WG, Lassman LP, Pearce GW. The neuromyopathy of vincristine in man: clinical electrophysiological and pathological studies. J Neurol Sci 1970;10:107–131.

244. Casey EB, Jellife AM, Le Quesne PM, et al. Vincristine neuropathy, clinical and electrophysiological observations. Brain 1973;96:69–86.

245. Swain SM, Arezzo JC. Neuropathy associated with microtubule inhibitors: diagnosis, incidence, and management. Clin Adv Hematol Oncol 2008;6:455–467.

246. Park SB, Krishnan AV, Lin CS, et al. Mechanisms underlying chemotherapy-induced neurotoxicity and the potential for neuroprotective strategies. Curr Med Chem 2008;15:3081–3094.

247. Gilliland P, Holguin M. Phrenic nerve paralysis due to vincristine. Leuk Lymphoma 2007;48:2452–2453.

248. Greig NH, Soncrant TT, Shetty HU, et al. Brain uptake and anticancer activities of vincristine and vinblastine are restricted by their low cerebrovascular permeability and binding to plasma constituents in rats. Cancer Chemother Pharmacol 1990;26:263–268.

249. Carpentieri U, Lockhart LH. Ataxia and athetosis as side effects of chemotherapy with vincristine in non-Hodgkin's lymphomas. Cancer Treat Rep 1978;62:561–562.

250. Riga M, Psarommatis I, Korres S, et al. Neurotoxicity of vincristine on the medial olivocochlear bundle. Int J Pediatr Otorhinolaryngol 2007;71:63–69.

251. Hirvonen HE, Salmi TT, Heinonen E, et al. Vincristine treatment of acute lymphoblastic leukemia induces transient autonomic cardioneuropathy. Cancer 1988;64:801–805.

252. Gottlieb RJ, Cuttner J. Vincristine-induced bladder atony. Cancer 1971;28:674–675.

253. Carmichael SM, Eagleton L, Ayers CR, et al. Orthostatic hypotension during vincristine therapy. Arch Intern Med 1970;126:290–293.

254. Charisius J, Stiefel M, Merkel N, et al. Critical illness polyneuropathy: a rare but serious adverse event in pediatric oncology. Pediatr Blood Cancer 2010;54:161–165.

255. Burns BV, Shotton JC. Vocal fold palsy following vinca alkaloid treatment. J Laryngol Otol 1998;112:485–487.

256. Kuruvilla G, Perry S, Wilson B, et al. The natural history of vincristine-induced laryngeal paralysis in children. Arch Otolaryngol Head Neck Surg 2009;135:101–105.

257. Choi BS, Robins HI. Reversible paclitaxel-induced vocal cord paralysis with later recall with vinorelbine. Cancer Chemother Pharmacol 2008;61:345–346.

258. Woods WG, O'Leary M, Nesbit ME. Life-threatening neuropathy and hepatotoxicity in infants during induction therapy for acute lymphoblastic leukemia. J Pediatr 1981;98:642–645.

259. Orejana-Garcia AM, Pascual-Huerta J, Perez-Melero A. Charcot-Marie-Tooth disease and vincristine. J Am Pediatr Med Assoc 2003;93:229–233.

260. Olek MJ, Bordeaux B, Leshner RT. Charcot-Marie-Tooth disease type I diagnosed in a 5-year old boy after vincristine neurotoxicity, resulting in maternal diagnosis. J Am Osteopath Assoc 1999;99:165–167.

261. McGuire SA, Gospe SM Jr, Dahl G. Acute vincristine neurotoxicity in the presence of hereditary motor and sensory neuropathy type I. Med Pediatr Oncol 1989;17:520–523.

262. Trobaugh-Lotrario AD, Smith AA, Odom LF. Vincristine neurotoxicity in the presence of hereditary neuropathy. Med Pediatr Oncol 2003;40:39–43.

263. Nishikawa T, Kawakami K, Kumamoto T, et al. Severe neurotoxicities in a case of Charcot-Marie-Tooth disease type 2 caused by vincristine for acute lymphoblastic leukemia. J Pediatr Hematol Oncol 2008;30:519–521.

264. Desai ZR, Van den Berg HW, Bridges JM, et al. Can severe vincristine neurotoxicity be prevented? Cancer Chemother Pharmacol 1982;8:211–214.

265. Jackson DV Jr, McMahan RA, Pope EK, et al. Clinical trial of folinic acid to reduce vincristine neurotoxicity. Cancer Chemother Pharmacol 1986;17:281–284.

266. Grush OC, Morgan SK. Folinic acid rescue for vincristine toxicity. Clin Toxicol 1979;14:71–78.

267. Helmann K, Hutchinson GE, Henry K. Reduction of vincristine toxicity by Cronassial. Cancer Chemother Pharmacol 1987;20:21–25.

268. Boyle FM, Wheeler HR, Shenfield GM. Glutamate ameliorates experimental vincristine neuropathy. J Pharmacol Exp Ther 1996;279:410–415.

269. Jackson DV, Wells HB, Atkins JN, et al. Amelioration of vincristine neurotoxicity by glutamic acid. Am J Med 1988;84:1016–1022.

270. Amara S. Oral glutamine for the prevention of chemotherapy-induced peripheral neuropathy. Ann Pharmacother 2008;42:1481–1485.

271. Binet S, Fellous A, Lataste H, et al. In situ analysis of the action of Navelbine on various types of microtubules using immunofluorescence. Semin Oncol 1989;16(Suppl 4):5–8.

272. Lobert S, Ingram JW, Hill B, et al. A comparison of thermodynamic parameters for vinorelbine and vinflunine induced tubulin self-association by sedimentation velocity. Mol Pharmacol 1998;53:908–915.

273. Okouneva T, Hill BT, Wilson L, et al. The effects of vinflunine, vinorelbine and vinblastine on centromere dynamics. Mol Cancer Ther 2003;2:427–436.

274. Le Chevalier T, Brisgand D, Douillard J-Y, et al. Randomized study of vinorelbine and cisplatin versus vindesine and cisplatin versus vindesine and cisplatin versus vinorelbine alone in non-small cell lung cancer: results of a European multicenter trial including 612 patients. J Clin Oncol 1994;12:360–367.

275. Bunn PA, Ford SS, Shackney SE. The effects of colcemide on hematopoiesis in the mouse. J Clin Invest 1975;58:1280–1285.

276. Sharma RK. Vincristine and gastrointestinal transit. Gastroenterology 1988;95:1435–1436.

277. Tester W, Forbes W, Leighton J. Vinorelbine-induced pancreatitis: a case report. J Natl Cancer Inst 1997;89:1631.

278. Subar M, Muggia FM. Apparent myocardial ischemia associated with vinblastine administration. Cancer Treat Rep 1986;70:690–691.

279. Hansen SW, Helweg-Larsen S, Trajoborg W. Long-term neurotoxicity in patients treated with cisplatin, vinblastine, and bleomycin for metastatic germ cell cancer. J Clin Oncol 1989;7:1457–1461.

280. Hantel A, Rowinsky EK, Donehower RC. Nifedipine and oncologic Raynaud's phenomenon. Ann Intern Med 1988;108:767.

281. Ballen KK, Weiss ST. Fatal acute respiratory failure following vinblastine and mitomycin administration for breast cancer. Am J Med Sci 1988;295:558–560.

282. Hohneker JA. A summary of vinorelbine (Navelbine) safety data from North American clinical trials. Semin Oncol 1994;21(Suppl 10):42–46.

283. Dorr RT, Alberts DS. Vinca alkaloid skin toxicity: antidote and drug disposition studies in the mouse. J Natl Cancer Inst 1985;74:113–120.

284. Bellone JD. Treatment of vincristine extravasation. JAMA 1981;245:343.

285. Dorr T. Antidotes to vesicant chemotherapy extravasation. Blood Rev 1990;4:41–60.

286. Pattison J. Managing cytotoxic extravasation. Nurs Times 2002;98:32–34.

287. Goolsby TV, Lombardo FA. Extravasation of chemotherapeutic agents: prevention and treatment. Semin Oncol 2006:33:139–143.

288. Kuroda H, Kawamura M, Hato T, et al. Syndrome of inappropriate secretion of antidiuretic hormone after chemotherapy with vinorelbine. Cancer Chemother Pharmacol 2008;62:331–333.

289. Blain PG. Adverse effects of drugs on skeletal muscle. Adverse Drug React Bull 1984;104:384.

290. Hoff PM, Valero V, Ibrahim N, et al. Hand-foot syndrome following prolonged infusion of high doses of vinorelbine. Cancer 1998;85:965–969.

291. Stefanou A, Dooley M. Simple method to eliminate the risk of inadvertent intrathecal vincristine administration. J Clin Oncol 2002;20:4705–4712.

292. Rowinsky EK, Donehower RC. Drug Therapy: paclitaxel (Taxol). N Engl J Med 1995;332:1004–1014.

293. Wani MC, Taylor HL, Wall ME, et al. Plant antitumor agents: VI. The isolation and structure of Taxol, a novel antileukemic and antitumor agent from Taxus brevifolia. J Am Chem Soc 1971;93:2325–2327.

294. Schiff PB, Fant J, Horwitz SB. Promotion of microtubule assembly in vitro by taxol. Nature 1979;22:665–667.

295. Schiff PB, Horwitz SB. Taxol stabilizes microtubules in mouse fibroblast cells. Proc Natl Acad Sci USA 1980;77:1561–1565.

296. Manfredi JJ, Parness J, Horwitz SB. Taxol binds to cellular microtubules. J Cell Biol 1982;94:688–696.

297. Cortes JE, Pazdur R. Docetaxel. J Clin Oncol 1995;13:2643–2655.

298. Rowinsky EK, Calvo E. Novel agents that target tublin and related elements. Semin Oncol 2006;33:421–435.

299. McGuire WP, Hoskins WJ, Brady MF, et al. Cyclophosphamide and cisplatin compared with paclitaxel and cisplatin in patients with stage III and IV ovarian cancer. N Engl J Med 1996;334:1–6.

300. Piccart-Bebhart MJ, Burzkowski T, Buyse, M, et al. Taxanes alone or in combination with anthracyclines as first-line therapy of patients with metastatic breast cancer. J Clin Oncol 2008:26:1980–1986.

301. Citron ML, Berry DA, Cirrincione C, et al. Randomized trial of dose-dense vs conventionally scheduled and sequential vs concurrent combination chemotherapy as postoperative adjuvant treatment of nodepositive primary breast cancer: first report of Intergroup Trial C9741/Cancer and Leukemia Group B Trial 9741. J Clin Oncol 2003;21:1432–1439.

302. Henderson IC, Berry D, Demetri G, et al. Improved outcomes from adding sequential paclitaxel but not from escalating doxorubicin dose in an adjuvant chemotherapy regimen for patients with nodetic inpositive primary breast cancer. J Clin Oncol 2003;21:976–983.

303. Mamounas EP, Bryant J, Lembersky B, et al. Paclitaxel after doxorubicin plus cyclophosphamide as adjuvant chemotherapy for node-positive breast cancer: results from NSABP B-28. J Clin Oncol 2005;23:3686–3696.

304. Dent S, Messersmith H, Trudeau M. Gemcitabine in the management of metastatic breast cancer: a systematic review. Breast Cancer Res Treat 2008;108:319–331.

305. Miller K, Wang M, Gralow J, et al. Paclitaxel plus bevacizumab versus paclitaxel alone for metastatic breast cancer. N Engl J Med 2007;357:2666–2676.

306. Slamon DJ, Leyland-Jones B, Shak S, et al. Use of chemotherapy plus a monoclonal antibody against HER2 for metastatic breast cancer that overexpresses HER2. N Engl J Med 2001;344:783–792.

307. Sparano JA, Wang M, Martino S, et al. Weekly paclitaxel in the adjuvant treatment of breast cancer. N Engl J Med 2008;358:1663–1671.

308. Seidman AD, Berry D, Cirrincione C, et al. Randomized phase III trial of weekly compared with every-3-weeks paclitaxel for metastatic breast cancer, with trastuzumab for all HER-2 overexpressors and random assignment to trastuzumab or not in HER-2 nonoverexpressors: final results of Cancer and Leukemia Group B protocol 9840. J Clin Oncol 2008;26:1642–1649.

309. Seidman AD, Hudis CA, Albanel J, et al. Dose-dense therapy with weekly 1-hour paclitaxel infusions in the treatment of metastatic breast cancer. J Clin Oncol 1998;16:3353–3361.

310. Jie C, Tulpule A, Zheng T, et al. Treatment of epidemic AIDS-related Kaposi's sarcoma. Curr Opin Oncol 1997;9:433–439.

311. Bonomi P, Kim K, Fariclough D, et al. Comparison of survival and quality of life in advanced non-small cell lung cancer patients treated with two dose levels of paclitaxel combined with cisplatin versus etoposide with cisplatin: results from an Eastern Cooperative Oncology Group trial. J Clin Oncol 2000;18:623–631.

312. Sandler A, Gray R, Perry MC, et al. Paclitaxel-carboplatin alone or with bevacizumab for non-small-cell lung cancer. N Engl J Med 2006;355:2542–2550.

313. Martin M, Pienkowski T, Mackey J, et al. Breast Cancer International Research Group 001 Investigators. Adjuvant docetaxel for node-positive breast cancer. N Engl J Med 2005;352:2302–2313.

314. Fossella F, Pereira JR, von Pawel J, et al. Randomized, multinational, phase III study of docetaxel plus platinum combinations versus vinorelbine plus cisplatin for advanced non-small-cell lung cancer: the TAX 326 study group. J Clin Oncol 2003;21:3016–3024.

315. Tannock IF, de Wit R, Berry WR, et al. Docetaxel plus prednisone or mitoxantrone plus prednisone for advanced prostate cancer. N Engl J Med 2004;351:1502–1512.

316. Petrylak DP, Tangen CM, Hussain MH, et al. Docetaxel and estramustine compared with mitoxantrone and prednisone for advanced refractory prostate cancer. N Engl J Med 2004;351:1513–1520.

317. Posner MR, Hershock DM, Blajman CR, et al. Cisplatin and fluorouracil alone or with docetaxel in head and neck cancer. N Engl J Med 2007;357:1705–1715.

318. Van Cutsem E, Moiseyenko VM, Tjulandin S, et al. Phase III study of docetaxel and cisplatin plus fluorouracil compared with cisplatin and fluorouracil as first-line therapy for advanced gastric cancer: a report of the V325 Study Group. J Clin Oncol. N Engl J Med 2006;24:4991–4997.

319. Gradishar WJ, Tjulandin S, Davidson N, et al. Phase III trial of nanoparticle albumin-bound paclitaxel compared with polyethylated castor oil-based paclitaxel in women with breast cancer. J Clin Oncol 2005;23:7794–7803.

320. Lataste H, Senilh V, Wright M, et al. Relationships between the structures of Taxol and baccatine III derivatives and their in vitro action of the disassembly of mammalian brain and Pysarum amoebal microtubules. Proc Natl Acad Sci USA 1984;81:4090–4094.

321. Gueritte-Voegelein F, Guenard D, Lavelle F, et al. Relationships between the structures of Taxol analogues and their antimitotic activity. J Med Chem 1991;34:992–998.

322. Rao S, Krauss NE, Heerding JM, et al. 3′-(p-Azidobenzamido) taxol photolabels the N-terminal 31 amino acids of β-tubulin. J Biol Chem 1994;269:3132–3134.

323. Rao S, Orr GA, Chaudhary AG, et al. Characterization of the Taxol binding site on the microtubule: 2-(m-azidobenzoyl)taxol photolabels a peptide (amino acids 217–231) of beta tubulin. J Biol Chem 1995;270:20235–20238.

324. Ojima I, Chakravarty S, Inoue T, et al. A common pharmacophore for cytotoxic natural products that stabilize microtubules. Proc Natl Acad Sci USA 1999;96:4256–4261.

325. Nogales E, Wolf SG, Downing KH. Structure of the alpha beta tubulin dimer by electron crystallography. Nature 1998;391:199–203.

326. Jordan A, Hadfield JA, Lawrence NJ, et al. Tubulin as a target for anticancer drugs which interact with the mitotic spindle. Med Res Rev 1998;18:259–296.

327. Diaz JF, Andreu JM. Assembly of purified GDP-tubulin into microtubules induced by taxol and taxotere: reversibility, ligand stoichiometry and competition. Biochemistry 1993;32:2747–2755.

328. Caplow M, Shanks J, Ruhlen R. How taxol modulates microtubule disassembly. J Biol Chem 1994;269:23399–23402.

329. Vanhoerfer U, Cao S, Harstrict A, et al. Comparative antitumor efficacy of docetaxel and paclitaxel in nude mice bearing human tumor xenografts that overexpress the multidrug resistant protein. Ann Oncol 1997;8:1221–1228.

330. Valero V, Jones SE, Von Hoff DD, et al. A phase II study of docetaxel in patients with paclitaxel-resistant metastatic breast cancer. J Clin Oncol 1998;16:3362–3368.

331. Ravdin P, Erban J, Overmoyer B, et al. Phase III comparison of docetaxel (D) and paclitaxel (P) in patients with metastatic breast cancer (MBC). Proc Eur Cancer Conference 2003;12:670.

332. Blum JL, Savin MA, Edelman G, et al. Phase II study of weekly albumin-bound paclitaxel for patients with metastatic breast cancer heavily pretreated with taxanes. Clin Breast Cancer 2007;7:850–856.

333. Jordan MA, Toso RJ, Thrower D, et al. Mechanism of mitotic block and inhibition of cell proliferation by taxol at low concentrations. Proc Natl Acad Sci USA 1993;90:9552–9556.

334. Derry WB, Wilson L, Jordan MA. Substoichiometric binding of taxol suppresses microtubule dynamics. Biochemistry 1995;34:2203–2211.

335. Horwitz SB, Cohen D, Rao S, et al. Taxol: mechanisms of action and resistance. Monogr Natl Cancer Inst 1993;15:55–61.

336. Chen J-G, Horwitz SB. Differential mitotic responses to microtubule-stabilizing and -destabilizing drugs. Cancer Res 2002;62:1935–1938.

337. Abal M, Andreu JM, Barasoain I. Taxanes microtubule and centrosome targets, and cell cycle dependent mechanisms of action. Curr Cancer Drug Targets 2003;3:193–203.

338. Derry WB, Wilson L, Jordan MA. Low potency of taxol at microtubule minus ends: implications for its antimitotic and therapeutic mechanism. Cancer Res 1998;58:1177–1184.

339. Jordan MA, Wilson L. Use of drugs to study the role of microtubule assembly dynamics in living cells. Methods Enzymol 1998;298:252–276.

340. Ringel I, Horwitz SB. Studies with RP56976 (Taxotere): a semisynthetic analogue of taxol. J Natl Cancer Inst 1991;83:288–291.

341. Bhalla K, Ibrado AM, Tourkina E, et al. Taxol induces internucleosomal DNA fragmentation associated with programmed cell death in human myeloid leukemia cells. Leukemia 1993;7:563–568.

342. Poruchynsky MS, Wang EE, Rudin CM, et al. Bcl-xL is phosphorylated in malignant cells following microtubule disruption. Cancer Res 1998;58:3331–3338.

343. Wang LG, Liu XM, Kreis W, et al. The effect of antimicrotubule agents on signal transduction pathways of apoptosis: a review. Cancer Chemother Pharmacol 1999;44:355–361.

344. Dumontet C, Sikic B. Mechanism of action and resistance to antitubulin agents: microtubule dynamics, drug transport, and cell death. J Clin Oncol 1999;17:1061–1070.

345. Zhang CC, Yang JM, Bash-Babula J, et al. DNA damage increases sensitivity to vinca alkaloids and decreases sensitivity to taxanes through p53-dependent repression of microtubule-associated protein 4. Cancer Res 1999;59:3663–3670.

346. Strobel T, Swanson L, Korsmeyer S, et al. BAX enhances paclitaxel-induced apoptosis through a p53-independent pathway. Proc Natl Acad Sci USA 1996;93:14094–14099.

347. Scatena CD, Stewart ZA, Mays D, et al. Mitotic phosphorylation of Bcl-2 during normal cell cycle progression and Taxol-induced cell growth arrest. J Biol Chem 1998;273:30777–30784.

348. Torres K, Horwitz SB. Mechanisms of Taxol-induced cell death are concentration dependent. Cancer Res 1998;58:3620–3626.

349. Ferlini C, Raspaglio G, Mozzetti S. Bcl-2 down-regulation is a novel mechanism of paclitaxel resistance. Mol Pharmacol 2003;64:51–58.

350. Moos PJ, Fitzpatrick FA. Taxane-mediated gene induction is independent of microtubule stabilization: induction of transcription regulators and enzymes that modulate inflammation and apoptosis. Proc Natl Acad Sci USA 1998;95:3896–3901.

351. Griffon-Etienne G, Boucher Y, Brekken C, et al. Taxane-induced apoptosis decompresses blood vessels and lowers interstitial fluid pressure in solid tumors: clinical implications. Cancer Res 1999;59:776–782.

352. Milross CG, Mason KA, Hunter NR, et al. Relationship of mitotic arrest and apoptosis to antitumor effect of paclitaxel. J Natl Cancer Inst 1996;88:1308–1314.

353. Paoletti A, Giocanti N, Favaudon V, et al. Pulse treatment of interphasic HeLa cells with nanomolar doses of docetaxel affects centrosome organization and leads to catastrophic exit of mitosis. J Cell Sci 1997;110:2403–2415.

354. Hernández-Vargas H, Palacios J, Moreno-Bueno G. Telling cells how to die: docetaxel therapy in cancer cell lines. Cell Cycle 2007;6:780–783.

355. Hernández-Vargas H, Palacios J, Moreno-Bueno G. Molecular profiling of docetaxel cytotoxicity in breast cancer cells: uncoupling of aberrant mitosis and apoptosis. Oncogene 2007;26:2902–2913.

356. Ganansia-Leymarie V, Bischoff P, Bergerat JP. Signal transduction pathways of taxanes-induced apoptosis. Curr Med Chem Anti-Cancer Agents 2003;291–306.

357. Blagosklonny MV, Schulte TW, Nguyen P, et al. Taxol-induction of p21 WAF1 and p53 requires c-raf-1. Cancer Res 1995;55:4623–4626.

358. Blagosklonny MV. Unwinding the loop of Bcl-2 phosphorylation. Leukemia 2001;15:869–874.

359. Konishi Y, Lehtinen M, Donovan N, et al. Cdc2 phosphorylation of BAD links the cell cycle to the cell death machinery. Mol Cell 2002;9:1005–1016.

360. Mielgo A, Torres VA, Clair K, et al. Paclitaxel promotes a caspase 8-mediated apoptosis through death effector domain association with microtubules. Oncogene 2009;28:3551–3562.

361. Xu M, Takanashi M, Oikawa K, et al. USP15 plays an essential role for caspase-3 activation during paclitaxel-induced apoptosis. Biochem Biophys Res Commun 2009;388:366–371.

362. Impens F, Van Damme P, Demol H, et al. Mechanistic insight into taxol-induced cell death. Oncogene 2008;27:4580–4591.

363. Ho LH, Read SH, Dorstyn L, et al. Caspase-2 is required for cell death induced by cytoskeletal disruption. Oncogene 2008;27:3393–3404.

364. Rodi DJ, Janes RW, Sanganee HJ, et al. Screening of a library of phage-displayed peptides identifies human bcl-2 as a taxol-binding protein. J Mol Biol 1999;285:197–203.

365. Ferlini C, Cicchillitti L, Raspaglio G, et al. Paclitaxel directly binds to Bcl-2 and functionally mimics activity of Nur77. Cancer Res 2009;69:6906–6914.

366. Kitagawa K, Niikura Y. Caspase-independent mitotic death (CIMD). Cell Cycle 2008;7:1001–1005.

367. Rowinsky EK, Donehower RC, Jones RJ, et al. Microtubule changes and cytotoxicity in leukemic cell lines treated with taxol. Cancer Res 1988;48:4093–4100.

368. Burkhart CA, Berman JW, Swindell CS, et al. Relationship between taxol and other taxanes on induction of tumor necrosis factor-alpha gene expression and cytotoxicity. Cancer Res 1994;54:5779–5782.

369. Creane M, Seymour CB, Colucci S. Radiobiological effects of docetaxel (Taxotere): a potential radiation sensitizer. Int J Radiat Biol 1999;75:731–737.

370. Fetell MR, Grossman SA, Fisher J, et al. Pre-irradiation paclitaxel in glioblastoma multiforme (GBM): efficacy, pharmacology, and drug interactions. J Clin Oncol 1997;15:3121–3128.

371. Tishler RB, Geard CR, Hall EJ, et al. Taxol sensitizes human astrocytoma cells to radiation. Cancer Res 1992;52:3595–3597.

372. Mason KA, Hunter NR, Milas M, et al. Docetaxel enhances tumor radioresponse in vivo. Clin Cancer Res 1997;3:2431–2438.

373. Niero A, Emiliani E, Monti G, et al. Paclitaxel and radiotherapy: sequence-dependent efficacya preclinical model. Clin Cancer Res 1999;5:2213–2222.

374. Belotti D, Vergani V, Drudis T, et al. The microtubule-affecting drug paclitaxel has antiangiogenic activity. Clin Cancer Res 1996;2:1843–1849.

375. Klauber N, Paragni S, Flynn E, et al. Inhibitor of angiogenesis and breast cancer in mice by the microtuble inhibitors 2-methoxyestradiol and taxol. Cancer Res 1997;57:81–86.

376. Wang J, Lou P, Lesniewski R. Paclitaxel at ultra low concentrations inhibits angiogenesis without affecting cellular microtubule assembly. Anticancer Drugs 2003;14:13–19.

377. Pasquier E, Honore S, Pourroy B, et al. Antiangiogenic concentrations of paclitaxel induce an increase in microtubule dynamics in endothelial cells but not in cancer cells. Cancer Res 2005;65:2433–2440.

378. Muta M, Yanagawa T, Sai Y, et al. Effect of low-dose Paclitaxel and docetaxel on endothelial progenitor cells. Oncology 2009;77:182–191.

379. Roberts JR, Allison DC, Dooley WC, et al. Effects of Taxol on cell cycle traverse: taxol-induced polyploidization as a marker for drug resistance. Cancer Res 2990;50:710–716.

380. Quillen M, Castello C, Krishan A, et al. Cell surface tubulin in leukemic cells: molecular structure surface binding, turnover, cell cycle expression, and origin. J Cell Biol 1985;101:2345–2354.

381. Ding AH, Porteu F, Sanchez E, et al. Shared actions of endotoxin and Taxol on TNF receptors and TNF release. Science 1990;248:370–372.

382. Van Bockxmeer FM, Martin CE, Thompson DE, et al. Taxol for the treatment of proliferative vitreoretinopathy. Invest Ophthalmol Vis Sci 1985;26:1140–1147.

383. Sollott SJ, Cheng L, Pauly RR, et al. Taxol inhibits neointimal smooth muscle cell accumulation after angioplasty in the rat. J Clin Invest 1995;95:1869–1876.

384. Laroia ST, Laroia AT. Drug-eluting stents. A review of the current literature. Cardiol Rev 2004;12:37–43.

385. Robinson DM, Keating GM. Albumin bound paclitaxel: in metastatic breast cancer. Drugs 2006;66:941–948.

386. Ibrahim NK, Desai N, Legha S, et al. Phase I and pharmacokinetic study of ABI-007, a Cremophor-free, protein-stabilized, nanoparticle formulation of paclitaxel. Clin Cancer Res 2002;8:1038–1044.

387. Desai N, Trieu V, Yao Z, et al. Increased antitumor activity, intratumor paclitaxel concentrations, and endothelial cell transport of cremophor-free, albumin-bound paclitaxel, ABI-007, compared with cremophor-based paclitaxel. Clin Cancer Res 2006;12:1317–1324.

388. Gradishar WJ. Albumin-bound paclitaxel: a next-generation taxane. Expert Opin Pharmacother 2006;7:1041–1053.

389. Desai N, Trieu V, Damascelli B, et al. SPARC Expression correlates with tumor response to albumin-bound paclitaxel in head and neck cancer patients. Transl Oncol 2009;2:59–64.

390. Desai NP, Trieu V, Hwang LY, et al. Improved effectiveness of nanoparticle albumin-bound (nab) paclitaxel versus polysorbate-based docetaxel in multiple xenografts as a function of HER2 and SPARC status. Anticancer Drugs 2008;19:899–909.

391. Roy SN, Horwitz SB. A phosphoglycoprotein with taxol resistance in J774. 2 cells. Cancer Res 1985;45:3856–3863.

392. Cole SP, Sparks KE, Fraser K, et al. Pharmacological characterization of multidrug resistant MRP-transfected human tumor cells. Cancer Res 1994;54:5902–5910.

393. Lorico A, Rappa G, Flavell RA, et al. Double knockout of the MRP gene leads to increased drug sensitivity in vitro. Cancer Res 1996;56:5351–5355.

394. Geney R, Ungureanu M, Li D. Overcoming multidrug resistance in taxane chemotherapy. Clin Chem Lab Med 2002;40:918–925.

395. Rowinsky EK, Smith L, Chaturvedi P, et al. Pharmacokinetic and toxicologic interactions between the multidrug resistance reversal agent VX-710 and paclitaxel in cancer patients. J Clin Oncol 1998;16:2964–2976.

396. Webster LK, Cosson EJ, Stokes KH, et al. Effect of the paclitaxel vehicle, Cremophor EL, on the pharmacokinetics of doxorubicin and doxorubicinol in mice. Br J Cancer 1996;73:522–524.

397. Rowinsky EK. Pharmacology and metabolism. In: McGuire WG, Rowinsky EK, eds. Paclitaxel in Cancer Treatment. New York: Marcel Dekker, 1995;91–122.

398. Patnaik A, Warner E, Michael M, et al. A phase I dose-finding and pharmacokinetic study of paclitaxel and carboplatin with oral oral valspodar in patients with advanced solid tumors. J Clin Oncol 2000;18:3677–3689.

399. Cabral F, Wible L, Brenner S, et al. Taxol-requiring mutants of Chinese hamster ovary cells with impaired mitotic spindle activity. J Cell Biol 1983;97:30–39.

400. Drukman S, Kavallaris M. Microtubule alterations and resistance to tubulin-binding agents. Int J Oncol 2002;21:621–628.

401. Haber M, Burkhart CA, Regl DL, et al. Altered expression of Mb2, the class II b-tubulin isotype, in a murine J774.2 cell line with a high level of taxol resistance. J Biol Chem 1995;270:31269–31273.

402. Kavallaris M, Kuo DYS, Burkhart CA, et al. Taxol-resistant ovarian tumors are associated with altered expression of specific beta-tubulin isotypes. J Clin Invest 1997;100:1282–1293.

403. Ranganathan S, Dexter DW, Benetatos CA, et al. Increase of beta(III)- and beta(IVa)- tubulin isotopes in human prostate carcinoma cells as a result of estramustine resistance. Cancer Res 1996;56:2584–2586.

404. Giannakakou P, Sackett DL, Kang YK, et al. Paclitaxel-resistant human ovarian cancer cells have mutant beta-tubulins that exhibit impaired paclitaxel-driven polymerization. J Biol Chem 1997;272:17118–17125.

405. Gonzalez-Garay ML, Chang L, Blade K, et al. A β-tubulin leucine cluster involved in microtubule assembly and paclitaxel resistance. J Biol Chem 1999;274:23875–23882.

406. Monzo M, Rosell R, Sánchez JJ, et al. Paclitaxel resistance in nonsmall cell lung cancer associated with beta tubulin gene mutations. J Clin Oncol 1999;17:1786–1793.

407. Kelley MJ, Li S, Harpole DH. Genetic analysis of the beta-tubulin gene, TUBB, in non-small cell lung cancer. J Natl Cancer Inst 2001;93:1886–1888.

408. Verrills NM, Po'uha ST, Liu ML, et al. Alterations in gamma-actin and tubulin-targeted drug resistance in childhood leukemia. J Natl Cancer Inst. 2006;98:1363–1374.

409. Dumontet C, Jaffrezou JP, Tsuchiya E, et al. Resistance to microtubule-targeted cytotoxins in a K562 leukemia cell variant associated with altered tubulin expression and polymerization. Bull Cancer 2004;91:E81–E112.

410. Blade K, Menick DR, Cabral F. Overexpression of class I, II, or IVb beta-tubulin isotypes in CHO cells is insufficient to confer resistance to paclitaxel. J Cell Sci 1999;112:2213–2221.

411. Hari M, Yang H, Zeng C, et al. Expression of class III beta-tubulin reduces microtubule assembly and confers resistance to paclitaxel. Cell Motil Cytoskeleton 2003;56:45–56.

412. Ranganathan S, Benetatos CA, Colarusso PJ, et al. Altered beta-tubulin isotype expression in paclitaxel-resistant human prostate carcinoma cells. Br J Cancer 1998;77:562–569.

413. Sève P, Dumontet C. Is class III beta-tubulin a predictive factor in patients receiving tubulin-binding agents? Lancet Oncol 2008;9:168–175.

414. Sève P, Reiman T, Lai R, et al. Class III beta-tubulin is a marker of paclitaxel resistance in carcinomas of unknown primary site. Cancer Chemother Pharmacol 2007;60:27–34.

415. Tommasi S, Mangia A, Lacalamita R, et al. Cytoskeleton and paclitaxel sensitivity in breast cancer: the role of beta-tubulins. Int J Cancer 2007;120:2078–2085.

416. Rosell R, Fossella F, Milas L. Molecular markers and targeted therapy with novel agents: prospects in the treatment of non-small cell lung cancer. Lung Cancer 2002;38(Suppl 4):43–49.

417. Kavallaris M, Burkhart CA, Horwitz SB. Antisense oligonucleotides to class III beta-tubulin sensitize drug resistant cells to taxol. Br J Cancer 1999;80:1020–1025.

418. Gooch JL, Van Den Berg CL, Yee D, et al. Insulin-like growth factor (IGF)-I rescues breast cancer cells from chemotherapy-induced cell death-proliferative and anti-apoptotic effects. Breast Cancer Res Treat 1999;56:1–10.

419. Chang MC, Chen CA, Hsieh CY, et al. Mesothelin inhibits paclitaxel-induced apoptosis through the PI3-kinase pathway. Biochem J 2009;424:449–448.

420. Kim SH, Juhnn YS, Song YS. Akt involvement in paclitaxel chemoresistance of human ovarian cancer cells. Ann NY Acad Sci 2007;1095:82–89.

421. McGrogan BT, Gilmartin B, Carney DN, et al. Taxanes, microtubules and chemoresistant breast cancer. Biochim Biophys Acta 2008;1785:96–132.

422. Ishibashi M, Nakayama K, Yeasmin S, et al. A BTB/POZ gene, NAC-1, a tumor recurrence-associated gene, as a potential target for Taxol resistance in ovarian cancer. Clin Cancer Res 2008;14:3149–3155.

423. Schmidt M, Lu Y, Liu B, et al. Differential modulation of paclitaxel-mediated apoptosis by p21^{Waf1} and p27^{Kip1}. Oncogene 2000;19:2423–2429.

424. Li W, Fan J, Banerjee D, et al. Overexpression of p21^{waf1} decreases G2-M arrest and apoptosis induced by paclitaxel in human sarcoma cells lacking both p53 and functional rb protein. Mol Pharmacol 1999;55:1088–1093.

425. Alli E, Yang JM, Ford JM, et al. Reversal of stathmin-mediated resistance to paclitaxel and vinblastine in human breast carcinoma cells. Mol Pharmacol 2007;71:1233–1240.

426. Yu D, Liu B, Jing T, et al. Overexpression of both p185^{c-erB2} and p170^{mdr-1} renders breast cancer cells highly resistant to Taxol. Oncogene 1998;16:2087–2094.

427. Yu D, Liu B, Tan M, et al. Overexpression of c-erbB-2/neu in breast cancer cells confers increased resistance to Taxol via mdr-1-independent mechanisms. Oncogene 1996;13:1359–1365.

428. Hayes DF, Thor AD, Dressler LG, et al. Cancer and Leukemia Group B (CALGB) Investigators. HER2 and response to paclitaxel in node-positive breast cancer. N Engl J Med 2007;357:1496–1506.

429. Konecny GE, Thomssen C, Luck HJ, et al. Her-2/neu gene amplification and response to paclitaxel in patients with metastatic breast cancer. J Natl Cancer Inst 2004;96:1141–1151.

430. Hamel E, Lin CM, Johns DG. Tubulin-dependent biochemical assay for the antineoplastic agent Taxol and applications to measurements of the drug in the serum. Cancer Treat Rep 1982;66:1381–1386.

431. Leu J-G, Chen B-X, Schiff PB, et al. Characterization of polyclonal and monoclonal anti-Taxol antibodies and measurement of Taxol in serum. Cancer Res 1993;53:1388–1391.

432. Mortier KA, Verstraete AG, Zhang GF, et al. Enhanced method performance due to a shorter chromatographic run-time in a liquid chromatography-tandem mass spectrometry assay for paclitaxel. J Chromatogr A 2004;1041:235–238.

433. Gustafson DL, Long ME, Zirrolli JA, et al. Analysis of docetaxel pharmacokinetics in humans with the inclusion of later sampling time-points afforded by the use of a sensitive tandem LCMS assay. Cancer Chemother Pharmacol 2003;52:159–166.

434. Zhang SQ, Chen GH. Determination of paclitaxel in human plasma by ultra-performance liquid chromatography-tandem mass spectrometry. J Chromatogr Sci 2008;46:220–224.

435. Malingre MM, Beijnen JH, Schellens JHM. Oral delivery of the taxanes. Invest New Drugs 2001;19:155–162.

436. Huizing MT, Keung AC, Rosing H, et al. Pharmacokinetics of paclitaxel and metabolites in a randomized comparative study in platinum-pretreated ovarian cancer patients. J Clin Oncol 1993;11:2127–2135.

437. Ohtsu T, Sasaki Y, Tamura T, et al. Clinical pharmacokinetics and pharmacodynamics of paclitaxel: a 3-hour infusion versus a 24-hour infusion. Clin Cancer Res 1995;1:599–606.

438. Gianni L, Kearns C, Gianni A, et al. Nonlinear pharmacokinetics and metabolism of paclitaxel and its pharmacokinetic/pharmacodynamic relationships in humans. J Clin Oncol 1995;13:180–190.

439. Sonnichsen D, Hurwitz C, Pratt C, et al. Saturable pharmacokinetics and paclitaxel pharmacodynamics in children with solid tumors. J Clin Oncol 1994;12:532–538.

440. Van Tellingen O, Huizing MT, Panday VR, et al. Cremophor EL causes (pseudo) nonlinear pharmacokinetics of paclitaxel in patients. Br J Cancer 1999;81:330–335.

441. Sparreboom A, van Zuylen L, Brouwer E, et al. Cremophor EL-mediated alterations of paclitaxel distribution in human blood: clinical pharmacokinetic implications. Cancer Res 1999;59:1454–1457.

442. Gelderblom H, Mross K, ten Tije AJ, et al. Comparative pharmacokinetics of unbound paclitaxel during 1- and 3-hour infusions. J Clin Oncol 2002;20:574–581.

443. Spartlin J, Sawyers, MB. Pharmacogenetics of paclitaxel metabolism. Crit Rev Oncol Hematol 2007:61:222–229.

444. Kumar GN, Walle UK, Bhalla KN, et al. Binding of taxol to human plasma, albumin, and alpha 1-acid glycoprotein. Res Commun Chem Pathol Pharmacol 1993;80:337–344.

445. Henningsson A, Sparreboom A, Sandstrom M, et al. Population pharmacokinetic modelling of unbound and total plasma concentrations of paclitaxel in cancer patients. Eur J Cancer 2003;39:1105–1114.

446. Lesser G, Grossman SA, Eller S, et al. The neural and extra-neural distribution of systemically administered [3H]paclitaxel in rats: a quantitative autoradiographic study. Cancer Chemother Pharmacol 1995;34:173–178.

447. Smorenburg CH, Sparreboom A, Bontenbal M, et al. Randomized crossover evaluation of body-surface area-based dosing versus flat-fixed dosing of paclitaxel. J Clin Oncol 2003;21:197–202.

448. Glantz MJ, Choy H, Kearns CM, et al. Paclitaxel disposition in plasma and central nervous systems of humans and rats with brain tumors. J Natl Cancer Inst 1995;87:1077–1081.

449. Monsarrat B, Alvinerie P, Dubois J, et al. Hepatic metabolism and biliary clearance of taxol in rats and humans. Monograph Natl Cancer Inst 1993;15:39–46.

450. Cresteil T, Monsarrat B, Alvinerie P, et al. Taxol metabolism by human liver microsomes: identification of cytochrome P450 isoenzymes involved in its biotransformation. Cancer Res 1994;54:386–392.

451. Nallani SC, Goodwin B, Maglich JM. Introduction of cytochrome P450 3A by paclitaxel in mice: pivotal role of the nuclear xenobiotic receptor, pregnane X receptor. Drug Metab Dispos 2003;31:681–684.

452. Harris JW, Rahman A, Kim B-R, et al. Metabolism of taxol by human hepatic microsomes and liver slices: participation of cytochrome P450 3A4 and an unknown P450 enzyme. Cancer Res 1994;15:4026–4035.

453. Kerns CM, Gianni L, Egorin M. Paclitaxel pharmacokinetics and pharmacodynamics. Semin Oncol 1995;22:16–23.

454. Monsarrat B, Chatelut E, Royer I, et al. Modification of paclitaxel metabolism in a cancer patient by induction of cytochrome P450 3A4. Drug Metab Dispos 1998;26:229–233.

455. Sparreboom A, Huizing MT, Boesen JJ, et al. Isolation, purification, and biological activity of mono- and dihydroxylated paclitaxel metabolites from human feces. Cancer Chemother Pharmacol 1995;36:299–304.

456. Mielke S. Individualized pharmacotherapy with paclitaxel. Curr Opin Oncol 2007;19:586–589.

457. Steed H, Sawyer MB. Pharmacology, pharmacokinetics, and phamracogenomics of paclitaxel. Pharmacogenomics 2007;8:803–815.

458. Van Schaik RH. CYP450 pharmaocogenetics for personalizing cancer therapy. Drug Resist Updat 2008;11:77–98.

459. Rahman A, Korzekwa KR, Grogan J, et al. Selective biotransformation of taxol to 6 alpha-hydroxytaxol by human cytochrome P450 2C8. Cancer Res 1994;54:5543–5546.

460. Dai D, Zeldin DC, Blaisdell JA, et al. Polymorphisms in human CYP2C8 decrease metabolism of the anticancer drug paclitaxel and arachidonic acid. Pharmacogenetics 2001;11:597–607.

461. Henningsson A, Marsh S, Loos WJ, et al. Association of CYP2C8, CYP3A4, CYP3A5, and ABCB1 polymorphisms with the pharmacokinetics of paclitaxel. Clin Cancer Res 2005;11:8097–8104.

462. Daily EB, Aquilante CL. Cytochrome P450 2C8 pharmacogenetics: a review of clinical studies. Pharmacogenomics 2009;10:1489–1510.

463. Green H. Pharmacogenomics of importance for paclitaxel chemotherapy. Pharmacogenomics 2008;9:671–674.

464. Gianni L, Munzone E, Capri G, et al. Paclitaxel by 3-hour infusion in combination with bolus doxorubicin in women with untreated metastatic breast cancer: high antitumor efficacy and cardiac effects in a dose-finding and sequence- finding study. J Clin Oncol 1995;13:2688–2699.

465. Rowinsky EK, Jiroutek M, Bonomi P, et al. Paclitaxel steady-state plasma concentration as a determinant of disease outcome and toxicity in lung cancer patients treated with paclitaxel and cisplatin. Clin Cancer Res 1999;5:767–774.

466. Clarke SJ, Rivory LP. Clinical pharmacokinetics of docetaxel. Clin Pharmacokinet 1999;36:99–114.

467. Bruno R, Hille D, Riva A, et al. Population pharmacokinetic/pharmacodynamics of docetaxel in phase II studies in patients with cancer. J Clin Oncol 1998;16:186–196.

468. Bruno R, Vivier N, Veyrat-Follet C, et al. Population pharmacokinetics and pharmacokinetic-pharmadynamic relationships for docetaxel. Invest New Drugs 2001;19:163–169.

469. McLeod HL, Kearns CM, Kuhn JG, et al. Evaluation of the linearity of docetaxel pharmacokinetics. Cancer Chemother Pharmacol 1998;42:155–159.

470. Marland M, Gaillard C, Sanderink G, et al. Kinetics, distribution, metabolism and excretion of radiolabeled Taxotere (14C-RPR 56976) in mice and dogs. Proc Am Assoc Cancer Res 1993;34:393.

471. Sparreboom A, Van Tellingen O, Scherrenburg EJ, et al. Isolation, purification and biological activity of major docetaxel metabolites from human feces. Drug Metab Dispos 1996;24:655–658.

472. Baker SD, Zhao M, Lee CK, et al. Comparative pharmacokinetics of weekly and every-three-weeks docetaxel. Clin Cancer Res 2004;10:1976–1983.

473. Ten Tije AJ, Loos WJ, Zhao M, et al. Limited cerebrospinal fluid penetration of docetaxel. Anticancer Drugs 2004;15:715–718.

474. Royer I, Monsarrat B, Sonnier M, et al. Metabolism of docetaxel by human cytochromes P450: interactions with paclitaxel and other antineoplastic agents. Cancer Res 1996;56:58–65.

475. Shou M, Martinet M, Korzekwa KR, et al. Role of cytochrome P450 3A4 and 3A5 in the metabolism of taxotere and its derivatives: enzyme specificity, interindividual distribution and metabolic contribution in human liver. Pharmacogenetics 1998;8:8391–8401.

476. Hirth J, Watkins PB, Strawderman M, et al. The effect of an individual's cytochrome CYP3A4 activities on docetaxel clearance. Clin Cancer Res 2000;6:1255–1258.

477. Tran A, Jullien V, Alexandre J, et al. Pharmacokinetics and toxicity of docetaxel: role of CYP3A, MDR1, and GST polymorphisms. Clin Pharmacol Ther 2006;79:570–580.

478. Bosch TM, Huitema AD, Doodeman VD, et al. Pharmacogenetic screening of CYP3A and ABCB1 in relation to population pharmacokinetics of docetaxel. Clin Cancer Res 2006;12:5786–5793.

479. Sissung TM, Danesi R, Price DK, et al. Association of the CYP1B1*3 allele with survival in patients with prostate cancer receiving docetaxel. Mol Cancer Ther 2008;7:19–26.

480. Tsai SM, Lin CY, Wu SH, et al. Side effects after docetaxel treatment in Taiwanese breast cancer patients with CYP3A4, CYP3A5, and ABCB1 gene polymorphisms. Clin Chim Acta 2009;404:160–165.

481. Johnatty SE, Beesley J, Paul J, et al. ABCB1 (MDR 1) polymorphisms and progression-free survival among women with ovarian cancer following paclitaxel/carboplatin chemotherapy. Clin Cancer Res 2008;14:5594–5601.

482. Sissung TM, Baum CE, Deeken J, et al. ABCB1 genetic variation influences the toxicity and clinical outcome of patients with androgen-independent prostate cancer treated with docetaxel. Clin Cancer Res 2008;14:4543–4549.

483. Goh BC, Lee SC, Wang LZ, et al. Explaining interindividual variability of docetaxel pharmacokinetics and pharmacodynamics in Asians through phenotyping and genotyping strategies. J Clin Oncol 2002;20:3683–3690.

484. Ng SS, Sparreboom A, Shaked Y, et al. Influence of formulation vehicle on metronomic taxane chemotherapy: albumin-bound versus cremophor EL-based paclitaxel. Clin Cancer Res 2006;12(14 Pt 1):4331–4338.

485. Sparreboom A, Scripture CD, Trieu V, et al. Comparative preclinical and clinical pharmacokinetics of a cremophor-free, nanoparticle albumin-bound paclitaxel (ABI-007) and paclitaxel formulated in Cremophor (Taxol). Clin Cancer Res 2005;11:4136–4143.

486. Gardner ER, Dahut WL, Scripture CD, et al. Randomized crossover pharmacokinetic study of solvent-based paclitaxel and nab-paclitaxel. Clin Cancer Res 2008;14:4200–4205.

487. Vigano L, Locatelli A, Grasselli G, et al. Drug interactions of paclitaxel and docetaxel and their relevance for the design of combination therapy. Invest New Drugs 2001;19:179–196.

488. Rowinsky EK, Gilbert M, McGuire WP, et al. Sequences of taxol and cisplatin: a phase I and pharmacologic study. J Clin Oncol 1991;9:1692–1703.

489. Rowinsky EK, Citardi M, Noe DA, et al. Sequence-dependent cytotoxicity between cisplatin and the antimicrotubule agents taxol and vincristine. J Cancer Res Clin Oncol 1993;119:727–733.

490. Belani CP, Kearns CM, Zuhowski EG, et al. Phase I trial, including pharmacokinetic and pharmacodynamic correlations, of combination paclitaxel and carboplatin in patients with metastatic non-small-cell lung cancer. J Clin Oncol 1999;17:676–684.

491. Kearns CM, Egorin MJ. Considerations regarding the less-than-expected thrombocytopenia encountered with combination paclitaxel/carboplatin chemotherapy. Semin Oncol 1997;24 (Suppl 2):91–96.

492. Daga H, Isobe T, Miyazaki M, et al. Investigating the relationship between serum thrombopoietin kinetics and the platelet-sparing effect: a clinical pharmacological evaluation of combined paclitaxel and carboplatin in patients with non-small cell lung cancer. Oncol Rep 2004;11:2225–2231.

493. Holmes FA, Madden T, Newman RA, et al. Sequence-dependent alteration of doxorubicin pharmacokinetics by paclitaxel in a phase I study of paclitaxel and doxorubicin in patients with metastatic breast cancer. J Clin Oncol 1996;14:2713–2721.

494. Gianni L, Vigano L, Locatelli A, et al. Human pharmacokinetic characterization and in vitro study of the interactions between doxorubicin and paclitaxel in patients with breast cancer. J Clin Oncol 1997;15:1906–1915.

495. Kennedy MJ, Zahurak ML, Donehower RC, et al. Phase I and pharmacologic study of sequences of paclitaxel and cyclophosphamide supported by granulocyte colony-stimulating factor in women with previously treated metastatic breast cancer. J Clin Oncol 1995;14:783–791.

496. Shou M, Martinet M, Korzekwa KR, et al. Role of cytochrome P450 3A4 and 3A5 in the metabolism of Taxotere and its derivatives: enzyme specificity, interindividual distribution and metabolic contribution in human liver. Pharmacogenetics 1998;8:8391–8401.

497. Perotti A, Cresta S, Grasselli G. Cardiotoxic effects of anthracycline-taxane combinations. Expert Opin Drug Saf 2003;2:59–71.

498. Gennari A, Salvadori B, Donati S, et al. Cardiotoxicity of epirubicin/paclitaxel-containing regimens: role of cardiac risk factors. J Clin Oncol 1999;11:3596–3602.

499. Sawada N, Ishikawa T, Fukase Y, et al. Induction of thymidine phosphorylase activity and enhancement of capecitabine efficacy by taxol/taxotere in human cancer xenografts. Clin Cancer Res 1998;4:1013–1019.

500. Prados MD, Schold SC, Spence AM, et al. Phase II study of paclitaxel in patients with recurrent malignant glioma. J Clin Oncol 1996;14:2316–2321.

501. Desai PB, Duan JZ, Zhu YW, et al. Human liver microsomal metabolism of paclitaxel and drug interactions. Eur J Drug Metab Pharmacokinet 1998;23:417–424.

502. Bun SS, Ciccolini J, Bun H. Drug interactions of paclitaxel metabolism in human liver microsomes. J Chemother 2003;15:266–274.

503. Nallani SC, Goodwin B, Buckley AR, et al. Differences in the induction of cytochrome P450 3A4 by taxane anticancer drugs, docetaxel, and paclitaxel, assessed by employing primary human hepatocytes. Cancer Chemother Pharmacol 2004;54:219–229.

504. Van Veldhuizen PJ, Reed G, et al. Docetaxel and ketoconazole in advanced hormone-refractory prostate carcinoma: a phase I and pharmacokinetic study. Cancer 2003;98:1855–1862.

505. Slichenmyer W, McGuire W, Donehower R, et al. Pretreatment H2 receptor antagonists that differ in P450 modulation activity: comparative effects on paclitaxel clearance rates. Cancer Chemother Pharmacol 1995;36:227–232.

506. Jamis-Dow CA, Klecker RW, Katki AG, et al. Metabolism of Taxol by human and rat liver in vitro. A screen for drug interactions and interspecies differences. Cancer Chemother Pharmacol 1995;36:107–114.

507. Klecker RW, Jamis-Dow CA, Egorin MJ, et al. Effect of cimetidine, probenecid, and ketoconazole on the distribution, biliary secretion, and metabolism of ^{3}H-Taxol in the Sprague-Dawley rat. Drug Metab Dispos Biol Fate 1994;22:254–258.

508. Thompson ME, Highley MS. Interaction between paclitaxel and warfarin. Ann Oncol 2003;14:500.

509. Jerian S, Keegan P. Cardiotoxicity associated with paclitaxel/trastuzumab combination chemotherapy. J Clin Oncol 1999;17:1647–1648.

510. Rowinsky EK. The taxanes: dosing and scheduling considerations. Oncology 1997;11(3 Suppl 2):7–19.

511. Seidman AD, Hochhauser D, Gollub M, et al. Ninety-six-hour paclitaxel infusion after progression during short taxane exposure: a phase II pharmacokinetic and pharmacodynamic study in metastatic breast cancer. J Clin Oncol 1996;14:1877–1884.

512. Markman M, Rose PG, Jones E, et al. Ninety-six-hour infusional paclitaxel as salvage therapy of ovarian cancer patients previously failing treatment with 3-hour or 24-hour paclitaxel infusion. J Clin Oncol 1998;16:1849–1851.

513. Spriggs DR, Brady MF, Vaccarello L, et al. Phase III randomized trial of intravenous cisplatin plus a 24- or 96-hour infusion of paclitaxel in epithelial ovarian cancer: a Gynecologic Oncology Group Study. J Clin Oncol 2007;25:4466–4471.

514. Holmes FA, Valero V, Buzdar AU, et al. Final results: randomized phase III trial of paclitaxel by 3-hr versus 96-hr infusion in patients with metastatic breast cancer. Proc Am Soc Clin Oncol 1999;18:110A.

515. Wilson WH, Berg S, Bryant G, et al. Paclitaxel in doxorubicin-refractory or mitoxantrone-refractory breast cancer: a phase I/II trial of 96 hour infusion. J Clin Oncol 1994;12:1621–1629.

516. Greco FA, Thomas M, Hainsworth JD. One-hour paclitaxel infusions: review of the safety and efficacy. Cancer Sci Am 1999;5:179–191.

517. Hainsworth JD, Burris HA, Greco FA. Weekly administration of docetaxel (Taxotere): summary of clinical data. Semin Oncol 1999;26(Suppl 10):19–24.

518. Green MC, Buzdar AU, Smith T, et al. Weekly paclitaxel improves pathologic complete remission in operable breast cancer when compared with paclitaxel once every 3 weeks. J Clin Oncol 2005;23:5983–5992.

519. Smith RE, Brown AM, Mamounas EP, et al. Randomized trial of 3-hour versus 24-hour infusion of high-dose paclitaxel in patients with metastatic or locally advanced breast cancer: National Surgical Adjuvant Breast and Bowel Project Protocol B-26. J Clin Oncol 1999;17:3403–3411.

520. Winer EP, Berry DA, Woolf S, et al. Failure of higher-dose paclitaxel to improve outcome in patients with metastatic breast cancer: cancer and leukemia group B trial 9342. J Clin Oncol 2004;22:2061–2068.

521. Francis P, Rowinsky E, Schneider J, et al. Phase I feasibility and pharmacologic study of intraperitoneal paclitaxel: a Gynecologic Oncology Group study. J Clin Oncol 1995;13:2961–2967.

522. Armstrong DK, Bundy B, Wenzel L, et al. Intraperitoneal cisplatin and paclitaxel in ovarian cancer. N Engl J Med 2006;354:34–43.

523. Bookman MA, Kloth DD, Kover PE, et al. Short-course intravenous prophylaxis for paclitaxel-related hypersensitivity reactions. Ann Oncol 1997;8:611–614.

524. Kloover JS, den Bakker MA, Gelderblom H, et al. Fatal outcome of a hypersensitivity reaction to paclitaxel: a critical review of premedication regimens. Br J Cancer 2004;90:304–305.

525. Zidan J, Hussein O, Abzah A, et al. Oral premedication for the prevention of hypersensitivity reactions to paclitaxel. Med Oncol 2008;25:274–278.

526. Baker SD, Ravdin P, Aylesworth C, et al. A phase I and pharmacokinetic study of docetaxel in cancer patients with liver dysfunction due to malignancies. Proc Am Soc Clin Oncol 1998;17:192.

527. Venook AP, Egorin MJ, Rosner GL, et al. Phase I and pharmacokinetic trial of paclitaxel in patients with hepatic dysfunction. Cancer and leukemia group B 9264. J Clin Oncol 1998;16:1811–1819.

528. Joerger M, Huitema AD, Huizing MT, et al. Safety and pharmacology of paclitaxel in patients with impaired liver function: a population pharmacokinetic-pharmacodynamic study. Br J Clin Pharmacol 2007;64:622–633.

529. Woo MH, Gregornik D, Shearer PD, et al. Pharmacokinetics of paclitaxel in an anephric patient. Cancer Chemother Pharmacol 1999;43:92–96.

530. Salminen E, Bergman M, Huhtala S, et al. Docetaxel: standard recommended dose of 100 mg/m^2 is effective but not feasible for some metastatic breast cancer patients heavily pretreated with chemotherapy—A phase II single-center study. J Clin Oncol 1999;17:1127.

531. Piccart MJ, Klijn J, Paridaens R, et al. Corticosteroids significantly delay the onset of docetaxel-induced fluid retention: final results of a randomized study of the European Organization for Research and Treatment of Cancer, Investigational Drug Branch for Breast Cancer. J Clin Oncol 1997;15:3149–3155.

532. Markman M. Managing taxane toxicities. Support Care Cancer 2003;11:144–147.

533. Rowinsky EK, Eisenhauer EA, Chaudhry V, et al. Clinical toxicities encountered with taxol. Semin Oncol 1993;20(Suppl 3):1–15.

534. Eisenhauer E, ten Bokkel Huinink W, Swenerton KD, et al. European-Canadian randomized trial of taxol in relapsed ovarian cancer: high vs low dose and long vs. short infusion. J Clin Oncol 1994;12:2654–2666.

535. Weiss R, Donehower RC, Wiernik PH, et al. Hypersensitivity reactions from taxol. J Clin Oncol 1990;8:1263–1268.

536. Peereboom D, Donehower RC, Eisenhauer EA, et al. Successful retreatment with taxol after major hypersensitivity reactions. J Clin Oncol 1993;11:885–890.

537. Price KS, Castells MC. Taxol reactions. Allergy Asthma Proc 2002;23:205–208.

538. Olson JK, Sood AK, Sorosky JJ, et al. Taxol hypersensitivity: rapid pretreatment is safe and cost effective. Gynecol Oncol 1996;68:25–28.

539. Szebeni J, Muggia FM, Alving CR. Complement activation by Cremophor EL as a possible contributor to hypersensitivity to paclitaxel: an in vitro study. J Natl Cancer Inst 1998;90:300–306.

540. Chaudhry V, Rowinsky EK, Sartorious SE, et al. Peripheral neuropathy from taxol and cisplatin combination chemotherapy: clinical and electrophysiological studies. Ann Neurol 1994;35:304–311.

541. Rowinsky EK, Chaudhry V, Cornblath DR, et al. The neurotoxicity of taxol. Monogr Natl Cancer Inst 1993;15:107–115.

542. Gelmon K, Eisenhauer E, Bryce C, et al. Randomized phase II study of high-dose paclitaxel with or without amifostine in patients with metastatic breast cancer. J Clin Oncol 1999;17:3038–3047.

543. Loven D, Levavi H, Sabach G, et al. Long-term glutamate supplementation failed to protect against peripheral neurotoxicity of paclitaxel. Eur J Cancer Care (Engl) 2009;18:78–83.

544. Vahdat L, Papadopoulos K, Lange D, et al. Reduction of paclitaxel-induced periperial neuropathy with glutamine. Clin Cancer Res 2004;7:1192–1197.

545. Garrison JA, McCune JS, Livingston RB, et al. Myalgias and arthralgias associated with paclitaxel. Oncology 2003;17:271–277.

546. Capri G, Munzone E, Tarenzi E, et al. Optic nerve disturbances: a new form of paclitaxel neurotoxicity. J Natl Cancer Inst 1994;86:1099–1101.

547. Hofstra LS, de Vries EG, Willemse PH. Ophthalmic toxicity following paclitaxel infusion. Ann Oncol 1997;8:1053.

548. Nieto Y, Cagnoni PJ, Bearman SI, et al. Acute encephalopathy: a new toxicity associated with high-dose paclitaxel. Clin Cancer Res 1999;5:501–506.

549. Ziske CG, Schottker B, Gorschluter M, et al. Acute transient encephalopathy after paclitaxel infusion: report of three cases. Ann Oncol 2002;13:629–631.

550. Markman M, Kennedy A, Webser K, et al. Paclitaxel administration to gynecologic cancer patients with major cardiac risk factors. J Clin Oncol 1998;16:3483–3485.

551. Rowinsky EK, McGuire WP, Guarnieri T, et al. Cardiac disturbances during the administration of taxol. J Clin Oncol 1991;9:170412.

552. Arbuck SG, Strauss H, Rowinsky EK, et al. A reassessment of the cardiac toxicity associated with taxol. Monogr Natl Cancer Inst 1993;15:117–130.

553. Della Torre P, Imondi AR, Bernardi C, et al. Cardioprotection by dexrazoxane in rats treated with doxorubicin and paclitaxel. Cancer Chemother Pharmacol 1999;44:138–142.

554. Sparano JA, Speyer J, Gradishar WJ, et al. Phase I trial of escalating doses of paclitaxel plus doxorubicin and dexrazoxane in patients with advanced breast cancer. J Clin Oncol 1999;17:880–886.

555. Rowinsky EK, Burke PJ, Karp JE, et al. Phase I and pharmacodynamic study of taxol in refractory adult acute leukemia. Cancer Res 1989;49:4640–4647.

556. Pestalozzi BC, Sotos GA, Choyke PL, et al. Typhlitis resulting from treatment with taxol and doxorubicin in patients with metastatic breast cancer. Cancer 1993;71:1797–1800.

557. Seewaldt VL, Cain JM, Goff BA, et al. A retrospective review of paclitaxel-associated gastrointestinal necrosis in patients with epithelial ovarian cancer. Gynecol Oncol 1997;67:137–140.

558. Feenstra J, Vermeer RJ, Stricker BH. Fatal hepatic coma attributed to paclitaxel. J Natl Cancer Inst 1997;16:582–584.

559. Ramanathan RK, Reddy VV, Holbert JM, et al. Pulmonary infiltrates following administration of paclitaxel. Chest 1996;110:289–292.

560. Ayoub JP, North L, Greer J, et al. Pulmonary changes in patients with lymphoma who receive paclitaxel. J Clin Oncol 1997;15:2476.

561. Minisini AM, Tosti A, Soberero AF, et al. Taxane-induced nail changes: incidence, clinical presentation and outcome. Annal Oncol 2003;14:333–337.

562. Schrijvers D, Wanders J, Dirix L, et al. Coping with toxicities of docetaxel (Taxotere). Ann Oncol 1993;4:610–611.

563. Bernstein BJ. Docetaxel as an alternative to paclitaxel after acute hypersensitivity reactions. Ann Pharmacother 2000;34:1332–1335.

564. Semb KA, Aamdal S, Oian P. Capillary protein leak syndrome appears to explain fluid retention in cancer patients who receive docetaxel treatment. J Clin Oncol 1998;16:3426–3432.

565. Zimmerman GC, Keeling JH, Barris HA, et al. Acute cutaneous reactions to docetaxel, a new chemotherapeutic agent. Arch Dermatol 1995;131:202–206.

566. Vukeljia SJ, Baker WJ, Burris HA III, et al. Pyridoxine therapy for palmar-plantar erythrodysesthesia associated with Taxotere. J Natl Cancer Inst 1993;85:1432–1433.

567. Zimmerman GC, Keeling JH, Lowry M, et al. Prevention of docetaxel-induced erythrodysesthesia with local hypothermia. J Natl Cancer Inst 1994;86:557–558.

568. Wasner G, Hilpert F, Schattschneider J. Docetaxel-induced nail changes-a neurogenic mechanism: a case report. J Neurooncol 2002;58:167–174.

569. Hilkens PH, Verweij J, Stoter G, et al. Peripheral neurotoxicity induced by docetaxel. Neurology 1996;46:104–108.

570. Vasey PA. Survival and long-term toxicity results of the SCOTROC study: docetaxel-carboplatin (DC) vs. paclitaxel-carboplatin (PC) in epithelial ovarian cancer. Proc Am Soc Clin Oncol 1992;21:202A.

571. Roglio I, Bianchi R, Camozzi F, et al. Docetaxel-induced peripheral neuropathy: protective effects of dihydroprogesterone and progesterone in an experimental model. J Peripher Nerv Syst 2009;14:36–44.

572. Esmaeli B, Hortobagyi G, Esteva F. Canalicular stenosis secondary to weekly docetaxel: a potentially preventable side effect. Ann Oncol 2002;13:1188–1191.

573. Stachel SJ, Biswas K, Danishefsky SJ. The epothilones, eleutherobins, and related types of molecules. Curr Pharm Des 2001;7:1277–1290.

574. Kingston DG. Tubulin-interactive natural products as anticancer agents. J Nat Prod 2009;72:507–515.

575. Risinger AL, Giles FJ, Mooberry SL. Microtubule dynamics as a target in oncology. Cancer Treat Rev 2009;35:255–261.

576. Honore S, Kamath K, Braguer D, et al. Synergistic suppression of microtubule dynamics by discodermolide and paclitaxel in non-small cell lung carcinoma cells. Cancer Res 2004;64:4957–4964.

577. Mita AA, Lockhart C, Chen T-L, et al. A phase I pharmacokinetic (PK) trial of XAA296A (Discodermolide) administered every 3 wks to adult patients with advanced solid malignancies [abstract 205]. Proc Am Soc Clin Oncol 2004;23:133.

578. Buzdar AU. Clinical experience with epothilones in patients with breast cancer. Clin Breast Cancer 2008;8(Suppl 2):S71–S78.

579. Thomas ES, Gomez HL, Li RK, et al. Ixabepilone plus capecitabine for metastatic breast cancer progressing after anthracycline and taxane treatment. J Clin Oncol 2007;25:5210–5217.

580. Lee JJ, Kelly WK. Epothilones: tubulin polymerization as a novel target for prostate cancer therapy. Nat Clin Pract Oncol 2009;6:85–92.

581. Larkin JM, Kaye SB. Potential clinical applications of epothilones: a review of phase II studies. Ann Oncol 2007;18(Suppl 5):28–34.

582. Lee JJ, Swain SM. The epothilones: translating from the laboratory to the clinic. Clin Cancer Res 2008;14:1618–1624.

583. Bollag DM, McQueney PA, Zhu J, et al. Epothilones, a new class of microtubule-stabilizing agents with a Taxol-like mechanism of action. Cancer Res 1995;55:2325–2333.

584. Goodin S, Kane MP, Rubin EH. Epothilones: mechanism of action and biologic activity. J Clin Oncol 2004;22:2015–2025.

585. Bode CJ, Gupta ML Jr, Reiff EA, et al. Epothilone and paclitaxel: unexpected differences in promoting the assembly and stabilization of yeast microtubules. Biochemistry 2002;41:3870–3874.

586. Giannakakou P, Gussio R, Nogales E, et al. A common pharmacophore for epothilone and taxanes: molecular basis for drug resistance conferred by tubulin mutations in human cancer cells. Proc Natl Acad Sci USA 2000;97:2904–2909.

587. Dumontet C, Jordan MA, Lee FF. Ixabepilone: targeting betaIII-tubulin expression in taxane-resistant malignancies. Mol Cancer Ther 2009;8:17–25.

588. Dabydeen DA, Florence GJ, Paterson I, et al. A quantitative evaluation of the effects of inhibitors of tubulin assembly on polymerization induced by discodermolide, epothilone B, and paclitaxel. Cancer Chemother Pharmacol 2004;53:397–403.

589. Kowalski RJ, Giannakakou P, Hamel E. Activities of the microtubule-stabilizing agents epothilones A and B with purified tubulin and in cells resistant to paclitaxel (Taxol). J Biol Chem 1997;272:2534–2541.

590. Chen JG, Horwitz SB. Differential mitotic responses to microtubule-stabilizing and -destabilizing drugs. Cancer Res 2002;62:1935–1938.

591. Lee FY, Borzilleri R, Fairchild CR, et al. BMS-247550: a novel epothilone analog with a mode of action similar to paclitaxel but possessing superior antitumor efficacy. Clin Cancer Res 2001;7:1429–1437.

592. Nettles JH, Li H, Cornett B, et al. The binding mode of epothilone A on alpha,beta-tubulin by electron crystallography. Science 2004;305:866–869.

593. Kamath K, Jordan MA. Suppression of microtubule dynamics by epothilone B is associated with mitotic arrest. Cancer Res 2003;63:6026–6031.

594. Ioffe ML, White E, Nelson DA, et al. Epothilone induced cytotoxicity is dependent on p53 status in prostate cells. Prostate 2004;;61:243–247.

595. Sakaushi S, Nishida K, Fukada T, et al. Differential responses of mitotic spindle pole formation to microtubule-stabilizing agents epothilones A and B at low concentrations. Cell Cycle 2008;7:477–483.

596. Wang Y, O'Brate A, Zhou W, Giannakakou P. Resistance to microtubule-stabilizing drugs involves two events: beta-tubulin mutation in one allele followed by loss of the second allele. Cell Cycle 2005;4:1847–1853.

597. Mozzetti S, Iantomasi R, De Maria I, et al. Molecular mechanisms of patupilone resistance. Cancer Res 2008;68:10197–10204.

598. Hopper-Borge E, Xu X, Shen T, et al. Human multidrug resistance protein 7 (ABCC10) is a resistance factor for nucleoside analogues and epothilone B. Cancer Res 2009;69:178–184.

599. Lee FY, Smykla R, Johnston K, et al. Preclinical efficacy spectrum and pharmacokinetics of ixabepilone. Cancer Chemother Pharmacol 2009;63: 201–212.

600. Goel S, Goldberg GL, Kuo DY, et al. Novel neurosensory testing in cancer patients treated with the epothilone B analog, ixabepilone. Ann Oncol 2008;19:2048–2052.

601. Lee JJ, Low JA, Croarkin E, et al. Changes in neurologic function tests may predict neurotoxicity caused by ixabepilone. J Clin Oncol 2006;24: 2084–2091.

602. Alimonti A, Nardoni C, Papaldo P, et al. Nail disorders in a woman treated with ixabepilone for metastatic breast cancer. Anticancer Res 2005;25:3531–3532.

603. Poncet J. The dolastatins, a family of promising antineoplastic agents. Curr Pharm Des 1999;5:139–162.

604. Ray A, Okouneva T, Manna T, et al. Mechanism of action of the microtubule-targeted antimitotic depsipeptide tasidotin (formerly ILX651) and its major metabolite tasidotin C-carboxylate. Cancer Res 2007;67: 3767–3776.

605. Watanabe J, Natsume T, Kobayashi M. Comparison of the antivascular and cytotoxic activities of TZT-1027 (Soblidotin) with those of other anticancer agents. Anticancer Drugs 2007;18:905–911.

606. Shnyder SD, Cooper PA, Millington NJ, et al. Auristatin PYE, a novel synthetic derivative of dolastatin 10, is highly effective in human colon tumour models. Int J Oncol 2007;31:353–360.

607. Jimeno A. Eribulin: rediscovering tubulin as an anticancer target. Clin Cancer Res 2009;15:3903–3905.

608. Jordan MA, Kamath K, Manna T, et al. The primary antimitotic mechanism of action of the synthetic halichondrin E7389 is suppression of microtubule growth. Mol Cancer Ther 2005;4:1086–1095.

609. Okouneva T, Azarenko O, Wilson L, et al. Inhibition of centromere dynamics by eribulin (E7389) during mitotic metaphase. Mol Cancer Ther 2008;7:2003–2011.

610. Towle MJ, Salvato KA, Budrow J, et al. In vitro and in vivo anticancer activities of synthetic macrocyclic ketone analogues of halichondrin B. Cancer Res 2001;61:1013–1021.

611. Loganzo F, Discafani CM, Annable T, et al. HTI-286, a synthetic analogue of the tripeptide hemiasterlin, is a potent antimicrotubule agent that circumvents P-glycoproteinmediated resistance in vitro and in vivo. Cancer Res 2003;63:1838–1845.

612. Loganzo F, Hari M, Annable T, et al. Cells resistant to HTI-286 do not overexpress P-glycoprotein but have reduced drug accumulation and a point mutation in alpha tubulin. Mol Cancer Ther 2004;3:1319–1327.

613. Poruchynsky MS, Kim JH, Nogales E, et al. Tumor cells resistant to a microtubule depolymerizing hemiasterlin analogue, HTI-286, have mutations in alpha- or beta tubulin and increased microtubule stability. Biochemistry 2004;43:13944–13954.

614. Tozer GM, Kanthou C, Baguley BC. Disrupting tumour blood vessels. Nat Rev Cancer 2005;5:423–435.

615. Sarli V, Giannis A. Targeting the kinesin spindle protein: basic principles and clinical implications. Clin Cancer Res 2008;14:7583–7587.

616. Wood KW, Cornwell WD, Jackson JR. Past and future of the mitotic spindle as an oncology target. Curr Opin Pharmacol 2001;4:370–377.

617. Goldstein LS, Philp AV. The road less traveled: emerging principles of kinesin motor utilization. Annu Rev Cell Dev Biol 1999;15:141–183.

618. Sakowicz R, Finer JT, Beraud C, et al. Antitumor activity of a kinesin inhibitor. Cancer Res 2004;64:3276–3280.

619. Wood KW, Chua P, Sutton D, Jackson JR. Centromere-associated protein E: a motor that puts the brakes on the mitotic checkpoint. Clin Cancer Res 2008;14:7588–7592.

620. Kim Y, Heuser JE, Waterman CM, Cleveland DW. CENP-E combines a slow, processive motor and a flexible coiled coil to produce an essential motile kinetochore tether. J Cell Biol 2008;181:411–419.

621. Lapenna S, Giordano A. Cell cycle kinases as therapeutic targets for cancer. Nat Rev Drug Discov 2009;8:547–566.

622. Warner SL, Stephens BJ, Von Hoff DD. Tubulin-associated proteins: Aurora and Polo-like kinases as therapeutic targets in cancer. Curr Oncol Rep. 2008;10:122–129.

623. Gautschi O, Heighway J, Mack PC, et al. Aurora kinases as anticancer drug targets. Clin Cancer Res 2008;14:1639–1648.

624. Tew KD. The mechanism of action of estramustine. Semin Oncol 1983;10:21–27.

625. Benson R, Hartley-Asp B. Mechanisms of action and clinical uses of estramustine. Cancer Invest 1990;8:375–380.

626. Tew KD, Glusker JP, Hartley-Asp B, et al. Preclinical and clinical perspectives on the use of estramustine as an antimitotic drug. Pharmacol Ther 1992;56:323–339.

627. Fex H, Hogberg B, Konyves I. Estramustine phosphate historical overview. Urology 1984;23:4–5.

628. Forsberg JG, Hoisaeter PA. Effects of hormone-cytostatic complexes on the rat ventral prostate in vivo and in vitro. Vitam Horm 1975;33:137–154.

629. Lindberg B. Treatment of rapidly progressing prostatic carcinoma with estracyt. J Urol 1972;108:303–306.

630. Machiels JP, Mazzeo F, Clausse M, et al. Prospective randomized study comparing docetaxel, estramustine, and prednisone with docetaxel and prednisone in metastatic hormone-refractory prostate cancer. J Clin Oncol 2008;26:5261–5268.

631. Savarese DM, Halabi S, Hars V, et al. Phase II study of docetaxel, estramustine and low-dose hydrocortisone in men with hormone-refractory prostate cancer: a final report of CALGB 9780. J Clin Oncol 2001;19:2509–2516.

632. Hudes G, Haas N, Yeslow G, et al. Phase I clinical and pharmacologic trial of intravenous estramustine phosphate. J Clin Oncol 2002;20:1115–1127.

633. Basch EM, Somerfield MR, Beer TM, et al. American Society of Clinical Oncology. American Society of Clinical Oncology endorsement of the Cancer Care Ontario Practice Guideline on nonhormonal therapy for men with metastatic hormone-refractory (castration-resistant) prostate cancer. J Clin Oncol 2007;25:5313–5318.

634. Fizazi K, Le Maitre A, Hudes G, et al. Meta-analysis of Estramustine in Prostate Cancer (MECaP) Trialists' Collaborative Group. Addition of estramustine to chemotherapy and survival of patients with castration-refractory prostate cancer: a meta-analysis of individual patient data.: Lancet Oncol 2007;8:994–1000.

635. Kanje M, Deinum J, Wallin M, et al. Effect of estramustine phosphate on the assembly of isolated bovine brain microtubules and fast axonal transport in the frog sciatic nerve. Cancer Res 1985;45:2234–2239.

636. Hartley-Asp B. Estramustine-induced mitotic arrest in two human prostatic carcinoma cell lines DU 145 and PC-3. Prostate 1984;5:93–100.

637. Stearns ME, Tew KD. Antimicrotubule effects of estramustine, an antiprostatic tumor drug. Cancer Res 1985;45:3891–3897.

638. Stearns ME, Wang M, Tew KD, et al. Estramustine binds a MAP-1-like protein to inhibit microtubule assembly in vitro and disrupt microtubule organization in DU 145 cells. J Cell Biol 1998;107:2647–2656.

639. Dahllof B, Billstrom A, Cabral F, et al. Estramustine depolymerizes microtubules by binding to tubulin. Cancer Res 1993;53:4573–4581.

640. Friden B, Wallin M. Dependency of microtubule-associated proteins (MAPs) for microtubule stability and assembly: use of estramustine phosphate in the study of microtubules. Mol Cell Biol 1991;105:149–158.

641. Laing N, Dahllof B, Hartley-Asp B, et al. Interaction of estramustine with tubulin isotypes. Biochemistry 1997;36:871–878.

642. Panda D, Miller HP, Islam K, et al. Stabilization of microtubule dynamics by estramustine by binding to a novel site in tubulin: a possible mechanistic basis for its antitumor action. Proc Natl Acad Sci USA 1997;94:10560–10564.

643. Mohan R, Panda D. Kinetic stabilization of microtubule dynamics by estramustine is associated with tubulin acetylation, spindle abnormalities, and mitotic arrest. Cancer Res 2008;68:6181–6189.

644. Eklov S, Mahdy E, Wester K, et al. Estramustine-binding protein (EMBP) content in four different cell lines and its correlation to estramustine induced metaphase arrest. Anticancer Res 1996;16:1819–1822.

645. Walz PH, Bjork P, Gunnarsson PO, et al. Differential uptake of estramustine phosphate metabolites and its correlation with the levels of estramustine binding protein in prostate tumor tissue. Clin Cancer Res 1998;4:2079–2084.

646. Yoshida D, Cornell-Bell A, Piepmeier JM. Selective antimitotic effects of estramustine correlate with its antimicrotubule properties on glioblastoma and astrocytes. Neurosurgery 1994;34:863–867.

647. Vallbo C, Bergenheim AT, Bergstrom P, et al. Apoptotic tumor cell death induced by estramustine in patients with malignant glioma. Clin Cancer Res 1998;4:87–91.

648. Johansson M, Bergenheim AT, D'Argy R, et al. Distribution of estramustine in the BT4C rat glioma model. Cancer Chemother Pharmacol 1998;41:317–325.

649. Bergenheim AT, Zackrisson B, Elfverson J, et al. Radiosensitizing effect of estramustine in malignant glioma in vitro and in vivo. J Neurooncol 1995;23:191–200.

650. Yoshida D, Piepmeier J, Weinstein M. Estramustine sensitizes human glioblastoma cells to irradiation. Cancer Res 1994;54:1415–1417.

651. Ståhlberg K, Kairemo K, Erkkilä K, et al. Radiation sensitizing effect of estramustine is not dependent on apoptosis. Anticancer Res 2005;25:2873–2878.

652. Ranganathan S, McCauley RA, Dexter DW, Hudes GR. Modulation of endogenous-tubulin isotype expression as a result of human III cDNA transfection into prostate carcinoma cells. Br J Cancer 2001;85:735–740.

653. Sangrajrang S, Denoulet P, Millot G, et al. Estramustine resistance correlates with tau over-expression in human prostatic carcinoma cells. Int J Cancer 1998;77:625–631.

654. Stearns ME, Tew KD. Estramustine binds MAP-2 to inhibit microtubule assembly in vitro. J Cell Sci 1988;89:331–342.

655. Speicher LA, Barone LR, Chapman AE, et al. P-glycoprotein binding and modulation of the multidrug-resistant phenotype by estramustine. J Natl Cancer Inst 1994;86:688–694.

656. Speicher LA, Sheridan VR, Godwin AK, et al. Resistance to the antimitotic drug estramustine is distinct from the multidrug resistant phenotype. Br J Cancer 1991;267–273.

657. Yang CP, Shen HJ, Horwitz SB. Modulation of the function of P-glycoprotein by estramustine. J Natl Cancer Inst 1994;86:723–725.

658. Laing NM, Belinsky MG, Kruh GD, et al. Amplification of the ATP-binding cassette 2 transporter gene is functionally linked with enhanced efflux of estramustine in ovarian carcinoma cells. Cancer Res 1998;58:1332–1337.

659. Mack JT, Townsend DM, Beljanski V, et al. The ABCA2 transporter: intracellular roles in trafficking and metabolism of LDL-derived cholesterol and sterol-related compounds. Curr Drug Metab 2007;8:47–57.

660. Gunnarsson PO, Andersson SB, Johansson SA, et al. Pharmacokinetics of estramustine phosphate (Estracyt) in prostatic cancer patients. Eur J Clin Pharmacol 1984;26:113–119.

661. Forshell GP, Muntzing J, Ek A, et al. The absorption, metabolism, and excretion of Estracyt (NSC 89199) in patients with prostatic cancer. Invest Urol 1976;14:128–131.

662. Dixon R, Brooks M, Gill G. Estramustine phosphate: plasma concentrations of its metabolites following oral administration to man, rat and dog. Res Commun Chem Pathol Pharmacol 1980;27:17–29.

663. Gunnarsson PO, Forshell GP. Clinical pharmacokinetics of estramustine phosphate. Urology 1984;23:22–27.

664. Yamazaki H, Shaw PM, Guengerich FP, et al. Roles of cytochromes P450 1A2 and 3A4 in the oxidation of estradiol and estrone in human liver microsomes. Chem Res Toxicol 1998;11:659–665.

665. Gunnarsson PO, Davidsson T, Andersson SB, et al. Impairment of estramustine phosphate absorption by concurrent intake of milk and food. Eur J Clin Pharmacol 1990;38:189–193.

666. Kamata Y, Iwamoto M, Kamimura T, et al. Repeated massive tongue swelling due to the combined use of estramustine phosphate and angiotensin-converting enzyme inhibitor. J Investig Allergol Clin Immunol 2006;16:388–390.

667. Ozeki T, Takeuchi M, Suzuki M, et al. Single nucleotide polymorphisms of 17beta-hydroxysteroid dehydrogenase type 7 gene: mechanism of estramustine-related adverse reactions? Int J Urol 2009;16:836–841.

668. Von Schoultz B, Carlstrom K, Collste L, et al. Estrogen therapy and liver function-metabolic effects of oral and parenteral administration. Prostate 1989;14:389–395.

669. Smith PH, Suciu S, Robinson MR, et al. A comparison of the effect of diethylstilbestrol with low dose estramustine phosphate in the treatment of advanced prostatic cancer: final analysis of a phase III trial of the European Organization for Research on Treatment of Cancer. J Urol 1986;136:619–623.

670. Madison DL, Beer TM. Acute estramustine induced hypocalcemia unmasking severe vitamin D deficiency. Am J Medicine 2002;112:680–681.

671. Park DS, Vassilopoulou Sellin R, Tu S-M. Estramustine-related hypocalcemia in patients with prostate carcinoma and osteoblastic metastases. Urology 2001;58:105.

672. Ferrari AC, Chachoua A, Singh H, et al. A phase I/II study of weekly paclitaxel and 3 days of high dose oral estramustine in patients with hormone-refractory prostate carcinoma. Cancer 2001;91:2039–2045.

673. Sinibaldi VJ, Carducci MA, Moore-Cooper S, et al. Phase II evaluation of docetaxel plus one-day oral estramustine phosphate in the treatment of patients with androgen independent prostate carcinoma. Cancer 2002;94:1457–1465.

674. Kamata Y, Iwamoto M, Kamimura T, et al. Repeated massive tongue swelling due to the combined use of estramustine phosphate and angiotensin-converting enzyme inhibitor. J Investig Allergol Clin Immunol 2006;16:388–390.

Alkylating Agents

PART A CLASSICAL ALKYLATING AGENTS

Stanton L. Gerson, Alina D. Bulgar, Lachelle D. Weeks, and Bruce A. Chabner

The alkylating agents are antitumor drugs that act through the covalent binding of alkyl groups to cellular molecules. This binding is mediated by reactive intermediates formed from a more parent alkylating compound. Historically, the alkylating agents have played an important role in the development of cancer chemotherapy. The nitrogen mustards mechlorethamine (HN_2, "nitrogen mustard") and tris(β-chloroethyl)amine (HN_3) were the first nonhormonal agents to show significant antitumor activity in humans.[1,2] The clinical trials of nitrogen mustards in patients with lymphomas evolved from the observation that lymphoid atrophy, in addition to lung and mucous membrane irritation, was produced by sulfur mustard during World War I. Antitumor evaluation[3] showed that the related but less reactive nitrogen mustards, the bischloroethylamines (Fig. 14A-1), were less toxic and caused regression of lymphoid tumors in mice. The first clinical studies produced dramatic tumor regressions in some patients with lymphoma, and the antitumor effects were confirmed by an organized multi-institution study.[1,2] This demonstration of efficacy encouraged further efforts to find chemical agents with antitumor activity, leading to the wide variety of antitumor agents in use today. Nonclassical alkylating agents include methylating agents such as procarbazine and temozolomide and are discussed later in this chapter. Alkylating agents, despite the enthusiastic development of targeted agents, continue to occupy a central position in cancer chemotherapy, both in conventional combination regimens and in high-dose protocols with hematopoietic cell transplantation (HCT). Because of their linear dose-response relationship in cell culture experiments,[4] these drugs have become primary tools used in HCT for a variety of diseases. Better appreciation of resistance mechanisms and development of targeting agents to block these resistance pathways promise to improve the efficacy of alkylating agents.

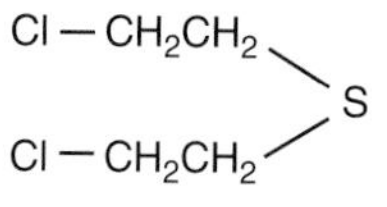

Alkylating Reactions

An alkylation reaction can occur by two mechanisms: S_N1 and S_N2. In S_N1 reactions, the rate-limiting step is the formation of a carbonium ion that can react rapidly with a nucleophile. This reaction follows first-order kinetics with a rate that depends solely on the concentration of the alkylating agent. In contrast, S_N2 reactions follow second-order kinetics and depend on the concentrations of both the alkylating agent and the nucleophile. Such reactions involve a transition-state entity formed by both reactants that decomposes to form the alkylated cellular constituent. Agents such as chloroethylnitrosoureas, through a S_N1-type of mechanism, can form covalent adducts with oxygen and nitrogen atoms in DNA. Compounds with S_N2 predominant mechanisms, such as busulfan, tend to react more slowly, with little alkylation of oxygen sites. Because alkylating agents are designed to produce reactive intermediates, the parent compounds typically have short elimination half-lives of less than 5 hours.

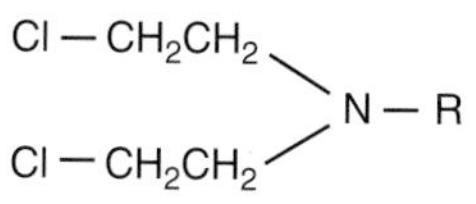

As a class, the alkylating agents share a common target (DNA) and are cytotoxic, mutagenic, and carcinogenic. The activity of most alkylating agents is enhanced by radiation, hyperthermia, nitroimidazoles, glutathione depletion, and inhibition of DNA repair. They differ greatly, however, in their toxicity profiles and antitumor activity. These differences are undoubtedly the result of differences in pharmacokinetic features, lipid solubility, ability to penetrate the central nervous system (CNS), membrane transport properties, detoxification reactions, and specific enzymatic reactions capable of repairing alkylation sites on DNA.[5-7] Application of techniques such as magnetic resonance imaging and mass spectrometry to the

A
Bischloroethylsulfide (sulfur mustard).

B
Bischloroethylamine (nitrogen mustard general
structure). —R = —CH₃ in mechlorethamine. —R = —CH₂CH₂Cl
in tris(β-chloroethyl)amine.

FIGURE **14A-1** Structures of bischloroethylsulfide and bischloroethylamine. **A.** Bischloroethylsulfide (sulfur mustard). **B.** Bischloroethylamine (nitrogen mustard general structure).

TABLE **14A.1**   Key features of selected alkylating agents

	Cyclophosphamide	Ifosfamide	Melphalan	BCNU	Busulfan	Bendamustine
Mechanism of action	All agents produce alkylation of DNA through the formation of reactive intermediates that attack nucleophilic sites.					
Mechanisms of resistance	Increased capacity to repair alkylated lesions, for example, guanine O^6-alkyl transferase (nitrosoureas, busulfan). Increased expression of glutathione-associated enzymes, including γ-glutamyl cysteine synthetase, γ-glutamyl transpeptidase, and glutathione-S-transferases. Increased ALDH (cyclophosphamide). Decreased expression or mutation of p53					
Dose/schedule (mg/m²)	400–2,000 IV; 100 PO qd	1,000–4,000 IV	8 PO qd×5 d	200 IV	2–4 mg qd	70–100 mg daily, on day 1 and 2 of a 28-day cycle
Oral bioavailability	100%	Unavailable	30% (variable)	Not known	50% or greater	?
Pharmacokinetics Primary elimination $t_{1/2}$ (h)	3–10 (parent); 1.6 (aldophosphamide); 8.7 (phosphoramide mustard)	7–15 (parent)	1 (parent)	0.25–0.75[a] (nonlinear increase with dose from 170 to 720 mg/m²)	2–3 h	0.5 (parent)
Metabolism and excretion	Microsomal hydroxylation activates, then chemical decomposition. Hydrolysis to phosphoramide mustard (active) and acrolein. Excretion as inactive oxidation products	Microsomal hydroxylation activates, then chemical decomposition. Hydrolysis to iphosphoramide mustard and acrolein. Excretion as inactive oxidation and dechloroethylated products	Spontaneously decomposes. 20%–35% excreted unchanged in urine	Decomposes to active and inert products; also P450-mediated inactivation	Enzymatic conjugation with glutathione	Chemical decomposition. Excretion primarily in feces
Toxicity						
Bone Marrow	Acute, platelets spared	Acute but mild	Delayed, nadir at 4 wk	Delayed, nadir 4–6 wk	Acute and delayed marrow aplasia	Acute but mild
Other	Hemorrhagic cystitis, cardiac toxicity, IADH	Hemorrhagic cystitis, encephalopathy	—	Pulmonary fibrosis, renal failure, hypotension	Addisonian syndrome, seizures, pulmonary fibrosis, venoocclusive disease	Mucositis, infections, tumor lysis syndrome
Precautions	Use MESNA with high-dose therapy	Always coadminister MESNA	Decomposes if administered over <1 h	—	Monitor AUC with high-dose therapy Induces phenytoin metabolism	

[a]See reference 296.

AUC, area under the concentration time curve; BCNU, bischloroethylnitrosourea; IADH, inappropriate antidiuretic hormone syndrome; IV, intravenously; MESNA, 2-mercaptoethane sulfonate; PO, per os; $t_{1/2}$, plasma half-life.

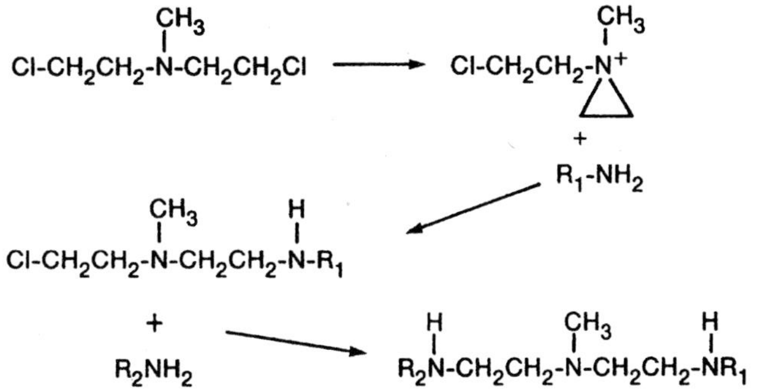

FIGURE **14A-2**   Alkylation mechanism of nitrogen mustards. (From Colvin M. Molecular pharmacology of alkylating agents. In: Cooke ST, Prestayko AW. Cancer and Chemotherapy, vol 3. New York: Academic Press, 1981:291.)

study of the alkylation mechanism and the chemical nature of the intermediates involved have led to a detailed understanding of these reactions.[8,9] Such approaches, coupled with improved techniques for studying cellular damage[10,11] and for determining mechanisms of detoxification,[12] make it possible to predict sites of alkylation of an agent and allow scientists to understand and modify the biologic consequences of such alkylations.

Alkylating Agents Used Clinically

The important pharmacologic properties of the clinically useful alkylating agents are summarized in Table 14A-1.

Nitrogen Mustards

The prototypic alkylating agents have been the bischloroethylamines or nitrogen mustards. The first nitrogen mustard to be used extensively in the clinic was *mechlorethamine* (*mustine*) (Fig. 14A-1), sometimes referred to by its original code name HN_2 or by the term *nitrogen mustard*. The mechanism of alkylation by the nitrogen mustards is shown in Figure 14A-2. In the initial step, chlorine is lost and the β-carbon reacts with the nucleophilic nitrogen atom to form the cyclic, positively charged, and very reactive aziridinium moiety. Reaction of the aziridinium ring with a nucleophile (electron-rich atom) yields the initial alkylated product. Formation of a

second aziridinium by the remaining chloroethyl group allows for a second alkylation, which produces a cross-link between the two alkylated nucleophiles.

Numerous analogs of mechlorethamine were synthesized in which the methyl group was replaced by a variety of chemical groups that stabilized the molecule. Most of these compounds proved to have less antitumor activity than mechlorethamine, but many other derivatives have a higher therapeutic index, a broader range of clinical activity, and can be administered both orally and intravenously. These drugs, which for the most part have replaced mechlorethamine in clinical use, are *melphalan* (L-phenylalanine mustard), *chlorambucil*, *bendamustine*, *cyclophosphamide*, and *ifosfamide* (Fig. 14A-3). The latter two agents are unique in that they require metabolic activation and undergo a complex series of activation and degradation reactions (to be described in detail later in this chapter).

These derivatives have electron-rich groups substituted on the nitrogen atom. This alteration reduces the electrophilicity of the nitrogen and renders the molecules less reactive. Melphalan and chlorambucil retain alkylating activities and seem to be more tumor selective than nitrogen mustard. Cyclophosphamide and ifosfamide, on the other hand, possess no intrinsic alkylating activity and must be metabolized to produce alkylating compounds.

Cyclophosphamide remains the most widely used alkylating agent.[13] It is an essential component of drug regimens for non-Hodgkin's lymphoma (NHL) (CHOP—cyclophosphamide, doxorubicin, vincristine (oncovin), prednisone), other lymphoid malignancies, and solid tumors in children. Additionally, it is used in combination treatments for breast cancer, and in high-dose chemotherapy with bone marrow restoration.

Ifosfamide, an isomeric analog of cyclophosphamide, was introduced into clinical use in 1972. It is currently approved for the treatment of relapsed testicular germ cell tumors[14] and for the treatment of both pediatric and adult soft tissue sarcomas.[15,16] It is used in combination with etoposide and carboplatin for relapsed lymphomas.

Melphalan is primarily employed in multiple myeloma,[17] occasionally in malignant melanoma and in high-dose chemotherapy with marrow transplantation.

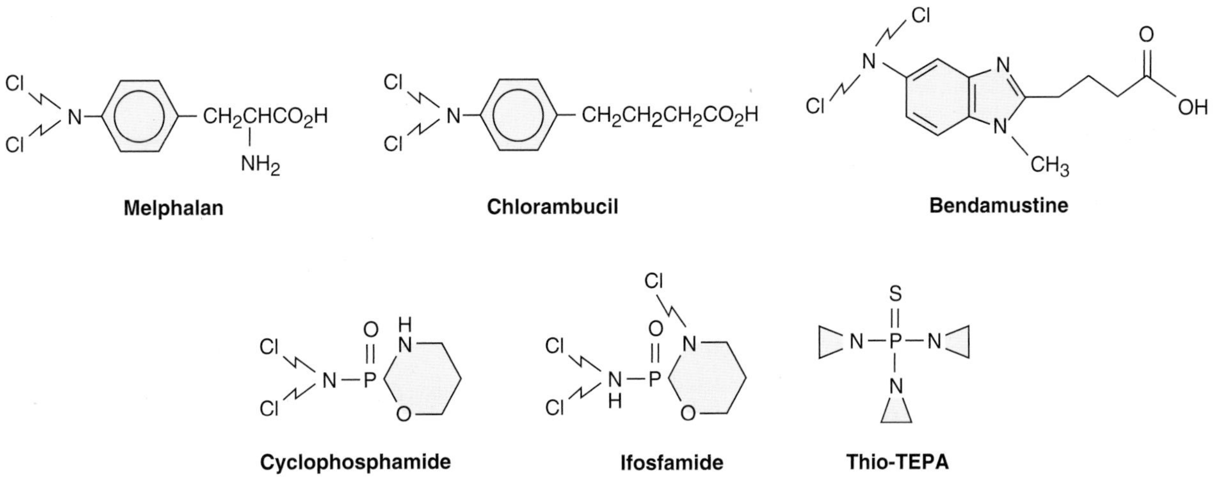

FIGURE **14A-3**   Alkylating agent structures.

Chlorambucil, an oral medication, has single agent activity against chronic lymphocytic leukemia (CLL) and small B-cell lymphomas.[18]

Originally described in 1963, *bendamustine* (Fig. 14A-3) has emerged as an effective treatment for patients with CLL and indolent NHL.[19–27]

Aziridines

The stable aziridines are analogs of the reactive ring-closed intermediates of the nitrogen mustards. Compounds bearing two or more aziridine groups, such as *thiotepa* (Fig. 14A-3; [thiotepa, triethylenethiophosphoramide]), have clinical activity against breast and ovarian cancer,[28] but thiotepa is currently used as an occasional component of high-dose regimens.[29] It was originally tested for antitumor activity because the nitrogen mustards alkylate through an aziridine intermediate. Both thiotepa and its primary desulfurated metabolite *TEPA* (triethylenephosphoramide) have cytotoxic activity in vitro.

Altretamine, with hydroxymethylmelamine as the active metabolite, is only rarely used as salvage therapy in recurrent ovarian cancer.[30] It is less toxic than other alkylating drugs but has a low level of antitumor activity for this disease. Although the mechanism of action of these compounds has not been explored thoroughly, they presumably alkylate through opening of the aziridine rings, as shown for the nitrogen mustards. The reactivity of the aziridine groups is increased by protonation and thus is enhanced at the low pH more characteristic of tumors than normal tissues.

Alkyl Alkane Sulfonates

The major clinical representative of the alkyl alkane sulfonates is *busulfan*, which is widely used in high-dose regimens for the treatment of acute myelogenous leukemia.[31] Of the alkyl alkane sulfonates, compounds with one to eight methylene units between the sulfonate groups have antitumor activity, but maximal cross-linking and activity are achieved by compounds with four units.[32] The mechanism of action of the alkyl alkane sulfonates is shown in Figure 14A-4.

Busulfan exhibits second-order alkylation kinetics. The compound reacts more extensively with thiol groups of amino acids and proteins[33] than do the nitrogen mustards, and these findings have prompted the suggestion that the alkyl alkane sulfonates may exert their cytotoxic activities through such thiol reactions along with interactions with DNA.[33,34] Brookes and Lawley[35,36] were able to demonstrate the reaction of busulfan with the N-7 position of guanine. The cytotoxic potential of busulfan correlates with adenine-to-guanine cross-linking.[37] Busulfan is markedly cytotoxic to hematopoietic stem cells. This effect is seen clinically in the prolonged aplasia that may follow busulfan administration and can be shown experimentally in stem cell cloning systems.[38] The pharmacologic basis for this property of busulfan is not well understood but may involve damage to the mesenchymal stem cells in the microenvironment. In recent years, an intravenous formulation has simplified the dose appropriate administration of busulfan to achieve optimal blood levels during high-dose myeloablative treatments.

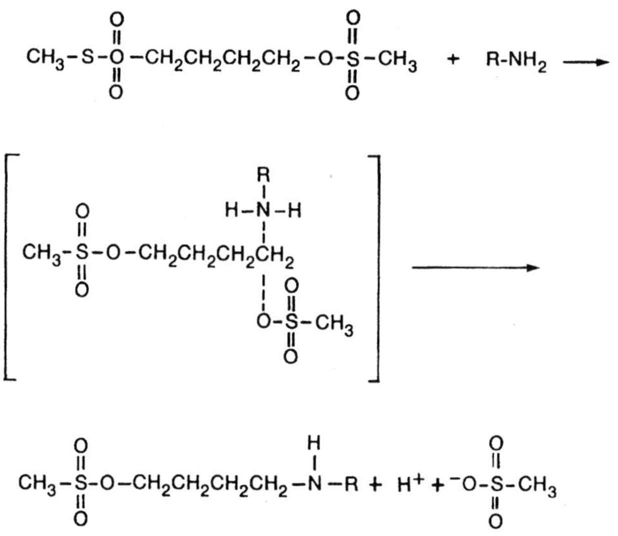

FIGURE 14A-4 Structure and alkylating mechanism of busulfan, an alkane sulfonate. (From Colvin M. Molecular pharmacology of alkylating agents. In: Cooke ST, Prestayko AW. Cancer and Chemotherapy, vol 3. New York: Academic Press, 1981:291.)

Nitrosoureas

The nitrosourea antitumor agents were discovered in a drug screening effort that focused on analogues of methylnitrosoguanidine and methylnitrosourea.[39] Chloroethyl derivatives such as *chloroethylnitrosourea* and *BCNU (carmustine)* (Fig. 14A-5) possess marked antitumor activity and had activity against tumor in the CNS.[39,40] In addition to chloroethyl alkylating activity, the available nitrosoureas can also carbamoylate nucleophiles.[41] Closely related methylating agents, *procarbazine*, *temozolomide*, and *dacarbazine (DTIC)*, are lipophilic and penetrate the CNS (see nonclassical alkylating agents, this chapter).

The nitrosoureas exhibit only partial cross-resistance with other alkylating agents,[40] and a number of studies established unique aspects of the mechanism of the alkylation reaction for these compounds (Fig. 14A-6). BCNU cross-links DNA after the formation of initial monoadducts, particularly at the N-7 position of guanine. As shown

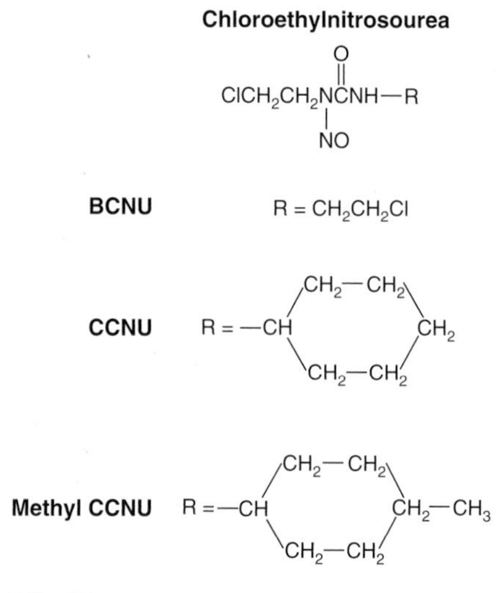

FIGURE 14A-5 Structures of nitrosoureas. BCNU, bischloroethylnitrosourea; CCNU, cyclohexylchloroethylnitrosourea.

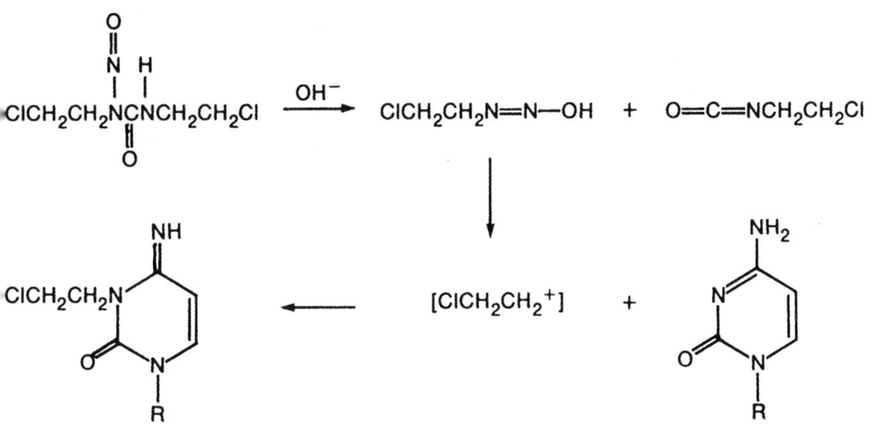

FIGURE **14A-6** Alkylation of nucleoside by bis-chloroethylnitrosourea (BCNU).

in Figure 14A-6, the diazonium hydroxide intermediate formed during BCNU hydrolysis decomposes to form a 2-chloroethyl carbonium ion (or equivalent), a strong electrophile, capable of alkylation of guanine, cytidine, and adenine bases.[42] In a subsequent step occurring over hours, the chloride is displaced by electron-rich nitrogen on the complementary DNA strand base to form a cross-link. DNA-protein cross-links are also possible by initiating chloroethylation at the amino or sulfhydryl group of protein.[43]

Isocyanates resulting from the spontaneous breakdown of many of the methyl- and chloroethylnitrosoureas are also shown in Figure 14A-6. The role of isocyanate-mediated carbamoylation in antitumor effects is incompletely understood, but this activity may be responsible for some toxicities associated with nitrosourea therapy.[44]

High-dose BCNU, etoposide, and cisplatin comprise the BEP regimen used for autologous stem-cell transplantation in patients with refractory or relapsed lymphoma.[45] Another high-dose BCNU-containing regimen, BEAM (BCNU, etoposide, cytarabine, melphalan), has also been used with success with autologous hematopoietic stem-cell transplant in patients with NHL.[46] In the 1980s, BCNU attracted interest as an adjuvant to radiation therapy in the treatment of patients with grade III and IV astrocytoma[47] but has been replaced by temozolomide.[48] BCNU-impregnated polymer wafers implanted in the tumor bed at the time of surgical resection provide a controlled release form of local chemotherapy.[49]

Streptozotocin is a unique methylnitrosourea with methylating activity that lacks carbamoylating activity. It is used exclusively in the treatment of metastatic islet cell carcinoma of the pancreas and malignant carcinoid tumors.[50] The dose-limiting toxicities in humans have been gastrointestinal and renal, but not hematopoietic.

Alkylating Agent–Steroid Conjugates

Steroid receptors may serve to localize and concentrate appended drug species in hormone-responsive cancers. A number of synthetic conjugates of mustards and steroids have been developed. Of these drugs, two have made the transition into clinical application. *Prednimustine*, an ester-linked conjugate and slow release form of chlorambucil and prednisolone, is no longer available for clinical use.[51] *Estramustine* is a carbamate ester–linked conjugate of nornitrogen mustard and estradiol but functions as an inhibitor of tubulin polymerization (see Chapter 13).

Prodrugs of Alkylating Agents

Therapy with alkylating agents is compromised by a high level of toxicity to normal tissues and a lack of tumor selectivity. Cyclophosphamide and ifosfamide were prodrugs synthesized in the hope that high levels of phosphamidases in epithelial tumors would selectively activate the drugs.[52] Strategies for more selective delivery of alkylating agent to tumor have been explored including cleavable tumor-directed antibody-alkylating agent conjugates,[53] alkylating agent-glutathione conjugates (which might be selectively cleaved by glutathione transferase (GST) P1 expressed in high levels in tumor cells)[54] or viral vectors delivering activating enzymes to tumor cells.[55]

Cellular Pharmacology

Cellular Uptake

The uptake of alkylating agents into cells is an important determinant of cellular specificity. Many are highly lipid soluble (including the active metabolites of the methylating agents, cyclophosphamide, and ifosfamide, as well as chlorambucil) and readily enter cells by passive diffusion. Mechlorethamine uptake depends upon the choline transport system.[56] Melphalan is transported into several cell types by at least two active transport systems, which also carry leucine and other neutral amino acids across the cell membrane.[57,58] High levels of leucine in the medium protect cells from the cytotoxic effects of melphalan by competing with melphalan for transport.[59] In contrast to mechlorethamine and melphalan, the highly lipid-soluble nitrosoureas BCNU and CCNU enter cells by passive diffusion.[60] Chlorambucil uptake also occurs through simple passive diffusion.

Studies of cellular uptake of alkylating agents that require metabolic activation (such as cyclophosphamide or ifosfamide) are hampered by uncertainty about which metabolite, or even parent drug, is the most critical moiety for transport.

Sites of Alkylation

Any alkylating agent producing reactive intermediates binds to a variety of cellular constituents[61] including nucleic acids, proteins, amino acids, and nucleotides. As an example, the active alkylating species from a nitrogen mustard demonstrates selectivity for nucleophiles in the following order: (a) oxygens of phosphates, (b) oxygens of bases, (c) amino groups of purines, (d) amino groups of proteins, (e) sulfur atoms of methionine, and (f) thiol groups of cysteinyl residues of glutathione.[62] This ranking, however, assumes there are no steric or hydrophilic/hydrophobic barriers to the tissue nucleophile, and this is seldom the case. In addition, glutathione conjugation is often favored in the presence of GSTs, which offer catalysis. Thus, generalizations about alkylating agent targets are fraught with difficulty. In addition, it seems likely that a matrix of biochemical targets of alkylating agents may contribute to cytotoxicity, though DNA is generally favored as the primary target. Proof of this hypothesis may be emerging from three areas of research where cytotoxicity correlates with (a) activity of DNA repair enzymes, perhaps best shown for BCNU and repair by alkyl guanine alkyltransferase (AGT),[63] (b) changes in a matrix of genetic and epigenetic events measured and analyzed by gene expression arrays,[64] and (c) specific DNA adducts shown by mass spectrometric analysis.[65] The stringency of such analyses requires that alternative toxic pathways not involving DNA must be excluded, a difficult requirement to meet. For this reason, mechanistic understanding of alkylating agent activity must be considered incomplete.

In the DNA molecule, the phosphoryl oxygens of the sugar phosphate backbone are obvious electron-rich targets for alkylation. Alkylation of the phosphate groups occurs[66,67] and can result in strand breakage from hydrolysis of the resulting phosphotriesters. Although the biologic significance of the strand breakage caused by phosphate alkylation remains uncertain, the process is so slow that it seems unlikely to be a major determinant of cytotoxicity, even for monofunctional agents.[68]

Extensive studies with carcinogenic alkylating agents such as methyl methane sulfonate have shown that virtually all the oxygen and nitrogen atoms of the purine and pyrimidine bases of DNA can be alkylated to varying degrees. The relative significance of these sites of alkylation of specific bases and of specific sites on DNA in determining cytotoxicity, specific organ toxicities, or carcinogenesis remains uncertain. Alkylation of the O-6 atom and of the extracyclic nitrogen of guanine appears to be particularly important for carcinogenesis.[69–71]

> Studies of the base specificity of alkylation by the chemotherapeutic alkylating agents have been much less extensive. Busulfan and mechlorethamine alkylate the N-7 position of guanine. Guanine cross-links (two guanine molecules abridged at the N-7 position by an alkylating agent) have been isolated from acid hydrolysates of the reaction mixtures.[35,36]
>
> Reaction of the nitrogen mustard with native DNA, however, produces alkylation of the N-1 position of adenine in addition to N-7–alkylated guanine. The enhanced alkylation of the N-7 position of guanine may result from base stacking and charge transfer that enhance the nucleophilic character of the N-7 position.[72] Melphalan preferentially alkylates guanine N-7 or adenine N-3.[65]
>
> Base sequence influences the alkylating reaction. The N-7 position of guanine is most electronegative and, therefore, most vulnerable to attack by the aziridinium cation intermediate of the nitrogen mustards when the base is flanked by guanines on its 5′ and 5′ sides. The key site of DNA attack for the nitrosoureas as well as nonclassic methylating agents

such as procarbazine and dacarbazine seems to be the O-6 methyl group of guanine.[7] Enhanced repair of this site is associated with drug resistance.[73] Thus, the preferred sites for alkylation vary by alkylating agent and chemical environment around the DNA base in question.

DNA Cross-Linking

On the basis of their isolation of the guanines linked at N-7 by alkylating agents, Brookes and Lawley[72,74] postulated that the bifunctional alkylating agents such as the nitrogen mustards produced interstrand and intrastrand DNA-DNA cross-links and that these cross-links were responsible for the inactivation of the DNA and cytotoxicity. On the basis of the Watson-Crick DNA model, these authors suggested that appropriate spatial relationships for cross-linking by nitrogen mustards or sulfur mustard occurred between the N-7 positions of guanine residues in complementary DNA strands (Fig. 14A-7).

The importance of cross-linking is supported by the fact that the bifunctional alkylating agents, with few exceptions, are much more effective antitumor agents than the analogous monofunctional agents. Furthermore, increasing the number of alkylating units on the molecule beyond two does not usually increase the antitumor activity of the compound.

Direct evidence that DNA cross-linking occurs as the result of treatment of DNA or cells with bifunctional alkylating agents was provided initially by relatively insensitive physical techniques, including sedimentation velocity studies and denaturation-renaturation studies.[75] These techniques, however, could not detect DNA interstrand cross-linking in mammalian cells exposed to therapeutic levels of alkylating agents in vitro or in tissues after in vivo drug administration. In 1976, a more sensitive assay for DNA interstrand cross-linking in cells, the alkaline elution method,[76] was reported and had the necessary sensitivity to detect DNA cross-linking in cells and tumor-bearing animals exposed to minimal cytotoxic levels of alkylating agents.[77,78] These studies and others using ethidium bromide fluorescence to detect cross-links have shown that DNA cross-linking by bifunctional alkylating agents correlates with cytotoxicity and that DNA in drug-resistant cells has lower levels of cross-linkage.[79,80] The alkaline elution technique also detects DNA-protein as well as DNA-DNA cross-links.[81] DNA-protein cross-links likely do not play a major role in cytotoxicity and may be repaired by replication bypass mechanisms.[81]

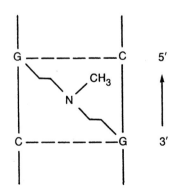

FIGURE 14A-7   Cross-linking of DNA by nitrogen mustard. (Modified and reproduced from Brookes P, Lawley PD. The reaction of monofunctional and difunctional alkylating agents with nucleic acids. Biochem J 1961;80:486, with permission.)

In addition to these target effect-response studies, silencing of the AGT promoter in gliomas correlates with improved antitumor activity and survival in patients treated with BCNU.[82] Because AGT repairs guanine alkylation products produced by BCNU, decreased enzyme activity would be expected to increase DNA alkylation, implying that DNA is a critical target for BCNU effects. Thus, evidence increasingly supports the hypothesis that DNA adduct formation is the major mechanism of alkylating agent cytotoxicity.

Chloroethylnitrosoureas cross-link via a unique mechanism.[43] The spontaneous decomposition of the chloroethylnitrosoureas generates a chloroethyldiazonium hydroxide entity that can alkylate DNA bases to produce an alkylating chloroethylamine group on the nucleotide in the DNA strand. This group could then alkylate an adjacent nucleotide on the complementary DNA strand in a slower step, producing an interstrand cross-link. The mechanism of alkylation by thiophosphates such as thiotepa likely begins with protonation of the aziridine N, which leads to ring opening. Cross-linking can proceed by one of several mechanisms, either activation of the free chloroethyl carbon or activation of a second aziridine ring on the original molecule. Although interstrand cross-links are important mediators of the cytotoxic effects of alkylating agents, the monofunctional DNA alkylations exceed cross-links in number and are potentially cytotoxic. This hypothesis is supported by the fact that certain clinically effective agents, such as procarbazine and dacarbazine, are monofunctional alkylating compounds and do not produce cross-links in experimental systems. The basis of the cytotoxic effects of monofunctional alkylation appears to be through mismatch repair–mediated processes, since cells lacking mismatch repair are often methylating agent tolerant. The futile cycling of repair reactions through mismatch repair efficiently removes bases opposite O^6-methylguanine and reinserts a thymine, with repeated attempt to repair the O^6-mG:T mismatch and further futile repair. This produces single and double strand breaks that are cytotoxic, especially in the second round of DNA synthesis, after formation of the O^6-mG:T mismatch.

Data suggest that alkylation is nonuniform along the DNA strand and may be concentrated in specific regions. One determinant of regional specificity of DNA alkylations may be chromatin structure[11,83]; areas of active transcription seem to be most vulnerable. Additionally, evidence shows that nitrogen mustards such as mechlorethamine preferentially cross-link at 5′-GNC sequence.[84]

In summary, the preponderance of evidence supports the hypothesis that the major factor in the cytotoxicity of most clinically effective alkylating agents is interstrand DNA cross-linking, which results in inactivation of the DNA template, cessation of DNA synthesis, and ultimately cell death. Cell-cycle checkpoint proteins, including most prominently p53, are responsible for the recognition of DNA alkylation and strand breaks. Recognition of DNA damage leads to a halt in cell-cycle progression and initiation of programmed cell death. Cells containing mutated p53 have greater resistance to alkylating agents.[85]

An increased knowledge of alkylation mechanisms and targets may make it possible to improve the therapeutic index of these agents. For example, the therapeutic index of alkylating agents should improve if the alkylation of tumor cells were increased without a simultaneous increase in normal tissue alkylation. This might be accomplished by maneuvers designed to inhibit drug activation by glutathione or GST P1,[86] or by blocking the repair processes, as discussed below.

Tumor Resistance

The emergence of alkylating agent–resistant tumor cells is a major problem that limits the clinical effectiveness of these drugs. Cellular resistance mechanisms identified in preclinical experimental settings include drug uptake, enhanced anti-apoptosis pathways, activation of survival pathways, enhanced intratumoral drug inactivation, and changes in DNA repair.

Decreased Cellular Uptake of Selected Alkylating Agents

Several of the drugs (melphalan, nitrogen mustard) of this class require active transport into cells. One mechanism for drug resistance is decreased drug entry into the cell. This mechanism was best demonstrated in L5178Y lymphoblast cells resistant to mechlorethamine.[56] The extracellular domain of the leucine-melphalan transporter expresses CD98. Reduced expression of CD98 on human myeloma cells is associated with melphalan resistance.[87] The glutathione-dependent efflux transporters MRP1 and MRP2 can confer resistance to chlorambucil.[89]

Resistance due to Inactivation by Glutathione or GSTs

Intracellular inactivation of alkylating agents has been implicated in human tumor resistance. Early studies showed increased levels of sulfhydryls associated with resistance in experimental tumors, and increased nonprotein sulfhydryl content, particularly in the form of glutathione, in resistant tumor cell lines.[88] While increased intracellular glutathione content may be found in resistant cells, elevated GST activity may also play a role[90] and increased aldehyde dehydrogenase (ALDH) activity, which converts aldophosphamide to the inactive carboxyphosphamide, was present in cells resistant to cyclophosphamide.[91–93]

Alterations in the GSH/GST system found in alkylating agent resistance phenotypes include increased intracellular GSH levels, elevation of GST activity, and changes in the expressed levels of one or more GST isozymes. Currently, several GSH-related mechanisms may explain the observed tumor cell resistance to alkylating agents, including (a) enhanced inactivation of electrophilic alkylating agents, such as melphalan[94] by direct conjugation to GSH; (b) GSH-dependent denitrosation of nitrosoureas, a reaction that is preferentially catalyzed by one of the rat liver GST μ enzymes in the case of BCNU; (c) scavenging for reactive organic peroxidases, a process that is catalyzed by GSH peroxidase;[95] and (d) quenching of chloroethylated-DNA monoadducts.[96]

Inherited polymorphisms of functional significance have been reported in genes that encode glutathione-S-transferases (GSTs) and may contribute to resistance (see Chapter 6). There are four cytosolic families of GSTs, including GST α, GST μ, GST θ, and GST π.[97] Gene clusters of GST μ (GSTM1, M2, M3, M4, and M5) and GST θ (GSTT1 and T2) are located on chromosomes 1 and 22, respectively.[98] Independent gene deletions at GSTM1 and GSTT1 loci result in a lack of active protein in ≈50% and 20% of Caucasians, respectively.[99] GST π or GSTP1, encoded by a single locus (GSTP1) on chromosome 11, is also subject to polymorphic variation.[100] Codon 105 residue forms part of the GSTP1 active site for binding of hydrophobic electrophiles,[101] and the Ile–Val substitution affects substrate-specific catalytic activity and thermal stability of the encoded protein.[102] Reactive metabolites of ifosfamide, busulfan, and chlorambucil are substrates for GSTP1-mediated glutathione conjugation in vitro. Allelic variants of GSTP1 differ significantly in their efficacy in catalyzing the GSH conjugation and hence their ability to detoxify alkylating agents.[103] The effect of these polymorphisms on clinical conjugation, toxicity, and antitumor response is uncertain, and the studies to date are summarized in Chapter 6.

Resistance to Cyclophosphamide due to Elevated Aldehyde Dehydrogenase Activity

Resistance to cyclophosphamide may also be determined by the activity of cellular ALDH.[93,104] ALDH is an enzyme responsible for the oxidation of intracellular aldehydes.[105] The cytoplasmatic ALDH isozyme converts activated cyclophosphamide to the inactive excretory product, carboxyphosphamide, in both murine and human cell lines.[106] There is no clear evidence that ALDH activity confers resistance in human tumors.

> ALDH may have an important role in early differentiation of hematopoietic stem cells by oxidizing retinol to retinoic acid.[107] It is hypothesized that cancer stem cells survive cyclophosphamide treatment due to ALDH. Murine and human hematopoietic and neural stem and progenitor cells

have high ALDH activity.[108,109] Increased ALDH activity has also been found in malignant stem cell populations in multiple myeloma and acute myeloid leukemia.[110]

DNA repair and Alkylating Agent Resistance

Enhanced repair of DNA lesions generated by alkylation plays a clearly established role in resistance of experimental and human tumor cells to alkylating agents. Because DNA appears to be the most critical target for the alkylating agents, its repair has been a major focus of study and several mechanisms involved in repairing alkylation and strand breaks are summarized in Figure 14A-8.

Enhanced excision of alkylated nucleotides from DNA as a mechanism of resistance to alkylating agents was first demonstrated in bacteria[75] and later in mammalian cells. Bacterial, fungal, and mammalian cells are capable of excising and repairing sites of alkylation, as well as removing cross-links and repairing single- and double-strand breaks.

Alkylguanine DNA Alkyltransferase Mediated repair

Repair of DNA alkylation products and cross-links involves multiple systems, each composed of one or several distinct enzymes.

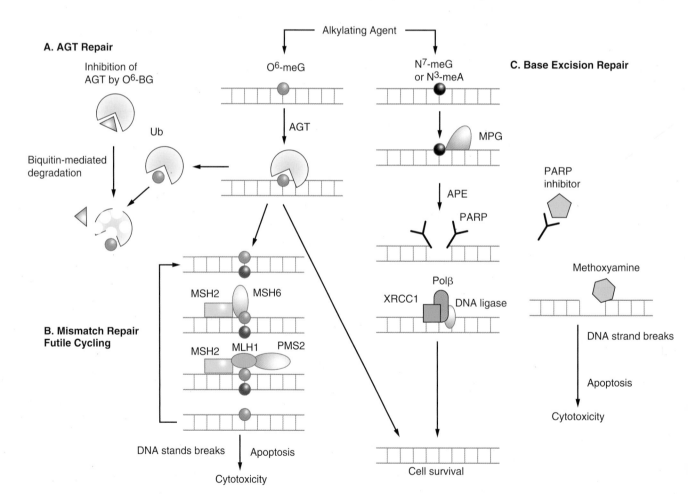

Figure 14A-8 DNA repair pathways that play an important role in resistance to alkylating agents. **A.** AGT. **B.** Mismatch repair. **C.** Base excision repair. Targeted therapies to improve tumor sensitivity including *O*⁶-benzylguanine, PARP inhibition, and methoxyamine are indicated. AGT, alkylguanine transferase; O6-meG, *O*⁶-methylguanine; N7-meG, N7-methylguanine; N3-meA, N3-methyladenine; O6-BG, *O*⁶-benzylguanine; Ub, ubiquitin; PARP, Poly-ADP-ribose polymerase; Polβ, DNA Polymerase β; MPG, methylpurine glycosylase. Not shown are components of the double-strand break repair complexes. (Adapted from Sarkaria JN, Kitange GJ, James CD, et al. Mechanisms of chemoresistance to alkylating agents in malignant glioma Clin Cancer Res 2008;14:2900–2908, with permission.)

(see Fig. 14A-8). The simplest of these catalyzes the transfer of alkyl substituents (methyl-, ethyl-, benzyl-, 2-chloroethyl-, and pyridyloxobutyl-) from the O^6-position of guanine to an active cysteine acceptor site within the protein in a single enzyme repair process. This enzyme, alkylguanine-O^6-alkyl transferase (AGT), is encoded by the MGMT (O^6-methylguanine methyltransferase) gene in humans and is homologous to the bacterial alkyltransferase gene, ada.

Several clinical trials have established an inverse correlation between AGT content in brain tumors and the response to treatment of brain tumor patients receiving BCNU, temozolomide, and other alkylating agents.[111–113] Lower levels of AGT activity result from epigenetic silencing due to MGMT promoter methylation. Tumors with methylated MGMT are highly responsive to these agents, while those with fully expressed AGT tend to be resistant. The availability of 5′ cytosine methylation–specific PCR (MSP) provides a facile assessment of MGMT promoter methylation and has value as a predictive assay for response to alkylating agent–based chemotherapy. MGMT promoter methylation has been correlated with survival in patients with glioma treated with nitrosoureas and temozolomide[82,114] and prolonged progression-free survival (PFS) in patients treated with temozolomide.[115,116] Together, these data illustrate a role for MGMT gene function in glioma chemoresistance to alkylating agents. Clinical trials attempting to modulate AGT activity are discussed below.[111,117,118]

Mismatch Repair

A second DNA repair system, mismatch repair (MMR), recognizes the mismatch created by alkylation of DNA bases, and, after unsuccessful attempts at repair, triggers cell-cycle arrest and apoptosis. For example, O^6 alkylation of guanine leads to mispairing of the damaged base with thymine, creating a distortion in the DNA double helix, which is recognized by components of the MMR complex. MMMR deficiency has been associated with resistance to alkylating agents owing to the inability to recognize the mismatch and initiate the cycle of futile repair attempts, cell-cycle arrest, and apoptosis.[119,120] Several proteins comprise the MMR pathway (hMLH1, hPMS2, hMSH2, hMSH3, and hMSH6), which is programmed to correct erroneous DNA base pairing.

> In MMR competent cells during DNA replication, DNA polymerase mispairs unresolved O^6-methylguanine with thymine. The mismatch triggers attempts to remove the mispaired thymine. If repair is successful, subsequent rounds of replication continue to mispair O^6-methylguanine with thymine, resulting in repetitive futile cycles of MMR. This futile cycle may induce double-strand breaks, which in turn, trigger p53-dependent cell-cycle arrest and apoptosis.[121] Loss of MMR competence creates tolerance to the mispaired bases and allows cell replication and survival, provided the DNA lesions are compatible with viability. The loss of MLH6 is a frequent event in glioma cells selected by resistance to temozolomide.[122]

Specific interactions of MMR proteins with cell-cycle checkpoint proteins have been implicated in apoptosis. hMLH1 has been associated with signaling ATR-dependent G2 cell-cycle arrest in response to DNA methylation,[123] and MMR proteins may initiate degradation of cyclin D1 following alkylation to promote cell-cycle arrest in response to alkylation.[124] Functional MSH2 and hMLH1 are also believed to activate p73-dependent apoptosis pathways via c-Abl.[125]

Resistance to alkylating agents conferred by MMR deficiency is further illustrated by hereditary nonpolyposis colon cancer, which is caused by mutations in hMLH1 or hMSH2 genes. Colon cancer cells harboring these mutations are resistant to alkylating agents,[126] as are other cell lines deficient in hMLH1.[127]

DNA Excision Repair

NA excision repair pathways provide a comprehensive mechanism for recognizing and removing damaged bases or nucleotide segments from a single DNA strand and then resynthesizing the new DNA segment, using the opposing undamaged strand as a template. Excision repair complexes includes base excision repair (BER) and nucleotide excision repair (NER).

Base Excision Repair

In response to DNA alkylation, BER is initiated by the action of damage-specific DNA glycosylases that recognize and excise single base lesions such as N^3 methyladenine and N^7-methylguanine. Release of the damaged base produces an apurinic/apyrimidinic (AP) site, which is excised by the APE endonuclease (Fig. 14A-9). The missing segment is then resynthesized by DNA polymerase and sealed by DNA ligase. Persistent AP sites are recognized by topoisomerase I and II and these may form cleavable complexes that induce apoptotic signals. The enzyme PARP plays a pivotal role in the recognition of strand breaks and in the formation of DNA strand break intermediates that attract repair complexes. The N^3-methyladenine and N^7-methylguanine are the most common adducts created by alkylation and account for greater than 80% of all methylation events. However, these lesions contribute modestly to the cytotoxicity of alkylating agents due to the efficiency of the BER pathway. Perturbation of BER capacity through alterations of glycosylase expression or through pathway inhibition greatly decreases the efficiency of N^3 and N^7 methyl adduct repair.[128] Targeting of BER, as described below, is particularly effective in enhancing the sensitivity to platinating agents in various cell lines tumors, especially breast cancers deficient in BRCA 1 and BRCA 2, and to alkylating agents in MMR-deficient tumors.[129]

Nucleotide Excision Repair

NER is an additional mechanism for excising bulky alkylation products and DNA intrastrand cross-links. The pathway includes multiple proteins that recognize DNA adducts, such as those produced by alkyl lesions and incise 3′ and 5′ to the damaged base(s), causing release of the damaged nucleotides and surrounding segments of DNA. Excision is followed by resynthesis of the missing segment, using the opposing strand as a template. Components of the NER complex also have a role in repair of double-strand breaks. NER-deficient mammalian cells, such as those derived form patients with xeroderma pigmentosum (XP), are hypersensitive to alkylating and cross-linking agents.[130,131] Studies of the effects of NER deficiency

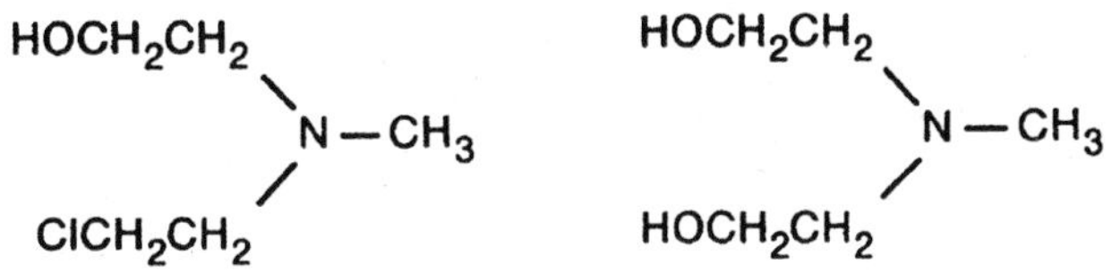

FIGURE **14A-9**   Hydrolysis products of mechlorethamine.

on the toxicity of alkylating agents are most extensive in rodent models, but there is evidence that polymorphic variants of ERCC1 confer increased alkylating agent sensitivity for both normal and malignant tissues, influence response to treatment, and greater toxicity.[132] The role of NER in alkylating agent sensitivity and resistance in clinical cancer treatment is under active investigation.

Cross-Link Repair

Interstrand cross-links covalently tether strands of DNA, preventing unwinding of duplex DNA and prohibiting polymerase access. Both strands of DNA are involved in this lesion, precluding straightforward excision repair and gap-filling pathways. Consequently, the repair of interstrand DNA cross-links is complex, integrating elements of the NER pathway, a variety of less well-understood activities to form a double-strand break, insertion of new bases, and homologous recombination (HR). Though mechanisms are incompletely understood several, mammalian cell types have extreme sensitivity to cross-linking agents. Faconi anemia[133] and Bloom's (BLM) syndrome cells[134] are both hypersensitive to alkylating agents that cause interstrand cross-links. The Fanconi anemia pathway and the BLM helicase are believed to be activated in response to replication stalling due to cross-linked DNA; their dysfunction in the inherited disorders accounts for alkylating agent sensitivity.[135,136] Furthermore, mutations in excision repair genes ERCC1 and ERCC4 (XPF) also render cells sensitive to cross-linking by alkylating agents, suggesting these genes play a role in the repair of cross-links in addition to their role in NER.[137]

Akt

The Akt family in humans is comprised of three genes (Akt1, Akt2, and Akt3) encoding for serine/threonine protein kinases (PKB). Akt activation occurs downstream of various receptor tyrosine kinases and phosphatidylinositol 3-kinase (PI3K). The PI3K/Akt pathway is frequently activated in human cancer and has been implicated in tumor cell proliferation, cellular survival, and chemotherapy resistance (see Chapter 30). In response to alkylation by the agent temozolomide, Akt is induced in lymphoblastoid, colon, and breast cancer cells in a mismatch repair–dependent manner.[138,139]

> Upon activation, PI3K/Akt signaling confers resistance to chemotherapy through its antiapoptotic effects as mediated by phosphorylation of several downstream targets. Activated Akt is thought to inhibit apoptosis by phosphorylating molecules upstream and downstream of the mitochondrial apoptotic pathway. Akt-dependent phosphorylation of proapoptotic BH3 family members such as Bad, Bax and Bim-EL decreases the ability of these proteins to hold mitochondria in an open configuration, resulting in a reduction in cytochrome c release. Akt can phosphorylate caspase-9 to inhibit its ability to activate executioner caspase 3.[140,141] Akt reduces cytochrome c release through modification of the antiapoptotic Bcl-2 homologous Mcl-1.[142,143] Akt exerts indirect inhibition of apoptosis through effects on p53, the most important regulator of apoptosis.[144]
>
> Akt also drives chemoresistance by promoting cell growth. Akt is involved in the survival pathway of mammalian target of rapamycin (mTOR), a serine/threonine kinase that is implicated in protein synthesis control.[145] Akt activates mTOR complex 1 (mTORC1; or mTOR-raptor complex) indirectly by inhibiting phosphorylation of tuberous sclerosis complex 2, thereby allowing Ras-related small G protein (Rheb)-GTP to activate mTORC1 signaling.[146]

Defects in Cell Cycle Arrest and Apoptosis

In addition to the mechanisms described above, mutation or silencing of genes that induces cell-cycle arrest and apoptosis may lead to alkylator resistance.

In cells that experience genotoxic stress during replication, activation of these factors triggers the signaling cascades, leading to delayed progression through S-phase in order to allow time for DNA repair.[147] In the presence of DNA damage, an S-phase cell-cycle checkpoint is activated by the checkpoint kinases ataxia-telangectasia mutated (ATM) and ATM- and Rad3-related (ATR). Activation depends on the type of DNA damage: ATM is recruited to DNA double-strand breaks (DSBs) induced by agents such as ionizing radiation (IR), whereas ATR is recruited to sites of replication protein A (RPA)-coated single-stranded DNA (ssDNA). These sites accumulate at stalled replication forks or at sites of single-strand damage.[148,149] The involvement of ATM and ATR in the response to carcinogen-induced DNA damage has been established,[150] by showing an enhanced sensitivity of ATM- and ATR-defective cells to methylating agents.

> Two parallel branches of the DNA damage-dependent S-phase checkpoint are thought to cooperate by inhibiting distinct steps of DNA replication. One branch is activated by the phosphorylation of structural maintenance of chromosomes 1 (SMC1), a cohesin that is activated by ATM or ATR.[151] The second branch, consisting of the ATR-Chk1- or ATM-Chk2-complexes, regulates turnover of CDC25A, a phosphatase that regulates Cdk2 and consequently blocks the initiation of replication.[152]

Defects in damage recognition or apoptotic signaling may lead to relative resistance.[153] For example, loss of normal p53 function, up-regulation of the antiapoptotic proteins, Bcl-2 or Bcl-X$_L$, or overexpression of the epidermal-growth factor receptor (EGFR) can disrupt the normal apoptotic response to DNA damage caused by alkylating agents.[154,155] As mentioned previously, apoptotic cell death after DNA damage is mediated through p53, which blocks cell-cycle progression, initiates attempts to repair damage, and ultimately activates apoptotic pathways.

Summary

Cellular resistance may arise through alterations in drug uptake, through enhancement of drug inactivation, through changes in checkpoint function, or through alterations in DNA repair. Multiple changes may occur in a given tumor cell population and may lead to the phenotype of drug resistance observed clinically. Varying degrees of cross-resistance between alkylating agents are observed for each of their mechanisms so that a tumor that is resistant to one alkylating agent may remain significantly responsive to another. This finding forms the rational basis for the use of combinations of alkylating agents in high-dose chemotherapy regimens.[156]

Reversal of Resistance

Exposure to alkylating agents leads to induction of a series of compensatory defensive responses in cell-cycle drug-activating and drug-inactivating enzymes and induction of DNA-repair capacity. Efforts to prevent or reverse tumor cell resistance have involved modulation of glutathione detoxification, as well as inhibition of DNA repair (Fig. 14A-9).

Glutathione Inhibition

Because of the pivotal importance of GSH in alkylating agent detoxification, three pharmacological approaches to modulation have been adopted: (a) precursors of GSH or other sulfhydryls replete sulfhydryls content in normal tissues, thus reducing the host toxicity; (b) specific inhibitors of GSH biosynthetic enzymes selectively decrease intracellular GSH in tumors; (c) inhibitors of detoxifying enzymes (GSTs) decrease the tumor cell's ability to protect itself against alkylating metabolites.

1. Because GSH cannot readily cross cell membranes, early efforts to increase intracellular GSH relied on administration of a precursor, L-2-oxothiazolidine-4-carboxylate, that must be enzymatically metabolized to L-cysteine, one of the three constituents of GSH. More recently, membrane permeable monoesters of GSH have been synthesized, such as GSH-monoethyl ester, which is activated by intracellular hydrolysis.[157] In animal studies, the GSH-monoethyl ester successfully reduced the toxicity of BCNU, cyclophosphamide, and mitomycin C.[158] Primarily, the ester protected liver, lungs, and spleen.

2. A number of agents, including diethylmaleate, phorone, and dimethylfumarate, have been used to deplete GSH by chemical interaction but proved too toxic clinically. Direct interference with GSH synthetase results in the buildup of 5-oxoproline, and this causes marked acidosis in patients.[159] By far the most effective approach in reducing the GSH biosynthetic capacity of a tumor cell has been achieved by administering amino acid sulfoximines,[160,161] which inhibit γ-glutamylcysteine synthetase. The lead compound to emerge from these studies was L-buthionine (SR)-sulfoximine (BSO), the R-stereoisomer of which inhibits γ-glutamylcysteine synthetase.[162] GSH levels are low in unperturbed tumor cells adding to the rationale for BSO to improve the therapeutic index of alkylating agents. Although BSO caused differential sensitization of tumors in animal models,[163] trials in humans failed to clearly demonstrate therapeutic index improvement[164,165] and enthusiasm for clinical use of BSO has waned.

3. An alternative approach to decreasing GSH effects is to inhibit the enzymes that use GSH as a cofactor. GST overexpression was determined to be at least one contributing mechanism to the alkylating agent–resistant phenotype, providing a rationale for the use of GST inhibitors as modulating agents. Because GST P1 often dominates in tumors whereas other subtypes are most prominent in normal tissues, inhibitors specific for GST P1 might offer a better therapeutic index. Initial studies employed a relatively nonspecific inhibitor of GSTs, ethacrynic acid, a common diuretic. Preclinical studies were promising,[163] but dose escalation in human subjects was limited by diuretic complications. Poor specificity for tumor-associated GST has deterred further development. Specific inhibitors of GST P1 have now been developed and are being studied clinically but with inconclusive clinical results.[166,167]

4. A very different approach to modulation of alkylator toxicity was suggested in studies by the United States Army, which examined over 4,000 synthetic thiol derivatives as radioprotectors.[168] One of these compounds, WR2721, 5-2-(3-aminopropylamino)-[H$_2$N(CH$_2$)$_3$NH(CH$_2$)$_2$-S-PO$_3$H$_2$], has been shown to dephosphorylate selectively in normal tissues through catalysis by alkaline phosphatase.[169] This agent, with the generic name of amifostine, is approved for ameliorating renal toxicity in patients receiving cisplatin, and for reducing xerostomia in patients receiving head and neck irradiation. In experimental tumors, it enhanced the antitumor activity of many alkylating agents,[170] and in clinical trials, it showed some modest effect on the neutropenia caused by cyclophosphamide but failed to produce measurable benefit in patients receiving combined radiochemotherapy (with cisplatin and cyclophosphamide) and those with head and neck cancer.[171] Similarly, its ability to reduce toxicity of high-dose chemotherapy with HCT remains unproven.[172]

Inhibition of DNA Alkyl Adduct Repair

As discussed previously, silencing of MGMT by methylation of its promoter ablates expression of AGT, a key repair enzyme for alkylation adducts of O^6-guanine, and correlates with sensitivity of human gliomas to treatment with various drugs, including BCNU and temozolomide.[82,173] Preclinical data support the concept that inhibition of AGT sensitizes human glioma xenograft to the same drugs and that resistance can be restored by mutations in AGT that decrease binding of inhibitors to the enzyme. AGT binds irreversibly to these guanine adducts and is permanently inactivated in the process. Small molecular weight analogs of O^6-methyl guanine can inactivate AGT and sensitize tumor cells. The most potent of these inhibitors is O^6-benzyl guanine (OBG), a compound that has reached clinical development. Its evaluation has been slowed by uncertainty regarding the optimal dose in combination with chemotherapy drugs. A trial with BCNU and OBG (120 mg/m^2) in patients with multiple myeloma depleted AGT by 94% in bone marrow tumor cells but produced responses in only 4 of 17 patients.[174] OBG clearly enhances BCNU toxicity, but clinical evidence for sensitization of tumors is still lacking.[175]

Inhibition of BER

BER is one of the fundamental mechanisms for removing nonbulky DNA adducts, as created by oxidative stress and reactive molecules. This multistep pathway begins when alkylated bases are excised by lesion-specific glycosylases to create apurinic/apyrimidinic (AP) sites. These sites are then substrates for endonuclease cleavage of the phosphodiester backbone, creating single-strand breaks. The single-strand break is identified by poly-adenosine diphosphate-ribose polymerase (PARP, an essential component of BER. Binding of PARP to strand breaks promotes poly(ADP) ribosylation of nuclear accessory proteins, forming negatively charged branch polymers that recruit enzymes that accomplish repair of the gap. The gap is filled by reading off the complementary DNA strand, and the single strand is resealed. If the BER system is blocked by inhibitors of one of the important components in the pathway, single-strand breaks accumulate and may be converted into double-strand breaks by an encounter with a replication fork.

Inhibitors of various steps in BER have been identified. The first of these was methoxyamine, an orally available compound that binds to the aldehydic oxygen of the AP site and prevents access of BER enzymes.[176] In model systems, methoxyamine leads to accumulation of DNA breaks and potentiates the cytotoxicity of alkylating agents. It has entered clinical trials, with temozolomide. Potent inhibitors of PARP have been discovered by several pharmaceutical companies and have entered advanced stages of clinical evaluation. By inactivating BER, these compounds create a flurry of single-strand and ultimately double-strand breaks (dsb) in cells deficient in dsb repair. In preclinical experiments, they enhance the activity of methylating agents and sensitize cells to DNA damage, even in the presence of high levels of expression of AGT,[177–182] and are particularly effective against cells defective in dsb repair. One compound, olaparib, has clear single-agent activity in ovarian cancer patients who have mutations in the BRCA 1 or BRCA 2 gene, which are components of the dsb complex.[177] Another compound of this class, BSI201, dramatically enhanced activity of chemotherapy and prolonged survival of triple negative breast cancer patients (negative for estrogen and progesterone receptors and negative for HER 2/neu amplification) who received carboplatin and gemcitabine.[178] These promising agents will undergo extensive evaluation with temozolomide, cyclophosphamide, and the platinum analogs.

Inhibition of AKT

Based on experimental evidence that the PI3Kinase pathway, including AKT, promotes survival and DNA repair, inhibitors of AKT and the downstream mTOR have been evaluated as chemosensitizers for alkylating agents.[183–186] Akt inhibitors such as LY294002 and wortmannin, and inhibitors of mTOR (the rapamycin analogs) enhanced sensitivity to temozolomide, the nitrosoureas, and cisplatin in various human tumor cell lines. Inhibitors of the PI3K pathway are in early stages of clinical development as single agents, and the rapamycin analogs, approved for single-agent treatment of renal cell cancer, are being evaluated in combination with alkylating agents and platinum analogs.

Clinical Pharmacology

The primary pharmacokinetics properties of standard alkylating agents are given in Table 14A-1. Although some agents are too reactive chemically to provide more than momentary exposure of tumor cells to parent drug (the best examples are mechlorethamine and BCNU), others are stable in their parent form and even others require metabolic activation, as in the case of cyclophosphamide and ifosfamide. Doses of some alkylating agents may need to be adjusted for organ dysfunction and may require pharmacokinetic monitoring in individual patients, as with high-dose busulfan, to execute rational treatment regimens.

Activation, Decomposition, and Metabolism

Decomposition Versus Metabolism

A principal route of degradation of most of the reactive alkylating agents is spontaneous hydrolysis of the alkylating entity (i.e., alkylation by water). For example, mechlorethamine rapidly undergoes reaction to produce 2-hydroxyethyl-2-chloroethylmethylamine and bis-2-hydroxyethylmethylamine (Fig. 14A-9). Likewise, both melphalan and chlorambucil undergo similar hydrolysis to form the monohydroxyethyl and bishydroxyethyl products, although less rapidly than the aliphatic nitrogen mustards.[187,188] The mono hydroxylated products are less active alkylators than their chloroalkyl precursors.

Most alkylating agents also undergo some degree of enzymatic metabolism. For example, if mechlorethamine radiolabeled in the methyl group is administered to mice, approximately 15% of the radioactivity can be recovered as exhaled carbon dioxide, which indicates that enzymatic demethylation is occurring. For the phosphoramide mustards and nitrosoureas, enzymatic metabolism plays a significant role in determining their pharmacokinetic profile.

Cyclophosphamide and Ifosfamide

Cyclophosphamide is activated to alkylating and cytotoxic metabolites by cytochrome P450 isozymes 2B6, 2C9, and 3A4.[189] The complex metabolic transformations are illustrated in Figure 14A-10. The initial metabolic step is the oxidation of the ring carbon adjacent to the nitrogen to produce 4-hydroxycyclophosphamide, which establishes equilibrium with aldophosphamide. Aldophosphamide undergoes a spontaneous (nonenzymatic) elimination reaction to form phosphoramide mustard and acrolein. Phosphoramide mustard, which is generally believed to be the DNA cross-linking agent of clinical significance, is a circulating metabolite that does not enter cells easily due to its anionic form. Thus, the intracellular generation of phosphoramide mustard from aldophosphamide is believed to be important to a therapeutic result. A major detoxification route is the oxidation of aldophosphamide to the inactive carboxyphosphamide by ALDH1A1 and, to a much lesser extent, by ALDH3A1 and ALDH5A1 in liver and in red blood cells. The concentration of ALDH in a variety of cell types appears inversely proportional to cytotoxicity, supporting its crucial role in determining cytotoxicity.[93] The high enzyme concentration in hematopoietic progenitor cells may explain the ability of cyclophosphamide to produce major myelosuppression without myeloablation in patients receiving high doses without transplantation.[190] Likewise, cancer stem cells expressing ALDH may also be drug resistant.

Multiple metabolites can react with glutathione (GSH). Some of these reactions with GSH may be reversible while others are irreversible; the latter are associated with detoxification pathways. Several-fold differences in the extent of metabolite formation have been observed among patients and these interindividual differences may be due to polymorphisms in cytochrome P450 enzymes (see Chapter 4). CYP3A4 and 3A5 genotypes may influence response or survival in patients treated with cyclophosphamide.

A minor (~10%) alternative oxidative pathway leads to N-dechloroethylation and the formation of the neurotoxic chloroacetaldehyde. Cytochrome P450 3A4 is the main enzyme responsible for this undesirable secondary oxidation with a minor contribution from cytochrome P450 2B6.

The metabolism of ifosfamide (Fig. 14A-11) parallels that of cyclophosphamide but with some differences in isozyme specificities and reaction kinetics. Activation of ifosfamide to 4-hydroxyifosfamide is catalyzed by the hepatic cytochrome P450 isoform 3A4. Aldo-ifosfamide partitions between ALDH1A1-mediated detoxification to carboxyifosfamide and a spontaneous (nonenzymatic) elimination reaction to yield isophosphoramide mustard and acrolein. Isophosphoramide is the DNA cross-linking agent of clinical significance. Hydroxylation proceeds at a slower rate for ifosfamide than for cyclophosphamide, which results in a longer plasma half-life for the parent compound. Dechloroethylation of ifosfamide produces inactive metabolites (primarily mediated by cytochrome

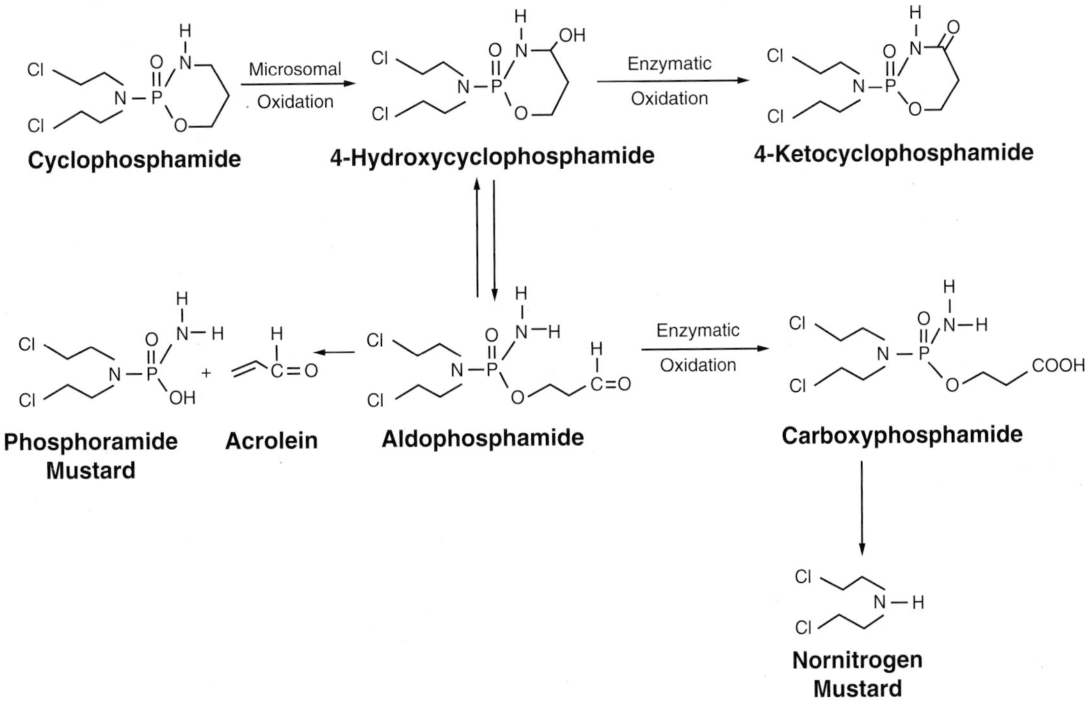

FIGURE **14A-10** Metabolism of cyclophosphamide.

P450 isozyme 2B6 and 3A4) and competes with the activation step as a major pathway of elimination.[191–194]

Both cyclophosphamide (above doses of 4 g/m^2) and ifosfamide (above doses of 5 g/m^2) exhibit dose-dependent nonlinear pharmacokinetics, with significant delays in elimination at higher doses.[195] Interestingly, both drugs also induce their own metabolism, resulting in significant shortening of the elimination half-life for the parent compound when the drugs are administered on multiple consecutive days.[196]

Both agents can undergo further chemical reaction to form acrolein, which is toxic to bladder. This compound may also form O^6G adducts, and these may be recognized and removed by AGT.

Nitrosoureas

The decomposition of nitrosoureas to generate the alkylating chloroethyldiazonium hydroxide entity has been mentioned, and the products generated by this decomposition in aqueous solution are illustrated in Figure 14A-12.

The nitrosoureas also undergo metabolic transformation. BCNU can be inactivated through denitrosation reactions catalyzed by both cytosolic and microsomal enzymes. Class μ glutathione S-transferase is a major catalyst of the cytosolic denitrosation reaction. Enhancement of P450 activity in vivo by phenobarbital abolished the therapeutic effect of BCNU against the 9L intracerebral rat tumor and decreased the therapeutic activity of CCNU and BCNU against this tumor.[197] The phenobarbital-treated rats had increased plasma clearance of BCNU. The plasma clearance of parent BCNU decreases and the plasma half-life increases as doses escalate from standard-dose (150 to 200 mg/m^2) to high-dose regimens (600 mg/m^2) (Table 14A-1).

CCNU and methyl-CCNU undergo hydroxylation of their cyclohexyl ring to produce a series of metabolites that represent

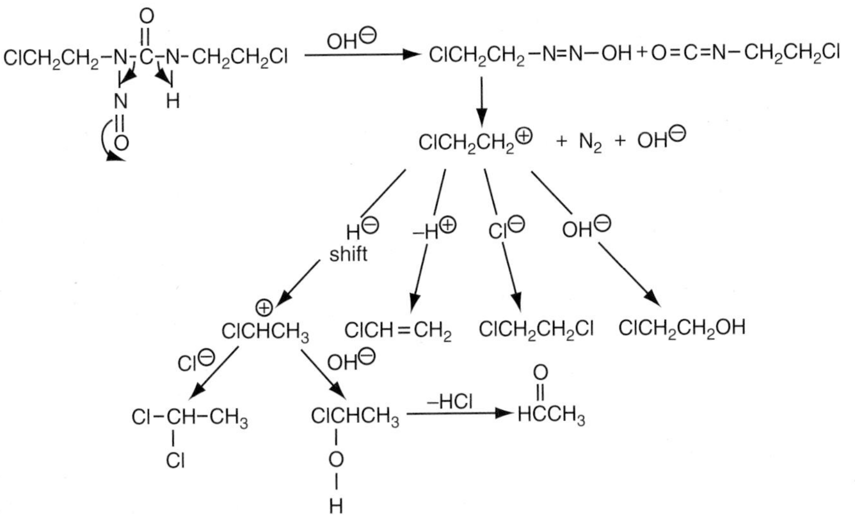

FIGURE **14A-11** Metabolic activation of ifosfamide to its active form, 4-hydroxyifosfamide, and further metabolic transformation to chloracetaldehyde and other end products. NADPH, reduced form of nicotinamide adenine dinucleotide phosphate.

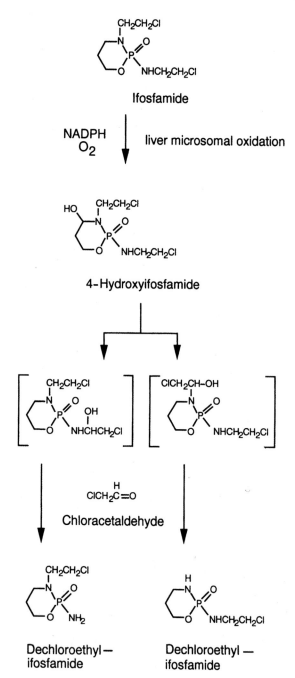

FIGURE 14A-12 Decomposition of bischloroethylnitrosourea (BCNU) in buffered aqueous solution.

the major circulating species after treatment with these drugs.[198] These metabolites have increased alkylating activity but diminished carbamoylating effects.[198]

Clinical Pharmacokinetics

Gas chromatography–mass spectrometry and high-pressure liquid chromatography (HPLC) have generated pharmacokinetic information (Table 14A-1) for alkylating agents and their metabolites.

Melphalan

In patients who received 0.6 mg/kg of the drug intravenously, the peak levels of melphalan, as measured by HPLC, were 4.5 to

13 μmol/L (1.4 to 4.1 μg/mL), and the mean terminal-phase half-life ($t_{1/2\beta}$) of the drug in the plasma was 1 hour. Dose adjustment is not indicated at conventional doses, but in high-dose regimens, there are conflicting data regarding adjustment for renal function.[199] The 24-hour urinary excretion of the parent drug averaged 13% of the administered dose. Inactive monohydroxy and dihydroxy metabolites appear in plasma within minutes of drug administration.[170]

Other studies have demonstrated low and variable systemic availability of the drug after oral dosing.[187,200] Food slows its absorption. After oral administration of melphalan, 0.6 mg/kg, much lower peak levels of drug of approximately 1 μmol/L (0.3 μg/mL) were seen. The time to achieve peak plasma levels varied considerably and occurred as late as 6 hours after dosing. The low bioavailability was caused by incomplete absorption of the drug from the gastrointestinal tract because 20% to 50% of an oral dose could be recovered in the feces.[200] Regional administration of melphalan is possible by both intracavitary[201] and limb perfusion methods.[202]

Chlorambucil

After the oral administration of 0.6 mg/kg of chlorambucil,[187,188] peak levels of 2.0 to 6.3 μmol/L (0.6 to 1.9 μg/mL) occur within 1 hour. Peak plasma levels of phenylacetic acid mustard, an oxidation product of chlorambucil with alkylating activity, range from 1.8 to 4.3 μmol/L (0.5 to 1.18 μg/mL), and the peak levels of this metabolite are achieved 2 to 4 hours after dosing. The terminal-phase half-lives for chlorambucil and phenylacetic acid mustard are 92 and 145 minutes, respectively. Less than 1% of the administered dose of chlorambucil is excreted in the urine as either chlorambucil (0.54%) or phenylacetic acid mustard (0.25%). Approximately 50% of the radioactivity from carbon-14–labeled chlorambucil administered orally is excreted in the urine in 24 hours. Of this material, over 90% appears to be the monohydroxy and dihydroxy hydrolysis products of chlorambucil and phenylacetic acid mustard.

Cyclophosphamide

Cyclophosphamide is well absorbed after oral administration to humans[196] The systemic availability of the unchanged drug after oral administration of 100-mg doses (1 to 2 mg/kg) was 97% of that after intravenous injection of the same dose.[196] Juma et al.[203] found the systemic availability of the drug to be somewhat less and more variable (mean, 74%; range, 34% to 90%) after oral administration of larger doses of 300 mg (3 to 6 mg/kg). A comparison of oral versus intravenous cyclophosphamide in the same patient revealed no difference in the AUC for the primary cytotoxic metabolites, hydroxycyclophosphamide and phosphoramide mustard.[204] After intravenous administration, the peak plasma levels of the parent compound are dose dependent. Peak levels are 4, 50, and 500 nmol/mL (Table 14A-2) after the administration of 1 to 2,[196] 6 to 15,[203] and 60 mg/kg,[205] respectively. The terminal-phase half-life of cyclophosphamide varies considerably among patients (3 to 10 hours). In patients less than 19 years of age, the plasma half-life of parent drug is 1.5 hours.[206] Less than 15% of the parent drug is eliminated in the urine; the major site of clearance is the liver. Peak alkylating levels are achieved 2 to 3 hours after drug administration and the terminal half-life of plasma alkylating activity is 7.7 hours with a plateau-like level of plasma alkylating activity maintained for at least 6 hours.

TABLE

14B.3 *Key features of dacarbazine [5-(3,3-dimethyl-1-triazeno) imidazole-4-carboxamide, DTIC, DIC, NSC-45388]*

Factor	Result
Mechanism of action	Metabolic activation probably required; methylation of nucleic acids; direct DNA damage; inhibition of purine synthesis.
Metabolism	Oxidative *N*-methylation to 5-aminoimidazole-4-carboxamide via formation of 5(3-hydroxymethyl-3-methyltriazen-1-yl) imidazole-4-carboxamide and 5-(3-methyltriazen-2-yl) imidazole-4-carboxamide.
	$t_{1/2}\alpha$ = 3 min; $t_{1/2}\beta$ = 41 min
	V_d = 0.6 L/kg; Cl = 15 mL/kg/min
	20% protein bound
	Variable oral absorption.
	Poor CSF penetration (plasma/CSF ratio = 7:1 at equilibrium).
Elimination	Renal excretion: 50% as unchanged dacarbazine and 9%–18% as 5-aminoimidazole-4-carboxamide.
	Minor hepatobiliary and pulmonary excretion.
Drug and food interactions	*Corynebacterium parvum* may prolong $t_{1/2}$.
Toxicity	Myelosuppression.
	Gastrointestinal (nausea and vomiting).
	Influenza-like syndrome (fever, myalgia, and malaise).
	Infrequent alopecia, cutaneous hypersensitivity, or photosensitivity.
	Rare hepatic vein thrombosis and hepatic necrosis.
	Possible carcinogenesis and teratogenesis.
Precautions	Dose modification may be necessary in hepatic and/or renal dysfunction.

Cl, clearance; CSF, cerebrospinal fluid; $t_{1/2}$, half-life; V_d, apparent volume of distribution.

for use in these two diseases. It is frequently used alone or in combination with agents such as nitrosoureas, bleomycin, and vinca alkaloids in melanoma,[85,88] and it is most commonly used as part of the doxorubicin, bleomycin, vinblastine, and DTIC (ABVD) and actinomycin D, bleomycin, and vincristine regimens for Hodgkin's disease.[89,90] In addition, DTIC has demonstrated activity in the treatment of sarcomas,[91–93] childhood neuroblastoma,[94,95] and primary brain tumors.[96] It may be the most active agent alone or in combination for the treatment of malignant amine precursor uptake and decarboxylation and other neuroendocrine tumors.[97–99] The key features of DTIC are summarized in Table 14B-3.

General Mechanism of Action and Cellular Pharmacology

The exact mechanism underlying DTIC's antitumor activity remains an enigma. Although DTIC was developed as a purine antimetabolite, there is abundant evidence that its antitumor activity does not result from interference with purine synthesis. The drug is active against several cell lines resistant to the purine analogs 6-thioguanine and 6-mercaptopurine, and it does not demonstrate cell-cycle schedule dependence observed with other antimetabolites.[81] Second, the AIC portion of the molecule is not necessary for antitumor activity.[100,101]

There is mounting evidence to suggest that, similar to PCB, the production of O^6-methylguanine is the primary cytotoxic event

after administration of DTIC. Xenografts, or cell lines with negligible levels of AGT, are more sensitive to DTIC than are xenografts or cell lines with high levels of AGT.[102–107] Furthermore, DTIC depletes AGT levels in human colon cancer HT 29 xenografts in athymic mice[108] and in human peripheral blood cells in patients treated for metastatic melanoma.[109]

The previously mentioned work[102–107] supporting O^6-methylguanine as the major cytotoxic lesion produced by DTIC strongly suggests that elevated levels of AGT may be responsible for resistance to this agent. The inverse relationship between AGT levels and response to DTIC in human xenografts also may be operational in clinical tumor resistance to DTIC.[102–107] Furthermore, resistance to all methylators, including DTIC, is seen in the setting of a deficiency of DNA mismatch repair.[34–36] Finally, Lev et al.[110] have reported DTIC resistance mediated by upregulation of interleukin-8 and vascular endothelial growth factor in melanoma cells.

Drug Interactions

At present, there are no known drug or food interactions with DTIC that are of clinical importance. Because DTIC has been used in conjunction with immune adjuvants in the treatment of malignant melanoma, there has been some interest in the influence of these agents on DTIC pharmacology. Farquhar and coworkers described an inhibition of DTIC *N*-demethylase in rats pretreated with bacillus Calmette-Guérin (BCG), suggesting that patients receiving both agents may be less able to activate DTIC. In four patients with melanoma, BCG did not seem to influence DTIC pharmacokinetics, although altered metabolism per se was not examined. In contrast, patients receiving *Corynebacterium parvum* adjuvant immunotherapy did show a prolongation of DTIC serum half-life consistent with the ability of *C. parvum* to depress hepatic microsomal N-demethylation of a variety of drugs. Although the initial step for metabolic activation of DTIC is catalyzed by microsomal cytochrome P-450, the interaction of phenobarbital, or other commonly used cytochrome P-450–inducing agents, with DTIC has not been reported.

DTIC activity against L1210 murine leukemia is potentiated by alkylating agents, such as melphalan, and by doxorubicin.[81] Activity is also enhanced when DTIC is combined with the nitrosoureas bischloromethyl-nitrosourea (BCNU) and chloroethylcyclohexylnitrosourea (CCNU). The mechanism(s) for the potentiation observed using these combinations may be related to the ability of nitrosoureas to deplete AGT and thereby sensitize cells to methylating agents.

Clinical Pharmacology

DTIC is supplied in sterile vials containing 100 or 200 mg DTIC for intravenous administration. As a single agent, a dose of up to 1,500 mg/m^2 of body surface area may be given as a single bolus as opposed to the more frequently used schedule of 250 mg/m^2 daily for 5 days every 3 to 4 weeks.[86,88,92,111] The latter schedule was developed in an attempt to minimize the gastrointestinal toxicity from DTIC, which tends to lessen with repeated administration. Most studies, however, fail to show any significant schedule dependency with respect to antitumor efficacy or toxicity.[86,88] DTIC also has been used by intra-arterial infusion for the regional treatment of malignant melanoma involving liver, pelvis, the maxillofacial region, and extremities with high response rates in uncontrolled series.[112–115] It is not known whether in situ melanoma cells in humans are capable of metabolizing DTIC[116]; otherwise, these results are difficult to interpret because DTIC requires metabolic activation for its antitumor activity.

Initial studies of DTIC pharmacokinetics and metabolism in rodents, dogs, and humans used radiochemical and colorimetric methods. More recently, improved experimental methods, such as HPLC and mass spectroscopy, have been used to study triazine pharmacology. Because of the scarcity of clinical studies using adequately sensitive and specific techniques, knowledge of DTIC pharmacology in humans remains incomplete. After oral administration, the drug is absorbed slowly and variably; therefore, intravenous administration is the preferred route. Intravenous boluses of 2.65 to 6.85 mg/kg (~120 to 300 mg/m^2) produced peak plasma concentrations of nearly 10 to over 30 μg/mL, respectively. After intravenous administration of DTIC, Breithaupt et al. found a biphasic plasma disappearance of the parent drug consistent with a two-compartment model with an initial half-life of 3 minutes and a terminal half-life of 41 minutes (Fig. 14B-3). This is in contrast to a terminal half-life of 3.2 hours found in an earlier study using HPLC[117] analysis. Approximately 20% of DTIC is loosely bound to plasma protein.[118] In humans, the mean volume of distribution for DTIC was 0.6 L/kg, and the total-body clearance was 15.4 mL/kg/min. In one study, approximately 50% of an intravenous dose of DTIC was recovered in the urine as parent drug, and the renal clearance was calculated to be between 5 and 10 mL/kg/min, confirming earlier reports that tubular secretion may be involved in the renal excretion of DTIC. Altered schedules of intravenous drug administration did not change the area under the curve (concentration × time), confirming a lack of schedule dependence for DTIC pharmacokinetics.[119]

In dogs[118] and humans,[86] DTIC penetrates poorly into the CSF. At equilibrium, the ratio between plasma and spinal fluid was 7:1. This finding may explain the lack of DTIC activity against intracranial L1210 leukemia.[81] It fails to explain, however, the observations that DTIC has activity against transplantable murine ependymoblastoma[120] and against primary and metastatic brain tumors in humans.[83,87,96]

The major metabolite of DTIC found in plasma and urine is AIC (Fig. 14B-3) with cumulative excretion in the urine accounting for 9% to 20% of parent compound in several patients studied. AIC is also formed from DTIC in the presence of liver microsomes and by some tumor cells. After the intraperitoneal administration of [^{14}CO-methyl]DTIC to rats or mice, 4% of the dose is recovered as respiratory ^{14}CO$_2$ in 6 hours, and 9% of the dose is recovered as ^{14}CO$_2$ in 24 hours. Presumably, the expired radiolabeled ^{14}CO$_2$ is derived from the formaldehyde produced after N-demethylation of DTIC. These findings, as well as the identification of 5-(3-hydroxymethyl-3-methyltriazen-1-yl) imidazole-4-carboxamide (HMTIC) as a urinary metabolite of DTIC in rats, are consistent with a metabolic pathway for DTIC, as shown in Figure 14B-4, in which MTIC is the primary active metabolite, responsible for transferring its methyl group to DNA.

Toxicity

The most frequent toxic reaction to DTIC treatment is moderately severe nausea and vomiting, which occurs in 90% of patients.[92] These symptoms appear soon after infusion and may persist for up to 12 hours. The severity of gastrointestinal toxicity decreases with successive doses when the drug is given on a 5-day schedule and if the initial dose is decreased. Above 1,200 mg/m^2 as a rapid intravenous bolus, DTIC frequently causes severe, but short-lived, watery diarrhea.[86] After rapid infusion of a high-dose (>1,380 mg/m^2) of DTIC, hypotension may occur.

Myelosuppression is a common dose-related toxicity of DTIC, although the degree of leukopenia and thrombocytopenia is variably mild to moderate. Significant myelosuppression occurs when more than 1,380 mg/m^2 is given as a single intravenous bolus, whereas studies using a 5-day administration schedule reported increasing frequency of myelosuppression above a total of 1,000 mg/m^2.[86,92] In the latter, nadir leukopenia and thrombocytopenia occurred on day 25, with complete recovery by day 40. This delayed bone marrow recovery is not common, however, and usually there is sufficient recovery so that DTIC may be administered every 21 to 28 days.

Less frequent toxic reactions include a flulike syndrome of fever up to 39°C, myalgias, and malaise lasting several days after DTIC treatment. Headache, facial flushing, facial paresthesias, pain along the injection vein, alopecia, and abnormal hepatic and renal function tests rarely occur. Photosensitivity to DTIC has been reported in several patients, especially after high-dose therapy.[121] Therefore, patients should be advised to avoid sunlight exposure for several days after DTIC therapy. Cases of hepatic vein occlusion associated

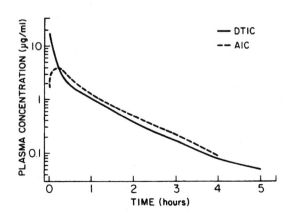

DACARBAZINE

uv

5-DIAZOIMIDAZOLE-4-CARBOXAMIDE

+ $HN(CH_3)_2$

CYT. P-450

5-(3-HYDROXYMETHYL-3-METHYLTRIAZEN-1-YL)IMIDAZOLE-4-CARBOXAMIDE

2-AZAHYPOXANTHINE

5-(3-METHYLTRIAZEN-2-YL)IMIDAZOLE-4-CARBOXAMIDE

+ CH_2O

5-AMINOIMIDAZOLE-4-CARBOXAMIDE

+ $N \equiv N^+ CH_3$

$N_2 + [^+CH_3]$

FIGURE 14B-3 Plasma concentrations of dacarbazine (DTIC) and 5-aminoimidazole-4-carboxamide (AIC) in a patient after administration of dacarbazine, 6.34 mg/kg, intravenously. (From Breithaupt H, Dammann A, Aigner K. Pharmacokinetics of dacarbazine [DTIC] and its metabolite 5-aminoimidazole-4-carboxamide [AIC] following different dose schedules. Cancer Chemother Pharmacol 1982;9:103.)

with fever, eosinophilia, and hepatic necrosis and resulting in death have been attributed to DTIC as a distinct clinical pathologic syndrome.[122–126] The mechanism for this toxicity is unknown, but an allergic etiology has been suggested.[122,126]

FIGURE 14B-4 Light-activated and metabolic reactions of dacarbazine, leading to the generation of reactive intermediates. CYT, cytochrome; UV, ultraviolet.

DTIC causes a number of immunologic effects in vitro and in vivo. The drug markedly depresses antibody responses and allograft rejection in mice for up to 60 days after a single injection. This is probably a specific effect of DTIC because structure activity studies showed different patterns of immunodepression depending on which phenyltriazene analog was tested. DTIC apparently does not directly suppress natural killer cell activity in mice. After DTIC treatment, L1210 or L5178 lymphomas were found to be highly immunogenic such that large inocula of the DTIC-resistant tumors were rejected by immunocompetent animals. DTIC-treated cells were actually less susceptible to natural killer cell cytolysis in vitro.

DTIC has mutagenic, carcinogenic, and teratogenic properties in experimental systems.[127,128] In rodents, DTIC causes lymphoma and tumors of the thymus, lung, uterus, or mammary glands when given orally or by single or multiple injections.[101] MTIC treatment also caused similar tumors but in a lower frequency compared with DTIC.[129] It is not firmly established whether DTIC is carcinogenic for humans. In a retrospective analysis of patients receiving either MOPP or ABVD (plus or minus radiation therapy) for Hodgkin's disease, Valagussa et al.[130] reported no treatment-associated secondary malignancies in patients receiving ABVD. Subsequently, isolated cases of acute leukemia occurring after DTIC therapy have been reported,[131,132] but these remain rare. Finally, DTIC causes dose-dependent fetal malformations and fetal resorptions when administered to pregnant rats and rabbits.[133,134] Teratogenic effects were observed in the urogenital system, skeleton, eye, and cardiovascular system.

Temozolomide

History

Several series of 1,2,4-triazines and 1,2,4-triazinones were synthesized in England in the 1960s and 1970s, and selected compounds proved to have activity against murine tumors.[135–139] The most promising was mitozolomide, which was active against a broad spectrum of murine tumors,[137] but it produced severe and unpredictable thrombocytopenia in clinical trials and was abandoned as a clinical candidate.[138]

Selection of the next generation of imidazotetrazinones focused on TMZ, the 3-methyl derivative of mitozolomide (Fig. 14B-5). This compound, with a different spectrum of activity against murine tumors,[140] was less active and considerably less toxic than mitozolomide and displayed superb delivery to all body tissues, including the brain;[141,142] TMZ was rationally advanced to clinical trial, partly based on the realization that under physiologic conditions, the ring opens with resulting generation of the monomethyl triazine MTIC, the same metabolite formed by metabolic dealkylation of DTIC.[143] The inefficient demethylation of DTIC in humans (despite rapid demethylation in mice) coupled with the conversion of TMZ to MTIC without need for this metabolic step suggested a potential benefit for the use of TMZ. Table 14B-4 lists the key features of TMZ.

Phase 1 trials of intravenous and subsequently oral TMZ began in 1987 with a single-dose schedule and demonstrated the dose-limiting toxicity to be myelosuppression with trivial clinical benefits observed.[144] However, based on preclinical data supporting a multiple-dose regimen, another phase 1 trial using a 5-day schedule was conducted, with myelosuppression again the dose-limiting toxicity. Greater clinical activity was noted with four responses (two partial and two complete) in 23 patients with metastatic melanoma and two partial responses in four patients with high-grade glioma.[144]

Further evaluation in 28 patients with primary brain tumors revealed five radiographic responses in 10 patients with recurrent

TABLE **14B.4**	*Key features of temozolomide {8-carbamoyl-3-methylimidazo [5,1-D]-1,2,3,5-tetrazin-4(3H)-one}*
Factor	**Result**
Mechanism of action	Methylation of nucleic acids
Metabolism	Chemical conversion of 5(3-methyltriazeno) imidazole-4-carboxamide
Pharmacokinetics (IV or PO)	Volume of distribution: 28.3 L
	Elimination half-life: 1.8 h
	Distribution half-life: 0.26 h
	Clearance: 11.76 L/h[253]
Drug and food interactions	Unknown
Toxicity	Myelosuppression
	Nausea and vomiting
	Elevated hepatic transaminases

IV, intravenously; PO, per os.

astrocytoma (the majority of which were high-grade type). Similarly, four radiographic responses were seen in seven patients with newly diagnosed high-grade glioma.[145] It should be noted that radiographic criteria for response were not the conventionally accepted partial or complete response criteria. Nevertheless, these results are provocative and justified further studies in patients with CNS tumors, particularly gliomas.

This study of O'Reilly et al.[145] was extended to 75 patients (48 with recurrent disease and 27 with new diagnoses).[146] Improvements on computed tomography (CT) were seen in 12 (25%) of the patients with recurrent disease and in eight (30%) of the patients with new diagnoses. Twenty-two percent of patients with recurrences and 43% of those with newly diagnosed tumors survived to 1 year.

The Cancer Research Campaign (CRC) conducted a multicenter phase 2 study in which TMZ demonstrated activity in patients with recurrent and progressive high-grade glioma.[147] Objective responses, measured by improvement in neurologic status, were seen in 11 of 103 patients (11%) who received TMZ; five of these patients had improvement on CT or magnetic resonance imaging (MRI) scans.[147] Objective responses were observed in patients in whom anaplastic astrocytoma, glioblastoma multiforme (grade IV), and unclassified high-grade astrocytoma (grades III–IV) were diagnosed.

The Schering-Plough Research Institute conducted a randomized, multicenter, open-label phase 2 study of TMZ and PCB in 225 patients with glioblastoma multiforme (GBM) at first relapse.[148] The primary objectives were to compare the progression-free survival at 6 months and safety of TMZ and PCB in adult patients with GBM who had failed conventional treatment. The 6-month progression-free survival rate was significantly higher for patients who received TMZ (21%) than for those who received PCB (8%) ($P = 0.008$). Median progression-free survival for TMZ patients (12.4 weeks) was significantly longer than for PCB patients (8.32 weeks; $P = 0.0063$). The 6-month overall survival rate for TMZ patients was 60% versus 44% for PCB patients ($P = 0.019$).

The Schering-Plough Research Institute also conducted an open-label, multicenter phase 2 trial comprising 162 patients with malignant astrocytoma at first relapse.[149] The primary protocol end point, progression-free survival at 6 months, was 46% [95% confidence limit (CL), 38% to 54%]. The median progression-free survival was 5.4 months, and 24% of patients remained progression-free at 12 months based on Kaplan-Meier estimates. Additional studies have extended these results in newly diagnosed patients.[150,151]

Duke University participated in a Schering-Plough Research Institute multicenter phase II trial evaluating the activity of TMZ *before* radiation therapy in the treatment of newly diagnosed high-grade glioma.[152] Eligibility criteria included residual enhancing disease on postoperative MRI and a Karnofsky performance score (KPS) ≥70%. Thirty-three patients with GBM evaluated for tumor response revealed 3 with complete response, 14 with partial response, 4 with stable disease, and 12 with progressive disease. Five patients with anaplastic astrocytoma evaluated for response revealed one with partial response, two with stable disease, and two with progressive disease. These results with patients with glioblastoma multiforme have been extended to phase 3 trials, confirming an increase in survival when TMZ is used in an adjuvant setting.[153,154]

This latter trial was a randomized phase 3 trial for newly diagnosed adults with glioblastoma conducted by the European Organization for Research and Treatment of Cancer (EORTC) and the National Cancer Institute of Canada. The addition of TMZ given during and after radiotherapy (for 6 months) increased median survival from 12 (radiotherapy alone) to 14.5 months (radiotherapy plus TMZ). The survival rate at 2 years increased from 10% with radiotherapy alone to 27% with radiotherapy plus TMZ. This overnight became the gold standard for patients with newly diagnosed glioblastoma. A subsequent analysis utilizing the RTOG recursive partitioning analysis (RPA) criteria[155] revealed that as the RPA class increased from 3 to 4 to 5, the 2-year survival rate of the combined therapy fell from 43.4% to 27.9% to 16.5%.[156] Accordingly, TMZ is most effective in patients with better prognostic features.

A more recent update showed that the benefits of TMZ with radiotherapy lasted at least for 5 years with occasional patients surviving longer than 5 years.[157]

Furthermore, TMZ has been shown to be active in the treatment of other primary brain tumors, including low-grade glioma,[158,159] oligodendroglioma,[160,161] and meningioma.[162]

The efficacy of TMZ has also been evaluated in a study of patients with advanced metastatic melanoma, including patients with brain metastases.[163] Among 56 patients (49 with evaluable lesions), complete responses occurred in 3, all with lung metastases only, and partial responses occurred in 9, yielding a response rate of 21%. Stable disease was observed in an additional eight patients. A more recent review demonstrated responses but no increase in overall survival.[164]

General Mechanism of Action and Cellular Pharmacology

The spontaneous conversion of TMZ is initiated by the effect of water at the highly electropositive C^4 position of TMZ. This activity opens the ring, releases CO_2, and generates the reactive methylating agent MTIC. The initial proposal was that this effect of water was catalyzed in the close environment of the major groove of DNA,[165,166] but confirming this mechanism has been difficult, and it is known that TMZ converts readily to MTIC in free solution in the absence of DNA.[167] MTIC degrades to the methyldiazonium cation, which transfers the methyl group to DNA and to the final degradation product AIC, which is excreted via the kidneys.[168,169] The methylation of DNA appears to be the principal mechanism responsible for the cytotoxicity of TMZ to malignant cells (see following discussion). The methyldiazonium cation can also react with RNA and with soluble and cellular proteins.[170] However, the methylation of RNA and the methylation or carbamoylation of protein do not appear to have any known significant role in the antitumor activity of TMZ.[170] Further studies are required to clarify the role of these targets in the biochemical mechanism of action of TMZ.

The spontaneous conversion of TMZ and MTIC depends on pH. Under acidic conditions, TMZ is stable; however, its chemical stability decreases at a pH of greater than 7.0 and is converted rapidly to MTIC in that environment.[168] In contrast, MTIC is more stable under basic conditions and rapidly degrades to the methyldiazonium cation and AIC at a pH of less than 7.0.[168] A comparison of the half-life of TMZ in phosphate buffer (pH, 7.4; $t_{1/2} = 1.83$ hours)[144,168] indicates that the conversion of TMZ to MTIC is a chemically controlled reaction with little or no enzymatic component. The spontaneous conversion of TMZ may contribute to its highly reproducible pharmacokinetics in comparison with other alkylating agents such as DTIC and PCB, which must undergo metabolic conversion in the liver and are thus subject to interpatient variation in metabolic rates of conversion.[166,168]

Among the lesions produced in DNA after treatment of cells with TMZ, the most common is methylation at the N^7 position of guanine, followed by methylation at the O^3 position of adenine and the O^6 position of guanine.[168] Although the N^7-methylguanine and O^3-methyladenine adducts probably contribute to the antitumor activity of TMZ in some, if not all, sensitive cells, their role is controversial.[171] The critical role of the O^6-methylguanine adduct, which accounts for 5% of the total adducts formed by TMZ,[168] in the agent's antitumor activity is supported by the correlation between the sensitivity of tumor cell lines to TMZ and the activity of the DNA repair protein AGT, which specifically removes alkyl groups at the O^6 position of guanine. Cell lines that have low levels of AGT are sensitive to the cytotoxicity of TMZ, whereas cell lines that have high levels of this repair protein are much more resistant to it.[172–175] This correlation also has been observed in human glioblastoma xenograft models.[176–178] The preferential alkylation of guanine and adenine and the correlation of sensitivity to the drug with the ability to repair the O^6-alkylguanine lesion also have been seen with triazine, DTIC, and the nitrosourea alkylating agents BCNU and CCNU.[173,179,180]

The cytotoxic mechanism of TMZ appears to be related to the failure of the DNA mismatch repair system to find a complementary base for methylated guanine. This system involves the formation of a complex of proteins that recognize, bind to, and remove methylated guanine.[181–183] The proposed hypothesis is that when this repair process is targeted to the DNA strand opposite the O^6-methylguanine, it cannot find a correct partner, thus resulting in long-lived nicks in the DNA.[184] These nicks accumulate and persist into the subsequent cell cycle, where they ultimately inhibit initiation of replication in the daughter cells, blocking the cell cycle at the G_2M boundary.[184–188] In murine[188] and human[189] leukemia cells, sensitivity to TMZ correlates with increased fragmentation of DNA and apoptotic cell death. More recent work has shown that TMZ induces G_2-M arrest through activation of Chk1 kinase with subsequent phosphorylation of Ccd 25 phosphatase and cdc2.[190,191] This has been shown to be p53 independent, although p53 status impacts on G_2-M arrest duration and outcome. Specifically, p53 wild-type cells undergo prolonged G_2-M arrest and senescence, whereas p53-deficient cells bypass cell-cycle arrest and die by mitotic catastrophe. Since p53-proficient cells were less sensitive than p53-deficient cells to TMZ, it is possible that targeting the G_2 checkpoint might enhance TMZ-induced antitumor activity.[190,191] Additionally, O^6-methylguanine-induced apoptosis is executed by the mitochondrial damage pathway, requires DNA replication, and is mediated by p53 and Fas/CD95/Apo-1.[192] Nevertheless, studies confirming that base excision repair mediates TMZ resistance have not yet been conclusively demonstrated.

DNA adducts formed by TMZ and the subsequent DNA damage or alteration of specific genes may cause cell death or reduce the metastatic potential of tumor cells. For example, mutations caused by adduct formation may result in altered surface antigens on tumor cells that contribute enhanced immunogenicity in the host.[193,194] The effects of enhanced immunologic response range from complete tumor rejection to reduced growth rates and reduced metastatic potential.[195] Additional evidence suggests that TMZ can reduce the metastatic potential of Lewis lung carcinoma cells[196] and induce differentiation in the K562 erythroleukemia cell line.[197] It has been postulated that TMZ-induced DNA damage and subsequent cell-cycle arrest may reduce the metastatic properties of some tumor cells.[197]

Mechanism of Resistance

AGT DNA Repair Protein

Several studies have shown that AGT is the primary mechanism of resistance to TMZ and other alkylating agents.[103,198] AGT functions as the first line of defense against TMZ by removing the alkyl groups from the O^6 position of guanine, in effect reversing the cytotoxic lesion of TMZ. AGT levels can be correlated with the sensitivity of tumor cell lines to TMZ and the alkylating agents BCNU and DTIC.[179,189,199–202] The role of AGT in resistance to TMZ is also evidenced by the ability of the virally transfected human AGT gene to confer a high level of resistance to TMZ and other methylating and chloroethylating agents on cells that are devoid of endogenous AGT activity.[203]

AGT levels in human tumor tissues and normal tissue specimens derived from brain, lung, and ovary vary widely over a 100-fold range, with some human tumors having no detectable activity.[204–207] Some specimens from all tumor types examined in these studies have demonstrated a complete absence of AGT activity: as many as 22% of primary brain tumor specimens have no detectable AGT

activity.[205] Similar findings with respect to AGT levels in brain tumor cells have been observed in in vitro models.[208] AGT activity has been localized to both the cytoplasm and the nucleus of the cell, although the function of cytoplasmic AGT and its mechanism of transport to the nucleus are unknown.[204] AGT transfers the methyl group to an internal cysteine residue, acting as methyltransferase and methyl acceptor protein. In the process, AGT becomes irreversibly inactivated, and new AGT must be synthesized to restore AGT activity.[31] Therefore, the number of O^6-methylguanine adducts that can be repaired is limited by the number of AGT molecules of the protein available.[31] Recent work has confirmed that elevated AGT levels (measured by immunohistochemistry or implied by methylation of the promoter of the gene) in newly diagnosed glioblastoma multiforme directly correlated with lack of response to TMZ[152] or survival following adjuvant therapy with this methylator.[209,210]

Deficiency in Mismatch Repair Pathway

Although AGT is clearly important in the resistance of cells to TMZ, some cell lines that express low levels of AGT are nevertheless resistant, indicating that other resistance mechanisms may be involved.[211,212] A deficiency in the mismatch repair pathway as a result of mutations in any one of the proteins that recognize and repair DNA (i.e., including GTBP, hMSH2, hPMS2, hMLH1, and MSH6) can render cells tolerant to methylation and the cytotoxic effects of TMZ. This deficiency in the mismatch repair pathway results in a failure to recognize and repair the O^6-methylguanine adducts produced by TMZ and other methylating agents.[34,174,213] The DNA damage that results from failure to repair the O^6-methylguanine adducts produces a particular type of genomic instability, microsatellite instability, that is associated with some familial and sporadic cancers, such as hereditary nonpolyposis colorectal cancer.[214,215] The high level of resistance in tumor cells that are deficient in mismatch repair is unrelated to the level of AGT and is, therefore, unaffected by AGT inhibitors. Recent studies suggest that while MSH6 mutations do not occur commonly in newly diagnosed glioblastoma, they are seen in approximately 26% of glioblastoma that have recurred after treatment with alkylating agents, notably temozolomide.[216–219] These data, while not definite proof that mismatch repair deficiency is a clinically relevant mechanism of temozolomide resistance in glioblastoma, which have received the following treatment with this alkylator, are suggestive and bear further explanation.

Base Excision Repair

A series of studies have shown that two Temodar-initiated adducts, N^7-methylguanine and N^3-methyladenine, are not susceptible to AGT and produce cytotoxicity (particularly N^3-methyladenine), independently of DNA mismatch repair activity.[171,212,220,221] These lesions are promptly repaired by a series of enzymatic steps including N-methylpurine-DNA glycosylase, AP endonuclease, poly (ADP-ribose) polymerase (PARP) DNA polymerase β, x-ray repair cross complementing 1, and ligase III. Tumor cells resistant to Temodar because of DNA mismatch repair deficiency have been rendered susceptible to this methylator by inhibition of base excision repair. Strategies have included inhibition of PARP[212,220–227] and use of methoxyamine.[171] Intriguingly, moderate enhancement of Temodar activity following base excision repair disruption was also seen in DNA mismatch repair–proficient cells.[171,212,220,221] Nevertheless, conclusive evidence confirming that base excision repair mediates TMZ resistance or that a Parp inhibitor or methoxyamine can reverse TMZ resistance in patients has not yet been published.

Drug Interactions

There are no known adverse reactions with other drugs. It is expected that compounds that deplete AGT will increase TMZ toxicity.

Clinical Pharmacology and Toxicity

TMZ is supplied in capsules containing 5, 25, 100, or 250 mg for oral use although an intravenous formulation has recently been approved for commercial use. In the initial phase 1 trial in the United Kingdom, TMZ was administered as a single intravenous dose at doses of 50 to 200 mg/m² and subsequently was given orally to fasted patients as a single dose, up to a total dose of 200 to 1,200 mg/m². Additionally, oral doses of 750 to 1,200 mg/m² were divided into five equal doses and administered daily for 5 days at 4-week intervals.

The pharmacokinetics of TMZ were evaluated in the United Kingdom phase 1 trials.[144] After intravenous administration, plasma TMZ concentrations declined biexponentially consistent with a two-compartment open model and a terminal elimination half-life of 1.8 hours. After oral administration, plasma TMZ concentrations were consistent with a one-compartment oral model, with rapid absorption and maximum plasma concentrations occurring 0.7 hour after treatment. The clearance of TMZ was 11.8 L/h, and the pharmacokinetics were independent of the dosage (with a linear relationship between dose and area under the time × concentration curve). Oral bioavailability was considered to be complete.

In 1993, Schering-Plough began the worldwide development of TMZ using machine-filled capsules that were prepared according to good manufacturing practices, which differed from the hand-filled capsules used in the initial study. Several phase 1 studies have evaluated the safety and tolerability of that new TMZ formulation (Temodar). Data from these studies have confirmed the safety, tolerability, and pharmacokinetics of TMZ reported in the CRC phase 1 study (Table 14B-3).[228–235]

Phase 1 studies of TMZ also were expanded to include pediatric cancer patients. A phase 1 study was conducted to define the multiple-dose pharmacokinetics of TMZ in this population. In this study, 19 patients between 3 and 17 years old were given TMZ over a dosage range of 100 to 240 mg/m²/d. TMZ was absorbed rapidly, had an AUC that increased in a dosage-related manner, and showed no evidence of accumulation. The plasma half-life, whole-body clearance, and volume of distribution were independent of dosage (Table 14B-4).[231] Compared with adult patients treated with 200 mg/m²/d, children appeared to have a higher AUC (48.7 versus 34.5 mg/h/mL), most likely because children have a larger ratio of body surface area to volume. Despite higher concentrations at dosages equivalent to those used in adult patients, the bone marrow function in pediatric patients appears to allow greater exposure to the drug before dose-limiting bone marrow toxicity develops.[231]

The effects of food and gastric pH on the pharmacokinetics and bioavailability of orally administered TMZ also have been evaluated.

TABLE 14B.5	Key features of temozolomide {8-carbamoyl-3-methylimidazo [5,1-D]-1,2,3,5-tetrazin-4(3H)-one}
Mechanism of action	Methylation of nucleic acids
Metabolism	Chemical conversion of 5(3-methyltriazeno) imidazole-4-carboxamide
Pharmacokinetics (IV or PO)	Volume of distribution: 28.3 L Elimination half-life: 1.8 h Distribution half-life: 0.26 h Clearance: 11.76 L/h[253]
Drug and food interactions	Unknown
Toxicity	Myelosuppression Nausea and vomiting Elevated hepatic transaminases

Administration of TMZ after ingestion of food resulted in a small decrease in its oral bioavailability.[234] When TMZ was taken after a meal, a slight (9%), but statistically significant, reduction occurred in the rate and extent of its absorption (Table 14B-5). Because AUC confidence levels were within the bioequivalence guidelines of 80% to 125%, it is unlikely that the slight reduction observed in the oral bioavailability of TMZ in the presence of a meal has any clinical effect on the antitumor activity of TMZ.

The oral bioavailability, maximum plasma concentration, and half-life of TMZ were not affected by an increase in gastric pH of 1 to 2 units, resulting from the administration of ranitidine every 12 hours on either the first 2 or the last 2 days of the 5-day TMZ dosing schedule.[235]

Subsequent phase 1 trials sponsored by Schering-Plough in adult[229,230,232–235] and pediatric patients[231,236] with advanced cancer also have confirmed that hematologic toxicity, specifically thrombocytopenia and neutropenia, is dose limiting. Neutropenia or thrombocytopenia appeared 21 to 28 days after the first dose of each cycle and recovered to grade 1 myelosuppression within 7 to 14 days. Grade 4 toxicity occurred at cumulative oral dosages of more than 1,000 mg/m² over 5 days, but little other toxicity was seen.[232] Grade 3 or 4 myelosuppression occurred in less than 10% of patients studied.

The effect of prior treatment with chemotherapy, radiation, or both, on the maximum tolerated dose (MTD) of TMZ has been evaluated.[230,233] In one of these studies,[233] 24 patients stratified according to prior exposure to chemotherapy and radiation were given a dosage of 100 mg/m²/d of TMZ for 5 days, which was escalated to 150 and 200 mg/m²/d in the absence of myelosuppression. The MTD for TMZ was established as 150 mg/m²/d.[233] The other similar phase 1 study, reported by the National Cancer Institute, evaluated the safety of TMZ in patients who were stratified on the basis of prior exposure to nitrosourea.[230] The MTD for patients with prior exposure to nitrosourea was 150 mg/m²/d, and the MTD for patients without such prior exposure was 250 mg/m²/d. An evaluation of the pharmacokinetics of TMZ showed that its clearance from the plasma was significantly less in patients with prior exposure to nitrosourea than it was in patients without such prior exposure.[230] This may have contributed to the lower dose of TMZ that was tolerated by these patients and had a notable effect on the dosing recommendation for these patients.[230]

The results of these studies indicated that a dosage of 200 mg/m^2 of TMZ given on a 5-day schedule and repeated every 28 days is appropriate for patients who are not pretreated with radiation, chemotherapy, or both. Patients who are pretreated with chemotherapy receive a lower starting dose of TMZ (i.e., 150 mg/m^2), which can be escalated to 200 mg/m^2 in subsequent courses in the absence of grade 3 or 4 myelosuppression.[233] Other schedules including 21 days out of 28 and 7 days on/7 days off have also been evaluated, though they have not yet produced convincing changes in activity.[237]

References

1. Newell D, Gescher A, Harland S, et al. N-methyl antitumour agents. A distinct class of anticancer drugs? Cancer Chemother Pharmacol 1987;19: 91–102.
2. Zeller P, Gutmann H, Hegedus B, et al. Methylhydrazine derivatives, a new class of cytotoxic agents. Experientia 1963;19:129.
3. Bollag W. The tumor-inhibitory effects of the methylhydrazine derivative Ro 4–6467/1 (Nsc-77213). Cancer Chemother Rep 1963;33:1–4.
4. Bollag W, Grunberg E. Tumour inhibitory effects of a new class of cytotoxic agents: methylhydrazine derivatives. Experientia 1963;19:130–131.
5. Brunner KW, Young CW. A Methylhydrazine Derivative in Hodgkin's Disease and Other Malignant Neoplasms. Therapeutic and Toxic Effects Studied in 51 Patients. Ann Intern Med 1965;63:69–86.
6. Martz G, D AA, Keel HJ, et al. Preliminary clinical results with a new antitumor agent Ro 4–6467 (Nsc-77213). Cancer Chemother Rep 1963;33:5–14.
7. Mathe G, Schweisguth O, Schneider M, et al. Methyl-hydrazine in treatment of Hodgkin's disease and various forms of haematosarcoma and leukaemia. Lancet 1963;2:1077–1080.
8. Samuels ML, Leary WV, Alexanian R, et al. Clinical trials with N-isopropyl-alpha-(2-methylhydrazino)-p-toluamide hydrochloride in malignant lymphoma and other disseminated neoplasia. Cancer 1967;20:1187–1194.
9. Spivack SD. Drugs 5 years later: procarbazine. Ann Intern Med 1974;81: 795–800.
10. DeVita VT, Jr., Hubbard SM, Longo DL. The chemotherapy of lymphomas: looking back, moving forward–the Richard and Hinda Rosenthal Foundation award lecture. Cancer Res 1987;47:5810–5824.
11. DeVita VT Jr, Canellos GP, Chabner B, et al. Advanced diffuse histiocytic lymphoma, a potentially curable disease. Lancet 1975;1:248–250.
12. Devita VT Jr, Serpick AA, Carbone PP. Combination chemotherapy in the treatment of advanced Hodgkin's disease. Ann Intern Med 1970;73:881–895.
13. Stolinsky DC, Solomon J, Pugh RP, et al. Clinical experience with procarbazine in Hodgkin's disease, reticulum cell sarcoma, and lymphosarcoma. Cancer 1970;26:984–990.
14. Daniels JR, Chak LY, Sikic BI, et al. Chemotherapy of small-cell carcinoma of lung: a randomized comparison of alternating and sequential combination chemotherapy programs. J Clin Oncol 1984;2:1192–1199.
15. Pedersen AG, Sorenson S, Aabo K, et al. Phase II study of procarbazine in small cell carcinoma of the lung. Cancer Treat Rep 1982;66:273–275.
16. Samuels ML, Leary WV, Howe CD. Procarbazine (NSC-77213) in the treatment of advanced bronchogenic carcinoma. Cancer Chemother Rep 1969;53:135–145.
17. Carmo-Pereira J, Costa FO, Henriques E. Combination cytotoxic chemotherapy with procarbazine, vincristine, and lomustine (POC) in disseminated malignant melanoma: 8 years' follow-up. Cancer Treat Rep 1984;68:1211–1214.
18. Luce JK. Chemotherapy of malignant melanoma. Cancer 1972;30:1604–1615.
19. Gutin PH, Wilson CB, Kumar AR, et al. Phase II study of procarbazine, CCNU, and vincristine combination chemotherapy in the treatment of malignant brain tumors. Cancer 1975;35:1398–1404.
20. Levin VA, Rodriguez LA, Edwards MS, et al. Treatment of medulloblastoma with procarbazine, hydroxyurea, and reduced radiation doses to whole brain and spine. J Neurosurg 1988;68:383–387.
21. Vasantha Kumar AR, Renaudin J, Wilson CB, et al. Procarbazine hydrochloride in the treatment of brain tumors. Phase 2 study. J Neurosurg 1974;40:365–371.
22. Newton HB, Bromberg J, Junck L, et al. Comparison between BCNU and procarbazine chemotherapy for treatment of gliomas. J Neurooncol 1993;15:257–263.
23. Newton HB, Junck L, Bromberg J, et al. Procarbazine chemotherapy in the treatment of recurrent malignant astrocytomas after radiation and nitrosourea failure. Neurology 1990;40:1743–1746.
24. Rodriguez LA, Prados M, Silver P, et al. Reevaluation of procarbazine for the treatment of recurrent malignant central nervous system tumors. Cancer 1989;64:2420–2423.
25. Meer L, Schold SC, Kleihues P. Inhibition of the hepatic O6-alkylguanine-DNA alkyltransferase in vivo by pretreatment with antineoplastic agents. Biochem Pharmacol 1989;38:929–934.
26. Bedell MA, Lewis JG, Billings KC, et al. Cell specificity in hepatocarcinogenesis: preferential accumulation of O6-methylguanine in target cell DNA during continuous exposure to rats to 1,2-dimethylhydrazine. Cancer Res 1982;42:3079–3083.
27. Rossi SC, Conrad M, Voigt JM, et al. Excision repair of O6-methylguanine synthesized at the rat H-ras N-methyl-N-nitrosourea activation site and introduced into Escherichia coli. Carcinogenesis 1989;10:373–377.
28. Swenberg JA, Bedell MA, Billings KC, et al. Cell-specific differences in O6-alkylguanine DNA repair activity during continuous exposure to carcinogen. Proc Natl Acad Sci U S A 1982;79:5499–5502.
29. Hall J, Kataoka H, Stephenson C, et al. The contribution of O6-methylguanine and methylphosphotriesters to the cytotoxicity of alkylating agents in mammalian cells. Carcinogenesis 1988;9:1587–1593.
30. Schold SC, Jr., Brent TP, von Hofe E, et al. O6-alkylguanine-DNA alkyltransferase and sensitivity to procarbazine in human brain-tumor xenografts. J Neurosurg 1989;70:573–577.
31. Pegg AE. Mammalian O6-alkylguanine-DNA alkyltransferase: regulation and importance in response to alkylating carcinogenic and therapeutic agents. Cancer Res 1990;50:6119–6129.
32. Gutterman J, Huang AT, Hochstein P. Studies on the mode of action of N-isopropyl-alpha-(2-methylhydrazino)-p-toluamide (MIH). Proc Soc Exp Biol Med 1969;130:797–802.
33. Huang AT, Gutterman J, Hochstein P. Cytogenetic changes induced by 1-(N1-methylhydrazinomethyl)-N-isopropyl benzamide in Ehrlich ascites tumor cells. Experientia 1969;25:203–204.
34. Friedman HS, Johnson SP, Dong Q, et al. Methylator resistance mediated by mismatch repair deficiency in a glioblastoma multiforme xenograft. Cancer Res 1997;57:2933–2936.
35. Kat A, Thilly WG, Fang WH, et al. An alkylation-tolerant, mutator human cell line is deficient in strand-specific mismatch repair. Proc Natl Acad Sci U S A 1993;90:6424–6428.
36. Koi M, Umar A, Chauhan DP, et al. Human chromosome 3 corrects mismatch repair deficiency and microsatellite instability and reduces N-methyl-N'-nitro-N-nitrosoguanidine tolerance in colon tumor cells with homozygous hMLH1 mutation. Cancer Res 1994;54:4308–4312.
37. Eade NR, MacLeod SM, Renton KW. Inhibition of hepatic microsomal drug metabolism by the hydrazines Ro 4–4602, MK 486, and procarbazine hydrochloride. Can J Physiol Pharmacol 1972;50:721–724.
38. Lee IP, Lucier GW. The potentiation of barbiturate-induced narcosis by procarbazine. J Pharmacol Exp Ther 1976;196:586–593.
39. Oliverio VT, Denham C, Devita VT, et al. Some pharmacologic properties of a new antitumor agent, N-isopropyl-alpha-(2-methylhydrazino)-P-toluamide, hydrochloride (Nsc-77213). Cancer Chemother Rep 1964;42:1–7.
40. Reed DJ. Effects in vivo of lymphoma ascites tumors and procarbazine, alone and in combination, upon hepatic drug-metabolizing enzymes of mice. Biochem Pharmacol 1976;25:153–156.
41. Berneis K, Kofler M, Bollag W, et al. The degradation of deoxyribonucleic acid by new tumour inhibiting compounds: the intermediate formation of hydrogen peroxide. Experientia 1963;19:132–133.
42. Hande KR, Noone RM. Cimetidine prolongs the half-life of PCB and hexamethylmelamine. Proc Am Assoc Cancer Res 1983;24:287.

43. Schwartz DE. Comparative metabolic studies with Natulan, methylhydrazine and methylamine in rats. Experientia 1966;22:212–213.

44. Shiba DA, Weinkam RJ. The in vivo cytotoxic activity of procarbazine and procarbazine metabolites against L1210 ascites leukemia cells in CDF1 mice and the effects of pretreatment with procarbazine, phenobarbital, diphenylhydantoin, and methylprednisolone upon in vivo procarbazine activity. Cancer Chemother Pharmacol 1983;11:124–129.

45. De Vita VT, Hahn MA, Oliverio VT. Monoamine oxidase inhibition by a new carcinostatic agent, N-isopropyl-a92-methylhydrazino)-p-toluamide (MIH). Proc Soc Exp Biol Med 1965;120:561–565.

46. Chabner BA, DeVita VT, Considine N, et al. Plasma pyridoxal phosphate depletion by the carcinostatic procarbazine. Proc Soc Exp Biol Med 1969;132:1119–1122.

47. DeVita VT, Serpick A, Carbone PP. Preliminary clinical studies with ibenzmethyzin. Clin Pharmacol Ther 1966;7:542–546.

48. Hoagland HC. Hematologic complications of cancer chemotherapy. Semin Oncol 1982;9:95–102.

49. Sponzo RW, Arseneau JC, Canellos GP. Procabazine induced oxidative haemolysis: relationship in vivo red cell survival. Br J Haematol 1974;27:587–595.

50. Weiss HD, Walker MD, Wiernik PH. Neurotoxicity of commonly used antineoplastic agents (first of two parts). N Engl J Med 1974;291:75–81.

51. Casimir A, Kavanaugh J, Liu F. Phase 1 trial of intravenous PCB administered as a 5 day continuous infusion: correlation with plasma levels of pyridoxal phosphate. Proc Am Assoc Cancer Res 1983;24:144.

52. Chabner BA, Sponzo R, Hubbard S, et al. High-dose intermittent intravenous infusion of procarbazine (NSC-77213). Cancer Chemother Rep 1973;57:361–363.

53. Dunagin WG. Clinical toxicity of chemotherapeutic agents: dermatologic toxicity. Semin Oncol 1982;9:14–22.

54. Garbes ID, Henderson ES, Gomez GA, et al. Procarbazine-induced interstitial pneumonitis with a normal chest x-ray: a case report. Med Pediatr Oncol 1986;14:238–241.

55. Jones SE, Moore M, Blank N, et al. Hypersensitivity to procarbazine (Matulane) manifested by fever and pleuropulmonary reaction. Cancer 1972;29:498–500.

56. Lokich JJ, Moloney WC. Allergic reaction to procarbazine. Clin Pharmacol Ther 1972;13:573–574.

57. Weiss RB. Hypersensitivity reaction to cancer chemotherapy. Semin Oncol 1982;9:5–13.

58. Liske R. A comparative study of the action of cyclophosphamide and procarbazine on the antibody production in mice. Clin Exp Immunol 1973;15:271–280.

59. Parvinen LM. Early effects of procarbazine (N-isopropyl-L-(2-methylhydrazino)-p-toluamide hydrochloride) on rat spermatogenesis. Exp Mol Pathol 1979;30:1–11.

60. Chryssanthou CP, Wallach RC, Atchison M. Meiotic chromosomal changes and sterility produced by nitrogen mustard and procarbazine in mice. Fertil Steril 1983;39:97–102.

61. Chaube S, Murphy ML. Fetal malformations produced in rats by N-isopropyl-alpha-(2-methylhydrazino)-p-toluamide hydrochloride (procarbazine). Teratology 1969;2:23–31.

62. Gatehouse DG, Paes DJ. A demonstration of the in vitro bacterial mutagenicity of procarbazine, using the microtitre fluctuation test and large concentrations of S9 fraction. Carcinogenesis 1983;4:347–352.

63. Pueyo C. Natulan induces forward mutations to L-arabinose-resistance in Salmonella typhimurium. Mutat Res 1979;67:189–192.

64. Kelly MG, O'Gara RW, Yancey ST, et al. Comparative carcinogenicity of N-isopropyl-alpha-(2-methylhydraziono)-p-toluamide. HCI (procarbazine hydrochloride), its degradation products, other hydrazines, and isonicotinic acid hydrazide. J Natl Cancer Inst 1969;42:337–344.

65. Sieber SM, Correa P, Dalgard DW, et al. Carcinogenic and other adverse effects of procarbazine in nonhuman primates. Cancer Res 1978;38:2125–2134.

66. Chapman RM. Effect of cytotoxic therapy on sexuality and gonadal function. Semin Oncol 1982;9:84–94.

67. Horning SJ, Hoppe RT, Kaplan HS, et al. Female reproductive potential after treatment for Hodgkin's disease. N Engl J Med 1981;304:1377–1382.

68. Schilsky RL, Lewis BJ, Sherins RJ, et al. Gonadal dysfunction in patients receiving chemotherapy for cancer. Ann Intern Med 1980;93:109–114.

69. Schilsky RL, Sherins RJ, Hubbard SM, et al. Long-term follow up of ovarian function in women treated with MOPP chemotherapy for Hodgkin's disease. Am J Med 1981;71:552–556.

70. Waxman JH, Terry YA, Wrigley PF, et al. Gonadal function in Hodgkin's disease: long-term follow-up of chemotherapy. Br Med J (Clin Res Ed) 1982;285:1612–1613.

71. Johnson JM, Thompson DJ, Haggerty GC, et al. The effect of prenatal procarbazine treatment on brain development in the rat. Teratology 1985;32:203–212.

72. Andrieu JM, Ochoa-Molina ME. Menstrual cycle, pregnancies and offspring before and after MOPP therapy for Hodgkin's disease. Cancer 1983;52:435–438.

73. Lacher MJ, Toner K. Pregnancies and menstrual function before and after combined radiation (RT) and chemotherapy (TVPP) for Hodgkin's disease. Cancer Invest 1986;4:93–100.

74. Glicksman AS, Pajak TF, Gottlieb A, et al. Second malignant neoplasms in patients successfully treated for Hodgkin's disease: a Cancer and Leukemia Group B study. Cancer Treat Rep 1982;66:1035–1044.

75. Grunwald HW, Rosner F. Acute myeloid leukemia following treatment of Hodgkin's disease: a review. Cancer 1982;50:676–683.

76. Henry-Amar M. Quantitative risk of second cancer in patients in first complete remission from early stages of Hodgkin's disease. NCI Monogr 1988;65–72.

77. Goldstein LS. Dominant lethal mutations induced in mouse spermatogonia by mechlorethamine, procarbazine and vincristine administered in 2-drug and 3-drug combinations. Mutat Res 1987;191:171–176.

78. Yost GS, Horstman MG, el Walily AF, et al. Procarbazine spermatogenesis toxicity: deuterium isotope effects point to regioselective metabolism in mice. Toxicol Appl Pharmacol 1985;80:316–322.

79. Horstman MG, Meadows GG, Yost GS. Separate mechanisms for procarbazine spermatotoxicity and anticancer activity. Cancer Res 1987;47:1547–1550.

80. Prough RA, Tweedie DJ. PCB. In: Metabolism and Action of Anti-Cancer Drugs. Powis G, Prough RA, eds. London: Taylor & Francis, 1987;29.

81. Montgomery JA. Experimental studies at Southern Research Institute with DTIC (NSC-45388). Cancer Treat Rep 1976;60:125–134.

82. Shealy YF, Montgomery JA, Laster WR Jr. Antitumor activity of triazenoimidazoles. Biochem Pharmacol 1962;11:674–676.

83. Comis RL. DTIC (NSC-45388) in malignant melanoma: a perspective. Cancer Treat Rep 1976;60:165–176.

84. Frei E III, Luce JK, Talley RW, et al. 5-(3,3-dimethyl-1-triazeno)imidazole-4-carboxamide (NSC-45388) in the treatment of lymphoma. Cancer Chemother Rep 1972;56:667–670.

85. Carey RW, Anderson JR, Green M, et al. Treatment of metastatic malignant melanoma with vinblastine, dacarbazine, and cisplatin: a report from the Cancer and Leukemia Group B. Cancer Treat Rep 1986;70:329–331.

86. Cowan DH, Bergsagel DE. Intermittent treatment of metastatic malignant melanoma with high-dose 5-(3,3-dimethyl-1-triazeno)imidazole-4-carboxamide (NSC-45388). Cancer Chemother Rep 1971;55:175–181.

87. Einhorn LH, Furnas B. Combination chemotherapy for disseminated malignant melanoma with DTIC, vincristine, and methyl-CCNU. Cancer Treat Rep 1977;61:881–883.

88. Pritchard KI, Quirt IC, Cowan DH, et al. DTIC therapy in metastatic malignant melanoma: a simplified dose schedule. Cancer Treat Rep 1980;64:1123–1126.

89. Bonadonna G, Valagussa P, Santoro A. Alternating non-cross-resistant combination chemotherapy or MOPP in stage IV Hodgkin's disease. A report of 8-year results. Ann Intern Med 1986;104:739–746.

90. Bonadonna G, Zucali R, Monfardini S, et al. Combination chemotherapy of Hodgkin's disease with adriamycin, bleomycin, vinblastine, and imidazole carboxamide versus MOPP. Cancer 1975;36:252–259.

91. Gottlieb JA, Benjamin RS, Baker LH, et al. Role of DTIC (NSC-45388) in the chemotherapy of sarcomas. Cancer Treat Rep 1976;60:199–203.

92. Luce JK, Thurman WG, Isaacs BL, et al. Clinical trials with the antitumor agent 5-(3,3-dimethyl-1-triazeno)imidazole-4-carboxamide(NSC-45388). Cancer Chemother Rep 1970;54:119–124.

93. Vogel CL, Primack A, Owor R, et al. Effective treatment of Kaposi's sarcoma with 5-(3,3-dimethyl-1-triazeno)imidazole-4-carboxamide (NSC-45388). Cancer Chemother Rep 1973;57:65–71.

94. Finklestein JZ, Albo V, Ertel I, et al. 5-(3,3-Dimethyl-1-triazeno)imidazole-4-carboxamide (NSC-45388) in the treatment of solid tumors in children. Cancer Chemother Rep 1975;59:351–357.

95. Finklestein JZ, Klemperer MR, Evans A, et al. Multiagent chemotherapy for children with metastatic neuroblastoma: a report from Childrens Cancer Study Group. Med Pediatr Oncol 1979;6:179–188.

96. Eyre HJ, Eltringham JR, Gehan EA, et al. Randomized comparisons of radiotherapy and carmustine versus procarbazine versus dacarbazine for the treatment of malignant gliomas following surgery: a Southwest Oncology Group Study. Cancer Treat Rep 1986;70:1085–1090.

97. Altimari AF, Badrinath K, Reisel HJ, et al. DTIC therapy in patients with malignant intra-abdominal neuroendocrine tumors. Surgery 1987;102:1009–1017.

98. Averbuch SD, Steakley CS, Young RC, et al. Malignant pheochromocytoma: effective treatment with a combination of cyclophosphamide, vincristine, and dacarbazine. Ann Intern Med 1988;109:267–273.

99. Kessinger A, Foley JF, Lemon HM. Therapy of malignant APUD cell tumors. Effectiveness of DTIC. Cancer 1983;51:790–794.

100. Clarke DA, Barclay RK, Stock CC, et al. Triazenes as inhibitors of mouse sarcoma 180. Proc Soc Exp Biol Med 1955;90:484–489.

101. Schmid FA, Hutchison DJ. Chemotherapeutic, carcinogenic, and cell-regulatory effects of triazenes. Cancer Res 1974;34:1671–1675.

102. Catapano CV, Broggini M, Erba E, et al. In vitro and in vivo methazolastone-induced DNA damage and repair in L-1210 leukemia sensitive and resistant to chloroethylnitrosoureas. Cancer Res 1987;47:4884–4889.

103. D'Incalci M, Citti L, Taverna P, et al. Importance of the DNA repair enzyme O6-alkyl guanine alkyltransferase (AT) in cancer chemotherapy. Cancer Treat Rev 1988;15:279–292.

104. Foster BJ, Newell DR, Lunn JM. Correlation of dacarbazine and CB10-277 activity against human melanoma xenografts with O6-alkyltransferase. Proc Am Assoc Cancer Res 1990;31:401.

105. Gibson NW, Hartley J, La France RJ, et al. Differential cytotoxicity and DNA-damaging effects produced in human cells of the Mer+ and Mer- phenotypes by a series of alkyltriazenylimidazoles. Carcinogenesis 1986;7:259–265.

106. Hayward IP, Parsons PG. Comparison of virus reactivation, DNA base damage, and cell cycle effects in autologous human melanoma cells resistant to methylating agents. Cancer Res 1984;44:55–58.

107. Lunn JM, Harris AL. Cytotoxicity of 5-(3-methyl-1-triazeno)imidazole-4-carboxamide (MTIC) on Mer+, Mer+Rem- and Mer- cell lines: differential potentiation by 3-acetamidobenzamide. Br J Cancer 1988;57:54–58.

108. Mitchell RB, Dolan ME. Effect of temozolomide and dacarbazine on O6-alkylguanine-DNA alkyltransferase activity and sensitivity of human tumor cells and xenografts to 1,3-bis(2-chloroethyl)-1-nitrosourea. Cancer Chemother Pharmacol 1993;32:59–63.

109. Lee SM, Thatcher N, Dougal M, et al. Dosage and cycle effects of dacarbazine (DTIC) and fotemustine on O6-alkylguanine-DNA alkyltransferase in human peripheral blood mononuclear cells. Br J Cancer 1993;67:216–221.

110. Lev DC, Ruiz M, Mills L, et al. Dacarbazine causes transcriptional up-regulation of interleukin 8 and vascular endothelial growth factor in melanoma cells: a possible escape mechanism from chemotherapy. Mol Cancer Ther 2003;2:753–763.

111. Buesa JM, Gracia M, Valle M, et al. Phase I trial of intermittent high-dose dacarbazine. Cancer Treat Rep 1984;68:499–504.

112. Aigner K, Hild P, Henneking K, et al. Regional perfusion with cis-platinum and dacarbazine. Recent Results Cancer Res 1983;86:239–245.

113. Einhorn LH, McBride CM, Luce JK, et al. Intra-arterial infusion therapy with 5-(3,3-dimethyl-1-triazeno) imidazole-4-carboxamide (NSC 45388) for malignant melanoma. Cancer 1973;32:749–755.

114. Jortay AM, Lejeune FJ, Kenis Y. Regional chemotherapy of maxillofacial malignant melanoma with intracarotid artery infusion of DTIC. Tumori 1977;63:299–302.

115. Savlov ED, Hall TC, Oberfield RA. Intra-arterial therapy of melanoma with dimethyl triazeno imidazole carboxamide (NSC-45388). Cancer 1971;28:1161–1164.

116. Mizuno NS, Humphrey EW. Metabolism of 5-(3,3-dimethyl-1-triazeno) imidazole-4-carboxamide (NSC-45388) in human and animal tumor tissue. Cancer Chemother Rep 1972;56:465–472.

117. Benvenuto JA, Stewart DJ, Benjamin RS, et al. High-performance liquid chromatographic analysis of pentamethylmelamine and its metabolites in biological fluids. J Chromatogr 1981;222:518–522.

118. Loo TL, Luce JK, Jardine JH, et al. Pharmacologic studies of the antitumor agent 5-(dimethyltriazeno)imidazole-4-carboxamide. Cancer Res 1968;28:2448–2453.

119. Breithaupt H, Dammann A, Aigner K. Pharmacokinetics of dacarbazine (DTIC) and its metabolite 5-aminoimidazole-4-carboxamide (AIC) following different dose schedules. Cancer Chemother Pharmacol 1982;9:103–109.

120. Venditti JM. Antitumor activity of DTIC (NSC-45388) in animals. Cancer Treat Rep 1976;60:135–140.

121. Beck TM, Hart NE, Smith CE. Photosensitivity reaction following DTIC administration: report of two cases. Cancer Treat Rep 1980;64:725–726.

122. Ceci G, Bella M, Melissari M, et al. Fatal hepatic vascular toxicity of DTIC. Is it really a rare event? Cancer 1988;61:1988–1991.

123. Feaux de Lacroix W, Runne U, Hauk H, et al. Acute liver dystrophy with thrombosis of hepatic veins: a fatal complication of dacarbazine treatment. Cancer Treat Rep 1983;67:779–784.

124. Frosch PJ, Czarnetzki BM, Macher E, et al. Hepatic failure in a patient treated with dacarbazine (DTIC) for malignant melanoma. J Cancer Res Clin Oncol 1979;95:281–286.

125. Greenstone MA, Dowd PM, Mikhailidis DP, et al. Hepatic vascular lesions associated with dacarbazine treatment. Br Med J (Clin Res Ed) 1981;282:1744–1745.

126. McClay E, Lusch CJ, Mastrangelo MJ. Allergy-induced hepatic toxicity associated with dacarbazine. Cancer Treat Rep 1987;71:219–220.

127. Singh B, Gupta RS. Mutagenic responses of thirteen anticancer drugs on mutation induction at multiple genetic loci and on sister chromatid exchanges in Chinese hamster ovary cells. Cancer Res 1983;43:577–584.

128. Tamaro M, Dolzani L, Monti-Bragadin C, et al. Mutagenic activity of the dacarbazine analog p-(3,3-dimethyl-1-triazeno)benzoic acid potassium salt in bacterial cells. Pharmacol Res Commun 1986;18:491–501.

129. Beal DD, Skibba JL, Croft WA, et al. Carcinogenicity of the antineoplastic agent, 5-(3,3-dimethyl-1-triazeno)-imidazole-4-carboxamide, and its metabolites in rats. J Natl Cancer Inst 1975;54:951–957.

130. Valagussa P, Santoro A, Fossati Bellani F, et al. Absence of treatment-induced second neoplasms after ABVD in Hodgkin's disease. Blood 1982;59:488–494.

131. Brusamolino E, Papa G, Valagussa P, et al. Treatment-related leukemia in Hodgkin's disease: a multi-institution study on 75 cases. Hematol Oncol 1987;5:83–98.

132. Carey RW, Kunz VS. Acute non-lymphocytic leukemia (ANLL) following treatment with dacarbazine for malignant melanoma. Am J Hematol 1987;25:119–121.

133. Chaube S, Swinyard CA. Urogenital anomalies in fetal rats produced by the anticancer agent 4(5)-(3,3-dimethyl-1-triazeno) imidazole-4-carboxamide. Anat Rec 1976;186:461–469.

134. Thompson DJ, Molello JA, Strebing RJ, et al. Reproduction and teratology studies with oncolytic agents in the rat and rabbit. II. 5-(3,3-dimethyl-l-triazeno)imidazole-4-carboxamide (DTIC). Toxicol Appl Pharmacol 1975;33:281–290.

135. Baldwin RW, Partridge MW, Stevens MFG. Pyrazolotriazines: a new class of tumour-inhibitory agents. J Pharm Pharmacol 1966;18S:1S.

136. Harrap KA, Connors TA, Stevens MFG. Second-generation azolotetrazinones. In: New Avenues in Developmental Cancer Chemotherapy. London: Academic Press, 1987:335.

137. Hickman JA, Stevens MF, Gibson NW, et al. Experimental antitumor activity against murine tumor model systems of 8-carbamoyl-3-(2-chloroethyl)imidazo[5,1-d]-1,2,3,5-tetrazin-4(3 H)-one (mitozolomide), a novel broad-spectrum agent. Cancer Res 1985;45:3008–3013.

138. Newlands ES, Blackledge G, Slack JA, et al. Phase I clinical trial of mitozolomide. Cancer Treat Rep 1985;69:801–805.

139. Stevens MF, Hickman JA, Stone R, et al. Antitumor imidazotetrazines. 1. Synthesis and chemistry of 8-carbamoyl-3-(2-chloroethyl)imidazo[5,1-d]-1,2,3,5-tetrazin-4(3 H)-one, a novel broad-spectrum antitumor agent. J Med Chem 1984;27:196–201.

140. Horspool KR, Stevens MF, Newton CG, et al. Antitumor imidazotetrazines. 20. Preparation of the 8-acid derivative of mitozolomide and its utility in the preparation of active antitumor agents. J Med Chem 1990;33:1393–1399.

141. Stevens MF, Hickman JA, Langdon SP, et al. Antitumor activity and pharmacokinetics in mice of 8-carbamoyl-3-methyl-imidazo[5,1-d]-1,2,3,5-tetrazin-4(3H)-one (CCRG 81045; M & B 39831), a novel drug with potential as an alternative to dacarbazine. Cancer Res 1987;47:5846–5852.

142. Stevens MF, Newlands ES. From triazines and triazenes to temozolomide. Eur J Cancer 1993;29A:1045–1047.

143. Tsang LL, Quarterman CP, Gescher A, et al. Comparison of the cytotoxicity in vitro of temozolomide and dacarbazine, prodrugs of 3-methyl-(triazen-1-yl)imidazole-4-carboxamide. Cancer Chemother Pharmacol 1991;27:342–346.

144. Newlands ES, Blackledge GR, Slack JA, et al. Phase I trial of temozolomide (CCRG 81045: M&B 39831: NSC 362856). Br J Cancer 1992;65:287–291.

145. O'Reilly SM, Newlands ES, Glaser MG, et al. Temozolomide: a new oral cytotoxic chemotherapeutic agent with promising activity against primary brain tumours. Eur J Cancer 1993;29A:940–942.

146. Newlands ES, O'Reilly SM, Glaser MG, et al. The Charing Cross Hospital experience with temozolomide in patients with gliomas. Eur J Cancer 1996;32A:2236–2241.

147. Bower M, Newlands ES, Bleehen NM, et al. Multicentre CRC phase II trial of temozolomide in recurrent or progressive high-grade glioma. Cancer Chemother Pharmacol 1997;40:484–488.

148. Yung WK, Albright RE, Olson J, et al. A phase II study of temozolomide vs. procarbazine in patients with glioblastoma multiforme at first relapse. Br J Cancer 2000;83:588–593.

149. Yung WK, Prados MD, Yaya-Tur R, et al. Multicenter phase II trial of temozolomide in patients with anaplastic astrocytoma or anaplastic oligoastrocytoma at first relapse. Temodal Brain Tumor Group. J Clin Oncol 1999;17:2762–2771.

150. Mikkelsen T, Doyle T, Anderson J, et al. Temozolomide single-agent chemotherapy for newly diagnosed anaplastic oligodendroglioma. J Neurooncol 2009;92:57–63.

151. Vogelbaum MA, Berkey B, Peereboom D, et al. Phase II trial of preirradiation and concurrent temozolomide in patients with newly diagnosed anaplastic oligodendrogliomas and mixed anaplastic oligoastrocytomas: RTOG BR0131. Neuro Oncol 2009;11:167–175.

152. Friedman HS, McLendon RE, Kerby T, et al. DNA mismatch repair and O6-alkylguanine-DNA alkyltransferase analysis and response to Temodal in newly diagnosed malignant glioma. J Clin Oncol 1998;16:3851–3857.

153. Stupp R, Dietrich PY, Ostermann Kraljevic S, et al. Promising survival for patients with newly diagnosed glioblastoma multiforme treated with concomitant radiation plus temozolomide followed by adjuvant temozolomide. J Clin Oncol 2002;20:1375–1382.

154. Stupp R, Mason WP, van den Bent MJ, et al. Radiotherapy plus concomitant and adjuvant temozolomide for glioblastoma. N Engl J Med 2005;352:987–996.

155. Curran WJ, Jr., Scott CB, Horton J, et al. Recursive partitioning analysis of prognostic factors in three Radiation Therapy Oncology Group malignant glioma trials. J Natl Cancer Inst 1993;85:704–710.

156. Mirimanoff RO, Gorlia T, Mason W, et al. Radiotherapy and temozolomide for newly diagnosed glioblastoma: recursive partitioning analysis of the EORTC 26981/22981-NCIC CE3 phase III randomized trial. J Clin Oncol 2006;24:2563–2569.

157. Stupp R, Hegi ME, Mason WP, et al. Effects of radiotherapy with concomitant and adjuvant temozolomide versus radiotherapy alone on survival in glioblastoma in a randomised phase III study: 5-year analysis of the EORTC-NCIC trial. Lancet Oncol 2009;10:459–466.

158. Chamberlain MC. Temozolomide for recurrent low-grade spinal cord gliomas in adults. Cancer 2008;113:1019–1024.

159. Quinn JA, Reardon DA, Friedman AH, et al. Phase II trial of temozolomide in patients with progressive low-grade glioma. J Clin Oncol 2003;21:646–651.

160. Kesari S, Schiff D, Drappatz J, et al. Phase II study of protracted daily temozolomide for low-grade gliomas in adults. Clin Cancer Res 2009;15:330–337.

161. van den Bent MJ, Taphoorn MJ, Brandes AA, et al. Phase II study of first-line chemotherapy with temozolomide in recurrent oligodendroglial tumors: the European Organization for Research and Treatment of Cancer Brain Tumor Group Study 26971. J Clin Oncol 2003;21:2525–2528.

162. Chamberlain MC, Tsao-Wei DD, Groshen S. Temozolomide for treatment-resistant recurrent meningioma. Neurology 2004;62:1210–1212.

163. Bleehen NM, Newlands ES, Lee SM, et al. Cancer Research Campaign phase II trial of temozolomide in metastatic melanoma. J Clin Oncol 1995;13:910–913.

164. Quirbt I, Verma S, Petrella T, et al. Temozolomide for the treatment of metastatic melanoma. Curr Oncol 2007;14:27–33.

165. Clark AS, Stevens MF, Sansom CE, et al. Anti-tumour imidazotetrazines. Part XXI. Mitozolomide and temozolomide: probes for the major groove of DNA. Anticancer Drug Des 1990;5:63–68.

166. Lowe PR, Sansom CE, Schwalbe CH, et al. Antitumor imidazotetrazines. 25. Crystal structure of 8-carbamoyl-3-methylimidazo[5,1-d]-1,2,3,5-tetrazin-4(3H)-one (temozolomide) and structural comparisons with the related drugs mitozolomide and DTIC. J Med Chem 1992;35:3377–3382.

167. Clark AS, Deans B, Stevens MF, et al. Antitumor imidazotetrazines. 32. Synthesis of novel imidazotetrazinones and related bicyclic heterocycles to probe the mode of action of the antitumor drug temozolomide. J Med Chem 1995;38:1493–1504.

168. Denny BJ, Wheelhouse RT, Stevens MF, et al. NMR and molecular modeling investigation of the mechanism of activation of the antitumor drug temozolomide and its interaction with DNA. Biochemistry 1994;33:9045–9051.

169. Spassova MK, Golovinsky EV. Pharmacobiochemistry of arylalkyltriazenes and their application in cancer chemotherapy. Pharmacol Ther 1985;27:333–352.

170. Bull VL, Tisdale MJ. Antitumour imidazotetrazines–XVI. Macromolecular alkylation by 3-substituted imidazotetrazinones. Biochem Pharmacol 1987;36:3215–3220.

171. Liu L, Taverna P, Whitacre CM, et al. Pharmacologic disruption of base excision repair sensitizes mismatch repair-deficient and -proficient colon cancer cells to methylating agents. Clin Cancer Res 1999;5:2908–2917.

172. D'Atri S, Bonmassar E, Franchi F. Repair of DNA methyl adducts and sensitivity to temozolomide of acute myelogenous leukemia (AML) cells. Proc Soc Hema Stem Cells 1991;19:530.

173. Dolan ME, Mitchell RB, Mummert C, et al. Effect of O6-benzylguanine analogues on sensitivity of human tumor cells to the cytotoxic effects of alkylating agents. Cancer Res 1991;51:3367–3372.

174. Wedge SR, Porteous JK, Newlands ES. 3-aminobenzamide and/or O6-benzylguanine evaluated as an adjuvant to temozolomide or BCNU treatment in cell lines of variable mismatch repair status and O6-alkylguanine-DNA alkyltransferase activity. Br J Cancer 1996;74:1030–1036.

175. Wedge SR, Porteus JK, May BL, et al. Potentiation of temozolomide and BCNU cytotoxicity by O(6)-benzylguanine: a comparative study in vitro. Br J Cancer 1996;73:482–490.

176. Friedman HS, Dolan ME, Pegg AE, et al. Activity of temozolomide in the treatment of central nervous system tumor xenografts. Cancer Res 1995;55:2853–2857.

177. Plowman J, Waud WR, Koutsoukos AD, et al. Preclinical antitumor activity of temozolomide in mice: efficacy against human brain tumor xenografts and synergism with 1,3-bis(2-chloroethyl)-1-nitrosourea. Cancer Res 1994;54:3793–3799.

178. Wedge SR, Porteous JK, Newlands ES. Effect of single and multiple administration of an O6-benzylguanine/temozolomide combination: an evaluation in a human melanoma xenograft model. Cancer Chemother Pharmacol 1997;40:266–272.

179. D'Atri S, Piccioni D, Castellano A, et al. Chemosensitivity to triazene compounds and O6-alkylguanine-DNA alkyltransferase levels: studies with blasts of leukaemic patients. Ann Oncol 1995;6:389–393.

180. Dolan ME, Moschel RC, Pegg AE. Depletion of mammalian O6-alkylguanine-DNA alkyltransferase activity by O6-benzylguanine provides a means to evaluate the role of this protein in protection against carcinogenic and therapeutic alkylating agents. Proc Natl Acad Sci U S A 1990;87:5368–5372.

181. Drummond JT, Li GM, Longley MJ, et al. Isolation of an hMSH2-p160 heterodimer that restores DNA mismatch repair to tumor cells. Science 1995;268:1909–1912.

182. Li GM, Modrich P. Restoration of mismatch repair to nuclear extracts of H6 colorectal tumor cells by a heterodimer of human MutL homologs. Proc Natl Acad Sci U S A 1995;92:1950–1954.

183. Palombo F, Gallinari P, Iaccarino I, et al. GTBP, a 160-kilodalton protein essential for mismatch-binding activity in human cells. Science 1995;268:1912–1914.

184. Karran P, Macpherson P, Ceccotti S, et al. O6-methylguanine residues elicit DNA repair synthesis by human cell extracts. J Biol Chem 1993;268:15878–15886.

185. Ceccotti S, Dogliotti E, Gannon J, et al. O6-methylguanine in DNA inhibits replication in vitro by human cell extracts. Biochemistry 1993;32:13664–13672.

186. Karran P, Bignami M. Self-destruction and tolerance in resistance of mammalian cells to alkylation damage. Nucleic Acids Res 1992;20:2933–2940.

187. Karran P, Hampson R. Genomic instability and tolerance to alkylating agents. Cancer Surv 1996;28:69–85.

188. Taverna P, Catapano CV, Citti L, et al. Influence of O6-methylguanine on DNA damage and cytotoxicity of temozolomide in L1210 mouse leukemia sensitive and resistant to chloroethylnitrosoureas. Anticancer Drugs 1992;3:401–405.

189. Tentori L, Graziani G, Gilberti S, et al. Triazene compounds induce apoptosis in O6-alkylguanine-DNA alkyltransferase deficient leukemia cell lines. Leukemia 1995;9:1888–1895.

190. Hirose Y, Berger MS, Pieper RO. Abrogation of the Chk1-mediated G(2) checkpoint pathway potentiates temozolomide-induced toxicity in a p53-independent manner in human glioblastoma cells. Cancer Res 2001;61:5843–5849.

191. Hirose Y, Berger MS, Pieper RO. p53 effects both the duration of G2/M arrest and the fate of temozolomide-treated human glioblastoma cells. Cancer Res 2001;61:1957–1963.

192. Roos W, Baumgartner M, Kaina B. Apoptosis triggered by DNA damage O6-methylguanine in human lymphocytes requires DNA replication and is mediated by p53 and Fas/CD95/Apo-1. Oncogene 2004;23:359–367.

193. Bianchi R, Citti L, Beghetti R, et al. O6-methylguanine-DNA methyltransferase activity and induction of novel immunogenicity in murine tumor cells treated with methylating agents. Cancer Chemother Pharmacol 1992;29:277–282.

194. Puccetti P, Romani L, Fioretti MC. Chemical xenogenization of experimental tumors. Cancer Metastasis Rev 1987;6:93–111.

195. Allegrucci M, Fuschiotti P, Puccetti P, et al. Changes in the tumorigenic and metastatic properties of murine melanoma cells treated with a triazene derivative. Clin Exp Metastasis 1989;7:329–341.

196. Tentori L, Leonetti C, Aquino A. Temozolomide reduces the metastatic potential of Lewis lung carcinoma (3LL) in mice: role of alpha-6 integrin phosphorylation. Eur J Cancer 1995;31A:746–754.

197. Tisdale MJ. Antitumour imidazotetrazines-X. Effect of 8-carbamoyl-3-methylimidazo[5,1-d]-1,2,3,5-tetrazin-4-(3H)-one (CCRG 81045; M & B 39831; NSC 362856) on DNA methylation during induction of haemoglobin synthesis in human leukaemia cell line K562. Biochem Pharmacol 1986;35:311–316.

198. Pegg AE, Dolan ME, Moschel RC. Structure, function, and inhibition of O6-alkylguanine-DNA alkyltransferase. Prog Nucleic Acid Res Mol Biol 1995;51:167–223.

199. Baer JC, Freeman AA, Newlands ES, et al. Depletion of O6-alkylguanine-DNA alkyltransferase correlates with potentiation of temozolomide and CCNU toxicity in human tumour cells. Br J Cancer 1993;67:1299–1302.

200. Franchi A, Papa G, D'Atri S, et al. Cytotoxic effects of dacarbazine in patients with acute myelogenous leukemia: a pilot study. Haematologica 1992;77:146–150.

201. Redmond SM, Joncourt F, Buser K, et al. Assessment of P-glycoprotein, glutathione-based detoxifying enzymes and O6-alkylguanine-DNA alkyltransferase as potential indicators of constitutive drug resistance in human colorectal tumors. Cancer Res 1991;51:2092–2097.

202. Tisdale MJ. Antitumor imidazotetrazines–XV. Role of guanine O6 alkylation in the mechanism of cytotoxicity of imidazotetrazinones. Biochem Pharmacol 1987;36:457–462.

203. Wang G, Weiss C, Sheng P, et al. Retrovirus-mediated transfer of the human O6-methylguanine-DNA methyltransferase gene into a murine hematopoietic stem cell line and resistance to the toxic effects of certain alkylating agents. Biochem Pharmacol 1996;51:1221–1228.

204. Belanich M, Randall T, Pastor MA, et al. Intracellular Localization and intercellular heterogeneity of the human DNA repair protein O(6)-methylguanine-DNA methyltransferase. Cancer Chemother Pharmacol 1996;37:547–555.

205. Citron M, Decker R, Chen S, et al. O6-methylguanine-DNA methyltransferase in human normal and tumor tissue from brain, lung, and ovary. Cancer Res 1991;51:4131–4134.

206. Frosina G, Rossi O, Arena G, et al. O6-alkylguanine-DNA alkyltransferase activity in human brain tumors. Cancer Lett 1990;55:153–158.

207. Wiestler O, Kleihues P, Pegg AE. O6-alkylguanine-DNA alkyltransferase activity in human brain and brain tumors. Carcinogenesis 1984;5:121–124.

208. Yarosh DB. The role of O6-methylguanine-DNA methyltransferase in cell survival, mutagenesis and carcinogenesis. Mutat Res 1985;145:1–16.

209. Hegi ME, Diserens AC, Godard S, et al. Clinical trial substantiates the predictive value of O-6-methylguanine-DNA methyltransferase promoter methylation in glioblastoma patients treated with temozolomide. Clin Cancer Res 2004;10:1871–1874.

210. Hegi ME, Diserens AC, Gorlia T, et al. MGMT gene silencing and benefit from temozolomide in glioblastoma. N Engl J Med 2005;352:997–1003.

211. Bobola MS, Tseng SH, Blank A, et al. Role of O6-methylguanine-DNA methyltransferase in resistance of human brain tumor cell lines to the clinically relevant methylating agents temozolomide and streptozotocin. Clin Cancer Res 1996;2:735–741.

212. Tentori L, Leonetti C, Scarsella M, et al. Combined treatment with temozolomide and poly(ADP-ribose) polymerase inhibitor enhances survival of mice bearing hematologic malignancy at the central nervous system site. Blood 2002;99:2241–2244.

213. Liu L, Markowitz S, Gerson SL. Mismatch repair mutations override alkyltransferase in conferring resistance to temozolomide but not to 1,3-bis (2-chloroethyl)nitrosourea. Cancer Res 1996;56:5375–5379.

214. Aaltonen LA, Peltomaki P, Leach FS, et al. Clues to the pathogenesis of familial colorectal cancer. Science 1993;260:812–816.

215. Ionov Y, Peinado MA, Malkhosyan S, et al. Ubiquitous somatic mutations in simple repeated sequences reveal a new mechanism for colonic carcinogenesis. Nature 1993;363:558–561.

216. Cancer Genome Atlas Research Network. Comprehensive genomic characterization defines human glioblastoma genes and core pathways. Nature 2008;455:1061–1068.

217. Cahill DP, Codd PJ, Batchelor TT, Curry WT, Louis DN. MSH6 inactivation and emergent temozolomide resistance in human glioblastomas. Clin Neurosurg 2008;55:165–171.

218. Maxwell JA, Johnson SP, Quinn JA, et al. Quantitative analysis of O6-alkylguanine-DNA alkyltransferase in malignant glioma. Mol Cancer Ther 2006;5:2531–2539.

219. Yip S, Miao J, Cahill DP, et al. MSH6 mutations arise in glioblastomas during temozolomide therapy and mediate temozolomide resistance. Clin Cancer Res 2009;15:4622–4629.

220. Tentori L, Leonetti C, Scarsella M. Systemic administration of the PARP inhibitor GPI 15427 increases the anti-tumor activity of temozolomide in melanoma, glioma and lymphoma preclinical models in vivo. Proc Am Assoc Cancer Res 2003;44:1253.

221. Tentori L, Portarena I, Torino F, et al. Poly(ADP-ribose) polymerase inhibitor increases growth inhibition and reduces G(2)/M cell accumulation induced by temozolomide in malignant glioma cells. Glia 2002;40:44–54.

222. Boulton S, Pemberton LC, Porteous JK, et al. Potentiation of temozolomide-induced cytotoxicity: a comparative study of the biological effects of poly(ADP-ribose) polymerase inhibitors. Br J Cancer 1995;72:849–856.

223. Bowman KJ, White A, Golding BT, Griffin RJ, Curtin NJ. Potentiation of anti-cancer agent cytotoxicity by the potent poly(ADP-ribose) polymerase inhibitors NU1025 and NU1064. Br J Cancer 1998;78:1269–1277.

224. Calabrese CR, Batey MA, Thomas HD, et al. Identification of potent non-toxic poly(ADP-Ribose) polymerase-1 inhibitors: chemopotentiation and pharmacological studies. Clin Cancer Res 2003;9:2711–2718.

225. Curtin NJ, Wang LZ, Yiakouvaki A, et al. Novel poly(ADP-ribose) polymerase-1 inhibitor, AG14361, restores sensitivity to temozolomide in mismatch repair-deficient cells. Clin Cancer Res 2004;10:881–889.

226. Miknyoczki SJ, Jones-Bolin S, Pritchard S, et al. Chemopotentiation of temozolomide, irinotecan, and cisplatin activity by CEP-6800, a poly(ADP-ribose) polymerase inhibitor. Mol Cancer Ther 2003;2:371–382.

227. Tentori L, Turriziani M, Franco D, et al. Treatment with temozolomide and poly(ADP-ribose) polymerase inhibitors induces early apoptosis and increases base excision repair gene transcripts in leukemic cells resistant to triazene compounds. Leukemia 1999;13:901–909.

228. Baker SD, Wirth P, Statkevich P. Absorption, metabolism and excretion of 14C-temozolomide in patients with advanced cancer. Proc Am Soc Clin Oncol 1997;16:214a.

229. Brada M, Judson I, Beale P, et al. Phase I dose-escalation and pharmacokinetic study of temozolomide (SCH 52365) for refractory or relapsing malignancies. Br J Cancer 1999;81:1022–1030.

230. Dhodapkar M, Rubin J, Reid JM, et al. Phase I trial of temozolomide (NSC 362856) in patients with advanced cancer. Clin Cancer Res 1997;3:1093–1100.

231. Estlin EJ, Lashford L, Ablett S, et al. Phase I study of temozolomide in paediatric patients with advanced cancer. United Kingdom Children's Cancer Study Group. Br J Cancer 1998;78:652–661.

232. Hammond LA, Eckardt JR, Baker SD, et al. Phase I and pharmacokinetic study of temozolomide on a daily-for-5-days schedule in patients with advanced solid malignancies. J Clin Oncol 1999;17:2604–2613.

233. Reidenberg P, Statkevich P, Judson I. Effect of food on the oral bioavailability of temozolomide, a new chemotherapeutic agent Proc Am Soc Clin Pharmacol Thera 1996;59:70.

234. Reidenberg P, Willalona M, Eckhardt G. Phase 1 clinical and pharmacokinetic study of temozolomide in advanced cancer patients stratified by extent of prior therapy Proc European Soc Med Oncol 1996;7:99.

235. Statkevich P, Judson I, Batra V. Effect of ranitidine (R) on the pharmacokinetics (PK) of temozolomide (T). Proc Am Soc Clin Pharmacol Thera 1997;61:72.

236. Nicholson HS, Krailo M, Ames MM, et al. Phase I study of temozolomide in children and adolescents with recurrent solid tumors: a report from the Children's Cancer Group. J Clin Oncol 1998;16:3037–3043.

237. Perry JR, Rizek P, Cashman R, Morrison M, Morrison T. Temozolomide rechallenge in recurrent malignant glioma by using a continuous temozolomide schedule: the "rescue" approach. Cancer 2008;113:2152–2157.

Platinum Analogues

Eddie Reed and Bruce A. Chabner

Collectively, cisplatin, carboplatin, and oxaliplatin are major contributors to systemic therapy, for a very broad range of malignancies—with the exception of taxanes, the most active class of anticancer agents. Cisplatin was discovered when Rosenberg and colleagues[1,2] in a set of experiments involving *Escherichia coli* observed the dramatic inhibitory effects of platinum compounds on cellular replication. Following those seminal studies, a rapid series of basic, preclinical, and clinical studies resulted in Food and Drug Administration (FDA) approval for the treatment of testicular cancer. Within 15 years, cisplatin's effectiveness in testicular, ovarian, lung, head and neck, and bladder cancer was established; new analogues (oxaliplatin) and more recent studies have established the value of this class of drugs in important subset of patients with ovarian cancer, colorectal cancer, breast cancer, lymphoma, childhood malignancies, and numerous rarer cancers.

Because of the particularly troublesome toxicities of renal damage, nausea and vomiting, deafness, and peripheral neuropathy, major efforts were undertaken to identify analogs of cisplatin that have equivalent clinical effectiveness but without the toxicities of the parent compound. Carboplatin, the first such analog to meet achieve widespread clinical use (Fig. 15-1), proved to be equally effective as cisplatin in ovarian cancer, lung cancer, and several other malignancies but, for unclear reasons, less effective than cisplatin in the treatment of germ cell malignancy. Carboplatin is less neurotoxic, emetogenic, and nephrotoxic than cisplatin but more myelosuppressive.

Among newer platinum analogs, only oxaliplatin (Fig. 15-1) has received FDA approval. For unclear reasons, oxaliplatin is particularly effective in colorectal cancer (in combination with 5-fluorouracil (Chapter 9). Colon cancer is a disease for which neither cisplatin nor carboplatin shows meaningful benefit. Understanding the molecular basis for these peculiarities for these three compounds could potentially unlock a treasure trove of new insights as to how cancer cells escape the effects of DNA-damaging agents.

Chemistry

Cisplatin and carboplatin are divalent inorganic complexes and are highly water soluble and readily activated by water displacement of their chloride or carboxylate groups. Oxaliplatin is a divalent oxalate salt, and not entirely cross-resistant with carboplatin and cisplatin in model tumor systems. The more complex leaving groups of carboplatin and oxaliplatin tend to reduce reactivity in aqueous solution, decrease renal toxicity and hearing loss, and the cyclohexyl substitution on oxaliplatin may alter susceptibility to repair of DNA adducts, as will be explained below. The structures of the three FDA-approved analogues are shown in Figure 15-1, and important aspects of their chemistry are summarized in Table 15-1 and in previous reviews.[3,4]

The most exciting of new developments in the chemistry of platinum analogues is the discovery and characterization of cisplatin and carboplatin nanocapsules.[5-8] Cisplatin nanocapsules were a product of efforts to develop better methods for enclosing cisplatin in liposomes. For cisplatin, such nanoparticles have approximate bidimensional measurements of 50 to 120 nm. The cisplatin-to-lipid molar ratio is about eleven to one. The solid core of the nanoparticle is 90% the dichloride species of cisplatin, and the outer lipid bilayer is very different from that of conventional liposomes. A slight modification of the cisplatin nanocapsule method was used to develop carboplatin nanocapsules, including modest differences in molar ratios of drug to lipid. Most importantly, when comparing the IC50 values of cisplatin nanocapsules to cisplatin, and that of carboplatin nanocapsules to carboplatin, in both cases, the nanocapsules are two orders of magnitude more cytotoxic than their parent drug against IGROV-1 human ovarian cancer cells.

Thus, platinum compounds may possibly become even more effective through the use of nanotechnology.

Subcellular Pharmacology

The cellular pharmacology of platinum compounds has been extensively studied.[3,4] Cisplatin is able to cross cellular barriers because of its simple chemistry. However, work by a number of laboratories strongly suggests that simple diffusion of cisplatin across cell membranes does not fully explain transmembrane trafficking of platinum drugs.[9-13] Specific transmembrane transport proteins may promote influx and efflux of the drug, such as the CTR1, ATP7A, and ATP7B transporters.[9,10] At physiologic pH of 7.4, dissociation of its chlorides and their replacement by -OH molecules result in cisplatin having a neutral charge (Fig. 15-2). This makes it possible for ready diffusion across the cellular membrane.

As suggested above, there is good evidence that CTR1, a copper transporter in the cell membrane, is a significant contributor to the active uptake of platinum drugs by cells, including cisplatin, carboplatin, and oxaliplatin.[9,11] Also, ATP7A and ATP7B, normal copper efflux proteins in the cell membrane, are major contributors to the efflux of platinum drugs in cancer cells.[10] In addition, the human organic cation transporters 1, 2, and 3, have been implicated in

Whereas many institutions give cisplatin over 30 minutes, this shorter infusion may be associated with a higher rate of severe side effects. These authors recommend a 1-hour infusion time.

Carboplatin is now most commonly dosed by the selecting the desired AUC for the drug and determining dose according to renal function. The most common and well-tolerated AUCs are 5 or 6. The AUC dose is calculated using the Calvert formula:

$$\text{Carboplatin dose} = \text{Target AUC (GFR} + 25)^{3,4}$$

An older approach, though currently a less well-accepted alternative, is to use 300 mg/m² per dose when the drug is given in combination with a taxane or 400 mg/m² per dose as a single agent. This is based on the clinical observation that, in terms of antitumor efficacy, 1 mg of cisplatin appears to be equivalent to 4 mg of carboplatin; that is, a 75-mg dose of cisplatin is therapeutically equivalent to 300-mg of carboplatin.

Whether one bases dose on AUC or the milligrams per square meter method, the calculated total milligram dosage for any individual tends to be similar if the creatinine clearance is nearly normal. The carboplatin dose should be administered every 21 or 28 days, depending on blood count recovery. In a percentage of patients, cumulative thrombocytopenia will result in dose reductions, or dosing delays, by the fourth or fifth cycle of therapy.

Oxaliplatin dosing guidelines are provided in Table 15-6. When given in combination with other agents, as in the treatment of colorectal cancer, these doses should never be exceeded. A number of oxaliplatin-based combination therapy regimens are under investigation in a range of diseases.

Clinical Concepts of Platinum Resistance

In the treatment of gynecologic malignancies, specifically in ovarian cancer, the disease may be clinically platinum sensitive or clinically platinum resistant.[100,101] Data show that if a patient with ovarian cancer is more than 2 years out from the most recent dose of platinum (having responded to that therapy), there is a greater than 70% likelihood that the disease will respond to re-treatment with cisplatin- or carboplatin-based therapy.[100]

The percentage of patients who will respond decreases with the shortening of the disease-free period. Persons who have disease recurrence within the first 6 months after the most recent dose of platinum have a low likelihood of response to re-treatment with cisplatin or carboplatin and are considered to have platinum-resistant disease. This concept is firmly established for cases of epithelial ovarian cancer. The applicability of this concept to other diseases commonly treated with platinum-based therapy is uncertain.

As discussed above, there are strong data that in non–small cell lung cancer, clinical treatment decisions can be made based on whether a tumor specimen expresses detectable levels of ERCC1 protein or not.[87] At a growing number of institutions, if ERCC1 protein is not detected in the lung cancer specimen, platinum-based therapy is begun. Clinical data suggest that these tumors are platinum sensitive, and the patient will benefit from platinum-based chemotherapy. If ERCC1 protein in easily detected, a nonplatinum regimen is utilized instead. These tumors are likely to be platinum resistant. It is not clear how useful this approach will be in the long-term, or, whether this approach may apply to other malignancies.

Common Clinical Uses

The platinum compounds constitute the mainstay of therapy for a wide range of malignancies. This includes potentially curative therapies for advanced-stage testicular and ovarian germ cell tumors, epithelial ovarian cancer, upper aerodigestive tumors, and small cell and non–small cell lung cancer. Effective oxaliplatinum-based therapies also are in place for advanced stages and for adjuvant therapy of colorectal cancer. Cisplatin, in conjunction with radiation, is curative for locally advanced head and neck malignancies and cervical cancer. There is a rapidly growing interest in cisplatin as an effective agent in BRCA-1 and BRCA-2 mutant breast cancer, and in triple negative (HER2/neu, estrogen receptor, and progesterone receptor–negative) breast cancers, which share similar gene expression profiles and exhibit striking clinical sensitivity to cisplatin as neoadjuvant chemotherapy.[83,102,103] Eighteen of twenty eight (64%) of triple negative patients responded partially or completely to single agent cisplatin, including two of two complete responses in BRCA-1 mutant tumors,[102] while 10 of 12 BRCA-1 mutant tumors responded completely to cisplatin in a second neoadjuvant trial.[103] Whether the basis for this sensitivity is a common underlying defect in double-strand break repair has not been established, but the hypothesis is intriguing.

Table 15-7 is a summary of the current use of platinum analogs in several major malignancies. An extensive review of the data is beyond the scope of this text but is easily obtained in major texts, or online. Generally, in most circumstances where the cisplatin and carboplatin have been tested in phase III trials, cisplatin is clearly the more toxic agent. Cisplatin commonly causes renal toxicity, neurotoxicity, auditory toxicity, and a range of other side effects. That said, there are several diseases where cisplatin remains the mainstay of therapy because of the strong advantage in clinical efficacy. Those diseases include testicular, bladder, small cell lung, esophageal, gastric, basal type breast, and cervical cancer. In several of these malignancies (cervix, head and neck), cisplatin's utility is due in part to its role as a radiation sensitizer. In non–small cell lung cancer and in head and neck cancers, cisplatin and carboplatin are both highly effective.

In ovarian cancer, cisplatin and carboplatin are viewed as having equivalent clinical efficacy, with carboplatin associated with a much lower rate of observed toxicities. For this reason, carboplatin has supplanted cisplatin in this disease. In colorectal cancer, the level of efficacy seen for oxaliplatin in phase II clinical trials far exceeded the historical phase II data for cisplatin and carboplatin. Its lack of dependence on MMR may account for this difference. Oxaliplatin is, therefore, considered much more efficacious in this disease than the other two compounds, even though direct comparisons are mostly lacking.

A potentially promising new analog of cisplatin is satraplatin (bisaceto-ammine-dichloro-cyclohexylamine platinum IV, or JM-216).[104] Satraplatin is an orally active platinum analogue, which has preclinical activity in tumor cell lines resistant to cisplatin, taxanes, and/or anthracyclines. This drug appears to be particularly active in prostate cancer. A recent phase III randomized trial compared satraplatin plus prednisone to prednisone plus placebo in castrate resistant prostate cancer.[105] Satraplatin was orally administered at 80mg/m2, as a single daily dose, on days 1 to 5 of a 35-day treatment cycle. All study participants received prednisone at 5 mg, PO, twice daily.

TABLE

15.7 *Disease comparisons of platinum analogues*

Ovarian cancer	Prospective randomized trials showed clinical equivalency for cisplatin and carboplatin. Cisplatin was more toxic.
Testicular cancer	Prospective randomized trials showed clinical superiority for cisplatin combinations over carboplatin combinations.
Non-small cell lung cancer	Meta-analyses suggest that cisplatin-based regimens MAY offer improved efficacy over carboplatin-based regimens.
Small cell lung cancer	Recent randomized trials suggest that carboplatin-based regimens may have equal efficacy and less toxicity.
Colorectal cancer	Phase II data for oxaliplatin are strongly superior over historical phase II data for cisplatin or carboplatin.
Bladder cancer	Prospective randomized trials showed clinical superiority for cisplatin combinations over carboplatin combinations.
Cervix cancer	Cisplatin is optimal radiosensitizer. Carboplatin is active. Oxaliplatin is much less active than cisplatin or carboplatin.
Gastric cancer	Cisplatin-based regimens appear superior. Oxaliplatin-based regimens may be equivalent to cisplatin-based regimens. Carboplatin less active.
Esophageal cancer	Cisplatin is optimal radiosensitizer. Carboplatin is active. Generally, cisplatin/5FU is used concurrent with radiation.
Head and neck cancers	Cisplatin is optimal radiosensitizer. Carboplatin is active.

When the satraplatin group was compared to the placebo treated group, the satraplatin-treated group showed statistically significant improvement in progression free-survival, time to progression, PSA responses, and pain responses. But there was similar overall survival comparing satraplatin to placebo. One subset analysis of this study was an assessment of satraplatin performance in patients who had previously received docetaxel chemotherapy. In this subgroup, it was observed that satraplatin treatment was associated with prolonged progression-free survival and a trend toward improved overall survival ($P = 0.06$). Further studies are indicated.

A better understanding of the molecular processes that underlie the clinical differences between cisplatin, carboplatin, and oxaliplatin may open the door for the development of future agents in this class, with an even better therapeutic index and broader efficacy. It is possible that satraplatin, and/or other platinum analogues such as the canocapsular formulations, may join the group of FDA-approved medications in the foreseeable future.

References

1. Rosenberg B, Van Camp L, Krigas T. Inhibition of cell division in *Escherichia coli* by electrolysis products from a platinum electrode. Nature 1965;205:698.

2. Rosenberg B, Van Camp L, Trosko JE, et al. Platinum compounds: a new class of potent antitumor agents. Nature 1969;222:385–386.

3. Reed E, Dabholkar M, Chabner BA. Platinum analogues. In: Chabner BA, Longo DL, eds. Cancer Chemotherapy, 2nd ed. Philadelphia: Lippincott-Raven Publishers, 1996:357–378.

4. Reed E. Cisplatin and analogs. In: Chabner BA, Longo DL, eds. Cancer Chemotherapy and Biotherapy: Principles and Practice, 3rd ed. Philadelphia: Lippincott Williams & Wilkins, 2001:447–465.

5. Burger KN, Staffhorst RW, Vijlder HC, et al. Nanocapsules: lipid coated aggregates of cisplatin with high toxicity. Nat Med 2002;8:81–84.

6. Chupin V, de Kroon AI, de Kruijff B. Molecular architecture of nanocapsules, bilayer enclosed solid particles of cisplatin. J Am Chem Soc 2004;126:13816–13821.

7. Hamelers IH, de Kroon AI. Nanocapsules: a novel formulation technology for platinum-based anticancer drugs. Future Lipidol 2007;2:445–453.

8. Hamelers IH, van Loenen E, Staffhorst RW, et al. Carboplatin nanocapsules: a highly cytotoxic, phospholipid-based formulation of carboplatin. Mol Cancer Ther 2006;5:2007–2012.

9. Kruh GD. Lustrous insights into cisplatin accumulation: copper transporters. Clin Cancer Res 2003;9:5807–5809.

10. Samini G, Katano K, Holzer AK, et al. Modulation of the cellular pharmacology of cisplatin and its analogs by the copper exporters ATP7A and ATP7B. Mol Pharmacol 2004;66:25–32.

11. Holzer AK, Manorek GH, Howell SB. Contribution of the major copper influx transporter CTR1 to the cellular accumulation of cisplatin, carboplatin, and oxaliplatin. Mol Pharmacol 2006;70:1390–1394.

12. Zhang S, Levejoy KS, Shima JE, et al. Organic cation transporters are determinants of oxaliplatin cytoxicity. Cancer Res 2006;66:8847–8857.

13. Ciarimboli G, Ludwig T, Lang D, et al. Cisplatin nephrotoxicity is critically mediated via the human organic cation transporter 2. Am J Pathol 2005;167:1477–1484.

14. Eastman A. Reevaluation of interaction of cis-dichloro (ethylene-diammine) platinum(II) with DNA. Biochemistry 1986;25:3912–3915.

15. Eastman A, Schulte N, Sheibani N, et al. Mechanisms of resistance to platinum drugs. In: Nicolini M, ed. Platinum and Other Metal Coordination Compounds in Cancer Chemotherapy. Boston: Martinus Nijhoff, 1988:178–196.

16. Fichtinger-Schepman AM, van der Veer JL, den Hartog JH, et al. Adducts of the antitumor drug cis-diamminedichloroplatinum (II), with DNA: formation, identification and quantitation. Biochemistry 1985;24:707–713.

17. Fichtinger-Schepman AMJ, van Oosterom AT, Lohman PHM, et al. Cis-diamminedichloroplatinum(II)-induced adducts in peripheral leukocytes from seven cancer patients: quantitative immunochemical detection of the adduct induction and removal after a single dose of cis-diamminedichloroplatinum(II). Cancer Res 1987;47:3000–3004.

18. Fichtinger-Schepman AMJ, van Oosterom AT, Lohman PHM, et al. Interindividual human variation in cisplatinum sensitivity, predictable in an in vitro assay? Mutat Res 1987;190:59–62.

19. Fichtinger-Schepman AM, van Dijk-Knijnburg HC, van der Velde-Visser SD, et al. Cisplatin and carboplatin DNA adducts: is PT-AG the cytotoxic lesion? Carcinogenesis 1995;16:2447–2453.

20. Gelasco A, Lippard SJ. NMR solution structure of a DNA dodecamer duplex containing a cis-diammineplatinum(II) d(GpG) intrastrand cross-link, the major adduct of the anti-cancer drug cisplatin. Biochemistry 1998;37:9230–9239.

21. Sancar A. Mechanisms of DNA excision repair. Science 1994;266:1954–1956.

22. De Laat WL, Jaspers NG, Hoeijmakers JH. Molecular mechanism of nucleotide excision repair. Genes Dev 1999;13:768–785.

23. Reed E. Platinum-DNA adduct, nucleotide excision repair, and platinum based anti-cancer chemotherapy. Cancer Treat Rev 1998;24:331–344.

24. Micetich K, Barnes D, Etickson LC. A comparative study of the cytotoxicity and DNA-damaging effects of cis-diammino(1,1 cyclobutanedicarboxylato)-platinum(II) and cisdiamminedichloroplatinum (II) on LI210 cells. Cancer Res 1985;45:4043–4047.

25. Reardon JT, Vaisman A, Chaney SG, et al. Efficient nucleotide excision repair of cisplatin, oxaliplatin, and bis-aceto-amminedichloro-cyclohexylamine-platinum(IV) (JM216) platinum intrastrand DNA diadducts. Cancer Res 1999;59:3968–3971.

26. Luo FR, Wyrick SD, Chaney SG. Cytotoxicity, cellular uptake, and cellular biotransformations of oxaliplatin in human colon carcinoma cells. Oncol Res 1998;10:595–603.

27. Saris CP, van de Vaart PJ, Rietbrock RC, et al. In vitro formation of DNA adducts by cisplatin, lobaplatin and oxaliplatin in calf thymus DNA in solution and in cultured human cells. Carcinogenesis 1996;17:2763–2769.

28. Raymond E, Faivre S, Chaney SG, et al. Cellular and molecular pharmacology of oxaliplatin. Mol Cancer Ther 2002;1:227–235.

29. Olivero OA, Semino C, Kassim A, et al. Preferential binding of cisplatin to mitochondrial DNA of Chinese hamster ovary cells. Mutat Res 1995;346:221–230.

30. Olivero OA, Chang PK, Lopez-Larraza DM, et al. Preferential formation and decreased removal of cisplatin-DNA adducts in Chinese hamster ovary cell mitochondrial DNA as compared to nuclear DNA. Mutat Res 1997;391:79–86.

31. Giurgiovich AJ, Diwan BA, Olivero OA, et al. Elevated mitochondrial cisplatin-DNA adduct levels in rat tissues after transplacental cisplatin exposure. Carcinogenesis 1997;18:93–96.

32. Deyoung MP, Ellisen LW. p63 and p73 in human cancer: defining the network. Oncogene 2007;26:5169–5183.

33. Aebi S, Fink D, Gordon R, et al. Resistance to cytotoxic drugs in DNA mismatch repair-deficient cells. Clin Cancer Res 1997;3:1763–1767.

34. Drummond JT, Anthoney A, Brown R, et al. Cisplatin and adriamycin resistance are associated with MutL-alpha and mismatch repair deficiency in an ovarian tumor cell line. J Biol Chem 1996;271:19645–19648.

35. Nehma A, Baskaran R, Nebel S, et al. Induction of JNK and c-Abl signalling by cisplatin and oxaliplatin in mismatch repair proficient and -deficient cells. Br J Cancer 1999;79:1104–1110.

36. Vaisman A, Varchenko M, Umar A, et al. The role of hMLH1, hMSH3, and hMSH6 defects in cisplatin and oxaliplatin resistance: correlation with replicative bypass of platinum-DNA adducts. Cancer Res 1998;58:3579–3585.

37. Siemer S, Ornskov D, Guerra B, et al. Determination of mRNA and protein levels of p53, MDM2, and protein kinase CK2 subunits in F9 cells after treatment with the apoptosis-inducing drugs cisplatin and carboplatin. Int J Biochem Cell Biol 1999;31:661–670.

38. Arriola EL, Rodriguez-Lopez AM, Hickman JA, et al. Bcl-2 overexpression results in reciprocal downregulation of Bcl-X(L) and sensitizes human testicular germ cell tumors to chemotherapy-induced apoptosis. Oncogene 1999;18(7):1457–1464.

39. Henkels KM, Turchi JJ. Cisplatin-induced apoptosis proceeds by caspase-3-dependent and -independent pathways in cisplatin-resistant and -sensitive human ovarian cancer cell lines. Cancer Res 1999;59:3077–3083.

40. Sharma S, Gong P, Temple B, et al. Molecular dynamic simulations of cisplatin- and oxaliplatin-d(GG) intrastrand cross-links reveal differences in their conformational dynamics. J Mol Biol 2007;373:1123–1140.

41. Rothenberg ML, Oza AM, Bigelow RH, et al. Superiority of oxaliplatin and fluorouracil-leucovorin compared with either therapy alone in patients with progressive colorectal cancer after irinotecan and fluorouracil-leucovorin: interim results of a phase III trial. J Clin Oncol 2003;21:2059–2069.

42. Villella J, Marchetti D, Odunsi K, et al. Response of combination platinum and gemcitabine chemotherapy for recurrent epithelial ovarian carcinoma. Gynecol Oncol 2004;95:539–545.

43. Engblom P, Rantanen V, Kulmala J, et al. Additive and supra-additive cytotoxicity of cisplatin-taxane combinations in ovarian carcinoma cell lines. Br J Cancer 1999;79:286–292.

44. Donawho CK, Luo Y, Luo Y, et al. ABT-888, an orally active poly(ADP-ribose) polymerase inhibitor that potentiates DNA-damaging agents in preclinical tumor models. Clin Cancer Res 2007;13:2728–2737.

45. Altaha R, Liang X, Yu JJ. Reed Excision repair cross complementing-group-1: gene expression and platinum resistance. Int J Mol Med 2004;14:959–970.

46. Li Q, Bostick-Bruton F, Reed. E. Modulation of ERCC-1 mRNA expression by pharmacological agents in human ovarian cancer cells. Biochem Pharmacol 1999;57:347–353.

47. Li Q, Bostick-Bruton F, Reed E. Effect of interleukin-1 and tumor necrosis factor on cisplatin-induced ERCC1 mRNA expression in a human ovarian carcinoma cell line. Anticancer Res 1998;18:2283–2287.

48. Mimnaugh EG, Yunmbam MK, Li Q, et al. Proteasome inhibitors prevent cisplatin-DNA adduct repair and potentiate cisplatin-induced apoptosis in ovarian carcinoma cells. Biochem Pharmacol 2000;60:1343–1354.

49. Bonovich M, Olive M, Reed E, et al. Adenoviral delivery of A FOS, an AP-1 dominant negative, selectively inhibits drug resistance in two human cancer cell lines. Cancer Gene Ther 2002;9:62–70.

50. Von Knethen A, Lotero A, Brune B. Etoposide and cisplatin induced apoptosis in activated RAW 264.7 macrophages is attenuated by cAMP-induced gene expression. Oncogene 1998;17:387–394.

51. Kleinerman ES, Zwelling L A, Howser D, et al. Defective monocyte killing in patients with malignancies and restoration of function during chemotherapy. Lancet 1980;2(8204):1102–1105.

52. Kleinerman ES, Zwelling LA, Muchmore AV. Enhancement of naturally occurring human spontaneous monocyte mediated cytotoxicity by cis-diamminedichloroplatinum(II). Cancer Res 1980;40:3099–3102.

53. Merritt RE, Mahtabifard A, Yamada RE, et al. Cisplatin augments cytotoxic T lymphocyte mediated antitumor immunity in poorly immunogenic murine lung cancer. J Thorac Cardiovasc Surg 2003;126:1609–1617.

54. Li Q, Gardner K, Zhang L, et al. Cisplatin induction of ERCC1 mRNA expression in A2780/CP70 human ovarian cancer cells. J Biol Chem 1998;273:23419–23425.

55. Li Q, Tsang B, Gardner K, et al. Phorbol ester exposure activates an AP-1 associated increase in ERCC1 mRNA expression in human ovarian cancer cells. Cell Mol Life Sci 1999;55:456–466.

56. Gupta S, Natarajan R, Payne SG, et al. Deoxycholic acid activates the c-Jun N-terminal kinase pathway via Fas receptor activation in primary hepatocytes. Role of acidic sphingomyelinase-mediated ceramide generation in Fas receptor activation. J Biol Chem 2004;279:5821–5828.

57. Schwabe RF, Uchinami H, Qian T, et al Differential requirement for c-Jun NH2-terminal kinase in TNF alpha-Fas-mediated apoptosis in hepatocytes. FASEB J 2004;18:720–722.

58. Shangary S, Lerner EC, Zhan Q, et al. Lyn regulates the cell death response to ultraviolet radiation through c-Jun N terminal kinase-dependent Fas ligand activation. Exp Cell Res 2003;289:67–76.

59. Toh U, Sudo T, Kido K, et al. Intraarterial cellular immunotherapy for patients with inoperable liver metastases of esophageal cancer. Gan To Kagaku Ryoho 2002;29:2152–2156.

60. Berghmans T, Paesmans M, Lalami Y, et al. Activity of chemotherapy and immunotherapy on malignant mesothelioma; a systematic review of the literature with meta-analysis. Lung Cancer 2002;38:111–121.

61. Yoshikawa T, Tsuburaya A, Kobayashi O, et al. A combination immunochemotherapy of 5-fluorouracil, cisplatin, leucovorin, and OK-432 for advanced and recurrent gastric carcinoma. Hepatogastroenterology 2003;50:2259–2263.

62. Lens MB, Eisen TG. Systemic chemotherapy in the treatment of malignant melanoma. Expert Opin Pharmacother 2003;4:2205–2211.

63. Ohtsukasa S, Okabe S, Yamashita H, et al. Increased expression of ECA and MHC class I in colorectal cancer cells exposed to chemotherapy drugs. J Cancer Res Clin Oncol 2003;129:719–726.

64. Wilailak S, Dangprasert S, Srisupundit S. Phase I clinical trial of chemoimmunotherapy in combination with radiotherapy in stage IIIB cervical cancer patients. Int J Gynecol Cancer 2003;13:652–656.

65. Godwin A, Meister A, O'Dwyer P, et al. High resistance to cisplatin in human ovarian cacer cell lines is associated with marked increase in glutathione systhesis. Proc Natl Acad Sci U S A 1992;89:3070–3074.

66. Hosking LK, Whelan RDH, Shellard SA, et al. An evaluation of the role of glutathione and its associated enzymes in the expression of differential sensitivities to antitumor agents shown by a range of human tumour cell lines. Biochem Pharmacol 1990;40:1833–1842.

67. Pattaniak A, Bachowski G, Laib J, et al. Properties of the reaction of cis-dichlorodiammineplatinum(II) with metallothionein. J Biol Chem 1992;267:16121.

68. Kelley S, Basu A, Teicher B, et al. Overexpression of metallothionein confers resistance to anticancer drugs. Science 1988;241:1813–1815.

69. Reed E, Ozols RF, Tarone R, et al. Platinum-DNA adducts in leukocyte DNA correlate with disease response in ovarian cancer patients receiving platinum-based chemotherapy. Proc Natl Acad Sci U S A 1987;84:5024–5028.

70. Reed E, Ostchega Y, Steinberg S, et al. An evaluation of platinum-DNA adduct levels relative to known prognostic variables in a cohort of ovarian cancer patients. Cancer Res 1990;50:2256–2260.

71. Darcy KM, Tian C, Reed E. A Gynecologic Oncology Group study of platinum-DNA adducts and excision repair complementation group 1 expression in optimal, stage III epithelial ovarian cancer treated with platinum-taxane chemotherapy. Cancer Res 2007;67:4474–4481.

72. Dabholkar M, Bostick-Bruton F, Weber C, et al. ERCC1 and ERCC2 expression in malignant tissues from ovarian cancer patients. J Natl Cancer Inst 1992;84:1512–1517.

73. Dabholkar M, Vionnet JA, Bostick-Bruton F, et al. mRNA Levels of XPAC and ERCC1 in ovarian tumor tissue correlates with response to platinum containing chemotherapy. J Clin Invest 1994;94:703–708.

74. Metzger R, Leichman CG, Danenberg KD, et al. ERCC1 mRNA levels complement thymidylate synthase mRNA levels in predicting response and survival for gastric cancer patients receiving combination cisplatin and fluorouracil chemotherapy. J Clin Oncol 1998;16:309–316.

75. Shirota Y, Stoehlmacher J, Brabender J, et al. ERCC1 and thymidylate synthase mRNA levels predict survival for colorectal cancer patients receiving combination oxaliplatin and fluorouracil chemotherapy. J Clin Oncol 2001;19:4298–4304.

76. Lord RV, Brabender J, Gandara D, et al. Low ERCC1 expression correlates with prolonges survival after cisplatin plus gemcitabine chemotherapy in non-small cell lung cancer. Clin Cancer Res 2002;8:2286–2291.

77. Rosell R, Taron M, Barnadas A, et al. Nucleotide excision repair pathways involved in cisplatin resistance in non-small-cell lung cancer. Cancer Control 2003;10:297–305.

78. Li Q, Yu JJ, Mu C, et al. Association between the level of ERCC1 expression and the repair of cisplatin-induced DNA damage in human ovarian cancer cells. Anticancer Res 2000;20(2A):645–652.

79. Wang G, Reed E, Li QQ. Molecular basis of cellular response to cisplatin chemotherapy in non-small cell lung cancer. Oncol Rep 2004;12:955–965.

80. Ferry K, Hamilton T, Johnson S. Increased nucleotide excision repair in cisplatin-resistant ovarian cancer cells: role for ERCC1-XPF. Biochem Pharmacol 2000;60:1305–1313.

81. Lee KB, Parker RJ, Bohr VA, et al. Cisplatin sensitivity/resistance in UV-repair deficient Chinese hamster ovary cells of complementation groups 1 and 3. Carcinogenesis 1993;14:2177–2180.

82. Taniguchi T, Tischkowitz M, Ameziane N, et al. Disruption of the Fanconi anemia–BRCA pathway in cisplatin-sensitive ovarian tumors. Nat Med 2003;9:568–574.

83. Rottenberg S, Jaspers JE, Kersbergen A, et. al. High sensitivity of BRCA 1-deficient mammary tumors to the PARP inhibitor ASD2281 alone and in combination with platinum drugs. Proc Natl Acad Sci U S A 2008;105:170794–170784.

84. Furuta T, Ueda T, Aune G, et al. Transcription-coupled nucleotide excision repair as a determinant of cisplatin sensitivity of human cells. Cancer Res 2002;62:4899–4902.

85. Zhen W, Link CJ Jr, O'Connor PM, et al. Increased genespecific repair of cisplatin interstrand crosslinks in cisplatin resistant human ovarian cancer cells. Mol Cell Biol 1992;12:3689–3698.

86. Jones JC, Zhen W, Reed E, et al. Preferential DNA repair of cisplatinum lesions in active genes in CHO cells. J Biol Chem 1991;266:7101–7107.

87. Olaussen KA, Dunant A, Fouret P, et al. DNA repair by ERCC1 in non-small-cell lung cancer and cisplatin-based adjuvant chemotherapy. N Engl J Med 2006;355:983–991.

88. Viguier J, Boige V, Miquel C, et al. ERCC1 codon 118 polymorphism is a predictive factor for the tumor response to oxaliplatin-5-fluorouracil combination chemotherapy in patients with advanced colorectal cancer. Clin Cancer Res 2005;11:6212–6217.

89. Cornelison TL, Reed E. Nephrotoxicity and hydration management for cisplatin, carboplatin, and ormaplatin: a review. Gynecol Oncol 1993;50:147–158.

90. Reed E, Jacob J. Carboplatin and renal dysfunction. Ann Intern Med 1989;110:409.

91. Reed E, Jacob J, Brawley O. Measures of renal function in cisplatin-related chronic renal disease. J Natl Med Assoc 1991;83:522–526.

92. Diaz-Rubio E, Sastre J, Zaniboni A. Oxaliplatin as a single agent in previously untreated colorectal carcinoma patients: a phase II multicentric study. Ann Oncol 1998;9:105–108.

93. Takimoto CH, Graham MA, Lockwood G, et al. Oxaliplatin pharmacokinetics and pharmacodynamics in adult cancer patients with impaired renal function. Clin Cancer Res 2007;13:4832–4839.

94. Extra JM, Espie M, Calvo F, et al. Phase I study of oxaliplatin in patients with advanced cancer. Cancer Chemother Pharmacol 1990;25(Suppl 5):299–303.

95. Hesketh PJ. Chemotherapy induced nausea and vomiting. N Engl J Med 2008;358:2482–2494.

96. Wiernik PH, Yeap B, Vogl SE, et al. Hexamethylmelamine and low or moderate dose cisplatin with or without pyridoxine for treatment of advanced ovarian carcinoma: a study of the Eastern Cooperative Oncology Group. Cancer Invest 1992;10:1–9.

97. Travis LB, Holowaty EJ, Bergfeldt K, et al. Risk of leukemia after platinum-based chemotherapy for ovarian cancer. N Engl J Med 1999;340:351–357.

98. Burkard R, Trautwein P, Salvi R. The effects of click level, click rate, and level of background masking noise on the inferior caliculus potential (ICP) in the normal and carboplatin treated chinchilla. J Acoust Soc Am 1997;102(6):3620–3627.

99. Lenz HJ. Management and preparedness for infusion and hypersensitivity reactions. Oncologist 2007;12:601–609.

100. Markman M, Rothman R, Hakes T, et al. Second line platinum therapy in patients with ovarian cancer previously treated with cisplatin. J Clin Oncol 1991;9:389–393.

101. Reed E, Jacob J, Ozols RF, et al. 5-Fluouracil and leucovorin in platinum-refractory advanced stage ovarian cancer. Gynecol Oncol 1992;46:326–329.

102. Silver DP, Richardson AJ, Eklund AC, et al. Efficacy of neoadjuvant cisplatin in triple-negative breast cancer. J Clin Oncol 2010;28(Jan 25, 2010 online).

103. Byrski T, Gronwald J, Huzarski T, et. al. Pathologic complete response rates in young women with BRCA1-positive breast cancer after neoadjuvant chemotherapy. J Clin Oncol 2010;28:375–379.

104. Sternberg CN, Petrylak DP, Sartor O, et al. Multinational, double-blind, phase III study of prednisone and either satraplatin or placebo in patients with castrate-refractory prostate cancer pregressing after prior chemotherapy: the SPARC trial. J Clin Oncol 2009;27:5431–5438.

105. Kelland LR, Abel G, McKeage MJ, et al. Preclinical antitumor evaluation of bis-acetato-ammine-dichloro-cyclohexylamine platinum (IV): an orally active platinum drug. Cancer Res 1993;53:2581–2586.

106. Yang J, Parsons J, Nicolay NH, et al. Cells deficient in the base excision repair protein, DNA polymerase beta, are hypersensitive to oxaliplatin chemotherapy. Oncogene 2010;29:463–468.

groups remaining at the site of DNA single-strand cleavage may promote access of a second bleomycin molecule to the opposing strand, resulting in a double-strand break.

Analysis of the products of DNA cleavage, using either viral or mammalian DNA, has consistently shown a preferential release of thymine or thymine-propenal, with lesser amounts of the other three bases or their propenal adducts.[16,34] The propensity for attack at thymine bases probably results from the previously mentioned preference for partial intercalation of bleomycin between base pairs in which at least one strand contains the sequence 5'-GpT-3'. The specificity for cleavage of DNA at a residue located at the 3' side of G seems to be absolute.[35] A schematic representation of the intercalation and cleavage processes as conceived by Grollman and Takeshita[36] is given in Figure 16-4 and summarizes the structural and sequence specificities discussed in this chapter.

Cellular Pharmacology

The cellular uptake of bleomycin is slow, and large concentration gradients are maintained between extracellular and intracellular spaces.[37] ^{14}C-bleomycin accumulates at the cell membrane of murine tumor cells, with gradual appearance of labeling at the nuclear membrane only after 4 hours of exposure.[38] The plasma membrane acts as a barrier for the highly cationic bleomycins, which also have a significant size that limits their diffusion.[39] A bleomycin-binding membrane protein, which may participate in its internalization, has a molecular mass of 250 kD and becomes half-maximally saturated with a bleomycin concentration of 5 μmol/L.[8] Using a fluorescent mimic of bleomycin or agents that disrupt vacuoles, Mistry et al.[40] and Lazo et al.[7] concluded that the internalized bleomycin is sequestered in cytoplasmic organelles. The process by which the entrapped bleomycin is released from the vesicles is not known.

Once bleomycin is internalized, it either translocates to the nucleus to effect DNA damage or can be degraded by bleomycin hydrolase, which has been characterized and cloned from human sources.[41,42] This homomultimeric enzyme metabolizes and inactivates a broad spectrum of bleomycin analogs. The enzyme cleaves the carboxamide amine from the β-aminoalaninamide, yielding a weakly cytotoxic (<1/100) deaminobleomycin.[41] Both the primary amino acid sequence and higher-order structure determined by x-ray crystallography reveal that bleomycin hydrolase is a founding member of what is a growing class of self-compartmentalizing or sequestered intracellular proteases.[43,44] Both yeast and human enzymes are homohexamers with a ring or barrel-like structure that have the papain-like active sites situated within a central channel in a manner resembling the organization of the active sites in the 20S proteosome.[44] The central channel, which has a strong positive electrostatic potential in the yeast protein, is slightly negative in human bleomycin hydrolase. The yeast enzyme binds to DNA and RNA, but human bleomycin hydrolase lacks this attribute.[42,44,45] The C-terminus requires autoprocessing of the terminal amino acid, and the processed enzyme has both aminopeptidase and peptide ligase activities. The kinetic properties of bleomycin hydrolase, such as its pH optimum and salt requirements, are distinct from those of other cysteine proteinases, although the substrate specificity of bleomycin hydrolase is similar to that of cathepsin H. Human bleomycin hydrolase is located on chromosome band 17q11.2 and has one polymorphic site encoding either a valine or isoleucine.[46] Bleomycin hydrolase is found in both normal and malignant cells.[42,47] That this is the only enzyme responsible for metabolizing bleomycin was documented with bleomycin hydrolase–null or "knockout" mice.[48] This inactivating enzyme is present in relatively low concentrations in lung and skin, the two normal tissues most susceptible to bleomycin damage.[41,47] Interestingly, pulmonary bleomycin hydrolase levels are highest in animal species or strains resistant to the pulmonary toxicity of bleomycin.[41] Mice that lack the functional gene are more sensitive to the toxic effects of bleomycin.[48] A polymorphism, A1450G, in the coding region is found in 10% of patients with testicular cancer and is associated with a 20% decrease in survival in patients receiving a regimen containing bleomycin. These findings suggest that the G/G genotype is associated with an increased hydrolytic activity.[49]

DNA is more sensitive to DNA cleavage at the G_2-M and G_1 phases of the cell cycle than at S phase, which may reflect differences in chromatin structure.[50] The degree of chromatin compactness dramatically influences bleomycin-induced DNA damage.[51]

Despite the apparent increased toxicity for cells in G_2, no agreement exists regarding preferential kill of logarithmically growing cells as compared with plateau-phase cells; indeed, some workers have observed greater fractional cell kill for plateau-phase cells.[52] The possibility of enhancing cell kill by maximizing exposure during G_2 has led to a trial of bleomycin by continuous infusion, with unimpressive clinical results.

The intracellular lesions caused by bleomycin include chromosomal breaks and deletions and both single-strand and (less frequently) double-strand breaks. In nonmitotic cells, DNA is organized into nucleosomes, or small beads, which are joined by long strands, or linker regions. The primary point of attack seems to be in the linker regions of DNA, between nucleosomes.[53] Interestingly, the resulting 180- to 200-base-pair fragments are similar in size to those formed by endonucleases activated during apoptosis.[39] Cell kill and DNA strand breakage increase in proportion to the duration of drug exposure for at least 6 hours; this finding again implies a possible advantage for giving bleomycin as a prolonged infusion.

Cells are able to repair bleomycin-induced DNA breaks via a complex array of enzymes and pathways specific for both single-strand and double-strand breaks. A delay in plating cells after bleomycin exposure increases plating efficiency, presumably by allowing time for repair of potentially lethal damage.[54] Inhibitors of DNA repair, such as caffeine and 3'-aminobenzamide,[55] accentuate DNA strand breakage and cell kill by bleomycin. Indirect evidence suggests that repair processes similar to those required for repair of lesions induced by *ionizing radiation* play a role in limiting damage due to bleomycin.[56] Cells from patients with ataxia-telangiectasia, which arises from an inherited defect in DNA repair, have increased sensitivity to bleomycin,[57] as do cells deficient in BRCA1and in other components of repair pathways.[58,59]

Resistance

Several intracellular factors have been identified as contributors to bleomycin tumor resistance: increased drug inactivation, decreased drug accumulation, and increased repair of DNA damage, particularly double-strand breaks.[58,59] Early studies[60] demonstrated increased rates of bleomycin inactivation in two bleomycin-resistant rat hepatoma cell lines. Morris et al.[61] demonstrated an increased level of bleomycin hydrolase in cultured human head and neck carcinoma cells with acquired resistance to bleomycin. Metabolic inactivation of bleomycin also can contribute to intrinsic bleomycin resistance in human colon carcinoma cells.[62]

Increased bleomycin hydrolase activity is not the only mechanism of bleomycin resistance.[63] Some cells selected in culture for bleomycin resistance display enhanced DNA repair capacity.[64] Because Fe(III)·bleomycin requires reduction to Fe(II)·bleomycin, sulfhydryl groups on proteins and peptides are potential factors in drug resistance. Tumor lines with elevated levels of glutathione, selected for resistance to doxorubicin, are collaterally sensitive to bleomycin.[65] The evidence for glutathione enhancement of bleomycin activity is not entirely clear, as buthionine sulfoxamine, a glutathione-depleting agent, enhances tumor sensitivity to bleomycin.[66] Increasing the major protein thiol metallothionein produces a small increase in bleomycin sensitivity, consistent with the proposal that this cysteine-rich protein may assist in the removal of Cu(I) from bleomycin.[9] Bleomycin is not affected by P-glycoprotein, the product of the multidrug resistance gene.

Clinical Pharmacokinetics

A number of techniques have been developed for assay of bleomycin in biologic fluids, including microbiologic methods,[67] HPLC,[68] biochemical techniques (degradation of DNA),[69] and radioimmunoassay methods,[70] which, using bleomycin labeled with iodine-125 or ^{57}Co, may be the most rapid and simple. The antibodies described by Broughton and Strong[70] react quantitatively with the component peptides of the clinically used bleomycin formulation. The primary component peptides A_2 and B_2 give 75% to 100% reactivity compared with the mixture in standard curve determinations. HPLC, using the ion-pairing technique, allows resolution of the component peptides but is more time consuming.

The hallmark of bleomycin pharmacokinetics in patients with normal serum creatinine is a rapid two-phase drug disappearance from plasma; 45%[71] to 70%[72] of the dose is excreted in the urine within 24 hours. For intravenous bolus doses, the half-lives for plasma disappearance have varied somewhat among the published studies. Alberts et al.[73] reported α and β half-lives of 24 minutes and 4 hours, respectively, whereas Crooke et al.[74] estimated the β half-life to be approximately 2 hours. Peak plasma concentrations reach 1 to 10 mU/mL for intravenous bolus doses of 15 U/m^2.

For patients receiving bleomycin by continuous intravenous infusion, the postinfusion half-life is approximately 3 hours. Intramuscular injection of bleomycin (2 to 10 U/m^2) gave peak plasma levels of 0.13 to 0.6 mU/mL, or approximately one tenth the peak level achieved by the intravenous bolus doses.[75] The mean half-life after intramuscular injection was 2.5 hours, or approximately the same as that after intravenous injection. Peak serum concentrations were reached approximately 1 hour after injection (Fig. 16-6). Bleomycin pharmacokinetics also have been studied in patients receiving intrapleural or intraperitoneal injections. These routes have proved effective in controlling malignant effusions due to breast, lung, and

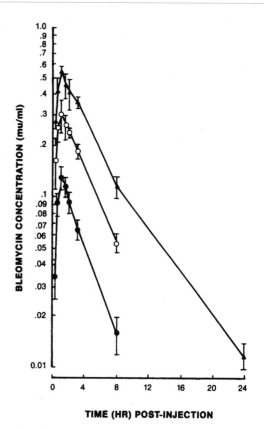

Figure 16-6   Pharmacokinetics of bleomycin after intramuscular administration of 2 (●), 5 (■), and 10 (▲) mg of bleomycin per meter square. (From Oken MM, Crooke ST, Elson MK, et al. Pharmacokinetics of bleomycin after IM administration in man. Cancer Treat Rep 1981;65:485.)

ovarian cancers.[76] Intracavitary bleomycin, in doses of 60 U/m^2, gives peak plasma levels of 0.4 to 5.0 mU/mL, with a plasma half-life of 3.4 hours after intrapleural doses and 5.3 hours after intraperitoneal injection.[77] Corresponding intracavitary levels are 10- to 22-fold higher than simultaneous plasma concentrations.[78] Approximately, 45% of an intracavitary dose is absorbed into the systemic circulation, and 30% is excreted in the urine as immunoreactive material.

As might be expected, bleomycin pharmacokinetics is markedly altered in patients with abnormal renal function, particularly those with creatinine clearance of less than 35 mL/min. Alberts et al.[73] noted a terminal half-life of approximately 10 hours in a patient with a slightly elevated creatinine clearance of 1.5 mg/dL, and Crooke et al.[71] reported a patient who showed a creatinine clearance of 10.7 mL/min and a β half-life of 21 hours. Others have reported a high frequency of pulmonary toxicity in patients with renal dysfunction secondary to cisplatin treatment.[72,79] One report described fatal pulmonary fibrosis that occurred after three doses of 20 U each given to a patient with chronic renal insufficiency (blood urea nitrogen, 48 mg/dL; creatinine, 4.8 mg/dL).[80] The available data are too limited to provide accurate guidelines for dosage adjustment in patients with renal failure. One retrospective study identified a glomerular filtration rate of less than 80 mL/min as conferring an increased risk of pulmonary toxicity.[81] The prudent course is to decrease dosages by 50% for patients with clearances below 80 mL/min or to give an alternative regimen such as vinblastine, ifosfamide, and cisplatin.[82]

Clinical Toxicity and Side Effects

The most important toxic actions of bleomycin affect the lungs and skin; usually little evidence of myelosuppression is apparent except in patients with severely compromised bone marrow function due to extensive previous chemotherapy.[83] In such patients, myelosuppression is usually mild and is seen primarily with high-dose therapy. Fever occurs during the 48 hours after drug administration in one quarter of patients. Some investigators advocate using a 1-U test dose of bleomycin in patients receiving their initial dose of drug,[84] because rare instances of fatal acute allergic reactions have been reported.

Pulmonary Toxicity

Pulmonary toxicity is manifest as a subacute or chronic interstitial pneumonitis complicated in its later stages by progressive interstitial fibrosis, hypoxia, and death.[85] Pulmonary toxicity, usually manifested with cough, dyspnea, and bibasilar pulmonary infiltrates on chest radiographs, occurs in 3% to 5% of patients receiving a total dose of less than 450 U bleomycin; it increases significantly to a 10% incidence in those treated with greater cumulative doses.[85] Toxicity is also more frequent in patients older than age 70, in those with underlying renal dysfunction or emphysema, and in patients receiving single doses greater than 25 U/m^2.[86] The use of bleomycin in single doses of more than 30 U should be discouraged because instances of rapid onset of fatal pulmonary fibrosis 7 to 8 weeks after high-dose bleomycin have been reported.[87] Previous radiotherapy to the chest predisposes to bleomycin-induced pulmonary toxicity.[88] Although the risk of lung toxicity increases with cumulative doses greater than 450 U, severe pulmonary sequelae have been observed at total doses below 100 U. In the standard regimen for treating testicular cancer, bleomycin is given in doses of 30 U/wk for 12 doses, and the incidence of fatal pulmonary toxicity in this low-risk population of young male patients is less than 2%.[89]

Pathogenesis of Pulmonary Toxicity

The potential for bleomycin A$_2$, A$_5$, A$_6$, or B$_2$ to cause pulmonary toxicity is easily demonstrated by intravenous infusion or by direct instillation of the parent molecule into the trachea of a rodent, where it induces an acute inflammatory response, epithelial apoptosis, an alveolar fibrinoid exudate, and, over a period of 1 to 2 weeks, progressive deposition of collagen.[90] The terminal amines of these bleomycins are sufficient, by themselves, to cause the toxicity in rodents, and the toxic potency of the bleomycins is directly correlated with the potency of their individual terminal amines, with the A$_2$ aminopropyl-dimethylsulfonium and the A$_5$ spermidine having greater effect than the B$_2$ agmatine.[91] These findings raise the possibility that modification of the terminal amine might allow selection of a less toxic analog for clinical use. Several such analogs have been tested, but clinical superiority has not been demonstrated.

The pathogenesis of bleomycin pulmonary toxicity in rodents serves as a model for understanding pulmonary fibrosis, an end result of a broad range of human diseases induced by drugs, autoimmunity, and infection.[90] The primary model has been the intratracheal instillation of bleomycin in mice or hamsters,[92] although in clinical drug use the agent is administered parenterally. The drug has direct toxicity to alveolar epithelial cells, causing induction of epithelial apoptosis, intra-alveolar inflammation, cytokine release by alveolar macrophages, fibroblast proliferation, and collagen deposition,[92,93] as well as endothelial cell damage in small pulmonary vessels.[94] As changes progress from acute inflammation to interstitial fibrosis, pulmonary function deteriorates, as indicated by a decrease in lung compliance, a decrease in carbon monoxide diffusion capacity, and terminal hypoxia.[95] Hydroxyproline deposition parallels the increase in collagen and serves as a quantitative measure of the progression of fibrosis in animal models.

A broad array of cytokines, produced by alveolar macrophages and by endothelial cells in response to bleomycin, have been implicated in the molecular pathogenesis of pulmonary fibrosis. These include transforming growth factor β (TGF-β),[96,97] tumor necrosis factor α (TNF-α),[98,99] interleukin 1β,[99] interleukins 2, 3, 4, 5, and 6,[100,101] and various chemokines. Bleomycin and TGF-β both stimulate the promoter that controls transcription of a collagen precursor.[97] Interleukin 1 augments TGF-β secretion stimulated by bleomycin, whereas TNF-α enhances prostaglandin secretion and fibroblast proliferation.[99]

Genetic experiments have provided further insight into factors that influence susceptibility to fibrosis[99–103] and into the central role of cytokines in bleomycin lung toxicity. They illustrate the importance of drug inactivation, fibrin deposition, and cytokine action in mediating lung injury. Travis et al. have shown that strains of mice with greatly increased susceptibility to bleomycin toxicity (and simultaneously to radiation toxicity) can be inbred, although the specific genetic defect is still unclear.[102,103] Other experiments have shown that specific genetic lesions do predispose to pulmonary fibrosis. Bleomycin hydrolase–knockout mice have significantly greater lung and epidermal toxicity than normal controls.[104] Mice lacking plasminogen activator inhibitor 1, a protein that blocks the activation of the major fibrinolytic protease in plasma and in the alveolar space, have decreased susceptibility to bleomycin pulmonary fibrosis,[105] as do mice lacking matrilysin, a matrix metalloproteinase.[106]

Perhaps the most compelling genetic experiments implicate the central role of TGF-β, which is secreted by alveolar macrophages in response to bleomycin.[107] TGF-β is secreted in a complex with a latency-associated peptide and is activated by binding of the complex to αvβ6 integrin found on alveolar epithelial cells and keratinocytes. This binding of the TGF-β complex to its integrin exposes cytokine-binding domains that allow interaction of TGF-β with its receptor(s) and stimulates the production of procollagen by fibroblasts.[108] Mice in which αvβ6 integrin has been knocked out develop an inflammatory alveolar response to bleomycin but do not develop progressive fibrosis.

The stimulus for cytokine and chemokine release is uncertain, although apoptosis of epithelial cells, alveolar macrophages, or lymphocytes may play an important role.[109,110] In mice, genetic deletion of either Fas, which is expressed on pulmonary epithelial cells, or Fas ligand, as expressed on T lymphocytes, does not prevent inflammation but does protect against pulmonary fibrosis.[110] Soluble Fas antigen or anti-Fas ligand antibody also provides protection against fibrosis, presumably by preventing Fas-mediated epithelial apoptosis. CXCL12, a potent chemokine, is secreted by inflammatory cells in response to lung injury and attracts bone marrow–derived stem cells that establish as fibrocytes in the damaged lung.[109] Anti-CXCL12 antibodies protect against bleomycin-induced pulmonary fibrosis. Lysophosphatidic acid may play a role in recruiting fibroblasts to the site of bleomycin lung injury.[111]

In addition to providing remarkable insights regarding the pathogenesis of pulmonary fibrosis, these experiments suggest a number of new approaches to the prevention of bleomycin toxicity. Thus, in various animal models, protection is provided by Fas antigen and anti-Fas ligand antibodies[110]; TNF-α–soluble receptor[112]; TGF-β antibodies[113]; granulocyte-macrophage colony–stimulating factor antibodies[114]; pirfenidone, an inhibitor of platelet-derived growth factor function and procollagen transcription[115]; the antioxidant amifostine[116]; relaxin, a collagen matrix–degrading protein that increases collagenase secretion and decreases procollagen synthesis[117]; transgenic expression of *Sh ble*, a yeast protein that binds the iron-bleomycin complex and protects against its toxicity[118]; dehydroproline, an inhibitor of procollagen synthesis[119,141]; indomethacin[120]; and anti-CXCL12 antibodies.[109] One can add to this list thalidolmide,[121] PPAR-gamma agonists,[122] and anti-HER 2 antibodies,[123] which attenuated bleomycin pulmonary toxicity in model systems. These findings may be applicable to the general problem of preventing drug-induced or idiopathic pulmonary fibrosis in humans,[124] although none of these agents has yet been shown to be efficacious in a clinical trial.

In general, in animal toxicology experiments, single high doses of bleomycin produce greater pulmonary inflammation and fibrosis than do smaller daily doses or continuous drug infusion,[125] but these findings have never been confirmed in humans.

Clinical Syndrome of Pulmonary Toxicity

Clinical symptoms of bleomycin pulmonary injury include a nonproductive cough, dyspnea, and occasionally fever and pleuritic pain. Physical examination usually reveals minimal auscultatory evidence of pulmonary alveolar infiltrates, and initial chest films are often negative or may reveal an increase in interstitial markings, especially in the lower lobes, with a predilection for subpleural areas. Chest radiographs, when positive, reveal patchy reticulonodular infiltrates, which in later stages may coalesce to form areas of apparent consolidation. In occasional patients, the initial radiographic changes may be discrete nodules indistinguishable from metastatic tumor; central cavitation of nodules may be present[126,127] (Fig. 16-7). Gallium-67 lung scans or computed tomographic scans (Fig. 16-8) may show the presence of a diffuse lung lesion at a time of minimal abnormality on plain films of the chest; computed tomographic scans are much more sensitive than posteroanterior chest films in revealing the extent of pulmonary fibrosis. Radiologic findings do not differentiate bleomycin lung toxicity from other forms of interstitial lung disease.[128] Arterial oxygen desaturation and an abnormal carbon monoxide diffusion capacity are present in symptomatic patients with bleomycin toxicity as well as in patients with other forms of interstitial pulmonary disease. Thus, open lung biopsy is usually required to distinguish between the primary differential diagnostic alternatives, specifically a drug-induced pulmonary lesion, an infectious interstitial pneumonitis, and neoplastic pulmonary infiltration. The findings on histologic examination of human lung after bleomycin treatment closely resemble those previously described in the experimental animal and include necrosis of Type I alveolar cells, an acute inflammatory infiltrate in the alveoli, interstitial and intra alveolar edema, pulmonary hyaline membrane formation, and intra alveolar and, later in the course, interstitial fibrosis. In addition, squamous metaplasia of Type II alveolar–lining

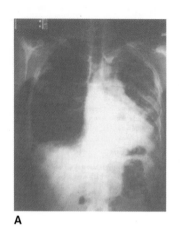
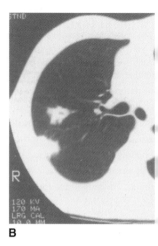

FIGURE 16-7   A: Typical interstitial pulmonary infiltrates, most obvious in left lung, observed during treatment of a patient with testicular carcinoma. **B:** Nodular variant of bleomycin pulmonary toxicity in a patient undergoing treatment for testicular cancer. Computed tomographic scan of chest showing a nodular density with central cavitation. On biopsy, the lesion was found to be composed of granulomas with associated interstitial pneumonitis. Appropriate stains and cultures did not reveal infectious agents. (From Talcott JA, Garnick MB, Stomper PC, et al. Cavitary lung nodules associated with combination chemotherapy containing bleomycin. J Urol 1987;138:619.)

cells has been described as a characteristic finding.[129] In rare cases, a true hypersensitivity pneumonitis may develop, characterized by underlying eosinophilic pulmonary infiltrates and a prompt clinical response to corticosteroids.[130]

Pulmonary function tests, particularly a rapid fall in the carbon monoxide–diffusing capacity, are of possible value in predicting a high risk of pulmonary toxicity. Most patients treated with bleomycin, however, show a progressive (10% to 15%) fall in diffusion capacity with increasing total dose and a more marked increase in changes above a 270-U total dose. Whether or not the diffusion capacity test can be used to predict which patients will subsequently develop clinically significant pulmonary toxicity is not clear.[131] Some investigators suggest that bleomycin should be halted if the diffusion capacity for carbon dioxide (DCO) falls below 40% of the initial value, even in the absence of symptoms. As mentioned earlier, at advanced stages in the evolution of bleomycin pulmonary toxicity, the diffusion capacity as well as arterial oxygen saturation and total lung capacity become markedly abnormal. Long-term assessment of pulmonary function in patients treated with bleomycin

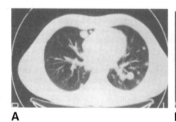
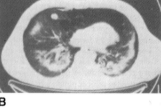

FIGURE 16-8   Computed tomographic scans of the chest before **(A)** and after **(B)** treatment for testicular cancer. The multiple metastatic pulmonary nodules partially regressed with therapy, but the posttreatment film shows dense bilateral pulmonary fibrosis as well as a large left pneumothorax and pneumomediastinum. The patient died of bleomycin pulmonary toxicity shortly afterward.

for testicular cancer has revealed a return to baseline normal values at a median of 4 years after treatment.[132]

Patients who have received bleomycin seem to be at greater risk of respiratory failure during the postoperative recovery period after surgery,[133] although others have questioned the association of perioperative oxygen and pulmonary toxicity.[134] In one study, five of five patients treated with 200 U/m² bleomycin (cumulative dose) for testicular cancer died of postoperative respiratory failure; a reduction in inspired oxygen to an inspired oxygen fraction of 0.24 and a decrease in the volume of fluids administered during surgery prevented mortality in subsequent patients.[133] The sensitivity of bleomycin-treated patients to high concentrations of inspired oxygen is intriguing in view of the molecular action of bleomycin, which is dependent on and mediated by the formation of oxygen-derived free radicals. Current safeguards for anesthesia of bleomycin-treated patients include the use of the minimum tolerated concentration of inspired oxygen and modest fluid replacement to prevent pulmonary edema.

No specific therapy is available for patients with bleomycin-induced lung toxicity. Discontinuation of the drug may be followed by a period of continued progression of the pulmonary findings, with partial reversal of the abnormalities in pulmonary function only after several months. The inflammatory component of the pathologic process does resolve in experimental models, and interstitial infiltrates regress clinically, but the reversibility of pulmonary fibrosis has not been documented. The value of corticosteroids in promoting recovery from bleomycin-induced lung toxicity remains controversial; beneficial effects have been described in isolated case studies.[135,136] Long-term follow-up of patients with clinical and radiographic evidence of bleomycin-induced pneumonitis suggests a complete resolution of radiographic, clinical, and pulmonary function abnormalities in a small series of eight patients 2 years after completion of treatment for testicular cancer.[137] However, in more severe cases, pulmonary fibrosis may be only partially reversible.

Cutaneous Toxicity

A more common but less serious toxicity of bleomycin is its effect on skin, which may relate to low bleomycin hydrolase levels in skin. Approximately, 50% of patients treated with conventional once-daily or twice-daily doses of this agent develop erythema, induration, and hyperkeratosis and peeling of skin that may progress to frank ulceration.[138] These changes predominantly affect digits, hands, joints, and areas of previous irradiation. Hyperpigmentation, alopecia, and nail changes also occur during bleomycin therapy. These cutaneous side effects do not necessitate discontinuation of therapy, particularly if clear benefit is being derived from the drug. Rarely, patients may develop Raynaud's phenomenon while receiving bleomycin.[139] Other toxic reactions to bleomycin include hypersensitivity reactions characterized by urticaria, periorbital edema, and bronchospasm.[138]

Schedules of Administration

Bleomycin has been administered using a number of different schedules and routes of administration. The most common route and schedule are bolus intravenous injection. An alternative regimen of continuous infusion of 25 U/d for 5 days produced the expected rapid onset of pulmonary toxicity, particularly in patients with previous chest irradiation,[88,140] but in addition caused hypertensive episodes in 17% of patients and hyperbilirubinemia in 30%.[86] These latter toxicities are rarely seen with conventional bolus doses.

Continuous intra-arterial infusion also has been used for patients with carcinoma of the cervix[141] and of the head and neck.[142] One study[141] noted a disappointing 12% response rate to infusion of 20 U/m²/wk for courses of up to 3 weeks. Pulmonary toxicity was observed in 20% of patients.

Bleomycin also has been applied topically as a 3.5% ointment in a xipamide (Aquaphor) base. Two-week courses of treatment produced complete regression of Paget's disease of the vulva in four of seven patients,[143] with no serious local toxicity.

As described previously in the discussion of pharmacokinetics, bleomycin can be used to sclerose the pleural space in patients with malignant effusions. After thorough evacuation of fluid from the pleural space, 40 U/m² is dissolved in 100 mL normal saline and instilled through a thoracostomy tube, which is clamped for 8 hours and then returned to suction. In approximately one third of patients thus treated, the effusion clears completely; this is about the same response rate as obtained with tetracycline instillation.[144,145] The only toxic reactions are fever and pleuritis, both of which resolve in 24 to 48 hours. The intraperitoneal instillation of bleomycin has been used in patients with ovarian cancer, mesothelioma, and other malignancy confined to the peritoneum[77] but with rare responses. Sixty milligrams of bleomycin per meter square was dissolved in 2 L of saline, and the solution was placed in the peritoneal cavity for a 4- to 8-hour dwell time. Side effects included abdominal pain, fever, rash, and mucositis. A limited pharmacokinetic advantage was observed (the peritoneal area under the concentration × time curve was sevenfold greater than the plasma area under the curve), which provides little justification for this route of administration.

Bleomycin has been instilled into the urinary bladder in doses of 60 U in 30 mL of sterile water.[146] Seven of twenty-six patients with superficial transitional cell carcinomas had complete disappearance of disease after 7 to 8 weekly treatments. The primary toxic reaction was cystitis. Plasma drug level monitoring revealed little systemic absorption.

Radiation and Drug Interaction

Bleomycin is used frequently in combination therapy regimens for treatment of lymphomas and less commonly for squamous carcinomas of the esophagus and head and neck, primarily because of its lack of myelosuppressive toxicity. The pharmacologic basis of synergism between bleomycin and radiation therapy has received considerable attention[147] but is poorly understood. Administration of bleomycin within 3 hours of irradiation, either before or after, produces greater than additive effects,[147] possibly owing to the production of free-radical damage to DNA by both agents. This interaction has been tested in a randomized clinical trial of radiation therapy plus or minus bleomycin, 5 mg twice weekly, in patients with head and neck cancer.[148] In this study, the group receiving bleomycin had a significantly higher complete response rate and a better 3-year disease-free survival rate. As mentioned earlier, synergistic pulmonary toxicity has been reported in patients receiving bleomycin after previous chest irradiation.

Other Antitumor Antibiotics

Over several decades, microbial fermentation has yielded many valuable compounds, such as the anthracyclines, the bleomycins, and nucleosides, which are discussed in separate chapters. In this chapter, we review two relatively long-standing antibiotics of diverse structure as well as one of the marine-originated ecteinascidins, namely, ecteinascidin-743 (Yondelis, trabectidin, ET-743). Dactinomycin (actinomycin D; DACT) remains a valuable drug in treating choriocarcinoma and pediatric sarcomas, whereas mitomycin C (MMC) is effective in treating anal carcinomas and as an inhibitor of fibrotic reactions in ophthalmologic surgery. Yondelis is a new and promising anticancer agent with a unique mechanism of action and is approved for treatment of soft-tissue sarcomas and ovarian cancer in Europe and soft-tissue sarcomas in Asia.

Dactinomycin

DACT, a product of the *Streptomyces* yeast species, was discovered in 1940;[149] it is a standard agent in combination therapy of Wilms tumor, neuroblastoma, childhood rhabdomyosarcoma, and Ewing's sarcoma. Its key pharmacological features are given in Table 16-2.

Mechanism of Action and Cellular Pharmacology

The structure of DACT[150] is shown in Figure 16-9. It is a chromopeptide consisting of a phenoxazinone planar chromophore to which are attached two pentapeptide rings. Naturally occurring actinomycins differ in the peptide chains but not in the phenoxazone ring. DACT is a strong DNA-binding drug and a potent inhibitor

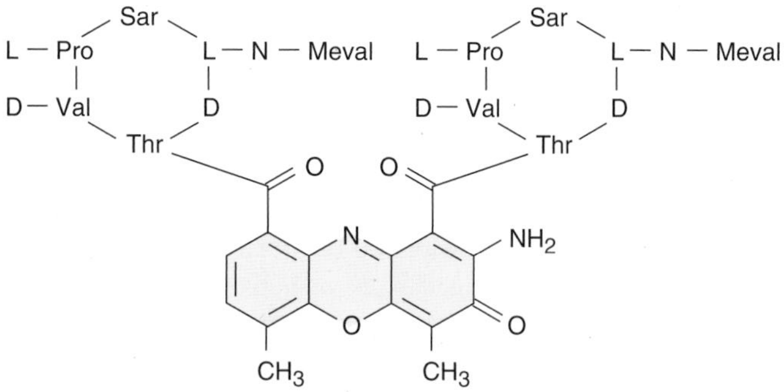

FIGURE 16-9 Structure of dactinomycin. D-Val, D-valine; L-N-Meval, methylvaline; L-Thr, L-threonine; L-Pro, L-proline; Sar, sarcosine.

of RNA and protein synthesis. Actual binding to DNA was shown to be intercalative: the chromophore inserts in between the DNA guanine-cytidine base pairs, while the two chains of the pentapeptide rest in the minor groove.[151,152] DACT can bind to both non-GpC and GpC-containing sequences. Interaction between GpC sequences leads to formation of two hydrogen bonds between each guanine and a pentapeptide.[151] Besides binding to double-strand DNA, DACT is also known to bind to single-strand DNA (ssDNA).[153] The overall association rate between DACT and DNA does not depend on polynucleotide sequence or length but probably reflects the summation of multiple sites of interaction.[154] When bound to ssDNA in a complex formed with polymerase, DACT prevents reannealing of ssDNA and stabilizes unusual ssDNA hairpins, leading to its potent inhibition of transcription.[155]

DACT enters cells by passive diffusion but may be subject to efflux by the P170 glycoprotein pump.[156] It causes cell death by apoptosis, as demonstrated in a variety of cells both in vitro and in vivo.[157] Although high doses of DACT inhibit growth and induce cytotoxicity, at low concentrations and in selected cell lines, the drug induces morphologic and phenotypic differentiation.[158]

Mechanism of Resistance

Resistance to DACT is related to increased efflux mediated by the P170 glycoprotein transporter.[159–163] For example, Chinese hamster ovary cells were found to be cross-resistant to DACT and to other drugs such as vinca alkaloids, anthracyclines, and epipodophyllotoxins.[160,161] Human tumor cell lines made resistant to DACT in vitro were found to amplify the P-glycoprotein–encoding MDR gene. Resistance is reversed in vitro by drugs that inhibit P-glycoprotein function.[163]

Drug Interactions

No pharmacokinetic interactions between DACT and other drugs are known.

Clinical Pharmacology

The pharmacokinetics of DACT have been studied in rat, monkey, and dog.[164] In these species, serum levels of DACT declined rapidly

TABLE 16.2	*Key features of dactinomycin*
Mechanism of action	Inhibition of RNA and protein synthesis
Metabolism	Unknown
Pharmacokinetics	$t_{1/2}$: 36 h
Elimination	Renal: 6%–30%, Bile: 5%–11%
Drug interactions	None
Toxicity	Myelosuppression
	Nausea and vomiting
	Mucositis
	Diarrhea
	Necrosis at extravasation site
	Radiation sensitization and recall reactions
Precautions	Avoid extravasation

$t_{1/2}$, half-life.

after administration, with concomitant accumulation of drug in the tissues. The mean drug half-life in tissues was 47 hours, and metabolites have not been identified. Urinary excretion varies from 6% to 31%, and bile excretion varies from 5% to 11%. A very limited and incomplete study in humans yielded similar results,[165] with a very short period of biodistribution and a long plasma elimination half-life (36 hours). Urinary excretion and fecal excretion were 20% and 14%, respectively, and only 3.3% of the urinary excretion consisted of metabolites.

Toxicity

At the usual clinical dosages of 10 to 15 mg/kg/d for 5 days, DACT causes nausea, vomiting, diarrhea, mucositis, and hair loss. The major and dose-limiting side effect is myelosuppression, with a white blood cell and platelet nadir occurring 8 to 14 days after drug administration.[166] Drug extravasation results in soft-tissue necrosis.[166] In rare cases, DACT treatment leads to severe hepatotoxicity with features of venoocclusive disease, as described in children treated for Wilms tumor.[167] DACT can act as a radiosensitizer and may cause radiation recall phenomena, in which patients receive DACT experience inflammatory reactions in previously irradiated sites.[168] The clinical consequences of such reactions may be serious, especially with the involvement of lung. Corticosteroids may ameliorate these reactions.

Mitomycin C

Mitomycin C (Mutamycin; MMC) was isolated from *Streptomyces caespitosus* in 1958.[169] The initial clinical studies used daily low-dose schedules, which resulted in unacceptably severe, cumulative myelosuppression. Later, an intermittent dosing schedule was introduced, using bolus injections every 4 to 8 weeks, which resulted in more manageable hematological toxicity. With the latter schedule, MMC was found to be active against a wide variety of solid tumors, including breast cancer, aerodigestive tract tumors, cervical cancer, and, with bladder instillation, superficial bladder cancer. In addition, MMC is used as a radiosensitizer with 5-fluorouracil for the treatment of epidermoid anal cancer.[170] Its key pharmacological features are given in Table 16-3.

Mechanism of Action and Cellular Pharmacology

MMC (Fig. 16-10) is a member of a drug family that has a unique chemical structure in which quinone, aziridine, and carbamate functions are arranged around a pyrrolo [l,2-*a*]indole nucleus.[171] Mitomycins are the only known naturally occurring compounds containing an aziridine ring. MMC is soluble in both aqueous and organic solvents. However, because of its chemical instability in solution, the clinical formulation of MMC is a lyophilized form containing mannitol (Mutamycin) or sodium chloride (Mitomycin Kyowa) as excipients. After dissolution in water, MMC is unstable and should be administered within several hours.

TABLE 16.3	Key features of mitomycin C
Mechanism of action	Alkylation of DNA
Metabolism	Hepatic
Pharmacokinetics	$t_{1/2}$ α: 2–10 min
	$t_{1/2}$ β: 25–90 min
Elimination	Renal: 1%–20%
Drug interaction	None
Toxicity	Myelosuppression
	Necrosis at extravasation
	Hemolytic uremic syndrome
	Interstitial pneumonitis
	Cardiomyopathy
Precautions	Avoid extravasation

$t_{1/2}$, half-life.

Formation of DNA Adducts

MMC not only cross-links complementary strands of DNA but also induces monofunctional alkylation, with attachment to a single DNA strand.[172] It primarily acts as a DNA replication inhibitor, and although monofunctional alkylation is by far the most frequently observed interaction, DNA interstrand cross-linking is considered to be the most lethal adduct. DNA cross-linking and alkylation require an initial chemical or enzymatic reduction of the quinone function. The primary mechanism of alkylation is accomplished by activation of the C-1 aziridine and the C-10 carbamate groups, although several additional reactive electrophiles derived from MMC, such as a quinone methide and the oxidized forms of aziridinomitosene and leuco-aziridinomitosene, may alkylate DNA as well.[173,174] Several MMC-induced DNA cross-links have been identified,[175] including 2,7-diaminomitosene, which specifically alkylates guanines in $(G)_n$ tracts of DNA. Selective removal of the aziridine function of MMC results in a switch from minor to major groove alkylation of DNA.[176]

Reductive Alkylation

MMC is considered the prototypical bioreductive alkylating agent. Two mechanisms exist through which reductive metabolism mediates the cytotoxic effects of MMC.[176–179] First, under anaerobic conditions, one- or two-electron reduction followed by spontaneous loss of methanol leads to the formation of reactive unstable intermediates.

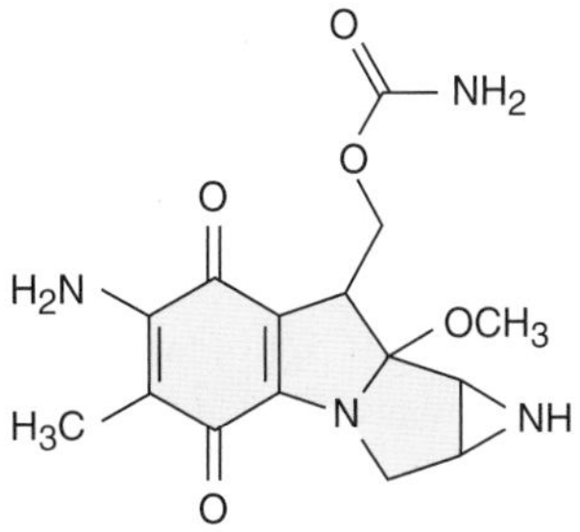

FIGURE 16-10 Structure of mitomycin C.

The suggested anaerobic mechanism begins with the formation of a hydroquinone and its rearrangement to yield a quinone-methide, which then engages in a nucleophilic attack leading to a mono-alkylation of DNA. Intramolecular displacement of the carbamate group would then result in a second reactive site that produces a cross-linked adduct. Although the cross-linking of MMC to DNA in viable cells and cell extracts is readily demonstrable, the mechanism is difficult to reproduce in cell-free systems. In vitro activation of MMC and binding to DNA can be demonstrated in the presence of reduced NADPH. The addition of a reducing agent stabilizes the semiquinone radical, the intermediate that is formed by the first electron uptake of MMC. It appears that one-electron reduction is sufficient to activate both the C-1 and C-10 electrophilic centers.[180]

Aerobic Activation

Under aerobic conditions, a second mechanism comes into play through which MMC develops its cytotoxic effect. Reductive metabolism again leads to the formation of reduced MMC; however, the aerobic fate of reduced MMC is different. Molecular oxygen reacts with either the short-lived semiquinone radical or the hydroquinone form to generate the superoxide radical anion, hydroxyl radicals, or hydrogen peroxide.[181] Formation of these highly reactive species may lead to cytotoxic effects such as lipid peroxidation or nucleic acid damage and can be prevented by free radical scavengers such as mannitol as well as by protective enzymes such as superoxide dismutase or catalase. Whether the reactive intermediate of MMC is formed through the radical semiquinone or the dianion (hydroquinone form) depends on the half-life of the radical anion. In an aprotic environment, the radical anion may have a considerable lifetime; in protic media, however, it exists only a few milliseconds, with rapid uptake of a second electron. Furthermore, oxygen definitely plays an important role, as it is a specific inhibitor of the two-electron pathway because of interaction with and inactivation of the semiquinone species by oxygen.

Several enzyme systems capable of activating MMC include NADPH-cytochrome P450 reductase, xanthine oxidase, and xanthine dehydrogenase.[177,181] However, a controversial aspect of the bioreductive activation of MMC concerns the role of an enzyme called DT-diaphorase (DTD).[173,176–179] DTD is an obligate two-electron reductase that is characterized by its ability to use both the reduced form of NADH and NADPH as electron donors and by its inhibition by dicumarol.[181] Both MMC-induced cytotoxicity and induction of DNA interstrand cross-links were found to be DTD dependent and could be inhibited by pretreatment of HT-29 colon carcinoma cell lines with dicumarol.[182] The ability of DTD to metabolize MMC to a reactive cytotoxic species suggests that the level of DTD may be an important determinant of the antitumor activity of MMC.

The NADPH-cytochrome P450 reductase, a flavoprotein containing 1 mole each of flavin mononucleotide and dinucleotide may play a role in aerobic MMC activation, although aerobic activation does occur in its absence.[183–185] It functions to transfer electrons from NADPH to the various forms of cytochrome P450. The enzyme is able to activate MMC to toxic species, with greatest cytotoxic potential under hypoxic conditions.[183,184] Cumulatively,

these various routes to activation suggest that the enzymes involved in the reduction of MMC under hypoxic conditions may not be the same as those observed under aerobic conditions and that the products of reduction in various pathways may differ.

Analysis of DNA Adducts

Several studies have been published on covalent interactions between MMC and DNA or DNA fragments.[175,186] The actual binding site of MMC in DNA is the N-6 position of adenine residues or either the N-2 or N-7 position of guanine residues. Acid-activated MMC was found to alkylate preferentially the guanine N-7 position, in contrast to reductively activated MMC, which preferentially alkylates the guanine N-2 position, possibly because of the different electronic structures of acid-activated and reduction-activated MMC. The activation mechanism of MMC can presumably now be evaluated from analysis of the DNA adducts formed in vivo.

Mechanism of Resistance

The mechanisms of resistance to MMC are incompletely understood but likely involve changes in drug accumulation, bioactivation, inactivation of the alkylating species, and DNA excision repair. In a series of Chinese hamster ovary cell mutants selected for MMC resistance, a progressive loss of MMC activation capacity and increased capacity for excision repair of DNA were found as cells became more drug resistant.[187] The specific bioactivation enzyme system deficient in the resistant cells was not identified in these studies, although the primary activation mechanism in the sensitive parent was sensitive to dicumarol and, therefore, probably DTD. Cells derived from subjects with Fanconi anemia, an inherited disease in which the nucleotide excision repair pathway is defective, are supersensitive to MMC.[188]

In some resistant cell lines, MMC shares in the MDR phenotype that encompasses doxorubicin, vincristine, and other natural products, as mediated by overexpression of the drug efflux protein P170.[189] On the other hand, several drugs known to reverse MDR induced by other drugs were not capable of reversing MMC-induced MDR, which suggests other pathways contributing to the process.[190]

Clinical Pharmacology

MMC has a biexponential decline of the plasma concentration time curves, which corresponds to a two-compartment model with linear pharmacokinetics up to doses as high as 60 mg/m^2.[191,192] After a rapid distribution half-life (2 to 10 minutes), the elimination half-life is 25 to 90 minutes (mean, 54 minutes). In two studies an unexplained increase in total-body clearance, and a decrease in the area under the plasma concentration time curve of MMC was observed in patients receiving combination chemotherapy that included 5-fluorouracil and doxorubicin,[191,193] an interaction not easily explained in terms of mechanisms of drug elimination.

Impaired liver or renal function does not seem to change the pharmacokinetic behavior of MMC. Urinary recovery of parent drug after intravenous administration ranged from 1% to 20%, which cannot explain the rapid plasma clearance. Therefore, the suggestion has been made that MMC is likely cleared from plasma by hepatic metabolism,[194] but the spleen, kidney, brain, and heart may also be involved in this process. The presence of oxygen markedly reduced the rate of metabolism of MMC in liver homogenates, compared with metabolism in a similar but anaerobic system. As biotransformation is required for activity, this supports the theory of a more pronounced metabolic activation under anaerobic conditions.

MMC is erratically absorbed after oral administration. Intravesical MMC therapy to treat superficial bladder cancer results in extremely low plasma levels, with virtually no systemic side effects and a significant exposure at the target site (bladder).[195–198] MMC uptake in bladder tissues is linearly related to drug concentration in the bladder fluid.[197] MMC administered intraperitoneally is rapidly absorbed through the serosal surface into plasma. Preliminary, uncontrolled studies suggest that intraperitoneal MMC may cause useful clinical benefit for patients with intraperitoneal carcinomatosis. In these studies, 10 to 12.5 mg MMC was dissolved in 1 L of 1.5% dextrose, instilled in the peritoneum for 23 hours, drained over a 1-hour period, and then followed by intraperitoneal 5-flurouracil.[199]

The drug is now used topically or by local injection to prevent fibrosis related to surgery of the conjunctiva, cornea, and other ophthalmologic structures.[200]

Toxicity

The most significant and frequent side effect of MMC is a delayed myelosuppression, which seems to be directly related to schedule and total dose.[201] Below a total dose of 50 mg/m², hematological toxicity is rare. At higher doses, thrombocytopenia is more frequent than leukocytopenia and anemia. Other toxic reactions usually include mild and infrequent anorexia, nausea, vomiting, and diarrhea. Alopecia, stomatitis, and rashes also occur infrequently. Extravasation results in tissue necrosis, with very disabling ulcers that may require plastic surgery. High doses of MMC may result in lethal venoocclusive liver disease.[202] Other more frequent and potentially lethal side effects include hemolytic uremic syndrome (HUS), interstitial pneumonitis, and cardiac failure. The incidence of MMC-induced HUS seems to be less than 10% and is dose dependent, mainly occurring at cumulative doses greater than 50 mg/m².[203,204] No consistently effective treatment for this syndrome is available. It may be noted that red blood cell transfusion should be avoided.

Pulmonary toxicity of MMC consists of an interstitial pneumonitis.[204] Discontinuation of MMC administration may occasionally lead to recovery, and corticosteroid treatment may be helpful in preventing progression of pulmonary dysfunction. The incidence of pulmonary toxicity is approximately 7% of the treated population.[205] Cardiac failure secondary to MMC occurs in a similar small percentage of patients, and the incidence rises with cumulative doses greater than 30 mg/m².[204]

Yondelis (Ecteinascidin, Trabectidin, ET-743)

In the late 1960s, extracts of the Caribbean marine tunicate *Ecteinascidia turbinata* were found to be active as inhibitors of cell proliferation. Twenty years later, the active compound, ecteinascinedin-743 (ET-743; Yondelis, trabectedin; NSC648766) was isolated, purified,

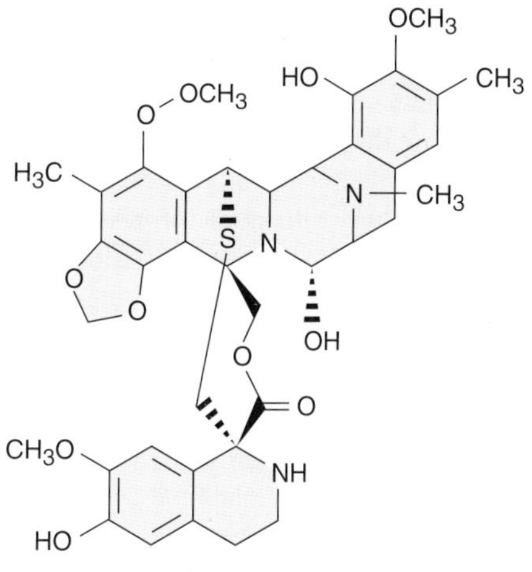

FIGURE **16–11**   Structure of ET-743.

and synthesized[206–208] (see Fig. 16-11). Yondelis belongs to the class of tetrahydro-isoquinolone compounds which includes saframycins, safracins, and naphthyridinomycins. It is produced by the marine tunicate *E. turbinata*.

Yondelis is extremely potent, producing cell death at picomolar or low nanomolar concentrations against animal tumors in vitro.[206] It displayed activity in preclinical tumor models of human ovarian, breast, non–small cell lung, melanoma, sarcoma, and renal cancer. Antitumor effects, particularly against soft-tissue sarcomas, ovarian cancer, and breast cancer, were observed in Phase I-II trials,[209–213] leading to approval in Europe for treatment of relapsed ovarian cancer and soft-tissue sarcomas and for soft-tissue sarcomas in many other countries but not the United States. Its key pharmacological features are given in Table 16-4.

Mechanism of Action

Yondelis exerts at least two separate actions that may contribute to its cytotoxicity: alkylation of DNA and inhibition of gene

TABLE 16.4	Key features of Yondelis
Mechanism of action	Alkylation of DNA, as well as synthesis inhibition of RNA, DNA, and protein
Metabolism	Desmethylation and CYP3A4-mediated oxidation
Pharmacokinetics	Terminal $t_{1/2}$: 40–50 h
Elimination	Primarily via bile (<2% in urine)
Drug interactions	None (doxorubicin does not affect PK)
Toxicity	Neutropenia
	Thrombocytopenia
	Hepatic toxicity
	Nausea and vomiting
	Fatigue
Precautions	Comedication with CYP3A4 substrates
	Care should be taken in case of bilirubin increase.

$t_{1/2}$, half-life.

transcription.[214–217] It binds to the minor groove of the DNA double helix, showing a preference for GG and GC-rich regions, and forms a covalent bond with the exocyclic N2 group of guanine. This alkylation step depends on the dehydration of the carbinolamine group of Yondelis, leading to the formation of a reactive iminium intermediate that attacks DNA.[216] Its mode of attack differs from that of other minor groove alkylators, such as CC1065 and tallimustine, which bind to the N3 of adenine in AT-rich regions. Two subunit of Yondelis (A and B) form the primary contacts with DNA, while the C subunit protrudes out of the minor groove and has been implicated in interactions with transcription factors.[218] Alkylation of DNA bends the helix toward its major groove, a structural change that may be important in inhibition of transcription.[219] The alkylation of DNA triggers recognition of the adduct and attempts to repair, with subsequent single strand breaks that are converted to double-strand breaks when encountered by the transcription-coupled nucleotide excision repair (TC-NER) complex.[220] The drug is most active against cells that have intact TC-NER, in contrast to cisplatin, which is most effective in cells with defective TC-NER.

A second important action of Yondelois is its ability to inhibit expression of a variety of transcription factions including oncogene products (myc, c-myb, and maf), cell cycle–related factors (E2F and SRF), and general transcriptions factors (TATA-binding protein, SCR, NF-Y, SXR, and Sp1), although high concentrations (>50 uM) were required in some experiments.[214,215] Of particular interest is its inhibition of the activation of the multidrug resistance gene (MDR1) and heat shock protein 70 (HSP70), which are both under the regulation of NF-Y. Constitutive expression of these genes is unaffected.[206,215,217,221] MDR1 transcription is under the control of the SXR transcription factor, the activation of which by paclitaxel is repressed by Yondelis. Both genes (MDR and HSP70) are important in promoting drug resistance. Thus these actions have implications for combination therapy with other cytotoxic agents.

Resistance Mechanisms

Although Yondelis inhibits the synthesis of MDR1, it is ineffective in cells that constitutively express high levels of the transporter.[206] The cytotoxicity of Yondelis is significantly influenced by the status of DNA repair pathways. Cells deficient in DNA mismatch repair are sensitive to the drug, but resistant to cisplatin, while those with inherited defects in double-strand break repair, such as Fanconi anemia or BRCA 1 or 2, are hypersensitive to Yondelis.[222–227] The presence of an intact DNA-dependent protein kinase, a component of the double-strand break repair pathway, is activated by irradiation or alkylating drugs and confers sensitivity to Yondelis,[225] as does intact TC-NER (Yondelis appears to trap NER proteins in a complex with DNA at adduct sites). Loss of a key component of TC-NER (the XPG protein) leads to resistance.[228] Conversely, loss of TC-NER leads to enhanced cisplatin sensitivity, thus providing a rationale for combination therapy with these agents, although clinical trials to date have not shown impressive Yondelis sensitivity in patients refractory to platinum-based regimens,[213] The drug has an inconsistent pattern of cross-resistance with other cytotoxics in cell culture studies, reflecting the presence of multiple different mechanisms of resistance in the cell lines tested.[229]

Cytokinetic Effects of Yondelis

Yondelis decreases the rate of progression of tumor cells through the S phase of the cell cycle, leading to a prolonged p53-independent blockage at the G2/M interface.[230] Cells in G1 are more sensitive than those in S or G2/M.[224]

Clinical Pharmacology

Yondelis is formulated as a lyophilized product. Each vial contains a 250 ug dosage unit in mannitol and 0.05 M phosphate buffer. This formulation, when reconstituted, is light sensitive and stable at room temperature for only a few hours. The usual dose is 1.3 mg/m^2 administered as a 24-hour infusion every 3 weeks. Quantitative bioanalytical methods utilize HPLC, combined with mass spectrometry.[209,231,232]

The predominant mechanism of drug clearance is hepatic metabolism by CYP3A4 as less than 2% of parent compound is excreted in the urine unchanged.[209] In vitro experiments with rat or human microsomes demonstrate conversion to N-desmethylyondelis and two oxidative products. Glucuronidation does not play an important role in its elimination.[233,234]

The favored schedule for drug administration is the 24-hour infusion, based on a randomized phase II trial (24 versus 3 hour infusion) in soft-tissue sarcoma, demonstrating a significantly improved time to tumor progression for the more prolonged schedule.[235] Other early trials have explored various durations of administration (1 to 72 hours).[209,236–239] There was no apparent advantage in terms of toxicity or response for the shorter schedules. With the 24-hour infusion, the drug clearance rate from plasma was 21 to 86 L/h and the terminal half-life in plasma was 26 to 89 hours. The area under the C × T curve (AUC) was 36 to 55 hours × ng/mL.[236–239]

Yondelis has a high volume of distribution (808 to 3,900 L), a slow redistribution from tissues, and a long elimination, with high inter-patient variability. Except for a decrease in clearance with increasing dose in 1-hour infusion regimens, and a disproportionate increase in AUC above doses of 1,050 mg/m in the 72-hour infusion, all phase I studies have shown dose-independent pharmacokinetics for a given infusion regimen.[209,210,238,241,242] A positive correlation between total plasma clearance and age was suggested in pharmacokinetic modeling of Phase II data, but no clear correlation of toxicity with age has been observed.[239,241]

Toxicity

The primary dose-limiting toxicities are myelosuppression and hepatic enzyme elevations. Myelosuppression (both platelet and neutrophils are affected) appears to be related to the Yondelis C_{max} in plasma, with greater myelosuppression with shorter infusions, while hepatic enzyme elevations are a function of the AUC. Hepatic toxicity consists of acute and rapidly reversible elevations of transaminases, to a lesser degree, alkaline phosphatase, and more rarely, bilirubin. Pretreatment with dexamethasone, 4 mg bid beginning 24 hours prior to infusion, effectively reverses toxicity in female rats and ameliorates clinical toxicity.[240–244]

Drug Interactions

Experience to date with Yondelis in combination therapy is limited. It has been combined with doxorubicin, with dose-limiting oxicity of myelosuppression. Doses of 700 ug/m² of Yondelis (as a ? hour infusion) and 60 mg/m² doxorubicin were well tolerated in n every 3-week regimen,[245] without evidence of pharmacokinetic interactions. Responses were observed in both metastatic breast ancer and soft-tissue sarcoma patients. A phase I trial of pegylated liposomal doxorubicin (PLD) and a 3-hour infusion of Yondelis established a well-tolerated regimen of 30 mg/m² of PLD and .1 mg/m² Yondelis, with dose-limiting toxicity of neutropenia and transaminase elevations.[246] This regimen was used to obtain marketing approval for the PDL/Yondelis combination versus elapsed ovarian cancer in Europe.

References

1. Umezawa H, Maeda K, Takeuchi T, et al. New antibiotics, bleomycin A and B. J Antibiot (Tokyo) 1966;19:200.

2. Levi JA, Raghavan D, Harvey V, et al. The importance of bleomycin in combination chemotherapy for good-prognosis germ cell carcinoma. J Clin Oncol 1993;11:1300.

3. Takita T, Umezawa Y, Saito S, et al. Total synthesis of bleomycin A₂. Tetrahedron Lett 1982;23:521.

4. Mistry JS, Sebti SM, Lazo JS. Separation of bleomycins and their deamido metabolites by high-performance cation-exchange chromatography. J Chromatogr 1990;514:86.

5. Stubbe J, Kozarich JW. Mechanisms of bleomycin-induced DNA degradation. Chem Rev 1987;87:1107.

6. Umezawa H. Advances in bleomycin studies. In: Hecht SM, ed. Bleomycin: Chemical, Biochemical, and Biological Aspects. New York: Springer-Verlag, 1979:24.

7. Lazo JS, Schisselbauer JC, Herring GM, et al. Involvement of the cellular vacuolar system with the cytotoxicity of bleomycin-like agents. Cancer Commun 1990;2:81.

8. Pron G, Belehradek J Jr, Mir LM. Identification of a plasma membrane protein that specifically binds bleomycin. Biochem Biophys Res Commun 1993;194:333.

9. Takahashi K, Takita T, Umezawa H. The nature of thiol compounds which trap cuprous ion reductively liberated from bleomycin-Cu(II) in cells. J Antibiot (Tokyo) 1987;40:348.

10. Dabrowiak JC, Greenaway FT, Santillo FS, et al. The iron complexes of bleomycin and tallysomycin. Biochem Biophys Res Commun 1979;91:721.

11. Takita T, Muraoka Y, Nakatani T, et al. Chemistry of bleomycin, XXI: metal-complex and its implication for the mechanism of bleomycin action. J Antibiot (Tokyo) 1978;31:1073.

12. Ehrenberg GM, Shipley JB, Heimbrook DC, et al. Copper dependent cleavage of bleomycin. Biochemistry 1987;26:931.

13. Hecht SM. The chemistry of activated bleomycin. Acc Chem Res 1986;19:383.

14. Sausville EA, Peisach J, Horwitz SB. Effects of chelating agents and metal ions on the degradation of DNA by bleomycin. Biochemistry 1978;17:2740.

15. Morgan MA, Hecht SM. Iron (II)·bleomycin-mediated degradation of a DNA-RNA heteroduplex. Biochemistry 1994;33:10286.

16. Burger RM. Cleavage of nucleic acids by bleomycin. Chem Rev 1998;98:1153.

17. Fulmer P, Pettering DH. Reaction of DNA-bound ferrous bleomycin with dioxygen: activation versus stabilization of dioxygen. Biochemistry 1994;33:5319.

18. Sausville EA, Peisach J, Horwitz SB. A role for ferrous ion and oxygen in the degradation of DNA by bleomycin. Biochem Biophys Res Commun 1976;73:814.

19. Ciriolo MR, Magliozzo RS, Peisach J. Microsome-stimulated activation of ferrous bleomycin in the presence of DNA. J Biol Chem 1987;262:6290.

20. Mahmutoglu I, Kappus H. Redox cycling of bleomycin-Fe(III) by an NADH-dependent enzyme, and DNA damage in isolated rat liver nuclei. Biochem Pharmacol 1987;36:3677.

21. Burger RM, Kent TA, Horwitz SB, et al. Mossbauer study of iron bleomycin and its activation intermediates. J Biol Chem 1983;258:1559.

22. Kasai H, Naganawa H, Takita T, et al. Chemistry of bleomycin, XXII: interaction of bleomycin with nucleic acids, preferential binding to guanine base and electrostatic effect of the terminal amine. J Antibiot (Tokyo) 1978;31:1316.

23. Umezawa H, Takita T, Sugiura Y, et al. DNA-bleomycin interaction: nucleotide sequence–specific binding and cleavage of DNA by bleomycin. Tetrahedron 1984;40:501.

24. Povirk LF, Hogan M, Dattagupta N. Binding of bleomycin to DNA: intercalation of the bithiazole rings. Biochemistry 1979;18:96.

25. Hertzberg RP, Caranfa MJ, Hecht SM. Degradation of structurally modified DNAs by bleomycin group antibiotics. Biochemistry 1988;27:3164.

26. Caspary WJ, Niziak C, Lanzo DA, et al. Bleomycin A₂: a ferrous oxidase. Mol Pharmacol 1979;16:256.

27. Kilkuskie RE, Macdonald TL, Hecht SM. Bleomycin may be activated for DNA cleavage by NADPH–cytochrome P450 reductase. Biochemistry 1984;23:6165.

28. Burger RM, Horwitz SB, Peisach J, et al. Oxygenated iron bleomycin: a short-lived intermediate in the reaction of ferrous bleomycin with O₂. J Biol Chem 1979;254:12299.

29. Sausville E, Stein R, Peisach J, et al. Properties and products of the degradation of DNA by bleomycin. Biochemistry 1978;17:2746.

30. Burger RM, Projan SJ, Horwitz SB, et al. The DNA cleavage mechanism of iron-bleomycin. J Biol Chem 1986;261:15955.

31. Rabow L, Stubbe J, Kozarich JW. Identification of the alkali-labile product accompanying cytosine release during bleomycin-mediated degradation of d(CGCGCG). J Am Chem Soc 1986;108:7130.

32. Grollman AP, Takeshita M, Pillai KM, et al. Origin and cytotoxic properties of base propenals derived from DNA. Cancer Res 1985;45:1127.

33. Keller TJ, Oppenheimer NJ. Enhanced bleomycin-mediated damage of DNA opposite charged nicks: a model for bleomycin-directed double strand scission of DNA. J Biol Chem 1987;262:15144.

34. Burger RM, Berkowitz AR, Peisach J, et al. Origin of malondialdehyde from DNA degraded by Fe(II)-bleomycin. J Biol Chem 1980;255:11832.

35. Takeshita M, Grollman AP, Ohtsubo E, et al. Interaction of bleomycin with DNA. Proc Natl Acad Sci USA 1978;75:5983.

36. Grollman AP, Takeshita M. Interactions of bleomycin with DNA. In: Weber G, ed. Advances in Enzyme Regulation. Vol 18. Oxford: Pergamon Press, 1980:67.

37. Roy SN, Horwitz SB. Characterization of the association of radiolabeled bleomycin A₂ with HeLa cells. Cancer Res 1984;44:1541.

38. Fugimito J, Higashi H, Kosaki G. Intracellular distribution of [¹⁴C]bleomycin and the cytokinetic effects of bleomycin in the mouse tumor. Cancer Res 1976;36:2248.

39. Touchekti O, Pron G, Belehradek J Jr, et al. Bleomycin, an apoptosis mimetic drug that induces two types of cell death depending on the number of molecules internalized. Cancer Res 1993;53:5462.

40. Mistry JS, Jani JP, Morris G, et al. Synthesis and evaluation of fluoromycin: a novel fluorescence-labeled derivative of talisomycin S₁₀b. Cancer Res 1992;52:709.

41. Lazo JS, Humphreys CJ. Lack of metabolism as the biochemical basis of bleomycin-induced pulmonary toxicity. Proc Natl Acad Sci USA 1983;80:3064.

42. Bršmme D, Rossi AB, Smeekens SP, et al. Human bleomycin hydrolase: molecular cloning, sequencing, functional expression, and enzymatic characterization. Biochemistry 1996;35:6706.

43. Joshua-Tor L, Xu HE, Johnston SA, et al. Crystal structure of a conserved protease that binds DNA: the bleomycin hydrolase, Gal6. Science 1995;269:945.

44. Farrell PA, Gonzalez F, Zheng W, et al. Crystal structure of human bleomycin hydrolase, a self-compartmentalizing cysteine protease. Structure 1999;7:619.

45. Koldamova RP, Lefterov IM, Gadjeva VG, et al. Essential binding and functional domains of human bleomycin hydrolase. Biochemistry 1998;37:2282.

46. Ferrando A, Pendas A, Elena L, et al. Gene characterization, promoter analysis, and chromosomal localization of human bleomycin hydrolase. J Biol Chem 1997;272:33298.

47. Takeda A, Nonaka M, Ishikawa A, et al. Immunohistochemical localization of the neutral cysteine protease bleomycin hydrolase in human skin. Arch Dermatol Res 1999;291:238.

48. Schwartz DR, Homanics GE, Hoyt DG. The neutral cysteine protease bleomycin hydrolase is essential for epidermal integrity and bleomycin resistance. Proc Natl Acad Sci USA 1999;96:4680.

49. de Haas EC, Zwart N, Meijer C, et al. Variation in bleomycin hydrolase gene is associated with reduced survival after chemotherapy for testicular germ cell cancer. J Clin Oncol 2008;26:1817–1823.

50. Olive PL, Banath JP. Detection of DNA double-strand breaks through the cell cycle after exposure to x-rays, bleomycin, etoposide and ^{125}IdUrd. Int J Radiat Biol 1993;64:349.

51. Lopez-Larraza DM, Bianchi NO. DNA response to bleomycin in mammalian cells with variable degrees of chromatin condensation. Environ Mol Mutagen 1993;21:258.

52. Twentyman PR. Bleomycin: mode of action with particular reference to the cell cycle. Pharmacol Ther 1983;23:417.

53. Kuo MT, Hsu TC. Bleomycin causes release of nucleosomes from chromatin and chromosomes. Nature 1978;271:83.

54. Barranco SC, Novak JK, Humphrey RM. Studies on recovery from chemically induced damage in mammalian cells. Cancer Res 1975;35:1194.

55. Nakatsugawa S, Dewey WC. The role in cancer therapy of inhibiting recovery from PLD induced by radiation or bleomycin. Int J Radiat Oncol Biol Phys 1984;10:1425.

56. Cramer P, Painter RB. Bleomycin-resistant DNA synthesis in ataxia telangiectasia cells. Nature 1981;291:671.

57. Taylor AMR, Rosney CM, Campbell JB. Unusual sensitivity of ataxia telangiectasia cells to bleomycin. Cancer Res 1979;39:1046.

58. Quinn JE, Kennedy RD, Mullan PB, et al. BRCA1 functions as a differential modulator of chemotherapy-induced apoptosis. Cancer Res 2003;63:6221.

59. Li HR, Shagisultanova EI, Yamashita K, et al. Hypersensitivity of tumor cell lines with microsatellite instability to DNA double strand break producing chemotherapeutic agent bleomycin. Cancer Res 2004;64:4760.

60. Mayaki M, Ono T, Hori S, et al. Binding of bleomycin to DNA in bleomycin-sensitive and resistant rat ascites hepatoma cells. Cancer Res 1975;35:2015.

61. Morris G, Mistry JS, Jani JP, et al. Neutralization of bleomycin hydrolase by an epitope-specific antibody. Mol Pharmacol 1992;42:57.

62. Jani JP, Mistry JS, Morris G, et al. In vivo circumvention of human colon carcinoma resistance to bleomycin. Cancer Res 1992;52:2931.

63. Brabbs S, Warr JR. Isolation and characterization of bleomycin-resistant clones of OHO cells. Genet Res 1979;34:269.

64. Zuckerman JE, Raffin TA, Brown JM, et al. In vitro selection and characterization of a bleomycin-resistant subline of B16 melanoma. Cancer Res 1986;46:1748.

65. Tsuruo T, Hamilton TC, Louie KG, et al. Collateral susceptibility of Adriamycin-, melphalan- and cisplatin-resistant human ovarian tumor cells to bleomycin. Jpn J Cancer Res 1986;77:941.

66. Russo A, Mitchell JB, McPherson S, et al. Alteration of bleomycin cytotoxicity by glutathione depletion or elevation. Int J Radiat Oncol Biol Phys 1984;10:1675.

67. Umezawa H, Takeuchi T, Hori S, et al. Studies on the mechanism of antitumor effect of bleomycin on squamous cell carcinoma. J Antibiot (Tokyo) 1972;25:409.

68. Shiu GK, Goehl TJ. High-performance liquid chromatographic determination of bleomycin A$_2$ in urine. J Chromatogr 1980;181:127.

69. Galvan L, Strong JE, Crooke ST. Use of PM-2 DNA degradation as a pharmacokinetic assay for bleomycin. Cancer Res 1979;39:3948.

70. Broughton A, Strong JE. Radioimmunoassay of bleomycin. Cancer Res 1976;36:1418.

71. Crooke ST, Luft F, Broughton A, et al. Bleomycin serum pharmacokinetics as determined by a radioimmunoassay and a microbiologic assay in a patient with compromised renal function. Cancer 1977;39:1430.

72. Bennett WM, Pastore L, Houghton DC. Fatal pulmonary bleomycin toxicity in cisplatin-induced acute renal failure. Cancer Treat Rep 1980;64:921.

73. Alberts DS, Chen HSG, Liu R, et al. Bleomycin pharmacokinetics in man, I: intravenous administration. Cancer Chemother Pharmacol 1978;1:177.

74. Crooke ST, Comis RL, Einhorn LH, et al. Effects of variations in renal function on the clinical pharmacology of bleomycin administered as an IV bolus. Cancer Treat Rep 1977;61:1631.

75. Oken MM, Crooke ST, Elson MK, et al. Pharmacokinetics of bleomycin after IM administration in man. Cancer Treat Rep 1981;65:485.

76. Paladine W, Cunningham TJ, Sponzo R, et al. Intracavitary bleomycin in the management of malignant effusions. Cancer 1976;38:1903.

77. Alberts DS, Chen HSG, Mayersohn M, et al. Bleomycin pharmacokinetics in man, II: intracavitary administration. Cancer Chemother Pharmacol 1979;2:127.

78. Howell SB, Schiefer M, Andrews PA, et al. The pharmacology of intraperitoneally administered bleomycin. J Clin Oncol 1987;5:2009.

79. Dalgleish AG, Woods RL, Levi JA. Bleomycin pulmonary toxicity: its relationship to renal dysfunction. Med Pediatr Oncol 1984;12:313.

80. McLeod BF, Lawrence HJ, Smith DW, et al. Fatal bleomycin toxicity from a low cumulative dose in a patient with renal insufficiency. Cancer 1987;60:2617.

81. O'Sullivan JM, Huddart RA, Norman AR, et al. Predicting the risk of bleomycin lung toxicity in patients with germ-cell tumors. Ann Oncology 2003;14:91.

82. Hinton S, Catalano PJ, Einhorn LH, et al. Cisplatin, etoposide and either bleomycin or ifosfamide in the treatment of disseminated germ cell tumors. Cancer 2003;97:1869.

83. Hubbard SP, Chabner BA, Canellos GP, et al. High-dose intravenous bleomycin in treatment of advanced lymphomas. Eur J Cancer 1975;11:623.

84. Levy RL, Chiarillo S. Hyperpyrexia, allergic-type response, and death occurring with bleomycin administration. Oncology 1980;37:316.

85. Comis RL. Bleomycin pulmonary toxicity: current status and future directions. Semin Oncol 1992;19(Suppl 5):64.

86. Parvinen LM, Kikku P, Maekinen E, et al. Factors affecting the pulmonary toxicity of bleomycin. Acta Radiol Oncol 1983;22:417.

87. Dee GJ, Austin JH, Mutter GL. Bleomycin-associated pulmonary fibrosis: rapidly fatal progression without chest radiotherapy. J Surg Oncol 1987;35:135.

88. Samuels ML, Johnson DE, Holoye PH, et al. Large-dose bleomycin therapy and pulmonary toxicity: a possible role of prior radiotherapy. JAMA 1976;235:1117.

89. Williams SD, Birch R, Einhorn LA, et al. Treatment of disseminated germ cell tumors with cisplatin, bleomycin, and either vinblastine or etoposide. N Engl J Med 1987;316:1435.

90. Moeller A, Ask K, Warburton D et al. The bleomycin animal mode: a useful tool to investigate treatment option for idiopathic pulmonary fibrosis. IJBCB 2007;40:362–382.

91. Raisfeld IH. Role of terminal substituents in the pulmonary toxicity of bleomycins. Toxicol Appl Pharmacol 1981;57:355.

92. Huff RA, Bevan DR. Application of alkaline unwinding to analysis of breaks induced by bleomycin in hamster lung DNA in vivo. J Appl Toxicol 1991;11:359.

93. Phan SH, Varani J, Smith D. Rat lung fibroblast collagen metabolism in bleomycin-induced pulmonary fibrosis. J Clin Invest 1985;76:241.

94. Adamson IY, Bowden DH. The pathogenesis of bleomycin-induced pulmonary fibrosis in mice. Am J Pathol 1974;77:185.

95. Sikic BI, Young DM, Mimnaugh EG, et al. Quantification of bleomycin pulmonary toxicity in mice by changes in lung hydroxyproline content and morphometric histopathology. Cancer Res 1978;38:787.

96. Hoyt DG, Lazo JS. Alterations in pulmonary mRNA encoding procollagens fibronectin and transforming growth factor-β precede bleomycin-induced pulmonary fibrosis in mice. J Pharmacol Exp Ther 1988;246:765.

97. King SL, Lichter AC, Rowe SW, et al. Bleomycin stimulates pro-alpha (I) collagen promoter through transforming growth factor beta response element by intracellular and extracellular signaling. J Biol Chem 1994;269:13156.

98. Everson MP, Chandler DB. Changes in distribution, morphology, and tumor necrosis factor-alpha secretion of alveolar macrophage subpopulations during the development of bleomycin-induced pulmonary fibrosis. Am J Pathol 1992;140:503.

99. Piguet PF, Collart MA, Grau GE, et al. Tumor necrosis factor/cachectin plays a key role in bleomycin induced pneumopathy and fibrosis. J Exp Med 1989;170:655.

100. Scheule RK, Perkins RC, Hamilton R, et al. Bleomycin stimulation of cytokine secretion by the human alveolar macrophage. Am J Physiol 1992;262:L386.

101. Baecher AC, Barth RK. PCR analysis of cytokine induction profiles associated with mouse strain variation in susceptibility to pulmonary fibrosis. Reg Immunol 1993;5:207.

102. Haston CK, Amos CI, King TM, et al. Inheritance of susceptibility to bleomycin-induced pulmonary fibrosis in the mouse. Cancer Res 1996;56:2596.

103. Haston CK, Travis EL. Murine susceptibility to radiation-induced pulmonary fibrosis is influenced by a genetic factor implicated in susceptibility to bleomycin-induced pulmonary fibrosis. Cancer Res 1997;57:5286.

104. Schwartz DR, Homanics GE, Hoyt DG, et al. The neutral cysteine protease bleomycin hydrolase is essential for epidermal integrity and bleomycin resistance. Proc Natl Acad Sci USA 1999;96:4680.

105. Eitzman DT, McCoy RD, Zheng X, et al. Bleomycin-induced pulmonary fibrosis in transgenic mice that either lack or overexpress the murine plasminogen activator inhibitor-1 gene. J Clin Invest 1996;97:232.

106. Zuo F, Kaminski N, Eugui E, et al. Gene expression analysis reveals matrilysin as a key regulator of pulmonary fibrosis in mice and humans. PNAS 2002;99:6292.

107. Munger JS, Huang X, Kawakatsu H, et al. The integrin $\alpha v \beta 6$ binds and activates latent TGFβ1: a mechanism for regulating pulmonary inflammation and fibrosis. Cell 1999;96:319.

108. Coker RK, Laurent GJ, Shahzeidi S, et al. Transforming growth factors-β_1, -β_2, and -β_3 stimulate fibroblast procollagen production in vitro but are differentially expressed during bleomycin-induced lung fibrosis. Am J Pathol 1997;150:981.

109. Phillips RJ, Burdick MD, Hing K, et al. Circulating fibrocytes traffic to the lungs in response to CXL12 and mediate fibrosis. J Clin Invest 2004;114:438.

110. Kuwano K, Hagimoto N, Kawasaki M, et al. Essential roles of the fas-fas ligand pathway in the development of pulmonary fibrosis. J Clin Invest 1999;104:13.

111. Tager AM, LaCamera P, Shea BS, et al. The lysophosphatidic acid receptor LPA$_1$ links pulmonary fibrosis to lung injury by mediating fibroblast recruitment and vascular leak. Nat Med 2008;14:45–54.

112. Piguet PK, Besin C. Treatment by human recombinant soluble TNF receptor of pulmonary fibrosis induced by bleomycin or silica in mice. Eur Respir J 1994;7:515.

113. Giri SN, Hyde DM, Hollinger MA. Effect of antibody to transforming growth factor beta on bleomycin-induced accumulation of lung collagen in mice. Thorax 1993;48:959.

114. Piguet PF, Grau GE, deKossodo S. Role of granulocyte-macrophage colony stimulating factor in pulmonary fibrosis induced in mice by bleomycin. Exp Lung Res 1993;19:579.

115. Gurujeyalakshmi G, Hollinger MA, Giri SN. Pirfenidone inhibits PDGF isoforms in bleomycin hamster model of lung fibrosis at the translational level. Am J Physiol 1999;276:L311.

116. Nici L, Santos-Moore A, Kuhn C, et al. Modulation of bleomycin-induced pulmonary toxicity in the hamster by the antioxidant amifostine. Cancer 1998;83:2008–2014.

117. Unemori EN, Pickford LB, Salles AL, et al. Relaxin induces an extracellular matrix-degrading phenotype in human lung fibroblasts in vitro and inhibits lung fibrosis in a murine model in vivo. J Clin Invest 1996;98:2739.

118. Weinbach J, Camus A, Barra J, et al. Transgenic mice expressing the Sh ble bleomycin resistance gene are protected against bleomycin-induced pulmonary fibrosis. Cancer Res 1996;56:5659.

119. Phan SH, Thrall RS, Ward PA. Bleomycin-induced pulmonary fibrosis in rats: biochemical demonstration of increased rates of collagen synthesis. Am Rev Respir Dis 1980;121:501.

120. Thrau RS, McCormick JR, Jack RM, et al. Bleomycin-induced pulmonary fibrosis in the rat: inhibition by indomethacin. Am J Pathol 1979;95:117.

121. Tabata C, Tabata R, Kadokawa Y, et al. Thalidomide prevents bleomycin-induced pulmonary fibrosis in mice. J Immunol 2007;179:708–714.

122. Milam JE, Keshamouni VG, Phan SH, et al. PPAR-gamma agonists inhibit profibrotic phenotypes in human lung fibroblasts and bleomycin-induced pulmonary fibrosis. Am J Physiol Lung Cell Mol Physiol 2008;294:L891–L901.

123. Faress JA, Nethery DE, Kern EFO, et al. Bleomycin-induced pulmonary fibrosis is attenuated by a monoclonal antibody targeting HER2. J Appl Physiol 2007;103:2077–2083.

124. Witschi H. Exploitable biochemical approaches for the evaluation of toxic lung damage. Essays Toxicol 1975;6:125.

125. Sikic BI, Collins JM, Mimnaugh EG, et al. Improved therapeutic index of bleomycin when administered by continuous infusion in mice. Cancer Treat Rep 1978;62:2011.

126. Zucker PK, Khouri NF, Rosenshein NB. Bleomycin-induced pulmonary nodules: a variant of bleomycin pulmonary toxicity. Gynecol Oncol 1987;28:284.

127. Talcott JA, Garnick MB, Stomper PC, et al. Cavitary lung nodules associated with combination chemotherapy containing bleomycin. J Urol 1987;138:619.

128. Richman SD, Levenson SM, Bunn PA, et al. ^{67}Ga-accumulation in pulmonary lesions associated with bleomycin toxicity. Cancer 1975;36:1966.

129. Burkhardt A, Gebbers JO, Holtje WJ. Die bleomycin-lunge. Dtsch Med Wochenschr 1977;102:281.

130. Holoye PY, Luna MA, MacKay B, et al. Bleomycin hypersensitivity pneumonitis. Ann Intern Med 1978;88:47.

131. Comis RL, Kuppinger MS, Ginsberg SJ, et al. Role of single-breath carbon monoxide–diffusing capacity in monitoring the pulmonary effects of bleomycin in germ-free tumor patients. Cancer Res 1979;39:5076.

132. Osanto S, Bukman A, Van Hoek F, et al. Long-term effects of chemotherapy in patients with testicular cancer. J Clin Oncol 1992;10:574.

133. Goldiner PL, Carlon GC, Critkovic E, et al. Factors influencing postoperative morbidity and mortality in patients treated with bleomycin. Br Med J 1978;1:1664.

134. Donat SM, Levy DA. Bleomycin associated pulmonary toxicity: is preoperative oxygen restriction necessary? J Urology 1998;160:1397.

135. Yagoda A, Etwbanas E, Tan CTC. Bleomycin, an antitumor antibiotic: clinical experience in 274 patients. Ann Intern Med 1972;77:861.

136. Maher J, Daley PA. Severe bleomycin lung toxicity: reversal with high dose corticosteroids. Thorax 1993;48:92–4.

137. Van Barneveld PW, Sleijfer DT, van der Mark TW, et al. Natural course of bleomycin-induced pneumonitis: a follow-up study. Am Rev Respir Dis 1987;135:48.

138. Blum RH, Carter SK, Agre K. A clinical review of bleomycin—a new antineoplastic agent. Cancer 1973;31:903.

139. Berger CC, Bokemeyer C, Schneider M, et al. Secondary Raynaud's phenomenon and other late vascular complications following chemotherapy for testicular cancer. Eur J Cancer 1995;31A(13–14):2229–2238.

140. Einhorn L, Krause M, Hornbach N, et al. Enhanced pulmonary toxicity with bleomycin and radiotherapy in oat cell lung cancer. Cancer 1976;37:2414.

141. Morrow CP, DiSaia PJ, Mangan CF, et al. Continuous pelvic arterial infusion with bleomycin for squamous carcinoma of the cervix recurrent after irradiation therapy. Cancer Treat Rep 1977;61:1403.

142. Bitter K. Pharmacokinetic behaviour of bleomycin–cobalt-57 with special regard to intra-arterial perfusion of the maxillofacial region. J Maxillofac Surg 1976;4:226.

143. Watring WG, Roberts JA, Lagasse LD, et al. Treatment of recurrent Paget's disease of the vulva with topical bleomycin. Cancer 1978;41:10.

144. Kessinger A, Wigton RS. Intracavitary bleomycin and tetracycline in the management of malignant pleural effusions: a randomized study. J Surg Oncol 1987;36:81.

145. Maiche AG, Virkkunen P, Kantkanen T, et al. Bleomycin and mitoxantrone in the treatment of malignant pleural effusions. Am J Clin Oncol 1992;16:50.

146. Bracken RB, Johnson DE, Rodriquez L, et al. Treatment of multiple superficial tumors of bladder with intravesical bleomycin. Urology 1977;9:161.

147. Takabe Y, Miyamoto T, Watanabe M, et al. Synergism of x-ray and bleomycin on Ehrlich ascites tumour cells. Br J Cancer 1977;36:391.

148. Fu K, Phillips TL, Silverberg IJ, et al. Combined radiotherapy and chemotherapy with bleomycin and methotrexate for advanced inoperable head and neck cancer: update of a Northern California Oncology Group randomized trial. J Clin Oncol 1987;5:1410.

149. Waksman SA, Woodruff HB. Bacteriostatic and bactericidal substances produced by soil Actinomyces. Proc Soc Biol Med 1940;45:609–614.

150. Brockmann H. Structural differences of the actinomycins and their derivatives. Ann NY Acad Sci 1960;89:323–335.

151. Chen FM, Sha F, Chin K, et al. The nature of actinomycin C binding to d(AACCAXYG) sequence motifs. Nucleic Acids Res 2004;32:271–277.

152. Brockmann H. History and chemistry: modification of the actinomycin molecule. Cancer Chemother Rep 1974;58(1):9–20.

153. Yoo H, Rill RL. Actinomycin D binding to unsaturated, single-stranded DNA. J Mol Recognit 2001;14:145–150.

154. Brown SC, Shafer RH. Kinetic studies of actinomycin D binding to mono-, oligo- and polynucleotides. Biochemistry 1987;26:277–281.

155. Wadkins RM, Vlady B, Tung CS. Actinomycin D binds to metastable hairpins in single-stranded DNA. Biochemistry 1998;37:11915–11923.

156. Kessel D, Wodinsky I. Uptake in vivo and in vitro of actinomycin D by mouse leukemias as factors in survival. Biochem Pharmacol 1968;17:161–164.

157. Kleeff J, Kornmann M, Sawhney H, et al. Actinomycin C induces apoptosis and inhibits growth of pancreatic cancer cells. Int J Cancer 2000;86: 399–407.

158. Marchal JA, Prados J, Melguizo C. Actinomycin D treatment leads to differentiation and inhibits proliferation in rhabdomyosarcoma cells. J Lab Clin Med 1997;130:42–50.

159. Goldberg, IH, Beerman TA, Poor R. Antibiotics: nucleic acids as targets in chemotherapy. In: Becker FF, ed. Cancer. New York: Plenum Press, 1978.

160. Gupta RS. Podophyllotoxin-resistant mutants of Chinese hamster ovary cells: cross-resistance studies with various microtubule inhibitors and podophyllotoxic analogues. Cancer Res 1983;43:505–512.

161. Gupta RS. Cross-resistance of vinblastine- and taxol-resistant mutants of Chinese hamster ovary cells to other anticancer drugs. Cancer Treat Rep 1985;69:515–521.

162. Gupta RS. Cross resistance pattern towards anticancer drugs of a human carcinoma multidrug-resistant cell line. Br J Cancer 1988;58:441–447.

163. Hofsli E, Nissen-Meyer J. Reversal of multidrug resistance by lipophilic drugs. Cancer Res 1990;50:3997–4002.

164. Galbraith WM, Mellet LB. Tissue disposition of 3H-actinomycin C (NSC-3053) in the rat, monkey and dog. Cancer Chemother Rep 1975;59:1061–1069.

165. Tattersall MHM, Sodergen JE, Dengupta SL, et al. Pharmacokinetics of actinomycin D in patients with malignant melanoma. Clin Pharmacol Ther 1975;17:701–708.

166. Frei E. The clinical use of actinomycin. Cancer Chemother Rep 1974;58: 49–54.

167. Hazar V, Kutluk T, Akyuz C, et al. Veno-occlusive disease-like hepatotoxicity in two children receiving chemotherapy for Wilms' tumor and clear sarcoma of kidney. Pediatr Hematol Oncol 1998;15:85–89.

168. D'Angio GJ, Farber S, Maddock CI. Potentiation of x-ray effects by actinomycin D. Radiology 1959;73:175–177.

169. Wakaki S, Marumo H, Tomioka K. Isolations of new fractions of antitumor mitomycins. Antibiot Chemother 1958;8:228–240.

170. Ajani JA, Winter KA, Gunderson LL, et al. Fluorouracil, mitomycin, and radiotherapy vs fluorouracil, cisplatin, and radiotherapy for carcinoma of the anal canal: a randomized Controlled Trial. JAMA 2008;299: 1914–1921.

171. Stevens CL, Taylor KG, Munk KE, et al. Chemistry and structure of mitomycin C. J Med Chem 1964;8:1–10.

172. Tomasz M, Palom Y. The mitomycin bioreductive antitumor agents: crosslinking and alkylation of DNA as the molecular basis of their activity. Pharmacol Ter 1997;76:73–87.

173. Cummings JS, Spanswick VJ, Smyth JF. Re-evaluation of the molecular pharmacology of mitomycin C. Eur J Cancer 1995;31A:1918–1933.

174. Suresh Kumar G, Lipman R, Cummings J, et al. Mitomycin C-DNA adducts generated by DT-diaphorase: revised mechanism of the enzymatic reductive activation of mitomycin C. Biochemistry 1997;36:14128–14136.

175. Tomasz M, Lipman R, Chowdary D, et al. Isolation and structure of a covalent cross-link adduct between mitomycin C and DNA. Science 1987;235:1204–1208.

176. Nishiyama M. Suzuki K, Kumazaki T, et al. Molecular targeting of mitomycin C chemotherapy. Int J Cancer 1997;72:649–656.

177. Cummings J, Spanswick VJ, Tomasz M, et al. Enzymology of mitomycin C metabolic activation in tumour tissue. Biochem Pharmacol 1998;56: 405–414.

178. Spanswick VJ, Cummings J, Ritchie AA, et al. Pharmacological determinants of the antitumour activity of mitomycin C. Biochem Pharmacol 1998;56:1497–1503.

179. Spanswick VJ, Cummings J, Smyth J. Current issues in the enzymology of mitomycin C metabolic activation. Gen Pharmacol 1998;4:539–544.

180. Kohn H. Mechanistic studies on the mode of reaction of mitomycin C under catalytic and electrochemical reductive conditions. J Am Chem Soc 987;109:1833–1840.

181. Rooseboom M, Commandeur JN, Vermeulen NP. Enzyme-catalyzed activation of anticancer prodrugs. Pharmacol Rev 2004;56:53–102.

182. Siegel D, Gibson NW, Preusch PC, et al. Metabolism of mitomycin C by DT-diaphorase: role of mitomycin C-induced DNA damage and cytotoxicity in human colon carcinoma cells. Cancer Res 1990;50:7483–7489.

183. Belcourt MF, Hodnick WF, Rockwell S, et al. Differential toxicity of mitomycin C and porfiromycin to aerobic and hypoxic Chinese hamster ovary cells overexpressing human NADPH:cytochrome c (P-450) reductase. Proc Natl Acad Sci USA 1996;93:456–460.

184. Sawamura AO, Aoyama T, Tamakoshi K, et al. Transfection of human cytochrome P-450 reductase cDNA and its effects on the sensitivities to toxins. Oncology 1996;53:406–411.

185. Hoban PR, Walton MI, Robson CN, et al. Decreased NADPH:cytochrome P-450 reductase activity and impaired drug activation in a mammalian cell line resistant to mitomycin C under aerobic but not hypoxic conditions. Cancer Res 1990;50:4692–4697.

186. Tomasz M, Chowdary D, Lipman R, et al. Reaction with DNA with chemically or enzymatically activated DNA: isolation and structure of the major covalent adducts. Proc Natl Acad Sci USA 1986;83:6702–6706.

187. Dulhanty AM, Li M, Whitmore GF. Isolation of Chinese hamster ovary cell mutants deficient in excision repair and mitomycin C bioactivation. Cancer Res 1989;49:117–122.

188. Collins NB, Wilson JB, Bush T, et al. ATR-dependent phosphorylation of FANCA on serine 1449 after DNA damage is important for FA pathway function. Blood 2009;113:2181–2190.

189. Giavazzi R, Kartner N, Hart IR. Expression of cell surface p-glycoprotein by an adriamycin-resistant murine fibrosarcoma. Cancer Res 1983;43: 145–147.

190. Dorr RT, Liddil JD. Modulation of mitomycin C–induced multidrug resistance in vitro. Cancer Chemother Pharmacol 1991;27:290–294.

191. Den Hartigh J, McVie JG, van Oort WJ, et al. Pharmacokinetics of mitomycin C in humans. Cancer Res 1983;43:5017–5021.

192. Dorr RT. New findings in the pharmacokinetics, metabolic, and drug-resistance aspects of mitomycin C. Semin Oncol 1988;15:32–41.

193. Verweij J, Stuurman M, de Vries J, et al. The difference in pharmacokinetics of mitomycin C, given either as a single agent or as part of combination chemotherapy. J Cancer Res Clin Oncol 1986;112:282–284.

194. Fujita H. Comparative studies on the blood level, tissue distribution, excretion and inactivation of anticancer drugs. Jpn J Clin Oncol 1971;12:335–342.

195. Dalton JT, Wientjes MG, Pfeffer M. Studies on mitomycin C absorption after intravesical treatment of superficial bladder tumors. J Urol 1991;132:30–33.

196. Wientjes MG, Badalment RA, Wang RC. Penetration of mitomycin C in human bladder. Cancer Res 1993;53:3314–3320.

197. Gao X, Au JL, Gadalament RA. Bladder tissue uptake of mitomycin C during intravesical therapy is linear with drug concentration in urine. Clin Cancer Res 1998;4:139–143.

198. Colombo R, Da Pozzo JF, Lev A. Neoadjuvant combined microwave-induced local HT and topical chemotherapy versus chemotherapy alone for superficial bladder cancer. J Urol 1996;155:1227–1232.

199. da Silva RG, Sugarbaker PH. Analysis of prognostic factors in seventy patients having a complete cytoreduction plus perioperative interaperitoneal chemotherapy for carcinomatosis from colorectal cancer. J Am Coll Surg 2006;203:878–886.

200. Panda A, Pe'er J, Aggarwal A, et al. Effect of topical mitomycin C on corneal endothelium. Am J Ophthalmol 2008;145:635–638.

201. Crooke ST, Bradner WT. Mitomycin C: a review. Cancer Treat Res 1976;3:121–139.

202. Lazarus HM, Gottfried MR, Herzig RH. Veno-occlusive disease of the liver after high dose mitomycin C therapy and autologous bone marrow transplantation. Cancer 1982;49:1789–1795.

203. Verweij J, de Vries J, Pinedo HM. Mitomycin C-induced renal toxicity, a dose-dependent side effect? Eur J Cancer Clin Oncol 1987;23:195–199.

204. Verweij J, Van der Burg MEL, Pinedo HM. Mitomycin C induced hemolytic uremic syndrome: sic case reports and review of the literature on renal, pulmonary and cardiac side effect of the drug. Radiother Oncol 1987;8:33–41.

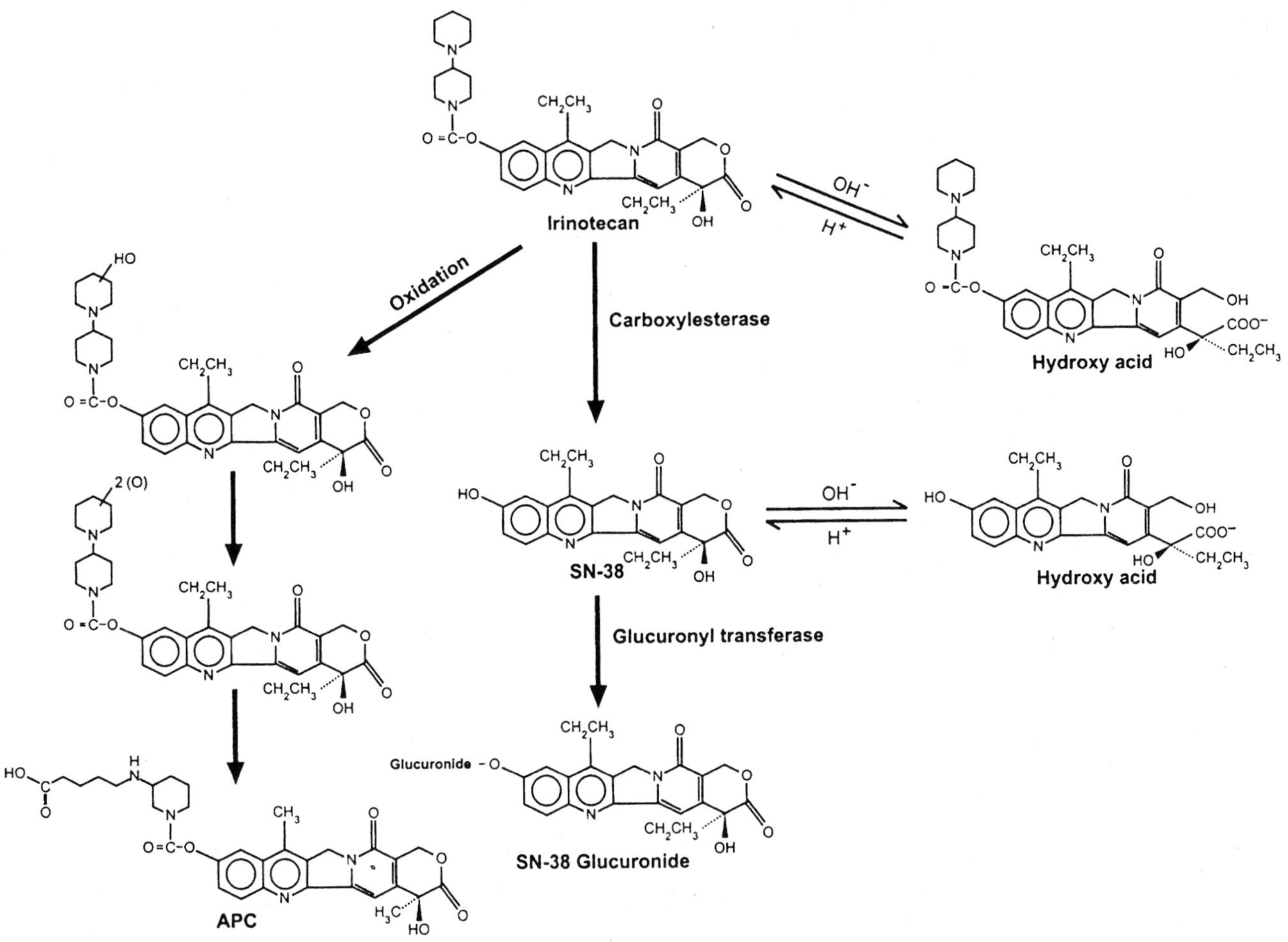

FIGURE **17-2**   Metabolic pathways of irinotecan (CPT-11).

became commercially available in Japan for treatment of lung cancer, cervical cancer, and ovarian cancer in 1994. In the United States, irinotecan was approved in 1996 for use in patients with advanced colorectal cancer refractory to 5-FU, and in 2000, it was approved as a component of first-line therapy in combination with 5-FU/LV for the treatment of metastatic colorectal cancer or for patients who have progressed following initial 5-FU-based chemotherapy. Key features of irinotecan are listed in Table 17-2.

Clinical Pharmacology

Systemic exposure to irinotecan can vary up to 10-fold among patients receiving standard doses.[38,39] Pharmacokinetic and pharmacodynamic properties of irinotecan can be affected by a variety of factors, including inherited genetic variability (see Chapter 24), age, sex, malnutrition, polypharmacy, complex physiological changes due to concomitant disease, organ dysfunction, and tumor invasion.

General Pharmacokinetics

Irinotecan is unique among camptothecin analogs in that it must first be converted by a carboxylesterase-converting enzyme to the active metabolite SN-38 (Fig. 17-2).[40] SN-38 is the major metabolite believed to be responsible for irinotecan's biologic effects, including efficacy and toxicity. SN-38 is predominantly detoxified

by a drug-metabolizing UDP-glucuronosyl transferase (UGT) 1A1 to form SN-38 glucuronide (SN-38G).[40] The relative AUC value of the active metabolite SN-38 to irinotecan varied from 0.9% to 11%. Irinotecan is also a substrate for metabolism by the CYP system, which creates an additional potential for drug interactions. Collectively, these studies demonstrate that the metabolic pharmacokinetics of irinotecan is complex and may be mediated by several different families of enzymes.

Carboxylesterase-Mediated Metabolism

Carboxylesterase-converting enzyme–specific activity is much lower in human serum and in comparable human tissues than that in rodents.[41] The main carboxylesterase responsible for the clinical activation of irinotecan in humans is carboxyl esterase 2 (CES2).[42] Carboxylesterase activity in human liver is found in the microsomal fractions, and this enzyme has been cloned and characterized.[41] In human and animal studies, no evidence exists that irinotecan induces hepatic or serum carboxylesterase activity.[43]

In most but not all studies, irinotecan and SN-38 plasma concentrations and AUC increased proportionally with increasing dose, which suggests linear pharmacokinetics.[40] The plasma half-life of SN-38 is relatively long compared with that of the other camptothecins, approximately 10 hours. The prolonged duration of exposure to SN-38 is probably a function of its sustained production from

TABLE

17.2 *Key features of irinotecan*

Mechanism of action	After metabolic activation to SN-38, the mechanism of action is the same as for topotecan.
Metabolism	Irinotecan is a prodrug that requires enzymatic cleavage of the C-10 side chain by an irinotecan carboxylesterase–converting enzyme to generate the biologically active metabolite SN-38. Irinotecan can also undergo hepatic oxidation of its dipiperidino side chain to form the inactive metabolite 7-ethyl-10-[4-*N*-(5-aminopentanoic acid)-1-piperidino]carbonyloxycamptothecin (APC).
Elimination	Elimination of irinotecan occurs by urinary excretion, biliary excretion, and hepatic metabolism. About 16.1% (range, 11.1%–20.9%) of an administered dose of irinotecan is excreted unchanged in the urine. SN-38 is glucuronidated, and both the conjugated and unconjugated forms are excreted in the bile.
Pharmacokinetics	Approximate terminal half-life of irinotecan lactone is 6.8 h (range, 5.0–9.6 h) and approximate clearance is 46.9 L/h/m^2 (range, 39.0–53.5 L/h/m^2). Approximate terminal half-life of SN-38 lactone is 11 h (range, 9.1–13.0 h).
Toxicity	Early-onset diarrhea within hours or during the infusion is associated with cramping, vomiting, flushing, and diaphoresis. Consider atropine 0.25–1.0 mg SC or IV in patients experiencing cholinergic symptoms. Late-onset diarrhea can occur later than 12 h after drug administration.
	Myelosuppression, predominantly neutropenia
	Alopecia
	Nausea and vomiting
	Mucositis
	Fatigue
	Elevated hepatic transaminases
	Pulmonary toxicity (uncommon) associated with a reticulonodular infiltrate, fever, dyspnea, and eosinophilia
Modifications for organ dysfunction	No definite recommendations are available for patients with impaired renal or hepatic dysfunction. Caution is warranted in patients with Gilbert's disease.
Precautions	Severe delayed-onset diarrhea may be controlled by high-dose loperamide given in an initial oral dose of 4 mg followed by 2 mg every 2 h during the day and 4 mg every 4 h during the night. High-dose loperamide should be started at the first sign of any loose stool and continued until no bowel movements occur for a 12-h period. Particular caution is also warranted in monitoring and managing toxicities in elderly patients (>64 y) or those who have previously received pelvic/abdominal irradiation.

irinotecan in tissues by CES2 because direct injection of SN-38 into rats resulted in extremely rapid plasma clearance, with a half-life of only 7 minutes.[44]

UGT-Mediated Metabolism of SN-38

The major metabolite of SN-38 is a glucuronidated derivative SN-38G, which is present in the plasma and bile of patients receiving irinotecan chemotherapy.[40] The decrease in plasma concentrations of SN-38G tends to parallel the decrease in SN-38 over time, suggesting that UGT is the rate-limiting step responsible for the elimination of SN-38.

The UGT1A isoforms UGT1A1, UGT1A3, UGT1A6, UGT1A7, and UGT1A9 have all been implicated in the glucuronidation of SN-38,[45] although UGT1A1 is believed to be predominantly responsible for SN-38 metabolism in humans.[46,47] UGT1A1 is known to be a highly polymorphic enzyme. Lines of evidence show that some of polymorphic variants are related to variability in the pharmacokinetics and toxicity (especially neutropenia in the every 3 week schedule) associated with irinotecan[48–51] and that

enzyme activity can be modulated by some prescription drugs such as ketoconazole[52] (see Chapter on "Pharmacogenetics").

CYP3A-Mediated Metabolism

Several additional metabolites of irinotecan have been identified and characterized in human matrices. They result from oxidation of the terminal piperidino ring.[53] CYP3A4 is thought to be responsible for the main oxidative irinotecan metabolites, known as APC and NPC.[40] APC is at least 100-fold less active than SN-38 as an inhibitor of topoisomerase I and is a poor substrate for conversion to SN-38 by human liver carboxylesterases. Nonetheless, formation of APC may represent an important metabolic pathway for irinotecan clearance.[54,55]

Transporter-Mediated Excretion

In addition to hepatic metabolism, elimination of irinotecan also occurs by urinary and fecal excretion. Up to 37% of the administered irinotecan dose is excreted unchanged in the urine over 48 hours after a short 90-minute infusion, with only less than 0.3%

being excreted as SN-38.[56] Biliary secretion of irinotecan, SN-38, and SN-38G also contributes substantially to drug elimination. The canalicular multispecific organic anion transporter ABCC2 (cMOAT; MRP2) is believed to be responsible for the biliary secretion of irinotecan carboxylate, SN-38 carboxylate, and the carboxylate and lactone forms of SN-38G.[57] SN-38 is also a substrate for other transport systems in the bile canaliculi such as ABCC1 (MRP1) and ABCG2 (BCRP; MXR), but not ABCB1.[40] OATP1B1 (OATP-C), which transports a variety of drugs and their metabolites from blood into hepatocytes, showed transport activity for SN-38 but not for irinotecan and SN-38G.[58]

Theoretically, another way of reducing gastrointestinal toxicity is by blocking biliary excretion of SN-38 and SN-38G. Cyclosporin A can reduce bile flow and inhibit bile canalicular active transport, and thus it is a potential modulator of SN-38–induced toxicity. Coadministration of cyclosporin A with irinotecan in rats increased the AUCs of irinotecan, SN-38, and SN-38G by 3.4-, 3.6-, and 1.9-fold, respectively,[59] suggesting this might be a possible strategy for reducing the gastrointestinal toxicities of irinotecan.

General Pharmacodynamics

Based on preclinical studies, it is likely that clinical outcome to irinotecan treatment might be altered by the three main mechanisms: (a) alterations in the target (topoisomerase I), (b) changes in the accumulation of drug in the tumor cells, and/or (c) alterations in the cellular response to the topoisomerase I.[60]

Alterations in Topoisomerase I

Various point mutations of topoisomerase I in different camptothecin-resistant cell lines have been associated with camptothecin resistance.[61] These point mutations result in decreased topoisomerase I catalytic activity or impaired binding of camptothecin to topoisomerase I. In some models, single amino acid changes resulted in partial resistance, while double mutation induced a synergistic resistance.

In clinical studies, point mutations were identified in patients treated with irinotecan that were located near a site in topoisomerase I previously identified as a position of a mutation in a camptothecin-resistant human lung cancer cell line.[62] In addition, amplification of topoisomerase I occurs in greater than 20% of colorectal cancers and was found to be associated with higher RNA and protein expression levels than the diploid tumors. This study suggests a potential pharmacogenomic influence of topoisomerase I copy-number alteration on its RNA/protein expressions.[63,64]

Altered Cellular Accumulation

The role of ABCB1-associated multidrug resistance (MDR) phenotypes in camptothecin resistance has still not been clearly defined. Nonetheless, irinotecan and SN-38 do not appear to interact significantly with ABCB1, and cross-resistance to irinotecan is not seen in P388 leukemia cells expressing pleiotropic drug resistance to vincristine and doxorubicin.[65]

In addition to active transport, cellular metabolism may be particularly important for irinotecan.[66] Indeed, increased levels of esterases are associated with increased sensitivity to irinotecan.[67] A large interindividual variation in expression of carboxylesterases in colon tumors may contribute to the variability of outcome of irinotecan therapy.[68,69]

Alternative Mechanisms

Other potential mechanisms of decreased sensitivity to camptothecins include a reduction in the number of cells in the S phase and increased expression of metallothionein.[70] Furthermore, double-stranded DNA break repair (DSBR) activity may also modulate camptothecin-induced cytotoxicity. For example, yeast mutants defective in the RAD52 DSBR gene are hypersensitive to camptothecin.[71,72] Whether up-regulated DSBR leads to resistance is not known.

Also important, but even less well understood, is the role of events downstream from the formation of cleavable complexes, such as DNA damage repair, the triggering of apoptosis, and alterations in the integrity of the G_2 cell-cycle checkpoint. It has been proposed by the Pharmacogenomics Knowledge Base (PharmGKB) resource that a handful of these proteins, including cell cycle division 45–like protein (CDC45L), nuclear factor-κB (p50 subunit; NFKB1), poly(ADP-ribose) polymerase I (PARP1), tyrosyl DNA phosphodiesterase (TDP1), and X-ray cross-complementation factor (XRCC1), are involved in the pharmacodynamic pathway of irinotecan (http://www.pharmgkb.org). Findings from studies using yeast or mammalian cancer cells suggest that these proteins influence the cytotoxic action of camptothecins.[73–77]

Adverse Reactions

The principal DLT for all irinotecan schedules used is delayed diarrhea and neutropenia. Severe, occasionally life-threatening toxicity occurs sporadically, even in relatively low-risk patients enrolled in well-controlled clinical trials.[78,79] The co-occurrence of diarrhea and neutropenia places patients at greatest risk.[79] The frequency of severe diarrhea (grade 3 or 4) can be reduced by more than 50% if an intensive treatment with loperamide is used. Neutropenia is typically dose related, is generally of brief duration and noncumulative, and occurs in 14% to 47% of patients treated once every 3 weeks and less frequently using the weekly schedule (12% to 19%). In approximately 3% of patients, the neutropenia is associated with fever. In one phase I study, where irinotecan was given as a 96-hour continuous infusion for 2 weeks every 3 weeks, thrombocytopenia was also dose limiting.[80] Due to inhibition of acetylcholinesterase activity by irinotecan within the first 24 hours after dosing of the drug, an acute cholinergic reaction can be observed. Interindividual variability in the pharmacokinetics of irinotecan is at least one of the major causes of irinotecan-induced severe toxicity.[81–83]

Antitumor Activity

Monotherapy

The most commonly used schedules of irinotecan administration are 30- or 90-minute IV infusions of 125 mg/m² given weekly for 4 of every 6 weeks or 350 mg/m² given every 3 weeks. In Japan, regimens of 100 mg/m² every week or 150 mg/m² every other week also have been used. The weekly times four schedule is more popular in North America, and the every-3-weeks schedule was developed predominantly in Europe. None of these regimens shows clear superiority with regard to antitumor efficacy in comparative clinical studies.[40] Remarkably, the dose intensity of all applied dosage regimens of irinotecan is approximately 100 mg/m²/wk, which suggests a schedule independency.

Phase II studies consistently revealed response rates of 10% to 35% to single-agent irinotecan in advanced or metastatic colorectal cancer independent of the applied schedules. There was no apparent difference between the various schedules with respect to the median remission duration and median survival time.[84] In a randomized phase III study comparing treatment with irinotecan given as an IV infusion at a dose of 300 to 350 mg/m^2 every 3 weeks to best supportive care in patients refractory to previous treatment with 5-FU–based chemotherapy, the 1-year survival rate was significantly greater for the irinotecan-treated group than for the control group, 36% and 14% ($P < 0.01$), respectively.[85] Another randomized phase III study, comparing treatment with irinotecan to three different continuous IV infusion schedules of 5-FU in patients with previously treated advanced colorectal cancer, revealed a survival advantage for the irinotecan-treated group in comparison to the 5-FU–treated group.[86] Apart from colorectal cancer antitumor activity, single-agent irinotecan was also moderately active in phase II studies in several other solid malignancies, including breast cancer, relapsed or refractory non-Hodgkin's lymphomas, and SCLC.

Short infusion schedules tested clinically include daily infusions for 3 days and infusions every 2 weeks, as well as 1-hour infusions of 20 mg/m^2/d daily for 5 days and a continuous infusion over 4 days, over 7 days, or over 14 days. The dose-limiting toxicity for all of these protracted administration schedules is diarrhea, with myelosuppression being less common than with the weekly or every-3-weeks short infusion schedules. Intraperitoneal, intra-arterial, and oral dosing of irinotecan have also been investigated.

Combination Therapy

5-FU Combinations

Based on the activity data in colorectal cancer derived from phase I/II studies on the combination of irinotecan with 5-FU/leucovorin (LV), two randomized phase III studies were performed comparing this combination to single-agent 5-FU/LV in the first-line treatment of metastatic colorectal cancer. Saltz et al.[87] randomized 683 patients to receive either a weekly times four regimen of irinotecan at a dose of 125 mg/m^2 and LV at a dose of 20 mg/m^2, followed by an IV bolus of 5-FU at 500 mg/m^2 (arm A); conventional low-dose 5-FU/LV (arm B); or irinotecan at a dose of 125 mg/m^2 for 4 consecutive weeks every 6 weeks (arm C). Arm A yielded a significantly longer overall survival (14.8 versus 12.6 months, $P = 0.04$) than arm B, although there was no difference between arm C and arm B.[87]

Douillard et al.[88] randomized 385 patients to the combination of irinotecan and an infusional schedule of 5-FU. The regimens were once weekly or every 2 weeks irinotecan 80 mg/m^2 with 5-FU (2,300 mg/m^2) by 24-hour infusion and LV (500 mg/m^2), irinotecan 180 mg/m^2 on day 1 with bolus 5-FU 400 and 600 mg/m^2 by 22-hour infusion, and LV 200 mg/m^2 on day 1 and 2 (arm A). For the control arm (arm B), the regimens were once weekly, 5-FU (2,600 mg/m^2) by 24-hour infusion and LV (500 mg/m^2), or every 2 weeks (called LVFU2).[88] The median time to disease progression (6.7 versus 4.4 months, $P < 0.001$) and overall survival (17.4 versus 14.1 months, $P < 0.031$) were statistically significant in favor of arm A compared with arm B.

The regimen of every 2 weeks, irinotecan 180 mg/m^2 on day 1 with 5-FU 400 mg/m^2 bolus and 600 mg/m^2 by 22-hour infusion,

and LV 200 mg/m^2 on day 1 and 2 is known as FOLFIRI. The treatment schedules used in both studies are approved by the FDA as first-line chemotherapy for patients with metastatic colorectal cancer. At present, there are modified FOLFIRI regimens. However, because of the higher toxicity seen in the Saltz regimen,[87] it is not further used in the clinical practice.

Oxaliplatin Combinations

The combination of irinotecan and oxaliplatin (85 mg/m^2) was evaluated in several studies using a once-every-2-weeks schedule and a once-every-3-weeks schedule. Interestingly, the interaction of both drugs produced acute cholinergic toxicities, the severity of which is potentiated by oxaliplatin. The combination showed an acceptable toxicity profile after dose-reduction of irinotecan to 150 mg/m^2 once every 3 weeks.[89]

A randomized study has shown that the combination of LVFU2 with oxaliplatin (FOLFOX4) prolonged progression-free survival.[90] Another phase III study has shown improved survival for FOLFOX4 over the combination of irinotecan and bolus 5-FU/LV.[91] The simplified LVFU2 regimen has been combined with irinotecan (FOLFIRI) and with oxaliplatin (FOLFOX6) and evaluated in second-line therapy.[92–94] A phase III study investigated two sequences: FOLFIRI followed by FOLFOX6; (arm A) and FOLFOX6 followed by FOLFIRI (arm B). Previously untreated patients were randomly assigned to receive a 2-hour infusion of *l*-LV 200 mg/m^2 or *dl*-LV 400 mg/m^2 followed by a FU bolus 400 mg/m^2 and 46-hour infusion of 2,400 to 3,000 mg/m^2 Fu every 2 weeks, either with irinotecan 180 mg/m^2 or with oxaliplatin 100 mg/m^2 as a 2-hour infusion on day 1. At progression, irinotecan was replaced by oxaliplatin (arm A) or oxaliplatin by irinotecan (arm B). Results of both arms were equivalent and impressive. Median survival was 21.5 months in 109 patients allocated to FOLFIRI then FOLFOX6 versus 20.6 months in 111 patients allocated to FOLFOX6 then FOLFIRI ($P = 0.99$). Median second progression-free survival was 14.2 months in arm A versus 10.9 in arm B ($P = 0.64$).

The FOCUS study randomly assigned 2,130 patients with advanced colorectal cancer to receive either first-line single-agent treatment or combination therapy.[95] Initially, the serial single-agent group received 5-FU/LV, then single-agent irinotecan. A second cohort began with 5-FU to which irinotecan or oxaliplatin was added upon progression. A third group received combination therapy with 5-FU plus irinotecan or oxaliplatin. The median overall survival was 13.9 months for sequential single-agent therapy, 15 months when single-agent therapy was followed by the addition of a second agent, and 15 to 16 months for sequential combination treatment. The only significant survival advantage was in the irinotecan combination arm as compared with the serial single-agent approach ($P = 0.01$).

Irinotecan Combined with a Monoclonal Antibody

Currently, two promising classes of targeted compounds have been introduced into the clinical management of advanced colorectal cancer: epidermal growth factor receptor (EGFR) antagonists and angiogenesis inhibitors.[96] For example, cetuximab (Erbitux, also known as C-225), a monoclonal antibody against the extracellular binding domain of EGFR, has single-agent activity against colorectal cancer and augments the effects of

63. Yu J, Miller R, Zhang W, et al. Copy-number analysis of topoisomerase and thymidylate synthase genes in frozen and FFPE DNAs of colorectal cancers. Pharmacogenomics 2008;9:1459–1466.

64. Braun MS, Richman SD, Quirke P, et al. Predictive biomarkers of chemotherapy efficacy in colorectal cancer: results from the UK MRC FOCUS trial. J Clin Oncol 2008;26:2690–2698.

65. Chen AY, Yu C, Potmesil M, et al. Camptothecin overcomes MDR1-mediated resistance in human KB carcinoma cells. Cancer Res 1991;51:6039–6044.

66. Danks MK, Potter PM. Enzyme-prodrug systems: carboxylesterase/CPT-11. Methods Mol Med 2004;90:247–262.

67. Danks MK, Morton CL, Pawlik CA, et al. Overexpression of a rabbit liver carboxylesterase sensitizes human tumor cells to CPT-11. Cancer Res 1998;58:20–22.

68. Sanghani SP, Quinney SK, Fredenburg TB, et al. Carboxylesterases expressed in human colon tumor tissue and their role in CPT-11 hydrolysis. Clin Cancer Res 2003;9:4983–4991.

69. Xu G, Zhang W, Ma MK, McLeod HL. Human carboxylesterase 2 is commonly expressed in tumor tissue and is correlated with activation of irinotecan. Clin Cancer Res 2002;8:2605–2611.

70. Chun JH, Kim HK, Kim E, et al. Increased expression of metallothionein is associated with irinotecan resistance in gastric cancer. Cancer Res 2004;64:4703–4706.

71. Eng WK, Faucette L, Johnson RK, et al. Evidence that DNA topoisomerase I is necessary for the cytotoxic effects of camptothecin. Mol Pharmacol 1988;34:755–760.

72. Nitiss J, Wang JC. DNA topoisomerase-targeting antitumor drugs can be studied in yeast. Proc Natl Acad Sci USA 1988;85:7501–7505.

73. Barthelmes HU, Habermeyer M, Christensen MO, et al. TDP1 overexpression in human cells counteracts DNA damage mediated by topoisomerases I and II. J Biol Chem 2004;279:55618–55625.

74. Cusack JC Jr, Liu R, Houston M, et al. Enhanced chemosensitivity to CPT-11 with proteasome inhibitor PS-341: implications for systemic nuclear factor-kappaB inhibition. Cancer Res 2001;61:3535–3540.

75. Malanga M, Althaus FR. Poly(ADP-ribose) reactivates stalled DNA topoisomerase I and Induces DNA strand break resealing. J Biol Chem 2004;279:5244–5248.

76. Park SY, Lam W, Cheng YC. X-ray repair cross-complementing gene I protein plays an important role in camptothecin resistance. Cancer Res 2002;62:459–465.

77. Reid RJ, Fiorani P, Sugawara M, et al. CDC45 and DPB11 are required for processive DNA replication and resistance to DNA topoisomerase I-mediated DNA damage. Proc Natl Acad Sci USA 1999;96:11440–11445.

78. Kudoh S, Fujiwara Y, Takada Y, et al. Phase II study of irinotecan combined with cisplatin in patients with previously untreated small-cell lung cancer. West Japan Lung Cancer Group. J Clin Oncol 1998;16:1068–1074.

79. Rothenberg ML, Meropol NJ, Poplin EA, et al. Mortality associated with irinotecan plus bolus fluorouracil/leucovorin: summary findings of an independent panel. J Clin Oncol 2001;19:3801–3807.

80. Takimoto CH, Morrison G, Harold N, et al. Phase I and pharmacologic study of irinotecan administered as a 96-hour infusion weekly to adult cancer patients. J Clin Oncol 2000;18:659–667.

81. Gupta E, Lestingi TM, Mick R, et al. Metabolic fate of irinotecan in humans: correlation of glucuronidation with diarrhea. Cancer Res 1994;54:3723–3725.

82. Gupta E, Mick R, Ramirez J, et al. Pharmacokinetic and pharmacodynamic evaluation of the topoisomerase inhibitor irinotecan in cancer patients. J Clin Oncol 1997;15:1502–1510.

83. Kudoh S, Fukuoka M, Masuda N, et al. Relationship between the pharmacokinetics of irinotecan and diarrhea during combination chemotherapy with cisplatin. Jpn J Cancer Res 1995;86:406–413.

84. Vanhoefer U, Harstrick A, Achterrath W, et al. Irinotecan in the treatment of colorectal cancer: clinical overview. J Clin Oncol 2001;19:1501–1518.

85. Cunningham D, Glimelius B. A phase III study of irinotecan (CPT-11) versus best supportive care in patients with metastatic colorectal cancer who have failed 5-fluorouracil therapy. V301 Study Group. Semin Oncol 1999;26:6–12.

86. Rougier P, Van Cutsem E, Bajetta E, et al. Randomised trial of irinotecan versus fluorouracil by continuous infusion after fluorouracil failure in patients with metastatic colorectal cancer. Lancet 1998;352:1407–1412.

87. Saltz LB, Cox JV, Blanke C, et al. Irinotecan plus fluorouracil and leucovorin for metastatic colorectal cancer. Irinotecan Study Group. N Engl J Med 2000;343:905–914.

88. Douillard JY, Cunningham D, Roth AD, et al. Irinotecan combined with fluorouracil compared with fluorouracil alone as first-line treatment for metastatic colorectal cancer: a multicentre randomised trial. Lancet 2000;355:1041–1047.

89. Scheithauer W, Kornek GV, Raderer M, et al. Randomized multicenter phase II trial of oxaliplatin plus irinotecan versus raltitrexed as first-line treatment in advanced colorectal cancer. J Clin Oncol 2002;20:165–172.

90. de Gramont A, Figer A, Seymour M, et al. Leucovorin and fluorouracil with or without oxaliplatin as first-line treatment in advanced colorectal cancer. J Clin Oncol 2000;18:2938–2947.

91. Goldberg RM, Sargent DJ, Morton RF, et al. A randomized controlled trial of fluorouracil plus leucovorin, irinotecan, and oxaliplatin combinations in patients with previously untreated metastatic colorectal cancer. J Clin Oncol 2004;22:23–30.

92. Andre T, Louvet C, Maindrault-Goebel F, et al. CPT-11 (irinotecan) addition to bimonthly, high-dose leucovorin and bolus and continuous-infusion 5-fluorouracil (FOLFIRI) for pretreated metastatic colorectal cancer. GERCOR. Eur J Cancer 1999;35:1343–1347.

93. Maindrault-Goebel F, de Gramont A, Louvet C, et al. Evaluation of oxaliplatin dose intensity in bimonthly leucovorin and 48-hour 5-fluorouracil continuous infusion regimens (FOLFOX) in pretreated metastatic colorectal cancer. Oncology Multidisciplinary Research Group (GERCOR). Ann Oncol 2000;11:1477–1483.

94. Maindrault-Goebel F, Louvet C, Andre T, et al. Oxaliplatin added to the simplified bimonthly leucovorin and 5-fluorouracil regimen as second-line therapy for metastatic colorectal cancer (FOLFOX6). GERCOR. Eur J Cancer 1999;35:1338–1342.

95. Seymour MT, Maughan TS, Ledermann JA, et al. Different strategies of sequential and combination chemotherapy for patients with poor prognosis advanced colorectal cancer (MRC FOCUS): a randomised controlled trial. Lancet 2007;370:143–152.

96. Meyerhardt JA, Mayer RJ. Systemic therapy for colorectal cancer. N Engl J Med 2005;352:476–487.

97. Cunningham D, Humblet Y, Siena S, et al. Cetuximab monotherapy and cetuximab plus irinotecan in irinotecan-refractory metastatic colorectal cancer. N Engl J Med 2004;351:337–345.

98. Jonker DJ, O'Callaghan CJ, Karapetis CS, et al. Cetuximab for the treatment of colorectal cancer. N Engl J Med 2007;357:2040–2048.

99. Raoul JL, Van Laethem JL, Peeters M, et al. Cetuximab in combination with irinotecan/5-fluorouracil/folinic acid (FOLFIRI) in the initial treatment of metastatic colorectal cancer: a multicentre two-part phase I/II study. BMC Cancer 2009;9:112.

100. Van Cutsem E, Peeters M, Siena S, et al. Open-label phase III trial of panitumumab plus best supportive care compared with best supportive care alone in patients with chemotherapy-refractory metastatic colorectal cancer. J Clin Oncol 2007;25:1658–1664.

101. Van Cutsem E, Nowacki M, Lang I, et al. Randomized phase III study of irinotecan and 5-FU/FA with or without cetuximab in the first-line treatment of patients with metastatic colorectal cancer: The CRYSTAL trial. J Clin Oncol 2007;25:164S.

102. Saltz L, Rubin M, Hochster H, et al. Cetuximab (IMC-C225) plus irinotecan (CPT-11) is active in CPT-11-refractory colorectal cancer (CRC) that expresses epidermal growth factor receptor (EGFR). J Clin Oncol 2001;20:3A.

103. Blanke CD. Dual-antibody therapy in advanced colorectal cancer: gather ye rosebuds while ye may. J Clin Oncol 2009;27:655–658.

104. Hurwitz H, Fehrenbacher L, Novotny W, et al. Bevacizumab plus irinotecan, fluorouracil, and leucovorin for metastatic colorectal cancer. N Engl J Med 2004;350:2335–2342.

105. Saltz LB, Lenz HJ, Kindler HL, et al. Randomized phase II trial of cetuximab, bevacizumab, and irinotecan compared with cetuximab and bevacizumab alone in irinotecan-refractory colorectal cancer: the BOND-2 study. J Clin Oncol 2007;25:4557–4561.

106. Fuchs CS, Marshall J, Mitchell E, et al. Randomized, controlled trial of irinotecan plus infusional, bolus, or oral fluoropyrimidines in first-line treatment of metastatic colorectal cancer: results from the BICC-C Study. J Clin Oncol 2007;25:4779–4786.

107. de Jonge MJ, Sparreboom A, Verweij J. The development of combination therapy involving camptothecins: a review of preclinical and early clinical studies. Cancer Treat Rev 1998;24:205–220.

108. Noda K, Nishiwaki Y, Kawahara M, et al. Irinotecan plus cisplatin compared with etoposide plus cisplatin for extensive small-cell lung cancer. N Engl J Med 2002;346:85–91.

109. Garcia-Carbonero R, Supko JG. Current perspectives on the clinical experience, pharmacology, and continued development of the camptothecins. Clin Cancer Res 2002;8:641–661.

110. Kerbusch T, Groenewegen G, Mathot RA, et al. Phase I and pharmacokinetic study of the combination of topotecan and ifosfamide administered intravenously every 3 weeks. Br J Cancer 2004;90:2268–2277.

111. Drummond DC, Meyer O, Hong K, et al. Optimizing liposomes for delivery of chemotherapeutic agents to solid tumors. Pharmacol Rev 1999;51:691–743.

112. Papahadjopoulos D, Allen TM, Gabizon A, et al. Sterically stabilized liposomes: improvements in pharmacokinetics and antitumor therapeutic efficacy. Proc Natl Acad Sci USA 1991;88:11460–11464.

113. D'Emanuele A, Attwood D. Dendrimer-drug interactions. Adv Drug Deliv Rev 2005;57:2147–2162.

114. Ouyang W, Chen H, Jones ML, et al. Artificial cell microcapsule for oral delivery of live bacterial cells for therapy: design, preparation, and in-vitro characterization. J Pharm Pharm Sci 2004;7:315–324.

115. Zamboni WC. Concept and clinical evaluation of carrier-mediated anticancer agents. Oncologist 2008;13:248–260.

116. Maeda H, Wu J, Sawa T, et al. Tumor vascular permeability and the EPR effect in macromolecular therapeutics: a review. J Control Release 2000;65:271–284.

117. Abraxane Package Insert 2005. http://www.abraxane.com

118. Krown SE, Northfelt DW, Osoba D, et al. Use of liposomal anthracyclines in Kaposi's sarcoma. Semin Oncol 2004;31:36–52.

119. Markman M, Gordon AN, McGuire WP, et al. Liposomal anthracycline treatment for ovarian cancer. Semin Oncol 2004;31:91–105.

120. Girard PM, Bouchaud O, Goetschel A, et al. Phase II study of liposomal encapsulated daunorubicin in the treatment of AIDS-associated mucocutaneous Kaposi's sarcoma. AIDS 1996;10:753–757.

121. DaunoXome Package Insert 1998. http://www.drugs.com

122. DepoCyt Package Insert 1999. http://www.drugs.com

123. Allen TM, Martin FJ. Advantages of liposomal delivery systems for anthracyclines. Semin Oncol 2004;31:5–15.

124. Rose PG. Pegylated liposomal doxorubicin: optimizing the dosing schedule in ovarian cancer. Oncologist 2005;10:205–214.

125. Abraham SA, McKenzie C, Masin D, et al. In vitro and in vivo characterization of doxorubicin and vincristine coencapsulated within liposomes through use of transition metal ion complexation and pH gradient loading. Clin Cancer Res 2004;10:728–738.

126. Laginha K, Mumbengegwi D, Allen T. Liposomes targeted via two different antibodies: assay, B-cell binding and cytotoxicity. Biochim Biophys Acta 2005;1711:25–32.

127. Park JW, Benz CC, Martin FJ. Future directions of liposome- and immunoliposome-based cancer therapeutics. Semin Oncol 2004;31:196–205.

128. Pridgen EM, Langer R, Farokhzad OC. Biodegradable, polymeric nanoparticle delivery systems for cancer therapy. Nanomed 2007;2:669–680.

129. Zamboni WC, Gervais AC, Egorin MJ, et al. Systemic and tumor disposition of platinum after administration of cisplatin or STEALTH liposomal-cisplatin formulations (SPI-077 and SPI-077 B103) in a preclinical tumor model of melanoma. Cancer Chemother Pharmacol 2004;53:329–336.

130. Laverman P, Carstens MG, Boerman OC, et al. Factors affecting the accelerated blood clearance of polyethylene glycol-liposomes upon repeated injection. J Pharmacol Exp Ther 2001;298:607–612.

131. Litzinger DC, Buiting AM, van Rooijen N, et al. Effect of liposome size on the circulation time and intraorgan distribution of amphipathic poly(ethylene glycol)-containing liposomes. Biochim Biophys Acta 1994;1190:99–107.

132. Woodle MC, Lasic DD. Sterically stabilized liposomes. Biochim Biophys Acta 1992;1113:171–199.

133. Kraut EH, Fishman MN, LoRusso PM, et al. Final results of a phase I study of liposome encapsulated SN-38 (LE-SN38): safety, pharmacogenomics, pharmacokinetics, and tumor response. Proc Am Soc Clin Oncol 2005;23:139S.

134. Lei S, Chien PY, Sheikh S, et al. Enhanced therapeutic efficacy of a novel liposome-based formulation of SN-38 against human tumor models in SCID mice. Anticancer Drugs 2004;15:773–778.

135. Pal A, Khan S, Wang YF, et al. Preclinical safety, pharmacokinetics and anti-tumor efficacy profile of liposome-entrapped SN-38 formulation. Anticancer Res 2005;25:331–341.

136. Zhang JA, Xuan T, Parmar M, et al. Development and characterization of a novel liposome-based formulation of SN-38. Int J Pharm 2004;270:93–107.

137. Dark GG, Calvert AH, Grimshaw R, et al. Randomized trial of two intravenous schedules of the topoisomerase I inhibitor liposomal lurtotecan in women with relapsed epithelial ovarian cancer: a trial of the national cancer institute of Canada clinical trials group. J Clin Oncol 2005;23:1859–1866.

138. Gelmon K, Hirte H, Fisher B, et al. A phase 1 study of OSI-211 given as an intravenous infusion days 1, 2, and 3 every three weeks in patients with solid cancers. Invest New Drugs 2004;22:263–275.

139. Giles FJ, Tallman MS, Garcia-Manero G, et al. Phase I and pharmacokinetic study of a low-clearance, unilamellar liposomal formulation of lurtotecan, a topoisomerase 1 inhibitor, in patients with advanced leukemia. Cancer 2004;100:1449–1458.

140. Kehrer DF, Bos AM, Verweij J, et al. Phase I and pharmacologic study of liposomal lurtotecan, NX 211: urinary excretion predicts hematologic toxicity. J Clin Oncol 2002;20:1222–1231.

141. Knight V, Koshkina NV, Waldrep JC, et al. Anticancer effect of 9-nitrocamptothecin liposome aerosol on human cancer xenografts in nude mice. Cancer Chemother Pharmacol 1999;44:177–186.

142. Koshkina NV, Gilbert BE, Waldrep JC, et al. Distribution of camptothecin after delivery as a liposome aerosol or following intramuscular injection in mice. Cancer Chemother Pharmacol 1999;44:187–192.

143. Verschraegen CF, Gilbert BE, Loyer E, et al. Clinical evaluation of the delivery and safety of aerosolized liposomal 9-nitro-20(s)-camptothecin in patients with advanced pulmonary malignancies. Clin Cancer Res 2004;10:2319–2326.

144. Drummond DC, Noble CO, Guo Z, et al. Development of a highly active nanoliposomal irinotecan using a novel intraliposomal stabilization strategy. Cancer Res 2006;66:3271–3277.

145. Messerer CL, Ramsay EC, Waterhouse D, et al. Liposomal irinotecan: formulation development and therapeutic assessment in murine xenograft models of colorectal cancer. Clin Cancer Res 2004;10:6638–6649.

146. Zamboni WC, Sidone BJ, Santory M, et al. Pharmacokinetic study of Optisomal topotecan (topotecan liposomal injection, TLI, OPTISOME) and non-liposomal topotecan in male Sprague-Dawley rats. Proc AACR-NCI-EORTC 2007;C113:292.

147. Zamboni WC, Whitner H, Potter DM, et al. Allometric scaling of STEALTH (R) liposomal anticancer agents. Proc Am Assoc Cancer Res Annu Meet 2005;46:326.

148. Zamboni WC, Strychor S, Joseph E, et al. Plasma, tumor, and tissue disposition of STEALTH liposomal CKD-602 (S-CKD602) and nonliposomal CKD-602 in mice bearing A375 human melanoma xenografts. Clin Cancer Res 2007;13:7217–7223.

149. Zamboni WC, Ramalingam S, Friedland DM, et al. Phase I and pharmacokinetic study of pegylated liposomal CKD-602 in patients with advanced malignancies. Clin Cancer Res 2009;15:1466–1472.

150. Drummond DC, Noble CO, Guo Z, et al. Development of a highly stable and targetable nanoliposomal formulation of topotecan. J Control Release 2010;141:13–21.

151. Chen L, Chang T, Cheng A, et al. Phase I study of liposomal encapsulated irinotecan (PEP02) in advanced solid tumor patients. J Clin Oncol 2008;26:2565.

152. Johnstone S, Harvie P, Shew C, et al. Synergistic antitumor activity observed for a fixed ratio liposome formulation of Cytarabine (Cyt):Daunorubicin (Daun) against preclinical leukemia models. Proc Am Assoc Cancer Res 2005;46:9.

153. Matsumura Y. Poly (amino acid) micelle nanocarriers in preclinical and clinical studies. Adv Drug Deliv Rev 2008;60:899–914.

154. Kato K, Hamaguchi T, Shirao K, et al. Interim analysis of phase I study of NK012, polymer micelle SN-38, in patients with advanced cancer. Gastrointestinal Cancers Symposium 2008;Abstract 485.

anthracycline and represent targeted anthracycline prodrugs that possess a unique spectrum of anticancer activity,[117,118] and they are significantly more cytotoxic and more efficient in producing apoptosis than the interaction of doxorubicin with top II.[119]

Finally, recent microarray-based investigations have revealed the broad range of changes in gene expression that follow doxorubicin exposure,[120–122] including alterations in multiple biochemical pathways such as DNA repair, RNA metabolism, reactive oxygen metabolism, chromatin remodeling, cell cycle and apoptotic programs, mitochondrial metabolism, and vacuolar function.

Drug Activation by One- and Two-Electron Reduction

During DNA intercalation and binding to top II, the anthracyclines act as chemically inert compounds that owe their activity to their ability to bind to key macromolecules and distort the three-dimensional geometry of these targets. However, the anthracyclines are also chemically reactive and capable of an extraordinarily rich chemistry that even now is not fully documented.[123,124]

One-Electron Reduction

The one-electron reduction of the anthracyclines was initially described in hepatic microsomal systems[125–127] but was later shown to play a central role in the cardiac toxicity of this class of drugs[128–130] and may be involved in antitumor activity as well.[131–135] All of the clinically active anthracyclines are anthraquinones. As is true of quinones in general,[136,137] the anthracyclines are able to undergo one- and two-electron reduction to reactive compounds that cause widespread damage to intracellular macromolecules including lipid membranes, DNA bases, and thiol-containing transport proteins (Fig. 18-3).[138–141] As outlined in Figure 18-4, the one-electron reduction of doxorubicin or daunorubicin may occur in essentially all intracellular compartments including the nuclear membrane and is catalyzed by flavin-centered dehydrogenases or reductases including cytochrome P-450 reductase, NADH dehydrogenase (complex I of the mitochondrial electron transport chain), xanthine oxidase, and cytochrome b_5 reductase.[142–144] In addition, all three isoforms of nitric oxide synthase (at their flavoprotein domains) are capable of catalyzing the one-electron reduction of doxorubicin with the subsequent production of superoxide and

a decrease in nitric oxide.[145,146] Furthermore, doxorubicin can directly inhibit nitric oxide synthase activity,[146,147] which could produce significant alterations in vascular tone both in the heart and in tumors.[148,149] It can also be metabolized by lactoperoxidase and nitrite.[150] These flavoenzymes are widely distributed in mammalian tissues, and anthracycline-mediated free-radical formation occurs in a wide range of organs and tumor cell lines. In addition to flavoproteins, doxorubicin can be reduced in the heart by oxymyoglobin, producing strong oxidant species.[151]

One-electron reduction of the anthracyclines leads to the formation of the corresponding semiquinone free radical. In the presence of oxygen, this free radical rapidly donates its electron to oxygen to generate superoxide anion (O_2^-). Although not highly toxic itself, the dismutation of superoxide yields hydrogen peroxide (H_2O_2).[152] Furthermore, in the presence of superoxide anion, the nitric oxide system can produce potentially toxic amounts of peroxynitrite.[153] Under biological conditions, the anthracycline semiquinone or reduced metal ions such as iron also reductively cleave hydrogen peroxide to produce the hydroxyl radical (•OH) or a higher oxidation state metal with the chemical characteristics of the hydroxyl radical, one of the most reactive and destructive chemical species known.[154,155] It is now commonly accepted that reduced metals are critical components in the formation of toxic free-radical intermediates and may well contribute to cell killing by the anthracyclines.[156] However, it is unclear how reduced metal species, including iron, become available for these free radical reactions.

Because oxygen radical formation occurs as a result of normal metabolic processes (including mitochondrial respiration) and is a common mechanism of action for several naturally occurring toxins, most mammalian cells have elaborate defenses against oxygen radical toxicity.[157] Superoxide dismutase, catalase, and glutathione peroxidase act in concert to reduce superoxide, hydrogen peroxide, and lipid hydroperoxides to water or nontoxic lipid alcohols without the formation of the hydroxyl or peroxyl radicals (Fig. 18-4). Glutathione, a sulfur-containing tripeptide, can react with many radicals. It also functions as a component of the glutathione peroxidase cycle to reduce peroxides to less reactive compounds.

There are also specific DNA repair systems to handle oxidative damage to DNA.[158–160] However, antioxidant defenses are not equally distributed in various tissues in the body. For example,

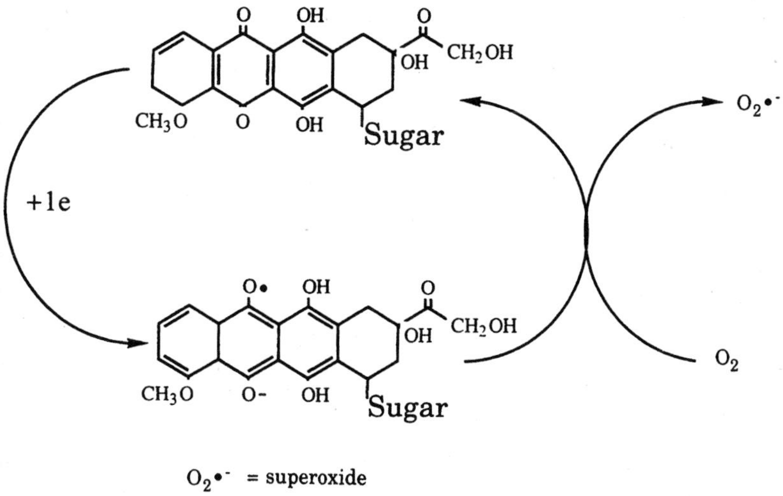

FIGURE **18-3** One-electron reduction of doxorubicin. This reduction occurs at the quinone oxygens of the chromophore. The semiquinones react rapidly with oxygen, when it is available, to yield the one-electron reduction product of oxygen, superoxide.

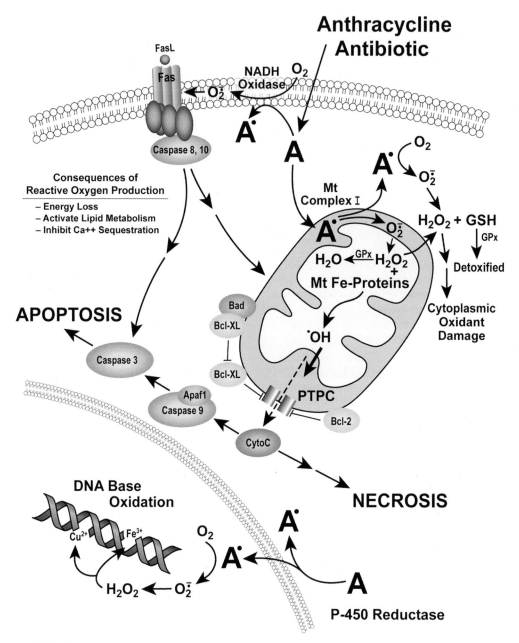

FIGURE 18-4 Anthracycline antibiotic cell death program. Anthracycline antibiotics can be metabolized at the cell surface, at complex I of the mitochondrial electron transport chain, in the cytosol, or at the nuclear envelop by flavin-containing dehydrogenases, leading to the production of reactive oxygen species with the potential to alter intracellular iron stores at multiple intracellular sites. This free-radical cascade can initiate both apoptotic and necrotic death programs associated with mitochondrial membrane injury, DNA base oxidation, altered calcium sequestration, energy loss, and altered proliferative potential. The effects of anthracycline-enhanced reactive oxygen production are modulated by intracellular antioxidant enzymes (glutathione peroxidase, catalase) and antiapoptotic proteins.

glutathione concentration is higher in the liver than in most other tissues and tumors. Catalase activity is lower in the heart than in the liver.[129,161] Likewise, the activity of several flavoproteins capable of activating the anthracyclines differs from tissue to tissue. These variations in drug activation and antioxidant defense provide ample opportunity for tissue specificity in terms of toxicity and antitumor activity. For example, the unique cardiac toxicity of the anthracyclines may result, in part, from the low level of cardiac catalase coupled with the extraordinary cardiac content of mitochondria and

myoglobin, both of which enhance drug activation. An additional contribution to cardiotoxicity may be the sensitivity of cardiac glutathione peroxidase to free radical attack;[129,162] free radicals destroy this critical enzyme at the same time that anthracyclines stimulate cardiac hydrogen peroxide formation.[163] In contrast, while anthracyclines can easily be activated to reactive intermediates by hepatic enzymes, the liver is infrequently damaged by anthracyclines in clinical chemotherapy, perhaps because it has an active free-radical defense system and is able to efflux anthracyclines and anthracycline metabolites. The importance of hepatic antioxidant systems is illustrated by the finding that pretreatment of rodents with agents (carmustine or acetaminophen) that significantly diminish the level of reduced glutathione dramatically sensitizes hepatocytes to injury by doxorubicin-induced free radicals.[164,165]

The role of oxygen radical formation in tumor cell killing.[166–170] Several lines of evidence support this hypothesis. First, doxorubicin resistance in tumor cell lines can frequently be reversed by agents which decrease glutathione concentration.[170–174] Second, anthracycline-enhanced free radical formation has been detected in many tumor cell lines.[131,152,175,176] The best studied are human breast cancer cell lines, in which both intracellular and extracellular reactive oxygen species were demonstrated.[132,177] Extracellular as well as intracellular antioxidants have also been demonstrated to decrease the cytotoxicity of the anthracyclines in normal and malignant cell lines.[132,133,156,178,180–182] In addition, some anthracycline-resistant cancer cell lines exhibit increases in various aspects of the oxygen free radical defense system, including increases in glutathione and the selenoprotein glutathione peroxidase.[169,174,183–186] Manipulation of glutathione peroxidase activity produced by changes in selenium status significantly affects tumor cell killing by doxorubicin.[187,188] Transfection of the human cytosolic glutathione peroxidase in the sense orientation produces doxorubicin resistance[189] while antisense expression sensitizes cells to doxorubicin cytotoxicity.[190] Finally, fourfold overexpression of the manganese superoxide dismutase in CHO cells produces 2.5-fold resistance to doxorubicin,[191] while inhibition of the copper-zinc superoxide dismutase with 1,25-dihydroxyvitamin D_3 significantly enhances doxorubicin cytotoxicity.[192]

Reservations about the role of oxygen radical formation in tumor cell killing arise from conflicting experimental evidence, although the balance suggests active redox cycling under conditions of tumor therapy. First, many studies demonstrating anthracycline-enhanced hydroxyl radical formation have utilized clinically irrelevant drug concentrations. This limitation is in part technical in that it was not possible in the early experiments to detect hydroxyl radicals at drug concentrations much below 10^{-7} M. However, fluorescent probes for hydrogen peroxide production by flow cytometry successfully demonstrated peroxide formation in colon cancer cells after treatment with 0.4 μM doxorubicin;[176] human breast cancer cells exposed to 0.05 μM doxorubicin exhibited enhanced oxidative respiration and reactive oxygen production as measured by chemiluminescent probes.[193] Second, many tumors for which doxorubicin has great clinical utility, such as breast cancer, are clearly hypoxic, and thus, the applicability of the redox chemistry outlined in Figures 18-3 and 18-4 might be questioned. However, under low partial pressures of oxygen, iron-mediated lipid peroxidation and DNA damage from the doxorubicin semiquinone are actually enhanced.[194] Third, glutathione depletion does not sensitize *all* tumor cell lines to the cytotoxic effect of doxorubicin,[195] and many doxorubicin-resistant cells have no alteration in antioxidant defense enzymes.[196] Fourth, a common presumption has been that oxygen radical–mediated effects on DNA are unlikely because intercalated drug could not be reduced. However, doxorubicin covalently bound to oligonucleotides can still be activated by cytochrome P-450 reductase,[197] and daunorubicin intercalated into calf thymus DNA can be reduced by a superoxide-generating system; under these circumstances the semiquinone is accessible to hydrogen peroxide for reaction, and the disproportionation of the semiquinone to the 7-deoxyaglycone may occur by intramolecular electron transfer with migration of electrons over several base pairs.[198–200] Finally, as outlined previously, oxidized DNA bases, by-products of anthracycline redox cycling, are present in both the urine[99] and peripheral blood mononuclear cells of patients receiving anthracycline therapy.[100,201] These reports provide evidence demonstrating the products of redox cycling in human tissues after anthracycline administration according to standard treatment schedules. Whether it is instrumental in cell killing of some or all human tumors is unclear.

Role of Iron

Although free radical formation was originally proposed as the basis for anthracycline cardiac toxicity in 1977 and various animal model studies suggested that hydroxyl radical scavengers could blunt doxorubicin-related heart damage, free radical scavengers were initially unsuccessful cardioprotective agents in humans.[202] These results suggested that some additional variable was involved. This variable proved to be the interaction of anthracyclines with iron. Because of its reactivity, free iron concentrations in the body are in the range of approximately 10^{-13} M, whereas total iron concentrations are between 10^{-4} and 10^{-5} M. Most iron in tissues is stored bound to ferritin. Doxorubicin releases iron from ferritin in two ways. The drug can slowly abstract iron from the ferritin shell[203]; a much more rapid release of iron follows conversion of the anthracycline to its semiquinone, which can release iron under hypoxic conditions or through the reducing power of the superoxide anion in air.[204,205] Doxorubicin can release nonheme, nonferritin iron from microsomes.[206–209] Doxorubicin can also increase the uptake of iron by a transferrin receptor–mediated process, enhancing intracellular iron availability.[210] The hydroxyquinone structure of doxorubicin or daunorubicin represents a powerful site for chelation of metal ions, especially ferric iron. Iron anthracycline complexes possess a wide range of interesting biochemical properties in vitro.[211,212] These complexes can bind DNA by a mechanism distinct from intercalation, cause oxidative destruction of membranes, and oxidize critical sulfhydryl groups. It remains unclear, however, whether these tightly bound iron-anthracycline complexes are stable and produce toxic effects intracellularly,[213,214] or whether the "delocalization" of catalytic amounts of protein-bound iron by anthracycline-stimulated free radical formation is responsible for hydroxyl radical formation in tissues.

These investigations suggested that the most effective way to interfere with the generation of highly reactive oxidants after anthracycline exposure would be to pretreat with a chelating agent that might withdraw iron from free radical reactions. This hypothesis has been confirmed; an iron chelator, dexrazoxane (ICRF-187), prevents doxorubicin-induced lipid peroxidation[215] and cardiac toxicity in a wide range of animal models.[216,217] Randomized, controlled clinical trials in humans have confirmed that this agent markedly reduces the cardiac toxicity of doxorubicin.[218,219] Dexrazoxane is a highly effective iron chelator in vivo; during phase I studies, it caused a tenfold increase in urinary iron clearance.[220,221] Dexrazoxane is itself a prodrug in that it must undergo hydrolysis to become an effective iron chelator (Fig. 18-5). This hydrolysis to ICRF-198, the major iron-binding metabolite of dexrazoxane, can occur spontaneously at physiologic pH but is markedly enhanced after uptake into cardiac myocytes with conversion of the parent

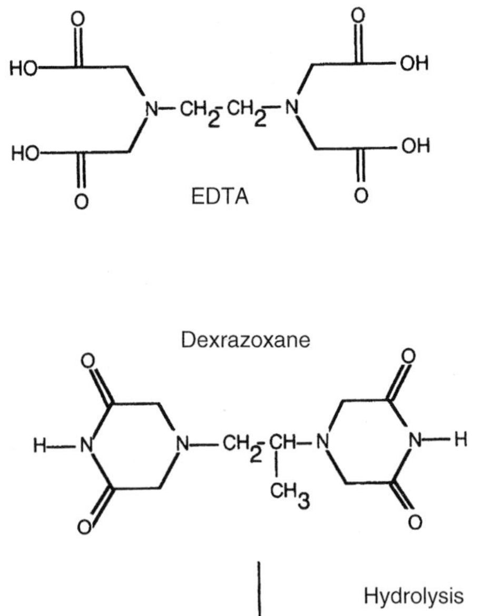

FIGURE 18-5 Dexrazoxane and its analogy to ethylenediaminetetra-acetic acid (EDTA). Dexrazoxane is much more nonpolar because the carboxylic acid groups have been fused into amide rings. This allows ready entry into the cell. Dexrazoxane can undergo hydrolysis to yield a carboxylamine that is able to bind iron.

drug to ICRF-198 in less than 60 seconds.[222] The parent drug is very lipid soluble and enters cells by passive diffusion. ICRF-198 has been demonstrated to efflux iron from iron-loaded myocytes; these studies suggest that the same chelating ability may remove iron that has been released from cardiac iron-storage proteins.[222]

Important additional studies have further elucidated the role of iron in free radical generation and other iron-dependent reactions that may contribute to the cardiac toxicity of the anthracyclines.[223–226] Down-regulation of cellular iron uptake by overexpression of the wild-type hemochromatosis gene in MCF-7 cells decreases doxorubicin-induced reactive oxygen production and apoptosis.[227] On the other hand, feeding rats a diet that is iron enriched dramatically enhances cardiac apoptosis and mitochondrial injury after treatment with doxorubicin.[228] Further, the alcohol metabolite of doxorubicin, doxorubicinol, which is produced by the two-electron reduction of the C-13 side chain carbonyl group, causes the delocalization of low molecular weight Fe(II) species from the iron-sulfur center of aconitase in a redox-dependent fashion. Further evidence supporting the role of alcohol metabolite in cardiotoxicity comes from a study of polymorphisms of carbonyl reductases. The CBRV244M variant of carbonyl reductase 3 is associated with an 8.5-fold increased risk of cardiotoxicity in children receiving doxorubicin. The recombinant variant had nearly three-fold greater activity in synthesizing doxorubicinol, as compared to

its more common counterpart.[613] The formation of a doxorubicin-iron-complex with aconitase interferes with critical interconversions of cytosolic aconitase with iron regulatory protein-1 (IRP-1); IRP-1 plays an essential role in iron homeostasis and, hence, in the regulation of critical intracellular metabolic processes (such as the action of mitochondrial electron transport proteins, myoglobin, and various cytochromes). These effects of doxorubicin metabolites suggest that iron-dependent reactions occur that may not be directly related to the formation of reactive oxygen species. This could help to explain the utility of dexrazoxane, compared to free radical scavengers that do not chelate iron, in the prevention of both acute and chronic anthracycline cardiotoxicity.[209]

> Doxorubicin is a powerful chelator of other metal ions, including Cu^{2+} and Al^{3+}. The chelation of aluminum by doxorubicin is so avid that a doxorubicin solution left in contact with aluminum foil for only 1 hour will change from the orange-red of doxorubicin to the bright cherry red of the aluminum complex. A similar reaction occurs with iron-containing alloys; doxorubicin left within a syringe needle for any significant period of time will also change color by virtue of chelation of metal from the needle. For this reason, every effort should be made in the clinic to keep anthracyclines from prolonged contact with any metal surface.

Two-Electron Reduction of the Anthracyclines

Two-electron reduction of doxorubicin (which may occur by sequential one-electron reductions or directly by strong reducing agents) results in the formation of an unstable quinone methide, which rapidly undergoes a series of reactions leading to the loss of the daunosamine sugar and formation of deoxyaglycone (Fig. 18-6).[123] Deoxyaglycone metabolites are formed in animals, and in human during clinical chemotherapy.[229,230] Deoxyaglycones exhibit far less cytotoxicity than the parent anthracycline for drug inactivation. It is likely that in the absence of oxygen the one-electron reduction product, the semiquinone, reacts with itself to yield parent drug and the two-electron reduction product. The quinone methide intermediate in this pathway may be a monofunctional alkylating agent; however, there is little evidence that this intermediate plays an important cytotoxic role in tumor cells. Finally, two-electron reduction of the anthracyclines using powerful reducing agents to convert doxorubicin to its inactive deoxyaglycone metabolite has been advocated as a means to reduce local tissue injury after anthracycline extravasation.[231] Direct enzymatic two-electron reduction is unlikely to occur under physiologic conditions.[232]

Signal Transduction, Membrane-Related Actions of the Anthracyclines, Apoptosis, and Cellular Senescence

Membrane Perturbations

It has been appreciated for more than two decades that the anthracycline antibiotics are membrane-active compounds that produce a myriad of effects at the cell surface.[233] It is now abundantly clear that events occurring at the cell surface, as well as in the nucleus, may contribute to anthracycline cytotoxicity and DNA damage. Doxorubicin alters the fluidity of both tumor cell plasma membranes[234,235] and cardiac mitochondria;[138] it binds avidly to phospholipids including cardiolipin,[236,237] causes an up-regulation of epidermal growth factor receptor (but not p185[HER-2/neu]),[238,239] inhibits the transferrin

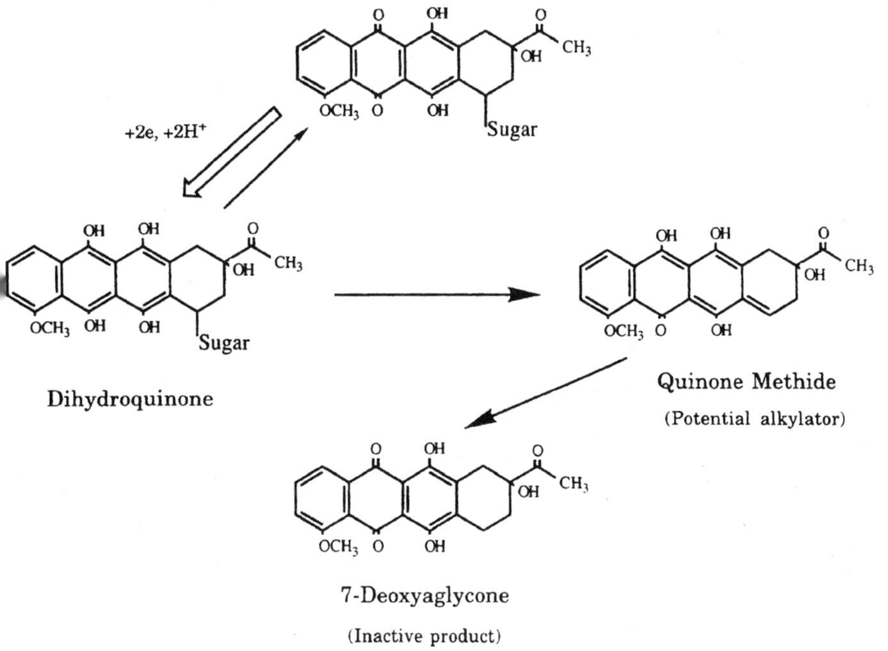

Dihydroquinone

Quinone Methide
(Potential alkylator)

7-Deoxyaglycone
(Inactive product)

FIGURE **18-6** Two-electron reduction of anthraquinones. The immediate product is the dihydroquinone, which is not stable. This undergoes rearrangement with loss of the sugar to yield the quinone methide. This structure has activity as an alkylator in pure chemical systems. The most likely fate, however, is progression, via a second arrangement, to yield the 7-deoxyaglycone. This final product is much less active than the parent drug.

reductase of the plasma membrane,[240] induces iron-dependent protein oxidation in erythrocyte plasma membranes in vivo,[241] and can be cytotoxic without entering the cell.[242,243] Furthermore, studies suggest that the presence of extracellular doxorubicin is of critical importance for membrane interactions that are important in tumor cell kill.[244] Doxorubicin cytotoxicity can be manipulated by membrane phospholipid alterations [245–247] that increase drug uptake but do not increase intracellular distribution. The confluence of these studies suggests that plasma membrane–associated events, modulated by lipid metabolism, may contribute to anthracycline cytotoxicity.

Signal Transduction and Anthracyclines

Communication between the cell surface and the nucleus plays a crucial role in growth control; important signal transduction pathways for mitogenic stimuli are initiated at the plasma membrane.[248–252] Anthracyclines impact signaling pathways in ways that may be important for cell survival and response to DNA damage.[253]

Anthracycline action affects specific signal transduction pathways, most importantly the protein kinase C(PKC) system. Anthracyclines inhibit PKC, but only at suprapharmacological concentrations (above $100 \mu M$)[254,255]; the doxorubicin-iron complex inhibits diacylglycerol stimulation of PKC at 10-fold lower concentrations.[256] Even lower concentrations of doxorubicin increase the turnover of phosphoinositide and phosphatidylcholine in Sarcoma 180 cells, which leads to the accumulation of diacylglycerol and inositol phosphates and a twofold increase in cytosolic PKC activity.[257] Furthermore, activation of the PKC pathway by phorbol esters enhances doxorubicin cytotoxicity and drug-related DNA-protein cross-links, whereas down-regulation of PKC reduces cell kill.[258] Since PKC can phosphorylate topoisomerase II,[259] it is possible that the initiation of membrane signaling by doxorubicin could be involved in the regulation of anthracycline-mediated DNA damage.

The importance of the sphingomyelin pathway in signal transduction has become increasingly clear.[248,260] In addition to participating in PKC-related signal transduction, sphingolipid metabolites transduce signals from cell surface molecules including interferon-γ, TNF-α, and Fas/APO-1. Activation of sphingomyelinase by cellular stresses, including exposure to the anthracyclines, leads to the release of the critical signaling intermediate ceramide from membrane sphingomyelin.[261–263] Intracellular ceramide accumulation can produce profound effects on cell cycle progression as well as on the effector arm of the cell death program.[264–266] Expression of glucosylceramide synthase (the enzyme that converts ceramide to glucosylceramide) in human MCF-7 cells blocks doxorubicin-induced increases in ceramide after drug exposure, leading to an 11-fold increase in IC_{50} concentration.[267]

Signal transduction pathways involving PKC and ceramide may contribute to the regulation of P170-glycoprotein function and the enhanced export of anthracyclines in drug-resistant cells[268–270]; inhibition of PKC down-regulates P170-glycoprotein function and enhances the sensitivity of myeloid leukemia cells to daunorubicin, providing a novel strategy for overcoming multidrug resistance.[271] Agents that reverse multidrug resistance, such as cyclosporin A and verapamil, may in part act by inhibiting ceramide glycosylation.[272]

As might be expected from the multiplicity of effects of anthracyclines on signaling pathways, doxorubicin alters activity of the phosphoinositide 3-kinase and AKT survival pathway, both in tumor cells and in the heart.[273–276] In malignant cells, doxorubicin exposure leads to increased phosphorylation of AKT, which, if blocked, increases tumor cell killing by the anthracycline. In related fashion, overexpression of PTEN, which dephosphorylates AKT, leads to an increase in the apoptotic program. In the heart, doxorubicin treatment decreases both AKT and ERK phosphorylation (critical for cell survival), an inhibition that is blocked by pretreatment with dexrazoxane.[277] Anthracyclines inhibit signaling through TGFβ1 and block activation of HIF-1α–mediated gene expression.[278–280]

Both of these latter effects may modify tumor-related angiogenesis by the anthracycline antibiotics.

Anthracyclines and Apoptosis

Anthracycline-related alterations in membrane biochemistry, signal transduction, mitochondrial metabolism, DNA damage, and free radical formation all contribute to apoptosis.[281–283]

Doxorubicin or daunorubicin exposure produces the morphological changes associated with apoptosis including chromatin condensation, internucleosomal DNA fragmentation, reduced cell volume, and cytoplasmic blebbing in many normal and malignant cell types.[284–291] In general, the degree of anthracycline-related apoptosis varies considerably between experimental model systems; in cell culture, the full expression of apoptotic morphology is often not observed until 48 to 120 hours after drug treatment. This variability is due, in part, to wide variations in the expression of both proapoptotic and antiapoptotic molecules in cultured tumor cells, including human tumor samples.[36,292–294]

Anthracycline-related apoptosis may involve biochemical interactions that produce several different initiating signals that produce apoptosis and/or necrotic cell kill. In selected cell lines, anthracyclines stimulate the interaction of the CD95 (APO-1/Fas) surface receptor with its natural ligand CD95L to form a signaling complex. This complex in turn activates proteases of the caspase family, resulting in apoptosis. The fas pathway, which plays a critical role in the regulation of lymphoid cell growth, is active in some solid tumors and leukemias. In some cell lines, doxorubicin produces apoptosis by inducing CD95L and CD95 receptor formation. CEM cells, Jurkat T cells, and neuroblastoma cells resistant to anti-CD95 antibody were resistant to doxorubicin-induced apoptosis.[295–297] Doxorubicin clearly appears to up-regulate CD95L expression after doxorubicin exposure in HeLa cells transfected with a CD95L reporter construct.[298] However, acquired resistance to CD95 by clonal selection or by treatment with other anti-CD95 antibodies that inhibit fas-mediated apoptosis does not concomitantly engender resistance to doxorubicin-related apoptosis.[299,300] Further, CD95 and CD95L are frequently not up-regulated following doxorubicin exposure,[301] and anthracycline-mediated activation of caspase 8, a component of the fas pathway, also occurs in the absence of signaling through the fas pathway.[302] These experiments suggest that doxorubicin and CD95 utilize common downstream effectors of apoptosis but that the CD95 pathway is not required for initiating death stimulus in all cell lines or tumors.

In other experimental systems, apoptosis due to the anthracyclines has also been clearly related to an alternative mediator of cell death, ceramide generation,[261,303] which links the plasma membrane biochemistry of doxorubicin with the induction of the cell death cascade. In these studies, ceramide generation following sphingomyelinase activation leads to increased mitochondrial permeability, the activation of proapoptotic caspases, and serine-threonine protein phosphatases.[248,264,304] It remains to be determined, however, whether ceramide production after anthracycline exposure is associated principally with the activation of cell death signals to the mitochondria or with the effector phase of apoptosis.[305]

One of the critical steps in translating a wide variety of apoptotic stimuli into either apoptotic or necrotic cell death is the induction of cytochrome c release from the space between the inner and outer mitochondrial membranes.[281,306,307] Cytochrome c release can lead to caspase activation or to altered mitochondrial electron transport with subsequent apoptosis or necrosis. Anthracyclines are fully capable of inducing cytochrome c release independent of DNA damage.[308–310] In light of the previously described extensive binding and metabolism of the anthracyclines by complex I of the mitochondrial electron transport chain,[143] it is likely that reactive oxygen species, produced by anthracycline-treated mitochondria, can damage mitochondrial membrane integrity and may play an important initiating role in doxorubicin-related apoptosis. Various free radical scavengers inhibit programmed cell death following anthracycline exposure.[93,168,180,181,311,312] Furthermore, cytokine-mediated induction of ceramide production is redox-sensitive, and overexpression of antioxidant genes in human tumor cells prevents ceramide production and partially blocks apoptosis.[313,314] These observations link many of the known but pleiotropic biochemical effects of the anthracyclines; further studies are likely to define the order of anthracycline-related death signals at the molecular level and the relationship of these signals to intracellular anthracycline metabolism.

Two major endogenous modulators of programmed cell death, Bcl-2 and p53, as well as their associated downstream effectors, play critical roles in regulating anthracycline-related apoptosis. The Bcl-2 protein functions in the outer membranes of mitochondria, nuclei, and the endoplasmic reticulum as an inhibitor of cell death; it blocks apoptosis following anthracycline exposure in many experimental systems.[315,316] Furthermore, in acute myelogenous leukemic blasts and HL-60 cells, the cytotoxicity of daunorubicin increases in cells treated with *bcl-2* antisense oligonucleotides.[317] Bcl-2 suppresses the p53-mediated transcriptional activation of several genes involved in the apoptotic process after doxorubicin exposure in MCF-7 cells.[318] The biochemical mechanisms through which Bcl-2 inhibits cell death continue to be elucidated; however, it is currently appreciated that Bcl-2 represses cytochrome c release from mitochondria, interferes with caspase activation, blocks the apoptotic effects of reactive oxygen species, and binds to transcription factors involved in doxorubicin-mediated apoptosis, such as NF-kappa B.[318–323]

The interaction between the anthracycline antibiotics and the NF-κB pathway has been the subject of intensive investigation.[324–328] In most cells, doxorubicin, and many other cytotoxic drugs, activate NF-κB, a key component of the response to cell stress and DNA damage; knockdown of components of the NF-κB complex impairs the NF-κB response and leads to increased apoptosis.[329,330] NF-κB expression is increased in cells resistant to doxorubicin and is associated with an increase in the antioxidant enzyme manganese superoxide dismutase.[312] NF-κB signaling also plays a role in regulating AKT phosphorylation in the heart after doxorubicin exposure.[331]

It appears that programmed cell death due to doxorubicin results from the balance of proapoptotic and antiapoptotic responses, and key players in this response are the antiapoptotic gene *bcl-2* and the *p53* tumor suppressor gene.[332] P53 functions as a transcription factor that causes cell cycle arrest or apoptosis after DNA damage; among the genes activated by p53 are the cyclin-dependent kinase inhibitor *p21, cyclin G*, and the apoptosis-inducing gene *bax*. Exposure to anthracyclines leads to elevated steady-state levels of p53 in cells expressing the wild type gene,[290,333] which produces cell cycle arrest or apoptosis depending on the conditions of drug exposure and the cell type studied. G_1 arrest is due to the induction of p21 in both p53-dependent and p53-independent contexts, and it leads to apoptosis or cellular senescence.[333–336] p53 induction after doxorubicin treatment also induces cyclin G expression with a consequent increase in the accumulation of cells in the G_2/M phase as well as G_1 phase of the cell cycle.[337] Finally, mutations in *p53*, found in almost half of human tumors, diminish apoptosis and promote doxorubicin resistance in many different tumor cell types.[338–340] Alternatively, up-regulation of expression of antiapoptotic factors, including bcl-2, bax, and bcl-long, is found in many human tumors and antagonizes the drive to apoptosis initiated by exposure to anthracyclines and other cytotoxics (see Chapter 1).

Cellular Senescence, and Other Mechanisms of Antitumor Action

In addition to necrotic or apoptotic death phenotypes, the anthracycline antibiotics may produce prolonged growth arrest that in morphologic and enzymatic terms resembles replicative senescence.[170,341] This response may occur whether or not p53 mutations are present and is characterized by the inability of cells undergoing terminal differentiation to form colonies, while at the same time remaining metabolically active but nonproliferative; furthermore, although not required for the initiation of cellular senescence, both p53 and p21 are positive regulators of the senescence phenotype.[342–344] cDNA microarray analysis shows that doxorubicin-related senescence is associated with the inhibition of genes associated with cell proliferation and the up-regulation of tumor suppressors.[345] The discovery of this novel antiproliferative pathway induced by the anthracycline antibiotics provides possible new approaches to enhancing their use in oncologic practice.[346]

Finally, the anthracyclines can produce direct antiangiogenic effects on endothelial cells and may be potent tumor stem cell poisons.[347,348] These findings, in light of the complex range of effects previously described for the anthracyclines, further broaden the spectrum of antineoplastic effects produced by these drugs.

Mechanisms of Resistance

Enhanced Drug Efflux

P170-Glycoprotein-Mediated Anthracycline Efflux. A majority of the doxorubicin-resistant cell lines developed in the laboratory exhibit increased expression of the P170-glycoprotein, an ATP-dependent exporter of the ABC-cassette family.[27,349] The evidence supporting its role in resistance includes (1) a strong correlation between the expression of this protein and a pattern of broad drug resistance that includes the anthracyclines, vinca alkaloids, actinomycin D, and the epipodophyllotoxins,[350] (2) transfer of the cloned *MDR*1 (ABCB1) gene for this protein conferring the full phenotype of multidrug resistance, including resistance to doxorubicin,[351] and (3) the reversal of anthracycline resistance by compounds (verapamil, cyclosporin A, calmodulin inhibitors, and tamoxifen) that block P170-mediated drug efflux by this protein.[352–356] The genetic mechanism behind this increased expression in selected lines in vitro is variable. Some cell lines with very high levels of anthracycline resistance have amplified the gene,

which is either present in double minute chromosome fragments or integrated within the chromosome as homogeneous staining regions; other lines show only increased message coding for the P170-glycoprotein.[357,358] The nature of the resistance that develops after prolonged exposure to doxorubicin in a human sarcoma cell line was evaluated using classic fluctuation analysis; induction of *MDR*1 expression was not demonstrated, but rather, resistance to doxorubicin spontaneously arose with an apparent frequency of 2×10^{-6} per cell generation.[359] However, transient and brief exposure of cells to doxorubicin leads to an acute increase in the expression of the *MDR*1 gene. The increase is mediated by induction of various transcription factors, including FOXO3A.[269,360–362]

The p170 glycoprotein is expressed in many normal tissues (colon mucosa, kidney, adrenal medulla, adrenal cortex, endothelium of the blood-brain barrier, hematopoietic and other stem cells and early myeloid precursors).[363–365] In addition, expression in liver is increased after both partial hepatectomy and exposure to carcinogens such as 2-acetylaminofluorene.[366] Based on this information, it has been postulated that the P170-glycoprotein is part of an integrated system for protecting cells, particularly those of stem cell status, against toxic xenobiotics.[367,368] Other components of this protective system include the mixed-function oxidases, glutathione transferases, glucuronyl transferases, glutathione, and glutathione peroxidase.

Human tumors have been examined before and after treatment with anthracyclines and other drugs that participate in the multidrug-resistance phenotype. Increased expression of the P170-glycoprotein is found before treatment in renal, colon, and adrenal carcinomas, some neuroblastomas and soft tissue sarcomas, and occasionally in tumors of lymphoid or myeloid origin(particularly in undifferentiated or secondary leukemias). For patients with acute lymphocytic and myelocytic leukemias, expression of P170-glycoprotein carries an adverse prognosis.[369,370] P170-glycoprotein expression is rarely found at significant levels either before or after therapy in small cell carcinoma of the lung, but expression is clearly increased posttreatment in some patients failing primary therapy for leukemia, lymphoma, or myeloma.[371,372] Expression in breast cancer is variable.[373,374]

Clinical trials have evaluated the effect of multidrug-reversal agents on the efficacy of anthracycline-containing chemotherapeutic programs but results are inconclusive.[375–377] In general, studies of this approach have demonstrated that clinical strategies to overcome P170-glycoprotein-mediated drug resistance are difficult to pursue and are most likely to be effective for patients with hematologic malignancies, and that better reversing agents, which can be administered at the appropriate dose, with an acceptable toxicity profile and without effects on anthracycline pharmacokinetics are urgently needed. Not unexpectedly, the pharmacokinetics of the anthracyclines may be significantly altered by P170 blocking drugs such as cyclosporin A, which markedly decreases the clearance of doxorubicin and doxorubicinol; this alteration of pharmacokinetics leads to higher levels of anthracycline exposure and clouds the interpretation of results.[378] A large randomized trial for patients with AML demonstrated significantly improved relapse free and overall survival when cyclosporin A was added to daunorubicin as part of a standard cytosine arabinoside and daunorubicin induction regimen.[379] A follow-up study of infusional daunorubicin Ara-C, designed to minimize the toxicity of peak drug levels, failed to show an improvement in response rates.[619] However, it is unclear whether these results reflect reversal of P-glycoprotein-mediated acquired resistance or are due to the increased levels of daunorubicin and its alcohol metabolite found in patients treated with cyclosporin A.

Multidrug Resistance Protein and Other ATP-Dependent Efflux Mechanisms

In some doxorubicin-resistant cell lines that exhibit decreased drug accumulation, P170-glycoprotein is not overexpressed and verapamil did not reverse resistance.[380,381] These results are explained by the selection of resistant cells that display other ATP-dependent efflux proteins. Members of the MRP subgroup have been associated with doxorubicin resistance, including MRP-1 and MRP-7.[618] The role of these exporters in clinical resistance is unproven, although many drug resistant tumor cell lines expressing various MRP family have been described.[31,382–386] MRP proteins may function coordinately with MDR1 to produce anthracycline resistance in patients with acute leukemia, suggesting that MRP may play an important role in the clinic.[387–391] These studies also suggest that critical tissue specificities may be involved in the evolution of the overexpression of different transport proteins.

When additional multidrug resistant tumor cell lines were discovered that relied on enhanced drug efflux but lacked either the P170 glycoprotein or overexpression of MRP, studies revealed other ATP-binding cassette transporters, initially in breast cancer cells resistant to the combination of doxorubicin and verapamil.[392–394] This transporter, a transmembrane protein with 7 intramembrane domains, as compared to the 14-domain P170, was initially described as a "half-transporter" and named the breast cancer resistance protein (BRCP; ABCG2) because it was cloned from MCF-7 breast cancer cells. Doxorubicin can, at variable levels, be transported by the BRCP; however, this depends on the presence of a specific mutation in BRCP at arginine 482, which increases drug efflux.[395] BRCP more effectively transports mitoxantrone, camptothecin-related topoisomerase I inhibitors, and quinazoline EGFR inhibitors. BRCP is expressed in acute myeloid leukemia cells, but its role in drug resistance is unproven.[396,397]

> Other ATP-dependent doxorubicin efflux pumps have also been characterized.[32,39,398] A 110 kDA lung resistance-related protein has been identified as the major vault protein, a critical component of subcellular organelles[37]; this protein has been associated with an adverse prognosis in patients with AML treated with anthracycline-containing chemotherapy.[36,38]

Altered Topoisomerase II Activity

A reduction or absence of top II activity has been implicated as a cause of resistance involving the anthracyclines. The resistance pattern of cells selected for top II–mediated drug insensitivity may differ from the classic profile of MDR1 substrates and includes anthracyclines and etoposide. Nonetheless, it is clear that doxorubicin resistance in P388 and L1210 cells, MCF-7 breast cancer cells, and small cell lung cancer and melanoma lines can be associated with reduced DNA top II activity and reduced drug-induced DNA cleavage.[62,399–402] When tumor cells are selected for anthracycline resistance in the presence of the cyclosporin A analogue PSC-833, which inactivates the P-glycoprotein, doxorubicin resis-

tance emerges, associated with significant reductions in top IIα mRNA and protein without overexpression of MDR1, MRP, or the lung resistance–associated protein.[403] It is relatively common for tumor cells selected with an anthracycline alone to exhibit both reduced top II activity and expression of the P170-glycoprotein or MRP.[402,404,405] The mechanism(s) of decreased top II activity forthcoming from in vitro studies include mutations in the topo IIα gene,[65] decreased top IIα gene copy number,[63] and transcriptional down-regulation of top II gene expression.[406] The most persuasive evidence that changes in top II activity are causally related to doxorubicin sensitivity and resistance comes from studies that demonstrate reversal of resistance after transfer of a fully functional top II gene into resistant cells.[407] In leukemia treatment, the role of top II activity is less certain; top II activity in AML cells is highly variable, with no obvious relationship between enzyme levels and drug sensitivity.[408]

Altered Free Radical Biochemistry, Sensitivity to Apoptosis, and Other Mechanisms of Anthracycline Resistance

The relationship between changes in intracellular free radical detoxifying species and doxorubicin resistance has been reviewed above. It is sufficient here to emphasize that there are considerable, and probably tissue specific, variations in the ability of cells to respond to a drug-induced free radical challenge through enhanced antioxidant defense.[409,410]

In addition to changes in drug export, top II activity, or defenses against free radicals, other resistance mechanisms are at work to prevent doxorubicin-related cell death. Clearly, overexpression of bcl-2 can significantly diminish the toxicity of doxorubicin, as can mutations in p53.[315,338,340] However, as described above, the varied downstream effectors of anthracycline-mediated programmed cell death may individually play critical roles in drug sensitivity beyond that produced by bcl-2 or p53 per se.[272,411–413] Furthermore, in light of the broad importance of these mediators of tumor cell killing for essentially all classes of antineoplastic agents,[414] it is also likely that alterations in components of the cell death cascade play an important role in resistance to the anthracyclines acquired in the clinic prior to anthracycline administration.[328,415]

Potent nuclear DNA repair systems also contribute substantially to the ability of tumor cells to withstand the cytotoxic effects of doxorubicin.[416] Attention has focused on the loss of DNA mismatch repair genes, such as MLH1, in the production of the doxorubicin-resistant phenotype, although the pathways to cell death that are interfered with remain unclear at present.[417–420] Mutations producing decreased levels of poly(ADP-ribose)polymerase (PARP) in V79 cells also dramatically decrease the efficacy of doxorubicin.[421] Since ADP-ribosylation is a well-established posttranslational modification of topoisomerase II and plays an important role in NAD$^+$ utilization, these results suggest that critical aspects of intermediary metabolism may modify the relationship between DNA cleavage reactions and tumor cell killing.[422–424] PARP inhibitors are also capable of producing doxorubicin resistance in human tumor cells.[425,426] These observations of antagonism between anthracyclines and PARP inhibitors have particular relevance to potential combination therapy as the PARP inhibitors have promising activity and are currently in advanced stages of clinical development in breast and ovarian cancers.

Additional mechanisms of DNA repair of relevance to the pharmacology of the anthracycline antibiotics are the activities of the

TABLE

18.4 Key features of anthracycline analogs

	Idarubicin	Epirubicin
Mechanism of action	DNA strand breakage mediated by topoisomerase II; free radical–induced injury; induction of apoptosis	Same
Mechanism of resistance	1. Multidrug resistance mediated by *MDR*1 or *MRP* 2. Topoisomerase II mutations 3. Altered apoptotic response	Same
Dose/schedule (mg/m^2)	10–15 IV q3wk 10 IV × 3 d (leukemia) 45 PO q3wk	90–110 IV q3wk
Pharmacokinetics Elimination half-life		
Parent compound	11.3 h	18.3 h
13-ol metabolite	40–60 h	21.1 h
Other metabolite		12.1 h (epiglucuronide)
Oral bioavailability	30%	
Metabolism	Primary metabolite, 13-epirubicinol, is cytotoxic and exceeds level of parent compound in plasma	Primary metabolites are glucuronides of parent and 13-ol
Excretion	80% excreted in urine as 13-ol	Primarily parent compound, 13-ol, and glucuronides
Toxicity	1. Leukopenia 2. Thrombocytopenia 3. Cardiotoxicity (less than doxorubicin)	1. Leukopenia 2. Thrombocytopenia 3. Cardiotoxicity equal to doxorubicin
Drug interactions	None established	None established
Precautions	None established	Possible dose reduction in hepatic dysfunction

a planar tetracyclic compound having two symmetrical aminoalkyl side arms but no glycosidic substituent as found in the active anthracyclines (Fig. 18-8). It is one of the most active agents tested against P388, yielding 500% increase in life span and a high percentage of cures.[561] Subsequent preclinical and clinical evaluation has demonstrated significant differences between this agent and the anthracyclines in terms of mechanism of action, the lesser cardiac toxicity of the anthracenediones, and their diminished potential for extravasation injury and for causing nausea and vomiting or alopecia. Their narrow spectrum of antitumor activity, confined to breast and prostate cancer,[562,563] the leukemias and lymphomas, has limited the opportunity to replace doxorubicin with mitoxantrone in clinical practice. It is infrequently used as an anticancer drug, although its immunosuppressive effects have led to its approval for patients with multiple sclerosis.[604,605] Its key features are given in Table 18-5.

Mechanism of Action

Like the anthracyclines, mitoxantrone binds avidly to nucleic acids and inhibits DNA and RNA synthesis. Its mode of binding to DNA includes intercalation between opposing DNA strands, with preference for GC base pairs.[564] Careful studies of the stoichiometry of binding and electron microscopic evaluation of the distortions produced in vitro in plasmid DNA indicate an additional type of binding that produces a compaction of chromatin[565] and, with plasmid DNA, lace-like intertwining of the DNA strands. These effects are dependent on the presence of the highly positively charged aminoalkyl side chains and probably represent electrostatic cross-linking of DNA strands. Also found are single- and double-strand breaks in DNA.[566] Because the drug has the basic quinone structure found in the anthracyclines, its ability to generate free radicals in a manner similar to that of doxorubicin has been examined. These studies revealed that the drug has a much reduced potential to undergo

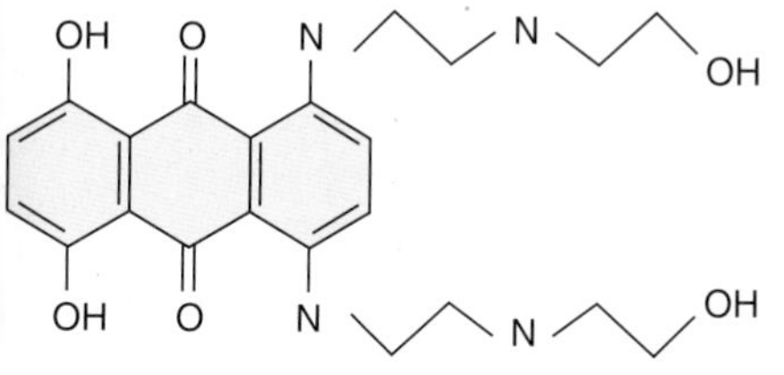

Mitoxantrone

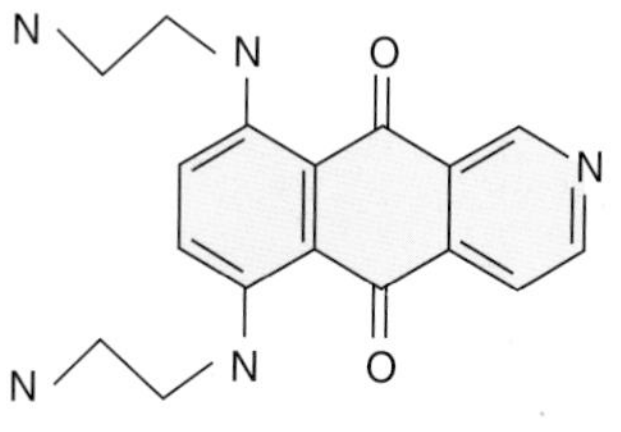

Pixantrone

Figure **18-8**   Structures of mitoxantrone and pixantrone.

18.5 *Key features of mitoxantrone*

Mechanism of action	Inhibition of top II; DNA intercalation
Pharmacokinetics Elimination Toxicity	Plasma $t_{1/2}$ = 23–42 h Hepatic metabolism (side chain oxidation) Acute myelosuppression Cardiac dysfunction (especially after doxorubicin) Blue tint to fingernails, sclerae
Precautions	Prior doxorubicin Hepatic dysfunction (reduce doses 50% for bilirubin elevation) Preexisting cardiac disease

one-electron reduction, compared to doxorubicin,[567,568] and is less readily reduced enzymatically.[569] Since the single-strand breaks are protein associated, they likely result from the formation of a cleavable complex with top II.[570] This possibility is heightened by the finding that there is little evidence for lipid peroxidation in cardiac tissue, modest stimulation of oxygen consumption in vitro, and, indeed, inhibition of doxorubicin-induced lipid peroxidation by mitoxantrone;[571] all of these findings argue against a free radical mechanism of tissue injury by mitoxantrone and favor enzyme-mediated DNA cleavage. The reduced potential for free radical formation may also explain the lesser cardiotoxicity of mitoxantrone, although this drug is able to oxidize critical sulfhydryl groups on the ryanodine receptor of the sarcoplasmic reticulum.[522,523,572] As is the case for the anthracyclines, mitoxantrone can also readily stimulate apoptosis in a variety of cell lines.[573–575] Ceramide-dependent pathways have been implicated as a contributor to mitoxantrone-induced programmed cell death.[263]

Mechanisms of Drug Resistance

As a planar anthraquinone analogue, mitoxantrone shares cross-resistance with many other natural products, including the vinca alkaloids and doxorubicin.[576–578] This resistance may be mediated by amplification of the P170-glycoprotein (classic *MDR*1); however, in some cell lines, decreased intracellular drug accumulation is related to the overexpression of members of the multidrug resistance protein (*MRP*) family, or to the BCRP transporter.[579,580] Mutations or decreased expression of top II have been associated with mitoxantrone resistance, sometimes accompanied by increased efflux.[581,582] Mitoxantrone resistance can occur in the absence of alterations in topoisomerase II or enhanced expression of *MDR*1 or *MRP*,[393,577,583,584] likely through induction of as yet unidentified efflux transporters. Additional mechanisms of mitoxantrone resistance have been related to altered intracellular pH in tumor cells[585] and to modifications in the cellular apoptotic program.

Drug Interactions

Mitoxantrone has been used in combination with arabinosylcytosine in the treatment of acute nonlymphocytic leukemia, and there is evidence for biochemical synergy

of the two agents. In studies of leukemic cells taken from patients during therapy, coadministration of mitoxantrone and arabinosylcytosine enhanced the accumulation of ara-CTP and single-strand DNA breaks in leukemic blast cells.[586] Like doxorubicin, mitoxantrone sensitizes cells to ionizing radiation.[587]

Dosage

The recommended dosage for bolus intravenous administration of mitoxantrone is $12 \, mg/m^2/d$ for 3 days for treatment of AML and 12 to $14 \, mg/m^2/d$ once every 3 weeks for patients with solid tumors. The drug has activity against breast cancer,[588] ovarian cancer,[589] non-Hodgkin's lymphoma,[590] and prostate cancer[562] in addition to acute leukemia but is rarely used in clinical practice in place of anthracyclines.[591] The drug is administered as a 30-minute infusion and rarely causes extravasation injury if infiltrated. Mitoxantrone should not be administered in solutions containing heparin.

Pharmacokinetics

Mitoxantrone is readily assayed in biological fluids by high performance liquid chromatography (HPLC) coupled with mass spectroscopy.[592,593] The plasma disappearance of mitoxantrone is characterized by a rapid preliminary phase distribution and cellular uptake followed by a long terminal half-life of 23 to 42 hours.[592,593] During this final phase of drug disappearance, drug concentrations in plasma approximate 1 ng/mL or 2 nM, a level at the margin of cytotoxicity. The pharmacokinetics of mitoxantrone is linear over the dose range from 8 to $14 \, mg/m^2$ administered as a short infusion.[594] Less than 30% of the drug can be accounted for by the fraction of drug that appears in the urine (<10%) or the stool (<20%). Like doxorubicin, the drug distributes in high concentrations into tissues (liver > bone marrow > heart > lung > kidney) and remains in these sites for weeks after therapy.[592] Although specific guidelines are not available for dose adjustment in patients with hepatic dysfunction, the terminal half-life may be prolonged to greater than 60 hours in patients with liver impairment.[593,595]

The specific metabolites of mitoxantrone have not been well characterized.[596] The side chains undergo oxidation, yielding the mono- and dicarboxylic acids of anthracenedione, and both have been recovered from urine.[597] Neither has antitumor activity.

As an alternative to intravenous infusion, mitoxantrone has been administered by hepatic intra-arterial infusion[598] and by intraperitoneal instillation.[599,600] These trials were based on the observation that mitoxantrone has a steep dose-response curve in vitro and that optimal concentrations of drug (1 to 10 μg/mL) are achieved only briefly during standard intravenous therapy. Local concentrations much higher than those realized in systemic administration can be achieved by either the intra-arterial or intraperitoneal routes. During intraperitoneal trials, patients with ovarian or colon cancer received 12 to $38 \, mg/m^2$ as a single dose every 4 weeks in 2 L of dialysate. An advantage of 1,400-fold was achieved in comparing intraperitoneal drug concentrations to simultaneous plasma levels. The terminal half-life for disappearance of drug from the intraperitoneal space was 9 hours. Toxicity was primarily leukopenia at the highest doses of drug. Abdominal discomfort and tenderness, as well as catheter dysfunction due to the formation of a fibrous sheath reflecting serositis, are not uncommon with intraperitoneal mitoxantrone.

Toxicity

The primary advantages of mitoxantrone, in comparison to doxorubicin, are its much reduced incidence of cardiac toxicity, the mild nausea and vomiting that follow intravenous administration, and minimal alopecia. Early trials of mitoxantrone revealed occasional episodes of cardiac failure,[601] primarily in patients who had received prior doxorubicin. A small percentage (1% to 5%) of patients will develop congestive heart failure after treatment with mitoxantrone in the absence of prior anthracycline exposure.[587,602,603] The potential for the cumulative cardiac toxicity of mitoxantrone has emerged from reports of heart damage occurring in patients with multiple sclerosis (for which mitoxantrone has been approved by the United States Food and Drug Administration).[604,605] In this setting, 5% of patients who receive over $100 \, mg/m^2$ of mitoxantrone develop an asymptomatic decrease in left ventricular ejection fraction. The risk of cardiac toxicity is greatest in cancer patients who have received prior anthracyclines or chest irradiation[606] and in those with underlying cardiac disease.[587,603,606]

Other toxicities include a reversible leukopenia, with recovery within 14 days of drug administration; mild thrombocytopenia; nausea and vomiting; and rarely abnormal liver enzymes in patients receiving dose levels appropriate for solid tumors.[607] One minor, and at times alarming, side effect of mitoxantrone is a bluish discoloration of the sclera, fingernails, and urine.[608]

Newer Anthracenedione Analogues

Attempts to find newer anthracenedione analogues have led to the discovery of pixantrone (see Fig. 18-8), an aza-analogue of mitoxantrone that lacks the hydroxy substitutions on the A ring and has a shortened side chain configuration. It has reduced capacity to generate free radicals because of the lack of the A ring hydroxyl substitutions. It retains the ability to intercalate DNA and likely interacts with top II. A phase III trial has disclosed significant response rates in previously treated non-Hodgkin lymphoma (NHL) (26% complete and partial responses in 70 patients, with a mean of 7 months to time of progression, as compared to a 7% response rate for best available second-line therapy). These promising results have led to a large randomized trial with pixantrone in combination with cyclophosphamide, vincristine, prednisone, and rituximab as primary therapy in NHL.[609]

Liposome Encapsulated Anthracyclines

In an effort to enhance tissue distribution and alter pharmacokinetics, doxorubicin has been encapsulated in a liposomal pegylated formation (Doxil) and in a non-pegylated liposome, Myocet. Pegylation (addition of multiple polyethylene glycol groups) extends the plasma half-life of drug released from the lipid capsule and restricts its distribution. Doxorubicin HCL liposome is approved for second-line treatment of ovarian cancer (for which doxorubicin has limited activity) and for Kaposi's sarcoma, a vascular endothelium tumor found frequently in AIDS patients. The drug has the same basic mechanism of action and toxicities of doxorubicin, with the notable exception of producing a plantar-palmar dysesthesia, a progressive accumulation of tender nodules, and erythematous desquamation on the palms and soles. This toxicity is found in approximately 25% of patients, leads to drug discontinuation in 3% to 5% of patients, and may recur in an exacerbated reaction with the use of other chemotherapy drugs that produce this toxicity.[616] There is no effective treatment for this condition other than drug discontinuation. Doxorubicin levels in plasma have an extended half-life (50 hours at doses of 10 to $20 \, mg/m^2$) due to slow release from the liposomes. It is unclear whether the risk of cardiotoxicity is less in patients receiving Doxorubicin HCL liposome rather than doxorubicin, although Doxorubicin HCL liposome-related cardiac dysfunction has been reported in Phase II and Phase III trials.[617]

Doxorubicin HCL liposome doses are $50 \, mg/m^2$ every 3 to 4 weeks in patients with ovarian cancer and $20 \, mg/m^2$ every 3 weeks in Kaposi's sarcoma. Doses should be reduced by 50% in patients with elevated bilirubin levels in plasma.

The nonpegylated doxorubicin, has shown equal antitumor activity to doxorubicin when used in equimolar doses, and possibly less cardiotoxicity, in breast cancer trials. When used in doses of $50 \, mg/m^2$ every 3 weeks, it produced a response rate of 98% in combination with paclitaxel and trastuzumab, with no episodes of clinical cardiotoxicity in 54 patients.[620] Further studies are required to fully access its cardiotoxicity and efficacy.

DaunoXome, a liposomal preparation of daunorubicin, is approved for treatment of AML in the United States but is not commonly used. In doses of $50 \, mg/m^2$, it produces tenfold higher AUCs than daunorubicin but has very limited distribution and equal intracellular AUCs (759 versus 715 $\mu M \times h$), as compared to the parent drug.[622] A randomized trial in patients older than 60 with AML showed than the liposomal preparation ($80 \, mg/m^2$ days 1 to 3) produced a higher incidence of early deaths but a lower late relapse rate and a possible late advantage in survival, as compared to daunorubicin ($45 \, mg/m^2$, days 1 to 3).[622] It is not clear that the improved recurrence rate and survival result from greater antitumor efficacy or simply a higher dose of drug.

References

1. Di Marco A, Gaetani M, Orezzi P, et al. "Daunomycin," a new antibiotic of the rhodomycin group. Nature 1964;201:706–707.

2. Arcamone F, Cassinelli G, Fantini G, et al. Adriamycin, 14-hydroxydaunomycin, a new antitumor antibiotic from *S. peucetius* var. *caesius*. Biotechnol Bioeng 1969;11:1101–1110.

3. Legha SS, Benjamin RS, Mackay B, et al. Adriamycin therapy by continuous intravenous infusion in patients with metastatic breast cancer. Cancer 1982;49:1762–1766.

4. Legha SS, Benjamin RS, Mackay B, et al. Role of adriamycin in breast cancer and sarcomas. In: Muggia FM, Young CW, Carter SK, eds. Anthracycline Antibiotics in Cancer Therapy. The Hague: Martinus Nijhoff Publishers, 1982:432–444.

5. Jones RB, Holland JF, Bhardwaj S, et al. A phase I-II study of intensive-dose adriamycin for advanced breast cancer. J Clin Oncol 1987;5:172–177.

6. Bronchud MH, Howell A, Crowther D, et al. The use of granulocyte colony-stimulating factor to increase the intensity of treatment with doxorubicin in patients with advanced breast and ovarian cancer. Br J Cancer 1989;60:121–125.

7. Citron ML, Berry DA, Cirrincione C, et al. Randomized trial of dose-dense versus conventionally scheduled and sequential versus concurrent combination chemotherapy as postoperative adjuvant treatment of node-positive primary breast cancer: first report of Intergroup Trial C9741/Cancer and Leukemia Group B Trial 9741. J Clin Oncol 2003;21:1431–1439.

8. Barlett JM, Munro AF, Dunn JA, et al. Predictive markers of anthracycline benefit: a prospectively planned analysis of the UK National Epirubicin Adjuvant Trial (NEAT/BR9601). Lancet Oncol 2010;11:266–274.

9. Dalmark M, Strom HH. A fickian diffusion transport process with features of transport catalysis: doxorubicin transport in human red blood cells. J Gen Physiol 1981;78:349–364.

10. Peterson C, Trouet A. Transport and storage of daunorubicin and doxorubicin in cultured fibroblasts. Cancer Res 1978;38:4645–4649.

11. Bachur NR, Steele M, Meriwether WD, et al. Cellular pharmocodynamics of several anthracycline antibiotics. J Med Chem 1976;19:651–654.

12. Gianni L, Corden B, Myers C. The biochemical basis of anthracycline toxicity and antitumor action. Rev Biochem Toxicol 1983;5:1–82.

13. Raghunand N, He X, van Sluis R, et al. Enhancement of chemotherapy by manipulation of tumour pH. Br J Cancer 1999;80:1005–1011.

14. Peterson C, Baurain R, Trouet A. The mechanism for cellular uptake, storage, and release of daunorubicin: studies on fibroblasts in culture. Biochem Pharmacol 1980;29:1687–1692.

15. Gerweck LE, Kozin SV, Stocks SJ. The pH partition theory predicts the accumulation and toxicity of doxorubicin in normal and low-pH-adapted cells. Br J Cancer 1999;79:838–842.

16. Schindler M, Grabski S, Hoff E, et al. Defective pH regulation of acidic compartments in human breast cancer cells (MCF-7) is normalized in adriamycin-resistant cells (MCF-7adr). Biochemistry 1996;35:2811–2817.

17. Vaupel PW, Frinak S, Bicher HI. Heterogeneous oxygen partial pressure and pH distribution in C3H mouse mammary adenocarcinoma. Cancer Res 1981;41:2008–2013.

18. Altan N, Chen Y, Schindler M, et al. Defective acidification in human breast tumor cells and implications for chemotherapy. J Exp Med 1998;187:1583–1598.

19. Simon SM, Schindler M. Cell biological mechanisms of multidrug resistance in tumors. Proc Natl Acad Sci USA 1994;91:3497–3504.

20. Johnson BA, Cheang MS, Goldenberg GJ. Comparison of adriamycin uptake in chick embryo heart and liver cells and murine L5178Y lymphoblasts in vitro: role of drug uptake in cardiotoxicity. Cancer Res 1986;46:218–223.

21. Peterson C, Paul C, Gahrton G. Studies on the cellular pharmacology of daunorubicin and doxorubicin in experimental systems and human leukemia. In: Mathe G, Maral R, De Jager R, eds. Anthracyclines: Current Status and Future Developments. New York: Masson Publishing USA, Inc., 1983:85–89.

22. Kiyomiya K, Matsuo S, Kurebe M. Proteasome is a carrier to translocate doxorubicin from cytoplasm into nucleus. Life Sci 1998;62:1853–1860.

23. Kiyomiya K, Matsuo S, Kurebe M. Mechanism of specific nuclear transport of adriamycin: the mode of nuclear translocation of adriamycin-proteasome complex. Cancer Res 2001;61:2467–2471.

24. Liu J, Zheng H, Tang M, et al. A therapeutic dose of doxorubicin activates ubiquitin-proteasome system-mediated proteolysis by acting on both the ubiquitination apparatus and proteasome. Am J Physiol Heart Circ Physiol 2008;295:H2541–H2550.

25. Kiyomiya K, Kurebe M, Nakagawa H, et al. The role of the proteasome in apoptosis induced by anthracycline anticancer agents. Int J Oncol 2002;20:1205–1209.

26. Cusack JC. Rationale for the treatment of solid tumors with the proteasome inhibitor bortezomib. Cancer Treat Rev 2003;29(Suppl 1):21–31.

27. Kartner N, Riordan JR, Ling V. Cell-surface P-glycoprotein associated with multidrug resistance in mammalian cell lines. Science 1983;221:1285–1288.

28. Ueda K, Cardarelli C, Gottesman MM, et al. Expression of a full-length cDNA for the human "MDR1" gene confers resistance to colchine, doxorubicin, and vinblastine. Proc Natl Acad Sci USA 1987;84:3004–3008.

29. Pastan I, Gottesman MM. Multidrug resistance. Annu Rev Med 1991;42:277–286.

30. Cole SPC, Bhardwaj G, Gerlach JH, et al. Overexpression of a transporter gene in a multidrug-resistant human lung cancer cell line. Science 1992;258:1650–1654.

31. Slovak ML, Ho JP, Bhardwaj G, et al. Localization of a novel multidrug resistance-associated gene in the HT1080/DR4 and H69AR human tumor cell lines. Cancer Res 1993;53:3221–3225.

32. Awasthi S, Singhal SS, Srivastava SK, et al. Adenosine triphosphate-dependent transport of doxorubicin, daunomycin, and vinblastine in human tissues by a mechanism distinct from the P-glycoprotein. J Clin Invest 1994;93:958–965.

33. Jedlitschky G, Leier I, Buchholz U, et al. ATP-dependent transport of glutathione S-conjugates by the multidrug resistance-associated protein. Cancer Res 1994;54:4833–4836.

34. Yi J-R, Lu S, Fernandez-Checa J, et al. Expression cloning of a rat hepatic reduced glutathione transporter with canalicular characteristics. J Clin Invest 1994;93:1841–1845.

35. Priebe W, Krawczyk M, Kuo MT, et al. Doxorubicin- and daunorubicin-glutathione conjugates, but not unconjugated drugs, competitively inhibit leukotriene C4 transport mediated by MRP/GS-X pump. Biochem Biophys Res Commun 1998;247:859–863.

36. Borg AG, Burgess R, Green LM, et al. Overexpression of lung-resistance protein and increased P-glycoprotein function in acute myeloid leukaemia cells predict a poor response to chemotherapy and reduced patient survival. Br J Haematol 1998;103:1083–1091.

37. Schroeijers AB, Scheffer GL, Flens MJ, et al. Immunohistochemical detection of the human major vault protein LRP with two monoclonal antibodies in formalin-fixed, paraffin-embedded tissues. Am J Pathol 1998;152:373–378.

38. Michieli M, Damiani D, Ermacora A, et al. P-glycoprotein, lung resistance-related protein and multidrug resistance associated protein in de novo acute non-lymphocytic leukaemias: biological and clinical implications. Br J Haematol 1999;104:328–335.

39. Singhal SS, Yadav S, Singhal J, et al. The role of PKCalpha and RLIP76 in transport-mediated doxorubicin-resistance in lung cancer. FEBS Lett 2005;579:4635–4641.

40. Frank NY, Margaryan A, Huang Y, et al. ABCB5-mediated doxorubicin transport and chemoresistance in human malignant melanoma. Cancer Res 2005;65:4320–4333.

41. Chaires JB, Fox KR, Herrera JE, et al. Site and sequence specificity of the daunomycin-DNA interaction. Biochemistry 1987;26:8227–8236.

42. Bailly C, Suh D, Waring MJ, et al. Binding of daunomycin to diaminopurine- and/or inosine-substituted DNA. Biochemistry 1998;37:1033–1045.

43. Trist H, Phillips DR. Invitro transcription analysis of the role of flanking sequence on the DNA sequence specificity of adriamycin. Nucl Acids Res 1989;17:3673–3688.

44. Evison BJ, Bilardi RA, Chiu FC, et al. CpG methylation potentiates pixantrone and doxorubicin-induced DNA damage and is a marker of drug sensitivity. Nucleic Acids Res 2009;37:6355–6370.

45. Tan HH, Porter AG. DNA methyltransferase I is a mediator of doxorubicin-induced genotoxicity in human cancer cells. Biochem Biophys Res Commun 2009;382:462–467.

46. Calendi E, Marco A, Reggiani M, et al. On physicochemical interactions between daunomycin and nucleic acids. Biochem Biophys Acta 1965;103:25–54.

47. Zeman SM, Phillips DR, Crothers DM. Characterization of covalent adriamycin-DNA adducts. Proc Natl Acad Sci USA 1998;95:11561–11565.

48. Zunino F, Ganbetta R, DiMarco A, et al. A comparison of the effects of daunomycin and adriamycin on various DNA polymerases. Cancer Res 1975;35:754–760.

49. Zunino F, Gambetta R, DiMarco A. The inhibition in vitro of DNA polymerase and RNA polymerase by daunomycin and adriamycin. Biochem Pharmacol 1975;24:309–311.

50. Siegfried JM, Sartorelli AC, Tritton TR. Evidence for the lack of relationship between inhibition of nucleic acid synthesis and cytotoxicity of adriamycin. Cancer Biochem Biophys 1983;6:137–142.

51. Ross WA, Glaubiger DL, Kohn KW. Protein-associated DNA breaks in cells treated with adriamycin and ellipticine. Biochim Biophys Acta 1978;519:23–30.

52. Zwelling LA, Michaels S, Erickson LC, et al. Protein-associated deoxyribonucleic acid strand breaks in L1210 cells treated with the deoxyribonucleic acid intercalating agents 4'-(9-acridinylamino)methanesulfon-m-anisidide and adriamycin. Biochemistry 1981;20:6553–6563.

53. Kohn KW. Beyond DNA cross-linking: history and prospects of DNA-targeted cancer treatment—fifteenth Bruce F. Cain Memorial Award Lecture. Cancer Res 1996;56:5533–5546.

54. Liu LF. DNA topoisomerase poisons as antitumor drugs. Annu Rev Biochem 1989;58:351–375.

55. Tewey KM, Chen GI, Nelson EM, et al. Intercalative antitumor drugs interfere with the breakage- reunion reaction of mammalian DNA topoisomerase. J Biol Chem 1984;259:9182–9187.

56. Pommier Y. DNA topoisomerase I and II in cancer chemotherapy: update and perspectives. Cancer Chemother Pharmacol 1993;32:103–108.

240. Sun IL, Navas P, Crane FL, et al. Diferric transferrin reductase in the plasma membrane is inhibited by adriamycin. Biochem Int 1987;14:119–127.

241. DeAtley SM, Aksenov MY, Aksenova MV, et al. Adriamycin induces protein oxidation in erythrocyte membranes. Pharmacol Toxicol 1998;83:62–68.

242. Tritton TR, Yee G. The anticancer agent adriamycin can be actively cytotoxic without entering cells. Science 1982;217:248–250.

243. Rogers KE, Carr BI, Tokes ZA. Cell surface-mediated cytotoxicity of polymer-bound adriamycin against drug-resistant hepatocytes. Cancer Res 1983;43:2741–2748.

244. Vichi P, Tritton TR. Adriamycin: protection from cell death by removal of extracellular drug. Cancer Res 1992;52:4135–4138.

245. Burns CP, Spector AA. Membrane fatty acid modification in tumor cells: a potential therapeutic adjunct. Lipids 1987;22:178–184.

246. Spector AA, Burns CP. Biological and therapeutic potential of membrane lipid modifications in tumors. Cancer Res 1987;47:4529–4537.

247. Burns CP, North JA, Petersen ES, et al. Subcellular distribution of doxorubicin: comparison of fatty acid- modified and unmodified cells. Proc Soc Exp Biol Med 1988;188:455–460.

248. Hannun YA. Functions of ceramide in coordinating cellular responses to stress. Science 1996;274:1855–1859.

249. Leevers SJ, Vanhaesebroeck B, Waterfield MD. Signalling through phosphoinositide 3-kinases: the lipids take centre stage. Curr Opin Cell Biol 1999;11:219–225.

250. Haimovitz-Friedman A. Radiation-induced signal transduction and stress response. Radiat Res 1998;150:S102–S108.

251. Bredel M, Pollack IF. The p21-Ras signal transduction pathway and growth regulation in human high-grade gliomas. Brain Res Brain Res Rev 1999;29:232–249.

252. Kyriakis JM. Making the connection: coupling of stress-activated ERK/MAPK (extracellular-signal-regulated kinase/mitogen-activated protein kinase) core signalling modules to extracellular stimuli and biological responses. Biochem Soc Symp 1999;64:29–48.

253. Tritton TR, Hickman JA. How to kill cancer cells: membranes and cell signaling as targets in cancer chemotherapy. Cancer Cells 1990;2:95–105.

254. Palayoor ST, Stein JM, Hait WN. Inhibition of protein kinase C by antineoplastic agents: implications for drug resistance. Biochem Biophys Res Commun 1987;148:718–725.

255. Donella-Deana A, Monti E, Pinna LA. Inhibition of tyrosine protein kinases by the antineoplastic agent adriamycin. Biochem Biophys Res Commun 1989;160:1309–1315.

256. Hannun YA, Foglesong RJ, Bell RM. The adriamycin-iron(III) complex is a potent inhibitor of protein kinase C. J Biol Chem 1989;264:9960–9966.

257. Posada J, Vichi P, Tritton TR. Protein kinase C in Adriamycin action and resistance in mouse sarcoma 180 cells. Cancer Res 1989;49:6634–6639.

258. Tritton TR. Cell death in cancer chemotherapy: the case of Adriamycin. In: Tomei LD, Cope FO, eds. Apoptosis: The Molecular Basis of Cell Death. Cold Spring Harbor: Cold Spring Harbor Laboratory Press, 1991;121–137.

259. Sahyoun N, Wolf M, Besterman J, et al. Protein kinase C phosphorylates topoisomerase II: topoisomerase activation and its possible role in phorbol ester-induced differentiation of HL-60 cells. Proc Natl Acad Sci USA 1986;83:1603–1607.

260. Sankala HM, Hait NC, Paugh SW, et al. Involvement of sphingosine kinase 2 in p53-independent induction of p21 by the chemotherapeutic drug doxorubicin. Cancer Res 2007;67:10466–10474.

261. Jaffrezou JP, Levade T, Bettaieb A, et al. Daunorubicin-induced apoptosis: triggering of ceramide generation through sphingomyelin hydrolysis. EMBO J 1996;15:2417–2424.

262. Bose R, Verheij M, Haimovitz-Friedman A, et al. Ceramide synthase mediates daunorubicin-induced apoptosis: an alternative mechanism for generating death signals. Cell 1995;82:405–414.

263. Bettaieb A, Plo I, Mansat-De M, V, et al. Daunorubicin- and mitoxantrone-triggered phosphatidylcholine hydrolysis: implication in drug-induced ceramide generation and apoptosis. Mol Pharmacol 1999;55:118–125.

264. Tepper AD, de Vries E, van Blitterswijk WJ, et al. Ordering of ceramide formation, caspase activation, and mitochondrial changes during CD95- and DNA damage-induced apoptosis. J Clin Invest 1999;103:971–978.

265. Mansat V, Bettaieb A, Levade T, et al. Serine protease inhibitors block neutral sphingomyelinase activation, ceramide generation, and apoptosis triggered by daunorubicin. Faseb J 1997;11:695–702.

266. Allouche M, Bettaieb A, Vindis C, et al. Influence of Bcl-2 overexpression on the ceramide pathway in daunorubicin-induced apoptosis of leukemic cells. Oncogene 1997;14:1837–1845.

267. Liu YY, Han TY, Giuliano AE, et al. Expression of glucosylceramide synthase, converting ceramide to glucosylceramide, confers adriamycin resistance in human breast cancer cells. J Biol Chem 1999;274:1140–1146.

268. Fine RL, Patel J, Chabner BA. Phorbol esters induce multidrug resistance in human breast cancer cells. Proc Natl Acad Sci USA 1988;85:582–586.

269. Yu G, Ahmad S, Aquino A, et al. Transfection with protein kinase Cα confers increased multidrug resistance to MCF-7 cells expressing P-glycoprotein. Cancer Commun 1991;3:181–189.

270. Budworth J, Gant TW, Gescher A. Co-ordinate loss of protein kinase C and multidrug resistance gene expression in revertant MCF-7/Adr breast carcinoma cells. Br J Cancer 1997;75:1330–1335.

271. Laredo J, Huynh A, Muller C, et al. Effect of the protein kinase C inhibitor staurosporine on chemosensitivity to daunorubicin of normal and leukemic fresh myeloid cells. Blood 1994;84:229–237.

272. Lavie Y, Cao H, Volner A, et al. Agents that reverse multidrug resistance, tamoxifen, verapamil, and cyclosporin A, block glycosphingolipid metabolism by inhibiting ceramide glycosylation in human cancer cells. J Biol Chem 1997;272:1682–1687.

273. Lupertz R, Chovolou Y, Unfried K, et al. The forkhead transcription factor FOXO4 sensitizes cancer cells to doxorubicin-mediated cytotoxicity. Carcinogenesis 2008;29:2045–2052.

274. Yu HG, Ai YW, Yu LL, et al. Phosphoinositide 3-kinase/Akt pathway plays an important role in chemoresistance of gastric cancer cells against etoposide and doxorubicin induced cell death. Int J Cancer 2008;122:433–443.

275. Li S, Zhou Y, Wang R, et al. Selenium sensitizes MCF-7 breast cancer cells to doxorubicin-induced apoptosis through modulation of phospho-Akt and its downstream substrates. Mol Cancer Ther 2007;6:1031–1038.

276. Pan L, Lu J, Wang X, et al. Histone deacetylase inhibitor trichostatin a potentiates doxorubicin-induced apoptosis by up-regulating PTEN expression. Cancer 2007;109:1676–1688.

277. Xiang P, Deng HY, Li K, et al. Dexrazoxane protects against doxorubicin-induced cardiomyopathy: upregulation of Akt and Erk phosphorylation in a rat model. Cancer Chemother Pharmacol 2009;63:343–349.

278. Filyak Y, Filyak O, Souchelnytskyi S, et al. Doxorubicin inhibits TGF-beta signaling in human lung carcinoma A549 cells. Eur J Pharmacol 2008;590:67–73.

279. Yamazaki Y, Hasebe Y, Egawa K, et al. Anthracyclines, small-molecule inhibitors of hypoxia-inducible factor-1 alpha activation. Biol Pharm Bull 2006;29:1999–2003.

280. Chen L, Feng P, Li S, et al. Effect of hypoxia-inducible factor-1alpha silencing on the sensitivity of human brain glioma cells to doxorubicin and etoposide. Neurochem Res 2009;34:984–990.

281. Reed JC. Dysregulation of apoptosis in cancer. J Clin Oncol 1999;17:2941–2953.

282. Wickremasinghe RG, Hoffbrand AV. Biochemical and genetic control of apoptosis: relevance to normal hematopoiesis and hematological malignancies. Blood 1999;93:3587–3600.

283. Hannun YA. Apoptosis and the dilemma of cancer chemotherapy. Blood 1997;89:1845–1853.

284. Skladanowski A, Konopa J. Adriamycin and daunomycin induce programmed cell death (apoptosis) in tumour cells. Biochem Pharmacol 1993;46:375–382.

285. Ling Y-H, Priebe W, Perez-Soler R. Apoptosis induced by anthracycline antibiotics in P388 parent and multidrug-resistant cells. Cancer Res 1993;53:1845–1852.

286. Lotem J, Sachs L. Hematopoietic cytokines inhibit apoptosis induced by transforming growth factor beta 1 and cancer chemotherapy compounds in myeloid leukemic cells. Blood 1992;80:1750–1757.

287. Thakkar NS, Potten CS. Inhibition of doxorubicin-induced apoptosis in vivo by 2-deoxy-d-glucose. Cancer Res 1993;53:2057–2060.

288. Onishi Y, Azuma Y, Sato Y, et al. Topoisomerase inhibitors induce apoptosis in thymocytes. Biochim Biophys Acta 1993;1175:147–154.

289. Zaleskis G, Berleth E, Verstovsek S, et al. Doxorubicin-induced DNA degradation in murine thymocytes. Mol Pharmacol 1994;46:901–908.

290. Chernov MV, Stark GR. The p53 activation and apoptosis induced by DNA damage are reversibly inhibited by salicylate. Oncogene 1997;14:2503–2510.

291. Wu XX, Jin XH, Zeng Y, et al. Low concentrations of doxorubicin sensitizes human solid cancer cells to tumor necrosis factor-related apoptosis-inducing ligand (TRAIL)-receptor (R) 2-mediated apoptosis by inducing TRAIL-R2 expression. Cancer Sci 2007;98:1969–1976.

292. Teixeira C, Reed JC, Pratt MAC. Estrogen promotes chemotherapeutic drug resistance by a mechanism involving bcl-2 proto-oncogene expression in human breast cancer cells. Cancer Res 1995;55:3902–3907.

293. Strobel T, Swanson L, Korsmeyer S, et al. BAX enhances paclitaxel-induced apoptosis through a p53- independent pathway. Proc Natl Acad Sci USA 1996;93:14094–14099.

294. Makris A, Powles TJ, Dowsett M, et al. Prediction of response to neoadjuvant chemoendocrine therapy in primary breast carcinomas. Clin Cancer Res 1997;3:593–600.

295. Friesen C, Herr I, Krammer PH, et al. Involvement of the CD95 (APO-1/FAS) receptor/ligand system in drug- induced apoptosis in leukemia cells. Nat Med 1996;2:574–577.

296. Fulda S, Sieverts H, Friesen C, et al. The CD95 (APO-1/Fas) system mediates drug-induced apoptosis in neuroblastoma cells. Cancer Res 1997;57:3823–3829.

297. Fulda S, Susin SA, Kroemer G, et al. Molecular ordering of apoptosis induced by anticancer drugs in neuroblastoma cells. Cancer Res 1998;58:4453–4460.

298. Mo YY, Beck WT. DNA damage signals induction of fas ligand in tumor cells. Mol Pharmacol 1999;55:216–222.

299. Eischen CM, Kottke TJ, Martins LM, et al. Comparison of apoptosis in wild-type and Fas-resistant cells: chemotherapy-induced apoptosis is not dependent on Fas/Fas ligand interactions. Blood 1997;90:935–943.

300. Landowski TH, Shain KH, Oshiro MM, et al. Myeloma cells selected for resistance to CD95-mediated apoptosis are not cross-resistant to cytotoxic drugs: evidence for independent mechanisms of caspase activation. Blood 1999;94:265–274.

301. McGahon AJ, Costa PA, Daly L, et al. Chemotherapeutic drug-induced apoptosis in human leukaemic cells is independent of the Fas (APO-1/CD95) receptor/ligand system. Br J Haematol 1998;101:539–547.

302. Wesselborg S, Engels IH, Rossmann E, et al. Anticancer drugs induce caspase-8/FLICE activation and apoptosis in the absence of CD95 receptor/ligand interaction. Blood 1999;93:3053–3063.

303. Come MG, Bettaieb A, Skladanowski A, et al. Alteration of the daunorubicin-triggered sphingomyelin-ceramide pathway and apoptosis in MDR cells: influence of drug transport abnormalities. Int J Cancer 1999;81:580–587.

304. Herr I, Wilhelm D, Bohler T, et al. Activation of CD95 (APO-1/Fas) signaling by ceramide mediates cancer therapy-induced apoptosis. EMBO J 1997;16:6200–6208.

305. Laurent G, Jaffrezou JP. Signaling pathways activated by daunorubicin. Blood 2001;98:913–924.

306. Garland JM, Rudin C. Cytochrome c induces caspase-dependent apoptosis in intact hematopoietic cells and overrides apoptosis suppression mediated by bcl-2, growth factor signaling, MAP-kinase-kinase, and malignant change. Blood 1999;92:1235–1246.

307. Kroemer G, Zamzami N, Susin SA. Mitochondrial control of apoptosis. Immunol Today 1997;18:44–51.

308. Green PS, Leeuwenburgh C. Mitochondrial dysfunction is an early indicator of doxorubicin-induced apoptosis. Biochim Biophys Acta 2002;1588:94–101.

309. Clementi ME, Giardina B, Di Stasio E, et al. Doxorubicin-derived metabolites induce release of cytochrome C and inhibition of respiration on cardiac isolated mitochondria. Anticancer Res 2003;23:2445–2450.

310. Munoz-Gamez JA, Martin-Oliva D, guilar-Quesada R, et al. PARP inhibition sensitizes p53-deficient breast cancer cells to doxorubicin-induced apoptosis. Biochem J 2005;386:119–125.

311. Doroshow JH, Matsumoto L, van Balgooy J. Modulation of doxorubicin-induced, oxygen radical mediated apoptosis by glutathione peroxidase and free radical scavengers in human breast cancer cells [abstract]. Proc Amer Assoc Cancer Res 1999;40:16.

312. Cho SJ, Park JW, Kang JS, et al. Nuclear factor-kappaB dependency of doxorubicin sensitivity in gastric cancer cells is determined by manganese superoxide dismutase expression. Cancer Sci 2008;99:1117–1124.

313. Singh I, Pahan K, Khan M, et al. Cytokine-mediated induction of ceramide production is redox- sensitive. Implications to proinflammatory

314. cytokine-mediated apoptosis in demyelinating diseases. J Biol Chem 1998;273:20354–20362.

314. Gouaze V, Mirault ME, Carpentier S, et al. Glutathione peroxidase-1 over-expression prevents ceramide production and partially inhibits apoptosis in doxorubicin-treated human breast carcinoma cells. Mol Pharmacol 2001;60:488–496.

315. Ohmori T, Podack ER, Nishio K, et al. Apoptosis of lung cancer cells caused by some anti-cancer agents (MMC, CPT-11, ADM) is inhibited by BCL-2. Biochem Biophys Res Commun 1993;192:30–36.

316. Reed JC. Bcl-2 and the regulation of programmed cell death. J Cell Biol 1994;124:1–6.

317. Campos L, Sabido O, Rouault J-P, et al. Effects of BCL-2 antisense oligodeoxynucleotides on in vitro proliferation and survival of normal marrow progenitors and leukemic cells. Blood 1994;84:595–600.

318. Froesch BA, Aime-Sempe C, Leber B, et al. Inhibition of p53 transcriptional activity by Bcl-2 requires its membrane-anchoring domain. J Biol Chem 1999;274:6469–6475.

319. Hockenbery DM, Oltvai ZN, Yin X-M, et al. Bcl-2 functions in an antioxidant pathway to prevent apoptosis. Cell 1993;75:241–251.

320. Decaudin D, Geley S, Hirsch T, et al. Bcl-2 and Bcl-XL antagonize the mitochondrial dysfunction preceding nuclear apoptosis induced by chemotherapeutic agents. Cancer Res 1997;57:62–67.

321. Boland MP, Foster SJ, O'Neill LA. Daunorubicin activates NFkappaB and induces kappaB-dependent gene expression in HL-60 promyelocytic and Jurkat T lymphoma cells. J Biol Chem 1997;272:12952–12960.

322. Wang CY, Mayo MW, Baldwin AS Jr. TNF- and cancer therapy-induced apoptosis: potentiation by inhibition of NF-kappaB. Science 1996;274:784–787.

323. Jeremias I, Kupatt C, Baumann B, et al. Inhibition of nuclear factor kappaB activation attenuates apoptosis resistance in lymphoid cells. Blood 1998;91:4624–4631.

324. Gangadharan C, Thoh M, Manna SK. Late phase activation of nuclear transcription factor kappaB by doxorubicin is mediated by interleukin-8 and induction of apoptosis via FasL. Breast Cancer Res Treat 2010;120:671–683.

325. Ma S, Tang J, Feng J, et al. Induction of p21 by p65 in p53 null cells treated with Doxorubicin. Biochim Biophys Acta 2008;1783:935–940.

326. Lin X, Li Q, Wang YJ, et al. Morphine inhibits doxorubicin-induced reactive oxygen species generation and nuclear factor kappaB transcriptional activation in neuroblastoma SH-SY5Y cells. Biochem J 2007;406:215–221.

327. Doublier S, Riganti C, Voena C, et al. RhoA silencing reverts the resistance to doxorubicin in human colon cancer cells. Mol Cancer Res 2008;6:1607–1620.

328. Gangadharan C, Thoh M, Manna SK. Inhibition of constitutive activity of nuclear transcription factor kappaB sensitizes doxorubicin-resistant cells to apoptosis. J Cell Biochem 2009;107:203–213.

329. Bednarski BK, Ding X, Coombe K, et al. Active roles for inhibitory kappaB kinases alpha and beta in nuclear factor-kappaB-mediated chemoresistance to doxorubicin. Mol Cancer Ther 2008;7:1827–1835.

330. Tapia MA, Gonzalez-Navarrete I, Dalmases A, et al. Inhibition of the canonical IKK/NF kappa B pathway sensitizes human cancer cells to doxorubicin. Cell Cycle 2007;6:2284–2292.

331. Ichihara S, Yamada Y, Kawai Y, et al. Roles of oxidative stress and Akt signaling in doxorubicin cardiotoxicity. Biochem Biophys Res Commun 2007;359:27–33.

332. Haldar S, Negrini M, Monne M, et al. Down-regulation of bcl-2 by p53 in breast cancer cells. Cancer Res 1994;54:2095–2097.

333. Bacus SS, Yarden Y, Oren M, et al. Neu differentiation factor (Heregulin) activates a p53-dependent pathway in cancer cells. Oncogene 1996;12:2535–2547.

334. Gartenhaus RB, Wang P, Hoffmann P. Induction of the WAF1/CIP1 protein and apoptosis in human T-cell leukemia virus type I-transformed lymphocytes after treatment with adriamycin by using a p53-independent pathway. Proc Natl Acad Sci USA 1996;93:265–268.

335. Michieli P, Chedid M, Lin D, et al. Induction of WAF1/CIP1 by a p53-independent pathway. Cancer Res 1994;54:3391–3395.

336. Wang Y, Blandino G, Givol D. Induced p21waf expression in H1299 cell line promotes cell senescence and protects against cytotoxic effect of radiation and doxorubicin. Oncogene 1999;18:2643–2649.

337. Shimizu A, Nishida J, Ueoka Y, et al. Cyclin G contributes to G2/M arresst of cells in response to DNA damage. Biochem Biophys Res Commun 1998;242:529–533.

338. Lowe SW, Ruley HE, Jacks T, et al. p53-dependent apoptosis modulates the cytotoxicity of anticancer agents. Cell 1993;74:957–967.

339. Lowe SW, Bodis S, McClatchey A, et al. p53 status and the efficacy of cancer therapy in vivo. Science 1994;266:807–810.

340. Aas T, Borresen AL, Geisler S, et al. Specific P53 mutations are associated with de novo resistance to doxorubicin in breast cancer patients. Nat Med 1996;2:811–814.

341. Chang BD, Broude EV, Dokmanovic M, et al. A senescence-like phenotype distinguishes tumor cells that undergo terminal proliferation arrest after exposure to anticancer agents. Cancer Res 1999;59:3761–3767.

342. Chang BD, Broude EV, Fang J, et al. p21Waf1/Cip1/Sdi1-induced growth arrest is associated with depletion of mitosis-control proteins and leads to abnormal mitosis and endoreduplication in recovering cells. Oncogene 2000;19:2165–2170.

343. Chang BD, Watanabe K, Broude EV, et al. Effects of p21Waf1/Cip1/Sdi1 on cellular gene expression: implications for carcinogenesis, senescence, and age-related diseases. Proc Natl Acad Sci USA 2000;97:4291–4296.

344. Chang BD, Xuan Y, Broude EV, et al. Role of p53 and p21waf1/cip1 in senescence-like terminal proliferation arrest induced in human tumor cells by chemotherapeutic drugs. Oncogene 1999;18:4808–4818.

345. Chang BD, Swift ME, Shen M, et al. Molecular determinants of terminal growth arrest induced in tumor cells by a chemotherapeutic agent. Proc Natl Acad Sci USA 2002;99:389–394.

346. Berns A. Senescence: a companion in chemotherapy? Cancer Cell 2002;1:309–311.

347. Wolf MB, Baynes JW. The anti-cancer drug, doxorubicin, causes oxidant stress-induced endothelial dysfunction. Biochim Biophys Acta 2006;1760:267–271.

348. Hirsch HA, Iliopoulos D, Tsichlis PN, et al. Metformin selectively targets cancer stem cells, and acts together with chemotherapy to block tumor growth and prolong remission. Cancer Res 2009;69:7507–7511.

349. Gros P, Croop J, Housman D. Mammalian multidrug resistance gene: complete cDNA sequence indicates strong homology to bacterial transport proteins. Cell 1986;47:371–380.

350. Endicott JA, Ling V. The biochemistry of P-glycoprotein-mediated multidrug resistance. Ann Rev Biochem 1989;58:137–171.

351. Sugimoto Y, Tsuruo T. DNA-mediated transfer and cloning of a human multidrug-resistant gene of adriamycin-resistant myelogenous leukemia K562. Cancer Res 1987;47:2620–2625.

352. Hamada H, Hagiwara T, Nakajma T, et al. Phosphorylation of Mr 170,000 to 180,000 glycoprotein species specific to multidrug-resistant tumor cells: effects of verapamil, trifluoroperazine and phorbol esters. Cancer Res 1987;47:2860–2865.

353. Coley HM, Twentyman PR, Workman P. The efflux of anthracyclines in multidrug-resistant cell lines. Biochem Pharmacol 1993;46:1317–1326.

354. Kang Y, Perry RR. Modulatory effects of tamoxifen and recombinant human α-interferon on doxorubicin resistance. Cancer Res 1993;53:3040–3045.

355. Merlin J-L, Guerci A, Marchal S, et al. Comparative evaluation of S9788, verapamil, and cyclosporine A in K562 human leukemia cell lines and in P-glycoprotein-expressing samples from patients with hematologic malignancies. Blood 1994;84:262–269.

356. Alvarez M, Pauli K, Monks A, et al. Generation of a drug resistance profile by quantitation of mdr-1/P-glycoprotein in the cell lines of the national cancer institute anticancer drug screen. J Clin Invest 1995;95:2205–2214.

357. Lemontt JF, Azzaria M, Gross P. Increased mdr gene expression and decreased drug accumulation in multidrug-resistant human melanoma cells. Cancer Res 1988;48:6348–6353.

358. Noonan KE, Beck C, Holzmayer TA, et al. Quantitative analysis of MDR1 (multidrug resistance) gene expression in human tumors by polymerase chain reaction. Proc Natl Acad Sci USA 1990;87:7160–7164.

359. Chen G, Jaffrezou J-P, Fleming WH, et al. Prevalence of multidrug resistance related to activation of the mdr1 gene in human sarcoma mutants derived by single-step doxorubicin selection. Cancer Res 1994;54:4980–4987.

360. Morton KA, Jones BJ, Sohn MH, et al. Enrichment for metallothionein does not confer resistance to cisplatin in transfected NIH/3T3 cells. J Pharmacol Exp Ther 1993;267:697–702.

361. Chaudhary PM, Roninson IB. Induction of multidrug resistance in human cells by transient exposure to different chemotherapeutic drugs. J Natl Cancer Inst 1993;85:632–639.

362. Hui RC, Francis RE, Guest SK, et al. Doxorubicin activates FOXO3a to induce the expression of multidrug resistance gene ABCB1 (MDR) in K562 leukemic cells. Mol Cancer Ther 2008;7:670–678.

363. Fojo AT, Ueda K, Siamon DJ, et al. Expression of a multidrug resistance gene in human tumors and tissues. Proc Natl Acad Sci USA 1987;84:265–269.

364. Sparreboom A, van Asperen J, Mayer U, et al. Limited oral bioavailability and active epithelial excretion of paclitaxel (Taxol) caused by P-glycoprotein in the intestine. Proc Natl Acad Sci USA 1997;94:2031–2035.

365. Egashira M, Kawamata N, Sugimoto K, et al. P-glycoprotein expression on normal and abnormally expanded natural killer cells and inhibition of P-glycoprotein function by cyclosporin A and its analogue PSC833. Blood 1999;93:599–606.

366. Fairchild CR, Ivy SP, Rushmore T, et al. Carcinogen-induced mdr overexpression is associated with xenobiotic resistance in rat preneoplastic liver nodules and hepatocellular carcinomas. Proc Natl Acad Sci USA 1987;84:7701–7705.

367. Myers CE, Cowan K, Sinha BK, et al. The phenomenon of pleiotropic drug resistance. In: De Vita VT, Jr., Hellman S, Rosenberg SA, eds. Important Advances in Oncology. Philadelphia: JB Lippincott Co., 1987:27–38.

368. Yeh GC, Lopaczynska J, Poore CM, et al. A new functional role for P-glycoprotein: efflux pump for benzo(a)pyrene in human breast cancer MCF-7 cells. Cancer Res 1992;52:6692–6695.

369. Marie J-P, Zittoun R, Sikic BI. Multidrug resistance (mdr1) gene expression in adult acute leukemias: correlations with treatment outcome and invitro drug sensitivity. Blood 1991;78:586–592.

370. Goasguen JE, Dossot J-M, Fardel O, et al. Expression of the multidrug resistance-associated P-glycoprotein (P-170) in 59 cases of de novo acute lymphoblastic leukemia: prognostic implications. Blood 1993;81:2394–2398.

371. Chabner BA, Fojo A. Multidrug resistance: P-glycoprotein and its allies - the elusive foes. J Natl Cancer Inst 1989;81:910–913.

372. Grogan TM, Spier CM, Salmon SE, et al. P-glycoprotein expression in human plasma cell myeloma: correlation with prior chemotherapy. Blood 1993;81:490–495.

373. Keith WN, Stallard S, Brown R. Expression of mdr1 and gst-π in human breast tumors: comparison to in vitro chemosensitivity. Br J Cancer 1990;61:712–716.

374. Verrelle P, Meissonnier F, Fonck Y, et al. Clinical relevance of immunohistochemical detection of multidrug resistance P-glycoprotein in breast carcinoma [see comments]. J Natl Cancer Inst 1991;83:111–116.

375. Miller TP, Grogan TM, Dalton WS, et al. P-glycoprotein expression in malignant lymphoma and reversal of clinical drug resistance with chemotherapy plus high-dose verapamil. J Clin Oncol 1991;9:17–24.

376. Wishart GC, Bissett D, Paul J, et al. Quinidine as a resistance modulator of epirubicin in advanced breast cancer: mature results of a placebo-controlled randomized trial. J Clin Oncol 1994;12:1771–1777.

377. Lum BL, Fisher GA, Brophy NA, et al. Clinical trials of modulation of multidrug resistance: pharmacokinetic and Pharmacodynamic Considerations. Cancer 1993;72:3502–3514.

378. Bartlett NL, Lum BL, Fisher GA, et al. Phase I trial of doxorubicin with cyclosporine as a modulator of multidrug resistance. J Clin Oncol 1994;12:835–842.

379. List AF, Kopecky KJ, Willman CL, et al. Benefit of cyclosporine (CsA) modulation of anthracycline resistance in high-risk AML: a southwest oncology group (SWOG) study [abstract]. Blood 1998;92(Suppl. 1):312a.

380. Slovak ML, Hoeltge GA, Dalton WS, et al. Pharmacological and biological evidence for differing mechanisms of doxorubicin resistance in two human tumor cell lines. Cancer Res 1988;48:2793–2797.

381. Mirski SE, Gerlach JH, Cole SP. Multidrug resistance in a human small cell line selected in adriamycin. Cancer Res 1987;47:2594–2598.

382. Krishnamachary N, Center MS. The MRP gene associated with a non-P-glycoprotein multidrug resistance encodes a 190-kDa membrane bound glycoprotein. Cancer Res 1993;53:3658–3661.

383. Eijdems EW, Zaman GJ, de Haas M, et al. Altered MRP is associated with multidrug resistance and reduced drug accumulation in human SW-1573 cells. Br J Cancer 1995;72:298–306.

384. Welters MJ, Fichtinger-Schepman AM, Baan RA, et al. Role of glutathione, glutathione S-transferases and multidrug resistance-related proteins in cisplatin sensitivity of head and neck cancer cell lines. Br J Cancer 1998;77:556–561.

385. Moran E, Cleary I, Larkin AM, et al. Co-expression of MDR-associated markers, including P-170, MRP and LRP and cytoskeletal proteins, in three resistant variants of the human ovarian carcinoma cell line, OAW42. Eur J Cancer 1997;33:652–660.

386. Slapak CA, Mizunuma N, Kufe DW. Expression of the multidrug resistance associated protein and p-glycoprotein in doxorubicin-selected human myeloid leukemia cells. Blood 1994;84:3113–3121.

387. Schneider E, Cowan KH, Bader H, et al. Increased expression of the multidrug resistance-associated protein gene in relapsed acute leukemia. Blood 1995;85:186–193.

388. Legrand O, Simonin G, Beauchamp-Nicoud A, et al. Simultaneous activity of MRP1 and Pgp is correlated with in vitro resistance to daunorubicin and with in vivo resistance in adult acute myeloid leukemia. Blood 1999;94:1046–1056.

389. Rappa G, Finch RA, Sartorelli AC, et al. New insights into the biology and pharmacology of the multidrug resistance protein (MRP. from gene knockout models. Biochem Pharmacol 1999;58:557–562.

390. Lorico A, Rappa G, Flavell RA, et al. Double knockout of the MRP gene leads to increased drug sensitivity in vitro. Cancer Res 1996;56:5351–5355.

391. Kool M, de Haas M, Scheffer GL, et al. Analysis of expression of cMoat, MRP2, MRP3, MRP4, and MRP5, homologues of the multidrug resistance-associated protein (MRP1), in human cancer cell lines. Cancer Res 1997;57:3537–3547.

392. Doyle LA, Ross DD. Multidrug resistance mediated by the breast cancer resistance protein BCRP (ABCG2). Oncogene 2003;22:7340–7358.

393. Doyle LA, Yang W, Abruzzo LV, et al. A multidrug resistance transporter from human MCF-7 breast cancer cells. Proc Natl Acad Sci USA 1998;95:15665–15670.

394. Calcagno AM, Fostel JM, To KK, et al. Single-step doxorubicin-selected cancer cells overexpress the ABCG2 drug transporter through epigenetic changes. Br J Cancer 2008;98:1515–1524.

395. Allen JD, Jackson SC, Schinkel AH. A mutation hot spot in the Bcrp1 (Abcg2) multidrug transporter in mouse cell lines selected for Doxorubicin resistance. Cancer Res 2002;62:2294–2299.

396. Plasschaert SL, Van Der Kolk DM, De Bont ES, et al. The role of breast cancer resistance protein in acute lymphoblastic leukemia. Clin Cancer Res 2003;9:5171–5177.

397. Sargent JM, Williamson CJ, Maliepaard M, et al. Breast cancer resistance protein expression and resistance to daunorubicin in blast cells from patients with acute myeloid leukaemia. Br J Haematol 2001;115:257–262.

398. Singhal SS, Yadav S, Singhal J, et al. Depletion of RLIP76 sensitizes lung cancer cells to doxorubicin. Biochem Pharmacol 2005;70:481–488.

399. Deffie AM, Batra JK, Goldenberg GG. Direct correlation between DNA topoisomerase II activity and cytotoxicity in adriamycin-sensitive and -resistant P388 leukemia cell lines. Cancer Res 1989;49:58–62.

400. Ramachandran C, Samy TS, Huang XL, et al. Doxorubicin-induced DNA breaks, topoisomerase II activity and gene expression in human melanoma cells. Biochem Pharmacol 1993;45:1367–1371.

401. Son YS, Suh JM, Ahn SH, et al. Reduced activity of topoisomerase II in an Adriamycin-resistant human stomach-adenocarcinoma cell line. Cancer Chemother Pharmacol 1998;41:353–360.

402. Wyler B, Shao Y, Schneider E, et al. Intermittent exposure to doxorubicin in vitro selects for multifactorial non-P-glycoprotein-associated multidrug resistance in RPMI 8226 human myeloma cells. Br J Haematol 1997;97:65–75.

403. Beketic-Oreskovic L, Duran GE, Chen G, et al. Decreased mutation rate for cellular resistance to doxorubicin and suppression of mdr1 gene activation by the cyclosporin PSC 833 [see comments]. J Natl Cancer Inst 1995;87:1593–1602.

404. Ganapathi R, Grabowski D, Ford J, et al. Progressive resistance to doxorubicin in mouse leukemia L1210 cells with multidrug resistance

phenotype: reductions in drug-induced topoisomerase II-mediated DNA cleavage. Cancer Commun 1989;1:217–224.

405. Friche E, Danks MK, Schmidt CA, et al. Decreased DNA topoisomerase II in daunorubicin-resistant Ehrlich ascites tumor cells. Cancer Res 1991;51:4213–4218.

406. Wang H, Jiang Z, Wong YW, et al. Decreased CP-1 (NF-Y) activity results in transcriptional down- regulation of topoisomerase IIalpha in a doxorubicin-resistant variant of human multiple myeloma RPMI 8226. Biochem Biophys Res Commun 1997;237:217–224.

407. McPherson JP, Deffie AM, Jones NR, et al. Selective sensitization of adriamycin-resistant P388 murine leukemia cells to antineoplastic agents following transfection with human DNA topoisomerase II alpha. Anticancer Res 1997;17:4243–4252.

408. Kaufman SH, Karp JE, Jones RJ, et al. Topoisomerase II levels and drug sensitivity in adult acute myelogenous leukemia. Blood 1994;83:517–530.

409. Lee FY, Vessey AR, Siemann DW. Glutathione as a determinant of cellular response to doxorubicin. Nci Monogr 1988;6:211–215.

410. Capranico G, Babudri N, Casciarri G, et al. Lack of effect of glutathione depletion on cytotoxicity, mutagenicity and DNA damage produced by doxorubicin in cultured cells. Chem Biol Interact 1986;57:189–201.

411. Yamamoto M, Maehara Y, Oda S, et al. The p53 tumor suppressor gene in anticancer agent-induced apoptosis and chemosensitivity of human gastrointestinal cancer cell lines. Cancer Chemother Pharmacol 1999;43:43–49.

412. Meng RD, Phillips P, el-Deiry WS. p53-independent increase in E2F-1 expression enhances the cytotoxic effects of etoposide and of adriamycin. Int J Oncol 1999;14:5–14.

413. Kuhl JS, Krajewski S, Duran GE, et al. Spontaneous overexpression of the long form of the Bcl-X protein in a highly resistant P388 leukaemia. Br J Cancer 1997;75:268–274.

414. Reed JC. Bcl-2 and the regulation of programmed cell death. J Cell Biol 1994;124:1–6.

415. Liu YY, Yu JY, Yin D, et al. A role for ceramide in driving cancer cell resistance to doxorubicin. Faseb J 2008;22:2541–2551.

416. Nielsen D, Maare C, Skovsgaard T. Cellular resistance to anthracyclines. Gen Pharmacol 1996;27:251–255.

417. Brown R, Hirst GL, Gallagher WM, et al. hMLH1 expression and cellular responses of ovarian tumour cells to treatment with cytotoxic anticancer agents. Oncogene 1997;15:45–52.

418. Durant ST, Morris MM, Illand M, et al. Dependence on RAD52 and RAD1 for anticancer drug resistance mediated by inactivation of mismatch repair genes. Curr Biol 1999;9:51–54.

419. Belloni M, Uberti D, Rizzini C, et al. Induction of two DNA mismatch repair proteins, MSH2 and MSH6, in differentiated human neuroblastoma SH-SY5Y cells exposed to doxorubicin. J Neurochem 1999;72:974–979.

420. Fink D, Aebi S, Howell SB. The role of DNA mismatch repair in drug resistance. Clin Cancer Res 1998;4:1–6.

421. Chatterjee S, Cheng MF, Berger NA. Hypersensitivity to clinically useful alkylating agents and radiation in poly(ADP-ribose. polymerase-deficient cell lines. Cancer Commun 1990;2:401–407.

422. Darby MK, Schmitt B, Jongstra-Bilen J, et al. Inhibition of calf thymus type II DNA topoisomerase by poly(ADP-ribosylation). EMBO J 1985;4:2129–2134.

423. Berger NA. Poly(ADP-ribose) in the cellular response to DNA damage. Radiat Res 1985;101:4–15.

424. Yamamoto K, Tsukidate K, Farber JL. Differing effects of the inhibition of poly(adp-ribose) polymerase on the course of oxidative cell injury in hepatocytes and fibroblasts. Biochem Pharmacol 1993;46:483–491.

425. Tanizawa A, Kubota M, Takimoto T, et al. Prevention of adriamycin-induced interphase death by 3- aminobenzamide and nicotinamide in a human promyelocytic leukemia cell line. Biochem Biophys Res Commun 1987;144:1031–1036.

426. Doroshow JH, Van Balgooy C, Akman SA. Effect of poly(ADP-ribose) polymerase inhibition on protein-associated DNA single-strand cleavage and cytotoxicity by anthracycline antibiotics. Proc Am Assoc Cancer Res 1995;36:444.

427. Chen JJ, Silver D, Cantor S, et al. BRCA1, BRCA2, and Rad51 operate in a common DNA damage response pathway. Cancer Res 1999;59:1752s–1756s.

428. MacLachlan TK, Dash BC, Dicker DT, et al. Repression of BRCA1 through a feedback loop involving p53. J Biol Chem 2000;275:31869–31875.

429. Su J, Ciftci K. Changes in BRCA1 and BRCA2 expression produced by chemotherapeutic agents in human breast cancer cells. Int J Biochem Cell Biol 2002;34:950–957.

430. Fedier A, Steiner RA, Schwarz VA, et al. The effect of loss of Brca1 on the sensitivity to anticancer agents in p53-deficient cells. Int J Oncol 2003;22:1169–1173.

431. Tassone P, Tagliaferri P, Perricelli A, et al. BRCA1 expression modulates chemosensitivity of BRCA1-defective HCC1937 human breast cancer cells. Br J Cancer 2003;88:1285–1291.

432. Egawa C, Motomura K, Miyoshi Y, et al. Increased expression of BRCA1 mRNA predicts favorable response to anthracycline-containing chemotherapy in breast cancers. Breast Cancer Res Treat 2003;78:45–50.

433. Reich SD, Bachur NR. Alterations in adriamycin efficacy by phenobarbital. Cancer Res 1976;36:3803–3806.

434. Innis JD, Meyer M, Hurwitz A. A novel acute toxicity resulting from the administration of morphine and adriamycin to mice. Toxicol Appl Pharmacol 1987;90:445–453.

435. Myrehaug S, Pintilie M, Tsang R, et al. Cardiac morbidity following modern treatment for Hodgkin lymphoma: supra-additive cardiotoxicity of doxorubicin and radiation therapy. Leuk Lymphoma 2008;49:1486–1493.

436. Holmes FA, Madden T, Newman RA, et al. Sequence-dependent alteration of doxorubicin pharmacokinetics by paclitaxel in a phase I study of paclitaxel and doxorubicin in patients with metastatic breast cancer. J Clin Oncol 1996;14:2713–2721.

437. Sparreboom A, van Tellingen O, Nooijen WJ, et al. Nonlinear pharmacokinetics of paclitaxel in mice results from the pharmaceutical vehicle Cremophor EL. Cancer Res 1996;56:2112–2115.

438. Legha SS, Benjamin RS, Mackay B, et al. Reduction of doxorubicin cardiotoxicity by prolonged continuous intravenous infusion. Ann Intern Med 1982;96:133–139.

439. Terasaki T, Iga T, Sugiyama Y, et al. Experimental evidence of characteristic tissue distribution of adriamycin: tissue DNA concentration as a determinant. Pharmacol Rev 1989;53:496–501.

440. Greene R, Collins J, Jenkins J, et al. Plasma pharmacokinetics of adriamycin and adriamycinol: implications for the design of in vitro experiments and treatment protocols. Cancer Res 1983;43:3417–3422.

441. Speth PAJ, Linssen PCM, Holdrinet RSG, et al. Plasma and cellular adriamycin concentrations in patients with myeloma treated with 96-hour continuous infusion. Clin Pharmacol Ther 1987;41:661–665.

442. Synold T, Doroshow JH. Anthracycline dose intensity: clinical pharmacology and pharmacokinetics of high-dose doxorubicin administered as a 96-hour continuous intravenous infusion. J Infus Chemother 1996;6:69–73.

443. Bronchud MH, Margison JM, Howell A, et al. Comparative pharmacokinetics of escalating doses of doxorubicin in patients with metastatic breast cancer. Cancer Chemother Pharmacol 1990;25:435–439.

444. Dobbs NA, Twelves CJ, Gillies H, et al. Gender affects doxorubicin pharmacokinetics in patients with normal liver biochemistry. Cancer Chemother Pharmacol. 1995;36:473–476.

445. Dobbs NA, Twelves CJ. What is the effect of adjusting epirubicin doses for body surface area? Br J Cancer. 1998;78:662–666.

446. Thompson PA, Rosner GL, Matthay KK, et al. Impact of body composition on pharmacokinetics of doxorubicin in children: a Glaser Pediatric Research Network study. Cancer Chemother Pharmacol 2009;64:243–251.

447. Huffman DH, Bachur NR. Daunorubicin metabolism in acute myelocytic leukemia. Blood 1972;39:637–643.

448. Gill P, Favre R, Durand A, et al. Time dependency of adriamycin and adriamycinol kinetics. Cancer Chemother Pharmacol 1983;10:120–124.

449. Lovless H, Arena E, Felsted RL, et al. Comparative mammalian metabolism of adriamycin and daunorubicin. Cancer Res 1978;38:593–598.

450. Felsted RL, Gee M, Bachur NR. Rat liver daunorubicin reductase. An aldo-keto reductase. J Biol Chem 1974;249:3672–3679.

451. Felsted RL, Richter DR, Bachur NR. Rat liver aldehyde reductase. Biochem Pharmacol 1977;26:1117–1124.

452. Felsted RL, Bachur NR. Mammalian carbonyl reductases. Drug Metab Rev 1980;11:1–60.

453. Forrest GL, Akman S, Doroshow J, et al. Genomic sequence and expression of a cloned human carbonyl reductase gene with daunorubicin reductase activity. Mol Pharmacol 1991;40:502–507.

454. Ozols RF, Willson JKV, Weltz MD, et al. Inhibition of human ovarian cancer colony formation by adriamycin and its major metabolites. Cancer Res 1980;40:4109–4112.

455. Gessner T, Preisler HD, Azarnia N, et al. Plasma levels of daunomycin metabolites and the outcome of ANLL therapy. Med Oncol Tumor Pharmacother 1987;4:23–31.

456. Lal S, Sandanaraj E, Wong ZW, et al. CBR1 and CBR3 pharmacogenetics and their influence on doxorubicin disposition in Asian breast cancer patients. Cancer Sci 2008;99:2045–2054.

457. Kassner N, Huse K, Martin HJ, et al. Carbonyl reductase 1 is a predominant doxorubicin reductase in the human liver. Drug Metab Dispos 2008;36:2113–2120.

458. Benjamin RS. A practical approach to adriamycin (NSC-123127) toxicology. Cancer Chemother Rep 1975;6:191–194.

459. Brenner DE, Wiernik PH, Wesley M, et al. Acute doxorubicin toxicity: relationship to pretreatment liver function, response and pharmacokinetics in patients with acute nonlymphocytic leukemia. Cancer 1984;53:1042–1048.

460. Chan KK, Chlebowski RT, Myron Tong H-S, et al. Clinical pharmacokinetics of adriamycin in hepatoma patients with cirrhosis. Cancer Res 1980;40:1263–1268.

461. Ackland SP, Ratain MJ, Vogelzang NJ, et al. Pharmacokinetics and pharmacodynamics of long-term continuous -infusion doxorubicin. Clin Pharmacol Ther 1989;45:340–347.

462. Twelves CJ, Dobbs NA, Gillies HC, et al. Doxorubicin pharmacokinetics: the effect of abnormal liver biochemistry tests. Cancer Chemother Pharmacol 1998;42:229–234.

463. Doroshow J and Chan K. Relationship between doxorubicin clearance and indocyanine green dye pharmacokinetics in patients with hepatic dysfunction. Proc Amer Soc Clin Oncol 1982;1:11.

464. Dekaney CM, Gulati AS, Garrison AP, et al. Regeneration of intestinal stem/progenitor cells following doxorubicin treatment of mice. Am J Physiol Gastrointest Liver Physiol 2009;297:G461–G470.

465. Kim EJ, Lim KM, Kim KY, et al. Doxorubicin-induced platelet cytotoxicity: a new contributory factor for doxorubicin-mediated thrombocytopenia. J Thromb Haemost 2009;7:1172–1183.

466. Sonneveld P, Wassenaar HA, Nooter K. Long persistence of doxorubicin in human skin after extravasation. Cancer Treat Rep 1984;68:895–896.

467. Dorr RT, Dordal MS, Koenig LM, et al. High levels of doxorubicin in the tissues of a patient experiencing extravasation during a 4-day infusion. Cancer 1989;64:2462–2464.

468. Andersson AP, Dahlstrom KK, Dahlstrm KK. Clinical results after doxorubicin extravasation treated with excision guided by fluorescence microscopy. Eur J Cancer 1993;29A:1712–1714.

469. Heitmann C, Durmus C, Ingianni G. Surgical management after doxorubicin and epirubicin extravasation. J Hand Surg [Br] 1998;23:666–668.

470. Bertelli G, Gozza A, Forno GB, et al. Topical dimethylsulfoxide for the prevention of soft tissue injury after extravasation of vesicant cytotoxic drugs: a prospective clinical study. J Clin Oncol 1995;13:2851–2855.

471. Disa JJ, Chang RR, Mucci SJ, et al. Prevention of adriamycin-induced full-thickness skin loss using hyaluronidase infiltration. Plast Reconstr Surg 1998;101:370–374.

472. El Saghir N, Otrock Z, Mufarrij A, et al. Dexrazoxane for anthracycline extravasation and GM-CSF for skin ulceration and wound healing. Lancet Oncol 2004;5:320–321.

473. Doroshow JH. Doxorubicin-induced cardiac toxicity. N Engl J Med 1991;324:843–845.

474. Singal PK, Iliskovic N. Doxorubicin-induced cardiomyopathy. N Engl J Med 1998;339:900–905.

475. Axim H, Azim HA Jr, Escudier B. Trastuzumab versus lapatinib: the cardiac side of the story. Cancer Treat Rev 2009;35:633–8.

476. Perez EA, Suman VJ, Davidson NE, et al. Cardiac safety analysis of doxorubicin and cyclophosphamide followed by paclitaxel with or without trastuzumab in the North Central Cancer Treatment Group N9831 adjuvant breast cancer trial. J Clin Oncol 2008;26:1231–1238.

477. Cobleigh MA, Vogel CL, Tripathy D, et al. Efficacy and safety of Herceptin™ (humanized anti-HER2 antibody. as a single agent in 222 women with HER2 overexpression who relapsed following chemotherapy for metastatic breast cancer [abstract]. Proc Amer Soc Clin Oncol 1998;17:97a.

478. Paik S, Bryant J, Park C, et al. erbB-2 and response to doxorubicin in patients with axillary lymph node-positive, hormone receptor-negative breast cancer [see comments]. J Natl Cancer Inst 1998;90:1361–1370.

479. Lipshultz SE, Colan SD, Gelber RD, et al. Late cardiac effects of doxorubicin (Adriamycin. therapy for childhood acute lymphoblastic leukemia. N Engl J Med 1991;324:808–815.

480. Schwartz CL, Hobbie WL, Truesdell S, et al. Corrected QT interval prolongation in anthracycline-treated survivors of childhood cancer. J Clin Oncol 1993;11:1906–1910.

481. Wexler LH, Andrich MP, Venzon D, et al. Randomized trial of the cardioprotective agent ICRF-187 in pediatric sarcoma patients treated with doxorubicin. J Clin Oncol 1996;14:362–372.

482. Kremer LC, Caron HN. Anthracycline cardiotoxicity in children. N Engl J Med 2004;351:120–121.

483. Bristow MR, Thompson PD, Martin RP, et al. Early anthracycline cardiotoxicity. Am J Med 1978;65:823–832.

484. Bristow MR, Minobe WA, Billingham ME, et al. Anthracycline-associated cardiac and renal damage in rabbits. Lab Invest 1981;45:157–168.

485. Billingham ME, Mason JW, Bristow MR, et al. Anthracycline cardiomyopathy monitored by morphologic changes. Cancer Treat Rep 1978;62:865–872.

486. Bristow MR, Mason JW, Billingham ME, et al. Doxorubicin cardiomyopathy: evaluation by phonocardiography, endomyocardial biopsy, and cardiac catheterization. Ann Intern Med 1978;88:168–175.

487. Von Hoff DD, Rozencweig M, Layard M, et al. Daunomycin-induced cardiotoxicity in children and adults: a review of 110 cases. Am J Med 1977;62:200–208.

488. Von Hoff DD, Layard MW, Basa P, et al. Risk factors for doxorubicin-induced congestive heart failure. Ann Intern Med 1979;91:710–717.

489. Swain SM. Adult multicenter trials using dexrazoxane to protect against cardiac toxicity. Semin Oncol 1998;25:43–47.

490. Cottin Y, Touzery C, Dalloz F, et al. Comparison of epirubicin and doxorubicin cardiotoxicity induced by low doses: evolution of the diastolic and systolic parameters studied by radionuclide angiography. Clin Cardiol 1998;21:665–670.

491. Perez EA, Suman VJ, Davidson NE, et al. Effect of doxorubicin plus cyclophosphamide on left ventricular ejection fraction in patients with breast cancer in the North Central Cancer Treatment Group N9831 Intergroup Adjuvant Trial. J Clin Oncol 2004;22:3700–3704.

492. Swain SM, Whaley FS, Gerber MC, et al. Delayed administration of dexrazoxane provides cardioprotection for patients with advanced breast cancer treated with doxorubicin- containing therapy. J Clin Oncol 1997;15:1333–1340.

493. Swain SM, Whaley FS, Gerber MC, et al. Cardioprotection with dexrazoxane for doxorubicin-containing therapy in advanced breast cancer. J Clin Oncol 1997;15:1318–1332.

494. Moreb JS, Oblon DJ. Outcome of clinical congestive heart failure induced by anthracycline chemotherapy. Cancer 1992;70:2637–2641.

495. Haq MM, Legha SS, Choksi J, et al. Doxorubicin-induced congestive heart failure in adults. Cancer 1985;56:1361–1365.

496. Hershman DL, McBride RB, Eisenberger A, et al. Doxorubicin, cardiac risk factors, and cardiac toxicity in elderly patients with diffuse B-cell non-Hodgkin's lymphoma. J Clin Oncol 2008;26:3159–3165.

497. Buzdar AU, Marcus C, Smith TL, et al. Early and delayed clinical cardiotoxicity of doxorubicin. Cancer 1985;55:2761–2765.

498. Lipshultz SE, Lipsitz SR, Sallan SE, et al. Long-term enalapril therapy for left ventricular dysfunction in doxorubicin-treated survivors of childhood cancer. J Clin Oncol 2002;20:4517–4522.

499. Alexander J, Dainiak N, Berger HJ, et al. Serial assessment of doxorubicin cardiotoxicity with quantitative radionuclide angiocardiography. N Engl J Med 1979;300:278–283.

500. Dresdale A, Bonow RO, Wesley R, et al. Prospective evaluation of doxorubicin-induced cardiomyopathy resulting from postsurgical adjuvant treatment of patients with soft tissue sarcomas. Cancer 1983;52:51–60.

501. Swain SM, Whaley FS, Ewer MS. Congestive heart failure in patients treated with doxorubicin: a retrospective analysis of three trials. Cancer 2003;97:2869–2879.

502. Billingham ME, Bristow MR, Glatstein E, et al. Adriamycin cardiotoxicity endomyocardial biopsy evidence of enhancement by irradiation. Am J Surg Pathol 1977;1:17–23.

503. Torti FM, Bristow MR, Howes AE, et al. Reduced cardiotoxicity of doxorubicin delivered on a weekly schedule: assessment by endomyocardial biopsy. Ann Intern Med 1983;99:745–749.

504. Goorin AM, Chauvenet AR, Perez-Atayde AR, et al. Initial congestive heart failure, six to ten years after doxorubicin chemotherapy for childhood cancer. J Pediatr 1990;116:144–147.

505. Lipshultz SE, Rifai N, Dalton VM, et al. The effect of dexrazoxane on myocardial injury in doxorubicin-treated children with acute lymphoblastic leukemia. N Engl J Med 2004;351:145–153.

506. Lipshultz SE, Giantris AL, Lipsitz SR, et al. Doxorubicin administration by continuous infusion is not cardioprotective: the Dana-Farber 91–01 Acute Lymphoblastic Leukemia protocol. J Clin Oncol 2002;20:1677–1682.

507. Ducroq J, Moha Ou MH, Guilbot S, et al. Dexrazoxane protects the heart from acute doxorubicin-induced QT prolongation: a key role for I(Ks). Br J Pharmacol 2009;159:93–101.

508. Lopez M, Vici P, Di Lauro K, et al. Randomized prospective clinical trial of high-dose epirubicin and dexrazoxane in patients with advanced breast cancer and soft tissue sarcomas. J Clin Oncol 1998;16:86–92.

509. Venturini M, Michelotti A, Del Mastro L, et al. Multicenter randomized controlled clinical trial to evaluate cardioprotection of dexrazoxane versus no cardioprotection in women receiving epirubicin chemotherapy for advanced breast cancer. J Clin Oncol 1996;14:3112–3120.

510. Singal PK, Pierce GN. Adriamycin stimulates low-affinity Ca^{2+} binding and lipid peroxidation but depresses myocardial function. Am J Physiol 1986;250:H419-H425.

511. Singal PK, Deally CMR, Weinberg LE. Subcellular effects of adriamycin in the heart: a concise review. J Mol Cell Cardiol 1987;19:817–828.

512. Singal PK, Forbes MS, Sperelakis N. Occurrence of intramitochondrial Ca^{2+} granules in a hypertrophied heart exposed to adriamycin. Can J Physiol Pharmacol 1984;62:1239–1244.

513. Villani F, Piccinini F, Merelli P, et al. Influence of adriamycin on calcium exchangeability in cardiac muscle and its modification by ouabain. Biochem Pharmacol 1978;27:985–987.

514. Milei J, Boveris A, Llesuy S, et al. Amelioration of adriamycin-induced cardiotoxicity in rabbits by prenylamine and vitamins A and E. Am Heart J 1986;111:95–102.

515. Emanuelov AK, Shainberg A, Chepurko Y, et al. Adenosine A(3) receptor-mediated cardioprotection against doxorubicin-induced mitochondrial damage. Biochem Pharmacol 2010;79:180–187.

516. Keung EC, Toll L, Ellis M, et al. L-type cardiac calcium channels in doxorubicin cardiomyopathy in rats: morphological, biochemical, and functional correlations. J Clin Invest 1991;87:2108–2113.

517. Doroshow JH. Effect of anthracycline antibiotics on oxygen radical formation in rat heart. Cancer Res 1983;43:460–472.

518. Davies KJ, Doroshow JH, Hochstein P. Mitochondrial NADH dehydrogenase-catalyzed oxygen radical production by adriamycin, and the relative inactivity of 5-iminodaunorubicin. Febs Lett 1983;153:227–230.

519. Jensen RA, Acton EM, Peters JH. Electrocardiographic and transmembrane potential effects of 5-iminodaunorubicin in the rat. Cancer Res 1984;44:4030–4039.

520. Feng W, Liu G, Xia R, et al. Site-selective modification of hyperreactive cysteines of ryanodine receptor complex by quinones. Mol Pharmacol 1999;55:821–831.

521. Kim SY, Kim SJ, Kim BJ, et al. Doxorubicin-induced reactive oxygen species generation and intracellular Ca2+ increase are reciprocally modulated in rat cardiomyocytes. Exp Mol Med 2006;38:535–545.

522. Abramson JJ, Salama G. Critical sulfhydryls regulate calcium release from sarcoplasmic reticulum. J Bioenerg Biomembr 1989;21:283–294.

523. Pessah IN, Durie EL, Schiedt MJ, et al. Anthraquinone-sensitized Ca2+ release channel from rat cardiac sarcoplasmic reticulum: possible receptor-mediated mechanism of doxorubicin cardiomyopathy. Mol Pharmacol 1990;37:503–514.

524. Papoian T, Lewis W. Adriamycin cardiotoxicity in vivo: selective alterations in rat cardiac mRNAs. Am J Pathol 1990;136:1201–1207.

525. Torti SV, Akimoto H, Lin K, et al. Selective inhibition of muscle gene expression by oxidative stress in cardiac cells. J Mol Cell Cardiol 1998;30:1173–1180.

526. Kurabayashi M, Dutta S, Jeyaseelan R, et al. Doxorubicin-induced Id2A gene transcription is targeted at an activating transcription factor/cyclic AMP response element motif through novel mechanisms involving protein kinases distinct from protein kinase C and protein kinase A. Mol Cell Biol 1995;15:6386–6397.

527. Jeyaseelan R, Poizat C, Baker RK, et al. A novel cardiac-restricted target for doxorubicin. CARP, a nuclear modulator of gene expression in cardiac progenitor cells and cardiomyocytes. J Biol Chem 1997;272:22800–22808.

528. Yoshida M, Shiojima I, Ikeda H, et al. Chronic doxorubicin cardiotoxicity is mediated by oxidative DNA damage-ATM-p53-apoptosis pathway and attenuated by pitavastatin through the inhibition of Rac1 activity. J Mol Cell Cardiol 2009;47:698–705.

529. Chandran K, Aggarwal D, Migrino RQ, et al. Doxorubicin inactivates myocardial cytochrome c oxidase in rats: cardioprotection by Mito-Q. Biophys J 2009;96:1388–1398.

530. Suliman HB, Carraway MS, Ali AS, et al. The CO/HO system reverses inhibition of mitochondrial biogenesis and prevents murine doxorubicin cardiomyopathy. J Clin Invest 2007;117:3730–3741.

531. Lyu YL, Kerrigan JE, Lin CP, et al. Topoisomerase IIbeta mediated DNA double-strand breaks: implications in doxorubicin cardiotoxicity and prevention by dexrazoxane. Cancer Res 2007;67:8839–8846.

532. Nakano E, Takeshige K, Toshima Y, et al. Oxidative damage in selenium deficient hearts on perfusion with adriamycin: protective role of glutathione peroxidase system. Cardiovasc Res 1989;23:498–504.

533. Kanter MM, Hamlin RL, Unverferth DV, et al. Effect of exercise training on antioxidant enzymes and cardiotoxicity of doxorubicin. J Appl Physiol 1985;59:1298–1303.

534. Gao J, Xiong Y, Ho YS, et al. Glutathione peroxidase 1-deficient mice are more susceptible to doxorubicin-induced cardiotoxicity. Biochim Biophys Acta 2008;1783:2020–2029.

535. Xiong Y, Liu X, Lee CP, et al. Attenuation of doxorubicin-induced contractile and mitochondrial dysfunction in mouse heart by cellular glutathione peroxidase. Free Radic Biol Med 2006;41:46–55.

536. Nicolay K, Fok JJ, Voorhout W, et al. Cytofluorescence detection of adriamycin-mitochondria interactions in isolated, perfused rat heart. Biochim Biophys Acta 1986;887:35–41.

537. Nohl H. Identification of the site of adriamycin-activation in the heart cell. Biochem Pharmacol 1988;37:2633–2637.

538. Goormaghtigh E, Pollakis G, Ruysschaert JM. Mitochondrial membrane modifications induced by adriamycin-mediated electron transport. Biochem Pharmacol 1983;32:889–893.

539. Nohl H, Gille L, Staniek K. The exogenous NADH dehydrogenase of heart mitochondria is the key enzyme responsible for selective cardiotoxicity of anthracyclines. Z Naturforsch [C] 1998;53:279–285.

540. Weiss RB. The anthracyclines: will we ever find a better doxorubicin. Semin Oncol 1992;19:670–686.

541. Lown JW. Anthracycline and anthraquinone anticancer agents: current status and recent developments. Pharmac Ther 1993;60:185–214.

542. LeBot MA, Begue JM, Kernaleguen D, et al. Different cytotoxicity and metabolism of doxorubicin, daunorubicin, epirubicin, esorubicin and idarubicin in cultured human and rat hepatocytes. Biochem Pharmacol 1988;37:3877–3887.

543. Bertelli G, Amoroso D, Pronzato P, et al. Idarubicin: an evaluation of cardiac toxicity in 77 patients with solid tumors. Anticancer Res 1988;8:645–646.

544. Dodion P, Sanders C, Rombaut W, et al. Effect of daunorubicin, carminomycin, idarubicin, and 4-demethoxydaunorubicinol against normal myeloid stem cells and human malignant cells in vitro. Eur J Cancer Clin Oncol 1987;23:1909–1914.

545. Tamassia V, Pacciarini MA, Moro E, et al. Pharmacokinetic study of intravenous and oral idarubicin in cancer patients. Int J Clin Pharmacol Res 1987;7:419–426.

546. Capranico G, Riva A, Tinelli S, et al. Markedly reduced levels of anthracycline-induced strand breaks in resistant P388 leukemia cells and isolated nuclei. Cancer Res 1987;47:3752–3756.

547. Tan CT, Hancock C, Steinherz P, et al. Phase I and clinical pharmacological study of 4- demethoxydaunorubicin (idarubicin. in children with advanced cancer. Cancer Res 1987;47:2990–2995.

548. Gillies HC, Herriott D, Liang R, et al. Pharmacokinetics of idarubicin (4-demethoxydaunorubicin; IMI-30; NSC 256439. following intravenous and oral administration in patients with advanced cancer. Br J Clin Pharmacol 1987;23:303–310.

549. Zwelling LA, Bales E, Altschuler E, et al. Circumvention of resistance by doxorubicin, but not by idarubicin, in a human leukemia cell line containing an intercalator-resistant form of topoisomerase II: evidence for a non-topoisomerase II-mediated mechanism of doxorubicin cytotoxicity. Biochem Pharmacol 1993;45:516–520.

550. Maessen PA, Mross KB, Pinedo HM, et al. Improved method for the determination of 4''-epidoxorubicin and seven metabolites in plasma by high-performance liquid chromatography. J Chromatogr 1987;417:339–346.

551. Hortobagyi GN, Yap HY, Kau SW, et al. A comparative study of doxorubicin and epirubicin in patients with metastatic breast cancer. Am J Clin Oncol 1989;12:57–62.

552. Havsteen H, Brynjolf I, Svahn T, et al. Prospective evaluation of chronic cardiotoxicity due to high- dose epirubicin or combination chemotherapy with cyclophosphamide, methotrexate, and 5-fluorouracil. Cancer Chemother Pharmacol 1989;23:101–104.

553. Robert J, Vrignaud P, Nguyen-Ngoc T, et al. Comparative pharmacokinetics and metabolism of doxorubicin and epirubicin in patients with metastatic breast cancer. Cancer Treat Rep 1985;69:633–640.

554. Camaggi CM, Strocchi E, Tamassia V, et al. Pharmacokinetic studies of 4'-epidoxorubicin in cancer patients with normal and impaired renal function and with hepatic metastases. Cancer Treat Rep 1982;66:1819–1824.

555. Vile GF, Winterbourn CC. Microsomal lipid peroxidation induced by Adriamycin, epirubicin, daunorubicin and mitoxantrone: a comparative study. Cancer Chemother Pharmacol 1989;24:105–108.

556. Fukushima T, Yamashita T, Yoshio N, et al. Effect of PSC 833 on the cytotoxicity of idarubicin and idarubicinol in multidrug-resistant K562 cells. Leuk Res 1999;23:37–42.

557. Chan EM, Thomas MJ, Bandy B, et al. Effects of doxorubicin, 4'-epirubicin, and antioxidant enzymes on the contractility of isolated cardiomyocytes. Can J Physiol Pharmacol 1996;74:904–910.

558. Bontenbal M, Andersson M, Wildiers J, et al. Doxorubicin vs epirubicin, report of a second-line randomized phase II/III study in advanced breast cancer. EORTC Breast Cancer Cooperative Group. Br J Cancer 1998;77:2257–2263.

559. Ryberg M, Nielsen D, Skovsgaard T, et al. Epirubicin cardiotoxicity: an analysis of 469 patients with metastatic breast cancer. J Clin Oncol 1998;16:3502–3508.

560. Murdock KC, Wallace RE, Durr FE, et al. Antitumor agents: I. 1,4-Bis((aminoalkyl)amino)-9,10- anthracenediones. J Med Chem 1979;22:1024–1030.

561. Johnson RK, Zee-Cheng RKY, Lee WW, et al. Experimental antitumor activity of aminoanthraquinones. Cancer Treat Rep 1979;63:425–439.

562. Moore MJ, Osoba D, Murphy K, et al. Use of palliative end points to evaluate the effects of mitoxantrone and low-dose prednisone in patients with hormonally resistant prostate cancer. J Clin Oncol 1994;12:689–694.

563. Bloomfield DJ, Krahn MD, Neogi T, et al. Economic evaluation of chemotherapy with mitoxantrone plus prednisone for symptomatic hormone-resistant prostate cancer: based on a Canadian randomized trial with palliative end points. J Clin Oncol 1998;16:2272–2279.

564. Foye WD, Vajragupta D, Sengupta SK. DNA binding specificity and RNA polymerase inhibitory activity of bis(aminoalkyl)anthraquinones and bis(methylthio)vinyl quinolinium iodides. J Pharm Sci 1982;71:253–257.

565. Lown JW, Hanstock CC, Bradley RD, et al. Interactions of the antitumor agents, mitoxantrone and bisantrene, with deoxyribonucleic acids studied by electron microscopy. Mol Pharmacol 1984;25:178–184.

566. Bowden GT, Roberts R, Alberts DS, et al. Comparative molecular pharmacology in leukemic L1210 cells of the anthracene anticancer drugs mitoxantrone and bisantrene. Cancer Res 1985;45:4915–4920.

567. Butler J, Hoey BM. Are reduced quinones necessarily involved in the antitumor activity of quinone drugs. Br J Cancer 1987;55(Suppl VIII): 53–59.

568. Nguyen B, Gutierrez PL. Mechanism(s) for the metabolism of mitoxantrone: electron spin resonance and electrochemical studies. Chem Biol Interact 1990;74:139–162.

569. Doroshow JH, Davies KJ. Comparative cardiac oxygen radical metabolism by anthracycline antibiotics, mitoxantrone, bisantrene, 4′-(9-acridinylamino)-methanesulfon-m-anisidide, and neocarzinostatin. Biochem Pharmacol 1983;32:2935–2939.

570. Crespi MO, Ivanier SE, Genovese J, et al. Mitoxantrone affects topoisomerase activities in human breast cancer cells. Biochem Biophys Res Commun 1986;136:521–528.

571. Kharasch ED, Novak RF. Inhibition of adriamycin-stimulated microsomal lipid peroxidation by mitoxantrone and ametantrone. Biochem Biophys Res Commun 1982;108:1346–1352.

572. Abramson JJ, Buck E, Salama G, et al. Mechanism of anthraquinone-induced calcium release from skeletal muscle sarcoplasmic reticulum. J Biol Chem 1988;263:18750–18758.

573. Bhalla K, Ibrado AM, Tourkina E, et al. High-dose mitoxantrone induces programmed cell death or apoptosis in human myeloid leukemia cells. Blood 1993;82:3133–3140.

574. Bellosillo B, Colomer D, Pons G, Gil J. Mitoxantrone, a topoisomerase II inhibitor, induces apoptosis of B- chronic lymphocytic leukaemia cells. Br J Haematol 1998;100:142–146.

575. Koceva-Chyla A, Jedrzejczak M, Skierski J, et al. Mechanisms of induction of apoptosis by anthraquinone anticancer drugs aclarubicin and mitoxantrone in comparison with doxorubicin: relation to drug cytotoxicity and caspase-3 activation. Apoptosis 2005;10:1497–1514.

576. Inaba M, Nagashima K, Sakurai Y. Cross-resistance of vincristine-resistant sublines of P388 leukemia to mitoxantrone with special emphasis on the relationship between in vitro and in vivo cross-resistance. Gann 1984;75:625–630.

577. Dalton WS, Cress AE, Alberts DS, et al. Cytogenetic and phenotypic analysis of a human colon carcinoma cell line resistant to mitoxantrone. Cancer Res 1988;48:1882–1888.

578. Bhalla K, Hindenburg A, Taub RN, et al. Isolation and characterization of an anthracycline-resistant human leukemic cell line. Cancer Res 1985;45:3657–3662.

579. Nakagawa M, Schneider E, Dixon KH, et al. Reduced intracellular drug accumulation in the absence of P- glycoprotein (mdr1. overexpression in mitoxantrone-resistant human MCF-7 breast cancer cells. Cancer Res 1992;52:6175–6181.

580. Satake S, Sugawara I, Watanabe M, et al. Lack of a point mutation of human DNA topoisomerase II in multidrug- resistant anaplastic thyroid carcinoma cell lines. Cancer Lett 1997;116:33–39.

581. Schneider E, Horton JK, Yang CH, et al. Multidrug resistance-associated protein gene overexpression and reduced drug sensitivity of topoisomerase II in a human breast carcinoma MCF7 cell line selected for etoposide resistance. Cancer Res 1994;54:152–158.

582. Hazlehurst LA, Foley NE, Gleason-Guzman MC, et al. Multiple mechanisms confer drug resistance to mitoxantrone in the human 8226 myeloma cell line. Cancer Res 1999;59:1021–1028.

583. Miyake K, Mickley L, Litman T, et al. Molecular cloning of cDNAs which are highly overexpressed in mitoxantrone-resistant cells: demonstration of homology to ABC transport genes. Cancer Res 1999;59:8–13.

584. Ross DD, Yang W, Abruzzo LV, et al. Atypical multidrug resistance: breast cancer resistance protein messenger RNA expression in mitoxantrone-selected cell lines. J Natl Cancer Inst 1999;91:429–433.

585. Kozin SV, Gerweck LE. Cytotoxicity of weak electrolytes after the adaptation of cells to low pH: role of the transmembrane pH gradient. Br J Cancer 1998;77:1580–1585.

586. Heinemann V, Murray D, Walters R, et al. Mitoxantrone-induced DNA damage in leukemia cells is enhanced by treatment with high-dose arabinosylcytosine. Cancer Chemother Pharmacol 1988;22:205–210.

587. Shenkenberg TD, VonHoff DD. Mitoxantrone: a new anticancer drug with significant clinical activity. Ann Intern Med 1986;105:67–81.

588. Neidhart JA, Gochnour D, Roach R, et al. A comparison of mitoxantrone and doxorubicin in breast cancer. J Clin Oncol 1986;4:672–677.

589. Lawton F, Blackledge G, Mould J, et al. Phase II study of mitoxantrone in epithelial ovarian cancer. Cancer Treat Rep 1987;71:627–629.

590. Coltman CAJ, McDaniel TM, Balcerzak SP, et al. Mitoxantrone hydrochloride (NSC-310739) in lymphoma. Invest New Drugs 1983;1:65–70.

591. Birot-Babapalle F, Catovsky D, Slocumbe G, et al. Phase II study of mitoxantrone and cytarabine in acute myeloid leukemia. Cancer Treat Rep 1987;71:161–163.

592. Alberts DS, Peng YM, Leigh S, et al. Disposition of mitoxantrone in cancer patients. Cancer Res 1985;45:1879–1884.

593. Smyth JF, Macpherson JS, Warrington PS, et al. The clinical pharmacology of mitoxantrone. Cancer Chemother Pharmacol 1986;17:149–152.

594. Repetto L, Vannozzi MO, Balleari E, et al. Mitoxantrone in elderly patients with advanced breast cancer: pharmacokinetics, marrow and peripheral hematopoietic progenitor cells. Anticancer Res 1999;19:879–884.

595. Savaraj N, Lu K, Manuel V, et al. Pharmacology of mitoxantrone in cancer patients. Cancer Chemother Pharmacol 1982;8:113–117.

596. Wolf CR, Macpherson JS, Smyth JF. Evidence for the metabolism of mitozantrone by microsomal glutathione transferases and 3-methylcholanthrene-inducible glucuronosyl transferases. Biochem Pharmacol 1986;35:1577–1581.

597. Chiccarelli FS, Morrison JA, Cosulich DB, et al. Identification of human urinary mitoxantrone metabolites. Cancer Res 1986;46:4858–4861.

598. Shepherd FA, Evans WK, Blackstein ME, et al. Hepatic arterial infusion of mitoxantrone in the treatment of primary hepatocellular carcinoma. J Clin Oncol 1987;5:635–640.

599. Alberts DS, Surwit EA, Peng YM, et al. Phase I clinical and pharmacokinetic study of mitoxantrone gien to patients by intraperitoneal administration. Cancer Res 1988;48:5874–5877.

600. Husain A, Sabbatini P, Spriggs D, et al. Phase II trial of intraperitoneal cisplatin and mitoxantrone in patients with persistent ovarian cancer. Gynecol Oncol 1999;73:96–101.

601. Yap HY, Blumenschein GR, Schell FC, et al. Dihydroanthracenedione: a promising new drug in the treatment of metastatic breast cancer. Ann Intern Med 1981;95:694–697.

602. Underferth DV, Underferth BJ, Balcerzak SP, et al. Cardiac evaluation of mitoxantrone. Cancer Treat Rep 1983;67:343–350.

603. Benjamin RS, Chawla SP, Ewer MS, et al. Evaluation of mitoxantrone cardiac toxicity by nuclear angiography and endomyocardial biopsy: an update. Invest New Drugs 1985;3:117–121.

604. Ghalie RG, Edan G, Laurent M, et al. Cardiac adverse effects associated with mitoxantrone (Novantrone) therapy in patients with MS. Neurology 2002;59:909–913.

605. Gonsette RE. Mitoxantrone in progressive multiple sclerosis: when and how to treat? J Neurol Sci 2003;206:203–208.

606. Prai GR, Reed NS, Ruddell NST. A case of mitoxantrone-associated cardiomyopathy without prior anthracycline therapy. Br J Radiol 1987;60:1125–1126.

607. Arlin ZA, Silver R, Cassileth P. Phase I-II trial of mitoxantrone in acute leukemia. Cancer Treat Rep 1985;69:61–64.

608. Speechly-Dick ME, Owen ERTC. Mitoxantrone-induced oncycholysis. Lancet 1988;1:113.

609. Borchmann P, Morschhauser F, Parry A., et al. Phase II study of new aza-anthracenedione, BBR 2778, in patients with relapsed aggressive non-Hodgkin's Lymphoma. Haematologica 2003;88:888–894.

610. Lipschultz SE, Alvarez JA, Scully RE. Anthracycline associated cardiotoxicity in survivors of childhood cancer. Heart 2008;94:525–531.

611. Mistry AR, Felix CA, Whitmarsh RJ, et al. DNA Topoisomerase II in Therapy-Related Acute Promyelocytic Leukemia. N Engl J Med 2005; 352:1529–1538.

612. Pedersen-Bjergaard J. Insights into leukemogenesis from therapy-related leukemia. N Engl J Med 2005;352:1591–1594.

613. Blanco JG, Leisenring WM, Gonzalez-Covarrubias VM, et al. Genetic polymorphism in the carbonyl redectase 3 gene CRB3 and the NAD (P) H: quinone oxireductase I Gene NQO1 in patients who developed anthracycline-related congestive heart failure after childhood cancer. Cancer 2008;112:2189–2139.

614. De Angelis A, Piegari E, Cappetta E, et al. Anthracycline cadiomyopathy is mediated by depletion of the cardiac stem cell pool and is rescued by restoration of progenitor cell function. Circulation 2010;121:276–292.

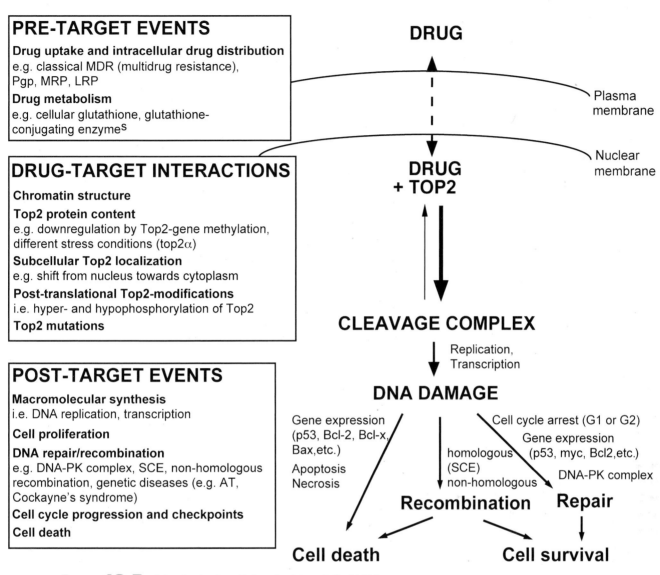

PRE-TARGET EVENTS

Drug uptake and intracellular drug distribution
e.g. classical MDR (multidrug resistance),
Pgp, MRP, LRP

Drug metabolism
e.g. cellular glutathione, glutathione-
conjugating enzyme^S

DRUG-TARGET INTERACTIONS

Chromatin structure

Top2 protein content
e.g. downregulation by Top2-gene methylation,
different stress conditions (top2α)

Subcellular Top2 localization
e.g. shift from nucleus towards cytoplasm

Post-translational Top2-modifications
i.e. hyper- and hypophosphorylation of Top2

Top2 mutations

POST-TARGET EVENTS

Macromolecular synthesis
i.e. DNA replication, transcription

Cell proliferation

DNA repair/recombination
e.g. DNA-PK complex, SCE, non-homologous
recombination, genetic diseases (e.g. AT,
Cockayne's syndrome)

Cell cycle progression and checkpoints

Cell death

DRUG

Plasma
membrane

Nuclear
membrane

**DRUG
+ TOP2**

CLEAVAGE COMPLEX

Replication,
Transcription

DNA DAMAGE

Gene expression
(p53, Bcl-2, Bcl-x,
Bax,etc.)

Cell cycle arrest (G1 or G2)

Gene expression
(p53, myc, Bcl2,etc.)

Apoptosis
Necrosis

homologous
(SCE)
non-homologous

DNA-PK complex

Recombination   **Repair**

Cell death   **Cell survival**

FIGURE **19-5**   Determinants of sensitivity and resistance to Top2 inhibitors.

the ATP binding site and the other around the catalytic tyrosine (Tyr 804 for human Top2) (Fig. 19-2). The presence of mutations near the catalytic tyrosine is consistent with the drug-stacking model at the interface of the enzyme-DNA complex.[34] The existence of the second mutation cluster near the putative ATP binding site suggests that Top2 folding brings this second region near the catalytic domain and that Top2 inhibitors bind at the interface of these two Top2 regions.[73,74] Some drug-resistant mutants are differentially resistant to epipodophyllotoxins, m-AMSA, and quinolones, a finding consistent with preferential interactions of each class of drug with certain Top2 amino acids and with the preferred DNA bases around the Top2 cleavage sites.

Changes in Top2 phosphorylation may also contribute to Top2-mediated drug resistance. However, in resistant cell lines, reduced cleavage complexes have been associated with both hyperphosphorylation and hypophosphorylation of Top2. Decreased Top2α protein levels were associated with hyperphosphorylation of the enzyme in VP-16-resistant cell lines.[75] Hypophosphorylated Top2α predominates in VP-16-resistant erythroleukemia[76] and HL-60 cells[77] and

in teniposide-resistant leukemia cell lines.[78] Top2 phosphorylation increases in parallel with the cellular need for the enzyme: during the S phase of the cell cycle, with a peak at the G2 phase.[79,80] Casein kinase II is probably the main kinase responsible for Top2 phosphorylation in cells.[81–84] Drug-induced cleavage complexes are reduced to approximately 50% after in vitro phosphorylation of Top2α by casein kinase II and protein kinase C.[85] This finding is in contrast with Top1 phosphorylation, which increases camptothecin activity.[86]

Since both normal and cancer cells express Top2, it is likely that drug-induced cleavage complexes are not sufficient for selective killing of cancer cells. DNA synthesis inhibition provides only partial protection against VP-16.[87] The interaction of transcription with cleavage complexes may play a prominent role in the activity of Top2 inhibitors since VP-16 cytotoxicity is decreased by RNA synthesis inhibitors.[88,89] The dependence of Top1 and Top2 inhibitor cytotoxicity on ongoing replication and transcription probably explains why simultaneous treatment with camptothecin and VP-16 has been found to be antagonistic.[88–90] VP-16 may suppress

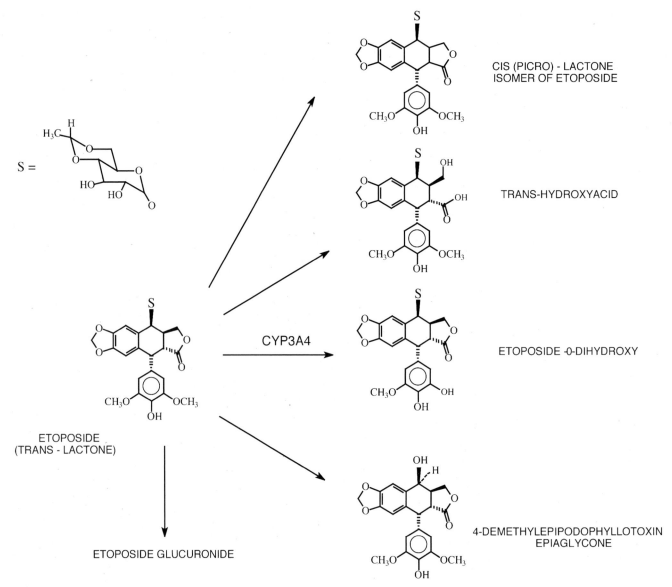

$S =$

CIS (PICRO) - LACTONE
ISOMER OF ETOPOSIDE

TRANS-HYDROXYACID

CYP3A4

ETOPOSIDE -0-DIHYDROXY

ETOPOSIDE
(TRANS - LACTONE)

ETOPOSIDE GLUCURONIDE

4-DEMETHYLEPIPODOPHYLLOTOXIN
EPIAGLYCONE

FIGURE 19-6   Metabolism of etoposide. Both etoposide-*o*-dihydroxy and 4-demethyl-epipodophyllotoxin aglycone are active against Top2.

camptothecin effects by inhibiting replication, and camptothecin may suppress the effects of VP-16 by inhibiting transcription.

Other conditions have been described in which the cytotoxicity of topoisomerase inhibitors can be abrogated without effect on cleavage complex formation. These include intracellular calcium depletion by EDTA[91] and protein synthesis inhibition by cycloheximide.[15,16] Poly(adenosine diphosphoribose) synthesis also may be important for cell killing since poly(adenosine diphosphoribose polymerase)-deficient Chinese hamster cells are resistant to VP-16 but hypersensitive to camptothecin.[92] These observations indicate that events downstream from the cleavage complexes are critical to cytotoxicity. Such events may involve the accumulation of genetic alterations, such as sister chromatid exchanges (SCE),[93] illegitimate recombinations,[94,95] and apoptosis.[96]

DNA repair must intervene to correct drug-induced and topoisomerase-mediated DNA damage. Yeast cells are usually resistant to topoisomerase inhibitors unless they are RAD52 mutants, for example, deficient in DNA double-strand break repair.[97] The ubiquitin proteolysis pathway has been reported to be responsible

for ubiquitination and degradation of Top1 and Top2 cleavage complexes.[98] Abnormal cell cycle control (checkpoints) has recently emerged as a key element in possibly explaining the differential responses of normal versus neoplastic cells to DNA damage. Therefore, alterations of cell cycle control may play a critical role in the cytotoxicity of topoisomerase inhibitors. Lack of arrest in G1, as in cells with mutated or absent p53 genes, may not provide the cell with the time required to repair damage and may lead to an accumulation of further damage. Hence, deregulation of cyclins, cell cycle–regulated kinases, and phosphatases and p53 mutations may sensitize cells to topoisomerase inhibitors.[99–102] Furthermore, pharmacological abrogation of drug induced S- and G2-phase checkpoints may provide a novel effective strategy for enhancing the chemotherapeutic activity of topoisomerase inhibitors.[103]

Another determinant of sensitivity to topoisomerase inhibitors is the predisposition of the cell to undergo apoptosis.[96] Some cells, such as human leukemia HL-60 cells, are known to be hypersensitive to a variety of injuries, including DNA damage by topoisomerase inhibitors. The underlying mechanism for this hypersensitivity may be the frequency in patients with HER2/neu amplification[203] as these reside in adjoining regions on chromosome 17. The response rate to anthracyclines is impressively greater in breast cancer patients with HER2 amplification in their tumors,[204] suggesting that high Top2α gene expression might become a biomarker for etoposide therapy in other tumors. Further clinical trials are required to answer this intriguing question.

References

1. Kohn KW. Beyond DNA cross-linking: history and prospects of DNA-targeted cancer treatment—fifteenth Bruce F. Cain Memorial Award Lecture. Cancer Res 1996;56:5533–5546.
2. Zwelling LA, Michaels S, Erickson LC, et al. Protein-associated deoxyribonucleic acid strand breaks in L1210 cells treated with the deoxyribonucleic acid intercalating agents 4′-(9-acridinylamino) methanesulfon-m-anisidide and adriamycin. Biochemistry 1981;20:6553–6563.
3. Pommier Y, Kerrigan D, Schwartz R, et al. The formation and resealing of intercalator-induced DNA strand breaks in isolated L1210 cell nuclei. Biochem Biophys Res Commun 1982;107:576–583.
4. Nelson EM, Tewey KM, Liu LF. Mechanism of antitumor drug action: poisoning of mammalian DNA topoisomerase II on DNA by 4′-(9-acridinylamino)-methanesulfon-m-anisidide. Proc Natl Acad Sci USA 1984;81:1361–1365.
5. Minford J, Pommier Y, Filipski J, et al. Isolation of intercalator-dependent protein-linked DNA strand cleavage activity from cell nuclei and identification as topoisomerase II. Biochemistry 1986;25:9–16.
6. Deweese JE, Osheroff N. The DNA cleavage reaction of topoisomerase II: wolf in sheep's clothing. Nucleic Acids Res 2009;37:738–748.
7. Nitiss JL. Targeting DNA topoisomerase II in cancer chemotherapy. Nat Rev Cancer 2009;9:338–350.
8. Nitiss JL. DNA topoisomerase II and its growing repertoire of biological functions. Nat Rev Cancer 2009;9:327–337.
9. Wang JC. Cellular roles of DNA topoisomerases: a molecular perspective. Nat Rev Mol Cell Biol 2002;3:430–440.
10. Levine C, Hiasa H, Marians KJ. DNA gyrase and topoisomerase IV: biochemical activities, physiological roles during chromosome replication, and drug sensitivities. Biochim Biophys Acta 1998;1400:29–43.
11. Hooper DC. Clinical applications of quinolones. Biochim Biophys Acta 1998;1400:45–61.
12. Berger JM. Type II DNA topoisomerases. Curr Opin Struct Biol 1998;8:26–32.
13. Wang JC. Moving one DNA double helix through another by a type II DNA topoisomerase: the story of a simple molecular machine. Q Rev Biophys 1998;31:107–144.
14. Pourquier P, Kohlhagen G, Ueng L-M, et al. Topoisomerase I and II activity assays. In: Brown R, Böger-Brown U, eds. Methods in Molecular Medicine: Cytotoxic Drug Resistance Mechanisms. Totowa: Humana Press, 1999:95–110.
15. Pommier Y, Leo E, Zhang H, et al. DNA topoisomerases and their poisoning by anticancer and antibacterial drugs. Chem Biol 2010;17:421–433.
16. Liu L. DNA Topoisomerases: Topoisomerase-Targeting Drugs. New York: Academic Press, 1994.
17. Burden DA, Osheroff N. Mechanism of action of eukaryotic topoisomerase II and drugs targeted to the enzyme. Biochim Biophys Acta 1998;1400:139–154.
18. Corbett AH, Osheroff N. When good enzymes go bad: conversion of topoisomerase II to a cellular toxin by antineoplastic drugs. Chem Res Toxicol 1993;6:585–597.
19. Subramanian D, Kraut E, Staubus A, et al. Analysis of topoisomerase I/DNA complexes in patients administered topotecan. Cancer Res 1995;55:2007–2103.
20. Pommier Y, Schwartz RE, Zwelling LA, et al. Effects of DNA intercalating agents on topoisomerase II induced DNA strand cleavage in isolated mammalian cell nuclei. Biochemistry 1985;24:6406–6410.
21. Tewey KM, Chen GL, Nelson EM, et al. Intercalative antitumor drugs interfere with the breakage-reunion reaction of mammalian DNA topoisomerase II. J Biol Chem 1984;259:9182–9187.
22. Roca J, Ishida R, Berger JM, et al. Antitumor bisdioxopiperazines inhibit yeast DNA topoisomerase II by trapping the enzyme in the form of a closed protein clamp. Proc Natl Acad Sci USA 1994;91:1781–1785.
23. Andoh T. Bis(2,6-dioxopiperazines), catalytic inhibitors of DNA topoisomerase II, as molecular probes, cardioprotectors and antitumor drugs. Biochimie 1998;80:235–246.
24. Zwelling LA, Michaels S, Kerrigan D, et al. Protein-associated deoxyribonucleic acid strand breaks produced in mouse leukemia L1210 cells by ellipticine and 2-methyl-9- hydroxyellipticinium. Biochem Pharmacol 1982;31:3261–3267.
25. Long BH, Musial ST, Brattain MG. Single- and double-strand DNA breakage and repair in human lung adenocarcinoma cells exposed to etoposide and teniposide. Cancer Res 1985;45:3106–3112.
26. Pommier Y, Orr A, Kohn KW, et al. Differential effects of amsacrine and epipodophyllotoxins on topoisomerase II cleavage in the human c-myc protooncogene. Cancer Res 1992;52:3125–3130.
27. Capranico G, Zunino F, Kohn KW, et al. Sequence-selective topoisomerase II inhibition by anthracycline derivatives in SV40 DNA: relationship with DNA binding affinity and cytotoxicity. Biochemistry 1990;29:562–569.
28. Capranico G, Kohn KW, Pommier Y. Local sequence requirements for DNA cleavage by mammalian topoisomerase II in the presence of doxorubicin. Nucleic Acids Res 1990;18:6611–6619.
29. Capranico G, De Isabella P, Tinelli S, et al. Similar sequence specificity of mitoxantrone and VM-26 stimulation of in vitro DNA cleavage by mammalian DNA topoisomerase II. Biochemistry 1993;32:3038–3046.
30. Capranico G, Binaschi M. DNA sequence selectivity of topoisomerases and topoisomerase poisons. Biochim Biophys Acta 1998;1400:185–194.
31. Freudenreich CH, Kreuzer KN. Mutational analysis of a type II topoisomerase cleavage site: distinct requirements for enzyme and inhibitors. Embo J 1993;12:2085–2097.
32. Jaxel C, Kohn KW, Wani MC, et al. Structure-activity study of the actions of camptothecin derivatives on mammalian topoisomerase I: evidence for a specific receptor site and a relation to antitumor activity. Cancer Res 1989;49:1465–1469.
33. Pommier Y, Capranico G, Orr A, et al. Local base sequence preferences for DNA cleavage by mammalian topoisomerase II in the presence of amsacrine or teniposide [published erratum appears in Nucleic Acids Res 1991 Dec 25;19(24):7003]. Nucleic Acids Res 1991;19:5973–5980.
34. Pommier Y, Kohn KW, Capranico G, et al. Base sequence selectivity of topoisomerase inhibitors suggests a common model for drug action. In: Andoh T, Ikeda H, Oguro M, eds. Molecular Biology of DNA Topoisomerases and its Application to Chemotherapy. Boca Raton: CRC Press, 1993:215.
35. Strumberg D, Nitiss JL, Dong J, et al. Molecular analysis of yeast and human type II topoisomerases: enzyme-DNA and drug interactions. J Biol Chem 1999;274:7292–7301.
36. Svejstrup JQ, Christiansen K, Gromova II, et al. New technique for uncoupling the cleavage and religation reactions of eukaryotic topoisomerase I. The mode of action of camptothecin at a specific recognition site. J Mol Biol 1991;222:669–678.
37. Robinson MJ, Osheroff N. Effects of antineoplastic drugs on the post-strand-passage DNA cleavage/religation equilibrium of topoisomerase II. Biochemistry 1991;30:1807–1813.
38. Strumberg D, Nitiss JL, Rose A, et al. Mutation of a conserved serine residue in a quinolone-resistant type II topoisomerase alters the enzyme-DNA and drug interactions. J Biol Chem 1999;274:7292–7301.
39. Pommier Y, Cherfils J. Interfacial protein inhibition: a nature's paradigm for drug discovery. Trends Pharmacol Sci 2005;28:136–145.
40. Bromberg KD, Burgin AB, Osheroff N. A two-drug model for etoposide action against human topoisomerase IIalpha. J Biol Chem 2003;278:7406–7412.
41. Khan QA, Kohlhagen G, Marshall R, et al. Position-specific trapping of topoisomerase II by benzo[a]pyrene diol epoxide adducts: implications for interactions with intercalating anticancer agents. Proc Natl Acad Sci USA 2003;100:12498–12503.
42. Gottesman MM, Fojo T, Bates SE. Multidrug resistance in cancer: role of ATP-dependent transporters. Nat Rev Cancer 2002;2:48–58.

43. Borrel MN, Fiallo M, Priebe W, et al. P-glycoprotein-mediated efflux of hydroxyrubicin, a neutral anthracycline derivative, in resistant K562 cells. FEBS Lett 1994;356:287–299.

44. Solary E, Ling YH, Perez-Soler R, et al. Hydroxyrubicin, a deaminated derivative of doxorubicin, inhibits mammalian DNA topoisomerase II and partially circumvents multidrug resistance. Int J Cancer 1994;58:85–94.

45. Cole SP, Bhardwaj G, Gerlach JH, et al. Overexpression of a transporter gene in a multidrug-resistant human lung cancer cell line [see comments]. Science 1992;258:1650–1654.

46. Scheffer GL, Wijngaard PL, Flens MJ, et al. The drug resistance-related protein LRP is the human major vault protein [see comments]. Nat Med 1995;1:578–582.

47. Ishikawa T. The ATP-dependent glutathione S-conjugate export pump [see comments]. Trends Biochem Sci 1992;17:463–468.

48. Leteurtre F, Madalengoitia J, Orr A, et al. Rational design and molecular effects of a new topoisomerase II inhibitor, azatoxin [published erratum appears in Cancer Res 1992 Nov 1;52(21):6136]. Cancer Res 1992;52:4478–4483.

49. Sinha BK, Eliot HM. Etoposide-induced DNA damage in human tumor cells: requirement for cellular activating factors. Biochim Biophys Acta 1991;1097:111–116.

50. Zwelling LA, Kerrigan D, Michaels S, et al. Cooperative sequestration of m-AMSA in L1210 cells. Biochem Pharmacol 1982;31:3269–3277.

51. Schuurhuis GJ, Broxterman HJ, de Lange JH, et al. Early multidrug resistance, defined by changes in intracellular doxorubicin distribution, independent of P-glycoprotein. Br J Cancer 1991;64:857–861.

52. Gervasoni JE Jr, Fields SZ, Krishna S, et al. Subcellular distribution of daunorubicin in P-glycoprotein-positive and -negative drug-resistant cell lines using laser-assisted confocal microscopy. Cancer Res 1991;51: 4955–4963.

53. Schuurhuis GJ, Broxterman HJ, Ossenkoppele GJ, et al. Functional multidrug resistance phenotype associated with combined overexpression of Pgp/MDR1 and MRP together with 1-beta-D-arabinofuranosylcytosine sensitivity may predict clinical response in acute myeloid leukemia. Clin Cancer Res 1995;1:81–93.

54. Hsiang YH, Wu HY, Liu LF. Proliferation-dependent regulation of DNA topoisomerase II in cultured human cells. Cancer Res 1988;48: 3230–3235.

55. Nelson WG, Cho KR, Hsiang YH, et al. Growth-related elevations of DNA topoisomerase II levels found in Dunning R3327 rat prostatic adenocarcinomas. Cancer Res 1987;47:3246–3250.

56. Nicklee T, Crump M, Hedley DW. Effects of topoisomerase I inhibition on the expression of topoisomerase II alpha measured with fluorescence image cytometry. Cytometry 1996;25:205–210.

57. Turley H, Comley M, Houlbrook S, et al. The distribution and expression of the two isoforms of DNA topoisomerase II in normal and neoplastic human tissues. Br J Cancer 1997;75:1340–1346.

58. Keith WN, Douglas F, Wishart GC, et al. Co-amplification of erbB2, topoisomerase II alpha and retinoic acid receptor alpha genes in breast cancer and allelic loss at topoisomerase I on chromosome 20. Eur J Cancer 1993;10:1469–1475.

59. Zwelling LA, Kerrigan D, Lippman ME. Protein-associated intercalator-induced DNA scission is enhanced by estrogen stimulation in human breast cancer cells. Proc Natl Acad Sci USA 1983;80:6182–6186.

60. Sorensen M, Sehested M, Jensen PB. Characterisation of a human small-cell lung cancer cell line resistant to the DNA topoisomerase I-directed drug topotecan. Br J Cancer 1995;72:399–404.

61. Tan KB, Mattern MR, Eng WK, et al. Nonproductive rearrangement of DNA topoisomerase I and II genes: correlation with resistance to topoisomerase inhibitors. J Natl Cancer Inst 1989;81:1732–1735.

62. Sandri MI, Isaacs RJ, Ongkeko WM, et al. p53 regulates the minimal promoter of the human topoisomerase IIalpha gene. Nucleic Acids Res 1996;24:4464–4470.

63. Wang Q, Zambetti GP, Suttle DP. Inhibition of DNA topoisomerase II alpha gene expression by the p53 tumor suppressor. Mol Cell Biol 1997; 17:389–397.

64. Yun J, Tomida A, Nagata K, et al. Glucose-regulated stresses confer resistance to VP-16 in human cancer cells through a decreased expression of DNA topoisomerase II. Oncol Res 1995;7:583–590.

65. Teicher BA, Holden SA, Rose CM. Effect of oxygen on the cytotoxicity and antitumor activity of etoposide. J Natl Cancer Inst 1985;75:1129–1133.

66. Shen JW, Subjeck JR, Lock RB, et al. Depletion of topoisomerase II in isolated nuclei during a glucose-regulated stress response. Mol Cell Biol 1989;9:3284–3291.

67. Luk CK, Veinot-Drebot L, Tjan E, et al. Effect of transient hypoxia on sensitivity to doxorubicin in human and murine cell lines. J Natl Cancer Inst 1990;82:684–692.

68. Hashimoto S, Chatterjee S, Ranjit GB, et al. Drastic reduction of topoisomerase II alpha associated with major acquired resistance to topoisomerase II active agents but minor perturbations of cell growth [published erratum appears in Oncol Res 1995;7(10–11):565]. Oncol Res 1995;7: 407–416.

69. Feldhoff PW, Mirski SE, Cole SP, et al. Altered subcellular distribution of topoisomerase II alpha in a drug-resistant human small cell lung cancer cell line. Cancer Res 1994;54:756–762.

70. Harker WG, Slade DL, Parr RL, et al. Alterations in the topoisomerase II alpha gene, messenger RNA, and subcellular protein distribution as well as reduced expression of the DNA topoisomerase II beta enzyme in a mitoxantrone-resistant HL-60 human leukemia cell line. Cancer Res 1995;55:1707–1716.

71. Dereuddre S, Frey S, Delaporte C, et al. Cloning and characterization of full-length cDNAs coding for the DNA topoisomerase II beta from Chinese hamster lung cells sensitive and resistant 9-OH-ellipticine. Biochim Biophys Acta 1995;1264:178–182.

72. Wessel I, Jensen PB, Falck J, et al. Loss of amino acids 1490Lys-Ser-Lys1492 in the COOH-terminal region of topoisomerase IIalpha in human small cell lung cancer cells selected for resistance to etoposide results in an extranuclear enzyme localization. Cancer Res 1997;57:4451–4454.

73. Liu Q, Wang JC. Similarity in the catalysis of DNA breakage and rejoining by type IA and IIA DNA topoisomerases. Proc Natl Acad Sci USA 1999;96:881–886.

74. Fass D, Bogden CE, Berger JM. Quaternary changes in topoisomerase II may direct orthogonal movement of two DNA strands. Nat Struct Biol 1999;6:322–326.

75. Matsumoto Y, Takano H, Fojo T. Cellular adaptation to drug exposure: evolution of the drug-resistant phenotype. Cancer Res 1997;57:5086–5092.

76. Ritke MK, Murray NR, Allan WP, et al. Hypophosphorylation of topoisomerase II in etoposide (VP-16)-resistant human leukemia K562 cells associated with reduced levels of beta II protein kinase C. Mol Pharmacol 1995;48:798–805.

77. Ganapathi R, Constantinou A, Kamath N, et al. Resistance to etoposide in human leukemia HL-60 cells: reduction in drug-induced DNA cleavage associated with hypophosphorylation of topoisomerase II phosphopeptides. Mol Pharmacol 1996;50:243–248.

78. Chen M, Beck WT. DNA topoisomerase II expression, stability, and phosphorylation in two VM-26-resistant human leukemic CEM sublines. Oncol Res 1995;7:103–111.

79. Heck MM, Hittelman WN, Earnshaw WC. In vivo phosphorylation of the 170-kDa form of eukaryotic DNA topoisomerase II. Cell cycle analysis. J Biol Chem 1989;264:15161–15164.

80. Taagepera S, Rao PN, Drake FH, et al. DNA topoisomerase II alpha is the major chromosome protein recognized by the mitotic phosphoprotein antibody MPM-2. Proc Natl Acad Sci USA 1993;90:8407–8411.

81. Cardenas ME, Dang Q, Glover CV, Gasser SM. Casein kinase II phosphorylates the eukaryote-specific C-terminal domain of topoisomerase II in vivo. Embo J 1992;11:1785–1796.

82. Ackerman P, Glover CV, Osheroff N. Phosphorylation of DNA topoisomerase II by casein kinase II: modulation of eukaryotic topoisomerase II activity in vitro. Proc Natl Acad Sci USA 1985;82:3164–3168.

83. Ackerman P, Glover CV, Osheroff N. Phosphorylation of DNA topoisomerase II in vivo and in total homogenates of Drosophila Kc cells. The role of casein kinase II. J Biol Chem 1988;263:12653–12660.

84. Bojanowski K, Filhol O, Cochet C, et al. DNA topoisomerase II and casein kinase II associate in a molecular complex that is catalytically active. J Biol Chem 1993;268:22920–22926.

85. DeVore RF, Corbett AH, Osheroff N. Phosphorylation of topoisomerase II by casein kinase II and protein kinase C: effects on enzyme-mediated DNA cleavage/religation and sensitivity to the antineoplastic drugs etoposide

and 4′-(9-acridinylamino)methane-sulfon-m-anisidide. Cancer Res 1992; 52:2156–2161.

86. Pommier Y, Kerrigan D, Hartman KD, et al. Phosphorylation of mammalian DNA topoisomerase I and activation by protein kinase C. J Biol Chem 1990;265:9418–9422.

87. Holm C, Covey JM, Kerrigan D, et al. Differential requirement of DNA replication for the cytotoxicity of DNA topoisomerase I and II inhibitors in Chinese hamster DC3F cells. Cancer Res 1989;49:6365–6368.

88. D'Arpa P, Beardmore C, Liu LF. Involvement of nucleic acid synthesis in cell killing mechanisms of topoisomerase poisons. Cancer Res 1990;50: 6919–6924.

89. Kaufmann SH. Antagonism between camptothecin and topoisomerase II-directed chemotherapeutic agents in a human leukemia cell line. Cancer Res 1991;51:1129–1136.

90. Bertrand R, O'Connor PM, Kerrigan D, et al. Sequential administration of camptothecin and etoposide circumvents the antagonistic cytotoxicity of simultaneous drug administration in slowly growing human colon carcinoma HT-29 cells. Eur J Cancer 1992:743–748.

91. Bertrand R, Kerrigan D, Sarang M, et al. Cell death induced by topoisomerase inhibitors. Role of calcium in mammalian cells. Biochem Pharmacol 1991;42:77–85.

92. Chatterjee S, Cheng MF, Berger NA. Hypersensitivity to clinically useful alkylating agents and radiation in poly(ADP-ribose) polymerase-deficient cell lines. Cancer Commun 1990;2:401–407.

93. Pommier Y, Zwelling LA, Kao-Shan CS, et al. Correlations between intercalator-induced DNA strand breaks and sister chromatid exchanges, mutations, and cytotoxicity in Chinese hamster cells. Cancer Res 1985;45: 3143–3149.

94. Pommier Y, Bertrand R. The mechanism of formation of chromosomal aberrations: role of eukaryotic DNA topoisomerases. In: Kirsch IR, ed. The Causes and Consequences of Chromosomal Aberrations. Boca Raton: CRC Press, 1993:277.

95. Zhu J, Schiestl RH. Topoisomerase I involvement in illegitimate recombination in Saccharomyces cerevisiae. Mol Cell Biol 1996;16:1805–1812.

96. Sordet O, Khan Q, Kohn KW, et al. Apoptosis induced by topoisomerase inhibitors. Curr Med Chem Anticancer Agents 2003;3:271–290.

97. Nitiss J, Wang JC. DNA topoisomerase-targeting antitumor drugs can be studied in yeast. Proc Natl Acad Sci USA 1988;85:7501–7505.

98. Desai SD, Liu LF, Vazquez-Abad D, et al. Ubiquitin-dependent destruction of topoisomerase I is stimulated by the antitumor drug camptothecin. J Biol Chem 1997;272:24159–24164.

99. Goldwasser F, Shimizu T, Jackman J, et al. Correlations between S and G2 arrest and the cytotoxicity of camptothecin in human colon carcinoma cells. Cancer Res 1996;56:4430–4437.

100. O'Connor PM, Kohn KW. A fundamental role for cell cycle regulation in the chemosensitivity of cancer cells? Semin Cancer Biol 1992;3: 409–416.

101. Shao RG, Cao CX, Zhang H, et al. Replication-mediated DNA damage by camptothecin induces phosphorylation of RPA by DNA-dependent protein kinase and dissociates RPA:DNA-PK complexes. Embo J 1999;18:1397–1406.

102. Gupta M, Fan S, Zhan Q, et al. Inactivation of p53 increases the cytotoxicity of camptothecin in human colon HCT116 and breast MCF-7 cancer cells. Clin Cancer Res 1997;3:1653–1660.

103. Shao RG, Cao CX, Shimizu T, et al. Abrogation of an S-phase checkpoint and potentiation of camptothecin cytotoxicity by 7-hydroxystaurosporine (UCN-01) in human cancer cell lines, possibly influenced by p53 function. Cancer Res 1997;57:4029–4035.

104. Bertrand R, Solary E, Jenkins J, et al. Apoptosis and its modulation in human promyelocytic HL-60 cells treated with DNA topoisomerase I and II inhibitors. Exp Cell Res 1993;207:388–397.

105. Kamesaki S, Kamesaki H, Jorgensen TJ, et al. bcl-2 protein inhibits etoposide-induced apoptosis through its effects on events subsequent to topoisomerase II-induced DNA strand breaks and their repair [published erratum appears in Cancer Res 1994 Jun 1;54(11):3074]. Cancer Res 1993;53:4251–4256.

106. Henneberry HP, Aherne GW, Marks V. An ELISA for the measurement of VP16 (etoposide) in unextracted plasma. J Immunol Methods 1988;107:205–209.

107. Hande KR, Wedlund PJ, Noone RM, et al. Pharmacokinetics of high-dose etoposide (VP-16-213) administered to cancer patients. Cancer Res 1984;44:379–382.

108. Rodman JH, Murry DJ, Madden T, et al. Altered etoposide pharmacokinetics and time to engraftment in pediatric patients undergoing autologous bone marrow transplantation. J Clin Oncol 1994;12:2390–2397.

109. Allen LM, Creaven PJ. Comparison of the human pharmacokinetics of VM-26 and VP-16, two antineoplastic epipodophyllotixin glucopyranoside derivatives. Eur J Cancer 1975;11:697–707.

110. Stewart CF, Arbuck SG, Fleming RA, et al. Changes in the clearance of total and unbound etoposide in patients with liver dysfunction. J Clin Oncol 1990;8:1874–1879.

111. Arbuck SG, Douglass HO, Crom WR, et al. Etoposide pharmacokinetics in patients with normal and abnormal organ function. J Clin Oncol 1986;4:1690–1695.

112. D'Incalci M, Rossi C, Zucchetti M, et al. Pharmacokinetics of etoposide in patients with abnormal renal and hepatic function. Cancer Res 1986;46: 2566–2571.

113. van Schaik RH. CYP450 pharmacogenetics for personalizing cancer therapy. Drug Resist Updat 2008;11:77–98.

114. Clark PI, Slevin ML. The clinical pharmacology of etoposide and teniposide. Clin Pharmacokinet 1987;12:223–252.

115. D'Incalci M, Farina P, Sessa C, et al. Pharmacokinetics of VP16-213 given by different administration methods. Cancer Chemother Pharmacol 1982;7:141–145.

116. Suzuki S, Koide M, Sakamoto S, et al. Pharmacokinetics of carboplatin and etoposide in a haemodialysis patient with Merkel-cell carcinoma. Nephrol Dial Transplant 1997;12:137–140.

117. Hande KR, Wolff SN, Greco FA, et al. Etoposide kinetics in patients with obstructive jaundice. J Clin Oncol 1990;8:1101–1107.

118. Stremetzne S, Jaehde U, Schunack W. Determination of the cytotoxic catechol metabolite of etoposide (□□□-demethyletoposide) in human plasma by high-performance liquid chromatography. J Chromatogr B Biomed Sci Appl 1997;703:209–215.

119. Mans DR, Lafleur MV, Westmijze EJ, et al. Formation of different reaction products with single- and double-stranded DNA by the ortho-quinone and the semi-quinone free radical of etoposide (VP-16-213). Biochem Pharmacol 1991;42:2131–2139.

120. Mans DR, Lafleur MV, Westmijze EJ, et al. Reactions of glutathione with the catechol, the ortho-quinone and the semi-quinone free radical of etoposide. Consequences for DNA inactivation. Biochem Pharmacol 1992;43:1761–1768.

121. Stewart CF, Fleming RA, Arbuck SG, et al. Prospective evaluation of a model for predicting etoposide plasma protein binding in cancer patients. Cancer Res 1990;50:6854–6856.

122. Vecht CJ, Wagner GL, Wilms EB. Interactions between antiepileptic and chemotherapeutic drugs. Lancet Neurol 2003;2:404–409.

123. Einhorn LH, Williams SD, Chamness A, et al. High-dose chemotherapy and stem-cell rescue for metastatic germ-cell tumors. N Engl J Med 2007; 357:340–348.

124. Leyvraz S, Pampallona S, Martinelli G, et al. A threefold dose intensity treatment with ifosfamide, carboplatin, and etoposide for patients with small cell lung cancer: a randomized trial. J Natl Cancer Inst 2008;100: 533–541.

125. Howell SB, Kirmani S, Lucas WE, et al. A phase II trial of intraperitoneal cisplatin and etoposide for primary treatment of ovarian epithelial cancer. J Clin Oncol 1990;8:137–145.

126. O'Dwyer PJ, LaCreta FP, Daugherty JP, et al. Phase I pharmacokinetic study of intraperitoneal etoposide. Cancer Res 1991;51:2041–2046.

127. Holoye PY, Jeffries DG, Dhingra HM, et al. Intrapleural etoposide for malignant effusion. Cancer Chemother Pharmacol 1990;26:147–150.

128. Fleischhack G, Reif S, Hasan C, et al. Feasibility of intraventricular administration of etoposide in patients with metastatic brain tumours. Br J Cancer 2001;84:1453–1459.

129. van der Gaast A, Sonneveld P, Mans DR, et al. Intrathecal administration of etoposide in the treatment of malignant meningitis: feasibility and pharmacokinetic data. Cancer Chemother Pharmacol 1992;29:335–337.

130. Savaraj N, Feun LG, Lu K, et al. Clinical pharmacology of intracarotid etoposide. Cancer Chemother Pharmacol 1986;16:292–294.

131. Toffoli G, Corona G, Basso B, et al. Pharmacokinetic optimisation of treatment with oral etoposide. Clin Pharmacokinet 2004;43:441–466.

132. Stewart DJ, Nundy D, Maroun JA, et al. Bioavailability, pharmacokinetics, and clinical effects of an oral preparation of etoposide. Cancer Treat Rep 1985;69:269–273.

133. Hande KR, Krozely MG, Greco FA, et al. Bioavailability of low-dose oral etoposide. J Clin Oncol 1993;11:374–377.

134. Harvey VJ, Slevin ML, Joel SP, et al. The effect of food and concurrent chemotherapy on the bioavailability of oral etoposide. Br J Cancer 1985;52:363–367.

135. Miller AA, Tolley EA, Niell HB. Therapeutic drug monitoring of 21-day oral etoposide in patients with advanced non-small cell lung cancer. Clin Cancer Res 1998;4:1705–1710.

136. Budman DR, Igwemezie LN, Kaul S, et al. Phase I evaluation of a water-soluble etoposide prodrug, etoposide phosphate, given as a 5-minute infusion on days 1, 3, and 5 in patients with solid tumors. J Clin Oncol 1994;12:1902–1909.

137. Millward MJ, Newell DR, Mummaneni V, et al. Phase I and pharmacokinetic study of a water-soluble etoposide prodrug, etoposide phosphate (BMY-40481). Eur J Cancer 1995;31A:2409–2411.

138. Fields SZ, Igwemezie LN, Kaul S, et al. Phase I study of etoposide phosphate (etopophos) as a 30-minute infusion on days 1, 3, and 5. Clin Cancer Res 1995;1:105–111.

139. Kaul S, Igwemezie LN, Stewart DJ, et al. Pharmacokinetics and bioequivalence of etoposide following intravenous administration of etoposide phosphate and etoposide in patients with solid tumors. J Clin Oncol 1995;13:2835–2841.

140. Sessa C, Zucchetti M, Cerny T, et al. Phase I clinical and pharmacokinetic study of oral etoposide phosphate. J Clin Oncol 1995;13:200–209.

141. de Jong RS, Mulder NH, Uges DR, et al. Randomized comparison of etoposide pharmacokinetics after oral etoposide phosphate and oral etoposide. Br J Cancer 1997;75:1660–1666.

142. Postmus PE, Smit EF, Berendsen HH, et al. Treatment of brain metastases of small cell lung cancer with teniposide. Semin Oncol 1992;19:89–94.

143. Smit EF, Ousterhuis BE, Berendsen HH, et al. Phase I study of oral teniposide (VM-26). Semin Oncol 1992;19:35–39.

144. Splinter TA, Holthuis JJ, Kok TC, et al. Absolute bioavailability and pharmacokinetics of oral teniposide. Semin Oncol 1992;19:28–34.

145. Mick R, Ratain MJ. Modeling interpatient pharmacodynamic variability of etoposide. J Natl Cancer Inst 1991;83:1560–1564.

146. Ratain MJ, Mick R, Schilsky RL, et al. Pharmacologically based dosing of etoposide: a means of safely increasing dose intensity. J Clin Oncol 1991;9:1480–1486.

147. Stewart CF, Arbuck SG, Fleming RA, et al. Relation of systemic exposure to unbound etoposide and hematologic toxicity. Clin Pharmacol Ther 1991;50:385–393.

148. Gentili D, Zucchetti M, Torri V, et al. A limited sampling model for the pharmacokinetics of etoposide given orally. Cancer Chemother Pharmacol 1993;32:482–486.

149. Lum BL, Lane KJ, Synold TW, et al. Validation of a limited sampling model to determine etoposide area under the curve. Pharmacotherapy 1997;17:887–890.

150. You B, Tranchand B, Girard P, et al. Etoposide pharmacokinetics and survival in patients with small cell lung cancer: a multicentre study. Lung Cancer 2008;62:261–272.

151. O'Dwyer PJ, Weiss RB. Hypersensitivity reactions induced by etoposide. Cancer Treat Rep 1984;68:959–961.

152. Karnaoukhova L, Moffat J, Martins H, Glickman B. Mutation frequency and spectrum in lymphocytes of small cell lung cancer patients receiving etoposide chemotherapy. Cancer Res 1997;57:4393–4407.

153. Armstrong GT, Liu Q, Yasui Y, et al. Late mortality among 5-year survivors of childhood cancer: a summary from the Childhood Cancer Survivor Study. J Clin Oncol 2009;27:2328–2338.

154. Felix CA. Secondary leukemias induced by topoisomerase-targeted drugs. Biochim Biophys Acta 1998;1400:233–255.

155. Smith MA, Rubinstein L, Anderson JR, et al. Secondary leukemia or myelodysplastic syndrome after treatment with epipodophyllotoxins. J Clin Oncol 1999;17:569–577.

156. Le Deley MC, Leblanc T, Shamsaldin A, et al. Risk of secondary leukemia after a solid tumor in childhood according to the dose of epipodophyllo-

157. Pui CH, Relling MV, Behm FG, et al. L-asparaginase may potentiate the leukemogenic effect of the epipodophyllotoxins. Leukemia 1995;9:1680–1684.

158. Pedersen-Bjergaard J, Rowley JD. The balanced and the unbalanced chromosome aberrations of acute myeloid leukemia may develop in different ways and may contribute differently to malignant transformation. Blood 1994;83:2780–2786.

159. Pedersen-Bjergaard J, Pedersen M, Roulston D, et al. Different genetic pathways in leukemogenesis for patients presenting with therapy-related myelodysplasia and therapy-related acute myeloid leukemia. Blood 1995;86:3542–3552.

160. Pedersen-Bjergaard J, Daugaard G, Hansen SW, et al. Increased risk of myelodysplasia and leukaemia after etoposide, cisplatin, and bleomycin for germ-cell tumours. Lancet 1991;338:359–363.

161. Pommier Y, Cockerill PN, Kohn KW, et al. Identification within the simian virus 40 genome of a chromosomal loop attachment site that contains topoisomerase II cleavage sites. J Virol 1990;64:419–423.

162. Mistry AR, Felix CA, Whitmarsh RJ, et al. DNA topoisomerase II in therapy-related acute promyelocytic leukemia. N Engl J Med 2005;352:1529–1538.

163. Azarova AM, Lyu YL, Lin CP, et al. From the cover: roles of DNA topoisomerase II isozymes in chemotherapy and secondary malignancies. Proc Natl Acad Sci USA 2007;104:11014–11019.

164. Hijiya N, Ness KK, Ribeiro RC, et al. Acute leukemia as a secondary malignancy in children and adolescents: current findings and issues. Cancer 2009;115:23–35.

165. Meyers M, Theodosiou M, Acharya S, et al. Cell cycle regulation of the human DNA mismatch repair genes hMSH2, hMLH1, and hPMS2. Cancer Res 1997;57:206–208.

166. Boothman DA, Fukunaga N, Wang M. Down-regulation of topoisomerase I in mammalian cells following ionizing radiation. Cancer Res 1994;54:4618–426.

167. Goldwasser F, Bae I, Pommier Y, et al. Evidence of a reduced DNA topoisomerase II mRNA expression after ionizing radiation. Anticancer Res 1999;19:3167–3171.

168. Albain KS, Crowley JJ, Turrisi AT III, et al. Concurrent cisplatin, etoposide, and chest radiotherapy in pathologic stage IIIB non-small-cell lung cancer: a Southwest Oncology Group phase II study, SWOG 9019. J Clin Oncol 2002;20:3454–3460.

169. Edelman MJ, Chansky K, Gaspar LE, et al. Phase II trial of cisplatin/etoposide and concurrent radiotherapy followed by paclitaxel/carboplatin consolidation for limited small-cell lung cancer: Southwest Oncology Group 9713. J Clin Oncol 2004;22:127–132.

170. Turrisi AT III, Kim K, Blum R, et al. Twice-daily compared with once-daily thoracic radiotherapy in limited small-cell lung cancer treated concurrently with cisplatin and etoposide. N Engl J Med 1999;340:265–271.

171. Hanna N, Neubauer M, Yiannoutsos C, et al. Phase III study of cisplatin, etoposide, and concurrent chest radiation with or without consolidation docetaxel in patients with inoperable stage III non-small-cell lung cancer: the Hoosier Oncology Group and U.S. Oncology. J Clin Oncol 2008;26:5755–5760.

172. Jackman DM, Johnson BE. Small-cell lung cancer. Lancet 2005;366:1385–1396.

173. Kanzawa F, Nishio K, Fukuoka K, et al. Evaluation of synergism by a novel three-dimensional model for the combined action of cisplatin and etoposide on the growth of a human small-cell lung-cancer cell line, SBC-3. Int J Cancer 1997;71:311–319.

174. Gentet JC, Brunat-Metigny M, Demaille MC, et al. Ifosfamide and etoposide in childhood osteosarcoma. A phase II study of the French Society of Paediatric Oncology. Eur J Cancer 1997;33:232–237.

175. Chou TC, Motzer RJ, Tong Y, Bosl GJ. Computerized quantitation of synergism and antagonism of taxol, topotecan, and cisplatin against human teratocarcinoma cell growth: a rational approach to clinical protocol design. J Natl Cancer Inst 1994;86:1517–1524.

176. Eder JP, Teicher BA, Holden SA, et al. Ability of four potential topoisomerase II inhibitors to enhance the cytotoxicity of cis-diamminedichloroplatinum (II) in Chinese hamster ovary cells and in an epipodophyllotoxin-resistant subline. Cancer Chemother Pharmacol 1990;26:423–428.

Proteasome Inhibitors

Igor Espinoza-Delgado, Monica G. Chiaramonte, Richard D. Swerdlow, and John J. Wright

The ubiquitin-proteasome pathway (UPP) is a tightly regulated process that, through the degradation of intracellular proteins, plays a major role in the cell biology and homeostasis of both normal cells and cancer cells.[1] Alterations in this pathway may lead to cell dysfunction.[2] Enormous efforts have been conducted over the last two decades to obtain a better understanding of this process. Given that intracellular proteolytic mechanisms are ubiquitous in all cells, it is easy to understand why early investigators thought that targeting such a process in tumor cells might be challenging due to both potential low therapeutic index and lack of tumor specificity. The FDA approval of bortezomib for the treatment of selected hematological malignancies has validated the proteasome as a therapeutic target and has prompted basic researchers and clinicians to identify and develop novel proteasome inhibitors (PIs) and also to define potential mechanisms of tumor resistance to the current PI. This chapter summarizes the molecular basis, preclinical development, and early clinical trials of investigational agents targeting the proteasome pathway.

Chemistry, Structure, and Function

Several classes of synthetic and natural products have the capacity to inhibit proteasomal activity through different mechanisms. Their structures have provided a model upon which many new analogs have been synthesized with better and more specific inhibitory effects against the 20S proteasome. Based on their inhibitory mechanisms, PI could be functionally divided into five classes (Fig. 21-1 and Table 21-1).

Class A (Peptide Aldehydes)

This class includes MG115 and MG132. They are tripeptide aldehydes and one of the most commonly used compounds of this class. They have potent inhibitory activity against the chymotryptic-like component of the 20S proteasome.[3] The N-terminal threonine of the proteasome interacts with the aldehyde moiety of the inhibitor forming a covalent hemiacetal adduct.[4] This is a reversible reaction and peptide aldehydes are rapidly oxidized into inactive compounds and transported out of the cell by the multidrug resistance (MDR) system. Most aldehyde-based PIs are relatively nonspecific.[5]

Class B (Peptide Boronates)

Sustained efforts to develop novel compounds with high specificity led to the identification of a new class of compounds that were synthetic reversible peptide amides and boronic acid derivatives. Bortezomib

(Figs. 21-1 and 21-5), a reversible PI, preferentially inhibits the β5-mediated chymotrypsin-like and β1-mediated peptidyl-glutamyl peptide hydrolyzing (PGPH)-like activities of the proteasome through interaction between the boronic acid on bortezomib and the threonine on β5 or β1 subunits on the proteasome.[6,7] The inhibitory potency and selectivity for the proteasome are excellent when compared to other PIs (Table 21-1). In contrast with class A compounds, boronates are not inactivated by oxidation and are not influenced by the MDR system. Bortezomib has been approved by the FDA for the treatment of multiple myeloma (MM) and mantle cell lymphoma (MCL).[8,9] CEP-18770 (Figs. 21-1 and 21-5), a novel orally active inhibitor of the chymotrypsin-like activity of the proteasome, inhibits nuclear factor kappa B (NF-κB)–mediated signaling pathways.[10] CEP-18770 induces apoptotic cell death in MM cell lines and in primary purified CD138-positive cells from untreated and bortezomib-treated MM patients. Compared to bortezomib, CEP-18770 exhibits a favorable cytotoxicity profile toward normal human endothelial cells, bone marrow progenitors, and bone marrow stromal cells. In vitro, CEP-18770 has a strong antiangiogenic activity and potently represses osteoclastogenesis compared with bortezomib, suggesting a potential benefit in managing the osteolytic-related morbidity and mortality associated with MM and other conditions with increased bone turnover.

Class C (β-Lactones)

To this class belongs lactacystin, one of the first identified natural PI.[11] Lactacystin and its active component clasto-lactacystin are structurally complex compounds, which makes its synthesis and clinical use difficult and expensive.[11–13] They have potent antitumor activity and induce cell cycle arrest in tumor cell lines.[14,15] However, lactacystin derivatives are not highly selective and inhibit several proteases, limiting their specificity and therapeutic potential. Another class member, salinosporamide A, also known as NPI-0052 (Figs. 21-1 and 21-5), was isolated from a marine bacterium.[16] Its structure is similar to clasto-lactacystin (Fig. 21-1) and inhibits chymotrypsin-like activity of the proteasome more potently than other β-lactones with an IC$_{50}$ of 0.7 nM. In contrast with bortezomib, salinosporamide A inhibits all three activities of the proteasome (chymotrypsin-like, trypsin-like, and caspase-like activities)[17] in an irreversible manner.[18–20] Salinosporamide A has strong synergistic activity in preclinical models[21] and is being evaluated in early clinical trials.[22–24]

Class D (Epoxyketones)

The first compounds of this class were originally isolated from an unidentified strain of actinomycete. Epoxomicin was identified and characterized as a highly specific inhibitor of the 20S proteasome.[25]

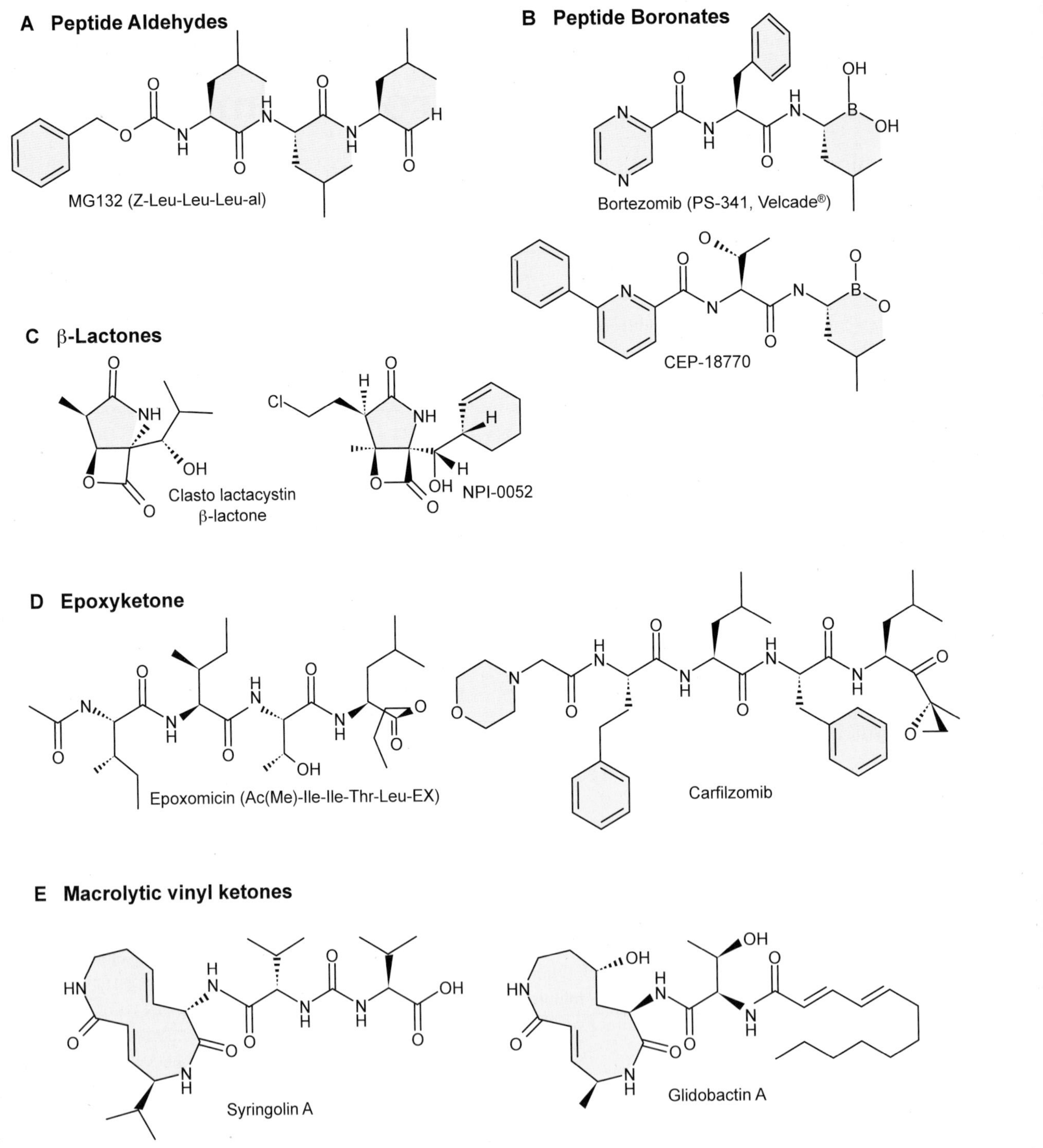

A   Peptide Aldehydes

MG132 (Z-Leu-Leu-Leu-al)

B   Peptide Boronates

Bortezomib (PS-341, Velcade®)

CEP-18770

C   β-Lactones

Clasto lactacystin
β-lactone

NPI-0052

D   Epoxyketone

Epoxomicin (Ac(Me)-Ile-Ile-Thr-Leu-EX)

Carfilzomib

E   Macrolytic vinyl ketones

Syringolin A

Glidobactin A

FIGURE **21-1**   Classes of PIs.

Carfilzomib (Figs. 21-1 and 21-5), structurally related to epoxomicin, has also been identified as an irreversible PI.[26] Carfilzomib has a major specificity for the chymotrypsin-like activity of the proteasome, is also more potent than bortezomib, and could even be active in the setting of bortezomib-resistant cells. Carfilzomib is being evaluated in early phase I and phase II clinical trials.[27–29]

Class E

Syringolin A was isolated from *Pseudomonas syringae* and irreversibly inhibits chymoptrypsin- trypsin- and caspase-like activity of

the proteasome.[30,31] Similarly, glidobactin A, also a bacterial product,[32] inhibits both chymotrypsin-like and trypsin-like activities of the proteasome.[30] These compounds have both antiproliferative and proapoptotic activities.

The Ubiquitin-Proteasome Pathway

The UPP has a major role in regulating a broad number of fundamental cellular pathways including apoptosis,[33] cell growth and

TABLE

21.1 *Proteasome inhibitors: specificity for 20S proteasome catalytic subunits*

Association constants ka ($M^{-1} s^{-1}$) or other values as indicated

Inhibitor Classes	CT-L	T-L	PGPH	In vivo	Cross-reactivity	Reference
A Peptide aldehydes						
MG132	K_i 4.0 nM	K_i 2,760 nM	K_i 900 nM	0.4 µM	Calpain, cathepsins	42, 186, 187
B Peptide boronates						
Bortezomib[a]	53,000 IC_{50} 0.62 nM	150	3,200	0.02 µM	None found	111, 188, 189
CEP-18770[b]	IC_{50} 3.8 nM	IC_{50} >100 nM	IC_{50} ~70 nM	1.2 mg/kg IV[c] 10 mg/kg PO		10
C β-Lactones						
Clasto-lactacystin	7,400	68	47	ND	Cathepsin A, TPPII	190
Salinosporamide A[b]	IC_{50} 3.5 nM	IC_{50} 28 nM	IC_{50} 430 nM	0.15 mg/kg IV[c]		19
D Epoxyketones						
Epoxomicin	20,000	300	40	0.03 µM	None found	191
Carfilzomib[b]	~170 nM[a]	~1,100 nM[a]	~1,800 µM[a]	ND		26
E Macrocyclic vinyl ketones						
Syringolin A	863 K_i 846 nM	94 K_i 6.7 nM	6 —	ND		30
Glidobactin A	3380 K_i 49 nM	141 K_i 2.0 µM	ND	ND		30

K_i: Inhibition constant; IC_{50}: 50% inhibition concentration; EC_{50}: Half saturated binding of inhibitor to active site;
[a] FDA approved.
[b] In clinical trials.
[c] Maximum tolerated dose (MTD) in mice.

proliferation,[34] DNA repair,[35] unfolded protein response (UPR),[33,36] and immune response.[37] Alterations in these pathways have been implicated in multiple diseases, particularly cancer. Therefore, compounds interfering with proteasome functions may have a major impact on cancer cell fate.

Broadly speaking, the UPP consists of two major components: the ubiquitinating enzyme complex (UEC) and the degradation system (26S proteasome). Three enzymes make up the UEC, the ubiquitin-activating enzyme (E1), the ubiquitin-conjugating enzyme (E2), and the ubiquitin-conjugating ligase (E3). E1 is a generic enzyme used

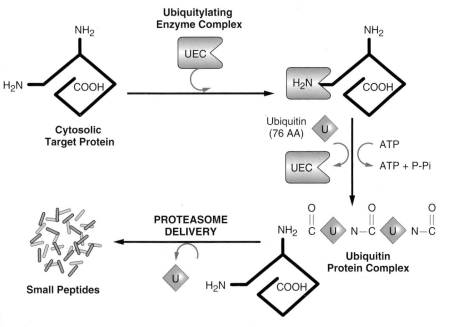

FIGURE **21-2** Schema of the ubiquitin-proteasome pathway.

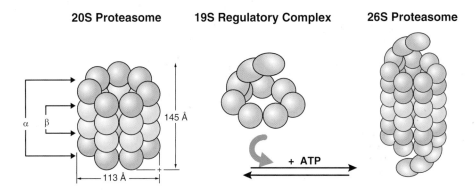

20S Proteasome

19S Regulatory Complex

26S Proteasome

145 Å

113 Å

+ ATP

- **STACK OF FOUR 7 MEMBERED RINGS; 700 kd; 2,000 kd**
- **700 kDa**
- **14 distinct subunits**
- **Broad substrate specificity**
- **Catalytic nucleophile: Thr of β subunit**

- **2,000 kDa**
- **Degrades ubiquitinated proteins**
- **Proteolysis is ATP-dependent**

FIGURE **21-3**   Structure of the 26S proteasome and its assembly.

by the pathways regardless of the protein substrate targeted. By contrast, there are 20 to 30 different ubiquitin-conjugating enzymes (E2) and likely hundreds of E3 ligases. The ligase steps are the points where the specificity of the ubiquitylation process is controlled, with most protein substrates having their own distinct ligase.[38,39] Each of these enzymes represents a potential therapeutic target offering unique ways to specifically inhibit the degradation of a very selective protein or groups of proteins. The initial step involves the binding of the UEC to the N-terminus of the target (Fig. 21-2). This enzyme complex catalyzes the covalent linkage of ubiquitin molecules to the ε-amino moieties of internal lysine residues in a processive manner. These ATP-dependent catalytic reactions eventually lead to the generation of a branched polyubiquitylated protein. This ubiquitylation process is the primary means by which the cells "tag" or "earmark" specific proteins for degradation at the 26S proteasome.

The second major component of the pathway includes the proteasome (Fig. 21-3), which is composed of two structures, the 20S proteasome and the 19S regulatory subunit. Collectively they form a complex called the 26S proteasome.[40] The isolated 20S proteasome does not exhibit proteolytic activity in the absence of the 19S regulatory subunit. The 19S subunit mediates the ATP-dependent process of denaturing and unfolding the ubiquitin conjugates. The 26S proteasome is a large structure with highly processive threonine proteolytic activity, and as a result it cleaves polypeptides at multiple sites, releasing very small peptides ranging in length from 2 to 24 amino acids.[41-43]

The 19S regulatory subunit includes multiple peptidases that disassemble and unfold the polyubiquitin conjugates. It also plays a major role in regulating and facilitating the multiple ATP-dependent processes used by the proteasome including 20S and 19S subunits assembly, protein unfolding, ubiquitylation, opening of the regulatory "gate" that allows the protein to enter the 26S lumen, and the action of the isopeptidases leading to the recycling of the ubiquitin molecules.[44]

The 20S proteasome consists of four rings, each containing seven individual globular proteins. As shown in Figure 21-3, the assembly of the rings forms a central lumen through which proteins are funneled. The two outer layers of the 20S proteasome are the

α-layers that allow anchorage of the 19S regulatory subunit. The two inner rings are the β-layers containing the proteolytic activity of the proteasome. The 19S subunit sits on top and bottom of the 20S subunit, controlling the entry of ubiquitylated proteins into the core of the proteasome.[44] Once the protein enters the lumen of the proteasome, the different proteases digest the protein into smaller peptides fragments. At least three different enzymatic activities have been ascribed to the β-layers, including (1) a peptidylglutamyl activity (β1) cleaving proteins near glutamate residues, (2) a tryptic-like function (β2) that cleaves proteins near lysine and arginine residues; and (3) a chymotryptic-like function (β5) that cleaves proteins near phenylalanine, tyrosine, and tryptophan.[40,45-48] Figure 21-4 shows the targets of several PIs that are in the clinic including bortezomib, carfilzomib, salinosporamide A, and CEP-18770.

Cross-sectional view of the β ring

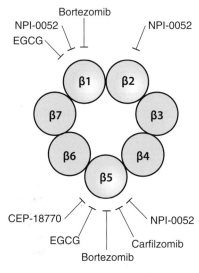

Bortezomib

NPI-0052

EGCG

NPI-0052

β1   β2

β7   β3

β6   β4

β5

CEP-18770

NPI-0052

EGCG   Carfilzomib

Bortezomib

FIGURE **21-4**   Cross-sectional view of the B-ring and the binding of PIs to the chymotryptic-like protease.

NF-κB, Endoplasmic Reticulum Stress, Unfolded Protein Response, and Apoptosis

One of the first observations suggesting the possibility that PIs could be used as anticancer agents was the early discovery that proteasome inhibition could lead to inactivation of NF-κB by stabilizing IκB and preventing the translocation of NF-κB to the nucleus.[49,50] NF-κB family is composed of several members including RELA, RELB, REL (cREL), NF-κB1, and NF-κB2. These proteins form heterodimeric and homodimeric complexes and their activities are regulated by two pathways known as the classical or canonical pathway and the alternative or noncanonical pathway.[51] In both pathways, ubiquitylation and degradation of critical components lead to translocation of RELA-p50 dimers (canonical pathway) and REL-p52 and REL-p50 (noncanonical) to the nucleus followed by binding to target gene DNA.[52–55] Abnormal regulation of NF-κB and the signaling pathways that control its activity are involved in cancer development and progression.[56] NF-κB activation affects all hallmarks of cancer through the transcription of genes involved in cell proliferation, angiogenesis, metastasis, inflammation, and suppression of apoptosis.[56–61] Constitutive activation of NF-κB has been described in several solid tumors as well as in a number of hematological malignancies including MM.[62–64] Moreover, leukemia, lymphoma, and MM cells have been reported to undergo apoptosis upon treatment with various inhibitors of NF-κB signaling including PIs.[65–69] Inhibition of NF-κB correlates with a decrease in the expression of antiapoptotic and antiproliferative genes such as BCL$_{XL}$, XIAP, cIAP2, interleukin (IL)-6, and cyclin D1.[62,70–72] Furthermore, interaction of bone marrow stromal cells with MM cells leads to NF-κB activation and promotes tumor growth.[73,74] Bortezomib is approved by the FDA for the treatment of MM and its efficacy is at least in part due to inhibition of NF-κB activity. Indeed, gene expression DNA microarray analysis has established a correlation between NF-κB signature and clinical outcome.[75]

The endoplasmic reticulum (ER) is an organelle that has an essential role in multiple cellular processes that are required for cell homeostasis and survival. ER stress (ERS), a condition typically associated with accumulation of misfolded or unfolded proteins in the lumen of the ER, triggers an evolutionarily conserved response termed the unfolded protein response (UPR).[76] Cell response to UPR is first to adapt and reestablish cell homeostasis by increasing the protein folding capacity of the ER.[77,78] The UPR-induced alarm refers to signal transduction events that are commonly associated with cellular stress, including activation of MAPKs, JNK, and p38 MAPK. In addition, kinases responsible for activation of NF-κB may be induced.[77] Finally, when the adaptive mechanisms put in place by the UPR fail to counteract the ERS, then cell death is induced through different mechanisms.[79–82] The important roles of ERS and the UPR in tumor biology make them novel therapeutic targets in cancer. Bortezomib induces ERS-mediated apoptosis in tumor cells.[83–86]

Interestingly, ERS has also been implicated in the antitumor effects of cisplatin and geldanamycin.[87–89] Bortezomib enhances ERS induced by both compounds, resulting in increased antitumor activity in an orthotopic pancreatic cancer xenograft model.[86] Cells exposed to bortezomib form aggregates of ubiquitin-conjugated proteins, or "aggresomes," *in vitro* and *in vivo*.[90] Bortezomib-induced aggresome formation may serve a cytoprotective role by allowing cells to dispose of accumulated unfolded proteins that result from proteasome dysfunction[91] and could represent a mechanism of resistance to bortezomib. Notably, bortezomib-induced aggresome formation could be disrupted using histone deacetylase (HDAC) 6 small interfering RNA or chemical HDAC inhibitors.[86,92,93] These events result in ERS and induction of apoptosis in pancreatic cancer cells, MM, and chronic myeloid leukemia (CML).[94–96] These results provided the rationale for the development of the combination of bortezomib and vorinostat in patients with refractory and relapsed MM patients.[97] The results of this phase I trial are encouraging and have prompted further development of the combination in other tumor histologies including non-Hodgkin's lymphoma (NHL), soft tissue sarcoma, and glioblastoma multiforme. ERS is probably related to the strong activity of bortezomib in MM patients where highly secretory plasma cells may overload the ER. The preclinical and early clinical results suggest that bortezomib-mediated disruption of the UPR represents a novel strategy to enhance the antitumor activity of agents that induce cell death via a classic ERS-dependent mechanism.

Effects on Cell Cycle Regulation

Control of cell cycle transition points depends heavily on both transcriptional and posttranscriptional mechanisms. The orderly degradation of key regulatory proteins though the UPP allows for the coordinated progression of cells through the different stages of the cell cycle, mitosis and proliferation. Inhibition of the degradation of any of the key proteins that control this well-orchestrated process can have profound consequences on cell cycle kinetics and tumor growth. Treatment of human colon cancer lines with the PI lactacystin leads to cell cycle arrest mediated by p21 accumulation.[98] Another well-established cell cycle control mechanism revolves around cyclin B, the synthesis of which begins early in the S phase, accumulating during G2 and early mitosis. Progression into and through anaphase is dependent on the degradation of cyclin B, which is regulated through ubiquitylation and proteolytic degradation by the proteasome.[99] Similarly, progression to S phase from G1 is regulated by the cyclin E-CDK2 complex. Association of this complex with p27 is responsible for inhibiting the kinase activity leading to cell cycle arrest.[100,101] P27 is also a target of the proteasome.[100,102,103] Therefore, a potential important mechanism of action of PIs is to disrupt normal regulation of cell cycle kinetics. The relevance of these findings is not completely clear; however, studies have shown that most MCLs have a decreased or lost expression of p27 with normal p27 mRNA.[104,105] Furthermore, overexpression of p53 and lost expression of p27 in patients with MCL correlate with a significant reduction in overall survival.[104]

Pharmacology

Preclinical models have extensively demonstrated that PIs have potent anticancer activities. Lactacystin induces cell death in leukemia cells at concentration of about 5 μM,[67] and bortezomib inhibits tumor growth in a broad variety of tumor models.[106–108] Normal cells were found to be more resistant to PIs than tumor cells.[109,110] Furthermore, within the dose range of bortezomib that induces tumor growth inhibition in xenograft models, normal hematopoietic cells seem not to be significantly affected by the cytotoxic effects of bortezomib. Boronate PIs have been shown to kill tumor cells in culture, as demonstrated by their activity in the tumor cell line screen.[111] Data from the NCI's algorithm COMPARE demonstrated that the mechanism of cytotoxicity of bortezomib was strikingly different from any of the other 60,000 compounds in the library. The average growth inhibition for bortezomib was 7 nM across the entire panel of cells. In prostate cancer cell lines, bortezomib induces G2-M growth arrest that was associated with the accumulation of p21 and p27. Cell death was noted at 20 nM for cells incubated for 24 hours with bortezomib.[111] Studies with radiolabeled bortezomib have shown that bortezomib is broadly distributed to all tissues in rats and cynomolgus monkeys and no detectable drug could be found crossing the blood-brain barrier.[111] *In vivo* models of drug-resistant human myeloma have shown that a twice weekly schedule of bortezomib administration resulted both in tumor shrinkage and prolonged median survival of treated mice.[112,113]

Clinical Pharmacology

Studies on nonhuman primates have shown that after a single intravenous dose of bortezomib, plasma concentrations decline in a classic biphasic manner with a $t_{1/2} \alpha$ of approximately 10 minutes.[114] The terminal elimination phase in humans has been estimated between 5 and 15 hours. Multiple doses of drug appear to result in some decrease in clearance, with a resulting increase in the terminal elimination half-life ($t_{1/2}$) and the area under the curve (AUC), but they have no effect on the estimated maximum plasma concentration (C_{max}) or distribution half-life. Similar pharmacokinetic profiles have also been observed in preclinical studies and do not appear to result in increased toxicity from accumulation of the drug with repeat dosing. The overall disposition of bortezomib is most consistent with a two-compartment pharmacokinetics (PK) model and the principal pathway of elimination is through oxidative deboronation. Based on *in vitro* studies, the major phase 1 metabolic reactions are mediated by cytochrome P450 isoforms 3A4 and 2C19.[115] Bortezomib exposure is increased in the presence of ketoconazole, a potent CYP3A inhibitor. On the other hand, omeprazole, a potent inhibitor of CYP2C19, has no significant effect on the exposure of bortezomib.

Pharmacokinetics of Bortezomib in Patients with Renal and Liver Dysfunction

A study by Mulkerin et al.[116] assessed the PK and pharmacodynamic profiles of bortezomib in patients with advanced malignancies and normal, mild, moderate, or severe renal insufficiency. The study was designed to evaluate safety and tolerability, as well as to determine the maximum tolerated dose (MTD) of bortezomib in this patient population.

Exposure to bortezomib was comparable among all groups and was not affected by the degree of renal impairment.

A PK study is being conducted, by the National Cancer Institute Organ Dysfunction Group, in patients with various degree of hepatic impairment who were classified according to the NCI classification of hepatic impairment (Table 21-2). Patients received bortezomib doses ranging from 05 to 1.3 mg/m². An interim analysis revealed that the exposure of bortezomib was increased in patients with moderate and severe hepatic impairment. Therefore, in this population, bortezomib should be started at lower dose and patients monitored closely.

Pharmacodynamics

Proteasome inhibition has been established as a critical pharmacodynamic endpoint for bortezomib. Bortezomib induces inhibition of the 20S proteasome in a dose-dependent manner.[117–119] The majority of the proteasome inhibition occurs within the 1st hour after administration and proteasome inhibition around 10% to 20% could be detected at 72 hours. This pharmacodynamic endpoint was the rationale for the scheduling of bortezomib once every 72 hours.

Bortezomib Single-Agent Phase I Experience

To date, several phase I studies with bortezomib in patients with hematological malignancies and solid tumors have been completed (Table 21-3). These phase I experiences have explored weekly and twice-weekly intravenous bolus schedules. In general, the pattern of toxicity paralleled what was noted in the preclinical findings. In the phase I study conducted by Papandreou et al.,[119] bortezomib was administered weekly for 4 weeks every 6 weeks establishing 1.6 mg/m² as the MTD on this schedule. The authors noted that hypotension and syncope were dose-limiting toxicities on the

---

TABLE

21.2   *NCI classification of hepatic impairment*

Liver function	Group A normal	Group B mild	Group B2 mild	Group C moderate	Group D severe
Bilirubin	≤ ULN	≤ ULN	>1.0–1.5 × ULN	>1.5–3 × ULN	>3 × ULN
SGOT/AST	≤ ULN	> ULN	Any	Any	Any

ULN: Upper limit of normal.

TABLE

21.5 Summary of select phase I combination studies of bortezomib

Disease	Agents (dose)	n	MTD	DLTs	CR	PR	Duration of response (mo)	Comments	Reference
NHL/CLL	Bortezomib (0.7–1.3 mg/m²); Fludarabine; Rituximab	24	Bortezomib 1.3 mg/m²; Fludarabine 25 mg/m²; Rituximab 375 mg/m²	Neutropenia, thrombocytopenia	3	8	3–36+	6 SDs	155
NSCLC	Bortezomib (1–1.3 mg/m²); Gemcitabine (Gem); Carboplatin	26	Bortezomib 1 mg/m²; Gem 1000 mg/m²; Carboplatin AUC 5	Febrile neutropenia, thrombocytopenia, hyponatremia		9		8 SDs Median PFS 4 mo; Median OS 9 mo	161
Ovarian/ peritoneal/ fallopian	Bortezomib (0.75–1.5 mg/m²); Carboplatin	14	Bortezomib 1.3 mg/m²; Carboplatin AUC 5	Diarrhea, rash, sensory neuropathy, constipation	2	5		4 SDs	120
MM	Bortezomib (1–1.3 mg/m²); Vorinostat	23	Bortezomib 1.3 mg/m²; Vorinostat 400 mg daily	Fatigue, QT prolongation		2 VGPR 7 PR		3 PRs in bortezomib-refractory pts	97
Advanced malignancies	Bortezomib (1 mg/m²); Oxaliplatin	30	Bortezomib 1 mg/m²; Oxaliplatin 85 mg/m²	Neurotoxicity		4		6 SDs	195
Advanced malignancies	Bortezomib (0.7–1.5 mg/m²); Vorinostat	22	Bortezomib 1.3 mg/m²; Vorinostat 400 mg daily	Fatigue, hyponatremia, elevated ALT		1	>9	PR in pt with soft tissue sarcoma	165
Advanced malignancies	Bortezomib (1.3 mg/m²); Vorinostat	29	Bortezomib 1.3 mg/m²; Vorinostat 300 mg BID	Fatigue, elevated ALT					196
Advanced malignancies	Bortezomib (0.7–1.7 mg/m²); Sorafenib	12	Bortezomib 1 mg/m²; Sorafenib 200 mg BID	Abdominal pain, lipase, vomiting		1		PR in pt with renal tumor and 4 SDs	197

n, number of patients; Pts, patients; MM, multiple myeloma; NHL, non-Hodgkin's lymphoma; CLL, chronic lymphocytic leukemia; NSCLC, non-small cell lung cancer; CR, complete response; PR, partial response; SD, stable disease; VGPR, very good partial response; mo, months; MTD, maximum tolerated dose; DLT, dose-limiting toxicity; OS, overall survival; PFS, progression-free survival; TTP, time-to-progression; NR, not reported; ND, not determined.

21.6 *Summary of select phase II combination studies of bortezomib*

Disease	Combination agent	N	ORR	CR	Comments	Reference
Advanced gastric adenocarcinoma	Irinotecan	28	44% versus 9% bortezomib alone	0%	Median PFS 1.9 mo versus 1.4 bortezomib alone Median OS 4.1 mo versus 5.4 bortezomib alone	166
Hepatocellular carcinoma	Doxorubicin	39	2.3%		10 SDs Median PFS 2.4 mo Median OS 5.7 mo	198
NSCLC	Gemcitabine, carboplatin	114	23%	NR	ORR + SD = 68% Median OS 11 mo Survival rates: at 1 y = 47%, at 2 y = 19%	162

n, number of patients; NSCLC, non-small cell lung cancer; ORR, overall response rate; CR, complete response; PR, partial response; SD, stable disease; mo, months; OS, overall survival; PFS, progression-free survival; TTP, time-to-progression; NR, not reported; ND, not determined.

with bortezomib. The primary endpoint was the time to disease progression. The time to progression among patients receiving bortezomib (bortezomib group) was 24 months, as compared with 16.6 months among those receiving melphalan-prednisone alone (control group) (hazard ratio for the bortezomib group, 0.48; $P < 0.001$). Patients with a PR or better were 71% in the bortezomib group and 35% in the control group; CR rates were 30% and 4%, respectively ($P < 0.001$). The median duration of the response was 19.9 months in the bortezomib group and 13.1 months in the control group. The hazard ratio for overall survival was 0.61 for the bortezomib group ($P = 0.008$). There were no significant differences in grade 4 events (28% and 27%, respectively) or treatment-related deaths (1% and 2%). This regimen is now labeled for first-line use.

Studies using cell line models of chronic lymphocytic leukemia have shown synergistic cytotoxicity with the combination of fludarabine and bortezomib.[153] Fludarabine is a potent cytotoxic agent that inhibits DNA polymerase and ribonucleotide reductase, thus terminating DNA strand replication. It is suggested that bortezomib may inhibit repair of the fludarabine-induced DNA lesions, thus potentiating the antineoplastic effect. In addition, bortezomib-induced down-regulation of NF-κB may counteract fludarabine resistance.[154] Using the combination of bortezomib, fludarabine, and rituximab, Barr et al.[155] reported significant antitumor activity in patients with relapsed and refractory indolent and mantle cell NHL. An overall response of 45% was observed in 11 of 24 evaluable patients, with a clinical benefit rate of 71%. Two of the three patients achieving CR have shown no relapse disease at 1 and 3 years, respectively. Moreover, the study showed that 5 of 12 patients who were refractory to their last therapy regimen achieved an objective response. The most notable adverse effects of this combination were neutropenia and thrombocytopenia, which caused treatment delays and interruptions; therefore, it is recommended that future studies using this combination include a hematopoietic growth factor.

Encouraging results were reported in patients with NSCLC treated with bortezomib in combination with gemcitabine and carboplatin, cytotoxic agents with demonstrated activity in this patient population. Bortezomib is already known to induce growth inhibition and apoptosis in lung cancer cells[156–158] and has shown mild activity in NSCLC.[118,140] The addition of bortezomib to gemcitabine *in vitro* has previously demonstrated synergistic activity[107,159] and showed no additive toxicity in phase I trials.[160] In a phase I combination trial, Davies et al.[161] reported data on 20 evaluable patients with advanced disease and demonstrated that the combination of bortezomib 1 mg/m^2, gemcitabine 1,000 mg/m^2, and carboplatin AUC 5.0 has manageable toxicities and significant antitumor activity in NSCLC, with nine PRs and eight stable diseases. Additionally, a phase II study with this combination[162] also showed significant results in chemotherapy-naïve patients with advanced NSCLC. A final analysis of 114 patients reported an ORR of 23%, with a disease control rate (response rate + stable disease) of 68%, with median survival rates of 47% and 19% at 1 and 2 years, respectively.

In a phase I study on solid tumors, Aghajanian et al.[120] reported data on 15 patients with recurrent or progressive epithelial ovarian cancer or primary peritoneal carcinoma treated with the combination of bortezomib and carboplatin. Four of the 15 patients were platinum-resistant. Among 14 evaluable patients, there were two CRs (one in a platinum-resistant patient) and five PRs (all in platinum-sensitive patients). An additional four patients experienced stable disease as their best response. The two patients who had CRs normalized their CA125. Of the five patients who experienced a PR, three had normalized CA125 and one had a greater than 50% decline in CA125. Of the four stable diseases, two had normalized CA125, one had a greater than 50% decline in CA125, and one had a stable CA125.

Preclinical data have also supported the potential synergistic activity of bortezomib with HDAC inhibitors, such as vorinostat.[95,96] HDAC inhibitors affect several cellular functions through different mechanisms, including modulation of chromatin structure,[163] upregulation of death receptors, induction of oxidative injury, disruption of chaperon protein function, and disruption of aggresome formation, among others.[92,93,164] The combination of bortezomib and vorinostat has been shown to diminish NF-κB activation and induction of p21CIP1,[94] as well as XIAP/Bcl-xL down-regulation.[71] Badros et al.[97] reported data on the first clinical trial of a regimen combining bortezomib with vorinostat in heavily pretreated relapsed and refractory MM patients. The MTD was determined to be vorinostat 400 mg daily for 8 days and bortezomib 1.3 mg/m^2 on days 1, 4, 8, and 11 of a 21-day cycle. The adverse effects were mild-to-moderate and included hematologic and gastrointestinal toxicities and fatigue. Prolonged QTc was noted in a number of patients, but it was not clinically significant. Interestingly, a limited number of patients (9 of 21, 42%) achieved objective responses, including two very good PRs and seven PRs. It is noteworthy that three of the nine responses occurred in bortezomib-refractory patients. Phase II clinical trials of this combination in relapsed and in bortezomib refractory patients are ongoing. These encouraging results warrant further evaluation of this combination in this patient population. Interestingly, a phase I study of this combination was conducted in patients with solid tumors and two PRs were observed: one in patient with NSCL cancer and one in a patient with refractory soft tissue sarcoma. Phase II studies on these two populations of patients are being conducted and will provide further information about efficacy of the combination in solid tumors.[165]

In a phase II study conducted by Ocean et al.[166] patients with adenocarcinoma of the stomach or gastroesophageal junction were treated with the combination of bortezomib with irinotecan, which has shown significant tumor shrinkage activity in previous preclinical studies. For previously treated patients, bortezomib was administered at 1.3 mg/m^2, and for previously untreated patients bortezomib 1.3 mg/m^2 was administered in combination with irinotecan at 125 mg/m^2. In 36 evaluable patients, the response rate was 44% for the combination versus 9% in patients receiving bortezomib alone, demonstrating that the combination is active in first-line therapy.

The future development of bortezomib will depend on the toxicity and efficacy of this agent in combination with other conventional and investigational agents. Preclinical data support the notion that PIs may be synergistic with other novel classes of drugs, including HDACs, cyclin-dependent kinase inhibitors like flavopiridol, and the bcl-2 targeting antisense molecule G3139 (Genasense).[70,145,167] What remains to be clarified from a pharmacologic perspective is the importance of scheduling these agents and defining the optimal concentrations of these drugs for inhibiting their principal targets. For example, in some in vivo models of NHL, the activity of the bcl-2 antisense molecule G3139 with cyclophosphamide and bortezomib was found to be very schedule dependent. Better results were seen using antisense bcl-2 first followed by cyclophosphamide and then followed 24 hours later by bortezomib.[145] Combinations of many standard chemotherapy drugs are often given together. Such approaches, while certainly more convenient for the patient, often disregard compelling preclinical evidence of schedule dependency. The burden is now on both laboratory and physician scientists to understand these scheduling phenomena and then to elucidate the biological basis for the schedule dependency. In addition to sorting out these critical pharmacologic questions with this new class of molecules, it is apparent that understanding the molecular basis for the response or nonresponse of certain patients will be absolutely critical in the development of new classes of drugs.

Bortezomib Resistance

Although the significant antitumor activity of bortezomib in MM patients has been extensively demonstrated, not all patients respond to therapy and most of the responders will ultimately relapse. The ability of bortezomib to overcome the poor prognosis of conventional anti-MM therapies strongly suggests that sensitivity versus resistance to bortezomib is determined by different molecular mechanisms than those determining responsiveness to conventional therapy. Extensive efforts have been put forward to identify specific molecular markers of resistance to bortezomib; however, to date, no predictive markers of resistance or sensitivity have been validated for clinical use.

Nevertheless, several studies have investigated gene expression profiles specific to MM patients treated with bortezomib, specifically in the phase 2 Summit and CREST trials and the APEX phase 3 trial.[126,128] Gene expression profiling in these patients revealed response and survival classifiers that were shown to be significantly associated with outcome via testing on independent data. In addition, predictive models and biologic correlates of response showed some specificity for bortezomib rather than dexamethasone.[75] While these studies provided interesting evidence regarding the molecular mechanisms behind bortezomib resistance, the heterogeneity of the patient population evaluated precluded a general application of these markers. Studies using acute lymphoblastic leukemia cell line models have suggested that mutations in the proteasome β5 subunit (PSMB5) protein might play a role in bortezomib resistance.[165] However, studies of this particular mutation have not confirmed a role in MM.[169,170]

A number of hypotheses have been proposed to account for resistance to bortezomib in solid tumors. One possibility could be related to the trial design targeting chemotherapy-exposed populations, including patients who have received the chemotherapeutic agent paired with bortezomib. A way to potentially reduce resistance to PIs would be by randomization of naïve patients to chemotherapy or a combination of chemotherapy with a PI.[171] Another way to enhance efficacy might involve the appropriate sequencing of bortezomib and the other combination agent. Indeed, a preclinical study has shown that synergy between bortezomib and cytarabine was sequence dependent,[172] while another study showed that bortezomib inhibited docetaxel activity in a p21-dependent fashion, when given prior to the chemotherapeutic agent.[173]

Another explanation of resistance to PIs could be found in bortezomib's greater activity against cyclin D–driven tumors[174]; therefore, trials designed to specifically target patients with these molecular patterns may prove beneficial. In addition, it has been postulated that activity of the NF-κB pathway predicted the highest response rate to bortezomib in MM,[175,176] particularly in tumors that contain activating NF-κB mutations; therefore, enriching for this population could also be of benefit. Consequently, the consensus appears to be that better results in solid tumors could be expected with an appropriate selection of patients with disease whose molecular determinants predict for responsiveness. The complexity of the mechanisms of action and resistance of bortezomib has been underscored by a report demonstrating that bortezomib significantly down-regulated IκBα expression and triggered NF-κB activation in MM cell lines and primary tumor cells from MM patients.[177] The study may represent a paradigm shift and implies that bortezomib-induced cytotoxicity cannot be fully attributed to inhibition of canonical NF-κB activity in MM cells.

Finally, secondary or acquired resistance is also emerging as an important issue to explore more extensively. Indeed, it has been demonstrated that the ability of bortezomib to reinduce a response in patients with previously sensitive disease is 31% to 60%,[178,179] with the higher rates reflecting the addition of other agents. In all, further preclinical and clinical studies are needed to find new strategies to overcome the resistance to PIs and outline the most efficient approaches in selective patient populations.

Novel Proteasome Inhibitors

To overcome some of the potential mechanisms of resistance to bortezomib, second-generation of PIs such as CEP-18770, salinosporamide A (NPI-0052), and carfilzomib have been developed and are in early clinical trials (Tables 21-7 and 21-8).

CEP-18770 is a novel orally active peptide boronate inhibitor of the proteasome (Fig. 21-5) that downmodulates NF-κB activity and the expression of several NF-κB downstream effectors.[10] CEP-18770 induces apoptotic cell death in both MM cell lines and in primary purified CD138-positive explant cultures from untreated and bortezomib-treated MM patients. It represses RANKL-induced osteoclastogenesis and exhibits a favorable cytotoxicity profile toward normal human epithelial cells, bone marrow progenitors, and bone marrow–derived stromal cells. Intravenous and oral administration of CEP-18770 resulted in a more sustained pharmacodynamic inhibition of proteasome activity in tumors relative to normal tissues, complete tumor regression of MM xenografts, and improved overall median survival in a systemic model of human MM. Two phase I clinical trials are recruiting patients to receive IV CEP-18770 in two different schedules (Table 21-7).

NPI-0052, a β-lactone similar to clasto-lactacystin (Fig. 21-5) inhibits all three activities of the proteasome enzyme activities[17] in an irreversible manner.[18–20] NPI-0052 A has shown strong synergistic activity in preclinical models[180] and is currently being evaluated in early clinical trials.[22–24] NPI-0052 was administered IV on days 1, 8 and 15 of 28-day cycles in a 3+3 design dose escalation to a recommended phase 2 dose (RP2D). Thirty patients were treated at doses ranging from 0.1 mg/m² to 0.9 mg/m²; 0.7 mg/m² was selected as the RP2D secondary to dose-limiting toxicities of visual disturbances and dizziness/unsteady gait at 0.9 mg/m². At the RP2D PK data showed $t_{1/2}$ = 31 ± 28 minutes; AUC_{total} = 270 ± 219 ng/mL*minute; C_{max} = 33.4 ± 34.2 ng/mL; CL = 7.17 ± 0.40 L/min; volume of distribution(V_d) = 223.3 ± 229.7 L. Proteasome inhibition assays indicated a dose-response relationship with mean inhibition of chymotrypsin-like activity up to of 88% on day 1 and 100% on day 15, and inhibition of caspase-like and trypsin-like activity of up to 51% and 72%, respectively. Stable disease was observed in 31% of patients, including one each with MCL, Hodgkin's lymphoma, follicular lymphoma, sarcoma, prostate carcinoma, and two with melanoma. This preliminary data demonstrate that NPI-0052 produces dose-dependent pharmacologic effects through the predicted efficacious range to an MTD, while producing a toxicity profile that is tolerable and dissimilar to bortezomib. Additional studies are being initiated in hematologic malignancies and solid tumors alone and in combination[181] (Table 21-7).

Carfilzomib, structurally related to epoxomicin, is an irreversible PI.[26] Therefore, proteasome inhibition is more sustained with carfilzomib than with bortezomib. Carfilzomib has a major specificity for the chymotrypsin-like activity of the proteasome and is also more potent than bortezomib and could even be active in the setting of bortezomib-resistant cells. Carfilzomib is being evaluated in early phase I and phase II clinical trials[27–29] (Table 21-8).

In a phase I trial evaluating the safety and efficacy of carfilzomib in relapsed or refractory hematologic malignancies, O'Connor et al. reported that patients received 5 consecutive days of carfilzomib IV push at doses ranging from 1 to 20 mg/m² within 14-day cycles.[28] The study recruited 29 patients who were relapsed or refractory after at least two prior therapies. Nonhematologic toxicities included fatigue, nausea, and diarrhea in more than one third of patients—mostly grade 1 or 2 in severity. At 20 mg/m², grade 3 febrile neutropenia and grade 4 thrombocytopenia were reported, establishing 15 mg/m² as the MTD. No grade 3 or 4 peripheral neuropathies were reported. Antitumor activity was observed at doses ≥11 mg/m²: one unconfirmed CR (MCL), one PR (MM), and two minimal responses (MM and Waldenström's macroglobulinemia). This is the first clinical use of carfilzomib that shows tolerability and clinical activity in multiple hematologic malignancies. The phase II results of a phase Ib/II study of carfilzomib assessed the MTD, safety, efficacy, PK, and pharmacodynamics of carfilzomib in patients with advanced metastatic solid tumors failing ≥2 prior treatments.[182] Patients received carfilzomib IV day 1, 2, 8, 9, 15 and 16 every 28 days for up to 12 cycles. There were 6 small cell lung cancer (SCLC), 10 NSCLC, 11 ovarian, 6 renal, and 18 other cancer patients enrolled. The most common AEs included fatigue headache, diarrhea, nausea, and constipation. Notable was the absence of grade 1 peripheral neuropathy and severe hematologic toxicities. The study shows that carfilzomib is active as a single agent in relapsed solid tumors demonstrating PR in both renal and SCLC; and SD >16 wks in mesothelioma, ovarian, renal, and NSCLC. The 20/36 mg/m² daily on day 1 and 2 dose schedule was well tolerated, which make carfilzomib an appealing agent to combine with chemotherapy or novel targeted agents.

New Strategies

In light of the therapeutic success of bortezomib in MM and MCL, new interest is shifting toward the possibility of targeting other components of the UPP. As the main driver of regulated protein degradation, it has become clear that defects in this pathway are responsible for a variety of human pathologies, including cancer and neurodegenerative diseases.[38] The ultimate goal is to develop inhibitors that target specific ubiquitylation pathways that are essential for tumor cell growth but not for normal cell growth.

As substrate selection in the UPP is driven by the ubiquitin ligases, they represent one of the most apparent targets for inhibition. The ubiquitin ligases are a diverse group of enzymes with very different catalytic mechanisms, providing both unique opportunities and challenges for small molecule-targeted therapy. Several alternatives are being pursued in preclinical studies, targeting different components of this pathway; however, a few of those are currently available for clinical trials.[38] One promising inhibitory strategy focuses on blocking binding of the ligases to the substrate, instead of inhibiting the catalytic domain of the proteasome. One

TABLE

21.7 *Active studies with new generation PIs CEP-18770 and NPI-0052*

Agent	Condition	Intervention	Phase/design	Objectives	Dose (mg/m²)	Schedule/cycle/ length treatment	Estimated accrual (n)	Status	Results
CEP-18770	Relapsed/refractory MM	Single agent (IV)	Phase 1/ nonrandomized open-label study	MTD, ORR, TTP, TTR	Starting dose: 1.5	Days 1, 8, 15/28-day cycle/8 cycles	67	Recruiting participants	
	Relapsed/refractory solid tumors/NHL	Single agent (IV)	Phase 1/ nonrandomized open-label study/ safety study	DLTs/MTD/PK/ efficacy	Starting dose: 0.1	Days 1, 4, 8, 11/21-day cycle/6 cycles	55	Recruiting participants	
NPI-0052	NSCLC, Pancreatic cancer, Melanoma, Lymphoma	NPI-0052 (IV) + vorinostat (PO)	Phase 1/ nonrandomized open-label study	MTD/RP2D/PK/ Pd safety/ efficacy		NPI-0052 weekly/ vorinostat daily	40	Recruiting participants	
	Solid tumors/ refractory lymphoma	Single agent (IV)	Phase 1/ nonrandomized open-label study	MTD/PK/Pd/ efficacy		3× every 28 d	50	Recruiting participants	39 pts treated. RP2D: 0.8 mg/m² DLTs: hallucinations, dizziness/ unsteady gait Response: SDs[23]
	MM	Single agent (IV)	Phase 1/ nonrandomized open-label study	MTD/RP2D/PK/ Pd/safety efficacy		Days 1, 8, 15/28-day cycle	35	Recruiting participants	

MM, multiple myeloma; NSCLC, non-small cell lung cancer; IV, intravenous; PO, orally; MTD, maximum tolerated dose; DLT, dose-limiting toxicities;; PK, pharmacokinetics; Pd, pharmacodynamics; RP2D, recommended phase 2 dose; ORR, overall response rate; TTP, time-to-progression; TTR, time-to-response; Pts, patients; SD, stable disease.

TABLE

21.8   *Active studies with new generation PI Carfilzomib (CFZ)*

Condition	Intervention	Phase/design	Objectives	Dose (mg/m²)	Schedule/cycle/length treatment	Estimated accrual (n)	Status	Results
Relapsed/RefractoryMM/Renal insufficiency	Single agent (IV)	Phase 2/nonrandomized open-label study	Safety/PK		Days 1,2,8,9,15,16/28-d cycle	36	Recruiting participants	
MM	CFZ (IV) + Len (PO) + Dex (IV or PO)	Phase 1b/2/nonrandomized open-label study/active control	Ph 1b: safety/MTD/Ph 2: ORR, PFS, TRP, OS	CFZ: Ph 1: dose escalation Ph 2: at MTD Len 25 mg Dex 40 mg	Ph 1 and Ph 2: CFZ: days 1,2,8,9,15,16 (cycles 1–8: induction); days 1, 2, 15, 16 (cycles 9+: maintenance) Len: Days 1–21 (cycles 1–8+); Dex between 30 min and 4 h preceding CFZ 28-d cycles	25	Recruiting participants	
Relapsed MM	CFZ (IV) + Len (PO) + Dex (IV or PO)	Phase 1b/nonrandomized open-label study	Safety/MTD PK	CFZ 15–20 Len 10–20 mg Dex 40 mg	First 12 cycles: CFZ 2x weekly for 3 wk/28-d cycle. Remaining six cycles: 2x weekly for wk 1 and 3/28-d cycle	55	Ongoing	No hem/renal DLTs; Responses: CFZ 15/Len 10 (n = 6): 3 PR/2 SD CFZ 15/Len 15 (n = 2): 1 PR/1 MR[199]
Relapsed MM	Arm 1 (active control): Len (PO) + Dex (IV or PO) Arm 2 (Exp): CFZ (IV) + Len (PO) + Dex (IV or PO)	Ph 3/randomized/open-label/active control	PFS/OS/ORR/DOR/TTP	Arm 1: Dex 40 mg/Len 25 mg Arm 2: Dex 40 mg Len 25 mg CFZ: 20, 27 mg/m²	Dex: Days 1, 8, 15, 22 Len: Days 1–21; CFZ: cycles 1–12: six doses/cycle; cycles 13–18: four doses/cycle 28-day cycle	700	Not yet open	

MM, multiple myeloma; CFZ, carfilzomib; Len, lenalidomide; Dex, dexamethasone; IV, intravenous; PO, orally; MTD, maximum tolerated dose; DLT, dose-limiting toxicities; PK, pharmacokinetics; Pd, pharmacodynamics; RP2D, recommended phase 2 dose; PFS, progression-free survival; ORR, overall response rate; TTP, time-to-progression; DOR, duration of response; Pts, patients; PR, partial response; MR, minor response; SD, stable disease.

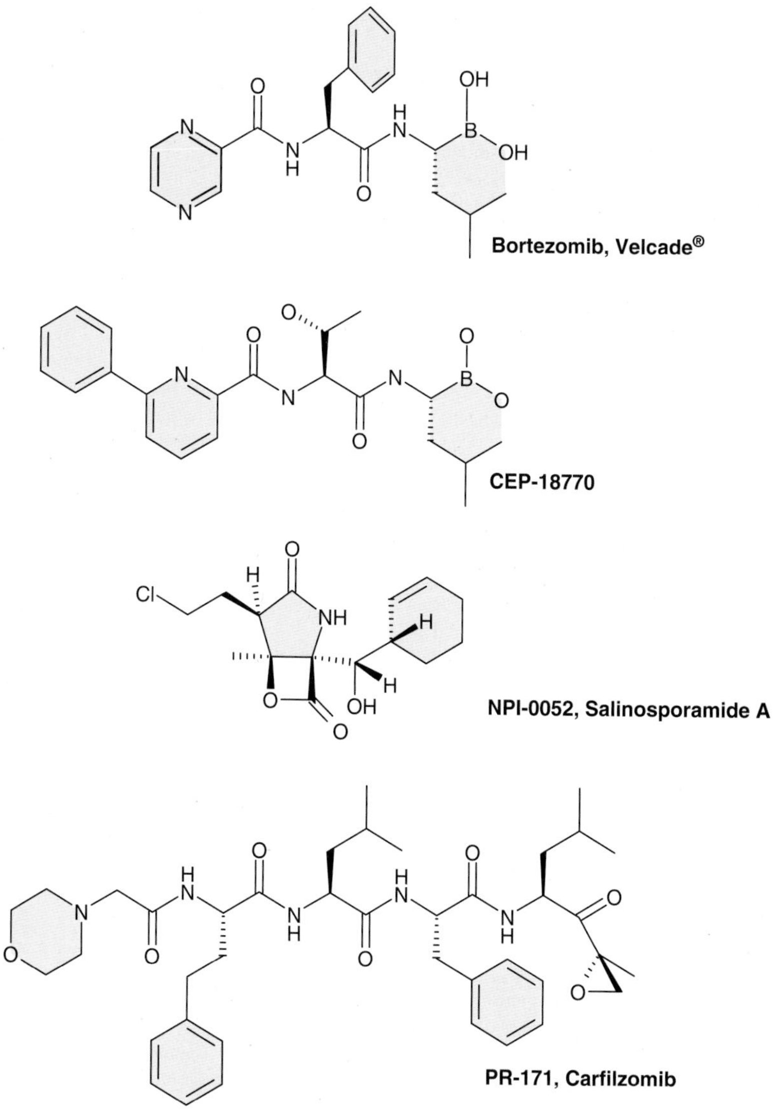

Bortezomib, Velcade®

CEP-18770

NPI-0052, Salinosporamide A

PR-171, Carfilzomib

FIGURE **21.5** PIs in clinical trials.

of the best characterized inhibitors using this approach are the Nutlins,[39] which particularly target the Mdm2-p53 binding and are currently most advanced in the drug development process. The precise mechanism of action of these compounds was revealed in a crystal structure showing the Nutlin binding to Mdm2 in a manner almost identical to p53.[38] This compound inhibits p53 degradation in cells and reduces tumor growth in an *in vivo* xenograft model. Compounds from this series are expected to be evaluated in early clinical trials.

Another interesting therapeutic target is the immunoproteasome.[183] The identification of specific immunoproteasome inhibitors[184,185] may allow for improvements in the selectivity and efficacy of this approach. In addition, the selective expression of the immunoproteasome in hematopoietic tissues could potentially alleviate the neurotoxicity or gastrointestinal effects induced by the regular PIs, since those tissues express lower levels of immunoproteasome subunits.

The extensive list of new PIs being evaluated preclinically brings promising prospects to the ultimate goal of finding efficient and selective agents for cancer therapy.

References

1. Hoeller D, Hecker CM, Dikic I. Ubiquitin and ubiquitin-like proteins in cancer pathogenesis. Nat Rev Cancer 2006;6(10):776–788.
2. Rubinsztein DC. The roles of intracellular protein-degradation pathways in neurodegeneration. Nature 2006;443(7113):780–786.
3. Rock KL, Gramm C, Rothstein L, et al. Inhibitors of the proteasome block the degradation of most cell proteins and the generation of peptides presented on MHC class I molecules. Cell 1994;78(5):761–771.
4. Tsukamoto S, Yokosawa H. Targeting the proteasome pathway. Expert Opin Ther Targets 2009;13(5):605–621.
5. Vinitsky A, Cardozo C, Sepp-Lorenzino L, et al. Inhibition of the proteolytic activity of the multicatalytic proteinase complex (proteasome) by substrate-related peptidyl aldehydes. J Biol Chem 1994;269(47):29860–29866.
6. Adams J. The development of proteasome inhibitors as anticancer drugs. Cancer Cell 2004;5(5):417–421.
7. Dou QP, Goldfarb RH. Bortezomib (millennium pharmaceuticals). IDrugs 2002;5(8):828–834.
8. Bross PF, Kane R, Farrell AT, et al. Approval summary for bortezomib for injection in the treatment of multiple myeloma. Clin Cancer Res 2004;10(12 Pt 1):3954–3964.
9. Kane RC, Dagher R, Farrell A, et al. Bortezomib for the treatment of mantle cell lymphoma. Clin Cancer Res 2007;13(18 Pt 1):5291–5294.

10. Piva R, Ruggeri B, Williams M, et al. CEP-18770: a novel, orally active proteasome inhibitor with a tumor-selective pharmacologic profile competitive with bortezomib. Blood 2008;111(5):2765–2775.

11. Fenteany G, Standaert RF, Lane WS, et al. Inhibition of proteasome activities and subunit-specific amino-terminal threonine modification by lactacystin. Science 1995;268(5211):726–731.

12. Corey EJ, Li WD. Total synthesis and biological activity of lactacystin, omuralide and analogs. Chem Pharm Bull (Tokyo) 1999;47(1):1–10.

13. Dick LR, Cruikshank AA, Grenier L, et al. Mechanistic studies on the inactivation of the proteasome by lactacystin: a central role for clasto-lactacystin beta-lactone. J Biol Chem 1996;271(13):7273–7276.

14. Fenteany G, Standaert RF, Reichard GA, et al. A beta-lactone related to lactacystin induces neurite outgrowth in a neuroblastoma cell line and inhibits cell cycle progression in an osteosarcoma cell line. Proc Natl Acad Sci U S A 1994;91(8):3358–3362.

15. Katagiri M, Hayashi M, Matsuzaki K, et al. The neuritogenesis inducer lactacystin arrests cell cycle at both G0/G1 and G2 phases in neuro 2a cells. J Antibiot (Tokyo) 1995;48(4):344–346.

16. Feling RH, Buchanan GO, Mincer TJ, et al. Salinosporamide A: a highly cytotoxic proteasome inhibitor from a novel microbial source, a marine bacterium of the new genus salinospora. Angew Chem Int Ed Engl 2003;42(3):355–357.

17. Groll M, Huber R, Potts BC. Crystal structures of Salinosporamide A (NPI-0052) and B (NPI-0047) in complex with the 20S proteasome reveal important consequences of beta-lactone ring opening and a mechanism for irreversible binding. J Am Chem Soc 2006;128(15):5136–5141.

18. Berkers CR, Verdoes M, Lichtman E, et al. Activity probe for in vivo profiling of the specificity of proteasome inhibitor bortezomib. Nat Methods 2005;2(5):357–362.

19. Chauhan D, Catley L, Li G, et al. A novel orally active proteasome inhibitor induces apoptosis in multiple myeloma cells with mechanisms distinct from Bortezomib. Cancer Cell 2005;8(5):407–419.

20. Groll M, Berkers CR, Ploegh HL, et al. Crystal structure of the boronic acid-based proteasome inhibitor bortezomib in complex with the yeast 20S proteasome. Structure 2006;14(3):451–456.

21. Chauhan D, Singh A, Brahmandam M, et al. Combination of proteasome inhibitors bortezomib and NPI-0052 trigger in vivo synergistic cytotoxicity in multiple myeloma. Blood 2008;111(3):1654–1664.

22. Hamlin PA, Aghajanian C, Hong D, et al. First-in-human phase 1 dose escalation study of NPI-0052, a novel proteasome inhibitor, in patients with lymphoma and solid tumor. ASH Annual Meeting Abstracts 2008;112(11):A4939.

23. Hamlin PA, Aghajanian C, Younes A, et al. First-in-human phase I study of the novel structure proteasome inhibitor NPI-0052. J Clin Oncol (Meeting Abstracts) 2009;27(15S):A3516.

24. Richardson P, Hofmeister CC, Zimmerman TM, et al. Phase 1 clinical trial of NPI-0052, a novel proteasome inhibitor in patients with multiple myeloma. ASH Annual Meeting Abstracts 2008;112(11):A2770.

25. Hanada M, Sugawara K, Kaneta K, et al. Epoxomicin, a new antitumor agent of microbial origin. J Antibiot (Tokyo) 1992;45(11):1746–1752.

26. Kuhn DJ, Chen Q, Voorhees PM, et al. Potent activity of carfilzomib, a novel, irreversible inhibitor of the ubiquitin-proteasome pathway, against preclinical models of multiple myeloma. Blood 2007;110(9):3281–3290.

27. Jagannath S, Vij R, Stewart AK, et al. Initial results of PX-171–003, an open-label, single-arm, phase II study of Carfilzomib (CFZ) in patients with relapsed and refractory multiple myeloma (MM). ASH Annual Meeting Abstracts 2008;112(11):A864.

28. O'Connor OA, Stewart AK, Vallone M, et al. A phase 1 dose escalation study of the safety and pharmacokinetics of the novel proteasome inhibitor carfilzomib (PR-171) in patients with hematologic malignancies. Clin Cancer Res 2009;15(22):7085–7091.

29. Vij R, Wang M, Orlowski R, et al. Initial results of PX-171–004, an open-label, single-arm, phase II study of Carfilzomib (CFZ) in patients with relapsed myeloma (MM). ASH Annual Meeting Abstracts 2008;112(11):A865.

30. Groll M, Schellenberg B, Bachmann AS, et al. A plant pathogen virulence factor inhibits the eukaryotic proteasome by a novel mechanism. Nature 2008;452(7188):755–758.

31. Hassa P, Granado J, Freydl E, et al. Syringolin-mediated activation of the Pir7b esterase gene in rice cells is suppressed by phosphatase inhibitors. Mol Plant Microbe Interact 2000;13(3):342–346.

32. Amrein H, Makart S, Granado J, et al. Functional analysis of genes involved in the synthesis of syringolin A by Pseudomonas syringae pv. syringae B301 D-R. Mol Plant Microbe Interact 2004;17(1):90–97.

33. Chen ZJ. Ubiquitin signalling in the NF-kappaB pathway. Nat Cell Biol 2005;7(8):758–765.

34. Reed SI. The ubiquitin-proteasome pathway in cell cycle control. Results Probl Cell Differ 2006;42:147–181.

35. Huen MS, Chen J. The DNA damage response pathways: at the crossroad of protein modifications. Cell Res 2008;18(1):8–16.

36. Kostova Z, Tsai YC, Weissman AM. Ubiquitin ligases, critical mediators of endoplasmic reticulum-associated degradation. Semin Cell Dev Biol 2007;18(6):770–779.

37. Wang J, Maldonado MA. The ubiquitin-proteasome system and its role in inflammatory and autoimmune diseases. Cell Mol Immunol 2006;3(4):255–261.

38. Eldridge AG, O'Brien T. Therapeutic strategies within the ubiquitin proteasome system. Cell Death Differ 2010;17(1):4–13.

39. Vassilev LT, Vu BT, Graves B, et al. In vivo activation of the p53 pathway by small-molecule antagonists of MDM2. Science 2004;303(5659):844–848.

40. Adams J, Palombella VJ, Elliott PJ. Proteasome inhibition: a new strategy in cancer treatment. Invest New Drugs 2000;18(2):109–121.

41. Holzl H, Kapelari B, Kellermann J, et al. The regulatory complex of Drosophila melanogaster 26S proteasomes. Subunit composition and localization of a deubiquitylating enzyme. J Cell Biol 2000;150(1):119–130.

42. Kisselev AF, Akopian TN, Woo KM, et al. The sizes of peptides generated from protein by mammalian 26 and 20S proteasomes. Implications for understanding the degradative mechanism and antigen presentation. J Biol Chem 1999;274(6):3363–3371.

43. Nussbaum AK, Dick TP, Keilholz W, et al. Cleavage motifs of the yeast 20S proteasome beta subunits deduced from digests of enolase 1. Proc Natl Acad Sci U S A 1998;95(21):12504–12509.

44. Voges D, Zwickl P, Baumeister W. The 26S proteasome: a molecular machine designed for controlled proteolysis. Annu Rev Biochem 1999;68:1015–1068.

45. Ciechanover A. The ubiquitin-proteasome pathway: on protein death and cell life. EMBO J 1998;17(24):7151–7160.

46. Lee DH, Goldberg AL. Proteasome inhibitors: valuable new tools for cell biologists. Trends Cell Biol 1998;8(10):397–3403.

47. Spataro V, Norbury C, Harris AL. The ubiquitin-proteasome pathway in cancer. Br J Cancer 1998;77(3):448–455.

48. Zwickl P, Baumeister W, Steven A. Dis-assembly lines: the proteasome and related ATPase-assisted proteases. Curr Opin Struct Biol 2000;10(2):242–250.

49. Orlowski RZ, Baldwin Jr AS. NF-kappaB as a therapeutic target in cancer. Trends Mol Med 2002;8(8):385–389.

50. Palombella VJ, Rando OJ, Goldberg AL, et al. The ubiquitin-proteasome pathway is required for processing the NF-kappa B1 precursor protein and the activation of NF-kappa B. Cell 1994;78(5):773–785.

51. Ghosh S, May MJ, Kopp EB. NF-kappa B and Rel proteins: evolutionarily conserved mediators of immune responses. Annu Rev Immunol 1998;16:225–260.

52. Dejardin E, Droin NM, Delhase M, et al. The lymphotoxin-beta receptor induces different patterns of gene expression via two NF-kappaB pathways. Immunity 2002;17(4):525–535.

53. Derudder E, Dejardin E, Pritchard LL, et al. RelB/p50 dimers are differentially regulated by tumor necrosis factor-alpha and lymphotoxin-beta receptor activation: critical roles for p100. J Biol Chem 2003;278(26):23278–23284.

54. Ghosh S, Karin M. Missing pieces in the NF-kappaB puzzle. Cell 2002;109(Suppl):S81–S96.

55. Xiao G, Harhaj EW, Sun SC. NF-kappaB-inducing kinase regulates the processing of NF-kappaB2 p100. Mol Cell 2001;7(2):401–409.

56. Basseres DS, Baldwin AS. Nuclear factor-kappaB and inhibitor of kappaB kinase pathways in oncogenic initiation and progression. Oncogene 2006;25(51):6817–6830.

57. Burstein E, Duckett CS. Dying for NF-kappaB? Control of cell death by transcriptional regulation of the apoptotic machinery. Curr Opin Cell Biol 2003;15(6):732–737.

58. Cilloni D, Martinelli G, Messa F, et al. Nuclear factor kB as a target for new drug development in myeloid malignancies. Haematologica 2007;92(9):1224–1229.

59. Dutta J, Fan Y, Gupta N, et al. Current insights into the regulation of programmed cell death by NF-kappaB. Oncogene 2006;25(51):6800–6816.

60. Jost PJ, Ruland J. Aberrant NF-kappaB signaling in lymphoma: mechanisms, consequences, and therapeutic implications. Blood 2007;109(7):2700–2707.

61. Luo JL, Kamata H, Karin M. The anti-death machinery in IKK/NF-kappaB signaling. J Clin Immunol 2005;25(6):541–550.

62. Bharti AC, Donato N, Singh S, et al. Curcumin (diferuloylmethane) down-regulates the constitutive activation of nuclear factor-kappa B and Ikap-

paBalpha kinase in human multiple myeloma cells, leading to suppression of proliferation and induction of apoptosis. Blood 2003;101(3):1053–1062.

63. Hideshima T, Chauhan D, Richardson P, et al. NF-kappa B as a therapeutic target in multiple myeloma. J Biol Chem 2002;277(19):16639–16647.

64. Ni H, Ergin M, Huang Q, et al. Analysis of expression of nuclear factor kappa B (NF-kappa B) in multiple myeloma: downregulation of NF-kappa B induces apoptosis. Br J Haematol 2001;115(2):279–286.

65. Delic J, Masdehors P, Omura S, et al. The proteasome inhibitor lactacystin induces apoptosis and sensitizes chemo- and radioresistant human chronic lymphocytic leukaemia lymphocytes to TNF-alpha-initiated apoptosis. Br J Cancer 1998;77(7):1103–1107.

66. Hideshima T, Neri P, Tassone P, et al. MLN120B, a novel IkappaB kinase beta inhibitor, blocks multiple myeloma cell growth in vitro and in vivo. Clin Cancer Res 2006;12(19):5887–5894.

67. Imajoh-Ohmi S, Kawaguchi T, Sugiyama S, et al. Lactacystin, a specific inhibitor of the proteasome, induces apoptosis in human monoblast U937 cells. Biochem Biophys Res Commun 1995;217(3):1070–1077.

68. Jourdan M, Moreaux J, Vos JD, et al. Targeting NF-kappaB pathway with an IKK2 inhibitor induces inhibition of multiple myeloma cell growth. Br J Haematol 2007;138(2):160–168.

69. Shinohara K, Tomioka M, Nakano H, et al. Apoptosis induction resulting from proteasome inhibition. Biochem J 1996;317(Pt 2):385–388.

70. Dai Y, Pei XY, Rahmani M, et al. Interruption of the NF-kappaB pathway by Bay 11–7082 promotes UCN-01-mediated mitochondrial dysfunction and apoptosis in human multiple myeloma cells. Blood 2004;103(7):2761–2770.

71. Mitsiades N, Mitsiades CS, Poulaki V, et al. Biologic sequelae of nuclear factor-kappaB blockade in multiple myeloma: therapeutic applications. Blood 2002;99(11):4079–4086.

72. Sanda T, Iida S, Ogura H, et al. Growth inhibition of multiple myeloma cells by a novel IkappaB kinase inhibitor. Clin Cancer Res 2005;11(5):1974–1982.

73. Chauhan D, Uchiyama H, Akbarali Y, et al. Multiple myeloma cell adhesion-induced interleukin-6 expression in bone marrow stromal cells involves activation of NF-kappa B. Blood 1996;87(3):1104–1112.

74. Landowski TH, Olashaw NE, Agrawal D, et al. Cell adhesion-mediated drug resistance (CAM-DR) is associated with activation of NF-kappa B (RelB/p50) in myeloma cells. Oncogene 2003;22(16):2417–2421.

75. Mulligan G, Mitsiades C, Bryant B, et al. Gene expression profiling and correlation with outcome in clinical trials of the proteasome inhibitor bortezomib. Blood 2007;109(8):3177–3188.

76. Xu C, Bailly-Maitre B, Reed JC. Endoplasmic reticulum stress: cell life and death decisions. J Clin Invest 2005;115(10):2656–2564.

77. Kaneko M, Niinuma Y, Nomura Y. Activation signal of nuclear factor-kappa B in response to endoplasmic reticulum stress is transduced via IRE1 and tumor necrosis factor receptor-associated factor 2. Biol Pharm Bull 2003;26(7):931–935.

78. Wu J, Kaufman RJ. From acute ER stress to physiological roles of the Unfolded Protein Response. Cell Death Differ 2006;13(3):374–384.

79. Bernales S, McDonald KL, Walter P. Autophagy counterbalances endoplasmic reticulum expansion during the unfolded protein response. PLoS Biol 2006;4(12):e423.

80. Egger L, Schneider J, Rheme C, et al. Serine proteases mediate apoptosis-like cell death and phagocytosis under caspase-inhibiting conditions. Cell Death Differ 2003;10(10):1188–1203.

81. Levine B, Kroemer G. Autophagy in the pathogenesis of disease. Cell 2008;132(1):27–42.

82. Ogata M, Hino S, Saito A, et al. Autophagy is activated for cell survival after endoplasmic reticulum stress. Mol Cell Biol 2006;26(24):9220–931.

83. Fribley A, Zeng Q, Wang CY. Proteasome inhibitor PS-341 induces apoptosis through induction of endoplasmic reticulum stress-reactive oxygen species in head and neck squamous cell carcinoma cells. Mol Cell Biol 2004;24(22):9695–9704.

84. Landowski TH, Megli CJ, Nullmeyer KD, et al. Mitochondrial-mediated dysregulation of Ca2+ is a critical determinant of Velcade (PS-341/bortezomib) cytotoxicity in myeloma cell lines. Cancer Res 2005;65(9):3828–3836.

85. Lee AH, Iwakoshi NN, Anderson KC, et al. Proteasome inhibitors disrupt the unfolded protein response in myeloma cells. Proc Natl Acad Sci U S A 2003;100(17):9946–9951.

86. Nawrocki ST, Carew JS, Dunner K Jr, et al. Bortezomib inhibits PKR-like endoplasmic reticulum (ER) kinase and induces apoptosis via ER stress in human pancreatic cancer cells. Cancer Res 2005;65(24):11510–11519.

87. Mandic A, Hansson J, Linder S, et al. Cisplatin induces endoplasmic reticulum stress and nucleus-independent apoptotic signaling. J Biol Chem 2003;278(11):9100–9106.

88. Marcu MG, Doyle M, Bertolotti A, et al. Heat shock protein 90 modulates the unfolded protein response by stabilizing IRE1alpha. Mol Cell Biol 2002;22(24):8506–8513.

89. Mimnaugh EG, Xu W, Vos M, et al. Simultaneous inhibition of hsp 90 and the proteasome promotes protein ubiquitination, causes endoplasmic reticulum-derived cytosolic vacuolization, and enhances antitumor activity. Mol Cancer Ther 2004;3(5):551–566.

90. Hideshima T, Bradner JE, Wong J, et al. Small-molecule inhibition of proteasome and aggresome function induces synergistic antitumor activity in multiple myeloma. Proc Natl Acad Sci U S A 2005;102(24):8567–8572.

91. Garcia-Mata R, Gao YS, Sztul E. Hassles with taking out the garbage: aggravating aggresomes. Traffic 2002;3(6):388–396.

92. Bali P, Pranpat M, Bradner J, et al. Inhibition of histone deacetylase 6 acetylates and disrupts the chaperone function of heat shock protein 90: a novel basis for antileukemia activity of histone deacetylase inhibitors. J Biol Chem 2005;280(29):26729–26734.

93. Kawaguchi Y, Kovacs JJ, McLaurin A, et al. The deacetylase HDAC6 regulates aggresome formation and cell viability in response to misfolded protein stress. Cell 2003;115(6):727–738.

94. Mitsiades CS, Mitsiades NS, McMullan CJ, et al. Transcriptional signature of histone deacetylase inhibition in multiple myeloma: biological and clinical implications. Proc Natl Acad Sci U S A 2004;101(2):540–545.

95. Pei XY, Dai Y, Grant S. Synergistic induction of oxidative injury and apoptosis in human multiple myeloma cells by the proteasome inhibitor bortezomib and histone deacetylase inhibitors. Clin Cancer Res 2004;10(11):3839–3852.

96. Yu C, Rahmani M, Conrad D, et al. The proteasome inhibitor bortezomib interacts synergistically with histone deacetylase inhibitors to induce apoptosis in Bcr/Abl+ cells sensitive and resistant to STI571. Blood 2003;102(10):3765–3774.

97. Badros A, Burger AM, Philip S, et al. Phase I study of vorinostat in combination with bortezomib for relapsed and refractory multiple myeloma. Clin Cancer Res 2009;15(16):5250–5257.

98. Blagosklonny MV, Wu GS, Omura S, et al. Proteasome-dependent regulation of p21WAF1/CIP1 expression. Biochem Biophys Res Commun 1996;227(2):564–569.

99. Glotzer M, Murray AW, Kirschner MW. Cyclin is degraded by the ubiquitin pathway. Nature 1991;349(6305):132–138.

100. Polyak K, Lee MH, Erdjument-Bromage H, et al. Cloning of p27Kip1, a cyclin-dependent kinase inhibitor and a potential mediator of extracellular antimitogenic signals. Cell 1994;78(1):59–66.

101. Toyoshima H, Hunter T. p27, a novel inhibitor of G1 cyclin-Cdk protein kinase activity, is related to p21. Cell 1994;78(1):67–74.

102. Machiels BM, Henfling ME, Gerards WL, et al. Detailed analysis of cell cycle kinetics upon proteasome inhibition. Cytometry 1997;28(3):243–252.

103. Pagano M, Tam SW, Theodoras AM, et al. Role of the ubiquitin-proteasome pathway in regulating abundance of the cyclin-dependent kinase inhibitor p27. Science 1995;269(5224):682–685.

104. Chiarle R, Budel LM, Skolnik J, et al. Increased proteasome degradation of cyclin-dependent kinase inhibitor p27 is associated with a decreased overall survival in mantle cell lymphoma. Blood 2000;95(2):619–626.

105. Lim MS, Adamson A, Lin Z, et al. Expression of Skp2, a p27(Kip1) ubiquitin ligase, in malignant lymphoma: correlation with p27(Kip1) and proliferation index. Blood 2002;100(8):2950–2956.

106. Shah SA, Potter MW, McDade TP, et al. 26S proteasome inhibition induces apoptosis and limits growth of human pancreatic cancer. J Cell Biochem 2001;82(1):110–122.

107. Bold RJ, Virudachalam S, McConkey DJ. Chemosensitization of pancreatic cancer by inhibition of the 26S proteasome. J Surg Res 2001;100(1):11–17.

108. Pham LV, Tamayo AT, Yoshimura LC, et al. Inhibition of constitutive NF-kappa B activation in mantle cell lymphoma B cells leads to induction of cell cycle arrest and apoptosis. J Immunol 2003;171(1):88–95.

109. An B, Goldfarb RH, Siman R, et al. Novel dipeptidyl proteasome inhibitors overcome Bcl-2 protective function and selectively accumulate the cyclin-dependent kinase inhibitor p27 and induce apoptosis in transformed, but not normal, human fibroblasts. Cell Death Differ 1998;5(12):1062–1075.

110. Orlowski RZ, Eswara JR, Lafond-Walker A, et al. Tumor growth inhibition induced in a murine model of human Burkitt's lymphoma by a proteasome inhibitor. Cancer Res 1998;58(19):4342–4348.

111. Adams J, Palombella VJ, Sausville EA, et al. Proteasome inhibitors: a novel class of potent and effective antitumor agents. Cancer Res 1999;59(11):2615–2622.

112. Hideshima T, Mitsiades C, Akiyama M, et al. Molecular mechanisms mediating antimyeloma activity of proteasome inhibitor PS-341. Blood 2003;101(4):1530–1534.

113. LeBlanc R, Catley LP, Hideshima T, et al. Proteasome inhibitor PS-341 inhibits human myeloma cell growth in vivo and prolongs survival in a murine model. Cancer Res 2002;62(17):4996–5000.

114. Supko JG, Eder JP, Lynch TJ. Pharmacokinetics of gemcitabine and the proteasome inhibitor bortezomib (formerly PS-241) in adult patients with solid malignancies. Proc Am Soc Clin Oncol 2003;22:A544.

115. Nix D, Pien C, Newman R. Clinical Development of a proteasome inhibitor, PS-341, for the treatment of cancer. Proc Am Soc Clin Oncol 2001;20:A339.

116. Mulkerin D, Remick S, Ramanathan C, et al. A dose-escalating and pharmacologic study of bortezomib in adult cancer patients with impaired renal function. J Clin Oncol 2006;24:A2032.

117. Orlowski RZ, Stinchcombe TE, Mitchell BS, et al. Phase I trial of the proteasome inhibitor PS-341 in patients with refractory hematologic malignancies. J Clin Oncol 2002;20(22):4420–4427.

118. Aghajanian C, Soignet S, Dizon DS, et al. A phase I trial of the novel proteasome inhibitor PS341 in advanced solid tumor malignancies. Clin Cancer Res 2002;8(8):2505–2511.

119. Papandreou CN, Daliani DD, Nix D, et al. Phase I trial of the proteasome inhibitor bortezomib in patients with advanced solid tumors with observations in androgen-independent prostate cancer. J Clin Oncol 2004;22(11):2108–2121.

120. Aghajanian C, Dizon DS, Sabbatini P, et al. Phase I trial of bortezomib and carboplatin in recurrent ovarian or primary peritoneal cancer. J Clin Oncol 2005;23(25):5943–5949.

121. Cortes J, Thomas D, Koller C, et al. Phase I study of bortezomib in refractory or relapsed acute leukemias. Clin Cancer Res 2004;10(10):3371–3376.

122. Dy GK, Thomas JP, Wilding G, et al. A phase I and pharmacologic trial of two schedules of the proteasome inhibitor, PS-341 (bortezomib, velcade), in patients with advanced cancer. Clin Cancer Res 2005;11(9):3410–3416.

123. Phuphanich S, Supko J, Carson KA, et al. Phase I trial of bortezomib in adults with recurrent malignant glioma. J Clin Oncol (Meeting Abstracts) 2006;24(18s):A1567.

124. Horton TM, Pati D, Plon SE, et al. A phase 1 study of the proteasome inhibitor bortezomib in pediatric patients with refractory leukemia: a Children's Oncology Group study. Clin Cancer Res 2007;13(5):1516–1522.

125. Blaney SM, Bernstein M, Neville K, et al. Phase I study of the proteasome inhibitor bortezomib in pediatric patients with refractory solid tumors: a Children's Oncology Group study (ADVL0015). J Clin Oncol 2004;22(23):4804–4809.

126. Richardson PG, Barlogie B, Berenson J, et al. A phase 2 study of bortezomib in relapsed, refractory myeloma. N Engl J Med 2003;348(26):2609–2617.

127. Kane RC, Bross PF, Farrell AT, et al. Velcade: U.S. FDA approval for the treatment of multiple myeloma progressing on prior therapy. Oncologist 2003;8(6):508–513.

128. Jagannath S, Barlogie B, Berenson J, et al. A phase 2 study of two doses of bortezomib in relapsed or refractory myeloma. Br J Haematol 2004;127(2):165–172.

129. Kane RC, Farrell AT, Sridhara R, et al. United States Food and Drug Administration approval summary: bortezomib for the treatment of progressive multiple myeloma after one prior therapy. Clin Cancer Res 2006;12(10):2955–2960.

130. Richardson PG, Sonneveld P, Schuster MW, et al. Bortezomib or high-dose dexamethasone for relapsed multiple myeloma. N Engl J Med 2005;352(24):2487–2498.

131. Dispenzieri A, Zhang L, Fonseca R, et al. Single agent bortezomib is associated with a high response rate in patients with high risk myeloma: a phase II study from the Eastern Cooperative Oncology Group (E2A02). ASH Annual Meeting Abstracts 2006;108(11):3527.

132. O'Connor OA. The emerging role of bortezomib in the treatment of indolent non-Hodgkin's and mantle cell lymphomas. Curr Treat Options Oncol 2004;5(4):269–281.

133. O'Connor OA, Wright J, Moskowitz C, et al. Phase II clinical experience with the novel proteasome inhibitor bortezomib in patients with indolent non-Hodgkin's lymphoma and mantle cell lymphoma. J Clin Oncol 2005;23(4):676–684.

134. Goy A, Younes A, McLaughlin P, et al. Phase II study of proteasome inhibitor bortezomib in relapsed or refractory B-cell non-Hodgkin's lymphoma. J Clin Oncol 2005;23(4):667–675.

135. Fisher RI, Bernstein SH, Kahl BS, et al. Multicenter phase II study of bortezomib in patients with relapsed or refractory mantle cell lymphoma. J Clin Oncol 2006;24(30):4867–4874.

136. Belch A, Kouroukis CT, Crump M, et al. A phase II study of bortezomib in mantle cell lymphoma: the National Cancer Institute of Canada Clinical Trials Group trial IND.150. Ann Oncol 2007;18(1):116–121.

137. O'Connor O, Moskowitz C, Portlock C, et al. Patients with chemotherapy-refractory mantle cell lymphoma experience high response rates and identical progression-free survivals compared with patients with relapsed disease following treatment with single agent bortezomib: results of a multicentre phase 2 clinical trial. Br J Haematol 2009;145(1):34–39.

138. Kondagunta GV, Drucker B, Schwartz L, et al. Phase II trial of bortezomib for patients with advanced renal cell carcinoma. J Clin Oncol 2004;22(18):3720–3725.

139. Davis NB, Taber DA, Ansari RH, et al. Phase II trial of PS-341 in patients with renal cell cancer: a University of Chicago phase II consortium study. J Clin Oncol 2004;22(1):115–119.

140. Stevenson JP, Nho CW, Johnson SW. Effects of bortezomib (PS-341) on NF-κB activation in peripheral blood mononuclear cells (PBMCs) of advanced non-small cell lung cancer (NSCLC) patients: a phase II/pharmacodynamic trial. Proc Am Soc Clin Oncol 2004;23:A2346.

141. Cusack JC Jr, Liu R, Houston M, et al. Enhanced chemosensitivity to CPT-11 with proteasome inhibitor PS-341: implications for systemic nuclear factor-kappaB inhibition. Cancer Res 2001;61(9):3535–3540.

142. Wang CY, Cusack JC Jr, Liu R, et al. Control of inducible chemoresistance: enhanced anti-tumor therapy through increased apoptosis by inhibition of NF-kappaB. Nat Med 1999;5(4):412–417.

143. Desai SD, Liu LF, Vazquez-Abad D, et al. Ubiquitin-dependent destruction of topoisomerase I is stimulated by the antitumor drug camptothecin. J Biol Chem 1997;272(39):24159–24164.

144. Ma MH, Yang HH, Parker K, et al. The proteasome inhibitor PS-341 markedly enhances sensitivity of multiple myeloma tumor cells to chemotherapeutic agents. Clin Cancer Res 2003;9(3):1136–1144.

145. O'Connor OA, Wright J, Moskowitz C. Promising activity of the proteasome inhibitor bortezomib (Velcade®) in the treatment of indolent non-Hodgkin's lymphoma and mantle cell lymphoma. Blood 2003;102(11):A7145.

146. Teicher BA, Ara G, Herbst R, et al. The proteasome inhibitor PS-341 in cancer therapy. Clin Cancer Res 1999;5(9):2638–2645.

147. Orlowski RZ, Voorhees PM, Garcia RA, et al. Phase 1 trial of the proteasome inhibitor bortezomib and pegylated liposomal doxorubicin in patients with advanced hematologic malignancies. Blood 2005;105(8):3058–3065.

148. Orlowski RZ, Small GW, Shi YY. Evidence that inhibition of p44/42 mitogen-activated protein kinase signaling is a factor in proteasome inhibitor-mediated apoptosis. J Biol Chem 2002;277(31):27864–27871.

149. Small GW, Somasundaram S, Moore DT, et al. Repression of mitogen-activated protein kinase (MAPK) phosphatase-1 by anthracyclines contributes to their antiapoptotic activation of p44/42-MAPK. J Pharmacol Exp Ther 2003;307(3):861–869.

150. Blade J, Sonneveld P, San Miguel JF, et al. Pegylated liposomal doxorubicin plus bortezomib in relapsed or refractory multiple myeloma: efficacy and safety in patients with renal function impairment. Clin Lymphoma Myeloma 2008;8(6):352–355.

151. Orlowski RZ, Nagler A, Sonneveld P, et al. Randomized phase III study of pegylated liposomal doxorubicin plus bortezomib compared with bortezomib alone in relapsed or refractory multiple myeloma: combination therapy improves time to progression. J Clin Oncol 2007;25(25):3892–3901.

152. San Miguel JF, Schlag R, Khuageva NK, et al. Bortezomib plus melphalan and prednisone for initial treatment of multiple myeloma. N Engl J Med 2008;359(9):906–917.

153. Duechler M, Linke A, Cebula B, et al. In vitro cytotoxic effect of proteasome inhibitor bortezomib in combination with purine nucleoside analogues on chronic lymphocytic leukaemia cells. Eur J Haematol 2005;74(5):407–417.

154. Hewamana S, Alghazal S, Lin TT, et al. The NF-kappaB subunit Rel A is associated with in vitro survival and clinical disease progression in chronic

45. Krämer O, Baus D, Knauer S, et al. Acetylation of Stat1 modulates NF-kappaB activity. Genes Dev 2006;20:473–485.

46. Marks P, Xu W. Histone deacetylase inhibitors: Potential in cancer therapy. J Cell Biochem 2009;107:600–608.

47. Yu X, Guo ZS, Marcu MG, et al. Modulation of p53, ErbB1, ErbB2, and Raf-1 expression in lung cancer cells by depsipeptide FR901228. J Natl Cancer Inst 2002;94:504–513.

48. Fuino L, Bali P, Wittmann S, et al. Histone deacetylase inhibitor LAQ824 down-regulates Her-2 and sensitizes human breast cancer cells to trastuzumab, taxotere, gemcitabine, and epothilone B. Mol Cancer Ther 2003;2:971–984.

49. Nimmanapalli R, Fuino L, Bali P, et al. Histone deacetylase inhibitor LAQ824 both lowers expression and promotes proteasomal degradation of Bcr-Abl and induces apoptosis of imatinib mesylate-sensitive or -refractory chronic myelogenous leukemia-blast crisis cells. Cancer Res 2003;63:5126–5135.

50. Edwards A, Li J, Atadja P, et al. Effect of the histone deacetylase inhibitor LBH589 against epidermal growth factor receptor-dependent human lung cancer cells. Mol Cancer Ther 2007;6:2515–2524.

51. Nishioka C, Ikezoe T, Yang J, et al. MS-275, a novel histone deacetylase inhibitor with selectivity against HDAC1, induces degradation of FLT3 via inhibition of chaperone function of heat shock protein 90 in AML cells. Leuk Res 2008;32:1382–1392.

52. Rosato R, Almenara J, Maggio S, et al. Role of histone deacetylase inhibitor-induced reactive oxygen species and DNA damage in LAQ-824/fludarabine antileukemic interactions. Mol Cancer Ther 2008;7:3285–3297.

53. Adimoolam S, Sirisawad M, Chen J, et al. HDAC inhibitor PCI-24781 decreases RAD51 expression and inhibits homologous recombination. Proc Natl Acad Sci U S A 2007;104:19482–19487.

54. Geng L, Cuneo K, Fu A, et al. Histone deacetylase (HDAC) inhibitor LBH589 increases duration of gamma-H2AX foci and confines HDAC4 to the cytoplasm in irradiated non-small cell lung cancer. Cancer Res 2006;66:11298–11304.

55. Zhang F, Zhang T, Teng Z, et al. Sensitization to gamma-irradiation-induced cell cycle arrest and apoptosis by the histone deacetylase inhibitor trichostatin A in non-small cell lung cancer (NSCLC) cells. Cancer Biol Ther 2009;8:823–831.

56. Wang S, El-Deiry W. TRAIL and apoptosis induction by TNF-family death receptors. Oncogene 2003;22:8628–8633.

57. Guo F, Sigua C, Tao J, et al. Cotreatment with histone deacetylase inhibitor LAQ824 enhances Apo-2L/tumor necrosis factor-related apoptosis inducing ligand-induced death inducing signaling complex activity and apoptosis of human acute leukemia cells. Cancer Res. 2004;64:2580–2589.

58. Kwon S, Ahn S, Kim Y, et al. Apicidin, a histone deacetylase inhibitor, induces apoptosis and Fas/Fas ligand expression in human acute promyelocytic leukemia cells. J Biol Chem. 2002;277:2073–2080.

59. Kim Y, Park J, Lee J, et al. Sodium butyrate sensitizes TRAIL-mediated apoptosis by induction of transcription from the DR5 gene promoter through Sp1 sites in colon cancer cells. Carcinogenesis. 2004;25:1813–1820.

60. Park S, Kim M, Kim H, et al. Trichostatin A sensitizes human ovarian cancer cells to TRAIL-induced apoptosis by down-regulation of c-FLIPL via inhibition of EGFR pathway. Biochem Pharmacol 2009;77:1328–1336.

61. Rippo M, Moretti S, Vescovi S, et al. FLIP overexpression inhibits death receptor-induced apoptosis in malignant mesothelial cells. Oncogene 2004;23:7753–7760.

62. Jin Z, El-Deiry W. Overview of cell death signaling pathways. Cancer Biol Ther 2005;4:139–163.

63. Zhang X, Gillespie S, Borrow J, et al. The histone deacetylase inhibitor suberic bishydroxamate regulates the expression of multiple apoptotic mediators and induces mitochondria-dependent apoptosis of melanoma cells. Mol Cancer Ther 2004;3:425–435.

64. Fandy T, Shankar S, Ross D, et al. Interactive effects of HDAC inhibitors and TRAIL on apoptosis are associated with changes in mitochondrial functions and expressions of cell cycle regulatory genes in multiple myeloma. Neoplasia 2005;7:646–657.

65. Chen S, Dai Y, Pei X, et al. Bim upregulation by histone deacetylase inhibitors mediates interactions with the Bcl-2 antagonist ABT-737: evidence for distinct roles for Bcl-2, Bcl-xL, and Mcl-1. Mol Cell Biol. 2009;29:6149–6169.

66. Hideshima T, Bradner J, Wong J, et al. Small-molecule inhibition of proteasome and aggresome function induces synergistic antitumor activity in multiple myeloma. Proc Natl Acad Sci USA 2005;102:8567–8572.

67. Witt O, Deubzer H, Milde T, et al. HDAC family: What are the cancer relevant targets? Cancer Lett 2009;277:8–21.

68. Weichert W, Röske A, Niesporek S, et al. Class I histone deacetylase expression has independent prognostic impact in human colorectal cancer: specific role of class I histone deacetylases in vitro and in vivo. Clin Cancer Res 2008;14:1669–1677.

69. Huang B, Laban M, Leung C, et al. Inhibition of histone deacetylase 2 increases apoptosis and p21Cip1/WAF1 expression, independent of histone deacetylase 1. Cell Death Differ 2005;12:395–404.

70. Kawaguchi Y, Kovacs J, McLaurin A, et al. The deacetylase HDAC6 regulates aggresome formation and cell viability in response to misfolded protein stress. Cell 2003;115:727–738.

71. Demary K, Wong L, Spanjaard R. Effects of retinoic acid and sodium butyrate on gene expression, histone acetylation and inhibition of proliferation of melanoma cells. Cancer Lett 2001;163:103–107.

72. Davis T, Kennedy C, Chiew Y, et al. Histone deacetylase inhibitors decrease proliferation and modulate cell cycle gene expression in normal mammary epithelial cells. Clin Cancer Res 2000;6:4334–4342.

73. Phiel C, Zhang F, Huang E, et al. Histone deacetylase is a direct target of valproic acid, a potent anticonvulsant, mood stabilizer, and teratogen. J Biol Chem 2001;276:36734–36741.

74. Marks PA, Breslow R. Dimethyl sulfoxide to vorinostat: development of this histone deacetylase inhibitor as an anticancer drug. Nat Biotechnol 2007;25:84–90.

75. Richon VM, Emiliani S, Verdin E, et al. A class of hybrid polar inducers of transformed cell differentiation inhibits histone deacetylases. Proc Natl Acad Sci USA 1998;95:3003–3007.

76. Nakajima H, Kim YB, Terano H, et al. FR901228, a potent antitumor antibiotic, is a novel histone deacetylase inhibitor. Exp Cell Res 1998;241:126–133.

77. Ueda H, Nakajima H, Hori Y, et al. Action of FR901228, a novel antitumor bicyclic depsipeptide produced by Chromobacterium violaceum no. 968, on Ha-ras transformed NIH3T3 cells. Biosci Biotech Biochem 1994;58:1579–1583.

78. Lee JS, Paull K, Alvarez M, et al. Rhodamine efflux patterns predict P-glycoprotein substrates in the National Cancer Institute Drug Screen. Mol Pharmacol 1994;46:627–638.

79. Furumai R, Matsuyama A, Kobashi N, et al. FK228 (depsipeptide) as a natural prodrug that inhibits class I histone deacetylases. Cancer Res 2002;62:4916–4921.

80. Gore S, Carducci M. Modifying histones to tame cancer: clinical development of sodium phenylbutyrate and other histone deacetylase inhibitors. Expert Opin Investig Drugs 2000;9:2923–2934.

81. Atmaca A, Al-Batran SE, Maurer A, et al. Valproic acid (VPA) in patients with refractory advanced cancer: a dose escalating phase I clinical trial. Br J Cancer 2007;97:177–182.

82. Munster P, Marchion D, Bicaku E, et al. Phase I trial of histone deacetylase inhibition by valproic acid followed by the topoisomerase II inhibitor epirubicin in advanced solid tumors: a clinical and translational study. J Clin Oncol 2007;25:1979–1985.

83. Kelly WK, Richon VM, O'Connor O, et al. Phase I clinical trial of histone deacetylase inhibitor: suberoylanilide hydroxamic acid administered intravenously. Clin Cancer Res 2003;9:3578–3588.

84. Kelly WK, O'Connor OA, Krug LM, et al. Phase I study of an oral histone deacetylase inhibitor, suberoylanilide hydroxamic acid, in patients with advanced cancer. J Clin Oncol 2005;23:3923–3931.

85. Rubin E, Agrawal N, Friedman E, et al. A study to determine the effects of food and multiple dosing on the pharmacokinetics of vorinostat given orally to patients with advanced cancer. Clin Cancer Res 2006;12:7039–7045.

86. Steele N, Plumb J, Vidal L, et al. A phase 1 pharmacokinetic and pharmacodynamic study of the histone deacetylase inhibitor belinostat in patients with advanced solid tumors. Clin Cancer Res 2008;14:804–810.

87. Warren K, McCully C, Dvinge H, et al. Plasma and cerebrospinal fluid pharmacokinetics of the histone deacetylase inhibitor, belinostat (PXD101), in non-human primates. Cancer Chemother Pharmacol 2008;62:433–437.

88. Giles F, Fischer T, Cortes J, et al. A phase I study of intravenous LBH589, a novel cinnamic hydroxamic acid analogue histone deacetylase inhibitor, in patients with refractory hematologic malignancies. Clin Cancer Res 2006;12:4628–4635.

89. Ellis L, Pan Y, Smyth G, et al. Histone deacetylase inhibitor panobinostat induces clinical responses with associated alterations in gene expression profiles in cutaneous T-cell lymphoma. Clin Cancer Res 2008;14:4500–4510.

90. Prince H, Bishton M, Johnstone R. Panobinostat (LBH589): a potent pan-deacetylase inhibitor with promising activity against hematologic and solid tumors. Future Oncol 2009;5:601–612.

91. Woo S, Gardner E, Chen X, et al. Population pharmacokinetics of romidepsin in patients with cutaneous T-cell lymphoma and relapsed peripheral T-cell lymphoma. Clin Cancer Res 2009;15:1496–1503.

92. Fouladi M, Furman W, Chin T, et al. Phase I study of depsipeptide in pediatric patients with refractory solid tumors: a Children's Oncology Group report. J Clin Oncol 2006;24:3678–3685.

93. Shiraga T, Tozuka Z, Ishimura R, et al. Identification of cytochrome P450 enzymes involved in the metabolism of FK228, a potent histone deacetylase inhibitor, in human liver microsomes. Biol Pharm Bull 2005;28:124–129.

94. Berg S, Stone J, Xiao J, et al. Plasma and cerebrospinal fluid pharmacokinetics of depsipeptide (FR901228) in nonhuman primates. Cancer Chemother Pharmacol 2004;54:85–88.

95. Gore L, Rothenberg M, O'Bryant C, et al. A phase I and pharmacokinetic study of the oral histone deacetylase inhibitor, MS-275, in patients with refractory solid tumors and lymphomas. Clin Cancer Res 2008;14:4517–4525.

96. Ryan Q, Headlee D, Acharya M, et al. Phase I and pharmacokinetic study of MS-275, a histone deacetylase inhibitor, in patients with advanced and refractory solid tumors or lymphoma. J Clin Oncol 2005;23:3912–3922.

97. Acharya M, Karp J, Sausville E, et al. Factors affecting the pharmacokinetic profile of MS-275, a novel histone deacetylase inhibitor, in patients with cancer. Invest New Drugs 2006;24:367–375.

98. Siu L, Pili R, Duran I, et al. Phase I study of MGCD0103 given as a three-times-per-week oral dose in patients with advanced solid tumors. J Clin Oncol 2008;26:1940–1947.

99. Prince H, Bishton M, Harrison S. Clinical studies of histone deacetylase inhibitors. Clin Cancer Res 2009;15:3958–3969.

100. Bates S, Zhan Z, Steadman K, et al. Laboratory correlates for a phase II trial of romidepsin in cutaneous and peripheral T-cell lymphoma. Br J Haematol 2010;148:256–267.

101. Kummar S, Gutierrez M, Gardner ER, et al. Phase I trial of MS-275, a histone deacetylase inhibitor, administered weekly in refractory solid tumors and lymphoid malignancies. Clin Cancer Res 2007;13:5411–5417.

102. Fantin V, Loboda A, Paweletz C, et al. Constitutive activation of signal transducers and activators of transcription predicts vorinostat resistance in cutaneous T-cell lymphoma. Cancer Res 2008;68:3785–3794.

103. Garcia-Manero G, Yang H, Bueso-Ramos C, et al. Phase 1 study of the histone deacetylase inhibitor vorinostat (suberoylanilide hydroxamic acid [SAHA]) in patients with advanced leukemias and myelodysplastic syndromes. Blood 2008;111:1060–1066.

104. Schrump DS, Fischette MR, Nguyen DM, et al. Clinical and molecular responses in lung cancer patients receiving Romidepsin. Clin Cancer Res 2008;14:188–198.

105. Marquard L, Petersen K, Persson M, et al. Monitoring the effect of belinostat in solid tumors by H4 acetylation. APMIS 2008;116:382–392.

106. Sandor V, Bakke S, Robey RW, et al. Phase I trial of the histone deacetylase inhibitor, depsipeptide (FR901228, NSC 630176), in patients with refractory neoplasms. Clin Cancer Res 2002;8:718–728.

107. de Bono JS, Kristeleit R, Tolcher A, et al. Phase I pharmacokinetic and pharmacodynamic study of LAQ824, a hydroxamate histone deacetylase inhibitor with a heat shock protein-90 inhibitory profile, in patients with advanced solid tumors. Clin Cancer Res 2008;14:6663–6673.

108. Duvic M, Talpur R, Ni X, et al. Phase 2 trial of oral vorinostat (suberoylanilide hydroxamic acid, SAHA) for refractory cutaneous T-cell lymphoma (CTCL). Blood 2007;109:31–39.

109. Rowinsky EK, de Bono J, Deangelo DJ, et al. Cardiac monitoring in phase I trials of a novel histone deacetylase (HDAC) inhibitor LAQ824 in patients with advanced solid tumors and hematologic malignancies. J Clin Oncol (Meeting Abstracts) 2005;23:3131.

110. Beck J, Fischer T, George D, et al. Phase I pharmacokinetic (PK) and pharmacodynamic (PD) study of ORAL LBH589B: A novel histone deacetylase (HDAC) inhibitor. J Clin Oncol (Meeting Abstracts) 2005;23:3148.

111. Fischer T, Patnaik A, Bhalla K, et al. Results of cardiac monitoring during phase I trials of a novel histone deacetylase (HDAC) inhibitor LBH589 in patients with advanced solid tumors and hematologic malignancies. J Clin Oncol (Meeting Abstracts) 2005;23:3106.

112. Kelly WK, DeBono J, Blumenschein G, et al. Final results of a phase I study of oral belinostat (PXD101) in patients with solid tumors. J Clin Oncol (Meeting Abstracts) 2009;27:3531.

113. Kristeleit R, Fong P, Aherne G, et al. Histone deacetylase inhibitors: emerging anticancer therapeutic agents? Clin Lung Cancer 2005;7 Suppl 1:S19–S30.

114. Molife R, Fong P, Scurr M, et al. HDAC inhibitors and cardiac safety. Clin Cancer Res 2007;13:1068; author reply 1068–1069.

115. Piekarz RL, Frye AR, Wright JJ, et al. Cardiac studies in patients treated with depsipeptide, FK228, in a phase II trial for T-cell lymphoma. Clin Cancer Res 2006;12:3762–3773.

116. O'Mahony D, Piekarz R, Bandettini W, et al. Cardiac involvement with lymphoma: a review of the literature. Clin Lymphoma Myeloma 2008;8:249–252.

117. Olsen E, Kim Y, Kuzel T, et al. Phase IIb multicenter trial of vorinostat in patients with persistent, progressive, or treatment refractory cutaneous T-cell lymphoma. J Clin Oncol 2007;25:3109–3115.

118. Zhang L, Lebwohl D, Masson E, et al. Clinically relevant QTc prolongation is not associated with current dose schedules of LBH589 (panobinostat). J Clin Oncol 2008;26:332–333; discussion 333–334.

119. Shah MH, Binkley P, Chan K, et al. Cardiotoxicity of histone deacetylase inhibitor depsipeptide in patients with metastatic neuroendocrine tumors. Clin Cancer Res 2006;12:3997–4003.

120. Strevel E, Siu L. Cardiovascular toxicity of molecularly targeted agents. Eur J Cancer 2009;45(Suppl 1):318–331.

121. Fingert H, Varterasian M. Cardiac safety, risk management, and oncology drug development. Clin Cancer Res 2006;12:3646–3647.

122. Rock E, Finkle J, Fingert H, et al. Assessing proarrhythmic potential of drugs when optimal studies are infeasible. Am Heart J 2009;157:827–836; 836.e821.

123. Cabell C, Bates S, Piekarz R, et al. Systematic assessment of potential cardiac effects of the novel histone deacetylase (HDAC) inhibitor romidepsin. ASH Ann Meet Abst 2009;114:3709.

124. Munster P, Rubin E, Van Belle S, et al. A single supratherapeutic dose of vorinostat does not prolong the QTc interval in patients with advanced cancer. Clin Cancer Res 2009;15:7077–7084.

125. Ramalingam S, Belani C, Ruel C, et al. Phase II study of belinostat (PXD101), a histone deacetylase inhibitor, for second line therapy of advanced malignant pleural mesothelioma. J Thorac Oncol 2009;4:97–101.

126. Stadler WM, Margolin K, Ferber S, et al. A phase II study of depsipeptide in refractory metastatic renal cell cancer. Clin Genitourinary Cancer 2006;5:57–60.

127. Piekarz R, Frye R, Turner M, et al. Phase II multi-institutional trial of the histone deacetylase inhibitor romidepsin as monotherapy for patients with cutaneous T-cell lymphoma. J Clin Oncol 2009;27:5410–5417.

128. Kanji Z, Jung K. Evaluation of an electrolyte replacement protocol in an adult intensive care unit: a retrospective before and after analysis. Intensive Crit Care Nurs 2009;25:181–189.

129. Morgan M, Maloney D, Duvic M. Hypomagnesemia and hypocalcemia in mycosis fungoides: a retrospective case series. Leuk Lymphoma 2002;43:1297–1302.

130. Zain JM, Foss F, Kelly WK, et al. Final results of a phase I study of oral belinostat (PXD101) in patients with lymphoma. J Clin Oncol (Meeting Abstracts) 2009;27:8580.

131. Duvic M, Talpur R, Ni X, et al. Phase 2 trial of oral vorinostat (suberoylanilide hydroxamic acid, SAHA) for refractory cutaneous T-cell lymphoma (CTCL). Blood 2007;109:31–39.

132. Sherman EJ, Fury MG, Tuttle RM, et al. Phase II study of depsipeptide (DEP) in radioiodine (RAI)-refractory metastatic nonmedullary thyroid carcinoma. J Clin Oncol (Meeting Abstracts) 2009;27:6059.

133. Wise L, Turner K, Kerr J. Assessment of developmental toxicity of vorinostat, a histone deacetylase inhibitor, in Sprague-Dawley rats and Dutch Belted rabbits. Birth Defects Res B Dev Reprod Toxicol 2007;80:57–68.

134. Ritchie D, Piekarz R, Blombery P, et al. Reactivation of DNA viruses in association with histone deacetylase inhibitor therapy: a case series report. Haematologica 2009;94:1618–1622.

135. Edelstein L, Micheva-Viteva S, Phelan B, et al. Short communication: activation of latent HIV type 1 gene expression by suberoylanilide hydroxamic acid (SAHA), an HDAC inhibitor approved for use to treat cutaneous T cell lymphoma. AIDS Res Hum Retroviruses 2009;25:883–887.

136. Piekarz RL, Robey R, Sandor V, et al. Inhibitor of histone deacetylation, depsipeptide (FR901228), in the treatment of peripheral and cutaneous T-cell lymphoma: a case report. Blood 2001;98:2865–2868.

137. Pohlman B, Advani R, Duvic M, et al. Final results of a phase ii trial of belinostat (PXD101) in patients with recurrent or refractory peripheral or cutaneous t-cell lymphoma. ASH Ann Meet Abst 2009;114:920.

138. Piekarz R, Wright J, Frye R, et al. Final results of a phase 2 NCI multicenter study of romidepsin in patients with relapsed peripheral t-cell lymphoma (PTCL). ASH Ann Meet Abst 2009;114:1657.

139. Molife R, Patterson S, Riggs C, et al. Phase II study of FK228 in patients with metastatic hormone refractory prostate cancer. Am Soc Clin Oncol Prostate Cancer Symposium. 2006.

140. Whitehead RP, McCoy S, Wollner IS, et al. Phase II trial of depsipeptide (NSC-630176) in colorectal cancer patients who have received either one or two prior chemotherapy regimens for metastatic or locally advanced, unresectable disease: A Southwest Oncology Group study. J Clin Oncol 2006;24:170S–170S.

141. Mann B, Johnson J, Cohen M, et al. FDA approval summary: vorinostat for treatment of advanced primary cutaneous T-cell lymphoma. Oncologist 2007;12:1247–1252.

142. Mann B, Johnson J, He K, et al. Vorinostat for treatment of cutaneous manifestations of advanced primary cutaneous T-cell lymphoma. Clin Cancer Res 2007;13:2318–2322.

143. O'Connor O, Heaney M, Schwartz L, et al. Clinical experience with intravenous and oral formulations of the novel histone deacetylase inhibitor suberoylanilide hydroxamic acid in patients with advanced hematologic malignancies. J Clin Oncol 2006;24:166–173.

144. Crump M, Coiffier B, Jacobsen E, et al. Phase II trial of oral vorinostat (suberoylanilide hydroxamic acid) in relapsed diffuse large-B-cell lymphoma. Ann Onco. 2008;19:964–969.

145. Richardson P, Mitsiades C, Colson K, et al. Phase I trial of oral vorinostat (suberoylanilide hydroxamic acid, SAHA) in patients with advanced multiple myeloma. Leuk Lymphoma 2008;49:502–507.

146. Marshall J, Rizvi N, Kauh J, et al. A phase I trial of depsipeptide (FR901228) in patients with advanced cancer. J Exp Ther Oncol 2002;2:325–332.

147. Kim Y, Whittaker S, Demierre MF, et al. Clinically significant responses achieved with romidepsin in treatment-refractory cutaneous T-cell lymphoma: final results from a phase 2B, international, multicenter, registration study. ASH Ann Meet Abst 2008;112:263.

148. Whitehead R, Rankin C, Hoff P, et al. Phase II trial of romidepsin (NSC-630176) in previously treated colorectal cancer patients with advanced disease: a Southwest Oncology Group study (S0336). Invest New Drugs 2009;27:469–475.

149. Gojo I, Jiemjit A, Trepel JB, et al. Phase 1 and pharmacologic study of MS-275, a histone deacetylase inhibitor, in adults with refractory and relapsed acute leukemias. Blood 2007;109:2781–2790.

150. Hauschild A, Trefzer U, Garbe C, et al. Multicenter phase II trial of the histone deacetylase inhibitor pyridylmethyl-N-{4-[(2-aminophenyl)-carbamoyl]-benzyl}-carbamate in pretreated metastatic melanoma. Melanoma Res 2008;18:274–278.

151. Dickinson M, Ritchie D, DeAngelo D, et al. Preliminary evidence of disease response to the pan deacetylase inhibitor panobinostat (LBH589) in refractory Hodgkin Lymphoma. Br J Haematol 2009;147:97–101.

152. Ottmann OG, Spencer A, Prince HM, et al. Phase IA/II study of oral panobinostat (LBH589), a novel pan- deacetylase inhibitor (DACi) demonstrating efficacy in patients with advanced hematologic malignancies. ASH Ann Meet Abst 2008;112:958.

153. Crump M, Andreadis C, Assouline S, et al. Treatment of relapsed or refractory non-hodgkin lymphoma with the oral isotype-selective histone deacetylase inhibitor MGCD0103: interim results from a phase II study. J Clin Oncol (Meeting Abstracts) 2008;26:8528-.

154. Bots M, Johnstone R. Rational combinations using HDAC inhibitors. Clin Cancer Res 2009;15:3970–3977.

155. Badros A, Burger A, Philip S, et al. Phase I study of vorinostat in combination with bortezomib for relapsed and refractory multiple myeloma. Clin Cancer Res 2009;15:5250–5257.

156. Weber DM, Jagannath S, Mazumder A, et al. Phase I trial of oral vorinostat (suberoylanilide hydroxamic acid, SAHA) in combination with bortezomib in patients with advanced multiple myeloma. ASH Ann Meet Abst 2007; 110:1172.

157. Weber D, Badros AZ, Jagannath S, et al. Vorinostat plus bortezomib for the treatment of relapsed/refractory multiple myeloma: early clinical experience. ASH Ann Meet Abst 2008;112:871.

158. Nguyen DM, Schrump WD, Tsai WS, et al. Enhancement of depsipeptide-mediated apoptosis of lung or esophageal cancer cells by flavopiridol: activation of the mitochondria-dependent death-signaling pathway. J Thorac Cardiovasc Surg 2003;125:1132–1142.

159. Zhang Y, Jung M, Dritschilo A. Enhancement of radiation sensitivity of human squamous carcinoma cells by histone deacetylase inhibitors. Radiat Res 2004;161:667–674.

160. Camphausen K, Burgan W, Cerra M, et al. Enhanced radiation-induced cell killing and prolongation of gammaH2AX foci expression by the histone deacetylase inhibitor MS-275. Cancer Res 2004;64:316–321.

161. Camphausen K, Tofilon P. Inhibition of histone deacetylation: a strategy for tumor radiosensitization. J Clin Oncol 2007;25:4051–4056.

162. Kitazono M, Robey R, Zhan Z, et al. Low concentrations of the histone deacetylase inhibitor, depsipeptide (FR901228), increase expression of the Na(+)/I(-) symporter and iodine accumulation in poorly differentiated thyroid carcinoma cells. J Clin Endocrinol Metab 2001;86:3430–3435.

163. Chen J, Zhang M, Ju W, et al. Effective treatment of a murine model of adult T-cell leukemia using depsipeptide and its combination with unmodified daclizumab directed toward CD25. Blood 2009;113:1287–1293.

164. Piekarz RL, Robey RW, Zhan Z, et al. T-cell lymphoma as a model for the use of histone deacetylase inhibitors in cancer therapy: impact of depsipeptide on molecular markers, therapeutic targets, and mechanisms of resistance. Blood 2004;103:4636–4643.

165. Petrij F, Dauwerse H, Blough R, et al. Diagnostic analysis of the Rubinstein-Taybi syndrome: five cosmids should be used for microdeletion detection and low number of protein truncating mutations. J Med Genet 2000;37:168–176.

166. Taki T, Sako M, Tsuchida M, et al. The t(11;16)(q23;p13) translocation in myelodysplastic syndrome fuses the MLL gene to the CBP gene. Blood 1997;89:3945–3950.

167. Borrow J, Stanton VJ, Andresen J, et al. The translocation t(8;16)(p11;p13) of acute myeloid leukaemia fuses a putative acetyltransferase to the CREB-binding protein. Nat Genet. 1996;14:33–41.

168. Koshiishi N, Chong J, Fukasawa T, et al. p300 gene alterations in intestinal and diffuse types of gastric carcinoma. Gastric Cancer 2004;7:85–90.

169. Mattera L, Escaffit F, Pillaire M, et al. The p400/Tip60 ratio is critical for colorectal cancer cell proliferation through DNA damage response pathways. Oncogene 2009;28:1506–1517.

170. Grignani F, De Matteis S, Nervi C, et al. Fusion proteins of the retinoic acid receptor-alpha recruit histone deacetylase in promyelocytic leukaemia. Nature 1998;391:815–818.

171. Wang J, Hoshino T, Redner R, et al. ETO, fusion partner in t(8;21) acute myeloid leukemia, represses transcription by interaction with the human N-CoR/mSin3/HDAC1 complex. Proc Natl Acad Sci USA 1998;95:10860–10865.

172. Choi J, Kwon H, Yoon B, et al. Expression profile of histone deacetylase 1 in gastric cancer tissues. Jpn J Cancer Res 2001;92:1300–1304.

173. Song J, Noh J, Lee J, et al. Increased expression of histone deacetylase 2 is found in human gastric cancer. APMIS 2005;113:264–268.

174. Ashktorab H, Belgrave K, Hosseinkhah F, et al. Global histone H4 acetylation and HDAC2 expression in colon adenoma and carcinoma. Dig Dis Sci 2009;54:2109–2117.

175. Elsheikh S, Green A, Rakha E, et al. Global histone modifications in breast cancer correlate with tumor phenotypes, prognostic factors, and patient outcome. Cancer Res 2009;69:3802–3809.

176. Garcia-Manero G, Kantarjian H, Sanchez-Gonzalez B, et al. Phase 1/2 study of the combination of 5-aza-2′-deoxycytidine with valproic acid in patients with leukemia. Blood 2006;108:3271–3279.

177. Soriano AO, Yang H, Faderl S, et al. Safety and clinical activity of the combination of 5-azacytidine, valproic acid, and all-trans retinoic acid in acute myeloid leukemia and myelodysplastic syndrome. Blood 2007;110:2302–2308.

178. Gore S, Baylin S, Sugar E, et al. Combined DNA methyltransferase and histone deacetylase inhibition in the treatment of myeloid neoplasms. Cancer Res 2006;66:6361–6369.

179. Ramalingam S, Maitland M, Frankel P, et al. Carboplatin and paclitaxel in combination with either vorinostat or placebo for first-line therapy of advanced non-small-cell lung cancer. J Clin Oncol 2009;28:56–62.

180. Reguart N, Cardona AF, Isla D, et al. Phase I trial of vorinostat in combination with erlotinib in advanced non-small cell lung cancer (NSCLC) patients with EGFR mutations after erlotinib progression. J Clin Oncol (Meeting Abstracts) 2009;27:e19057.

181. Tredaniel J, Descourt R, Moro-Sibilot D, et al. Vorinostat in combination with gemcitabine and cisplatinum in patients with advanced non-small cell lung cancer (NSCLC): A Phase I dose-escalation study. J Clin Oncol (Meeting Abstracts) 2009;27:8049.

182. Fakih M, Pendyala L, Fetterly G, et al. A phase I, pharmacokinetic and pharmacodynamic study on vorinostat in combination with 5-fluorouracil, leucovorin, and oxaliplatin in patients with refractory colorectal cancer. Clin Cancer Res 2009;15:3189–3195.

183. Fouladi M, Park JR, Sun J, et al. A phase I trial and pharmacokinetic (PK) study of vorinostat (SAHA) in combination with 13 cis-retinoic acid (13cRA) in children with refractory neuroblastomas, medulloblastomas, primitive neuroectodermal tumors (PNETs), and atypical teratoid rhabdoid tumor. J Clin Oncol (Meeting Abstracts) 2008;26:10012.

184. Munster P, Marchion D, Thomas S, et al. Phase I trial of vorinostat and doxorubicin in solid tumours: histone deacetylase 2 expression as a predictive marker. Br J Cancer 2009;101:1044–1050.

185. Garcia-Manero G, Tambaro FP, Bekele BN, et al. Phase II Study of Vorinostat in Combination with Idarubicin (Ida) and Cytarabine (ara-C)

as Front Line Therapy in Acute Myelogenous Leukemia (AML) or Higher Risk Myelodysplastic Syndrome (MDS). ASH Ann Meet Abst 2009;114:1055.

186. Grant S, Kolla S, Sirulnik LA, et al. Phase I trial of vorinostat (SAHA) in combination with alvocidib (Flavopiridol) in patients with relapsed, refractory or (Selected) poor prognosis acute leukemia or refractory anemia with excess blasts-2 (RAEB-2). ASH Ann Meet Abst 2008;112:2986.

187. Dummer R, Hymes K, Sterry W, et al. Vorinostat in combination with bexarotene in advanced cutaneous T-cell lymphoma: a phase I study. J Clin Oncol (Meeting Abstracts) 2009;27:8572.

188. Harrison SJ, Quach H, Yuen K, et al. High response rates with the combination of bortezomib, dexamethasone and the pan-histone deacetylase inhibitor romidepsin in patients with relapsed or refractory multiple myeloma in a phase I/II clinical trial. ASH Ann Meet Abst 2008;112:3698.

189. Finkler NJ, Dizon DS, Braly P, et al. Phase II multicenter trial of the histone deacetylase inhibitor (HDACi) belinostat, carboplatin and paclitaxel (BelCaP) in patients (pts) with relapsed epithelial ovarian cancer (EOC). J Clin Oncol (Meeting Abstracts) 2008;26:5519.

190. Garcia-Manero G, Yang AS, Klimek V, et al. Phase I/II study of a novel oral isotype-selective histone deacetylase (HDAC) inhibitor MGCD0103 in combination with azacitidine in patients (pts) with high-risk myelodysplastic syndrome (MDS) or acute myelogenous leukemia (AML). J Clin Oncol (Meeting Abstracts) 2007;25:7062.

191. Hurwitz H, Nelson B, O'Dwyer PJ, et al. Phase I/II: The oral isotype-selective HDAC inhibitor MGCD0103 in combination with gemcitabine (Gem) in patients (pts) with refractory solid tumors. J Clin Oncol (Meeting Abstracts) 2008;26:4625.

192. Konduri K, Spira AI, Jotte RM, et al. Results from a phase I safety lead-in study investigating the combination of erlotinib and the histone deacetylase inhibitor entinostat in patients with advanced NSCLC. J Clin Oncol (Meeting Abstracts) 2009;27:e14545.

193. Juergens RA, Vendetti F, Coleman B, et al. Interim analysis of a phase II trial of 5-azacitidine (5AC) and entinostat (SNDX-275) in relapsed advanced lung cancer (NSCLC). J Clin Oncol (Meeting Abstracts) 2009;27:8055.

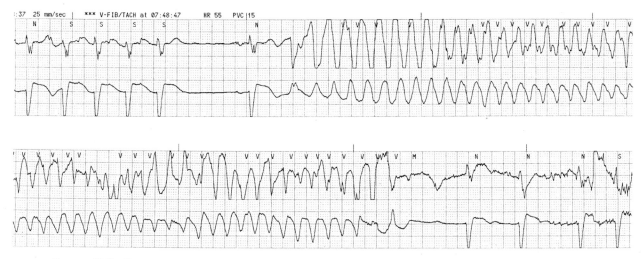

FIGURE **24-1**   Ventricular tachycardia with the features of torsade de pointes. QT is prolonged at baseline, with abrupt lengthening of the QT interval after the pause, followed by polymorphic ventricular tachycardia.

Clinical Toxicity

ATO has minimal acute toxic effects, aside from the lengthening of the QT interval and the risk of ventricular arrhythmias. Long-term follow-up of patients treated with the ATO/ATRA combination as primary therapy have revealed no significant long-term sequelae, despite fears of carcinogenesis, hepatic and cardiac toxicity, and no evidence of retention of arsenic in urine analyzed 2 years after treatment.[17] Patients may acutely experience fatigue, light-headedness, and numbness or tingling of the extremities, and serum chemistries may reveal electrolyte changes, hyperglycemia, and modest hepatic enzyme elevations, all of which are fully reversible with discontinuation of drug. Fewer than 10% of patients with APL develop a leukocyte maturation syndrome similar to that seen with ATRA, with pulmonary distress, effusions, and altered mental status. These symptoms abate with drug discontinuation, corticosteroids, oxygen, and diuretics.[18]

The most serious acute and subacute toxicity relates to prolongation of the QT interval. This toxicity has been ascribed to inhibition of the rapid K+ efflux channel, a change that slows ventricular repolarization and predisposes to ventricular instability.[19] Drugs that prolong conduction, such as macrolide antibiotics, quinidine, or methadone, should not be used with ATO. It is necessary to confirm a normal QT interval prior to treatment, to monitor the EKG and serum electrolytes at regular intervals (every 3 to 7 days) during therapy, and to correct abnormalities of serum K^+, Ca^+, and Mg^{2+} as necessary. In patients with QTc prolongation of greater than 0.47 seconds, treatment should be suspended until the electrolyte abnormalities are corrected and the QTc returns to normal.

Rarely, patients with prolongation of the QTc develop torsade de pointes (Fig. 24-1) or multifocal ventricular tachycardia, a potentially fatal arrhythmia. This event requires immediate defibrillation, treatment with intravenous magnesium sulfate, and correction of electrolyte abnormalities.[20] Extreme caution should be exercised in resuming ATO treatment in patients who have experienced a ventricular arrhythmia associated with a prolongation of the QTc.

Some investigators suggest resuming treatment at a lower dose of 0.10 mg/d, with close monitoring of the EKG and electrolytes.[16]

References

1. Hu J, Liu Y-F, Wu C-F, et al. Long-term efficacy and safety of all-trans retinoic acid/arsenic trioxide-based therapy in newly diagnosed acute promyelocytic leukemia. Proc Natl Acad Sci U S A 2009;106:3342–3327.
2. Shen ZX, Chen GQ, Ni JH, et al. Use of arsenic trioxide in the treatment of acute promyelocytic leukemia (APL). Blood 1997;89:3345–3353.
3. Leung J, Pang A, Yuen W-H, et al. Relationship of expression of aquaglyceroporin 9 with arsenic uptake and sensitivity in leukemia cells. Blood 2007;109:740–746.
4. Dilda PJ, Hogg PJ. Arsenical-based cancer drugs. Cancer Treat Rev 2007;33:542–564.
5. Lu J, Chew E-H, Holmgren A. Targeting thioredoxin reductase is a basis for cancer therapy by arsenic trioxide. 2007;104:12288–12293.
6. Wang J, Li L, Cang H, Shi G, et al. NADPH oxidase-derived reactive oxygen species are responsible for the high susceptibility to arsenic cytotoxicity in acute promyelocytic leukemia cells. Leuk Res 2008;32:429–436.
7. Han YH, Kim SZ, Kim SH, et al. Suppression of arsenic trioxide-induced apoptosis in HeLa cells by N-acetylcysteine. Mol Cells 2008;26:18–25.
8. Davison K, Mann KK, Waxman S, et al. JNK activation is a mediator of arsenic trioxide–induced apoptosis in acute promyelocytic leukemia cells. Blood 2004;103:3496–3502.
9. Mann KK, Colombo M, Miller WH Jr. Arsenic trioxide decreases AKT protein in a caspase-dependent manner. Mol Cancer Ther 2008;7:1680–1687.
10. Yoon P, Giafis N, Smith J, et al. Activation of mammalian target of rapamycin and the p70 S6 Kinase by arsenic trioxide in BCR-ABL-expressing cells. Mol Cancer Ther 2006;5:2815–2823.
11. Billottet C, Banerjee L, Vanhaesebroeck B, et al. Inhibition of class I phosphoinositide 3-kinase activity impairs proliferation and triggers apoptosis in acute promyelocytic leukemia without affecting ATRA-induced differentiation. Cancer Res 2009;69:1027–1036.
12. Kumar P, Gao Q, Ning Y, et al. Arsenic trioxide enhances the therapeutic efficacy of radiation treatment of oral squamous carcinoma while protecting bone. Mol Cell Ther 2008;7:2060–2069.
13. Lallemand-Breitenbach V, Jeanne M, Benhenda S, et al. Arsenic degrades PML or PML-RARalpha through a SUMO-triggered RNF4/ubiquitin-mediated pathway. Nat Cell Biol 2008;10:547–555.

14. Pelicano H, Carew JS, McQueen TJ, et al. Targeting Hsp9 by 17-AAG in leukemia cells: mechanisms for synergistic and antagonistic drug combinations with arsenic trioxide and Ara-C. Leukemia 2006;20:610–619.

15. Fox E, Razzouk BI, Widemann BC, et al. Phase 1 trial and pharmacokinetic study of arsenic trioxide in children and adolescents with refractory or relapsed acute leukemia, including acute promyelocytic leukemia or lymphoma. Blood 2008;111:566–573.

16. Liu J, Lu Y, Wu Q, et al. Mineral arsenicals in traditional medicines: orpiment, realgar, and arsenolite. J Pharmacol Exp Ther 2008;326: 363–368.

17. Soignet SL, Maslak P, Wang ZG, et al. Complete remission after treatment of acute promyelocytic leukemia with arsenic trioxide. N Engl J Med 1998;339:1341–1348.

18. Wang Z-Y, Chen Z. Acute promyelocytic leukemia: from highly fatal to highly curable. Blood 2008;111:2505–2515.

19. Drolet B, Simard C, Roden DM. Unusual effects of a QT-prolonging drug, arsenic trioxide, on cardiac potassium currents. Circulation 2004;109:26–29.

20. Gupta A, Lawrence AT, Krishnan K, et al. Current concepts in the mechanisms and management of drug-induced QT prolongation and torsade de pointes. Am Heart J 2007;153:891–899.

Inhibitors of Tumor Angiogenesis

Kari B. Wisinski and William J. Gradishar

Neoplasms occur when a normal cell acquires molecular changes that allow the cell to divide and metastasize in an unsupervised manner. This process requires a supply of nutrients, which is provided by the vasculature. In the early 1970s, Judah Folkman first proposed the theory of tumor angiogenesis, which he defined as the process of recruitment of new vessels to a tumor as it grows.[1] His hypothesis was that tumors are unable to grow beyond a certain size in the absence of a new vascular supply. Subsequent data have supported this hypothesis, indicating that angiogenesis is a critical step in tumor growth and metastases.[2,3] A concentrated effort is now underway to target angiogenesis as a component of cancer therapy.

The growth and maturation of new vasculature is a highly complex process involving interactions of multiple cellular pathways and communication between cells and the extracellular matrix. Many of the key molecules have been identified and have become potential therapeutic targets. As one of the first steps in this process, tumors produce signaling molecules that activate angiogenesis or down-regulate the expression of inhibitors of angiogenesis. This step alters the microenvironment to favor an "angiogenic switch."[4,5] This environment supports the proliferation of endothelial cells. In the normal microenvironment, endothelial cells are usually quiescent. In contrast, once the "angiogenic switch" occurs, proliferating endothelial cells form new blood vessels. These blood vessels are structurally abnormal with a leaky basement membrane, which allows tumor cells to become integrated into the vessel wall. This neo-vasculature is then responsible for the supply of nutrients to the tumor. Angiogenesis has been considered an ideal target for anti-neoplastic therapy, since it is a unique process that occurs only at tumor sites and not in normal human organs, a fact that may limit the toxicities related to these agents.

Three Food and Drug Association (FDA)-approved drugs target angiogenesis. This chapter reviews the process of angiogenesis and the rationale for the development of these angiogenesis inhibitors as antineoplastic therapies. The chemistry, pharmacology, and indications for each of the current FDA-approved angiogenesis inhibitors will be covered. In addition, an extensive discussion of the clinical studies leading to the FDA's approval will be presented. Finally, the common toxicities seen with these agents and their limitations in the treatment of malignancies will be discussed.

Tumor Angiogenesis

Since Judah Folkman initially proposed the concept of tumor angiogenesis in 1971, much work has been done to elucidate the key players in this critical event. Initiation of tumor angiogenesis leads to a cascade of events that must occur in concert in order for successful tumor angiogenesis to occur. Without angiogenesis, tumors cannot exceed a few cubic millimeters in size.[2]

Angiogenic Switch

The normal microenvironment has an anti-angiogenic disposition. As tumors grow they are initially dependent on the normal microenvironment for oxygen and other nutrients. However, since the diffusion limit of oxygen is around 100 μm, as tumors expand, those cells that are no longer within the oxygen diffusion perimeter become hypoxic.[6] In the setting of hypoxia, multiple intracellular molecules are activated. One well-characterized result of hypoxia is the activation of the hypoxia inducible factor-1 (HIF-1) transcriptional complex.[7] Activation of this complex leads to up-regulation of pro-angiogenic factors, such as vascular endothelial growth factor (VEGF), platelet-derived growth factor (PDGF), and nitric oxide synthase (NOS), which are released into the microenvironment. Consistent with this finding, HIF-1 is up-regulated in many cancers.[7] However, like most pathways in oncogenesis, redundancy is present and the HIF system is also influenced by many oncogenic pathways, including the insulin-like growth factor-1, epidermal growth factor (EGF), mutant Ras, and Src kinase pathways as well as tumor suppressor mutations, including PTEN, p53, p14ARF, and pVHL (von Hippel-Lindau).[7] The activation of HIF-1 is a critical step in initiation of the "angiogenic switch" in which the normal microenvironment changes from anti-angiogenic to pro-angiogenic and new blood vessel formation is started. Drugs targeting HIF-1 have been developed for clinical use and are currently being tested in early phase trials.

The Vascular Endothelial Growth Factor (VEGF) and VEGF Receptor Family

Activation of the VEGF pathway is critical in both physiologic and pathologic angiogenesis. The complexities of this system are beyond the scope of this chapter; therefore, only a brief overview is provided. Detailed reviews are available elsewhere.[8–10] The VEGF receptor family is made up of three tyrosine kinase receptors. Of these, only VEGFR-1 and VEGFR-2 bind the main ligand important in tumor angiogenesis, VEGF-A.[8,10] VEGF-A, usually referred to as VEGF, belongs to a family of genes including placenta growth factor (PLGF), VEGF-B, VEGF-C, and VEGF-D. The biology of VEGF and its primary receptors, VEGFR-1 and VEGFR-2, will be discussed in this chapter (Table 26-1).

TABLE

26.1	*The VEGF signaling family*

Receptor	Ligands	Role of receptor in angiogenesis
VEGFR-1 (Flt-1)	VEGF-A	Varies by developmental stage,
	VEGF-B	cell-type, and ligand binding
	PLGF	Little role in tumor angiogenesis
VEGFR-2 (KDR/Flk-1)	VEGF-A	Main mediator of endothelial cell
	VEGF-C	survival and proliferation as
	VEGF-D	well as vascular permeability
		Tumor angiogenesis primarily
		induced via VEGF-A
VEGFR-3 (Flt-4)	VEGF-C	Little role in tumor angiogenesis
	VEGF-D	Important for lymphangiogenesis

PLGF, placental growth factor.

The two circulating isoforms of VEGF, $VEGF_{121}$ and $VEGF_{165}$, are the major mediators of tumor angiogenesis.[9] One of the main inducers of VEGF expression is tumor hypoxia.[11] This is mediated in part by HIF-1.[12] Interestingly, loss of the von Hippel-Lindau (*vHL*) tumor suppressor gene in renal cell carcinomas results in constitutive overexpression of HIF-1 leading to elevated VEGF expression in these tumors.[13] Several other major growth factors including EGF, transforming growth factors alpha (TGF-α) and beta (TGF-β), keratinocyte growth factor, insulin-like growth factor-1, fibroblast growth factor (FGF), and PDGF also have been shown to up-regulate VEGF mRNA expression.[8] In addition, oncogenic mutations or amplifications of the Ras oncogene and inflammatory cytokines (IL-1α and IL-6) are associated with VEGF gene induction.[14,15] VEGF production can also originate from tumor-associated stromal cells[9] suggesting that paracrine or autocrine release of these factors cooperate with hypoxia to induce tumor angiogenesis via VEGF up-regulation. Vascular permeability is also mediated by VEGF, which forms fenestrations in blood vessels.[10] Therefore, agents targeting VEGF are also thought to exert antitumorigenic effects by allowing improved delivery of other agents, such as chemotherapy, to tumors.[16]

The VEGF-1 and VEGF-2 receptors are expressed normally on vascular endothelial cells engaged in angiogenesis as well as on bone marrow-derived cells. In addition, many solid and hematologic tumors also express the VEGF receptors, primarily VEGFR-1.[9] These receptors have a similar protein structure with seven immunoglobulin-like domains in the extracellular region, a single transmembrane region, and a consensus tyrosine kinase sequence that is interrupted by a kinase-insert domain.[8] Interestingly, the VEGF receptors can also be expressed inside the cell, where they can promote cell survival by an "intracrine" mechanism.[9]

VEGFR-1 (also known as Flt-1) was the first identified VEGF receptor; however, its role in angiogenesis remains controversial (Table 26-1). The data suggest that the function of VEGFR-1 differs depending on the developmental stage of the animal, the cell type on which it is being expressed, and the ligand to which it is

binding (VEGF-A, VEGF-B, or PLGF).[8,9] Studies linking VEGFR-1 to angiogenesis have found that expression of VEGFR-1 is up-regulated by hypoxia. Similar to the VEGF, this is mediated by HIF-1. However, VEGFR-1 has also been identified as a negative regulator of VEGF, especially in embryonic development. In addition, its signal transduction properties are very weak. In general, VEGFR-1 is thought to have little role in tumor angiogenesis.

VEGFR-2 (also known as KDR or Flk-1) is the main regulator of endothelial cell proliferation and survival, as well as vascular permeability (Table 26-1).[10] Upon VEGF ligand binding, the receptor undergoes dimerization and tyrosine phosphorylation. In endothelial cells, this VEGFR-2 activation leads to initiation of several signaling cascades.[9] This includes activation of the mitogen-activating protein kinase (MAPK) pathway, which involves phospholipase C-γ (PLC γ), protein kinase C (PKC), Raf kinase, and MEK. Activation of this pathway results in DNA synthesis and cell growth. Other pathways initiated by VEGFR-2 activation are the phosphatidylinositol 3′-kinase (PI3K)/Akt pathway that leads to increased endothelial cell survival and the Src family pathway that results in cell migration. Many of these pathways are abnormally expressed in tumors and have been targeted with specific inhibitors. In addition, the neuropilin (NRP) receptors also bind to VEGF and can act as co-receptors with VEGFR-2 to regulate angiogenesis; therefore, these receptors may be targeted by novel agents in the future.[9]

Other Molecular Pathways Important in Tumor Angiogenesis

Matrix metalloproteinases (MMPs) are a family of structurally related zinc-containing endopeptidases that are involved in the degradation of extracellular matrix components (ECM).[17] In angiogenesis, MMPs mediate remodeling and invasion of the ECM by new vessels by regulating endothelial cell attachment, proliferation, and migration. These observations suggest that matrix metalloproteinase inhibitors (MMPIs) could inhibit tumor progression at both the primary tumor site and sites of metastases. Several MMPIs have been developed for clinical use, but results in phase III clinical trials of patients with advanced malignancy were disappointing.[18,19]

Interaction between endothelial cells and the extracellular matrix is critical to tumor angiogenesis. The integrins are transmembrane receptors that bind to extracellular matrix proteins and play a significant role in this interaction. Studies have implicated a number of endothelial cell integrins in the regulation of endothelial cell growth, survival, and migration during angiogenesis.[20] In addition, integrin signaling is dysfunctional in cancer cells and their expression may correlate with prognosis.[21] Several inhibitors of these endothelial cell integrins have been developed and tested in early phase clinical trials.[20] Clinical studies indicate signs of potential therapeutic benefit from these agents; however, further testing is still needed.

Another receptor tyrosine kinase pathway involved in tumor angiogenesis involves the tie-2 receptor.[9] This receptor is expressed principally on the vascular endothelium. Its major ligands are angiopoietin-1 (ang-1) and angiopoietin-2 (ang-2). In concert with VEGF, this pathway stabilizes and matures new capillaries. Ang-1, ang-2, and tie-2 expression have been correlated with prognosis in several cancers, including early stage bladder cancers and breast cancer.[22,23] Peptibodies against ang-2 have been developed and are in early clinical development.

Another pathway that also appears to play an important role in tumor angiogenesis is the notch receptor pathway. The notch receptors are cell surface receptors implicated in cell fate, differentiation, and proliferation.[9,24] The ligands for these receptors are the transmembrane proteins, jagged and delta-like ligand (Dll), which are expressed on adjacent cells. Vascular endothelial cells express notch 1 and 4, as well as jagged 1, Dll-1, and Dll4. Notch-Dll4 signaling is essential for vascular development in the embryo and Dll4 is up-regulated in tumor vasculature. This is thought to be in part VEGF-mediated. Novel agents targeting this pathway are also currently in early phase clinical development.

Preclinical Development of VEGF Inhibitors

VEGF and its receptors are overexpressed in a number of tumor types, including colorectal, lung, breast, renal cell, and endometrial carcinomas, as well as hematologic malignancies, such as acute myelogenous leukemia.[8,9] The majority of retrospective studies correlating VEGF or VEGFR expression to prognosis suggest that high levels are associated with a worse prognosis.[25–27] Efforts to determine the prognostic significance of another marker of angiogenesis, microvascular density have had conflicting results, in part secondary to lack of standardized laboratory techniques. However, it appears that high microvascular density is a poor prognostic factor in several malignancies.[28,29]

In vitro and in vivo studies indicate the importance of VEGF signaling in enhancing proliferation and inhibiting apoptosis of endothelial cells. In addition to tumor angiogenesis, VEGF signaling is critical in developmental endothelial cell growth and in endothelial cell growth after normal tissue injury. However, established blood vessels are not VEGF-dependent. Therefore, agents targeting this pathway should have effects only in the peritumoral vasculature and not on the established vasculature critical for normal human physiology. Based on the data indicating the importance of VEGF signaling in tumor angiogenesis, animal studies were done and demonstrated that inhibition of VEGF signaling interrupts tumor growth and invasion.[30–33] The abundance of preclinical data supporting the antineoplastic potential of these agents led to the development of multiple drugs targeting the VEGF pathway.

Antibodies to Vascular Endothelial Growth Factor

Bevacizumab (Avastin)

Chemistry

Bevacizumab is a recombinant humanized monoclonal immunoglobulin G (IgG) antibody generated by engineering VEGF binding residues of a murine neutralizing antibody into the framework of a normal human IgG.[30] It consists of approximately 93% human and 7% murine protein sequences.[34] Bevacizumab has a molecular weight of approximately 149 kD (kilodaltons). It comes in a clear to slightly opalescent, colorless to pale brown, sterile, pH 6.2 solution for intravenous infusion.

Mechanism of Action

Bevacizumab binds and neutralizes the biologically active forms of VEGF by recognizing the binding sites for the VEGF receptors. This prevents the interaction of VEGF with its receptors on the surface of endothelial cells. Bevacizumab neutralizes all isoforms of human VEGF with a dissociation constant (K_d) of 1.1.[34] Inhibition of VEGF-induced proliferation of endothelial cells as well as tumor angiogenesis in vitro have been noted with bevacizumab. Preclinical studies showed that the administration of bevacizumab to mice with various tumor xenografts caused growth inhibition and decreased metastatic progression. Given that VEGF is produced and acts locally in a tumor site, the capacity of an antibody to interfere with its effects is somewhat surprising. Unlike antibodies targeting receptors, ligands can be difficult to sop up.

Absorption, Distribution, and Elimination

Bevacizumab is administered as an intravenous formulation. In a population pharmacokinetic analysis of 491 patients who received 1 to 20 mg/kg of bevacizumab weekly, every 2 weeks, or every 3 weeks, the estimated half-life of bevacizumab was approximately 20 days (range 11 to 50 days).[35] The predicted time to reach steady state was 100 days. The clearance of bevacizumab varied with body weight, sex, and tumor burden. Bevacizumab has been tested at doses from 3 to 20 mg/kg, but a clear dose-response relationship has not been identified. In colorectal cancer, a dose of 5 mg/kg was more effective than 10 mg/kg.[36] On the other hand, in renal cell cancer and non–small cell lung cancer, higher doses up to 15 mg/kg are more effective than lower doses.[37,38] Demographic data suggest that no dose adjustments are necessary for age or sex. No studies have been conducted to examine the pharmacokinetics of bevacizumab in patients with renal or hepatic impairment.

Drug Interactions

Bevacizumab has no known drug interactions. However, in a phase I study of bevacizumab and sunitinib in advanced renal cell carcinoma, two patients developed severe microangiopathic hemolytic anemia associated with hypertension, thrombocytopenia, renal insufficiency, and hemolysis. Evidence of less severe microangiopathic hemolytic anemia was also noted in three other patients on the study.[39] This combination should not be used outside of a clinical trial.

Pregnancy and Breast Feeding

Bevacizumab is a pregnancy category C agent. There are no studies of bevacizumab in pregnant women. Human IgG is known to cross the placental barrier; therefore, bevacizumab has the potential to cause fetal harm. Reproduction studies in rabbits treated with approximately 1 to 12 times the recommended human dose of bevacizumab resulted in teratogenicity, including an increased incidence of fetal skeletal alterations. It is not known whether bevacizumab is secreted in human milk. Although human IgG is excreted in human milk, some data suggest that breast milk antibodies do not enter the neonatal and infant circulation in substantial amounts. Recommendations for bevacizumab therapy during nursing must take into account the long half-life of the drug.

Special Considerations for Pediatric and Geriatric Populations

The safety, efficacy, and pharmacokinetic profile of bevacizumab in pediatric patients have not been established. Bevacizumab has been administered in the elderly population and no dose modifications are recommended in this group. The section on special populations has further details regarding the data on bevacizumab use in these groups of patients.

Therapeutic Uses

Renal Cell Carcinoma

Renal cell carcinoma was felt to be a potentially promising target disease for bevacizumab because most renal clear cell carcinomas have a mutation in the *vHL* tumor suppressor gene which leads to HIF-1–mediated VEGF production.[13] A randomized phase II trial of single-agent bevacizumab versus placebo was conducted in patients with metastatic renal clear cell carcinoma who had progressed after, or could not receive interleukin-2. A total of 116 patients were randomly assigned to placebo, bevacizumab 3 mg/kg every 2 weeks, or bevacizumab 10 mg/kg every 2 weeks. No responses were noted in the low-dose group, while a partial response was seen in 10% of patients in the higher dose group. Toxicities included proteinuria, hypertension, and epistaxis. There was a difference between PFS in the high-dose group compared with the placebo group (4.8 versus 2.5 months; $P < 0.001$), but no improvement in overall survival occurred in any of the cohorts.[40] Subsequent studies have been undertaken with various combination therapies.

The most promising combination in renal cell carcinoma has been with interferon. A multicenter, randomized, double-blind, placebo-controlled phase III study of 649 patients with previously untreated metastatic renal cell carcinoma was performed. Patients were randomly assigned to either interferon alpha-2a (9 million international units subcutaneously three times weekly) and bevacizumab (10 mg/kg every 2 weeks) or interferon alone.[37] Progression-free survival (PFS) was significantly longer in the combination group (10.2 versus 5.4 months; $P = 0.0001$). The combination group had a higher response rate as well (31% versus 13%; $P = 0.0001$). Hypertension (26% versus 9%), headaches (23% versus 16%), venous thromboembolism (3% versus <1%), and bleeding (33% versus 9%) of any grade were more frequent in the bevacizumab combination arm than with interferon alone. Adverse events included grade 3 or 4 gastrointestinal perforations or thromboembolic events in 1% and 3% of bevacizumab-treated patients, respectively (Table 26-2).

Other combinations with bevacizumab have also been evaluated in renal cell carcinoma. Thalidomide plus bevacizumab was not found to be effective.[41] A phase II trial combined bevacizumab with erlotinib, an epidermal growth factor receptor (EGFR) tyrosine kinase inhibitor.[42] All 63 patients were treated with bevacizumab 10 mg/kg every 2 weeks and erlotinib 150 mg orally daily. Of 59 evaluable patients, a partial response was seen in 15 (25%), and

---

TABLE

26.2 *Food and drug administration (FDA)-approved drugs targeting the VEGF signaling pathway*

Drug	Target(s)	FDA-approved indications
Bevacizumab[a]	Monoclonal antibody All isoforms of VEGF	Metastatic colorectal cancer with intravenous 5-FU–based chemotherapy for first- or second-line treatment. Nonsquamous NSCLC, with carboplatin and paclitaxel for first-line treatment of unresectable, locally advanced, recurrent, or metastastic disease. Metastatic breast cancer, with paclitaxel, for treatment of patients who have not received chemotherapy for metastatic HER-2 negative breast cancer. Glioblastoma, as a single agent for patients with progressive disease following prior therapy.
Sorafenib	Tyrosine kinase inhibitor VEGFR 1, 2, and 3 Raf kinase PDGFR Flt-3 KIT RET	Advanced renal cell carcinoma, single agent Unresectable hepatocellular carcinoma, single agent
Sunitinib	Tyrosine kinase inhibitor VEGFR 1, 2, and 3 PDGFR KIT Flt-3 CSF-1R RET	Advanced renal cell carcinoma, single agent Advanced GIST, as a single agent after progression on or intolerance to imatinib

[a]FDA approval for advanced renal cell carcinoma in combination with interferon alpha-2a is expected in 2009.
PDGFR, platelet-derived growth factor receptor; Flt-3, FMS-like tyrosine kinase 3; KIT, stem cell factor receptor; RET, glial cell-line derived neutrophic factor receptor; CSF-1R, colony-stimulating factor receptor type 1; 5-FU, 5-fluorouracil; NSCLC, non–small cell lung cancer; HER-2, human epidermal receptor-2; GIST, gastrointestinal stromal tumor.

Potential Molecular Targets

Discoveries of cancer biology continue to provide a number of potential targets. These include

(a) Mutation, amplification, or overexpression of growth factors or their receptors involved in proliferation and survival of various cancers, such as the EGFR family, including HER2/neu;

(b) Mutation or enhanced activity of intracellular signaling pathways that promote growth, impede cell death, or enhance metastasis, such as activation of the Ras-RAF-MEK or PI3K pathways;

(c) Antiapoptotic mechanisms that antagonize cell death, such as overexpression of bcl-2 or decreased bax expression;

(d) Pathways, such as chaperoning, ubiquination, and the proteosome, that protect mutant or oncogenic proteins or affect their turnover rates;

(e) Epigenetic factors such as methylation or acetylation of histones, or methylation of DNA, which regulate gene expression and differentiation;

(f) MicroRNAs (miRNAs) that promote malignant growth;

(g) Tumor promoting factors in the environment, such as angiogenic pathways (e.g., vascular endothelial growth factor [VEGF] or platelet-derived growth factor [PDGF]);

(h) Pathways involved in suppressing immune response to cancer.[1–7,19]

Somatic mutations provide particularly important and unique targets in cancer (c-KIT mutations in gastrointestinal stromal tumor [GIST], EGFR mutations and eml4-alk translocations in cases of non–small cell lung cancer (NSCLC), and BCR-ABL translocation in CML).[20–25] Important brakes on proliferation can be lost, such as by mutations that inhibit function of p53, RB, or the phosphate and tensin homolog (PTEN), which down-regulates the PI3 kinase pathway,[8–10,26] but replacing these missing functions has not been feasible. An alternative strategy, searching for a synthetic lethal target, has been demonstrated in the experimental setting, as discussed below.

A number of theoretical and practical questions must be answered in order to validate the target, before a large-scale investment is justified. Among the most relevant questions are the following:

(a) Are subject gene and its protein found in human tumors, and is there selective expression in tumors versus normal tissues?

(b) Is the subject protein's function essential to the survival and proliferation, and, indeed, the transformed behavior of the malignant cells?

(c) Does inhibition of the gene product change the phenotype of these cells and lead to the desired result (such as death or growth arrest of malignant cells or a decrease in metastasis) in an appropriate animal model? It is critical to establish that the gene and associated protein product are important for the biology of human tumors and not just an animal model. Short interfering RNAs (SiRNAs) have become invaluable tools for inhibiting the expression of target genes within cells and determining the role of the target.[8,27,28] SiRNAs also have potential as therapeutic agents and early evaluation in clinical trials has begun.

(d) Is the protein also expressed in key proliferating normal tissues, such as intestinal epithelium and/or bone marrow progenitors, or even nonproliferating tissues, such as heart, kidney, or brain,

and does targeting the protein therefore carry risks for significant toxicity?

(e) The profile of gene expression in normal tissues may provide helpful clues about potential toxicity of an agent directed against that gene, as in the case of trastuzumab, an inhibitor of Her2/neu, a growth factor expressed in myocardium. In this case, gene knockout in animal models had early and fatal consequences for the developing embryo, indicating that inhibition of that gene or its protein product might lead to significant toxicity.

(f) Are there closely related proteins and what is their physiological function? Are they essential for normal tissue function and survival of the host and might be cross-targeted by the agent producing unwanted toxicities?

(g) Are there appropriate biomarkers that can identify likely "responders" and can these be developed as a guides for drug development in early trials?

Identification and optimization of biomarkers that:

(1) Aid in selecting appropriate patients likely to respond to a specific agent (e.g., HER2 positivity for trastuzumab, EGFR mutations for erlotinib, and BRAF mutations for BRAF inhibitors);

(2) Help validate that the target is being modulated in vivo (e.g., decreased pERK phosphorylation with BRAF inhibitor);

(3) Aid in optimizing dose and schedule;

(4) Serve as surrogates for response (e.g., HER2 positivity in breast cancer patients treated with trastuzumab and early decline in PET avidity in GIST patients treated with imatinib).

These considerations are essential in determining choice of a target and probability of success. Obviously, even a well-validated target may not be amenable to a drug discovery strategy for a number of reasons. Unanticipated toxicities or pharmacokinetic or pharmacodynamic problems in drug uptake, distribution, or elimination may defeat the most rational strategy.

The reader is referred to excellent reviews of high-priority molecular targets for cancer therapy and the role of biomarkers in the development of targeted agents.[1–7] Angiogenesis inhibitors, mAbs, targeting the EGFR family (EGFRs including Her2) and the PI3K pathway (including mTOR inhibitors), and targeted endocrine therapies are covered elsewhere in this book. The following is a brief review of several of the growth factor receptors and downstream signaling pathways that have yielded substantial new leads for cancer treatment.

Examples of Specific Targets: Growth Factor Receptors

Growth factor receptors or their ligands are among the most attractive molecular targets for cancer therapy[1–7,14,20–22,29,30] (Fig. 29-1). Their presence on the cell surface makes them more readily accessible to antibodies. They are overexpressed in many malignancies and are mutationally activated in others. Their important role in cellular processes essential for angiogenesis, proliferation, and survival of cells has been demonstrated. Growth factors and their receptors (such as VEGF ligands, VEGFR family, EGF ligands, and EGFR family) promote metastatic potential.[29,30]

Members of the EGFR family of receptors, including HER2, are especially attractive targets.[30–32] Through either mutation or overexpression, EGFR family members drive cell survival and proliferation as well as the metastatic process in many epithelial tumors.

Inhibition of EGFR in certain preclinical models leads to death of malignant cells and significant antitumor response. HER2/neu is expressed in a subset of patients with breast and gastric cancers and has been successfully targeted.[30–33] Anti-EGFR mAbs or small molecules have successfully treated lung, colorectal, and head and neck cancers.[34,35] Finally, as discussed above, mutant proteins provide the most specific target in cancer. EGFRs are mutated in a subset of lung adenocarcinomas, primarily in nonsmokers or light smokers, and these are very sensitive to inhibition by small molecular inhibitors of the tyrosine kinase activity of the EGFR.[36]

Other growth factor receptors that have been successfully targeted clinically include c-KIT, platelet-derived growth factor receptor (PDGFR), and VEGFR.[1,2,4,23,29] Mutations in *c-KIT* are found frequently in GIST tumors, with mutant *PDGFR* found in a smaller subset, and targeting of both of these by imatinib or sunitinib has been very successful clinically.[23] The VEGFR family (critically involved in tumor angiogenesis) has been successfully targeted in a number of malignancies, including colorectal, lung, renal cell cancer (RCC), hepatocellular cancer (HCC), breast cancers, and glioblastoma.[1,2,4,29]

Signaling Pathways Downstream of Growth Factor Receptors

Signals from growth factors travel through multiple switches (Ras, PI3 kinase, MAP kinase, SMAD, and others; Fig. 29-1) to reach nuclear and cytoplasmic effectors. Studies continue to evaluate the potential for inhibiting these intracellular pathways either alone or in combination with each other or with anti–growth factor receptor agents as a means of treating cancer. The Ras and PI3 kinase pathways have been the two most extensively evaluated as potential targets to date. The RB pathway is essential in negatively controlling proliferation and various approaches are being pursued to modulating this function in malignant cells.

Ras Pathways

One of the first oncogenes to be recognized in human tumors was mutated *Ras* genes and the resultant constitutively activated Ras proteins[37–39] (Fig. 29-1). Ras proteins play central roles in transmitting signals important for a variety of critical processes in cells, including proliferation and differentiation. One of the key roles played by Ras proteins (products of the *KRAS, NRAS,* and *HRAS* genes) is in transmitting signals from growth factor receptors (such as the EGFR) to downstream signaling molecules. Normally, Ras proteins are activated by binding guanosine triphosphate (GTP), and they subsequently activate downstream targets in signaling cascades, including Raf kinases.[37–39] In the process, GTP is hydrolyzed to guanosine diphosphate and Ras is inactivated. Mutations at codons 12, 13, or 61 of the Ras genes activate Ras proteins by locking them in the GTP-bound state. This leads to constitutive signal transduction in the absence of growth factor stimulation. *Ras* mutations occur relatively frequently in a number of malignancies. For example, *KRAS* mutations are found in approximately 35% to 40% of colon cancers, 70% to 90% of pancreatic cancers, and 30% of adenocarcinomas of the lung.[40–42] *NRAS* is mutated in approximately 25% of acute nonlymphocytic leukemias and *KRAS* in another 15%.[42] *HRAS* is mutated in a minority of bladder and head and neck cancers. Thus, as a molecular target, Ras proteins have an essential role in maintaining the malignant state.

Attempts to inhibit the activated GTP binding site in mutant Ras have not been tractable to date so a number of other aproaches have been pursued. The unprocessed native protein is inactive and requires sequential extensive posttranslational modification to allow insertion in the plasma membrane, a step required for its active signaling function.[43] It must first be farnesylated (attachment of a 15-carbon, lipophilic group) by soluble prenylation enzymes. The carbon terminal (C-terminal) CAAX motif of Ras then directs the prenylated protein to the endoplasmic reticulum and Golgi, in which the C-terminal AAX residues are cleaved by a specific protease. The terminal prenylcysteine is then methylated by a prenyl cysteine methyl transferase found in the endomembrane system. The final product is exported to its active site in the plasma membrane. In the case of N- and H-RAS, this occurs after further lipid attachment (palmitic acid) to another cysteine or cysteines. KRAS, which possesses a polybasic region upstream from the C-terminal peptide, does not require palmitoylation to localize in the plasma membrane.[37,38,43] Initial attempts to develop compounds blocking Ras function focused attention on the farnesylation reaction,[43] although there has also been interest in exploring inhibition of prenyl cysteine methyl transferase and Ras proteases. The farnesyltransferase inhibitors lacked significant activity in the clinic, leading to new strategies that have examined inhibitors of downstream signaling (e.g., BRAF or the proteins in the MEK/ERK/MAP kinase pathway).[44,45] Plx4032, an inhibitor of BRAF kinase (another downstream target) has encouraging activity against melanomas harboring V600E BRAF mutations but only inhibits the mutant BRAF protein.[45] Engelman et al.[46] showed that the joint blockade of the MAP kinase and PI-3 kinase pathways kills Ras-mutant lung cancer cells, an approach that has entered clinical trials. Barbie et al.[47] found that KRAS mutation leads to synthetically lethal sensitivity to inhibition of BKT-1, a component of the NF-κB response to stress, providing another potential target for treating malignancies harboring KRAS mutations.

Ras and *BRAF* mutations also serve as important biomarkers for determining potential resistance to targeted therapies. Constitutive activation of Ras or Raf proteins in tumors negates the effect of inhibitors of upstream receptor proteins such as EGFR. For example, colorectal cancers that have mutations in KRAS are resistant to antibodies directed against the EGFR.[48] Although the data is not as mature, this is probably true for tumors harboring *BRAF* mutations as well.[49]

PI3K Pathway

The PI3K pathway also mediates signaling from growth factor receptors and is frequently activated in malignancies.[50,51] As mentioned above, many growth factor receptors signal through both MEK/MAP kinase and PI3K pathways and inhibiting both pathways may be necessary to optimally inhibit growth of certain malignant cells.[46] As mentioned above, combinations of MEK and PI3K pathway inhibitors are underway. PI3K inhibitors, including inhibitors of downstream mTOR signaling (temsirolimus and everolemis), are reviewed in Chapter 30.

Retinoblastoma Pathway

As opposed to the proliferative and cell survival signals mediated by the above two pathways, the RB pathway serves a critical role in negatively modulating proliferation.[9] The RB protein in its underphosphorylated state inhibits E2F, a transcription factor that promotes synthesis

Signaling Inhibitors: IGFR, PI3K Pathway, Embryonic Signaling Inhibitors, and Mitotic Kinase Inhibitors

Helen X. Chen, L. Austin Doyle, Naoko Takebe, William C. Timmer, and S. Percy Ivy

Significant progress has been made in understanding the molecular basis of cancer; this knowledge is being translated into the design and development of signal transduction inhibitors for cancer treatment. Multiple signaling pathways have been implicated in the development and persistence of cancer, including the (IGF-1R) and the phosphatidylinositol-3 kinase (PI3K)-protein kinase B (AKT) pathway, as well as several embryonic signaling pathways. In this review, we will examine the molecular targets within important signal transduction pathways, specifically IGF-1R, PI3K, AKT, Hedgehog (Hh), Notch, Wnt, kinesin spindle proteins (KSPs), polo-like kinases (PLKs), and aurora kinases, found to be responsible for cancer cell development, proliferation, maintenance, and malignancy. Furthermore, agents designed to target these pathways will also be discussed, as well as challenges facing the preclinical and clinical development of targeted therapies against these signaling pathways.

Inhibitors of IGF/IGF-1R Signaling

Overview

IGF-1R has been recognized for decades for its role in the tumorigenesis and growth.[1] Various approaches targeting this pathway have been explored in the laboratory, including monoclonal antibodies

(mAbs), small molecule tyrosine kinase inhibitors (TKIs), antisense, and insulin-like growth factor I (IGF-I) peptide mimetics.[2] Clinical development of IGF-1R inhibitors had, however, lagged until advances in medicinal chemistry and biotechnology. Currently, more than ten new IGF/IGF-1R-targeting agents have entered clinical trials. The two main classes of IGF-1R inhibitors in clinical development are mAbs and small molecule TKIs.

IGF-1R and IGF System

IGF-1R is a receptor tyrosine kinase (RTK) activated by binding to its ligands, IGF-I or insulin-like growth factor II (IGF-II). IGF-1R is expressed on the cell surface as preformed dimers and is composed of two extracellular α-chains and two membrane-spanning β-chains in a disulfide-linked β-α-α-β configuration.

IGF-1R shares extensive homology with the insulin receptor (IR) and belongs to the insulin receptor family that includes IR (homodimer), IGF-1R (homodimer), IGF-1R/IR (hybrid receptors), and the mannose-6-phosphate receptor (IGF-2R)[1] (Fig. 30-1). IGF-1R can be activated by IGF-I or IGF-II; IGF-1R/IR hybrids act like homodimers, preferentially binding and signaling with IGFs. IR exists in two isoforms: IR-B (traditional IRs) and IR-A (a fetal form that is re-expressed in selected tumors and preferentially binds IGF-II).[3] IGF-2R is a non–signaling receptor that acts as a "sink" for IGF-II.[4] These receptors may coexist in a given cell; however,

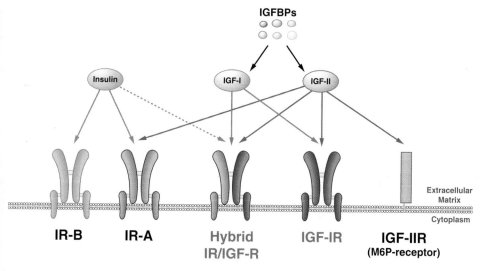

IGFBPs

Insulin   IGF-I   IGF-II

Extracellular Matrix
Cytoplasm

IR-B   **IR-A**   **Hybrid IR/IGF-R**   **IGF-IR**   **IGF-IIR (M6P-receptor)**

FIGURE 30-1 The insulin receptor family includes the IR (in isoforms IR-A and IR-B), the type 1 insulin-like growth factor (IGF-IR), and the mannose-6-phosphate receptor (IGF-IIR). IR and IGF-IR, both tyrosine kinase receptors, are expressed as preformed dimers, either as homodimers or heterodimers (IR/IGF-IR). IGF-IIR is a non-signaling receptor that acts as a "sink" for IGF-II. Insulin binds primarily to the two isoforms of the IR receptor, but also it has weak affinity for IR/IGF-IR heterodimer. IGF-I and IGF-II are ligands for the IGF-IR and IR/IGF-IR hybrid receptor; IGF-II also binds to IR-A isoform. IGF-BPs bind to and prevent IGF-I and -II from activating the receptor signaling cascades. (Please see Color Insert.)

individual receptors' relative abundance and activation status vary with specific cells, tissues, and physiological or pathological conditions.

The ligands, IGF-I and IGF-II, are abundant in the serum of adults.[5] IGF-I is secreted primarily by the liver upon stimulation by human growth hormone (HGH) but can also be produced in muscle and bone. IGF-II is not dependent upon HGH and is expressed in a variety of tissues. Six well-characterized IGF-binding proteins (IGFBP-1 through -6) can bind IGFs and prevent their action on the receptors. Only about 2% of IGF ligands exist in free-form in serum. Local bioavailability of IGF-I/II for IGF-1R signaling is also altered by IGF-BP protease and the presence of the non–signaling, IGF-II-binding IGF-2R.

Intracellular signaling of IGF-1R is triggered upon binding of IGF-I and IGF-II and mediated through IR substrates 1 to 4 (IRS 1 to 4) and Src-homology collagen protein (Shc).[6] This leads to activation of two main downstream pathways: the RAS-RAF-mitogen-activated protein kinase kinase (MEK)-extracellular signal-related kinase (ERK) pathway and the PI3K-AKT pathway.[4] It is generally accepted that PI3K-AKT is the more predominant signal transduction pathway for the IR family.

IGF-1R and IGF in Normal Tissues and Physiology

IGF-1R is ubiquitously expressed in normal tissues and plays an important role in growth and development and various organs' physiological functions including the cardiac and neurological systems. In addition, IGF-1R and IGF-I are also involved in glucose homeostasis, probably through the feedback downregulation of HGH by circulating IGF-I and the local effect of IGF-I on IGF-1R in muscles or kidneys to promote glucose uptake.[7,8]

IGF-1R in Cancer

In vitro and in vivo studies have implicated IGF-1R and IGF-I/II signaling in cancer development, maintenance, and progression. IGF-1R expression is critical for anchorage-independent growth, a well-recognized property of malignant cells. IGF-I and IGF-II are strong mitogens for a wide variety of cancer cell lines including prostate,[9] breast,[10–13] colon,[14,15] and myeloma.[16] High circulating levels of IGF-I have been associated with an increased risk of breast, prostate, and colon cancer.[1] IGF-1R signaling regulates a number of cellular processes including proliferation, apoptosis, and motility. Furthermore, the IGF/IGF-1R pathway has extensive cross talk with the estrogen receptor (ER), epidermal growth factor receptor (EGFR), and human epidermal growth factor receptor 2 (HER-2) signaling and plays an important role in the resistance mechanisms of cytotoxic drugs and EGFR/HER-2-targeted agents.[17]

Positive expression of IGF-1R is observed in most solid tumors and hematological malignancies examined to date, and IGF-II over-expression, IGF-BP modulations, and IGF-2R downregulation have also been seen in cancer cells.[6,18,19] However, unlike other growth factor receptors such as EGFR and HER-2, activation mutations of the IGF-1R gene have not been reported, and gene amplification is extremely rare in the tumors that have been tested.[20] Several genetic abnormalities can lead indirectly to IGF-1R-IGF overexpression and signaling. For example, in Ewing's sarcoma (EWS), the EWS/friend leukemia integration-1 (FLI-1) translocation product was found to interact with the IGF-BP3 promoter and repress its expression. IGF-1R is required for transformation by the EWS/FLI-1 fusion protein. Some tumor types, including hepatocellular carcinoma (HCC) and breast cancer, have been associated with deletion or loss of heterozygosity (LOH) of IGF-2R gene.[21] Loss of imprinting of the IGF-II (loss of methylation resulting in bi-allelic expression), first described in Wilms' tumor, has later been identified in adult tumors and is associated with an increased risk of colon cancer.[22,23] These genetic changes may increase IGF-II production or IGF-II bioavailability for IGF-1R signaling.

IGF/IGF-1R Pathway Inhibitors

Several approaches to inhibit the IGF-1R signaling have been investigated. Agents in current clinical development belong to three main classes (Tables 30-1 and 30-2): 1) mAbs against IGF-1R, 2)

TABLE 30.1 *Monoclonal antibodies IGF-1R or IGF (status as of 7/09) in clinical trials*

Target	Agent name	Sponsor	Status	Class	Phase 2 dose	Dose intensity (dose/wk)	Average $t_{1/2}$
IGF-1R	IMC-A12[29,321]	ImClone	Phase 2	IgG1	6 mg/kg qwk 10 mg/kg q2wk	5–6 mg/kg	8–9 d
IGF-1R	CP-751,871 (figitumumab)[26–28]	Pfizer	Phase 3	IgG2	20 mg/kg q3wk	6.7 mg/kg	12 d
IGF-1R	MK-0646 (h7C10)[33,322]	Pierre Fabre and Merck	Phase 3	IgG1	10 mg/kg q2wk	5 mg/kg	4 d
IGF-1R	AMG 479[32]	Amgen	Phase 2	IgG1	18 mg/kg q3wk	6 mg/kg	7–11 d
IGF-1R	R1507[30]	Roche	Phase 2	IgG1	9 mg/kg qwk	9 mg/kg	8 d
IGF-1R	SCH 717454 (19D12)[35]	Schering Plough	Phase 2	IgG1	NA	NA	NA
IGF-1R	AVE1642 (EM164)[31]	ImmunoGen/Sanofi	Phase 2	IgG1	8 mg/kg q4wk 12 mg/kg q3wk	2–3 mg/kg	9 d
IGF-1R	BIIB022[323,324]	Biogen-IDEC	Phase 1	IgG4	NA	NA	NA
IGF-I and IGF-II	MEDI-573[325,326]	MedImmune	Phase 1	IgG2	NA	NA	NA

$t_{1/2}$, half life; qwk, every week; q2wk, every 2 weeks; q3wk, every 3 weeks; q4wk, every 4 weeks; NA, not available.

TABLE

30.2 *Small molecule tyrosine kinase inhibitors against IGF-1R*

Agent	Sponsor	Class (route)	IC50 (µM) against			Status
			IGF-1R	InR	Other[a]	
OSI-906[39,40]	OSI	TKI (oral) ATP-competitive	0.018	0.054	None	Phase 1
BMS-754807[327]	BMS	TKI (oral) ATP-competitive	<2 nM	<2 nM	11 other kinases <100 nM	Phase 1
BVP 51004[328]	Biovitrum	Small molecule (oral) Non ATP-competitive	0.038 µM	No effect	None	Phase 1
XL228[329]	Exelixis	TKI (IV) ATP-competitive	1.6 nM (cellular)	NA*	• Bcr-abl: 5 nM • Bcr-abl T315I: 1.4 nM • Src: 6.1 nM • Aurora A: 3.1 nM • LYN: 2 nM (all cellular)	Phase 1
INSM-18 (NDGA)[330,331]	Insmed	Phenolic compound isolated from creosote bush *Larrea divaricatta*	31 µM (cellular)	NA*	HER-2: 15 µM (cellular)	Phase 1

*Not available.
[a]Targets for which IC50 is <50-fold of the IC50 for IGF-1R.
IC50, half maximal inhibitory concentration; IV, intravenous; NDGA, Nordihydroguaiaretic acid.

mAbs against the ligand (IGF-I and II), and 3) IGF-1R TKIs. Clinical data are available for IGF-1R mAbs and TKIs.

These IGF-IGF-1R-targeting agents share common effects on IGF/IGF-1R signaling but differ in mechanisms of action, spectrum of target inhibition, and pharmacological features (Table 30-3).

For example, anti-IGF-1R mAbs only block signaling through the IGF-1R and IGF-1R/IR hybrid, while the IGF-I/II-neutralizing mAb prevents IGF signaling through both homodimers and heterodimers of IGF-1R and IR-A, but spares insulin signaling. Due to the high homology between IGF-1R and IR, IGF-1R TKIs can

TABLE

30.3 *Main features of mAbs and small molecule TKIs against the IGF/IGF-1R pathway*

	mAb against IGF-1R	mAb against IGF-I and II	Small molecule TKI
Mechanism of action	• Block IGF-1R from ligand binding • Receptor degradation of IGF-1R homodimer and IGF-1R/IR hybrid • Possible ADCC (if IgG1)	• Neutralizing ligand from binding to IGF-1R and IR-A	• Kinase inhibition intracellular - (also inhibit ligand-independent activation, if relevant)
Signaling affected	• Specific • Inhibit signaling of: – IGF-1R – IGF-1R/IR-A hybrid • No effect on IR-A or IR-B	• Specific • Inhibit IGF-I or IGF-II signaling through – IGF-1R – IGF-1R/IRA – IRA • No effect on Insulin signaling	• Less specific • Inhibit signaling of RTKs (by any ligands): – IGF-1R – IGF-1R/IR – InR (to a lesser degree than for IGF-1R) • May inhibit targets beyond IGF-1R and IR (XL228; INSM-18)
PK	• Long $t_{1/2}$ (days to weeks) • PK interaction less likely in combination regimens • Poor CNS uptake	• Long $t_{1/2}$ (days to weeks) • PK interaction less likely in combination regimens • Poor CNS uptake	• Short $t_{1/2}$ (hours)

mAbs, monoclonal antibodies; TKIs, tyrosine kinase inhibitors; ADCC, antibody-dependent cell-mediated cytotoxicity; RTKs, receptor tyrosine kinases; PK, pharmacokinetics; $t_{1/2}$, half-life; CNS, central nervous system.

potentially block all receptors responsible for IGF/insulin signaling. The differing spectrum of target blockade may potentially translate into different toxicity and/or activity profiles.

Anti-IGF-1R Monoclonal Antibodies

At least eight human or humanized anti-IGF-1R mAbs are in clinical development, from phase 1 to phase 3 (Table 30-1). Treatment regimens being explored include monotherapy, combination with standard chemotherapies, and combination with other molecular-targeting agents. Table 30-1 depicts Immunoglobulin G (IgG) subclasses, stages in development, and average elimination half-lives $(t_{1/2})$. Since these mAbs' major mechanism of actions and pharmacokinetic (PK) features are similar, they are to be discussed as a group with selected examples.

These antibodies are highly specific to the target (IGF-1R) and do not bind IR. Although each antibody (Ab) may be unique in its epitope, common mechanisms of action include blockade of receptor from ligand binding and internalization/degradation of IGF-1R.[24] In addition, administration of anti-IGF-1R mAbs has also been shown to down-regulate the IGF-1R/IR hybrid receptor.[25] Most of the anti-IGF-1R mAbs are IgG1, except CP-751,871 (figitumumab) (IgG2), and BIB022 (IgG4). A potential mechanism of action of IgG1 is antibody-dependent cytotoxicity (ADCC); however, it is not known whether this is relevant to the anti-IGF-1R mAbs' antitumor activity patients.

Phase 1 Trials of Anti-IGF-1R mAbs

Phase 1 dose escalation trials with various anti-IGF-1R mAbs have been carried out using weekly, every 2-week (q2wk), every 3-week (q3wk), or every 4-week (q4wk) schedules. Various anti-IGF-1R mAbs' PK features are similar and consistent with humanized or human mAbs against other targets. For example, in the first-in-human phase 1 trial of CP751,871,[26] the agent was given q3wk at escalating dose levels from 0.025 to 20 mg/kg. The plasma concentration and the area under the curve (AUC) increased proportionally at dose levels beyond 1.5 mg/kg, with a $t_{1/2}$ of 10 to 12 days. The dose levels of 10 and 20 mg/kg q3wk were chosen as the recommended phase 2 doses (RP2Ds) for monotherapy or combination with chemotherapy.[27,28] Phase 1 studies with other anti-IGF-1R mAbs have average $t_{1/2}$ of about 7 to 9 days although the published data were based on limited number of patients (Table 30-1).[29-33]

The anti-IGF-1R mAbs are generally well tolerated as monotherapy. Common treatment-related adverse events (AEs), based on the Common Terminology Criteria for Adverse Events (CTCAE) version 3.0, include hyperglycemia, fatigue, anorexia, nausea, mild infusional reactions and rash. Thrombocytopenia and transaminase elevations may also occur, but their frequency and severity may depend on the clinical setting and prior therapies. Data from a larger number of patients in additional clinical studies are necessary to fully establish these toxicity profiles.

Hyperglycemia is considered the class side effect of all anti-IGF-1R mAbs. This AE is likely due to the blockade of IGF-I/IGF-1R interaction, which normally promotes glucose uptake and has a glucose-lowering effect.[7,8] Blockade of IGF-1R also significantly increases circulating HGH, which could lead to gluconeogenesis and hyperglycemia. The compensatory increase in insulin level, on the other hand, may be responsible for maintaining glucose homeostasis in most patients after anti-IGF-1R agents. In most phase 1 trials, which exclude patients with hyperglycemia at baseline (patients with history of diabetes were not excluded), the rate of mild/moderate hyperglycemia (grade 1 to 2) is around 20%, and grade 3 or higher hyperglycemia is very rare.[26,28] Risk of hyperglycemia may be increased in patients with history of glucose intolerance or concurrent use of glucocorticoids. In most patients, hyperglycemia can be controlled with oral diabetic medications.

The maximum tolerated doses (MTD) for monotherapy were not reached at the conclusion of the phase 1 trials for all anti-IGF-1R mAbs. Selection of the phase 2 dose was largely based on feasibility, and the target steady-state level was extrapolated from preclinical in vivo tumor models. Table 30-1 lists the recommended phase II doses for monotherapy for different IGF-1R mAbs.

Pharmacodynamic Changes and Preliminary Evidence of Antitumor Activity

Pharmacodynamic changes have been explored in early clinical trials with anti-IGF-1R mAbs. Downregulation of surface IGF-1R in granulocytes and circulating tumor cells has been reported with a number of mAbs, including AMG-479[32] and CP-751,871.[34] Anti-IGF-1R mAbs also induced a significant increase in HGH and IGF-I and a variable increase in the insulin level.[26,27,31,32,35] Decrease in the standardized uptake values of (18)F-fluoro-2-deoxy-D-glucose-positron emission tomography (FDG-PET) has also be observed in anecdotal cases[32]; however, these observations are too preliminary to provide information on the optimal dosing or correlation with clinical outcomes.

Anti-IGF-1R mAbs have demonstrated evidence of clinical activity in early trials. Most notable were reports of complete or partial responses (CRs or PRs) and prolonged stable disease (SD) in patients with EWS refractory to standard chemotherapies.[30,32,36,37] A number of phase 2 trials, including a pivotal registration trial with R1507, are ongoing to define the magnitude of activity with anti-IGF-1R mAbs in chemo-refractory EWS.

PRs and minor responses have also been observed in phase 1 trials in patients with neuroendocrine tumors,[38] and prolonged SD was seen in a patient with HCC, thymoma, and prostate cancer, although the clinical benefit in these indications was uncertain. The efficacy of monotherapy is being evaluated in phase 2 studies in a variety of tumor types including adult sarcomas, HCC, prostate cancer, breast cancer, neuroendocrine tumors, and multiple myeloma. A National Cancer Institute (NCI)/Cancer Therapy Evaluation Program (CTEP)–sponsored multistrata oncology trial is also evaluating the activity of an anti-IGF-1R mAb, IMC-A12, in a number of pediatric malignancies such as EWS, rhabdomyosarcoma, osteosarcoma, Wilms' tumor, and neuroblastoma.

IGF-1R Small Molecule TKIs

Several small molecule TKIs against the IGF-1R are under clinical investigation. Among them, OSI-906 and BMS 754-807 are the most specific, while others also inhibit RTKs beyond the IGF-1R and IR families (Table 30-2).

Because of the high degree of homology between IGF-1R and IR, even the most specific IGF-1R TKIs have some degree of inhibitory effect on the IR. For example, OSI-906 has a half maximal inhibitory concentration (IC_{50}) of 0.018 μM (micromolar) versus 0.054 μM against the IGF-1R and IR, respectively.[39,40] At the clinically relevant doses, this agent is expected to inhibit IGF-1R and IR simultaneously. Coinhibition of IR in addition to IGF-1R could confer therapeutic advantage and potentially increase toxicities. IR signaling by insulin or IGF-II has been implicated in a number of preclinical tumor models,[41] and IR overexpression is common in breast cancer.[42] Furthermore, when the IGF-1R signaling is disrupted, cells may respond with an increase in IR signaling.[43]

IGF-1R TKIs have demonstrated extensive antitumor activities in both in vitro and in vivo models as single agents and in combination with chemotherapy or targeted agents such as EGFR, mammalian target of rapamycin (mTOR), and HER2-inhibitors. Because IR inhibition is expected to be associated with toxicities, particularly hyperglycemia, the key question about IGF-1R TKIs is whether a therapeutic window can be achieved in patients.

Clinical Experience with IGF-1R TKIs

Phase 1 results for OSI-906 were reported at the American Society for Clinical Oncology (ASCO) Annual Meeting 2009[44,45] for two main schedules: continuous oral dosing (once or twice daily without interruption) and intermittent oral dosing (Day 1 to 3 every 14 days). At the dose range of 10 to 450 mg daily, 20 to 70 mg twice daily, or 10 to 450 mg on day 1 to 3 every 14 days, the treatment was well tolerated. Only mild (grade 1) and transient hyperglycemia were observed; one patient at 450 mg daily developed asymptomatic grade 3 hyperglycemia, which lasted for 5 hours.[45]

OSI-906's target effect was reflected by a dose-dependent increase in the insulin levels while glucose levels were relatively stable. SD (>12 weeks) was seen in patients with thymic, adrenocortical, and colorectal cancer (CRC). Most interestingly, in the phase 1 trial for the intermittent schedule,[44] one of the three patients with adrenocortical carcinoma had a confirmed PR in the primary and multiple lung metastases, while another patient had prolonged SD (32 weeks).

Daily dosing up to 300 mg indicated a linear PK, with median terminal $t_{1/2}$ of 2 to 4 hours, AUC from time 0 to infinity (AUC_{0-inf}) of 284 to 10,200 ng·h/mL and a maximum concentration (C_{max}) of 76.6 to 1,440 ng/mL.[45] At 450 mg in the intermittent schedule, the C_{max} was 3.2 μg/mL.[44] The plasma concentrations in the phase 1 trials exceeded the "efficacious" concentration (IC_{50}) in the in vitro models (1 μM). Additional data are needed to determine how the preclinical IC_{50} correlates with biologically and therapeutically relevant exposures in patients. Dose escalations for both schedules are ongoing.

Combination of IGF-1R Inhibitors with Other Anticancer Therapies

Combination of IGF-1R Inhibitors and Chemotherapy

IGF-1R signaling may protect tumor cells from chemotherapy and radiotherapy. Mechanistically, the enhanced activity of the combination of radiation and IGF-1R inhibition has been linked to the inactivation of the PI3K/AKT pathway. Inhibition of IGF-1R concurrently with chemotherapy enhances tumor cell apoptosis in several models, including cisplatin-treated ovarian cell lines,[46] gemcitabine-treated

pancreatic cancer xenografts,[47] and vinorelbine-treated breast and non–small cell lung cancer (NSCLC) xenografts.[48]

A number of clinical trials have tested combinations of anti-IGF-1R mAbs and standard chemotherapies in multiple tumor types. Data from a randomized phase 2 trial examining carboplatin and paclitaxel with or without CP-751,871 in patients with advanced untreated NSCLC have been reported.[28] The combination was feasible at the full dose of CP-751,871 for monotherapy (20 mg/kg q3wk) when administered with the chemotherapy. The rate of grade 3 to 4 hyperglycemia was increased and manageable with routine glucose-lowering medications. In comparison to chemotherapy alone, the addition of CP-751,871 was associated with an increase in the response rate, especially in the subset of patients with squamous cell histology. Two phase 3 confirmatory trials have been begun in NSCLC with chemotherapy and CP-751,871.

Combination with Antiestrogen Therapy

One key growth and survival mechanism of estrogen-dependent tumors is functional cross talk and codependence between the IGF/IGF-1R and ER.[17,49,50] IGF enhances the responsiveness of ER to estrogen and may also directly activate the ER. Anti-IGF-1R agents are highly active in estrogen-dependent, tamoxifen-responsive cell lines but generally ineffective in tamoxifen-resistant cells.[51] Furthermore, addition of anti-IGF-1R antibodies to tamoxifen enhanced the antitumor activity in T61 and MCF-7 tamoxifen-sensitive breast cancer models.[25,51,52]

These results support the clinical evaluation of addition of IGF-1R inhibitors to antiestrogen therapies. A number of clinical studies with several anti-IGF-1R mAbs in combination with aromatase inhibitors or estrogen antagonists are ongoing in hormonal therapy-naïve and therapy-resistant tumors. Given IRs' potential role in this cancer, evaluation of IGF-1R TKIs or IGF-I/II neutralizing mAbs would also be interesting.

IGF-1R Blockers and EGFR or HER-2 Inhibitors

IGF-1R signaling has been causally linked to de novo or acquired resistance to trastuzumab (Herceptin) and EGFR-targeting agents in numerous models, including breast cancer, CRC, and glioblastoma.[17] The mechanisms of IGF-related resistance to EGFR/HER-2 inhibitors have not been entirely elucidated, but are thought to be mediated through the PI3K/AKT pathway. In vitro and in vivo tumor models have also demonstrated direct interactions and cross talk between IGF-1R, EGFR, and HER-2.[17,50,53-55] In trastuzumab-resistant subclones of HER-2-overexpressing cell lines, unique colocalization of IGF-1R and HER-2 has been described.[55,56] Treatment of resistant cells with anti-IGF-1R antibodies or TKIs was shown to inhibit transactivation of HER-2 and restore sensitivity to trastuzumab.[17,55,56] Similarly, addition of anti-IGF-1R agents to EGFR TKIs or anti-EGFR antibodies has been shown to prevent, delay, or reverse resistance to these anti-EGFR agents.[53,54]

Taken together, these results suggest that combined inhibition of IGF-1R and EGFR or HER-2 may be a potentially useful strategy to enhance EGFR- or HER-2-targeting agents' therapeutic potential. Both anti-IGF-1R mAbs and TKIs (OSI-906) are being tested in combination with erlotinib (OSI-774, Tarceva) in NSCLC. Combinations of anti-IGF-1R and anti-EGFR mAbs [cetuximab (IMC-C225, Erbitux) or panitumumab (ABX-EGF, Vectibex)] are also ongoing in CRC, NSCLC, and head and neck cancer. In addition, NCI/CTEP is sponsoring randomized phase 2 trials for lapatinib (GSK-57216, Tykerb) with or without IMC-A12 in HER-2-positive (by gene amplification) breast cancer and erlotinib (OSI-774, Tarceva)/gemcitabine with or without IMC-A12 in patients with pancreatic cancer. Results of clinical testing are not yet available.

IGF-1R and mTOR Inhibitors

Treatment with mTOR inhibitors could lead to upregulation of AKT phosphorylation in tumors.[57,58] The feedback AKT activation was likely mediated by the IGF/IGF-1R pathway. Although it is not clear whether this AKT activation is related to mTOR inhibitors' escape/resistance mechanism, combination studies with rapamycin (sirolimus, Rapamune) and IGF-1R inhibitors suggest additive antitumor effects compared to single agents alone.[57,58] The most significant synergism in activity was observed in pediatric tumor EWS models and osterosarcoma, where the combination of an anti-IGF-1R mAb and rapamycin led to complete tumor regression, single-agent IGF-1R mAb, and rapamycin only induced modest growth delay.[59]

A number of proofs of principal clinical studies are ongoing to test the combination of IGF-1R and mTOR inhibitors in selected tumor types including sarcoma, breast, and prostate cancer. A phase 1 trial with IMC-A12 and temsirolimus (CCI-779, Torisel) has reported preliminary data indicating that the combination is feasible,[60] although the full safety profile in more patients with longer therapy remains to be established. Phase 1 and phase 2 trials for this combination have also been planned for the pediatric population.

Considerations in Predictive Markers for Sensitivity or Resistance

Preliminary experience with IGF-1R inhibitors indicates that the single-agent clinical benefit would be limited to a subset of tumors and a subset of patients. The potential reasons for de novo or acquired resistance would include absence or biological irrelevance of the intended target (IGF-1R), presence of redundant or compensatory pathways, or constitutively activated downstream effector molecules. Biomarker studies have the potential to elucidate the predictive markers for sensitivity or resistance and to provide guidance for rational combinations.

Currently, no predictive markers for IGF-1R inhibitors are available. In view of the complexity of the IGF-1R and IR family, as well as their extensive interaction with several other signal transduction pathways, it may be difficult to identify a uniform set of predictive markers for all tumor types and molecular contexts, and for all classes of the IGF/IGF-1R inhibitors. Biomarker studies are focusing on the following areas:

- Tumor genomic alternations within the IGF-1R axis;
- Genetic alterations outside the IGF-1R axis that may affect the IGF-1R signaling (e.g., chromosomal translocations resulting in transcriptional modulations of the IGF-ligand or receptors);
- Level and phosphorylation status of IGF-1R and IR;
- Bioavailability of the ligand (including IGFBP3, IGF-I/II, and decoy receptor IGF-2R);
- Activation mutations of the downstream molecules such as AKT, PI3K, RAS, and RAF; markers related to parallel pathways such as EGFR and vascular endothelial growth factor (VEGF); and
- Markers related to epithelial-mesenchymal transition.

Summary

The three classes of IGF/IGF-1R inhibitors—anti-IGF-1R mAbs, IGF-I/II-neutralizing mAbs, and IGF-1R TKIs—have distinctive mechanisms of actions and potentially different resistance/escape mechanisms. Given the complexity of the IGF-1R/IR receptor family, and the variable and dynamic predominance of each component in the physiologic conditions and tumor biology, each class of anti-IGF/IGF-1R agents may have unique advantages in selected tumor settings and different toxicity profiles. Clinical trials are under way in a variety of indications, including several pediatric malignancies, using single-agent or combination regimens with cytotoxic therapies and with other molecularly targeted agents.

Preliminary safety profiles with anti-IGF-1R mAbs and TKIs are favorable, with the main toxicity being mild-to-moderate and manageable hyperglycemia, although effects associated with prolonged therapy and combination regimens remain to be established. Clinical responses to monotherapy have been observed in certain tumors, providing proof of principle for IGF-1R as a valid target of cancer therapy. The most important task of the field is to explore predictive markers and to develop rational strategies for combination studies.

The PI3K/AKT/mTOR Signaling System

Overview

The PI3K/AKT/mTOR pathway is a cellular growth and survival pathway that is activated in a wide variety of human cancers. PI3K can be activated by tyrosine kinase growth factor receptors, integrins and other cell adhesion molecules, G-protein-coupled receptors, and intermediary proteins such as RAS[61] (Fig. 30-2). Activated tyrosine kinases recruit class Ia PI3K through binding of the Src-homology 2 (SH2) domain of the p85-regulatory subunit of PI3K to specific phosphotyrosine (YxxM) components of the signaling complex.[61,62] Activated PI3K causes phosphorylation of the D3 position of phosphoinositides to generate phosphatidylinositol-3,4,5-triphosphate (PIP_3). PIP_3 binds to the pleckstrin homology (PH) domain of the PH domain–containing kinase (PDK1) and the serine/threonine kinase AKT, anchoring both proteins to the cell membrane, leading to their activation. AKT1 is activated by phosphorylation of T308, in its catalytic domain, by PDK1 and then by subsequent phosphorylation of S473 by several kinases [including mTOR when bound to the rapamycin-insensitive companion of mTOR (Rictor) in the target of rapamycin complex 2 (TORC2)].[63,64] AKT is expressed in three different isoforms: AKT1, AKT2 and AKT3, which are variably expressed in most tissues and tumors.[65]

The membrane translocation and activation of AKT are opposed by the tumor suppressor phosphatase and tensin homolog on chromosome 10 (PTEN). PTEN is a phosphatase that antagonizes PI3K by dephosphorylating PIP_3, preventing activation of AKT and PDK-1.[66] Once activated, AKT phosphorylates the consensus sequence RXRXX(S/T) in many downstream targets,[67] leading to alterations in the expression of proteins important in cell-cycle progression, apoptosis, angiogenesis, cytoskeletal arrangement, and the regulation of ribonucleic acid (RNA) transcription and protein translation.

While AKT is undoubtedly a critical substrate of activated PI3K, the inhibition of PI3K also diminishes Rac activation and

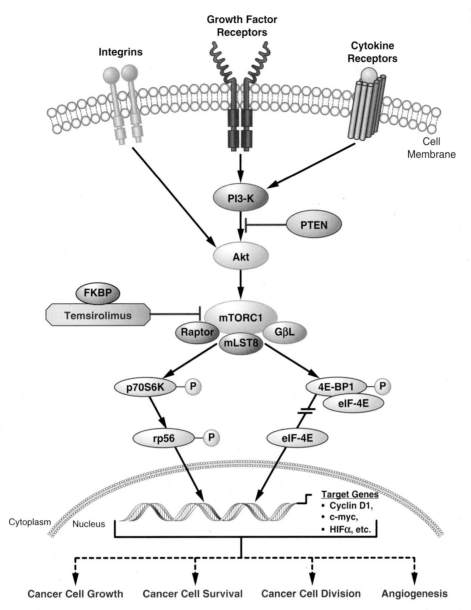

FIGURE **30-2** Activation of integrin receptors, growth factor receptors, and cytokine receptors activates the PI3K/AKT signaling pathway, leading to the activation of the mTOR (part of the mTORC1 complex). Activation of mTORC1 leads to the phosphorylation of S6K1 and 4E-BP1. S6K1 phosphorylates rpS6, while phosphorylated 4E-BP1 dissociates from eIF-4E. Both rpS6 and eIF-4E promote mRNA transcription and protein translation, leading to cell growth and proliferation, angiogenesis, and the prevention of apoptosis. mTOR inhibitors, such as temsirolimus, bind to FK506-binding protein (FKBP) and inhibit the kinase activity of the mTORC1 complex. (Please see Color Insert.)

other important downstream targets. Phosphoprotein profiling and functional genomic studies demonstrate that many cancer cell lines and human breast tumors with mutations of the catalytic (p110α) subunit of PI3K (PI3KCA) have only minimal AKT activation and little requirement of AKT for anchorage-independent growth.[68] These cells, instead, are characterized by robust PDK1 activation and have dependency on the PDK1 substrate serum/glucocorticoid regulated kinase 3 (SGK3). SGK3 undergoes PI3K- and PDK1-dependent activation in PIK3CA-mutant cancer cells. Therefore, PI3K activation may promote cancer through both AKT-dependent and -independent mechanisms, with important implications for the treatment of patients with these tumors.

Cell-cycle progression is influenced by AKT through inhibitory phosphorylation of the cyclin-dependent kinase inhibitors p21 and p27 and by the inhibition of glycogen synthase kinase 3β (GSK3β), which stabilizes cyclin D1.[69,70] AKT regulates apoptosis by inactivating the proapoptotic protein BAD, which controls the release of cytochrome c from mitochondria.[71,72] AKT phosphorylation of the FoxO family of transcription factors inhibits transcription of the proapoptotic genes Bim, Fas-L, and JGFBP-1.[73,74] AKT also phosphorylates IκB kinase (IKK), which increases the activity of nuclear factor-κB (NF-κB) and the transcription of prosurvival genes.[75] AKT phosphorylation of the human homologue of mouse double minute 2 (MDM2) leads to inhibition of p53, with effects on cell-cycle progression, apoptosis, and DNA repair.[76]

mTOR is a highly conserved 250-kD phosphoprotein, which is a critical convergence point in cellular signaling pathways for cell growth, metabolism, and proliferation.[77] mTOR is a serine/

threonine protein kinase, which acts to control protein translation in response to nutrients, hypoxia, energy levels, hormones, and growth factors, all modulated through the PI3K/AKT pathway. AKT can directly activate mTOR through phosphorylation but also causes indirect activation of mTOR by inhibitory phosphorylation of tuberous sclerosis complex 2 (TSC2). TSC2 inhibits mTOR through the guanosine triphosphate (GTP)–binding protein, Ras homolog enriched in brain (Rheb). Inhibitory phosphorylation of TSC2 by AKT results in conversion of Rheb to an active form that phosphorylates and activates mTOR. mTOR exists in two complexes: target of rapamycin complex 1 (TORC1) of mTOR, which is bound to the regulatory-associated protein of mTOR (Raptor), and the TORC2 complex, in which mTOR is bound to Rictor. The TORC1 complex includes a novel component, proline-rich AKT substrate (PRAS40), and TORC2 includes the proteins stress-activated map kinase–interacting protein 1 (SIN1) and proline-rich protein 5 (PRR5).[78] PRAS40 acts as an inhibitor of mTOR kinase activity in a phosphorylation-dependent manner.[77]

Activation of mTORC1 regulates cellular growth and proliferation through control of protein synthesis.[79] Components of this regulation include initiation of messenger RNA (mRNA) translation, organization of the actin cytoskeleton, ribosome biogenesis, and protein degradation. Phosphorylation of S6 kinase 1 (S6K1) at threonine 389 by mTORC1 leads to the subsequent phosphorylation of the ribosomal protein S6, eukaryotic initiation factor (eIF-4B), and eukaryotic elongation factor (eEF) 2 protein kinase, with critical effects on cellular protein translation.[80] The mTORC1 complex also phosphorylates 4E-binding protein 1 (4E-BP1), a translational repressor, causing 4E-BP1 to dissociate from eIF-4E, which is an mRNA cap-binding protein.[81] After dissociation from 4E-BP1, eIF-4E can then promote the translation of 5′-cap mRNA species, including cyclin D1, c-Myc, HIF-1α, and VEGF.[82]

The TORC2 complex can phosphorylate and activate AKT at serine 473 in a positive feedback mechanism.[64] However, TORC1 activation of S6K1 can inhibit the activation of AKT through a negative feedback mechanism, by catalyzing an inhibitory phosphorylation of IRS1 with resultant decreased activation of PI3K.[83]

The activity of mTOR is also regulated through a cellular energy–sensing pathway, sensitive to cellular levels of amino acids and adenosine triphosphate (ATP), and by the tumor suppressor protein LKB1, which is inactivated in Peutz-Jeghers syndrome.[83] LKB1 activates adenosine monophosphate (AMP)–activated kinase, which subsequently activates TSC1/2, thereby leading to mTOR inhibition.

Deregulation of the AKT Pathway in Human Cancer

The PI3k/AKT/mTOR pathway can be activated in cancer by loss of the tumor suppressor PTEN function, amplification or activating mutation of PI3K, amplification or mutation of AKT, or activation of upstream growth factor receptors (Table 30-4). Recent studies also demonstrate that mTOR signaling is inhibited by the p53 tumor suppressor gene, and that loss of p53 function results in mTOR activation.[84] Both PTEN phospholipase and PI3K3CA are frequently mutated across many human cancers.[68] PTEN mutations occur commonly in prostate cancer, renal cell cancer (RCC), HCC, melanoma, endometrial cancer, and glioblastoma. Activating mutations in the PI3KCA gene have been discovered in large numbers of human tumors, including 27% of breast and 19% of colon

TABLE 30.4 *Components of the mTOR pathway with evidence of involvement in human cancers*

Mutated/overexpressed protein	Types of cancer
PTEN	• Lung • Breast cancer • Prostate cancer • H&N cancer • Glioblastoma
AKT	• Breast cancer • Thyroid
PI3K	• Breast cancer • Endometrium • Colon • Liver
eIf4E	• H&N squamous carcinoma • Renal cancer • Lymphoma
TSC1/2	Benign tumor syndrome (hamartoma syndromes, including tuberous sclerosis complex, PTEN-related hamartoma syndromes and Peutz-Jeghers syndrome)
S6K1	Breast cancer
HIFα	• Renal cancer • Breast cancer • Prostate cancer

cancers, according to the Catalogue of Somatic Mutations in Cancer database. Three recurrent oncogenic "hotspot" mutations comprise the majority of somatic PI3KCA mutations.[85] Gene mutation in the p85 regulatory domain of PI3K has also been noted in colon and ovarian cancers.[86] Amplification of AKT1 has been described in human gastric carcinoma, and amplification of AKT2 has been reported in pancreatic, ovarian, gastric, head and neck, and breast carcinomas.[88–92]

Abnormal activation of the TSC/Rheb/mTOR pathway, through loss of tumor suppressor gene function, has been associated with the pathobiology of tumor predisposition syndromes such as tuberous sclerosis (TSC1/2), Cowden's syndrome (PTEN), and the Peutz-Jeghers syndrome (LKB1).[83] Loss of LKB1 function leads to hyperactivation of mTOR signaling.[87]

A number of downstream targets of mTOR are activated in human cancer. Overexpression or amplification of S6K1 or eIF-4E, with resultant effects on protein translation, has been associated with oncogenesis in breast, ovarian, and other human cancers.[88] Overexpression of eIF-4E has been shown in many human cancers and is linked to tumor progression and poor prognosis.[89] In contrast, expression of 4E-BP1 has an antitumorigenic effect, partly mediated through increased expression of the cell-cycle inhibitory protein p27Kip1, and appears to modulate the effect of eIF-4E overexpression.[90]

Deregulation of the PI3K/AKT/mTOR pathway has been consistently noted to be associated with high-risk or poor prognosis human cancers. PTEN genomic deletion is associated with pAKT expression and androgen receptor signaling in poorer outcome, hormone-refractory prostate cancer.[91]

Inhibitors of PI3K/AKT/mTOR Pathway

PI3K Inhibitors

It is not clear whether pan- versus isoform-specific inhibition of PI3K would have the greatest clinical utility in oncology. Inhibitors of all of the isoforms of PI3K effectively inhibit signaling from the great majority of all cell surface receptors and have pleiotropic effects on cell proliferation, apoptosis, angiogenesis, migration, and metastasis. The pharmacologic agents wortmannin and LY294002 are potent inhibitors of PI3KCA, but in vivo toxicity and poor solubility have prevented clinical development.[92–94]

LY294002 is an ATP-competitive pan-PI3K inhibitor that blocks all classes of PI3K at low μM concentrations.[95] Extensive preclinical evaluation demonstrates potent activity of LY294002 on cancer cells and on the tumor microenvironment. Wortmannin has been extensively tested with a variety of cytotoxic anticancer drugs, and it broadly increases apoptosis and inhibition of AKT in a wide variety of in vitro and in vivo cancer models.[96] While LY294002 and wortmannin are not suitable for human trials, a variety of PI3K inhibitors are in clinical trials, including SF1126, BEZ235, XL147, and TG100-115. SF1126 is an RGDS-conjugated prodrug of LY294002.[95] NVP-BEZ235 is a combined pan-PI3K/mTOR inhibitor, currently being tested in phase 1 and phase 2 trials of solid tumor patients.[97,98] TG100-115 is a $p110\gamma/\delta$ specific inhibitor of PI3K that has been demonstrated to reduce vascular permeability.[99]

PDK1 Inhibitors

PDK1 activates AKT through specific phosphorylation at Ser473 and Thr308 and has non–AKT-mediated mechanisms to promote the growth of cancer cells, leading to interest in PDK1 inhibitors.[68] UCN-01 (7-hydroxystaurosporine), a protein kinase C (PKC) inhibitor isolated from *Streptomyces*, is also a potent PDK1 inhibitor, and the subsequent inhibition of AKT is associated with apoptosis in cancer cells.[100] UCN-01 has had extensive clinical evaluation, but its toxicity and very long $t_{1/2}$ have limited development of the agent.[101] Newer PDK1 inhibitors, such as BX-795, BX-912, and BX-320, inhibit binding to the ATP-binding pocket of the catalytic domain of PDK1 and have potent inhibition of PDK1 and AKT activation in xenograft models.[102]

AKT Kinase Inhibitors

Perifosine (KRX-0401)

Perifosine is an orally bioavailable alkylphospholipid that interacts with the PH domain of AKT to prevent its translocation to the plasma membrane and subsequent activation.[103] Perifosine has demonstrated in vitro inhibition of the growth of breast, prostate, colon, and lung cancer cells, and potentiation of doxorubicin, etoposide, temozolomide (SCH52365, Temodar), and radiation therapy in cancer cell models.[104–106] Perifosine has been studied in phase 1 and 2 clinical trials, but limited data exist on its ability to inhibit AKT in clinical samples from these trials.[107]

TCN-P (triciribine)

TCN-P, also known as AKT/PKB signaling inhibitor 2 (API-2), is a tricyclic nucleoside that was initially shown to have antitumor activity in human clinical trials and later identified as an AKT inhibitor.[108] TCN-P was found to inhibit the growth of AKT2-transformed NIH3T3 cells, but not parental cells, and to selectively inhibit phosphorylation of AKT2.[109] TCN-P induced apoptosis in a number of cancer cell lines and inhibited the growth of xenograft tumors overexpressing AKT2 in nude mice. TCN-P has multiple toxicities including hyperglycemia, hepatotoxicity, hypertriglyceridemia, and thrombocytopenia, which have limited its clinical development.[108]

MK-2206

MK-2206 is an orally active, allosteric AKT inhibitor that inhibits all three AKT species in vitro.[110] The drug causes aggregation of the PH domain of AKT to the catalytic subunit, preventing membrane localization and activation of the protein. MK-2206 is highly selective and has inhibited tumor growth in several xenograft models, including A2780 human ovarian cancer, LNCaP human prostate cancer, and a spontaneous murine prostate tumor induced by organ-specific conditional PTEN knockout. MK-2206 caused complete tumor regressions of A2780 xenograft tumors when given on a weekly schedule following docetaxel. A phase 1 trial was completed, and MK-2206 was found to have a MTD of 60 mg orally every other day, with higher doses limited by rash.[111] The drug has also been associated with hyperinsulinemia and hyperglycemia, which represent pharmacodynamic effects, and have not been dose limiting. Phase 1 results have shown prolonged SD and minor antitumor effects, but no Response Evaluation Criteria in Solid Tumors (RECIST) responses to date. Evidence of potent inhibition of phosphorylated AKT by MK-2206, from pre- and posttreatment biopsies, has been seen in patients on the phase 1 trial.

mTOR inhibitors

Rapamycin (sirolimus, Rapamune)

Rapamycin is a macrolide antibiotic derived from the bacteria *S. hygroscopicus* isolated from a soil sample from Easter Island (Rapa Nui).[112] Rapamycin was initially found to have antifungal and immunosuppressive properties. Rapamycin was subsequently found to induce p53-independent apoptosis of rhabdomyosarcoma cell lines and decrease cyclin D1 expression and proliferation in pancreatic cancer cell lines.[113,114]

Rapamycin's pharmacologic action is mediated through its binding to the binding protein FK506, with subsequent inhibition of mTOR.[114] Researchers observed that rapamycin inhibited mTOR-mediated p70s6K and 4E-BP-1 phosphorylation; this suggested its antitumor effects were due to regulation of protein translation dependent on these targets. Rapamycin's effect on inhibiting cell cycling at the G1/S-phase transition point is related to the drug's effect on cyclin-dependent kinase activation and retinoblastoma protein phosphorylation, as well as on the accelerated cyclin D1 turnover and an increased association of p27[kip1] with cyclin E/cdk2.[115] Prolonged exposure to rapamycin may also lead to tissue-specific AKT inhibition, through depletion of mTORC2, which normally activates AKT.[116]

Poor aqueous solubility and chemical instability have limited the development of rapamycin as an intravenous (IV) anticancer drug.

It is currently being tested in oral formulations in several early phase trials in various cancers in daily and weekly dosing schedules.[117]

Temsirolimus (CCI-779, Torisel)

Temsirolimus is an ester analog of rapamycin that was developed by NCI in collaboration with Wyeth Ayerst due to favorable in vitro and in vivo efficacy and toxicity data. Temsirolimus was found to have a mechanism of action similar to rapamycin, and multiple human tumor cell lines were found to have sensitivity to temsirolimus with $IC_{50} < 10^{-8}$ M.[118] In vivo animal xenograft models demonstrated that temsirolimus induced significant tumor growth inhibition, using several intermittent dosing regimens. The efficacy of intermittent dosing with temsirolimus is of interest since the immunosuppressive effects of the drug resolve within 24 hours after dosing.

Early phase clinical trials with temsirolimus demonstrated prolonged SD and occasional tumor responses, particularly in RCC. Its toxicity included rash, mucositis, thrombocytopenia, hypertriglyceridemia, nausea, anorexia, edema, fatigue, and hypercholesterolemia.[119] The FDA approved temsirolimus for refractory RCC based on a phase 3 study of 626 patients who received either temsirolimus alone (25 mg IV weekly), interferon alpha alone, or a combination of the two agents.[120] Patients treated with temsirolimus had an improved median survival of 10.9 months compared to patients treated with interferon alpha, who had a median survival of 7.3 months ($P = 0.008$). Patients treated with the combination of agents survived a median of 8.4 months; therefore, combination therapy is not recommended.

Temsirolimus has demonstrated activity in mantle cell lymphoma, other B-cell lymphomas, breast cancer, endometrial cancer, and neuroendocrine cancers. In a phase 2 trial of metastatic or recurrent endometrial cancer, 5 of 19 evaluable patients (26%) had an objective response to 25 mg/week of temsirolimus, and 12 (63%) demonstrated SD.[121] Dose escalation above 25 mg IV weekly of temsirolimus has not been associated with improved clinical benefit, except in one Wyeth-sponsored phase 3 trial in mantle cell lymphoma, in which maintenance with 75 mg IV weekly was found to lead to improved progression-free survival (PFS).[120] More than 60 clinical trials are ongoing with temsirolimus, including 5 phase 3 trials. Temsirolimus in combination with cytotoxic chemotherapy frequently leads to significant problems with mucositis and other toxicity, but temsirolimus has been successfully combined with carboplatin and paclitaxel, at a modified dose of 25 mg IV Days 1 and 8 of a 3-week schedule, with promising activity in patients with refractory solid tumors.[122]

Everolimus (RAD001, Afinitor)

Everolimus is a hydroxyethyl ester of rapamycin developed for transplant and anticancer applications. Everolimus is rapidly absorbed after oral administration, and with a $t_{1/2}$ of approximately 30 hours, can be given on a daily schedule.[123,124] The FDA approved everolimus for relapsed advanced RCC based on results from the phase 3 RECORD-1 trial, in which treatment with everolimus more than doubled the time to progression relative to placebo (4.0 versus 1.9 months), and reduced the risk of disease progression by 70%.[125] Patients in the control arm were allowed to cross over to the everolimus arm upon disease progression.

Phase 2 data were reported for everolimus in patients with advanced neuroendocrine cancer.[126] Sixty patients with either islet cell or carcinoid tumors received depot octreotide and oral everolimus, either at 5 or 10 mg/d. The partial response rate was 17%, with an additional 75% of patients reported as having SD. Everolimus is being tested in a phase 3 placebo-controlled trial of patients with advanced neuroendocrine tumors. More than 80 everolimus trials, including 7 phase 3 trials, are ongoing in a wide variety of solid tumors and hematologic malignancies.[127] Everolimus is generally well tolerated but oral mucositis, rash, weakness, and the less common occurrence of grade 3 or 4 drug-related toxicities, such as pneumonitis, infection, and diarrhea, do occur.

Deferolimus (AP23573)

Deferolimus, another rapamycin anologue, can be given in a variety of IV schedules. Phase 1 testing found that the MTD was 18.75 mg daily when given 5 days per week, every 2 weeks.[128] Phase 2 studies have shown objective responses in patients with mantle cell lymphoma and agnogenic myeloid metaplasia, as well as hematologic improvement/SD in myelodysplastic syndrome and acute myelogenous leukemia (AML).[129] Deferolimus has been extensively tested in sarcoma, and objective responses, prolonged SD, and clinical benefit were noted.[130,131] Deferolimus is being evaluated in sarcoma with the phase 3 SUCCEED study (Sarcoma Multi-Centre Clinical Evaluation of the Efficacy of Deferolimus).

TORC1/TORC2 Inhibitors

Inhibition of mTORC1 by rapamycin analogues inhibits S6K and prevents an inhibitory phosphorylation of IRS1. This mechanism leads to increased PI3K activation and activating phosphorylation of AKT, which may allow survival of cancer cells treated with an mTOR inhibitor. Several agents inhibit both mTORC1 and mTORC2, preventing the second activating phosphorylation of AKT at Ser473 and countering the stimulatory effects of mTORC1 inhibition on AKT activation. AZD8055 is an ATP-competitive inhibitor of TORC1/TORC2 kinases.[132] AZD8055 was inactive in a counter screen against 260 other kinases. The drug inhibited downstream targets of mTORC1, such as phosphorylation of S6. It also inhibited the phosphorylation of Ser473 of AKT, a function of mTORC2. AZD8055 inhibited proliferation of a large number of malignant cell lines in vitro, with broader activity than rapamycin. It inhibited the growth of several xenograft models, and in a U87-MG glioblastoma xenograft model, a PK/pharmacodynamic relationship was found for total drug plasma concentrations greater than 30 nM with a 50% inhibitory phosphorylation of AKT in tumor tissue.

Toxicology studies demonstrated that AZD8055's dose-limiting toxicity (DLT) in animal models included emesis, enteritis, and weight loss, with hyperinsulinemia and hyperglycemia seen in a dog model.[132] AZD8055 is undergoing phase 1 testing on a twice-daily schedule.

OSI-027 is another TORC1/TORC2 kinase inhibitor. This agent is undergoing a multicenter phase 1 trial in patients with solid tumors and lymphoma in Europe.[98,133]

PI3K-PTEN Signaling Effects on Hypoxia and Angiogenesis

Hypoxia-induced factor 1-α (HIF1α) and VEGF are important antitumor targets expressed by cancer cells in response to hypoxia and to nutrient deficiency. The PTEN/PI3K balance of activity functions as a rheostat, integrating extracellular and cellular signal information to determine whether the cell needs to recruit a blood supply, as well as controlling the stromal response to angiogenic stimuli.[134] In prostate cancer biopsies, for example, microvessel density correlated inversely with PTEN status.[135] Activated mutants of PI3K expressed in chicken embryo cells were associated with VEGF signaling augmentation and increased angiogenesis.[136] The high vascularity of Cowden's disease, Peutz-Jeghers, and tuberous sclerosis complex may be related to the increased mTOR activity in these tumors. Regression of Kaposi sarcoma in renal transplant patients treated with rapamycin has demonstrated this approach's potential.[137]

The success of rapamycin analogues in clinical trials of hypervascularized human cancers, such as RCC and neuroendocrine tumors, may be related to their antiangiogenic effects. RCC frequently has loss of von Hippel-Lindau (VHL) tumor suppressor function, which functions to degrade HIF-1α.[138] In the absence of the VHL protein, RCC overexpresses HIF-1α, leading to an increase in VEGF, platelet-derived growth factor (PDGF), cyclin D levels, and transforming growth factor-α (TGF-α). mTOR regulates the mRNA translation of HIF-1α; therefore, inhibition of mTOR has antiangiogenic and antiproliferative properties through its regulation of HIF-1α. mTORC2 may have a complex role in modulating angiogenesis.[139]

Studies in glioblastomal cancer cells have demonstrated a correlation between activation of PI3K/AKT and the subsequent expression of HIF1α and its substrate VEGF.[140] Enforced expression of PTEN in cancer cells, or chemical inhibition of PI3K signaling with LY294002, inhibits expression of HIF1α.[140] Translation of both VEGF and HIF1α mRNA is regulated by mTOR signaling.[141] The inhibition of mTORC1 by CCI-779 has been shown to reduce expression of HIF1α and HIF2α under both normoxic and hypoxic conditions in mouse xenograft models. The antiangiogenic effects of rapamycin analogues through blocking VEGF/VEGFR and PDGF/PDGFR signaling pathways may be related in part to effects on endothelial cells and pericytes, and on the carcinoma cells themselves.[142]

Combinations with PI3K/AKT/mTOR

Combinations of mTOR Inhibitors and Inhibitors of Cell Signaling and Angiogenesis

mTOR functions as an integration system for a number of signaling pathways, and inhibition of mTOR may affect multiple pathways dysregulated in various cancers. mTOR inhibition can induce apoptosis and reduce cancer cell proliferation, angiogenesis, and metastasis. Preclinical studies suggested that mTOR inhibition could provide synergistic benefits when added to other targeted signal transduction inhibitors. Rapamycin synergizes with the EGFR inhibitor erlotinib in NSCLC, pancreatic, colon, and breast tumors.[143] In breast cancer, preclinical studies suggested that the aromatase inhibitor letrozole was synergistic with mTOR inhibition. A phase 3 international trial of advanced breast cancer, with patients randomly assigned to receive letrozole alone or in combination with intermittent CCI-779, was conducted.[144] No difference was found in the objective tumor responses and clinical benefit rate between the two arms of the study.

Antiangiogenic agents, such as bevacizumab (Avastin), sunitinib (Sutent), and sorafenib (Nexavar), could potentially complement the downstream antiangiogenic effects of an mTOR inhibitor. Phase 2 studies of temsirolimus and bevacizumab have shown promising activity, and an ongoing phase 3 trial is comparing bevacizumab combined with either temsirolimus or interferon as first-line therapy of advanced RCC. The BeST trial (bevacizumab, sorafenib, and temsirolimus) is a four-arm phase 2 study that will randomize 360 patients with advanced RCC to receive bevacizumab as a single agent, bevacizumab plus sorafenib, bevacizumab plus temsirolimus, or sorafenib plus temsirolimus.[145]

Combination of PI3K and MEK Inhibitors

The PI3K/AKT/mTOR pathway is interlinked with another crucial growth and survival signaling system, known as the MAP kinase (MAPK) pathway.[146] The MAPK pathway includes RAF kinases and their target kinase cascade, including MEK and ERK. Both the MAPK and PI3K/AKT/mTOR pathways are regulated by RAS, which directly stimulates the activation of both PI3K and RAF. The RAS pathway is constitutively activated in a sizable proportion of human cancers as a result of frequent activating mutation. Inhibition of mTORC1 has also been found to lead to MAPK pathway activation through a PI3K-dependent feedback loop in tumor biopsies from patients being treated with everolimus. These findings suggest a mechanism by which tumor cells may survive treatment with a rapamycin analogue but also indicate the potential of combined treatment with mTOR and MAPK inhibitors.

Tumors with constitutive activation of the RAS oncogene are frequently resistant to cytotoxic chemotherapy. In a mouse lung cancer model, driven by mutant KRAS, xenograft tumors did not respond substantially to the PI3K inhibitor NVP-BEZ235. When NVP-BEZ235 was combined with the MEK inhibitor AZD6244, however, marked synergy was noted in shrinking the KRAS-mutant xenograft tumors.[147]

Combination of mTOR and IGF-1R Inhibitors

Stimulation of the IGF-1R activates the PI3K/AKT/mTOR pathway in many cells. Activation of the mTOR substrate S6K leads to a feedback loss of IRS-1 expression, resulting in decreased signaling through the IGF-1R pathway.[57] mTOR inhibition induces IRS-1 expression in cancer cells and abrogates the feedback inhibition of the PI3K/AKT/mTOR pathway, leading to increased AKT phosphorylation. This phenomenon may explain cancer cell survival after mTOR inhibition and rapamycin analogues' limited efficacy in many human tumors. Preclinical studies have demonstrated that IGF-R1 inhibition prevents AKT activation induced by rapamycin, leading to sensitization of the tumor cell to mTOR inhibitors.[57] These findings suggest a therapeutic strategy of combining rapamycin analogues with small molecule or Ab inhibitors of IGF-1R signaling. Indeed, combinations of these agents are currently being tested in early-phase clinical trials.

AKT/mTOR Activation and the Cellular Stress Response

AKT-deficient cells are resistant to replicative senescence, oxidative stress, oncogenic RAS-induced premature senescence, and reactive oxygen species (ROS)–mediated apoptosis.[148] AKT activation in cancer cells induces premature senescence and sensitizes tumor cells to ROS-mediated apoptosis; it increases intracellular ROS by increasing oxygen consumption and inhibiting the expression of ROS scavengers that are regulated through the FoxO family of transcription factors. FoxO transcription factors decrease ROS and inhibit cellular senescence, while FoxO deficiency increases ROS and cellular senescence. The AKT-mediated increase in ROS levels could contribute to tumorigenesis by increasing the cancer cells' mutation rates and genetic instability. Tumor cells with increased intracellular ROS levels mediated by AKT are more susceptible to premature senescence unless they acquire an immortalizing genetic alteration, such as p53 loss.

While AKT inhibits apoptotic responses from many stimuli, it cannot inhibit ROS-mediated apoptosis.[148] This phenomenon may be a potentially exploitable treatment strategy to inhibit cancer cells with PI3K/AKT/mTOR signaling overexpression. Furthermore, since treatment of cancer cells with rapamycin analogues causes feedback activation of AKT, the rapamycin analogues may hypersensitize cancer cells to ROS-mediated apoptosis. A xenograft model treated with the ROS inducer PEITC and rapamycin showed complete eradication of tumor cells in which AKT is hyperactivated.

Oxygen deficiency in tumors is associated clearly with tumor heterogeneity, metastasis, and chemoresistance.[149] Hypoxia alters the tumor cell behavior through a variety of oxygen-sensitive pathways, most prominently through the HIF family of transcription factors. Hypoxia in tumors leads to activation of endoplasmic reticulum stress sensors and perturbs endoplasmic reticulum homeostasis. Hypoxia signaling through mTOR regulation of the translation of HIF transcription factors can lead to an unfolded protein response (UPR) in cancer cells. The UPR is a program of transcriptional and translational changes that occur as a consequence of endoplasmic reticulum stress and includes effects on protein production, maturation, and degradation, as well as effects on cellular metabolism, autophagy, and apoptosis. The emergence of the mTOR and UPR pathways as interlinked, important contributors to hypoxia tolerance, indicate new opportunities for targeted cancer therapy.

Inhibition of mTORC1 alone has a potential risk of increasing tumor hypoxia and tumor resistance to treatment by inhibiting angiogenesis or by promoting tumor thrombosis.[150] A number of TKIs and Abs that have had clinical value influence hypoxic cell signaling and improve tumor oxygenation through decreased VEGF expression and normalization of tumor vasculature.[151] Drugs such as bevacizumab, trastuzumab, erlotinib, imatinib (Gleevec), and tipifarnib all decrease tumor hypoxia, affect signaling to mTOR, and might have a rational basis for combination with mTOR inhibitors. Agents that increase endoplasmic reticulum stress in cancer cells by interfering with the UPR pathway, such as PS-341 (bortezomib, Velcade) and geldanomycin (17-AAG), also might reasonably be combined with agents that interfere with PI3K/AKT/mTOR signaling.[149] An interesting new drug, in this regard, is the protease inhibitor nelfinivar (Viracept), which is currently used in the treatment of human immunodeficiency virus (HIV) and affects hypoxia sensing and signaling. It is under evaluation in cancer clinical trials.[152,153] Nelfinivar increases endoplasmic reticulum stress in cancer cells, inhibits AKT signaling, impairs HIFα and VEGF expression, and induces apoptosis and autophagy. The combined effects of nelfinivar and radiation result in significant alteration of the tumor microenvironment, with less tumor hypoxia and improved radiation response.[153] Nelfinivar's clinical efficacy with other modulating

agents of PI3K/AKT/mTOR signaling or with cytotoxic chemotherapy has not yet been assessed.

Embryonic Stem Cell Signaling Inhibitors

Deregulation of Hedgehog, Wnt, and Notch Signaling Pathways in Cancer

Hh, Notch, and Wnt signaling pathways are required for normal embryonic development and function of many organs in addition to stem cells. These signal pathways regulate cell proliferation and apoptosis. In addition to the crucial role of these normal signaling pathways, increasing evidence suggests that deregulation of these pathways plays an important role in the development and progression of several malignancies. Therefore, Hh, Notch, and Wnt signaling pathways appear to represent novel therapeutic targets in cancer cells, including cancer stem cells (CSCs).

Hedgehog Signaling Pathway

The Hh signaling pathway is an essential mediator of normal tissue development.[154] The signaling mechanism of the Hh and the Wnt proteins (discussed later in this review) are similar despite their proteins being unrelated.[155] Hh protein has lipid-modified signals; the cell-surface receptor Smoothened (Smo) uses the protein kinases GSK3β and casein kinase I-alpha (Ck1α) to facilitate proteolysis of the key transcriptional effectors such as Cubitus interruptus (Ci), a *Drosophila* gene and glioma-associated (Gli) homologue, for Hh.[156] Moreover, Hh proteins are not glycosylated but acylated, carrying covalently attached palmitates at the N-terminus.[157,158] The Hh protein is made as a precursor molecule; it consists of a C-terminal protease domain that releases an active signaling domain (HhNp) by autocatalytic cleavage, followed by covalent binding of cholesterol.[155] The gene rasp is the enzyme that acylates Hh and is required for Hh production. Hh requires a devoted transport molecule called Dispatched, which is a multiple-pass transmembrane protein.

Hh binding it its receptor Patched (Ptch1) initiates signaling via the Sonic Hedgehog (Shh) pathway.[159] Hh binding to Ptch1 can also induce Hh inhibitor protein (Hip). Ptch inhibits the G-protein-coupled phosphoprotein receptor Smo by preventing its localization to the cell surface. In the presence of Shh, the ligand-Ptch complex is internalized and the repression of Ptch on Smo is relieved. Localization of Smo to the membrane primary cilium is thought to initiate a signaling cascade in mammals, leading to the activation of the Gli family of zinc finger transcription factors. In vertebrates, three Gli proteins are known, with Gli1 and Gli2 thought to activate Hh target genes and Gli3 thought to act mainly as a repressor. Hh signaling regulates tumor-related vascular formation and function[160]; the mechanism involved is associated with expression of Ptch1 in tumor-associated endothelial cells but not in normal tissue endothelial cells.[161]

Deregulated Hh Pathway in Cancer or CSCs

Aberrant activation of the Hh pathway in cancers is caused by mutations in the pathway including basal cell carcinoma (BCC) and medulloblastoma (ligand-independent). Alternatively, Hh overexpression can occur in pancreatic cancer, small cell lung cancer (SCLC), breast cancer, and digestive tract tumors (ligand-dependent).[159,162–164] A paracrine mechanism in Hh signaling in cancer was elegantly demonstrated in a xenograft model using a tumor and stromal cell coinjection procedure.[165] Tumors such as pancreatic cancer, CRC, ovarian cancer, and B-cell malignancies have an elevated level of Hh ligand expression that mediates Hh pathway activation through the stromal microenvironment, consistent with a paracrine signaling mechanism. Limited evidence in solid tumors demonstrates the association between Hh signaling and CSCs, such as the polycomb gene Bmi-1, which may regulate stem cell self-renewal by control of Gli transcription factor.[166] Hh signaling is essential for maintenance of CSCs in chronic myeloid leukemia (CML).[167]

Antagonism of excessive Hh signaling may provide a unique mechanism-based therapy, blocking tumor growth and stimulating tumor regression while sparing toxic effects on normal adjacent tissue. The prototype of Hh pathway-specific inhibitors is cyclopamine (11-deoxojervine), a plant-derived steroidal alkaloid from the herbaceous plant, *Veratrum californicum*, which directly binds to and inactivates Smo.[168] Synthetic small molecules with improved inhibiting activity against Smo were discovered and the other pathway inhibitors are also under investigation.[159,169] Results from in vitro studies must be interpreted with caution because high concentrations of an Hh antagonist were needed to inhibit cell proliferation, indicating the potential nonspecific or toxic effects of these compounds.[170,171]

Preclinical Investigational Agents Targeting Hh Pathway

Several natural and synthetic small molecule inhibitors of Smo targeting the Hh pathway may be suitable for therapeutic intervention (Table 30-5). These molecules are at the preclinical stage of development. The antagonists that bind to Smo include other plant alkaloids besides cyclopamine and their derivatives, such as jervine.[172] Cell-based high-throughput screening has revealed several distinct classes of antagonists, which also bind to Smo. These include KAAD cyclopamine,[168] SANTs1-4,[173] compound-5,[172] compound-Z,[172] and Curis compound CUR-61414,[178] an aminoproline. Moreover, small molecules that inhibit SHh signaling downstream of Smo such as GANT61 and GANT58 have been identified.[174] A small molecule that binds to the extracellular Shh protein, robotnikinin, was isolated from small-molecule microarray (SMM)–based screens.[175] Targeting Shh ligands may be an interesting approach since the tumor-derived Shh ligands directly activate signaling in stromal cells. This, in turn, stimulates tumor growth in a paracrine manner. Extracellular inhibitors of Hh and Wnt signaling have feedback loops as most

| | | | TABLE |
| | | | **30.5** *Hedgehog-targeted therapies* |

Agent	Target	Mechanism of action	Disease	Phase of development
Cyclopamine[168] • Natural compound	Smoothened	Antagonist	• Medulloblastoma • BCC • Pancreatic cancer • Prostate cancer • Breast cancer • GBM • MM • Ovarian cancer	Preclinical
IPI-926[332] • Synthetic small molecule			• Medulloblastoma • Pancreatic cancer • SCLC • Solid tumors	• Preclinical (medulloblastoma, pancreatic, and SCLC) • Phase 1 (solid tumors)
GDC-0449[333] (Cur-61414) • Synthetic small molecule			• BCC • Pancreatic cancer • Medulloblastoma • Ovarian cancer • SCLC • CRC	• Phase 1 (pancreatic) • Phase 2 (BCC, CRC, ovarian, medulloblastoma, and SCLC)
BMS-833923[334] • Synthetic small molecule			• Solid tumors • BCC • MM • SCLC	Phase 1–2
Robotnikinin (Broad Institute)[175] • Synthetic small molecule	Extracellular sHh	sHh inhibitor	Tumors overexpressing sHh ligand	Preclinical

signaling pathways are subject to negative regulation control.[176] In vertebrates, the Hh signal controls Ptch expression,[177] but it also induces the expression of cell surface proteins such as HP/HS interacting protein (HIP).

Clinical Development of Hh Pathway Inhibitors

With increasing enthusiasm for the development of Hh signaling inhibitors, especially Smo inhibitors, to block the aberrant signaling pathway, investigators have screened compound libraries with reporter and binding assays. This has yielded several promising compounds. GDC-0449 is a small molecule Smo inhibitor. In the first-in-human phase 1 study in advanced or metastatic solid tumors, no DLT was reached. The most common toxicities were dysgeusia, hair loss, nausea, vomiting, anorexia, dyspepsia, weight loss, hyponatremia, and fatigue, with the last two being grade 3.[178] The study included nine advanced BCC patients, six of whom had tumor regression. Three company-sponsored phase 2 trials are ongoing to evaluate the efficacy of the agent in ovarian cancer in remission, advanced CRC, and advanced BCC. One phase 1 and three phase 2 clinical trials are being sponsored by the NCI/CTEP. One phase 1 study in pancreatic carcinoma and other advanced solid tumors is evaluating a novel combination with GDC-0449 and EGFR inhibitor. Phase 2 trials include recurrent medulloblastoma studies in pediatric and adult populations, and a randomized study conducted by the Eastern Cooperative Oncology Group (ECOG) in SCLC comparing the cisplatin and etoposide chemotherapy backbone alone, with GDC-0449, or with an IGF-1R Ab.

Bristol-Myers Squibb and Exelixis initiated two phase 1 clinical trials with a small molecule Smo inhibitor, BMS-833923 (XL139): one single-agent trial in advanced solid tumor malignancies and one combination phase 1 study with either lenalidomide (Revlimid) or bortezomib in multiple myeloma. Two pending studies including the investigational agent with carboplatin and etoposide in extensive SCLC and advanced gastric or esophageal adenocarcinoma are planned.

IPI-926 is also in clinical trials for advanced stage solid tumors. The investigational compounds are shown in Table 30-5. In summary, most of these clinical trials are designed as "proof of concept" studies and to determine the safety and efficacy of the investigational agent.

Notch Signaling Pathway

The role of Notch signaling in cancer and progress in therapeutic development targeting Notch has been reviewed.[179,180] Investigational agents that inhibit Notch signaling are in early clinical development and preclinical development (Table 30-6).[180] In glioblastomas, Notch expression has been associated with high nestin levels and is linked to a poor prognosis.[181,182] Notch inhibition reduced the tumorigenicity of brain CSCs.[183] In breast cancer, Notch-1 and Jagged-1 expression correlates with poor prognosis, and Notch inhibitors can kill breast cancer cells in vitro and in vivo.[184–186] The activated Notch-1, Notch-4, and Notch target Hes-1 were expressed in mammospheres from ductal carcinoma in situ (DCIS) samples but not from normal breast tissue.[187] Notch inhibition with a γ-secretase

TABLE

30.6 *Notch-targeted therapeutics*

Agent	Targets	Mechanism of action	Phase of development
GSIs (γ-secretase inhibitors) • MK0752[202] • RO04929097[203]	• All 4 Notch paralogs • Notch ligands • Multiple other γ-secretase substrates	Inhibition of final Notch cleavage by γ-secretase	• Phase 1–2 for MK0752 • Phase 1 for RO04929097
GSMs (γ-secretase modifiers)[208]	Selective for specific γ-secretase substrates		• Phase 3 for β-amyloid-targeted GSMs • Discovery for Notch-targeted GSMs
MAML1 inhibitors • NOTCH-CSL-MAML[200] • ANTP/DN-MAML[201]	• All 4 Notch paralogs • Potentially other nuclear transcription factors that use MAML1	Interference with Notch nuclear coactivator MAML1	Preclinical
NRR mAbs[196]	Specific for individual Notch receptors	Interference with ligand-induced Notch subunit separation	Preclinical
DLL4 mAbs • OMP-21M18(OncoMed)[205] • Regeneron DLL4Ab[197] • Genentech DLL4[194]	Specific for DLL-4 ligand	Interference with ligand-receptor interaction	• Phase 1 for OMP-21M18 and Regeneron DLL4 Ab • Preclinical for Genentech DLL4
Notch soluble receptor decoys[199,335]	• Relatively specific for Notch paralogs • Potential pan-Notch inhibition		Preclinical

nhibitor or a neutralizing Notch-4 antibody reduced the ability of OCIS-derived cells to form mammospheres. In AML, a γ-secretase nhibitor inhibited the growth of leukemia stem cells (LSCs), which overexpress Jagged-2 in colony forming assays.[188] These results suggest that Notch inhibition may be able to preferentially target breast CSCs, glioblastoma CSCs, and possibly AML CSCs.

Deregulated Notch Signaling in Cancer and CSCs

Because Notch signaling has been associated with an oncogenic role n wide variety of solid tumors, targeting Notch has potential benefits in cancer therapeutics. For example, in breast cancer, Notch regulates survival and proliferation in "bulk" cancer cells[180] as well as CSCs.[187,189–192] At the same time, Notch plays a proangiogenic role in tumor endothelial cells, largely dependent on ligand Delta-4 (DLL-4).[193,194] Thus, pharmacologic inhibition of Notch signaling may have significant therapeutic effects in primary lesions, in recurrence and metastatic disease (in cases where self-renewal of CSCs is important), and in tumor angiogenesis.

At the molecular level, Notch signaling, like Hh and Wnt, is characterized by a great variety of effects on multiple proliferation, survival, and differentiation pathways.[195,196] Notch signaling is complex, with activation of receptor of Notch family members on one cell triggered by ligands expressed on the adjacent cell surface. While all signaling pathways are engaged in cross-talk interactions, inhibiting ancient developmental pathways such as Notch is likely to simultaneously affect numerous secondary therapeutic targets, resulting in so-called "multi-targeted" therapy with a single agent. Thus, Notch inhibitors may have the potential to synergize with multiple classes of drugs. Seeking the safest and most effective combinations with Notch inhibitors for specific indications is a promising strategy; however, Notch may have the opposite effect in some cancers since Notch effects are context dependent.

Preclinical Investigational Agents Targeting Notch Pathway

Table 30-6 summarizes Notch signaling inhibitors in preclinical and clinical development. Numerous γ-secretase inhibitors (GSIs) are commercially available for research, but we will not focus on them at this time. Several Notch inhibitors are in preclinical development, including inhibitors of DLL4 from Regeneron[197] and Genentech,[194] and a mAb against Notch-3[198] that prevents Notch activation by binding to the extracellular "negative regulatory region" (NRR). Two mAbs that target ligand DLL-4, preventing it from binding Notch receptors, are being developed as antiangiogenic agents. The mechanism of antiangiogenesis by these mAbs is inhibition of a negative-feedback regulator that restrains vascular sprouting and branching. Inhibition of DLL-4 results in excessive, nonproductive angiogenesis, which paradoxically decreases tumor growth even in tumors resistant to anti-VEGF therapies. Other possible ways of modulating Notch signaling have been reviewed.[180,195]

Other agents in preclinical development include Notch soluble receptor decoys that sequester Notch ligands or GSIs.[199] Newer agents, such as hydrocarbon-stapled peptide helices targeted against protein-protein interaction of Notch-CSL-mastermind-like 1 (MAML)[200] and the truncated version of MAML fused to a genetically engineered fusion protein consisted of *Drosophila* transcription

factor Antennapedia (ANTP), behave as a dominant negative inhibitors of Notch activation (ANTP/DN-MAML).[201]

GSIs are active in ERα-negative breast cancer xenografts and, in combination with endocrine therapy, in ERα-positive xenografts.[186] GSIs block the activation of all four human Notch homologues. This may be an advantage in indications like breast cancer, wherein at least three Notch homologues have prooncogenic effects.

Clinical Investigational Agents Targeting Notch Pathway

Based on the information from ClinicalTrials.gov, several investigational agents that block Notch signaling are being tested in patients. GSIs,[202] which were first developed as potential therapies for Alzheimer's disease, were adapted for use as Notch inhibitors. MK-0752 has been tested in early and advanced breast cancer, leukemia, T-cell acute lymphoblastic leukemia (ALL), and recurrent or refractory central nervous system (CNS) malignancies. RO4929097 will be soon tested in clinical trials among a wide range of tumors as a single agent and in combination with other oncology treatments in NCI/CTEP-sponsored investigator-initiated trials.[203] Non steroidal anti-inflammatory drugs (NSAIDs) and structurally related compounds that can allosterically modulate the substrate specificity of γ-secretase[204] may hold promise that more Notch-selective γ-secretase modifiers (GSM) could be developed in the near future.

OMP-21M18, a DLL4 Ab from OncoMed, shows anticancer activity in CRC and breast cancer models by disrupting tumor angiogenesis and reducing CSCs.[205] This investigational agent is currently in phase 1 clinical testing.

The use of a pan-GSI in initial clinical trials provided unique information in patients with T-cell ALL who developed diarrhea as the DLT.[202] It was likely to be an on-target side effect of Notch inhibition as Notch inhibition has been shown to alter intestinal crypt cells into mucous-secreting type goblet cells.[206] Fortunately, the severity of diarrhea is dependent on dosing schedule so that the continuous dosing schedule was modified in current clinical trials. In addition, concomitant use of glucocorticoids was proved to be a safe and effective approach to protect mice (T-cell ALL xenograft model) from developing the intestinal goblet cell metaplasia typically induced by inhibition of Notch signaling with GSIs.[207] Off-target effects are also potential concern with GSIs since γ-secretase has numerous substrates.[208] However, off-target effects are not necessarily an obstacle to clinical development, unless they are shown to reduce the safety or efficacy of these agents.

Due to some unique features of Notch signaling, targeting this pathway is of particular interest. First, because Notch-ligand interaction does not include an enzymatic amplification step, signal intensity can be modulated precisely by cellular regulatory mechanisms. Consequently, Notch activation downstream effects are particularly dose dependent.[196] This implies that complete Notch signaling blockade may not be necessary in targets to achieve therapeutic effect. Second, the duration of Notch signaling action at the cellular level is short, suggesting that intermittent or pulsatile pharmacologic inhibition may be sufficient in vivo. In fact, this concept was proved in animal toxicity studies without compromising the efficacy. Third, and most importantly, the effects of Notch are remarkably context dependent, that is, different Notch homologues have different effects in different cell types.

Wnt Signaling Pathway

Wnt was originally described as the Wingless (Wg) segment polarity gene in *Drosophila* and as the homologous *Int* gene in vertebrates.[209,210] The Wingless gene had been identified as a segment polarity gene in *D. melanogaster* that functions during embryogenesis.[211,212] Wnt proteins have been shown to play key roles in controlling cell proliferation, cell-fate determination, and differentiation both during embryonic development and in adult life.[213–216] While active during embryonic development, normal tissue regeneration, such as the epithelium of the small intestine, bone marrow, and osteoblasts, remains dependent upon the Wnt/β-catenin pathway in the adult. The Wnt/β-catenin signaling pathway is complex in nature and has cross talks with a number of other signaling pathways. The end result of Wnt signaling is transcription of a wide variety of target genes.

Wnt signaling has historically been divided into the canonical pathway, which is associated with the downstream activation of β-catenin and its subsequent accumulation in the cell nucleus, and the noncanonical pathway. In the noncanonical pathway, signaling events of β-catenin-independent pathways remain poorly defined.[217] In the canonical pathway, the signaling events associated with stabilization or the accumulation of β-catenin cause the transformation of breast cell lines on in vitro screening tests. Human Wnt isoforms that are potentially related to tumor development events are Wnt1, Wnt2, Wnt3, Wnt3a, Wnt6, Wnt7a, Wnt 9b, and Wnt11. The other known isoforms, such as Wnt4, Wnt5a, Wnt 5b, and Wnt7b, are categorized as "β-catenin-independent Wnts"; however, they do contribute to polarity regulation, asymmetric cell division, and morphogenic movements during vertebrate gastrulation. The rest of the Wnts (Wnt8a, Wnt 8b, Wnt9a, Wnt10a, Wnt10b, and Wnt16) are known to have a stabilization effect on β-catenin; transformation capability and the activation of PKC and Rho or Rac by these Wnt isoforms have not been determined. Wnt signaling pathways activated by a Wnt isoform can be highly dependent on cellular context and Wnt receptor cell surface components; therefore, such classification may not capture all events.

Wnt Protein Production

As described in Hh section, Wnt and Hh signaling are similar and include a ligand-lipid modification process.[155] Biochemical characterization of these proteins has been delayed by more than 20 years after the cloning of Wnt1 because of its insoluble nature and difficulty in isolating the protein and defining its structure. Willert et al.[158] purified the Wnt proteins, revealing the degree of palmitoylation and hydrophobicity, which was greater than previously predicted. As Wnts are lipid modified, acyltransferases are required for Wnt signaling and these genes, such as porcupine (Porc) in *Drosophila*[218] and mom-1 in *Caenorhabditis elegans*,[219] are found to be essential in Wnt-producing cells. Sequence similarities exist between Porc and membrane-bound acyltransferases, which are present in the endoplasmic reticulum membrane.[220] Porc was identified as the enzyme that is responsible for Wnt protein acylation.[158,221] Although a dedicated transport molecule Dispatched is required for Hh protein release, no evidence defines a similar transporter for Wnt molecules. Wnt or Wg (*Drosophila*) proteins are not secreted if palmitoylation is disrupted or Porc is absent.[158,222,223]

Wnt Signaling Cascade (Canonical Pathway)

Activation of Wnt signaling occurs when Wnt ligands bind to transmembrane receptors encoded by the *Frizzled* (Fzd) gene family, together with coreceptors such as LDL receptor protein (LRP) 5 and 6.[224] The Wnt-Fzd interaction leads to dephosphorylation of β-catenin, less degradation, and subsequent accumulation of β-catenin in the nucleus. Cell signaling outcome differences may be due to specific pairings of Wnt ligands with corresponding cellular receptors. For example, the mammalian genome codes for 19 Wnt proteins and 10 Fzd receptors; therefore, potentially 190 Wnt/Fzd pairing combinations exist. Wnt proteins are strongly hydrophobic and are mostly found on the surface of cell membranes and the extracellular matrix.[225]

Wnt and the Fzd/LRP membrane receptor interactions are regulated by secreted Fzd-related proteins (sFRPs), Dickkopfs (DKKs), and Wnt inhibitory factor-1 (WIF1).[226–228] In the nucleus, unphosphorylated β-catenin binds to T-cell factor/lymphoid enhancer factor (Tcf/Lef) proteins and with various cofactor recruitment, activates gene transcription. These events result in cellular proliferation and tumor growth.[229] Detecting the accumulation and nuclear localization of β-catenin is a useful means of examining Wnt/β-catenin signaling activation.[230]

In the absence of Wnt signaling, a cytoplasmic destruction complex leads to the phosphorylation of β-catenin[231]; β-catenin is ubiquinylated and targeted for proteasomal degradation. In the nucleus, β-catenin levels are kept low by its interaction with adenomatosis polyposis coli (APC) protein and axin, which cycles between the cytoplasmic and nuclear compartments preventing the accumulation of β-catenin in the nucleus.[232] In the nucleus, low levels of β-catenin allow the DNA-binding Tcf/Lef proteins to interact with transcriptional corepressors (Groucho/TLE) to inhibit target gene expression.[231,233] Wnt signaling increases the expression of HoxB4 and Notch-1 genes.[234]

Wnt/β-catenin Signaling and Tumorigenesis

Nuclear β-catenin has been detected in colorectal, gastric, esophageal, melanoma, lung, ovarian, cervical, endometrial, breast, prostate, thyroid, hepatoblastoma, HCC, medulloblastoma, and pancreatic malignancies,[235] suggesting a role of this signaling pathway in tumorigenesis. In addition, the pathway is activated in Wilms' tumor,[236] ALL,[237] and multiple myeloma cells.[238] Approximately 30% of CRCs[239] and 90% of human CRC have deregulated signaling pathway.[240]

APC mutations[241] have been reported in the majority of CRCs (75% to 80%), while the overall frequency of β-catenin mutations is low.[242] Unregulated β-catenin activity (due to mutated APC in a premalignant disease that usually progresses to malignancy) has been suggested as a key initiating factor in CRCs.[242] Aggressive desmoid tumors occur with increased frequency in patients with familial adenomatous polyposis (FAP) who carry APC mutations in their germline.[243] In an evaluation of 42 desmoid tumors, β-catenin mutations were found in more than half. Furthermore, β-catenin mutation has been described in colorectal, endometrial, prostate, endometrioid tumors of the ovary, and HCC.[244–247]

Wnt Signaling and CSCs

Wnt signaling in CRCs and stem cells has been summarized in a number of exceptional reviews.[215,248] Intestinal crypt stem cells form tumors rapidly following the deletion of the negative regulator *APC* gene.[249] Maintenance of cutaneous CSCs was shown to depend on the Wnt/β-catenin signaling pathway.[250] β-Catenin accumulates in granulocyte-macrophage progenitor cells during CML blast crisis, suggesting that molecular mechanisms can transform committed progenitors into LSCs.[251]

Wnt Pathway as Target for Anticancer Drug Development

Preclinical Agents Targeting Wnt Pathway

To block an activated Wnt β-catenin signaling pathway caused by any mutation below the receptor level, the choice of inhibitors includes compounds that can inhibit Tcf-β-catenin transcriptional activation (Table 30-7). ICG-001, identified by a high-throughput small-molecule library screening, is the first selective small molecule inhibitor of β-catenin-Tcf-mediated transcription.[252] ICG-001 was found to specifically target the transcriptional coactivator cyclic AMP response element binding (CREB)-binding protein (CBP). Despite CBP and p300 interacting with a large number of partners other

than β-catenin, ICG-001 selectively disrupts CBP-β-catenin interaction without affecting the highly homologous p300-β-catenin interaction. The switch from CBP-β-catenin to p300-β-catenin controls proliferation of CSCs to a differentiated state.[253] The novel compound AV65 has also shown activity in inducing apoptosis in a dose-dependent manner against CML cell lines.[254] AV65 has activity in both imatinib- (ST1571, Gleevec) and second-generation Abl TKI-resistant patients. AV65's mechanism of action is unclear at this point.

Two new classes of small molecule compounds were identified after a high-throughput synthetic chemical library screening.[255] One class inhibits the activity of Porc, whereas the other class abrogates destruction of Axin proteins. Compounds that disrupt the Wnt/β-catenin signaling cascade hold great promise for cancer therapeutics.

Clinical Investigational Agents Targeting Wnt Pathway

A variety of approved compounds have been evaluated for their ability to disrupt the Wnt/β-catenin signaling pathway in tumor cells (Table 30-7). These compounds include STI-571, which was

TABLE 30.7   *Wnt-targeted therapies*

Target	Agents in development	Mechanism of action	Disease	Phase of development
Wnt ligands	• Wnt1 mAb • Wnt2 mAb • Soluble Wnt receptor Frizzled8CRD-hFc Ab (decoy receptor— Genentech)	Bind to ligands extracellularlly resulting in apoptosis by decreased activity of the transcription factor	• CRC • Breast cancer • Melanoma • H&N cancer • NSCLC • Gastric cancer • Mesothelioma • Barrett's esophagus	Preclinical
Frizzled (Fzd) receptors	• Fzd1 receptor Ab • Fzd2 receptor Ab	Inhibit ligand-receptor interaction	• CRC • Breast cancer • H&N cancer • Gastric cancer • Synovial sarcomas	Preclinical
Disheveled (Dvl) family members	• NSC668036 • FJ9 (disrupts Fzd-7 and Disheveled)	Inhibition of Dvl causes stabilization of degradation complex, resulting in β-catenin degradation	• Mesothelioma • NSCLC • Cervical cancer	Preclinical
β-catenin reverse nuclear transport[265]	Thiazolidinedione (TZD) (antidiabetic drug)	Transport β-catenin from nuclear to plasma membrane		Preclinical in cancer settings
β-Catenin/TCF[252,258,259]	• PNU-74654 (β-catenin-Tcf) • ICG-001 (CBP-β-catenin) • NSAIDs (Cox2 inhibitor, Salmedix, etc.)	Inhibit protein-protein interaction, resulting in decreased β-catenin-dependent gene expression	• CRC • Gastric cancer • HCC • Hepatoblastoma • Wilms' tumor • Endometrial/ovarian cancer • Adrenocorticol tumors • Pilomatricomas	Preclinical (except for NSAIDs—Phase 2)

(continued)

TABLE

30.7 *Wnt-targeted therapies (continued)*

Target	Agents in development	Mechanism of action	Disease	Phase of development
Protein degradation process[254,255,336–338]	• AV65 • Artificial F-box protein • Sulindac	Exact mechanism is unknown. Thought to enhance proteasome degradation of β-catenin by directing to the ubiquitin-conjugated proteolysis	• CRC • CML	Preclinical (except for Sulindac—Phase 2)
Axin2[255]	• IWR (inhibitors of Wnt response)	IWR directly interacts with Axin2 to stabilize Axin proteins, causing β-catenin loss	• CRC (MSI) • HCC • Oligodontia	Preclinical
SFRP family members	Either Ab approach as above or small molecule inhibitors	Decrease ligands in extracellular level	• CRC • Breast cancer • Gastric cancer • Mesothelioma • NSCLC • Barrett's esophagus • Leukemia • Prostate cancer	Preclinical
WIF family members		Antagonize with ligands in extracellular level	• CRC • Breast cancer • Prostate cancer • Lung cancer • Bladder cancer • Mesothelioma	Preclinical
Porcupine (porc)[255]	IWP (inhibitors of Wnt production)	Block porc to cause inhibition of acylation of Wnt, resulting in inhibition of Wnt secretion	Tumors with Hh overexpression	Preclinical

originally identified as a PDGFR inhibitor.[256] STI-571 also inhibits the tyrosine phosphorylation of β-catenin.[257] Drugs currently available in the clinics include NSAIDs, such as FGN-1 (exisulind) or cyclooxygenase (COX) inhibitors.[258,259] Celecoxib (Celebrex), a COX-2 inhibitor, also was shown to inhibit β-catenin activity in human colon carcinoma cells by inducing its degradation.[260] Antisense inhibitors have been evaluated against colon, esophageal, and leukemia cells in vitro, resulting in decreased expression of β-catenin.[261–263] NSAIDs also have been shown to inhibit the Wnt/β-catenin signaling pathway. Both aspirin and indomethacin (Indocin) inhibited β-catenin transcription.[264] Thiazolidinedione (TZD) was reported to completely inhibit metastases in a colon cancer xenograft model by inducing the translocation of β-catenin from the nucleus to the plasma membrane.[265]

Summary/Future Directions

This brief review does not cover the area of signaling cross talk or novel regulatory proteins such as Musashi1, which is the RNA-binding protein identified as activators for Wnt and Notch pathways.[266]

The review also does not extend to the agents targeted at the additional signaling families involved in embryonic development such as the fibroblast growth factors and the bone morphogenic proteins. Developing embryonic signaling inhibitors for future clinical application will continue to be a challenge for several reasons. First, if the primary targets of their activities are CSCs, tumor volume may not be an appropriate efficacy endpoint in clinical trial. Second, because of the complicated cross talk of these pathways with each other and with other cell signaling pathways, inhibition of one pathway is likely to lead to feedback effects that counteract the effect of inhibitors. Combination regimens rationally designed based on thorough preclinical studies in specific indications are the most appropriate strategy for development of these agents, and these combination regimens should be conceived from the earliest stages of development, including novel-novel combinations. Third, appropriate biomarkers are absolutely needed to predict responses and for pharmacodynamic purposes at early stage of drug development. New classes of agents may hold promise for paradigm-shifting advances in cancer management, but their development requires sound preclinical science and innovative clinical trial designs to pilot the therapeutic potential of these agents correctly.

Targeting Mitosis and Microtubules for Chemotherapy

Overview

The cell cycle represents a fundamental biological process that ultimately results in the generation of two identical daughter cells. Cellular division, which occurs during the M-phase of the cell cycle, consists of two distinct steps: mitosis, in which the chromosomes condense and subsequently separate into two identical sets, and cytokinesis, which splits the cells into two identical daughter cells, each containing a full complement of chromosomes. The defining event of the five sequential step of mitosis—*prophase*, *prometaphase*, *metaphase*, *anaphase*, and *telophase*—is formation of microtubules, from the polymerization of tubulin, into the mitotic spindle (Fig. 30-3). Hence, the critical role of microtubules in cell division identifies them as potential targets for the development of chemotherapeutic drugs.

Microtubule-targeting agents are valid targets in cancer cells based on the successful use of the taxanes and vinca alkaloids as chemotherapeutic agents. These drugs, some of which have been in use for almost 50 years, disrupt microtubule function.[267] Between the individual steps of mitosis, specific proteins are identified as targets for drug development (Fig. 30-3). These potential targets are only expressed in dividing cells—both in healthy noncancerous cells and in rapidly dividing cancer cells. Molecular inhibitors of these targets, the aurora kinases (Aurora A, Aurora B), the PLKs, KSP, and centromere-associated protein E (CENP-E), have entered clinical trials and will be briefly surveyed. A useful reference for this purpose is ClinicalTrials.gov.

Kinesin Spindle Proteins

Kinesins consist of a superfamily of more than 600 motor proteins that are involved in a number of biological processes. In particular, the mitotic kinesins, consisting of at least 12 members, are intimately involved in the formation of the mitotic spindle, chromosome segregation, checkpoint control, and cytokinesis. Kinesins typically consist of a protein dimer, comprising two heavy chains and two light chains. The heavy chains consist of a globular head, which contains the highly conserved motor domain, followed by connection to a short neck linker that terminates in the tail region that is formed with the light chain. Each head has two separate binding sites: one for ATP and the other for the microtubule.[268] Kinesin movement is affected by hydrolysis of ATP and subsequent ADP release, which results in a conformational change that is transduced into either directional movement along microtubules or active polymerization of microtubules.[269] KSPs are highly expressed in breast, colon, lung, ovary, uterine, and retinoblastoma tumors.[270,271]

KSP Inhibitors

The first KSP inhibitor that was discovered was the small molecule monastrol, which was found to inhibit the mitotic kinesin Eg5, the *Xenopus laevis* homologue of human KSP. Crystallographic studies have identified two binding sites on the enzyme: the ATP-binding site and an allosteric binding pocket located a short distance away from the ATP site.[272] Monastrol is an allosteric inhibitor that, upon binding, affects a conformational change that allows ATP to bind but prevents the release of ADP, which ultimately arrests the cells in mitosis.[273] Subsequent studies have identified several other KSP inhibitors, most of which share the same allosteric binding pocket. Other inhibitors, such as the well-characterized thiazoles, compete with ATP for binding at the catalytic site. The mechanism of action of KSP inhibitors, regardless of the binding site, is the induction of apoptosis after prolonged mitotic arrest.[274]

Ispinesib (SB-715992)

Ispinesib (SB-715992), a polycyclic nitrogen containing heterocycle, was the first KSP inhibitor to enter clinical trials. Binding to the allosteric site, it is a highly selective inhibitor that prevents the formation of a bipolar mitotic spindle, causing cells to arrest in mitosis with unseparated chromosomes.[275] Phase 1 studies in patients with solid tumors have demonstrated that ispinesib was

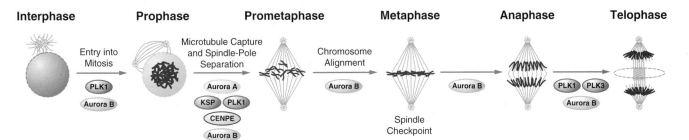

FIGURE **30-3**   Cellular division consists of two steps: mitosis, in which the chromosomes condense and subsequently separate into two identical sets, and cytokinesis, which splits the cells into two identical daughter cells, each containing a full complement of chromosomes. Mitosis is divided into five steps: prophase, prometaphase, metaphase, anaphase, and telophase. Certain proteins are only expressed during mitosis (both cancer cells and healthy non–cancerous cells); these proteins are excellent targets for drug development. Kinesin spindle protein (KSP) is required to establish mitotic spindle bipolarity through driving centrosome separation. Centromeric protein E (CENPE) is required for accurate chromosome pairing at metaphase. Aurora A is needed for centrosome maturation and separation during early prophase. Aurora B is involved in histone H3 phosphorylation, chromosomal condensation, chromosomal alignment of the metaphase plate, centromere-microtubule attachment, the spindle checkpoint, and cytokinesis. Polo-like kinases (PLKs) are involved in centrosome maturation and formation of the mitotic spindle. PLKs are also necessary for exit from mitosis and separation of sister chromotids during anaphase. (Please see Color Insert.)

generally well tolerated and had an acceptable safety profile, with a DLT of neutropenia.[276] Antitumor activity was noted in patients with locally advanced or metastatic breast cancer.[277] Moreover, combination therapy of ispinesib plus capecitabine had an acceptable tolerability profile with half the patients experiencing prolonged SD.[278]

Several phase 2 studies have been performed with ispinesib in patients with HCC, squamous cell carcinoma of the neck, and metastatic melanoma.[279–281] All three studies followed the same clinical protocol: ispinesib was administered as a 1-hour IV infusion at the MTD dose of 18 mg/m² once every 3 weeks. No objective responses were observed, with a best response of SD. Subsequent studies have demonstrated that single-agent ispinesib does not yield a significant response rate in CRC, ovarian, and RCC.[282–284] This clinical observation may be related to the fact that only a fraction of tumor cells are undergoing mitosis at any given time. Since ispinesib acts during mitosis, only actively dividing tumor cells would be affected. Ispinesib's efficacy could be increased by optimization of the dosing schedule; a greater therapeutic index may be achieved by repeated, or more prolonged, infusions, or by combination with other antitubulin agents.

Other KSP Inhibitors in Development

Several second-generation KSP inhibitors are now undergoing clinical trials. In a first-in-humans trial, SB-743921, a more potent analog of ispinesib was examined in a population of leukemia patients. The MTD was determined, and reversible neutropenia was determined to be the DLT. Two PRs, both in elderly patients with Hodgkin's lymphoma (Investigator communication), were observed.

ARRY-520, a selective KSP inhibitor, has shown potent activity in preclinical models of hematological cancers; it is being evaluated in a phase 1 trial in patients with advanced or refractory leukemias.[285] Two patients have, thus far, experienced a DLT of grade 3 mucositis. ARRY-520's promising signs of clinical activity include two patients with complete reductions in peripheral blasts; of these, one patient experienced a 70% reduction in bone marrow blasts while on study. Another KSP inhibitor, AZD4877, was also examined in an AML population.[286] Myelosuppression, generally the limiting toxicity in solid tumor studies, was not considered a DLT in this trial; instead, mucositis was the limiting toxicity. Bone marrow blasts decreased by 60% to 80% in two patients, and 30% to 50% in three patients. These results suggest possible clinical activity in AML. Finally, MK-0731, a competitive ATP inhibitor, was examined in a population of patients with solid tumors; treatment at the MTD showed some efficacy with a DLT of myelosuppression.[287]

Polo-like Kinases

PLKs constitute a highly conservative family of serine/threonine kinases that play a pivotal role in mitosis. The four mammalian PLKs (PLK-1 to PLK-4) share a considerable homology with the *polo* gene product of *D. melanogaster*, from which they derive the PLK name. PLKs are expressed at high levels in human tumors of diverse origin.[288] PLK-1, the most extensively studied PLK family member, controls critical steps in mitosis, including initiation of cells' entry into mitosis, centrosome maturation, metaphase to anaphase transition, and cytokinesis. Moreover, PLK-1 expression correlates with histological grade and clinical state in ovarian cancer[289] and high PLK-1

expression is an adverse prognostic factor in head and neck squamous cell carcinoma, NSCLC, and breast cancer.[288] PLKs are overexpressed in human tumors and are not expressed in healthy non–dividing cells; hence, they represent an attractive target for drug development.

PLK-1 Inhibitors

PLK inhibitors act directly on the microtubule spindle, resulting in metaphase arrest followed by induction of apoptosis. Numerous PLK-1 inhibitors are under development and in clinical trials; only a brief survey of agents in clinical trials is presented.

ON01910.Na

The PLK-1 inhibitor ON01910.Na is a synthetic benzyl styryl sulfone analogue that induces selective G_2-M arrest followed by apoptosis in a variety of tumor cells; in normal cells, however, treatment with ON01910.Na results in reversible cell arrest at the G_1 and G_2 stages *without* apoptosis. ON01910.Na inhibits PLK-1, and to some extent PLK-2 pathway activity in a substrate-dependent and ATP-independent manner. It induces spindle abnormalities (multipolar spindles) and abnormal centrosome localization and causes misalignment of the chromosomes, which do not attach securely to the spindle.[290] This results in a loss of cell viability, and apoptosis follows. The drug is not an ATP mimetic and is believed to compete for the substrate-binding site of the enzyme. ON01910.Na has shown broad-spectrum antitumor activity against both solid tumors and hematological malignancies.

ON01910.Na has been studied in two phase 1 studies; one study sought to determine the safety and efficacy of ON01910.Na using a weekly 24-hour continuous infusion (CIV),[291] the other administered the agent in 2-hour infusions on a 28-day cycle.[292] In the CIV study, maximum dose achieved was 2,750 mg/m²,[291] whereas in the other phase 1 study, dose levels up to 3,120 mg were evaluated in single-patient cohorts without any adverse effects.[292] This dose was determined to be the MTD when ON01910.Na was administered as a 2-hour infusion twice weekly for 3 consecutive weeks in a 4-week cycle. Overall, ON01910.Na was well tolerated, with the most common toxicities being fatigue, pain, nausea, vomiting, and an urge to defecate.[291,292] Antitumor activity was observed following ON01910.NA CIV in one patient with advanced epithelial ovarian cancer (SD for 36 weeks of treatment).[291] This effect is not unexpected since a moderate fraction (~25%) of these cancers have been shown to have high PLK-1 expression.[289] However, the activity of ON01910.Na may not be universal in ovarian cancer since two other ovarian cancer patients on the study experienced progressive disease. More studies are needed, as well as combination studies with platinum analogs.

GSK461364

GSK461364 is a selective thiophene amide PLK-1 inhibitor.[288] Preclinical studies have demonstrated that mitotic arrest by GSK461364 is concentration dependent: at high concentrations G_2-phase arrest is noted, while at lower concentrations arrest occurred. Mitotic arrest led to cell death, which was characterized by severe micronucleation. GSK461364 is an ATP-competitive inhibitor of PLK-1, and it forms a rapidly reversible complex with PLK-1. Antiproliferative activity was demonstrated in more than 120 cancer cell lines. In xenograft models, GSK461364 demonstrated antitumor activity at various stages of the tumor development from growth delay to complete tumor growth inhibition.

In the first-in-human phase 1 study, patients with advanced solid tumors received escalating doses of GSK461364 with the goal of determining the MTD and PK; secondary objectives included evaluation of antitumor activity.[293] Sequential cohorts of patients each received escalating doses of GSK461364 administered as a 4-hour IV infusion. DLTs observed, depending on the schedule and dose, were grade 4 sepsis (at the 225-mg dose) and grade 4 pulmonary embolism and neutropenia (at the 100 mg dose). The most common toxicities, regardless of dose level and schedule, were phlebitis, fatigue, nausea, anemia, anorexia, diarrhea, and infusion site reaction. Preliminary PK data indicated that AUC and C_{max} were proportional across doses. Phospho-histone H3, a marker of mitotic arrest, was detected in circulating tumor cells 24 hours after first dose. The MTD has not yet been reached, and dose escalation studies continue. Preliminary analysis reveals that two patients have had SD, including one patient with esophageal cancer on the weekly schedule and one patient with metastatic breast cancer on the twice weekly schedule.

BI 2536

Steegmaier reported the discovery of a potent small molecule, ATP-competitive, inhibitor of PLK-1, BI 2536.[294] BI 2536 induces G_2-M arrest and the formation of abnormal mitotic spindles. BI 2536 is highly potent with an IC_{50} of 0.8 nmol/L and has shown more than a 1,000-fold selectivity against a panel of kinases; in human tumor xenografts, treatment with BI 2536 resulted in tumor regression. The first clinical trial of BI 2536 was a dose-titration study in patients with advanced solid tumors.[295] Single doses of BI 2536 were administered as a 1-hour IV infusion. The MTD was defined at 200 mg ($n = 40$). The predominant DLT was reversible neutropenia with and without infection. This reversible toxicity could be the result of transient inhibition of the proliferation of bone marrow precursor cells. Other toxicities, such as fatigue, nausea, vomiting, and dizziness, were manageable. At the MTD, SD was reported as the best response for 42% of the patients, with 22.6% of patients treated at the MTD showing no progression for 3 or more months. A PR was observed after a second course in one patient with squamous head and neck cancer; however, the patient progressed after the fourth course.

An interesting aspect of this trial was that BI 2536 was administered as a flat dose, correlated to body surface area (BSA) and body weight. Since the PK profile indicated that drug exposure was independent of BSA or body weight, dose normalization to these parameters for future clinical trials is probably unnecessary. BI 2536 showed dose-proportional behavior, and the PK of BI 2536 was characterized by a high distribution into a tissue. The fraction bound to plasma proteins in vitro was approximately 94%. The clearance of BI 2536 was high and was mainly attributed to non-renal clearance; metabolism of BI 2536 was carried out by flavin-mono-oxygenases and cytochrome P450 enzymes.

Results of a phase 2 trial for BI 2536 were reported.[296] This open-label, single-arm phase 2 study was designed to investigate the antitumor efficacy of BI 2536 in SCLC patients with disease recurrence greater than 60 days after completion of first-line chemotherapy. Patients were dose-escalated to the MTD via a 1-hour IV infusion for a minimum of two courses. While no objective antitumor responses were observed, 30% of patients had SD as

best response, 60% had disease progression, and 9% were not evaluable. BI 2536 was well tolerated but did not demonstrate antitumor efficacy after stage 1 of the study. Therefore, the use of single-agent BI 2536 in SCLC seems unlikely, although combination of BI 2536 with other antimitotic agents may be worth investigating.

HMN-214

HMN-214 is an oral prodrug of HMN-176, a stilbene derivative that interferes with the spatial localization of PLK-1. HMN-176 has shown potent cytotoxic activity against several tumor cell lines with an average $IC_{50} = 118$ nmol/L. Exposure of mitotic cells to HMN-176 results in cell-cycle arrest at M-phase, with destruction of the spindle polar bodies, followed by DNA fragmentation. HMN-176 has shown antitumor activity in gastric, breast, lung, pancreas, and prostate cancers, and CRC human tumor xenografts.[297]

A phase 1 open-label, dose escalation trial of orally administered HMN-214 on days 1 to 21 of a 28-day dosing cycle was performed. HMN-214 was administered at a starting dose of 3 mg/m²/d, which was based on preclinical rat toxicology studies. DLT was principally defined as grade 4 neutropenia lasting more than 5 days. The MTD for the RP2D for HMN-214 was 8 mg/m²/d, based on dose-limiting musculoskeletal events such as bone pain, arthralgias, and myalgias. The clinical result is the arthralgia/myalgia syndrome seen with the taxanes. Due to the severity of these events, two patients treated at a high dose required hospitalization during the third week of dosing for further evaluation. Other nonhematologic toxicities related to HMN-214 were constitutional and gastrointestinal in nature.

PK analysis showed HMN-214 to be rapidly hydrolyzed to HMN-176, which was rapidly detected in the plasma after dosing. Dose-proportional increases were observed in AUC but not C_{max}. No appreciable differences were observed in terminal phase $t_{1/2}$ after single or multiple oral doses, suggesting no appreciable drug accumulation with continuous daily dosing over 21 days. In this patient population of advanced solid tumor patients who were not selected based on PLK-1 expression in tumor tissue, only very modest evidence of antitumor activity was noted, with 24% of patients having SD.[297] This included an observation of SD of 6-month duration in a patient with heavily pretreated breast cancer. Additionally, a transient decline in a tumor marker was observed in one patient with colon cancer. Further development of HMN-214 will focus on patient populations with high expression of PLK-1, such as prostate and pancreatic cancers.

Aurora Kinase Inhibitors

The Aurora kinases are composed of three mitotic kinases most homologous in their catalytic domains. Aurora A and Aurora B kinases appear to have a role in neoplastic transformation, while Aurora C expression appears to be limited to normal testicular tissue, with no clear relation to malignancy. Aurora A is a centrosomal protein involved in the formation of the bipolar mitotic spindle. Aurora A kinase accumulates and peaks at the G_2-M border and has a critical role in centrosome maturation, duplication, and separation.[298] By the G_2 phase through anaphase, Aurora A can be detected in pericentriolar material, as well as the mitotic spindle poles and midzone microtubules.[299] Aurora A phosphorylates and recruits several microtubule-associated proteins to the centrosomes to promote centrosomal maturation, and Aurora A also has other important cellular substrates such as p53 and BRCA1.

Aurora A kinase is overexpressed or amplified in hematological malignancies, and in solid tumors such as bladder, pancreas, breast, colon, head and neck, and ovarian cancers. Aurora A also has a critical role in the stabilization of N-Myc, which appears to be important to the growth and survival of neuroblastoma cells[300]; Aurora A expression in tumors is associated with genetic instability, poor histologic differentiation, and poor prognosis.[301] Aurora A kinase overexpression is associated with aneuploidy and centrosome amplification, and forced overexpression of Aurora A is transforming in some cultured cell models.[302] Aurora A overexpression also produces resistance to paclitaxel in human cancer cell lines. Aurora A inhibition leads to sensitization to taxanes, vinca alkaloids, and epothilones, as well as to cisplatin, inhibitors of kinesin spindles proteins and MEK, and other chemotherapeutic agents.[303,304]

Aurora B kinase is a chromosomal passenger protein found in the centromeric regions of chromosomes in early mitosis and relocalizing to the microtubules at the spindle-equator in anaphase. Aurora B kinase has an expression that increases at the G_2-M transition and high kinase activity throughout mitosis. Aurora B binds and activates other mitosis-regulatory proteins and has an important role in regulating the biorientation of the chromosome.[305] Aurora kinase B is critical for proper progression of cytokinesis and for spindle-assembly checkpoint signals.[306]

Aberrant expression of Aurora B kinase has been implicated in the development of human cancer, although Aurora B is not an oncogene in experimental systems. High expression of Aurora B has been associated with chromosomal instability.[307] Aurora B overexpression appears to correlate with nodal involvement of tumors in several clinical investigations.[308] Aurora B inhibitors have a distinct molecular mechanism of action in which exposed cells continue to cycle instead of arresting in mitosis. This phenotype suggests that Aurora B inhibitors could be given before other agents that require exposure during other phases of the cell cycle, and sequential combinations of Aurora B inhibitors and S-phase active cytotoxic therapies have been shown to be synergistic in leukemia.[309]

Inhibitors of Aurora Kinases

Aurora A and Aurora B kinases have significant sequence homology in the ATP-binding region of the catalytic domain, and many inhibitors of Aurora A also have significant inhibition of Aurora B as well. Dual inhibitors of Aurora A and Aurora B have a molecular phenotype similar to that of a pure Aurora B inhibitor and distinct from that of the less common pure inhibitors of Aurora A kinase.[310] Aurora B inhibitors induce misalignment of chromosomes, cell polyploidy, and inhibition of the paclitaxel-induced spindle checkpoint activation. It is not clear whether Aurora A or Aurora B is the better anticancer target, although one comparison of agents in pancreatic cancer cells showed more activity with Aurora A inhibition, with the induction of mitotic arrest and rapid induction of apoptosis.[311] At least nine Aurora kinase inhibitors have been developed and tried in clinical investigations, with common dose-limiting effects being granulocytopenia, nausea, and fatigue.

MK-0457 (VX-680)

MK-0457 is a pyrimidine derivative with nanomolar inhibition of Aurora A, B, and C kinases. In preclinical models, MK-0457 leads to polyploidy and in some models, extensive apoptosis. MK-0457 can induce regression in tumor xenografts.[310] In phase 1 trials, MK-0457 was administered as a 5-day CIV every 28 days, with neutropenia as the DLT. Preclinical activity has been seen in imatinib-resistant CML and in FLT3-mutant acute leukemia, suggesting activity in hematologic malignancies, although phase 2 studies are also ongoing for CRC and NSCLC.

AZD1152

AZD1152 is an ATP-competitive Aurora B inhibitor, which is a quinazoline prodrug converted in plasma to the active metabolite AZD1152-HQPA. AZD1152 was active in human xenograft models, with antitumor activity demonstrated in CRC and NSCLC. Two phase 1 studies of AZD1152 have been conducted, and prolonged SD has been seen in patients with melanoma, nasopharyngeal cancer, and adenocystic carcinoma. The primary toxicity of IV infusions of AZD1152 has been neutropenia.[312] Longer infusions of AZD1152 have demonstrated increased evidence of apoptosis in animal models; a phase 1/2 trial of AZD1152 is ongoing.

PHA-739358

PHA-739358 is a pan-Aurora kinase inhibitor currently in phase 2 studies in patients with CML who have relapsed after imatinib therapy. In vitro studies with PHA-739358 have demonstrated activity of the drug in imatinib-resistant BCR-ABL cells, especially with the T315I mutation. Two phase 1 studies of the agent, on different IV schedules, both showed a high proportion of patients with prolonged SD, although no objective responses were noted.[313]

MLN8237

MLN8237 is a selective Aurora A kinase inhibitor that shares a benzodiazepine chemical scaffold with a first-generation Aurora A inhibitor, MLN8054. MLN8237 causes less sedation than MLN8053, particularly if the drug is given twice a day rather than daily as sedation appears to correlate with peak levels of the agent. In addition, MLN8237 is more potent than MLN8054 and is given orally. MLN8237 causes tumor xenograft growth inhibition in multiple in vivo models and exerts additive to supra-additive effects in combination with docetaxel and rituximab in xenograft studies. MLN8237 demonstrated striking antitumor effects in ALL and neuroblastoma xenografts, with the latter possibly related to the destabilization of N-Myc by Aurora A inhibition.[314] MLN8237 has been tested in two phase 1 trials, with PRs noted in liposarcoma and ovarian cancer patients; a number of solid tumor patients have experienced prolonged SD.[315] With a RP2D of 50 mg orally twice daily, sedation has not been a significant problem, although granulocytopenia, thrombocytopenia, alopecia, and mucositis have been noted. A phase 1 pediatric oncology trial and phase 2 trials of MLN8237 in lymphoma, leukemia, and ovarian cancers are ongoing, and combination studies with taxanes are being initiated.

Centrosome-Associated Protein E

Centrosome-associated protein E (CENP-E) has been identified as a target for drug development. CENP-E has no function outside of mitosis, whereby it acts as a motor protein that serves to optimize chromosome alignment in the metaphase.[316] A second function performed by CENP-E during mitosis is modulation of the spindle checkpoint protein BubR1.[317] The loss of CENP-E affects chromosome alignment as well as the checkpoint mechanism that the cell uses to exit or delay exit from mitosis until damage can be repaired. CENP-E is overexpressed in a variety of human tumors relative to normal tissues, suggesting its role in tumor cell proliferation.[318] Thus, inhibition of CENP-E may ultimately result in cell-cycle arrest and subsequent apoptosis.

CENP-E Inhibitor GSK923295A

GSK923295A is the first drug candidate to enter human clinical trials that specifically targets CENP-E. The clinical trial uses a standard phase 1 design intended to determine MTD, DLT, and PK parameters. This trial is still in progress; however, an interim analysis revealed that the majority of patients experienced toxicities (typically grade 3).[319] A pediatric preclinical testing program was developed to examine GSK923295A in an in vitro panel of cell lines and an in vivo panel of xenografts representing most of the common childhood solid tumors as well as childhood ALL. Interestingly, GSK923295A demonstrated significant activity against the cell line panel; objective responses were noted in 13 of 35 xenografts, including 12 with CRs, and 1 with PR. Three of five EWS xenografts achieved CR, as did two of three rhabdoid tumors, and two of five rhabdomyosarcoma models. For the neuroblastoma panel, the best response was progressive disease with growth delay. Thus, the high level of activity for GSK923295A in these models, while promising, will need to be further evaluated in early phase pediatric clinical trials.[320]

Conclusion

This review outlines the current status of preclinical and clinical agents targeted at important cancer-related signaling pathways. While there are many promising compounds upcoming and already in the clinic, continual research in developing targeted compounds is warranted. Single-agent and combination regimens rationally designed, based on thorough preclinical studies in specific indications are the most appropriate strategy for development of these agents, and these combination regimens should be conceived from the earliest stages of development. In addition, appropriate biomarkers are absolutely necessary for predicting responses and for pharmacodynamic purposes at early stage of drug development. New class of agents may hold promise for paradigm-shifting advances in cancer management, but their development requires sound preclinical science for complexity and innovative clinical trial designs to correctly pilot the therapeutic potential of these agents.

References

1. Pollak M. Insulin and insulin-like growth factor signalling in neoplasia. Nat Rev Cancer 2008;8(12):915–928.

2. Sachdev D, Yee D. Disrupting insulin-like growth factor signaling as a potential cancer therapy. Mol Cancer Ther 2007;6(1):1–12.

3. Frasca F, Pandini G, Sciacca L, et al. The role of insulin receptors and IGF-I receptors in cancer and other diseases. Arch Physiol Biochem 2008;114(1):23–37.

4. Pollak MN, Schernhammer ES, Hankinson SE. Insulin-like growth factors and neoplasia. Nat Rev Cancer 2004;4(7):505–518.

5. Moschos SJ, Mantzoros CS. The role of the IGF system in cancer: from basic to clinical studies and clinical applications. Oncology 2002;63(4):317–332.

6. Baserga R. The IGF-I receptor in cancer research. Exp Cell Res 1999;253(1):1–6.

7. Clemmons DR. Involvement of insulin-like growth factor-I in the control of glucose homeostasis. Curr Opin Pharmacol 2006;6(6):620–625.

8. LeRoith D, Yakar S. Mechanisms of disease: metabolic effects of growth hormone and insulin-like growth factor 1. Nat Clin Pract Endocrinol Metab 2007;3(3):302–310.

9. Nickerson T, Chang F, Lorimer D, et al. In vivo progression of LAPC-9 and LNCaP prostate cancer models to androgen independence is associated with increased expression of insulin-like growth factor I (IGF-I) and IGF-I receptor (IGF-IR). Cancer Res 2001;61(16):6276–6280.

10. Cullen KJ, Yee D, Sly WS, et al. Insulin-like growth factor receptor expression and function in human breast cancer. Cancer Res 1990;50(1):48–53.

11. Gooch JL, Van Den Berg CL, Yee D. Insulin-like growth factor (IGF)-I rescues breast cancer cells from chemotherapy-induced cell death–proliferative and anti-apoptotic effects. Breast Cancer Res Treat 1999;56(1):1–10.

12. Lee AV, Yee D. Insulin-like growth factors and breast cancer. Biomed Pharmacother 1995;49(9):415–421.

13. Peyrat JP, Bonneterre J. Type 1 IGF receptor in human breast diseases. Breast Cancer Res Treat 1992;22(1):59–67.

14. Hassan AB, Macaulay VM. The insulin-like growth factor system as a therapeutic target in colorectal cancer. Ann Oncol 2002;13(3):349–356.

15. Wu Y, Yakar S, Zhao L, et al. Circulating insulin-like growth factor-I levels regulate colon cancer growth and metastasis. Cancer Res 2002;62(4):1030–1035.

16. Ge NL, Rudikoff S. Insulin-like growth factor I is a dual effector of multiple myeloma cell growth. Blood 2000;96(8):2856–2861.

17. Gee JM, Robertson JF, Gutteridge E, et al. Epidermal growth factor receptor/HER2/insulin-like growth factor receptor signalling and oestrogen receptor activity in clinical breast cancer. Endocr Relat Cancer 2005;12(Suppl 1):S99–S111.

18. Iravani S, Zhang HQ, Yuan ZQ, et al. Modification of insulin-like growth factor 1 receptor, c-Src, and Bcl-XL protein expression during the progression of Barrett's neoplasia. Hum Pathol 2003;34(10):975–982.

19. LeRoith D, Baserga R, Helman L, et al. Insulin-like growth factors and cancer. Ann Intern Med 1995;122(1):54–59.

20. Berns EM, Klijn JG, van Staveren IL, et al. Sporadic amplification of the insulin-like growth factor 1 receptor gene in human breast tumors. Cancer Res 1992;52(4):1036–1039.

21. De Souza AT, Hankins GR, Washington MK, et al. Frequent loss of heterozygosity on 6q at the mannose 6-phosphate/insulin-like growth factor II receptor locus in human hepatocellular tumors. Oncogene 1995;10(9):1725–1729.

22. Cui H, Cruz-Correa M, Giardiello FM, et al. Loss of IGF2 imprinting: a potential marker of colorectal cancer risk. Science 2003;299(5613):1753–1755.

23. Kaneda A, Feinberg AP. Loss of imprinting of IGF2: a common epigenetic modifier of intestinal tumor risk. Cancer Res 2005;65(24):11236–1140.

24. Burtrum D, Zhu Z, Lu D, et al. A fully human monoclonal antibody to the insulin-like growth factor I receptor blocks ligand-dependent signaling and inhibits human tumor growth in vivo. Cancer Res 2003;63(24):8912–8921.

25. Cohen BD, Baker DA, Soderstrom C, et al. Combination therapy enhances the inhibition of tumor growth with the fully human anti-type 1 insulin-like growth factor receptor monoclonal antibody CP-751,871. Clin Cancer Res 2005;1(5):2063–2073.

26. Lacy MQ, Alsina M, Fonseca R, et al. Phase I, pharmacokinetic and pharmacodynamic study of the anti-insulinlike growth factor type 1 receptor

monoclonal antibody CP-751,871 in patients with multiple myeloma. J Clin Oncol 2008;26(19):3196–3203.

27. Haluska P, Shaw HM, Batzel GN, et al. Phase I dose escalation study of the anti insulin-like growth factor-I receptor monoclonal antibody CP-751,871 in patients with refractory solid tumors. Clin Cancer Res 2007;13(19):5834–5840.

28. Karp DD, Paz-Ares LG, Novello S, et al. Phase II Study of the Anti-Insulin-Like Growth Factor Type 1 Receptor Antibody CP-751,871 in Combination With Paclitaxel and Carboplatin in Previously Untreated, Locally Advanced, or Metastatic Non-Small-Cell Lung Cancer. J Clin Oncol 2009;27(15):2516–2522.

29. Higano CS, Yu EY, Whiting SH, et al. A phase I, first in man study of weekly IMC-A12, a fully human insulin like growth factor-I receptor IgG1 monoclonal antibody, in patients with advanced solid tumors. ASCO Meeting Abstracts 2007;25(18 Suppl):3505.

30. Rodon J, Patnaik A, Stein M, et al. A phase I study of q3W R1507, a human monoclonal antibody IGF-1R antagonist in patients with advanced cancer. ASCO Meeting Abstracts 2007;25(18 Suppl):3590.

31. Tolcher AW, Patnaik A, Till E, et al. A phase I study of AVE1642, a humanized monoclonal antibody IGF-1R (insulin like growth factor1 receptor) antagonist, in patients(pts) with advanced solid tumor(ST). ASCO Meeting Abstracts 2008;26(15 Suppl):3582.

32. Tolcher AW, Rothenberg ML, Rodon J, et al. A phase I pharmacokinetic and pharmacodynamic study of AMG 479, a fully human monoclonal antibody against insulin-like growth factor type 1 receptor (IGF-1R), in advanced solid tumors. ASCO Meeting Abstracts 2007;25(18 Suppl):3002.

33. Hidalgo M, Tirado Gomez M, Lewis N, et al. A phase I study of MK-0646, a humanized monoclonal antibody against the insulin-like growth factor receptor type 1 (IGF1R) in advanced solid tumor patients in a q2 wk schedule. ASCO Meeting Abstracts 2008;26(15 Suppl):3520.

34. de Bono JS, Attard G, Adjei A, et al. Potential applications for circulating tumor cells expressing the insulin-like growth factor-I receptor. Clin Cancer Res 2007;13(12):3611–3616.

35. Seraj J, Tsai M, Wang Y, et al. Evaluation of pharmacodynamic properties of a fully human IGF-1 receptor antibody, SCH 717454, in healthy volunteers. AACR Meeting Abstracts 2009:A3615.

36. Patel S, Pappo A, Crowley J, et al. A SARC global collaborative phase II trial of R1507, a recombinant human monoclonal antibody to the insulin-like growth factor-1 receptor (IGF1R) in patients with recurrent or refractory sarcomas. ASCO Meeting Abstracts 2009;27(15S):10503.

37. Postel-Vinay S, Okuno S, Schuetze S, et al. Safety, pharmacokinetics and preliminary activity of the anti-IGF-IR antibody CP-751,871 in patients with sarcoma. EJC Suppl 2008;6(12):122.

38. Rothenberg ML, Tolcher A, Sarantopoulos J, et al. AMG479 monotherapy to treat patients with advanced GI carcinoid tumors: a subset analysis from the first-in-human study. 2009 Gastrointestinal Cancers Symposium, 2009:A386.

39. Ji Q-S, Mulvihill M, Franklin M, et al. Properties of small molecule IGF-IR kinase inhibitors in preclinical models. AACR Meeting Abstracts 2007;2007(1_Annual_Meeting):2373.

40. Ji Q-S, Mulvihill M, Rosenfeld-Franklin M, et al. Preclinical characterization of OSI-906: A novel IGF-1R kinase inhibitor in clinical trials. AACR Meeting Abstracts 2007;2007(3_Molecular_Targets_Meeting):C192.

41. Morrione A, Valentinis B, Xu SQ, et al. Insulin-like growth factor II stimulates cell proliferation through the insulin receptor. Proc Natl Acad Sci U S A 1997;94(8):3777–3782.

42. Milazzo G, Giorgino F, Damante G, et al. Insulin receptor expression and function in human breast cancer cell lines. Cancer Res 1992;52(14):3924–3930.

43. Zhang H, Pelzer AM, Kiang DT, et al. Down-regulation of type I insulin-like growth factor receptor increases sensitivity of breast cancer cells to insulin. Cancer Res 2007;67(1):391–397.

44. Carden CP, Frentzas S, Langham M, et al. Preliminary activity in adrenocortical tumor (ACC) in phase I dose escalation study of intermittent oral dosing of OSI-906, a small-molecule insulin-like growth factor-1 receptor (IGF-1R) tyrosine kinase inhibitor in patients with advanced solid tumors. ASCO Meeting Abstracts 2009;27(15S):3544.

45. Lindsay CR, Chan E, Evans TR, et al. Phase I dose escalation study of continuous oral dosing of OSI-906, an insulin like growth factor-1 receptor

(IGF-1R) tyrosine kinase inhibitor, in patients with advanced solid tumors. ASCO Meeting Abstracts 2009;27(15S):2559.

46. Gotlieb WH, Bruchim I, Gu J, et al. Insulin-like growth factor receptor I targeting in epithelial ovarian cancer. Gynecol Oncol 2006;100(2):389–396.

47. Maloney EK, McLaughlin JL, Dagdigian NE, et al. An anti-insulin-like growth factor I receptor antibody that is a potent inhibitor of cancer cell proliferation. Cancer Res 2003;63(16):5073–5083.

48. Goetsch L, Gonzalez A, Leger O, et al. A recombinant humanized anti-insulin-like growth factor receptor type I antibody (h7C10) enhances the antitumor activity of vinorelbine and anti-epidermal growth factor receptor therapy against human cancer xenografts. Int J Cancer 2005;113(2):316–328.

49. Klotz DM, Hewitt SC, Ciana P, et al. Requirement of estrogen receptor-alpha in insulin-like growth factor-1 (IGF-1)-induced uterine responses and in vivo evidence for IGF-1/estrogen receptor cross-talk. J Biol Chem 2002;277(10):8531–8537.

50. Nicholson RI, Hutcheson IR, Knowlden JM, et al. Nonendocrine pathways and endocrine resistance: observations with antiestrogens and signal transduction inhibitors in combination. Clin Cancer Res 2004;10(1 Pt 2):346S–54S.

51. Frogne T, Jepsen JS, Larsen SS, et al. Antiestrogen-resistant human breast cancer cells require activated protein kinase B/Akt for growth. Endocr Relat Cancer 2005;12(3):599–614.

52. Ye JJ, Liang SJ, Guo N, et al. Combined effects of tamoxifen and a chimeric humanized single chain antibody against the type I IGF receptor on breast tumor growth in vivo. Horm Metab Res 2003;35(11–12):836–842.

53. Camirand A, Zakikhani M, Young F, et al. Inhibition of insulin-like growth factor-1 receptor signaling enhances growth-inhibitory and proapoptotic effects of gefitinib (Iressa) in human breast cancer cells. Breast Cancer Res 2005;7(4):R570–R579.

54. Chakravarti A, Loeffler JS, Dyson NJ. Insulin-like growth factor receptor I mediates resistance to anti-epidermal growth factor receptor therapy in primary human glioblastoma cells through continued activation of phosphoinositide 3-kinase signaling. Cancer Res 2002;62(1):200–207.

55. Nahta R, Yuan LX, Zhang B, et al. Insulin-like growth factor-I receptor/human epidermal growth factor receptor 2 heterodimerization contributes to trastuzumab resistance of breast cancer cells. Cancer Res 2005;65(23):11118–11128.

56. Jones HE, Gee JM, Taylor KM, et al. Development of strategies for the use of anti-growth factor treatments. Endocr Relat Cancer 2005;12(Suppl 1):S173–S182.

57. O'Reilly KE, Rojo F, She QB, et al. mTOR inhibition induces upstream receptor tyrosine kinase signaling and activates Akt. Cancer Res 2006;66(3):1500–1508.

58. Wan X, Harkavy B, Shen N, et al. Rapamycin induces feedback activation of Akt signaling through an IGF-1R-dependent mechanism. Oncogene 2006;26(13):1932–1940.

59. Kurmasheva R, Boltz C, Phelps D, et al. Combination of CP-751871, a human monoclonal antibody against the IGF-1 receptor, with rapamycin results in a highly effective therapy for xenografts derived from childhood sarcomas. AACR Meeting Abstracts 2007;(3_Molecular_Targets_Meeting):C172.

60. Naing A, LoRusso P, Mills G, et al. Phase I study combining an IGFR inhibitor (IMC-A12) and an mTOR inhibitor (temsirolimus) in patients with solid tumors or lymphoma. ASCO Meeting Abstracts 2009;27(15S):e14535.

61. Wymann MP, Pirola L. Structure and function of phosphoinositide 3-kinases. Biochim Biophys Acta 1998;1436(1–2):127–150.

62. Maira SM, Voliva C, Garcia-Echeverria C. Class IA phosphatidylinositol 3-kinase: from their biologic implication in human cancers to drug discovery. Expert Opin Ther Targets 2008;12(2):223–238.

63. Bellacosa A, Chandra Kumar C, Di Cristofano A, Testa J. Activation of AKT Kinases in Cancer: Implications for Therapeutic Targeting. Advances in Cancer Research 2005; 94:29–86.

64. Sarbassov DD, Guertin DA, Ali SM, et al. Phosphorylation and regulation of Akt/PKB by the rictor-mTOR complex. Science 2005;307(5712):1098–1101.

65. Zinda MJ, Johnson MA, Paul JD, et al. AKT-1, -2, and -3 are expressed in both normal and tumor tissues of the lung, breast, prostate, and colon. Clin Cancer Res 2001;7(8):2475–2479.

66. Cantley LC, Neel BG. New insights into tumor suppression: PTEN suppresses tumor formation by restraining the phosphoinositide 3-kinase/AKT pathway. Proc Natl Acad Sci U S A 1999;96(8):4240–4245.

form homodimers or heterodimers and translocate to the nucleus. Two transcriptional complexes are formed, IFN-α-activated factor (AAF, IFN-γ-activated factor [GAF]) and IFN-stimulated gene factor-3 (ISGF3).[35] AFF is a homodimer of phosphorylated STAT1, which binds to the IFNγ activated sequence (GAS), and ISGF3 is a heterodimer of STAT1 and STAT2 complexed with IRF-9 (p48, ISGF3γ) that binds to the IFN-stimulated regulatory element (IRSE).[35–37] In addition to STAT dimers, CT10 oncogene homologue (avian)–like protein (CrkL) forms heterodimers with STAT5 upon receptor activation and binds with the GAS sequence.[38] Although the JAK/STAT pathway is the classic mediator of IFN signaling, a number of other signaling pathways play a critical role in IFN signaling.

The Type I IFN receptor activates the phosphatidylinositol 3-kinase (PI3K)/AKT pathway as well as members of the MAPK family.[39–41] PI3K activation generates the phosphatidylinositols, PIP2 and PIP3.[42] These second messengers activate downstream targets such as 3-phosphoinositide-dependent protein kinase 1 (PDK1) by recruitment or conformational change.[43] PDK1 in turn phosphorylates AKT (protein kinase B) on threonine 308, resulting in activation.[43] AKT is further activated by phosphorylation on serine 473 by a protein complex containing Tor.[44–46]

Torc 1 and 2 are enzymatic complexes of the mammalian target of rapamycin (mTor). Torc1, the rapamycin sensitive complex, consists of mTor, Raptor (regulatory associated protein of mTor), and mLST8 (mammalian lethal with sec18 protein 8). It regulates protein translation by phosphorylating ribosomal S6 kinases, S6K1 and S6K2, and the eIF4E (eukaryotic initiation factor 4E)-binding proteins, 4E-BP1 and 4E-BP2.[44–46] Torc1 regulates translation and has been implicated in autophagy.[47] Torc2, the rapamycin insensitive complex, consists of mTor, Rictor (rapamycin-insensitive companion of mTor), mLST8 (mammalian lethal with sec18 protein 8), and mSin1 (mammalian stress–activated protein kinase–interacting protein-1). This complex phosphorylates AKT on serine 473, leading to phosphorylation and inhibition of FOXO transcription factors. Torc2 in concert with PDK1 phosphorylates and stabilizes PKCα.[44–46] The PI3K/AKT/mTor pathway regulates apoptosis, gene expression, protein translation, and cytoskeletal organization.

Activation of the Type I and II IFN receptors activates the class I PI3K, which is composed of regulatory (p85) and catalytic subunits (p110).[41,48,49] Experiments using MEFs from p85 knockouts have shown that PI3K plays a role in the induction of IFN-stimulated genes (ISG) including ISG15, CXCL10, and IRF by regulating mRNA transcription through Torc1.[41] In addition, PI3K plays a role in phosphorylation of STAT1 on serine 727, which enhances STAT-dependent transcription.[50] A relatively small number of genes that are regulated by IFN are modulated by PI3K/mTor pathway.[51] The induction of IFN in pDC is also dependent on the PI3K/mTor pathway. These findings elucidate the molecular mechanism of immune suppression by rapamycin.[52]

The NF-*kappaB* (NFκB) transcription factors play a critical role in the suppression of apoptosis and regulation of the cell cycle. The NFκB family consists of p50, which is derived from the p105 precursor and p52, which is derived from the p100 precursor, RelA (p65), RelB, and cRel. The p50 and p52 subunits lack a transcription activation domain and as homodimers function as transcriptional repressors or form complexes with BCL-3 to activate transcription.[53,54] p50 is constitutively processed from p105, but the processing of p100 to p52 is tightly regulated by phosphorylation and ubiquitinylation.[53] In contrast, p65, cRel, and RelB have a transcription activation domain and thus, when complexed with p50 or p52, are capable of activating transcription.[53] NFκB homodimers and heterodimers are tightly regulated and are bound in the cytoplasm by inhibitors of NFκB (IκB). In the classical pathway of NFκB activation, IκB kinases (IKK) beta and gamma phosphorylate IκB, leading to IκB proteolytic degradation.[53] NFκB then freely moves into the nucleus and regulates transcriptional activity. In the alternative NFκB activation pathway, the TNF receptor–associated factors (TRAFs) activate MAP3K kinase and NFκB-inducing kinase (NIK), which leads to the processing of p100 to p52 in an IKKα-dependent manner.[53] The Type I IFN receptor activates NFκB through the classical and alternative pathways.[55,56] The classical pathway appears to be PI3K dependent, while the alternative pathway appears to be dependent on NIK.[55,56] NFκB binds to the promoter of a subset of IFN-induced genes that also have binding sites for IRFs and STATs.

The IRF transcription factors are intricately integrated into the regulation of IFN. Mouse knockouts have demonstrated that IRF-4 and IRF-8 are required for the generation of pDCs.[57] IRF-3 and IRF-7 along with NFκB directly regulated the expression of Type I IFNs.[58] ISGF3 complex, which contains IRF-9, is a signaling complex downstream from the Type I receptor that induces IRF-7 expression.[59] ISGF3 and IRF-1 both bind to the ISRE DNA sequence and IRF-1 acts as a positive regulator of Type I and Type II IFN-induced genes, whereas IRF-2 represses the effects of IRF-1.[60] The induction of ISGF3, NF-κB, and IRF-7 by the Type I IFN receptor provides a potential positive feedback mechanism for IFN in pDCs.[61–64]

In contrast to the positive regulators of IFN signaling (e.g., IRFs), activation of negative regulators attenuates IFN signaling. Phosphatases are the counter balance to kinase activity. Src-homology 2 domain–containing protein tyrosine phosphatase-1 (SHP-1) and SHP-2 are protein tyrosine phosphatases that contain SH2 domains. SHP-1 appears to be a negative regulator of signaling with multiple reported substrates.[65] SHP-1 can dephosphorylate JAK family kinases and terminate signaling.[66] SHP-2 appears to be a positive modulator of MAPK signaling, but it may also function as a negative effector.[67,68] Both phosphatases have been shown to have a negative regulatory role in IFN signaling as a heightened response to IFNs is observed in SHP-1- and SHP-2-deficient cells.[68,69] In addition, treatment of cells with stibogluconate, an inhibitor of both phosphatases, resulted in prolonged IFN signaling.[70] Thus, SHP-1 and SHP-2 would be potential pharmacologic targets to modulate the effect of IFNs.

STAT signaling is regulated by suppressor of cytokine signaling (SOCS) proteins and the protein inhibitor of activated STATs (PIAS) gene families. The SOCS proteins are induced by IFN and negatively regulate cytokine signaling through binding and inactivation of JAKs and STATs, targeting the protein for degradation, or both.[71–73] The PIAS proteins bind to STAT1 and STAT3 dimers, thereby blocking their DNA-binding activity. PIAS1 selectively regulates a subset of IFN-γ– or IFN-β–inducible genes by interfering with the recruitment of STAT1 to the gene promoter.[74] Both these pathways likely play critical roles in dampening the response to IFN in vivo.

Pharmaceutical Preparations

IFNα initially referred to as leukocyte IFN because of how it was originally isolated, is comprised of a group of at least 12 distinct proteins.[3] Recombinant IFNα-2a, IFNα-2b, and IFNα-2c differ by one to two amino acids and are the forms of IFNα that have been tested clinically.[3] In the United States, IFNα2a is sold under the trade name Roferon (Hoffmann-La Roche; Nutley, NJ) and IFNα-2b is available as Intron A (Schering; Kenilworth, NJ). IFNα-2c is available in Europe as Berofor (Bender; Vienna, Austria). These three compounds have never been compared in a randomized trial; however, their spectrum of activity is likely similar. The approved indications for these agents include treatment of viral diseases such as Hepatitis C and Kaposi's sarcoma (KS) as well as treatment of cancers such as melanoma and chronic myeloid leukemia (CML).[75–77] IFNα conjugated to polymer polyethylene glycol (PEG-IFN) has an increased half-life allowing for longer dosing intervals and long exposure times (see below).[78] Pegylated IFNα-2a (Pegasys, Hoffmann-La Roche) and pegylated IFNα-2b (Peg-Intron, Schering) are the two forms of PEG-IFN available in the United States.[79,80] These agents are widely used in combination with ribavirin in the treatment of Hepatitis C. The role of the PEG-IFNs as monotherapies for cancer is still under study.[81,82]

Clinical Pharmacology of Type I Interferons

Interferon-α

The pharmacokinetics of the IFNs was initially measured in serum using bioassays, which measure protection from viral cytopathic effect, prior to the development of direct immunological tests such as enzyme-linked immunosorbent assays. When given subcutaneously or intramuscularly to humans, approximately 80% of IFN-α is absorbed.[83] These routes of administration lengthen its distribution phase, with peak serum levels occurring at 1 to 8 hours. Clearance varies between 4.8 and 48 L/h, and the terminal elimination half-life is 4 to 16 hours.[83] The high-dose IFN-α2b regimen used for adjuvant therapy of melanoma may yield peak serum levels of 2,500 IU/mL at the end of the intravenous phase and 150 IU/mL after subcutaneous administration[83–85] (Table 31-1).

In order to improve the pharmacokinetic profile of IFN-α, these agents have been chemically modified by linkage to a PEG molecule.[78] The PEG modification increases the serum half-life, resulting in a less frequent dosing interval. A monopegylated IFN-α2b has been developed by Schering Plough (Kenilworth, NJ). This species has a 20-fold increase in serum half-life compared with native IFN-α2a.[86] Linkage of a 40-kD branched PEG molecule to IFN-α2a or a 12-kD linear PEG moiety to IFN-α2b markedly

TABLE

31.1 *Pharmacokinetics of interferons*

Route of administration	Dose (mU)	Serum concentration (U/mL)	Peak time	Duration (from–to)	IFN type	Reference
IFN-α						
IM	50	2,000 pg/mL	6 h	<0.5 to >24 h	α2a	286
	36	1,000 pg/mL	6 h	<0.5–24 h		
	18	500 pg/mL	6 h	<0.5–24 h		
Continuous SC infusion	2–5	20–60	Steady state	24–72 h	α2b	291
IV	4–10	10–300	30 min		Fibroblast β	292
	40–80	200–10,000	30 min			
	160–320	2,000–20,000	30 min			
IFN-β						
SC	90	10^2		1–8 h	β1b	246
IV	90	10^3	5 min	5 min–12 h		
IV 4-h infusion	0.01–1.00	<10			β1b	293
	10	25–30	6 h	0.5–24 h		
	30	140	4 h	0.05–24 h		
IV	45	350	5 min		β1b	294
	180	1,800	5 min			
SC	45	0				
	180	25				
IV 10-min infusion	0.01–20.00	0			γ	242
		30	15 min	<0.5–12 h		
		75	15 min	<0.5–24 h		
IFN-γ						
IV 6-h infusion	0.5 mg/m^2	3 ng/mL	6 h	2–8 h	γ	295
	1 mg/m^2	6 ng/mL	6 h	<1–8		
SC	1 mU	4 mg/mL	13 h		γ	296

TABLE **31.2** *Pharmacokinetics of pegylated parental IFN-ALPHAS*				
	IFN-α2a	PEG IFN-α2a	IFN-α2b	PEG IFN-α2b
Volume of distribution	31–73 L	8–12 L	1.4 L/kg	0.99 L/kg
Absorption $t_{1/2}$	2.3 h	50 h	2.3 h	4.6 h
Elimination $t_{1/2}$	3–8 h	65 h	4 h	~40 h
Time to max. conc.	7.3–12 h	80 h	7.3–12 h	15–44 h
Peak/trough		1.5		>10

$t_{1/2}$, half-life; max. conc., maximal concentration.

altered the pharmacokinetic profile and increased activity against hepatitis C in a direct clinical comparison of subcutaneous PEG-IFN with the parent compound.[87,88] The larger PEG moiety of PEG–IFN-α2a leads to the slowest absorption half-life and a longer elimination half-life[87,88] (Table 31-2)

PEG-IFN-α2b at 1 μg/kg/wk induced a biological response similar to that of IFN-α2b at 3 million IU administered subcutaneously three times a week.[89] Anticancer activity against solid tumors was demonstrated in a phase I/II trial of PEG–IFN-α2b, which determined 6 μg/kg/wk as the maximal tolerated dose (MTD) and showed evidence of drug accumulation with an area under the curve (AUC) of 374 pg/h/mL for week 1, compared with 480 pg/h/mL at week 4 for patients treated with the MTD.[90] PEG–IFN-α2b has been directly compared with the parent drug as initial treatment for chronic phase CML in a phase III study, where it showed efficacy and toxicity at 6 μg/kg/wk similar to those of IFN-α2b at 5 million IU/m²/d.[91] The toxicity of both agents appears comparable to historical controls treated with the parental compound.[81] Whether the alteration of IFN-α pharmacokinetics will increase antitumor activity must be addressed in future studies.

Interferon-β

A single species in humans, IFN-β, exists as a 25-kD glycoprotein containing 166 amino acids, and IFN-β appears to be metabolized primarily in the liver.[83] After intravenous injection, the terminal elimination half-life is about 1 to 2 hours, and IFN-β remains measurable for up to 4 hours (Table 31-1).[83] In contrast, after a single subcutaneous or intramuscular injection, serum IFN-β is barely detectable.[83] However, intravenous and subcutaneous administration of the same dose elicited similar pharmacodynamic responses, including 2 to 5 A synthetase induction—a known IFN response gene that has been correlated to dose and serum level in some studies.[83,92]

Three modifications of IFN-β to improve the pharmacokinetic profile have been developed. Albuferon is a recombinant protein resulting from fusion of the IFN-β peptide with albumin. In monkeys, the bioavailability of subcutaneous Albuferon was 87%, plasma clearance was reduced by 140-fold, and the terminal half-life increased 5-fold, while in vitro and in vivo activities were preserved.[93] Fusion of IFN-β to soluble recombinant Type I IFN receptor subunit (sIFNAR-2) prolonged the half-life and increased antitumor activity in mice.[94] Finally, pegylation of IFN-β1a with a linear 20-kD molecule increased the maximum serum

concentration achieved 4-fold, while the AUC increased 10-fold and the half-life increased 3-fold.[95]

Since IFNα and IFNβ signal through the same receptor, they would be expected to have similar biologic effects and have overlapping indications. However, this is not always the case. Although both IFNα and IFNβ have activities against gliomas, one small study suggests that IFNβ has a higher response rate compared to IFNα.[96] In contrast to IFNα, IFNβ has been reported to have no clinical activity against CML and no responses were seen in a phase I trial of 35 patients with metastatic solid tumors.[97,98] Two forms of IFNβ, originally named fibroblast IFN, have been approved for use in patients with relapsing multiple sclerosis—IFNβ-1a (Avonex, Biogen Idec; Cambridge, MA) and IFNβ-1b (Betaseron, Berlex; Montville, NJ). Their use in treatment of malignancy is currently limited to clinical trials.

IFNγ: Type II Interferon

IFNγ, also known as immune IFN, is the only Type II IFN and has effects on the innate and adaptive immune systems. IFNγ is secreted by NK cells, natural killer T cells (NKTs), Th1 CD4$^+$ T-cells, CD8$^+$ T-cells, antigen-presenting cells (APCs), and B cells.[99–102] IFNγ activates macrophages and stimulates up-regulation of MHC class I, MHC class II, and costimulatory molecules on APCs.[11,103–105] Additionally, IFNγ induces changes in the proteosome to enhance antigen presentation.[106–108] It promotes Th1 differentiation of CD4$^+$ T cells and blocks IL-4-dependent isotype switching in B cells.[103,109,110] Mice with targeted deletion of IFNγ or the Type II IFN receptor have an increased risk of spontaneous and chemically induced tumors compared to controls.[111–115] IFNγ is cytotoxic to some malignant cells and has antiangiogenic activity.[116–120]

IFNγ is located on chromosome 12q14 and activates the Type II IFN receptor composed of IFNGR1 and IFNGR2.[3,5–7] Like the Type I IFN receptor, IFNGR1 and IFNGR2 are constitutively associated with members of the JAK kinase, JAK1 and JAK2, respectively.[121] STAT1, 2, 3, and 5 are phosphorylated by the Type II IFN receptor, but STAT1 appears to be the critical mediator.[122–124] The Type II receptors also activate the PI3K/AKT and MAPK pathways as well as NFκB.[50,125,126] The activation of NFκB appears to be cell-type restricted, and its role in vivo is unclear.

Clinical Pharmacology of Type II Interferon (IFN-γ)

After subcutaneous or intramuscular administration, 30% to 70% of IFN-γ is absorbed, and the terminal elimination half-life is 25 to

35 minutes; after intravenous injection, IFN-γ remains detectable in serum up to 4 hours (Table 31-1). Like IFN-β, IFN-γ appears to be metabolized primarily by the liver.[83] A phase I trial in colon cancer patients achieved IFN-γ concentrations greater than 5 U/mL for more than 6.5 hours following subcutaneous administration of 100 $\mu g/m^2$.[83] Preclinical studies of PEG–IFN-γ show an increased elimination half-life activity with preserved activity, but this molecule has not yet been evaluated in patients.[83]

The antitumor effects of IFNγ suggested it would be effective against a wide spectrum of malignancies. Although IFNγ has demonstrated limited clinical utility in cancer, it likely plays a critical role in the in vivo effects of other cytokines.[127–129] Actimmune (Intermune; Brisbane, CA) is an IFNγ preparation that has been approved for the treatment of chronic granulomatous disease.[130] Clinically, significant benefit in treatment of malignancies has been largely restricted to Type I IFNs.

Type III Interferons

In 2003, two papers were published simultaneously describing novel cytokines designated IFNs λ/IL-28/29, which exhibited antiviral activity.[8,9] These genes, comprising five exons on chromosome 19, bind to a distinct dimeric membrane receptor, IFNLR1 and IL10R2.[8,9] These IFNs have antiviral activity, antiproliferative activity, and in vivo antitumor activity like the Type I IFNs. The receptor is associated with Jak1 and Tyk2 resulting in the activation of STAT1, 2, 3, 4, and 5, which results in expression of GAS and ISRE containing genes.[9] The signaling of the Type III IFNs appears to be quite similar to the Type I IFNs.[131] The differentiation appears to be at the level of the receptor. IL10R2 is ubiquitously expressed, while IFNLR1 is limited in its expression and inducible in some cell types such as pDC.[131–134] In pDC, TLR activation induces IFNλ just as it does the Type I IFNs; however, when IL-28R-deficient mice are exposed to a panel of different viruses, their immune response was unimpaired.[134] Type III IFNs have a positive feedback on either the Type III or Type I IFNs; the role of the Type III IFNs may be to regulate antiviral responses in epithelial cells.[134] Whether the Type III IFNs are a redundant system or have a unique role in IFN biology remains to be elucidated.

Clinical Indications

Hematologic Malignancies: Hairy Cell Leukemia

Type I IFNs have had their most clinical success against two hematologic malignancies: hairy cell leukemia (HCL) and CML. A regimen of IFNα-2b 2 million units/m² subcutaneously three times a week for 52 weeks produced an overall response rate of 77% with a complete response rate of 5% in patients with HCL.[135] The vast majority of these patients (61 out of 64) had undergone splenectomy but were otherwise untreated.[135] Subsequent studies demonstrated complete responses in 25% to 35% of patients who had not had splenectomies, leading to regulatory approval for IFN in this patient population.[136] Although IFN has a significant response rate and improves survival in HCL, the majority of patients relapse after discontinuation of therapy.[137] Subsequent studies demonstrated that 80% of patients who relapsed would respond to another course of IFN.[137] It is unclear whether the effects of IFN in HCL are mediated by immune mechanisms

or direct effects on the leukemic cells.[138–140] Although IFN was once considered first-line therapy, the introduction of the nucleoside analogs, which have a greater than 90% CR rate, has limited the use of IFN therapy to patients who have disease that is refractory to nucleosides or have contraindications to these agents.[141,142]

Hematologic Malignancies: Chronic Myeloid Leukemia

Initial trials of IFNα in CML noted complete hematologic responses in over 50% of patients and a complete cytogenic response in up to 25% of patients.[77,143] Follow-up randomized studies demonstrated that IFN was superior to hydroxyurea or busulfan or both.[144–148] Four studies demonstrated an improved overall survival (OS) for the IFN-treated patients.[144,145,147–150] A meta-analysis of the randomized trials demonstrated an improvement in the 5-year survival in the IFN-treated group of 12% over hydroxyurea and 20% over busulfan-treated patients.[151] Additionally, the meta-analysis showed the benefit extended to all risk groups. All three commercially available IFNα were used in the CML trials and although not formally compared, their activity in CML appeared similar.

The mechanism of response of CML to IFN has been extensively investigated. Reports that human leukocyte antigen (HLA) type and development of an immune response to Bcr-Abl correlate with a complete response suggest that IFN works through an immune mechanism in CML.[152] The observation that patients who obtain complete response correct abnormalities in the secretion of Th1 cytokines also supports an immune mechanism.[153] However, IFN also exerts a direct antiproliferative effect in CML through inhibition of DNA polymerase.[154] These data suggest the mechanism of action of IFN in CML is multifactorial.

In an effort to enhance the efficacy of IFN in CML, a number of trials were conducted using IFN combined with chemotherapy.[155] The combination of IFN and low-dose ara-C was shown to improve the number of cytogenetic remissions compared to IFN alone. However, the beneficial impact of the combination on OS is small and was achieved with a substantial increase in toxicity.[156–158] Although largely supplanted as first-line therapy by Bcr-Abl kinase inhibitors,[159] IFN and IFN-containing regimens remain a valid second-line therapeutic option for patients with CML.[159–162]

Hematologic Malignancies: Non-Hodgkin's Lymphoma

Early studies of IFNα monotherapy in follicular lymphomas demonstrated a response rate of over 50%.[163–165] Subsequently, several investigators combined IFN with chemotherapy in an induction regimen or as maintenance therapy. The results of these trials were mixed in terms of OS benefit. The Groupe d'Etude des Lymphoma Folliculaires (GELF) study demonstrated an advantage in response rate (85% versus 69%, $P < 0.001$) and OS (34 versus 19 months, $P = 0.02$) for chemotherapy plus IFNα 5 MIU thrice weekly for 18 months compared to chemotherapy alone using an anthracycline-based regimen.[166,167] These results were a major impetus for the approval of IFNα for the treatment of follicular lymphoma. A meta-analysis of the IFN trials supports a survival advantage for intensive chemotherapy regimens containing IFN.[168] Interestingly, a large SWOG trial did not show any survival advantage for IFNα at 2 MIU thrice weekly for 24 months versus observation.[169] These data suggest that the dose of IFNα used may be critical to the beneficial effect in patients with follicular lymphomas. IFN is approved for treatment of follicular lymphoma, but its use is limited due to its associated toxicities and the activity of a variety of other agents.

Melanoma

The natural history of some melanomas suggests that it may be an immune responsive tumor. Up to 25% of primary cutaneous melanomas show histologic regression at the time of biopsy.[170] All three IFNα's have been investigated in patients with metastatic (stage IV) melanoma. Multiple dose levels and schedules have been tested, and the overall response rate for single agent IFN in patients with metastatic melanoma is approximately 15%.[171–179] There is no clear most effective regimen; however, IFN administered thrice weekly is the most widely used schedule because it has a significantly better toxicity profile than daily administration with no diminution in response rates.[180,181] It is unknown if IFN provides a survival advantage because no randomized trials in metastatic melanoma compare IFN to either cytotoxic chemotherapy or best supportive care.[182] IFN appears to work best in patients with low metastatic tumor burden.[183]

IFNα has proved most useful in the management of melanoma in the adjuvant setting. Multiple IFN regimens have been used in the adjuvant setting for patients with intermediate- and high-risk melanoma (Tables 31-3 and 31-4).[184–194] IFNα was approved in Europe based on studies that used lower dose regimens. Two trials of low-dose IFNα-2a given for 12 to 18 months demonstrated a benefit in relapse-free survival (RFS) in patients with melanomas greater that 1.5 mm or locoregional disease, but neither trial showed an OS benefit.[185,189] Subsequent trials using low-dose IFNα-2a and

IFNα-2b have failed to demonstrate a durable RFS or an OS benefit (Table 31-3).[184,187,188,190,191,195]

In the United States, IFNα was approved for adjuvant therapy in patients with high-risk melanoma based on the results of the ECOG 1684 trial (Table 31-4).[84] In this trial, patients with high-risk melanoma, defined as primary tumors greater than 4 mm or pathologic or clinical regional lymph node involvement who had undergone lymphadenectomy, were randomized to receive 1 year of high-dose IFNα-2b (HDI) or observation.[84] The high-dose IFN regimen consisted of 20 million units/m^2/d 5 days/wk for 4 weeks followed by 10 million units/m^2/d thrice weekly for 48 weeks and demonstrated an overall improvement in median RFS from 1 to 1.7 years and median OS from 2.8 to 3.8 years.[84] In addition, risk of relapse was significantly (42%) reduced. In a subsequent intergroup trial, ECOG 1690, an improvement in median and overall RFS was seen in the HDI arm compared to observation, but there was no difference in OS (Table 31-4).[196] The reason for the lack of an OS advantage for the HDI in this trial appeared to be due to improved survival in patients on the observation arm following relapse (6 versus 2.8 years in ECOG 1984).[196] Multiple explanations for this disparity have been postulated. In contrast to E1684, patients on E1690 were not required to undergo elective node dissection before enrollment on study.[84,196] Consequently, many patients were enrolled with greater than 4 mm thick primary tumors that had no evaluation of their regional nodal basin.[196] Additionally, IFNα received FDA approval in 1996, while E1690 was ongoing. Consequently, many patients on the observation arm who relapsed in

TABLE

31.3 Adjuvant trials of low to intermediate dose IFN for melanoma

Trial	Number of patients	Dose	Population	RFS	OS
WHO-16	218	3 MIU SC 3×/wk × 3 y	>1.5 mm		
	208	Observation	Clinically node negative	NS	NS
NCCTG 83-7052	131	20 MIU/M² IM 3×/wk × 3 mo	>1.5 mm and/or		
	131	Observation	Resected regional disease	NS	NS
French Cooperative group	244	3 MIU SC 3×/wk × 18 mo	>1.5 mm		
	245	Observation	Clinically node negative	P = 0.04	NS
Austrian Melanoma Cooperative group	154	3 MIU/d × 3 wk then 3 MIU SQ/wk × 1 y	>1.5 mm		
	157	Observation	Clinically node negative	P = 0.02	NS
EORTC 18871	244	1MIU q od SQ x 1 y	>3.0 mm and/or		
	240	IFNg × 1 y	Resected regional disease	NS	NS
	244	Observation			
Scottish Melanoma Group	46	3 MIU SC 3×/wk × 6 mo	>3.0 mm and/or		
	49	Observation	Resected regional disease	NS	NS
EORTC 18952	553	10 MIU/d × 4 wk then 10 MIU sq 3×/wk × 1 yr	>4.0 mm and/or	NS	NS
	556	5 MIU sq 3×/wk × 2 y	Resected regional disease	NS	NS
	279	Observation			
AIM HIGH	338	3 MIU SQ 3×/wk × 2 y	>4.0 mm and/or		
	336	Observation	Resected regional disease	NS	NS

MIU, million international units.

TABLE

31.4   *Adjuvant trials of high-dose IFN for melanoma*

Trial	Number of patients	Dose	Population	RFS	OS
ECOG 1684	287	20MIU/M^2 5×/wk × 1 mo then 10MIU/M^2 3×/wk × 48 wk Observation	>4.0 mm and/or Resected regional disease	$P = 0.004$	$P = 0.046$
ECOG 1690	642	20MIU/M^2 5×/wk × 1 mo then 10MIU/M^2 3×/wk × 48 wk 3MIU SC 3×/wk × 3 y Observation	>4.0 mm and/or Resected regional disease	$P = 0.05$ $P = 0.17$	NS NS
ECOG 1694	385 389	20MIU/M^2 5×/wk × 1 mo then 10MIU/M^2 3×/wk × 48 wk GM2-KLH/QS-21 vaccine	>4.0 mm and/or Resected regional disease	$P = 0.0027$	$P = 0.0147$
EORTC 18991	627 629	6 µg/kg weekly × 8 wk then 3µg/kg weekly to 5 y Observation	Resected regional disease	$P = 0.01$	NS

MIU = million IUs

regional nodes received off protocol adjuvant IFN following therapeutic node dissection, perhaps contributing to their better than anticipated survival, while obscuring the survival benefit related to upfront IFN administration.[196]

No other trials have compared HDI to observation. However, ECOG 1694, a trial that compared HDI to the ganglioside GM2/keyhole limpet hemoycanin vaccine (GMK), showed an improvement in both RFS and OS for patients receiving HDI (Table 31-4).[192] Long-term follow-up of patients on ECOG 1684, 1690, and 1694 shows that the HDI arm of ECOG 1684 continues to demonstrate an improvement in RFS (HR = 1.38; $P = 0.02$) at a median follow-up of 12.6 years[193] (Fig. 31-3). The OS benefit also persisted (HR = 1.22; $P = 0.18$) but was no longer statistically significant.[193] Analysis of pooled data from both 1684 and 1690 (median follow-up 7.2 years) demonstrates a RFS benefit (HR = 1.30; $P < 0.006$) but no OS benefit.[193]

The ECOG adjuvant trials were stratified based on stage. Although not powered for subset analysis, these data were reviewed to determine if any populations disproportionately benefited from adjuvant IFN.[84,196] In ECOG 1684, the patients with microscopic involvement of their lymph nodes (Stage IIIaT4pN1) had the greatest improvement in their hazard ratio for relapse when treated with IFNα.[84,196] Since patients were not required to have lymphadenectomies, the group of patients who had microscopic disease was mixed in with the T4N0 subgroup in the E1690 trial.[84,196] In both studies, improvement in RFS was noted in node-positive disease that was proportionate to the patient's risk, while on E1694, the patients who benefited most were those with no evidence of nodal involvement. Taken together, the benefit of IFN appears to be proportionate to risk, with a 20% to 30% reduction in risk of relapse and 10% to 20% reduction in risk of death regardless of the extent of disease. Consideration of IFN therapy should take into account the patient's risk of relapse and comorbidities and potential side effects. Generally, IFNα treatment should be considered

in otherwise healthy patients whose risk of relapse is greater than 30%.[84,196]

EORTC 18991 was the first large study of pegylated IFNα for the treatment of melanoma in the adjuvant setting. This study randomly assigned 1,256 patients with stage III melanoma (with the exclusion in-transit metastases) to observation or 5 years of pegylated IFNα-2b.[197] During the first 8 weeks, pegylated IFNα-2b was administered at 6 µg/kg/wk for 8 weeks followed by 3µg/kg/wk maintenance therapy for up to 5 years. OS was not significantly different in the two groups; however, the IFN-treated patients showed a significant improvement in recurrence-free survival (HR 0.84; $P = 0.02$) with a median follow-up of 3.8 years. Subgroup analysis showed the greatest improvement in RFS was in the patients with microscopic nodal disease (HR 0.73; $P = 0.02$); those with macroscopic disease had no significant benefit (HR 0.86; $P = 0.12$).[197] A combined subset analysis of EORTC18952 and EORTC18991 showed improvement in DFS and OS in patients with ulcerated primaries. The prognostic value of ulceration in the adjuvant setting will be investigated prospectively in EORTC 18081.[198]

As with hematologic malignancies, combinations of IFN with chemotherapy have been studied in patients with metastatic melanoma in hopes of improving clinical benefit. One single institution, randomized phase II trial reported that combined IFNα and dacarbazine demonstrated an improved response rate (53% versus 20%) and improved OS (18 versus 10 months) relative to dacarbazine alone.[199] Unfortunately, this benefit could not be confirmed in a larger, multicenter randomized phase III trial (ECOG 3690).[182,200,201] In addition to chemotherapy, IFN has been combined with other cytokines. A trial testing the combination of a Type I IFN combined with IFNγ did not demonstrate any substantial benefit over Type I IFN alone.[202] Despite some controversy, IFNα remains the standard of care for adjuvant treatment of patients with high-risk melanoma, while its role in metastatic melanoma should be considered investigational.

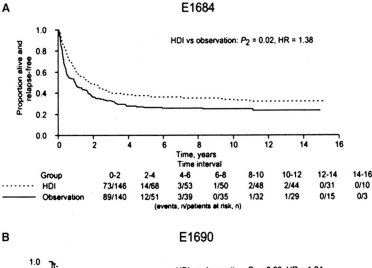

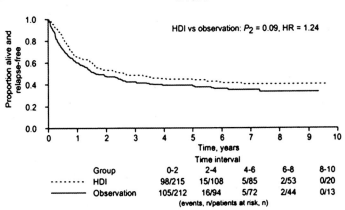

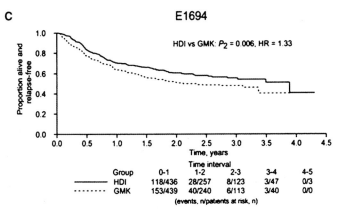

FIGURE **31-3**   Kaplan-Meier estimates of RFS based on long-term follow-up. **A.** ECOG 1684 (median follow-up 12.6 years), **B.** ECOG 1690 (median follow-up 6.6 years) and **C.** ECOG 1694 (median follow-up 2.1 years). (Adapted from Kirkwood JM, et al. A pooled analysis of eastern cooperative oncology group and intergroup trials of adjuvant high-dose interferon for melanoma. Clin Cancer Res 2004;10(5):1670–1677, with permission.)

Renal Cell Carcinoma

In advanced renal cell carcinoma (RCC), both recombinant IFNα2a and IFNα2b have undergone extensive clinical evaluation.[203–206] No clinically meaningful difference exists between these two IFNα products, and thus, the generic IFNα will be used to describe these data. Despite the use of a variety of preparations, doses, and schedules, most studies have shown modest antitumor activity, with the overall response rate being approximately 10% to 15%. Responses are often delayed in onset, with median time to response being about 4 months. Most responses are partial and short-lived (median response duration, 6 to 7 months). About 2% of patients have had complete responses, with only an occasional patient having a response persisting in excess of 1 year after therapy. Although

no clear dose-response relationship exists, daily doses in the 5- to 10-MU range appear to have the highest therapeutic index.[155,204–211]

In order to investigate a possible survival benefit to IFNα in RCC, several randomized trials have been performed. Table 31-5 is a summary of randomized trials that have investigated the effect of IFNα on OS in metastatic RCC patients. More recent studies have suggested the antitumor effects of IFNα are quite limited. For example, a French Immunotherapy Group Phase III trial, comparing IFNα to both IL-2 and IL-2 plus IFNα, reported a response rate of only 7.5% for the IFNα arm with a 1-year event-free survival rate of only 12%.[212] In addition, a Southwestern Oncology Group (SWOG) study comparing IFNα alone to debulking nephrectomy followed by IFNα reported tumor responses in less than 5% of patients receiving either treatment approach.[213]

TABLE

31.5   *IFN alpha in metastatic RCC*

Author	Trial design	No. of patients	Response rate advantage for IFN-α	OS impact
Ritchie	IFN-α versus medroxyprogesterone	335	10%	2.5 mo advantage for IFN-α ($P = 0.017$)
Pyrhonen	IFN-α plus vinblastine versus vinblastine	160	14%	7.0 mo advantage for IFN-α ($P = 0.0049$)
Coppin	Meta-analysis of randomized, controlled trials of IFN-α	4,216 (42 trials)	11%	3.8 mo advantage for IFN-α ($P = 0.0005$)

While the role of low-dose single agent cytokines is limited, combinations of cytokines with targeted therapy may have merit. Sorafenib and IFNα have been combined in two separate single-arm phase II trials.[214,215] These trials demonstrated objective response rates of 18% and 35%. Toxicity was typical of that observed with each single agent with a notable reduction in hand-foot syndrome compared to sorafenib monotherapy. This combination regimen will be examined in randomized trials. Two large phase III trials of IFNα plus bevacizumab versus IFNα alone have demonstrated superior efficacy with the combination regimen and suggest the potential of an additive effect.[216,217] Given the modest survival impact of IFNα seen in Phase III studies and its widespread application worldwide, regulatory agencies have supported the use of IFNα as a control arm for randomized trials with targeted therapies (e.g., sunitinib, temsirolimus) (see Chapters 26 and 34). The results of these investigations will likely narrow the future use of IFNα as a single agent.

Kaposi's Sarcoma

AIDS-related KS is a multifocal vascular proliferative disease associated with HIV and Kaposi's sarcoma herpes virus (KSHV)/human herpes virus-8 (HHV-8) coinfection.[218] Histologically, these lesions are composed of clusters of spindle-shaped cells (KS spindle cells) with prominent microvasculature. This angiogenic lesion is driven by autocrine and paracrine cytokine loops.[219,220] Because of the anti-angiogenic activity IFNα demonstrated in treating hemangiomas, it was tested in patients with KS.[221–223]

As a single agent for the treatment of KS, IFN has a response rate of 30% to 40% that appears to be dose dependent.[76,224–226] When combined with antiretroviral therapy, the response rate appears to be over 40%.[227,228] Although IFN is useful in KS, effective antiretroviral therapy, cytotoxic chemotherapy, and local therapy are currently the first-line treatments.[229]

Toxicities

The enthusiasm for IFN use is tempered by its side effects (Table 31-6). Nonetheless, the side effects are typically dose related and most resolve quickly with discontinuation of treatment. The toxicities can be broken down into five major categories—constitutional, neuropsychiatric, gastrointestinal, hematologic, and autoimmune.

Constitutional symptoms are the most common, with more than 80% of the patients in the high-dose IFN trials reporting fever and fatigue.[230] Additionally, more than half of patients report headache and myalgias.[230] The majority of these symptoms can be controlled with acetaminophen or NSAIDs; however, severe fatigue often requires a break from therapy with a subsequent dose reduction for amelioration. Fatigue is often underreported by patients because they accommodate to it. Many patients report not realizing how fatigued they felt until they stopped the drug.

Neuropsychiatric issues are not as common but are potentially life threatening. As many as 10% of patients complain of confusion and rarely (<1%) patients develop mania.[230,231] In some studies, up

TABLE

31.6   *IFN associated toxicities*

Acute effects
Fevers
Chills and rigors
Myalgias
Fatigue
Headache
Nausea/vomiting

Chronic effects
Constitutional
Anorexia
Fatigue
Weight loss
Headache
Nausea

Laboratory abnormalities
Transaminase elevations
Leukopenia/neutropenia
Thrombocytopenia
Anemia

Neuropsychiatric
Depression
Confusion
Dizziness/ataxia

Autoimmunity
Thyroiditis
Vitiligo

to 45% of patients reported depression, and suicides were occasionally reported.[232,233] In one small double-blind placebo-controlled trial in patients receiving HD IFN for high-risk melanoma, prophylactic use of antidepressants significantly reduced the risk of depression from 45% to 11% after 12 weeks.[232] These data suggest that at a minimum, patients with a history of depression should be treated with antidepressants if they are not currently taking them at the time of IFN initiation. All other patients should be monitored closely and antidepressant therapy instituted at the earliest sign of depression.

Gastrointestinal side effects are common with up to one third of patients having diarrhea, which is usually well controlled with over-the-counter antidiarrheal medications.[230] Two thirds of patients have problems with nausea and anorexia. Antiemetics often alleviate the nausea; however, the combination of nausea and anorexia can lead to significant weight loss.[230] Additionally, IFN can produce significant hepatic toxicity, which requires serial monitoring of liver function tests. In the early trials, some patients had fatal hepatic failure. Usually, a drug holiday until the liver function improves followed by dose reduction allows the majority of patients with liver toxicity to continue treatment.

IFN can affect all of the hematopoietic lineages. Thrombocytopenia, leukopenia, and neutropenia are common and are typically managed with dose reductions.[230] Anemia, if not hemolytic, can be treated with transfusions or dose reductions. Rarely, thrombotic thrombocytopenia purpura (TTP) has been reported in association with IFN.[234–237] Hemolytic anemia and TTP require permanent drug discontinuation.[238–241]

In addition to autoimmune hemolytic anemia and thrombocytopenia, other manifestations of immune dysfunction can also be observed. Thyroid dysfunction, either hyperthyroidism or hypothyroidism, occurs in about 15% of patients. Therefore, thyroid function tests should be routinely monitored in patients receiving IFN therapy.[242] The hyperthyroidism often presents as fatigue, restlessness, and/or significant weight loss and may be attributed to other causes if thyroid function tests are not checked. Sarcoid can occur in patients receiving IFN and can also present a diagnostic dilemma. It can present as skin lesions masquerading as subcutaneous metastases or as FDG-avid lymph nodes on PET scan.[243,244] Vitiligo, lupus, rheumatoid arthritis, polymyalgia rheumatica, and psoriasis are among the other autoimmune disorders that have been observed.[245,246] Of interest, patients who develop vitiligo or autoantibodies such as antithyroid and antinuclear antibodies during adjuvant IFN therapy for high-risk melanoma appear to have an improved RFS and OS relative to the total IFN-treated population, suggesting that IFN may mediate its antitumor effects in melanoma through an autoimmune mechanism.[247] The clinician using IFN should be aware that a change in symptomatology of a patient on long-term IFN might herald the development of an autoimmune disease.

Interleukins

Interleukins have pleiotropic effects on innate and cellular immunity as well as hematopoiesis. Studies of cytokines in animal tumor models suggested that they would have broad antitumor activity. Unfortunately, only IL-2 has shown sufficient activity to obtain regulatory approval.

Interleukin-2

Biology

IL-2's effects are mediated by the IL-2 receptor, a class I cytokine receptor.[248] The IL-2 receptor is composed of a α, β and γ chain. The β and γ chains are involved in signaling, while the α chain is only involved in cytokine binding.[248] These subunits form a high-, intermediate-, or low-affinity receptor depending on which of the chains are in the receptor complex (Fig. 31-1). The high-affinity receptor is a complex of all three subunits with a K_a of 10^{-11} M, and the intermediate-affinity receptor is composed of the β and γ chains with a K_a 10^{-9} M.[248] The alpha chain (CD25) is the low-affinity receptor with a K_a of 10^{-8} M; however, this receptor does not initiate intracellular signaling.[248] Although the β and γ chains are expressed on T cells, B cells, NK cells, and monocytes, the α chain (CD25) is inducible and expressed on T cells, B cells, monocytes, and some subsets of thymocytes.[248]

IL-2 has a myriad of effects on the immune system. When T cells are stimulated with antigen, IL-2 is produced resulting in autocrine and paracrine effects on T cells. Additionally, IL-2 stimulates release of other cytokines by T cells. NK-cells express the intermediate-affinity IL-2 receptor.[249] Exposure of NK cells to IL-2 results in enhanced cell proliferation, cytolytic activity, and secretion of other cytokines.[249] B cells also express intermediate-affinity IL-2 receptor and IL-2 in cooperation with other cytokines results in B-cell proliferation and differentiation.[250,251]

IL-2 may also play a critical role in suppressing immune responses. A subpopulation of CD4$^+$ T lymphocytes that coexpress CD25 function as T regulatory (Treg) cells and these cells suppress self-reactive T cells.[252] Depletion of CD4$^+$CD25$^+$ Tregs breaks tolerance to self-antigens and can lead to increased autoimmunity.[252] Additionally, depletion of CD4$^+$CD25$^+$ Tregs enhances tumor rejection and improves response to cancer vaccines by promoting the function of CD8$^+$ cytotoxic T-cell lymphocytes (CTLs) due to lack of inhibition by CD4$^+$CD25$^+$ lymphocytes.[253] The mechanism by which CD4$^+$CD25$^+$ lymphocytes inhibit the function of CD8$^+$ CTLs is poorly understood. Mice with targeted deletion of IL-2 and the IL-2 receptor develop a generalized inflammatory syndrome and often die of autoimmune colitis.[254–257] These data suggest that IL-2 not only activates immune responses but also participates in a negative feedback loop to limit immune responses.

IL-2 Signaling

The binding of IL-2 to its receptor induces the tyrosine phosphorylation of numerous cellular proteins, including the IL-2 receptor β chain itself (Fig. 31-4). Since all three chains of the IL-2 receptor lack intrinsic tyrosine kinase activity, these events must be transduced through kinases that physically associate with the cytoplasmic domains of the receptor subunits (Fig. 31-4). Indeed, the src family member p56lck associates with the β chain and its kinase activity is augmented by IL-2.[258] IL-2 also induces the recruitment and subsequent tyrosine phosphorylation of the adapter protein Shc to the IL-2R β chain. This particular association is thought to be largely responsible for the activation of p21ras and the downstream MAP kinases erk-1 and erk-2 in response to IL-2.[259] The IL-2 receptor γ chain is also essential for IL-2-induced signaling as mutant T cell lines expressing the α and β chains and a mutant version of the γ

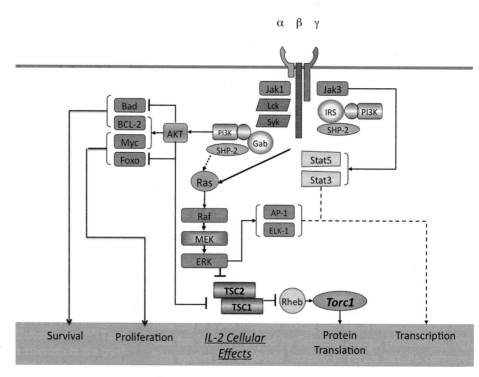

chain lacking the C-terminal 68 residues failed to express the proto-oncogenes c-fos, c-jun, and c-myc when stimulated with IL-2.[260]

The activation of the PI3K/mTor pathway by IL-2 is dependent on p56lck.[261,262] The recruitment of p85/p110 to the β and γ chains is mediated by the Gab and IRS scaffolding proteins[263–265]; IRS-1 and IRS-2 are associated with the common γ chain and phosphorylated in response to multiple cytokines.[264,265] Gab2 is associated with the β chain shared by IL-2 and IL-15 and is phosphorylated in response to both cytokines.[263] Inhibitors of PI3K have been shown to block MAPK signaling as well as STAT3 phosphorylation.[266] Inhibition of the Torc1 with rapamycin in the context of IL-2 stimulation appears to favor expansion of CD25⁺CD24⁺ "regulatory T cells."[267]

In addition to the association with src kinases and PI3K, both the β and γ receptor chains associate with members of the JAK family of tyrosine kinases.[259] JAK family member JAK3 associates with the C-terminus of the IL-2 receptor γ chain, and both JAK1 and JAK2 associate with the β chain. JAK1 has been shown to bind to a specific serine-rich domain present in the membrane proximal region of the β chain. JAKs activate various members of the STAT family of transcription factors. The binding of IL-2 to its receptor results in the activation of STAT1, STAT3, and STAT5 in T cells and an additional member, STAT4, in NK cells.[259]

Pharmacologic Preparations

Several recombinant preparations of IL-2 (rIL-2) have been used clinically; however; the only preparation currently available for clinical use in the United States is aldesleukin (Prometheus Therapeutics, San Diego, CA). Aldesleukin is a recombinant IL-2 that differs from natural human IL-2 in that a cysteine residue at amino acid 125 is replaced by serine, and it also lacks the N-terminal alanine.[268] Of historical interest is that the Hoffmann-La Roche rIL-2 preparation

lacks the amino acid substitution at position 125 and has an additional N-terminal methionine residue.[269] The measure of activity of IL-2 evolved during the development of these agents and understanding the differences are critical in reviewing the literature.

The International Unit (IU) is the accepted standard for calculating dose of IL-2. One IU of IL-2 is defined as the reciprocal of the dilution that produces 50% of the maximal proliferation of murine HT2 cells in a short-term tritium-labeled thymidine incorporation assay described by the World Health Organization.[270] 1.1 mg of aldesleukin contains 18 million IU of drug.[271] The Cetus unit was commonly used in the past to express doses of this cytokine, with 3×10^6 Cetus units equaling 1.1 mg of aldesleukin.[271] Hoffmann-La Roche rIL-2 contained 15×10^6 Cetus U/mg of protein.[271] Hank et al.[271] found that 3 to 6 IU of Chiron rIL-2 are required for induction of the same biologic effects as 1 IU of Hoffmann-La Roche rIL-2 and a dosage of 4.5×10^6 IU/m²/d of aldesleukin was equivalent in toxicity to a dose of 1.5×10^6 IU/m²/d of Roche rIL-2. Given these differences, care must be used in extrapolating date from the initial IL-2 literature.

Aldesleukin has a short half-life when administered as an intravenous (IV) bolus with a $t_{1/2}\alpha$ of 12.9 minutes, followed by a slower phase with a $t_{1/2}\beta$ of 85 minutes.[272] Injection of 6×10^6 IU/m² produces serum levels of 1,950 IU/mL, and reported clearance rate of 117 mL/min is consistent with renal filtration being the major route of elimination.[273] In an effort to simplify the dosing of IL-2, alternative routes of administration have been investigated.

Il-2 has been widely used by subcutaneous (SC) injection, and in this setting, peak serums concentrations occur at 120 to 360 minutes, the median peak serum levels of 32.1 to 42 IU/mL with SC doses of 6×10^6 IU/m², which are over 50-fold lower than the levels achieved with IV dosing.[272] The serum bioavailability of Il-2 administered by the SC route can be improved by split dosing. Kirchner et al.[274] demonstrated that the same dose of IL-2 given as two doses (10 MIU/m² twice daily) versus a single dose (20 MIU/m² daily) resulted in an almost twofold increase in the AUC of the twice daily regimen. Il-2 has also been administered by continuous infusion (c.i.), and steady-state levels are generally achieved within 2 hours.[272] Median steady-state levels of 123 IU/mL are produced by infusion of 6×10^6 IU/m² over 6 hours, and the levels then fall rapidly after termination of rIL-2 infusion. The clearance rate with c.i. administration is similar to that seen with bolus administration.[272] Although c.i. provides prolonged IL-2 levels, the high rate of catheter infections seen in studies has limited enthusiasm for this route of administration.[275,276]

Clinical Investigations Involving High-dose IL-2

Investigators at the NCI Surgery Branch developed a regimen that involved the administration of high-dose intravenous bolus IL-2.[277] In this regimen, IL-2 was administered at 600,000 to 720,000 IU/kg intravenously every 8 hours days 1 to 5 and 15 to 19 of a treatment course. A maximum of 28 to 30 doses per course was administered; however, doses were frequently withheld for excessive toxicity. Treatment courses were repeated at 8 to 12 week intervals in responding patients. During initial studies, patients underwent daily leukapheresis on days 8 to 12 during which large numbers of lymphocytes were obtained to be cultured in IL-2 for 3 to 4 days to generate lymphokine-activated killer (LAK) cells. These LAK cells were then reinfused into the patient during the second 5-day period of IL-2 administration. This high-dose IL-2 regimen with or without LAK cells produced overall tumor responses in 15% to 20% of patients with metastatic melanoma or renal cell cancer in clinical trials conducted either at the NCI Surgery Branch or within the Cytokine Working Group (formerly the Extramural IL-2 and LAK Working Group).[278] Complete responses were noted in 4% to 6% of patients with each disease and were frequently durable. Rare responses, usually partial and of shorter duration, were also noted in patients with either Hodgkin's or non–Hodgkin's lymphoma, or non–small cell lung, colorectal, or ovarian carcinoma.[279] Randomized and sequential clinical trials comparing IL-2 plus LAK cells with high-dose IL-2 alone failed to show sufficient benefit for the addition of LAK cells to justify their continued use.[280] Long-term follow-up data on patients with melanoma and renal cell cancer who were treated on the initial trials of high-dose bolus IL-2 have confirmed the durability of responses with median duration for complete responses yet to be reached, but exceeding 6 years and few, if any, relapses being observed in patients in complete remission for more than 30 months.[281,282] Several patients remain free of disease in excess of 10 years since initiating treatment. These data suggest that high-dose IL-2 treatment might actually have led to the cure of some patients with these previously incurable advanced malignancies.

Renal Cell Carcinoma

High-dose bolus interleukin-2 (IL-2) was granted Food and Drug Administration approval in 1992 based on its ability to produce durable complete responses in a small number of patients with metastatic RCC. However, the substantial toxicity and limited efficacy of IL-2 have narrowed its application to highly selected patients treated at specialized centers.[281,283–286] In an attempt to reduce toxicity, several investigators evaluated lower doses of IL-2.[287–289]

Attempts were also made to improve treatment efficacy by adding IFNα and then fluorouracil to lower-dose IL-2 regimens.[287–293] These regimens were reported to produce response rates and survival comparable to those reported for high-dose IL-2 with much less toxicity but possibly less durable responses. The relative merits of these low- and high-dose IL-2 regimens have been clarified by four randomized trials.[212,294–296] More significantly, laboratory investigations associated with this clinical research suggest that the potential exists for identifying predictors of response (or resistance) and limiting IL-2 therapy to those most likely to benefit.

Taken together, these studies suggest that high-dose IV bolus IL-2 is superior in response rate and possibly response quality to regimens that involve either low-dose IL-2 and IFN-α, intermediate- or low-dose IL-2 alone, or low-dose IFNα alone (Table 31-7). The superiority of high-dose IL-2 is particularly apparent in patients with tumor metastases in liver or bone, or who have their primary tumor in place, or who fall into the intermediate- or poor-risk groups defined by the French Immunotherapy Group. Consequently, although low-dose cytokine therapy has a limited role in metastatic RCC, high-dose IV IL-2 should remain the preferred therapy for appropriately selected patients with access to such therapy. However, given the toxicity and limited efficacy of high-dose IV IL-2 therapy, additional efforts should be directed at better defining the patient population for whom this therapy is appropriate.

Melanoma

HD IL-2 received regulatory approval for patients with advanced melanoma in 1998. This approval was also largely based on its demonstrated ability to produce durable complete responses in a minority of patients.[282] Data collected from multiple Phase II studies showed a response rate of 16% with 6% of patients achieving a CR and 10% a PR.[282] The median response duration was 11.2 months for all responders and exceeded 59 months for patients with a CR (Fig. 31-5).[282,297] No patient achieving a response lasting in excess of 30 months has relapsed. Given that follow-up on many of these patients exceeds 15 years, this remarkable durability suggests that some if not all of these patients may actually be cured (Fig. 31-5).

A variety of IL-2-containing regimens have been tested in patients with melanoma in an effort to improve the effectiveness of general applicability of IL-2. A study from the NCI Surgery Branch suggested the addition of a gp100 peptide vaccine to HD IL-2 might increase the response rate to 40%.[298,299] A randomized Phase III trial comparing high-dose IL-2+ gp-100 vaccine to high-dose IL-2 alone revealed significant improvements in both response rate and progression-free survival in patients receiving the combination.[300] This trial offered the first evidence of a clinical benefit with vaccination in patients with melanoma, although it is unclear whether it will become a new standard of care.

In the 1990s, biochemotherapy regimens were developed under the hypothesis that the combination of chemotherapy and cytokines would increase response rates and lead to an increase in the number of durable responses. The phase II data suggested these regimens had response rates in excess of 40% with up to 10% of patients achieving a durable.[301–305] Unfortunately, randomized trials showed no survival advantage to biochemotherapy compared to chemotherapy alone.[306–311] A study from the John Wayne Cancer Center administered IL-2/GM-CSF consolidation therapy to patients who

TABLE

31.7   *Select randomized trials of cytokine therapy in metastatic RCC*

Trial	Treatment regimens	N	Response rate	Durable complete response (%)	Overall survival (mo)	Overall survival difference
FIG[13]	CIV IL-2 18 MIU/m² CIV d 1–5, 12–16	138	6.5	1	12	NS
	LD SC IFN-α 18 MIU SC TIW	147	7.5	2	13	
	CIV IL-2 + IFN-α 18 MIU/m² CIV d 1–5, 12–16 6 × MIU SC TIW	140	18.6	5	17	
	MPA 200 mg PO QD	123	2.5	1	14.9	
FIG[17]	LD SC IFN-α 9 × MIU SC TIW	122	4.4	3	15.2	NS
	LD SC IL-2 9 MIU SC QD	125	4.1	0	15.3	
	SC IFN + SC IL-2 IFN 9 MIU SC TIW, IL-2 9 MIU SC QD	122	10.9	0	16.8	
NCI SB[14]	HD IV IL-2 720,000 IU/kg q8h D 1–5, 15–19 (max 28 doses)	156	21%	8	NR	NS
	LD IV IL-2 72,000 IU/kg q8h D 1–5, 15–19 (max 28 doses)	150	13%	3	NR	
	LD SC IL-2 250,000 IU/kg/QD × 5d wk 1, then 125,000 IU/kg/QD × 5d wk 2–6	94	10%	1	NR	
CWG[16]	LD SC IL-2/ IFN-α IL-2 5 MIU/m² SC Q8 h × 3 on day 1, then 5d/wk for 4 wk, IFN 5 MIU/m² SC Q8 h × 3 on day 1, then TIW for 4 wk	91	10%	2	13	NS
	HD IV IL-2 600,000 IU/kg q8h D 1–5, 15–19 (max 28 doses)	95	23%	9	17.5	

HD, high dose; LD, low dose; IV, intravenous; SC, subcutaneous; PO, orally; QD, once per day; IU, International Units; MIU, million IU; CIV, continuous IV infusion; NS, not statistically significant; TIW, three times per week; MPA, medroxyprogesterone acetate; NCI SB, National Cancer Institute Surgery Branch; CWG, Cytokine Working Group; FIG, French Immunotherapy Group; RR, response rate; CR, complete response.

were responding to biochemotherapy in an effort to obtain more durable responses.[312,313] A multicenter study using this regimen reported an overall response rate to biochemotherapy of 44% with 8% CRs.[314] However, almost 40% of the patients had CNS disease as their first or only site of progression. Although the data with maintenance IL-2 and GM-CSF were encouraging, the results from the randomized studies of biochemotherapy alone suggest it has a limited role outside of clinical trials.

Investigators have also continued to pursue IL-2 together with cellular therapy approaches. Combinations of IL-2 and tumor-infiltrating lymphocytes (TILs) were extremely promising in animal tumor models[315]; however, selection bias could not be excluded

as an explanation for the unusually high response rates. Interest in adoptive immunotherapy has been revived by an NCI Surgery Branch study involving the administration of clonally expanded, tumor antigen–specific CD8⁺ lymphocytes and IL-2 following chemotherapy and radiation-induced lymphodepletion that showed encouraging antitumor activity in patients with refractory melanoma.[316–318] The extent to which this approach can be streamlined and exported outside the NIH remains to be determined.

Toxicity

The utility of high-dose IL-2 has been limited by toxicity, many features of which resemble bacterial sepsis. Side effects are dose

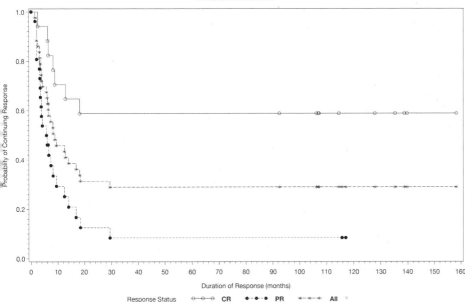

Response Duration for Complete Responders, Partial Responders, and All Responding Patients
Metastatic Melanoma

<small>Response Status ○—○—○ CR   ●—●—● PR   *—*—* All</small>

FIGURE **31-5** Kaplan-Meier estimates for the duration of response for patients with metastatic melanoma following HD IL-2 therapy for all responders, for the complete responders, and for the partial responders (median follow-up >7 years).

dependent and, fortunately, largely predictable and rapidly reversible. Common side effects include fever, chills, lethargy, diarrhea, nausea, anemia, thrombocytopenia, eosinophilia, diffuse erythroderma, hepatic dysfunction, and confusion.[319] Myocarditis also occurs in approximately 5% of patients. IL-2 therapy also commonly produces a "capillary leak syndrome," leading to fluid retention, hypotension, early adult respiratory distress syndrome, prerenal azotemia, and, occasionally, myocardial infarction. As a consequence of these side effects, few patients are able to receive all of the proposed therapy. IL-2 has also been shown to produce a neutrophil chemotactic defect that predisposes patients to infection with Gram-positive and occasionally Gram-negative bacteria.[320]

Early high-dose IL-2 studies were associated with 2% to 4% mortality, largely related to infection or cardiac toxicity.[282,319] The routine use of antibiotic prophylaxis, more extensive cardiac screening, and the more judicious IL-2 administration have greatly enhanced the safety of this therapy; since 1990, the mortality rates at experienced treatment centers have been less than 1% (Table 31-8).[321] Nonetheless, the considerable toxicity of the high-dose IL-2 regimen has continued to limit its application to highly selected patients with excellent performance status and adequate organ function treated at medical centers with considerable experience with this approach.

Laboratory studies have suggested that the toxicity of IL-2 appears to be in part mediated by the release of secondary cytokines such as TNF-α, IL-1, and IL-6.[322] Nonetheless, attempts to block the toxicity of IL-2 by the coadministration of soluble receptors of IL-1 or TNF, CNI-1493, an inhibitor of IL-1 and TNF signaling, or M40403, a non–peptidyl mimic of superoxide dismutase, have yielded only a modest reduction in the hypotension, vascular leak, and other serious side effects routinely observed in patients receiving high dose IL-2.[323–327]

Management of Patients Receiving High-Dose Interleukin-2

The safe administration of high-dose IL-2 requires a careful selection of patients capable of tolerating the fever, hypotension, and edema that often develops during treatment. As such, high-dose IL-2 should be considered a reasonable treatment option only in patients without significant cardiac disease (i.e., angina, congestive heart failure, arrhythmia, or prior myocardial infarction). Patients over 40 years of age should undergo stress testing and those found to have exercise-induced ischemia should be excluded. Patients should be specifically screened for CNS metastases and those with a positive head CT scan or MRI should not be given high-dose IL-2. Patients should also have adequate renal, hepatic, and pulmonary functions with a serum creatinine less than 1.6 mg/dL, bilirubin less than 1.5 mg/dL, and a forced expiratory volume (FEV1) of

TABLE

31.8 *Safety of high-dose IV bolus rIL-2 therapy (720,000 IU/kg q8h): The NCI experience*

- Incidence of grade 3–4 adverse events has been greatly reduced

Adverse event	1985 incidence	1997 incidence
Hypotension	81%	31%
Diarrhea	92%	12%
Neuropsychiatric toxicity	19%	8%
Line sepsis	18%	4%
Pulmonary complications	12%	3%

- With patient selection and experience managing side effects, high-dose rIL-2 is safe
- No treatment-related deaths in 809 consecutive patients treated at the NCI

Adapted from Kammula US, White DE, Rosenberg SA. Trends in the safety of high dose bolus interleukin-2 administration in patients with metastatic cancer. Cancer 1998;83(4):797–805, with permission.

greater than 2 L. They should also have an ECOG performance status of less than 2.

Once a decision is made to offer high-dose IL-2 to a patient, the various treatment-associated side effects can be ameliorated by the concomitant administration of acetaminophen and indomethacin to reduce fever and chills, H2 blockers to prevent gastritis, and pro-phylactic antibiotics to prevent central line–associated infections.[319] Patients should receive antiemetics and antidiarrheals as needed. IL-2-induced pruritus and dermatitis can be minimized with diphenhydramine, gabapentin, and various skin creams. Glucocorti-coids should be avoided since they antagonize the immunostimula-tory properties of IL-2. Hypotension is best managed initially with fluid replacement, but many patients require intravenous dopamine and, in some instances, both dopamine and phenylephrine. Most patients require supplemental IV sodium bicarbonate to prevent acidosis. In the event of life-threatening toxicity (e.g., hypoten-sion refractory to pressors), the IL-2 is discontinued but may be resumed after the resolution of the problem. Generally, doses of IL-2 withheld because of toxicity are not made up at the end of a treatment cycle. With careful patient selection and the appropri-ate use of concurrent medications, most patients can safely receive high-dose IL-2; however, the unusual array and severity of treatment side effects mandate that this form of immunotherapy be adminis-tered by a team of physicians and nurses experienced in the use of this agent.

Summary

While the clinical application of IL-2 has benefited only a small portion of patients with either melanoma or renal cancer to date, it remains the only treatment that can produce durable benefit in more than the anecdotal patient with these diseases. Unfortunately, efforts to build on the successes seen with high-dose IL-2 alone have been disappointing. However, correlative biomarker investigations associated with recent clinical trials suggest that the potential exists for identifying predictors of response (or resistance) and limiting IL-2 therapy to those most likely to benefit. This will be discussed in more detail below.

Granulocyte/Monocyte Colony–Stimulating Factor

GM-CSF was initially felt to be critical for hematopoiesis and was approved for clinical use in chemotherapy-related neutrope-nia. Investigations into the use of cytokines as adjuvants for vac-cines revealed the unexpected immunotherapeutic potential of GM-CSF.[328] In a murine melanoma model, injection of irradiated melanoma cells expressing GM-CSF provided protection to subse-quent tumor challenge in over 90% of mice.[328] Administration of irradiated melanoma cells expressing GM-CSF in mice with estab-lished tumors improved the survival by 40% to 60% depending on the initial tumor inoculum.[328] These initial data were validated in other animal model systems using various vaccination strategies. The antitumor activity of GM-CSF appears to be related to its abil-ity to activate macrophages and dendritic cells. GM-CSF-activated macrophages are cytotoxic to melanoma cells.[329] GM-CSF also matures DCs leading to up-regulation of costimulatory molecules

and CD1d receptors.[330–333] Initial studies suggested that CD4+ and CD8+ T cells mediated GM-CSF tumor immunity, but recent mod-els using CD1d-deficient mice support a critical role for NKT cells in GM-CSF antitumor immune responses.[334]

Clinical trials of GM-CSF have suggested activity as mono-therapy in patients with melanoma when injected intralesion-ally.[335–337] Additionally, multiple trials using autologous tumor vac-cines engineered to secrete GM-CSF have shown biologic activity, although few clinical responses have been observed.[338] Data from administration of GM-CSF in an adjuvant setting to patients with stage IV disease resected to NED suggested that GM-CSF pro-longed survival relative historical controls.[339,340] In an attempt to validate these observations, a phase III Intergroup trial compar-ing GM-CSF to placebo has been completed but these data are not yet mature. GM-CSF used in combination with IL-2 has been shown to have a CR rate of 15% in patients who had previously obtained SD or better on biochemotherapy.[312] These data as an aggregate demonstrate that GM-CSF has potential antitumor activ-ity; however, its role as an immunotherapeutic agent remains to be evaluated.

Predictors of Response to Cytokine Therapy

Cytokine therapy has produced durable responses in melanoma and RCC. The majority of patients, however, are exposed to substan-tial toxicity with only a small percentage obtaining clinical benefit. Potential predictive markers have been studied in an effort to pro-spectively identify the subset of patients most likely to benefit from cytokines.

In melanoma patients receiving high-dose IL-2, tumor responses were more likely in patients with melanoma who exhibited a good performance status (ECOG Performance Status 0) and who had not received prior systemic therapy.[341] Patients with cutaneous metastases and HLA Cw7 have been reported to be more likely to respond IL-2-containing therapy.[183,342,343] Response to HD IL-2 for melanoma also has been reported to be higher in patients with auto-immunity phenomenon such as thyroid dysfunction or vitiligo, low pretreatment IL-6 levels, and low pretreatment CRP levels.[343–346] More recently, response to IL-2 therapy has been correlated with pretreatment serum levels of vascular endothelial growth factors and fibronectin and tumor RNA expression of immune regulatory genes.[347,348] While these investigations have enhanced the under-standing of the mechanisms underlying the antitumor effects of IL-2 activity, for the most part, they do not aid in the selection of patients with melanoma for IL-2-based therapy as they lack pro-spective validation.

The development of autoimmunity during adjuvant IFN treat-ment for melanoma is associated with a dramatic improvement in survival.[247] These data combined with the observation that patients with ulcerated primaries have an improved outcome with adjuvant IFN therapy support the hypothesis that only a subgroup of patients benefit from IFN therapy.[198] Whether patients who present with ulcerated primaries and those who develop autoimmunity while receiving IFN represent groups of patients who have IFN responsive disease remains to be determined in prospective trials.

The correlation of autoimmunity with response has led to the investigation of polymorphisms of immune pathways as predictors of response. Single nucleotide polymorphisms (SNPs) may serve as prognostic or predictive markers due to their linkage to variable expression of critical genes. For example, SNPs that reportedly alter IL-10 and IFNγ expression are associated with response to biochemotherapy.[349] Perhaps paradoxically, SNPs related to increased IL-10 and decreased IFNγ expressions have been associated with good prognosis calling into question the mechanism of this linkage or the validity of these results.[349–352] Clearly, more research is needed to sort out the influence of genotype variations on the antitumor effects of various cytokine-based immunotherapies.

For patients with renal cancer, tumor response has been associated with ECOG performance status, number of metastatic sites, the degree of treatment-related thrombocytopenia, thyroid dysfunction, rebound lymphocytosis erythropoietin production, low pretreatment IL-6 levels, and posttreatment elevations of blood TNF alpha and IL-1 levels.[353] Additional retrospective studies suggested that the histologic pattern of the renal cancer also correlates with the probability of response to IL-2.[354] Response rates as high as 40% have been seen in patients whose primary tumors possessed favorable histologic features, clear cell histology with alveolar, but no papillary or granular cell components, while patients whose tumors displayed papillary or greater than 50% granular features were unlikely to respond. While this correlation was independently confirmed in an examination of metastatic lesions, prospective validation is lacking. Additional immunohistochemical studies have suggested that the expression of the G250 antigen (carbonic anhydrase IX) on a large percentage of renal cancer cells is also associated with an increased likelihood of benefit from IL-2 treatment.[355,356] A prospective trial is currently ongoing to validate these promising biomarkers in RCC. It is anticipated that additional molecular studies on tumor tissue obtained before therapy or sampled early on in therapy may ultimately lead to more definitive predictors of responsiveness to cytokine-based therapy and thereby limit this intensive and toxic therapy to those most likely to benefit.

Strategies for Overcoming Resistance to Immunotherapy

The immunosurveillance hypothesis suggests that tumors are constantly under attack from the immune system. The natural extension of this hypothesis, "immunoediting," suggests tumors are constantly under selective pressure that favors clones that can escape the onslaught of the immune system.[357] Thus, even when immune responses are seen in patients, they often do not correlate with clinical benefit since the tumors may have already undergone "immune escape."

Tumors utilize two broad strategies to escape immune surveillance—altered antigen presentation/T-cell response and immunosuppression. Tumor cells have down-regulated MHC class I molecules, CD80 (B7-1), CD86 (B7-2), and ICAM-1, which are important for antigen presentation and activation of CD8$^+$ CTLs.[358] In addition to tumor-specific defects, down-regulation of the T-cell signaling components, zeta chain and Lck, is seen in a number of malignancies.[359,360] The IFNs up-regulate MHC I and MHC II, and IL-2 has been shown to restore zeta chain and Lck expressions on T cells.[359,360]

Malignancies induce an immunosuppressive microenvironment by multiple mechanisms. Tumors secrete a number of cytokines that are potentially immunosuppressive such as IL-10, TGF-β, and IL-6.[361–365] Also nutrient-catabolizing enzymes such as indoleamine 2,3-dioxygenase (IDO) and arginase are thought to contribute to an immunosuppressive environment.[366,367] 1-Methyl-[D]-tryptophan (NewLinkGenetics) is a competitive inhibitor of IDO undergoing clinical investigation.[368]

Tumors cells are protected by mechanisms designed to prevent autoimmune disease. Expression of CLTA-4 on activated T cells limits the immune response. Invariant NKT (iNKT) cells, CD4$^+$CD25$^+$ T-regulatory (Tregs), Th3 cells, and Type I regulatory cells are all immunoregulatory T cells that are part of the natural course of an immune response. The fact that the induction of a tumor-focused immune response does not correlate with clinical benefit suggests that some of these of immune escape mechanisms are operating in vivo.

Treg numbers increase with HD IL-2 in most patients.[369,370] In one study, objective response in melanoma and RCC patients correlated with a subsequent decrease in Tregs 4 weeks after HD IL-2 therapy.[369] These data support the hypothesis that regulatory cells may inhibit responses to immunotherapy.

Efforts to deplete Tregs, Th3 cells, and Type I regulatory T cells have included the use of the anti-CD25 agent, denileukin diftitox (Ontak), and lymphodepletion. A single dose of Ontak has been shown to deplete circulating regulatory T-cell populations and enhances the antitumor response to DC-based vaccines.[371,372] Ontak as a single agent induced responses in 5 out of 16 melanoma patients who were associated with transient depletion of Tregs with the development of MART-1-specific CD8$^+$ T cells in one patient.[373] In contrast, investigators at the NCI using a different dosing schedule did not observe reductions in Tregs based on Foxp3 expression.[374] Whether these differences are due to patient selection or methodology remains to be determined. The NCI Surgery Branch piloted a strategy of lymphodepletion using fludarabine and cyclophosphamide to deplete immunoregulatory cells followed by adoptive transfer of T cells and IL-2 therapy. This regimen produces a response rate of 50% in patients who were previously resistant to IL-2-based immunotherapy.[316,317] The use of antibodies to block the activation of CTLA-4 has resulted in dramatic responses in early clinical trials.[375–377] The addition of this agent to HD IL-2 therapy in a phase Ib/II study resulted in a higher response than would have been expected with either agent alone but did not appear to be synergistic.[378] These early results suggest that strategies to disrupt the immunosuppressive microenvironment of the tumor may significantly enhance the efficacy of cytokines in the treatment of cancer.

Conclusion

Preclinical data suggested that cytokine base therapies would have efficacy against a broad spectrum of malignancies. Unfortunately, only IFN and IL-2 have found a place in the therapeutic armamentarium against cancer. IL-2 remains the only agent that reproducibly produces long-term remissions in patients with metastatic melanoma or RCC. Efforts focused on improved patient selection for IFN and IL-2 therapy have recently made progress and should allow patients with low likelihood of response to pursue other treatment options and avoid significant toxicity. Strategies for overcoming resistance to immunotherapy are under intense investigation and hold the promise of extending the clinical benefits of cytokines to larger populations of patients. While their success has been modest to date, immunoreactive cytokines will likely remain a critical component of a curative strategy for the treatment of metastatic solid tumors.

References

1. Isaacs A, Lindenmann J. Virus interference. I. The interferon. Proc R Soc Lond B Biol Sci 1957;147(927):258–267.
2. Abbas AK, Lichtman AH, Pober JS. Cellular and Moleuclar Immunology. Philadelphia, PA: W.B. Sanders, 2000.
3. Pestka S, Krause CD, Walter MR. Interferons, interferon-like cytokines, and their receptors. Immunol Rev 2004;202:8–32.
4. Pestka S, Langer JA, Zoon KC, et al. Interferons and their actions. Annu Rev Biochem 1987;56:727–777.
5. Stewart WE, II. Interferon nomenclature recommendations. J Infect Dis 1980;142(4):643.
6. Isaacs A, Lindenmann J. Virus interference. I. The interferon. J Interferon Res 1987;7(5):429–438.
7. Muller U, Steinhoff U, Reis LF, et al. Functional role of type I and type II interferons in antiviral defense. Science 1994;264(5167):1918–1921.
8. Kotenko SV, Gallagher G, Baurin VV, et al. IFN-lambdas mediate antiviral protection through a distinct class II cytokine receptor complex. Nat Immunol 2003;4(1):69–77.
9. Sheppard P, Kindsvogel W, Xu W, et al. IL-28, IL-29 and their class II cytokine receptor IL-28R. Nat Immunol 2003;4(1):63–68.
10. Basham TY, Bourgeade MF, Creasey AA, et al. Interferon increases HLA synthesis in melanoma cells: interferon-resistant and -sensitive cell lines. Proc Natl Acad Sci USA 1982;79(10):3265–3269.
11. Dolei A, Capobianchi MR, Ameglio F. Human interferon-gamma enhances the expression of class I and class II major histocompatibility complex products in neoplastic cells more effectively than interferon-alpha and interferon-beta. Infect Immun 1983;40(1):172–176.
12. Herberman RB, Ortaldo JR, Mantovani A, et al. Effect of human recombinant interferon on cytotoxic activity of natural killer (NK) cells and monocytes. Cell Immunol 1982;67(1):160–167.
13. Ortaldo JR, Mantovani A, Hobbs D, et al. Effects of several species of human leukocyte interferon on cytotoxic activity of NK cells and monocytes. Int J Cancer 1983;31(3):285–289.
14. Ortaldo JR, Mason A, Rehberg E, et al. Effects of recombinant and hybrid recombinant human leukocyte interferons on cytotoxic activity of natural killer cells. J Biol Chem 1983;258(24):15011–15015.
15. Dunn GP, Bruce AT, Sheehan KC, et al. A critical function for type I interferons in cancer immunoediting. Nat Immunol 2005;6(7):722–729.
16. Picaud S, Bardot B, De Maeyer E, et al. Enhanced tumor development in mice lacking a functional type I interferon receptor. J Interferon Cytokine Res 2002;22(4):457–462.
17. Wagner TC, Velichko S, Chesney SK, et al. Interferon receptor expression regulates the antiproliferative effects of interferons on cancer cells and solid tumors. Int J Cancer 2004;111(1):32–42.
18. Clemens MJ. Interferons and apoptosis. J Interferon Cytokine Res 2003;23(6):277–292.
19. Sidky YA, Borden EC. Inhibition of angiogenesis by interferons: effects on tumor- and lymphocyte-induced vascular responses. Cancer Res 1987;47(19):5155–5161.
20. Tsuruoka N, Sugiyama M, Tawaragi Y, et al. Inhibition of in vitro angiogenesis by lymphotoxin and interferon-gamma. Biochem Biophys Res Commun 1988;155(1):429–435.
21. Lesinski GB, Anghelina M, Zimmerer J, et al. The antitumor effects of IFN-alpha are abrogated in a STAT1-deficient mouse. J Clin Invest 2003;112(2):170–180.
22. Ronnblom L, Ramstedt U, Alm GV. Properties of human natural interferon-producing cells stimulated by tumor cell lines. Eur J Immunol 1983;13(6):471–476.
23. Cella M, Jarrossay D, Facchetti F, et al. Plasmacytoid monocytes migrate to inflamed lymph nodes and produce large amounts of type I interferon. Nat Med 1999;5(8):919–923.
24. Siegal FP, Kadowaki N, Shodell M, et al. The nature of the principal type 1 interferon-producing cells in human blood. Science 1999;284(5421):1835–1837.
25. Gilliet M, Cao W, Liu YJ. Plasmacytoid dendritic cells: sensing nucleic acids in viral infection and autoimmune diseases. Nat Rev Immunol 2008;8(8):594–606.
26. Noppert SJ, Fitzgerald KA, Hertzog PJ. The role of type I interferons in TLR responses. Immunol Cell Biol 2007;85(6):446–457.
27. Bjorck P. Isolation and characterization of plasmacytoid dendritic cells from Flt3 ligand and granulocyte-macrophage colony-stimulating factor-treated mice. Blood 2001;98(13):3520–3526.
28. Pulendran B, Banchereau J, Burkeholder S, et al. Flt3-ligand and granulocyte colony-stimulating factor mobilize distinct human dendritic cell subsets in vivo. J Immunol 2000;165(1):566–572.
29. Hu G, Mancl ME, Barnes BJ. Signaling through IFN regulatory factor-5 sensitizes p53-deficient tumors to DNA damage-induced apoptosis and cell death. Cancer Res 2005;65(16):7403–7412.
30. Karpova AY, Trost M, Murray JM, et al. Interferon regulatory factor-3 is an in vivo target of DNA-PK. Proc Natl Acad Sci USA 2002;99(5):2818–2823.
31. Pamment J, Ramsay E, Kelleher M, et al. Regulation of the IRF-1 tumour modifier during the response to genotoxic stress involves an ATM-dependent signalling pathway. Oncogene 2002;21(51):7776–7785.
32. Prost S, Bellamy CO, Cunningham DS, et al. Altered DNA repair and dysregulation of p53 in IRF-1 null hepatocytes. Faseb J 1998;12(2):181–188.
33. Colamonici OR, Domanski P. Identification of a novel subunit of the type I interferon receptor localized to human chromosome 21. J Biol Chem 1993;268(15):10895–10899.
34. Lutfalla G, Gardiner K, Proudhon D, et al. The structure of the human interferon alpha/beta receptor gene. J Biol Chem 1992;267(4):2802–2809.
35. Decker T, Lew DJ, Mirkovitch J, et al. Cytoplasmic activation of GAF, an IFN-gamma-regulated DNA-binding factor. Embo J 1991;10(4):927–932.
36. Decker T, Lew DJ, Darnell JE Jr. Two distinct alpha-interferon-dependent signal transduction pathways may contribute to activation of transcription of the guanylate-binding protein gene. Mol Cell Biol 1991;11(10):5147–5153.
37. Horvath CM, Stark GR, Kerr IM, et al. Interactions between STAT and non-STAT proteins in the interferon-stimulated gene factor 3 transcription complex. Mol Cell Biol 1996;16(12):6957–6964.
38. Fish EN, Uddin S, Korkmaz M, et al. Activation of a CrkL-stat5 signaling complex by type I interferons. J Biol Chem 1999;274(2):571–573.
39. David M, Petricoin E 3rd, Benjamin C, et al. Requirement for MAP kinase (ERK2) activity in interferon alpha- and interferon beta-stimulated gene expression through STAT proteins. Science 1995;269(5231):1721–1723.
40. Goh KC, Haque SJ, Williams BR. p38 MAP kinase is required for STAT1 serine phosphorylation and transcriptional activation induced by interferons. Embo J 1999;18(20):5601–5608.
41. Kaur S, Sassano A, Joseph AM, et al. Dual regulatory roles of phosphatidylinositol 3-kinase in IFN signaling. J Immunol 2008;181(10):7316–7323.
42. Auger KR, Serunian LA, Soltoff SP, et al. PDGF-dependent tyrosine phosphorylation stimulates production of novel polyphosphoinositides in intact cells. Cell, 1989. 57(1): p. 167–75.
43. Alessi, D.R., James SR, Downes CP, et al., Characterization of a 3-phosphoinositide-dependent protein kinase which phosphorylates and activates protein kinase Balpha. Curr Biol 1997;7(4):261–269.
44. Guertin DA, Stevens DM, Thoreen CC, et al. Ablation in mice of the mTORC components raptor, rictor, or mLST8 reveals that mTORC2 is required for signaling to Akt-FOXO and PKCalpha, but not S6K1. Dev Cell 2006;11(6):859–871.
45. Jacinto E, Facchinetti V, Liu D, et al. SIN1/MIP1 maintains rictor-mTOR complex integrity and regulates Akt phosphorylation and substrate specificity. Cell 2006;127(1):125–137.

310. Ridolfi R, Chiarion-Sileni V, Guida M, et al. Cisplatin, dacarbazine with or without subcutaneous interleukin-2, and interferon alpha-2b in advanced melanoma outpatients: results from an Italian multicenter phase III randomized clinical trial. J Clin Oncol 2002;20(6):1600–1607.

311. Rosenberg SA, Yang JC, Schwartzentruber DJ, et al. Prospective randomized trial of the treatment of patients with metastatic melanoma using chemotherapy with cisplatin, dacarbazine, and tamoxifen alone or in combination with interleukin-2 and interferon alfa-2b. J Clin Oncol 1999;17(3):968–975.

312. O'Day SJ, Boasberg PD, Piro L, et al. Maintenance biotherapy for metastatic melanoma with interleukin-2 and granulocyte macrophage-colony stimulating factor improves survival for patients responding to induction concurrent biochemotherapy. Clin Cancer Res 2002;8(9):2775–2781.

313. O'Day SJ, Atkins M, Weber J, et al. A phase II multi-center trial of maintenance biotherapy (MBT) after induction concurrent biochemotherapy (BCT) for patients (Pts) with metastatic melanoma (MM). ASCO Annual Meetings Proceedings 2005;23(16s):7503.

314. O'Day SJ, Atkins MB, Boasberg P, et al. Phase II multicenter trial of maintenance biotherapy after induction concurrent Biochemotherapy for patients with metastatic melanoma. J Clin Oncol 2009;27(36):6207–6212.

315. Rosenberg SA. A new era of cancer immunotherapy: converting theory to performance. CA Cancer J Clin 1999;49(2):70–73.

316. Dudley ME, Wunderlich JR, Robbins PF, et al. Cancer regression and autoimmunity in patients after clonal repopulation with antitumor lymphocytes. Science 2002;298(5594):850–854.

317. Dudley ME, Wunderlich JR, Yang JC, et al. A phase I study of nonmyeloablative chemotherapy and adoptive transfer of autologous tumor antigen-specific T lymphocytes in patients with metastatic melanoma. J Immunother 2002;25(3):243–251.

318. Dudley ME, Yang JC, Sherry R, et al. Adoptive cell therapy for patients with metastatic melanoma: evaluation of intensive myeloablative chemoradiation preparative regimens. J Clin Oncol 2008;26(32):5233–5239.

319. Margolin K. The clinical toxicities of high-dose interleukin-2. In: Atkins MB, ed. Therapeutic Applications of Interleukin-2. New York, Marcel Dekker Inc, 1993:331–362.

320. Klempner MS, Noring R, Mier JW, et al. An acquired chemotactic defect in neutrophils from patients receiving interleukin-2 immunotherapy. N Engl J Med 1990;322(14):959–965.

321. Kammula US, White DE, Rosenberg SA. Trends in the safety of high dose bolus interleukin-2 administration in patients with metastatic cancer. Cancer 1998;83(4):797–805.

322. Gemlo BT, Palladino MA Jr, Jaffe HS, et al. Circulating cytokines in patients with metastatic cancer treated with recombinant interleukin 2 and lymphokine-activated killer cells. Cancer Res 1988;48(20):5864–5867.

323. Atkins MB, Redman B, Mier J, et al. A phase I study of CNI-1493, an inhibitor of cytokine release, in combination with high-dose interleukin-2 in patients with renal cancer and melanoma. Clin Cancer Res 2001;7(3):486–492.

324. Du Bois JS, Trehu EG, Mier JW, et al. Randomized placebo-controlled clinical trial of high-dose interleukin-2 in combination with a soluble p75 tumor necrosis factor receptor immunoglobulin G chimera in patients with advanced melanoma and renal cell carcinoma. J Clin Oncol 1997;15(3):1052–1062.

325. Kilbourn RG, Fonseca GA, Trissel LA, et al. Strategies to reduce side effects of interleukin-2: evaluation of the antihypotensive agent NG-monomethyl-L-arginine. Cancer J Sci Am 2000;6 Suppl 1:S21–S30.

326. McDermott DF, Trehu EG, Mier JW, et al. A two-part phase I trial of high-dose interleukin 2 in combination with soluble (Chinese hamster ovary) interleukin 1 receptor. Clin Cancer Res 1998;4(5):1203–1213.

327. Samlowski WE, Petersen R, Cuzzocrea S, et al. A nonpeptidyl mimic of superoxide dismutase, M40403, inhibits dose-limiting hypotension associated with interleukin-2 and increases its antitumor effects. Nat Med 2003;9(6):750–755.

328. Dranoff G, Jaffee E, Lazenby A, et al. Vaccination with irradiated tumor cells engineered to secrete murine granulocyte-macrophage colony-stimulating factor stimulates potent, specific, and long-lasting anti-tumor immunity. Proc Natl Acad Sci USA 1993;90(8):3539–3543.

329. Grabstein KH, Urdal DL, Tushinski RJ, et al. Induction of macrophage tumoricidal activity by granulocyte-macrophage colony-stimulating factor. Science 1986;232(4749):506–508.

330. Yamasaki S, Okino T, Chakraborty NG, et al. Presentation of synthetic peptide antigen encoded by the MAGE-1 gene by granulocyte/macrophage-colony-stimulating-factor-cultured macrophages from HLA-A1 melanoma patients. Cancer Immunol Immunother 1995;40(4):268–271.

331. Hanada K, Tsunoda R, Hamada H. GM-CSF-induced in vivo expansion of splenic dendritic cells and their strong costimulation activity. J Leukoc Biol 1996;60(2):181–190.

332. Armstrong CA, Botella R, Galloway TH, et al. Antitumor effects of granulocyte-macrophage colony-stimulating factor production by melanoma cells. Cancer Res 1996;56(9):2191–2198.

333. Mach N, Gillessen S, Wilson SB, et al. Differences in dendritic cells stimulated in vivo by tumors engineered to secrete granulocyte-macrophage colony-stimulating factor or Flt3-ligand. Cancer Res 2000;60(12):3239–3246.

334. Hu HM, Winter H, Urba WJ, et al. Divergent roles for CD4+ T cells in the priming and effector/memory phases of adoptive immunotherapy. J Immunol 2000;165(8):4246–4253.

335. Ridolfi L, Ridolfi R. Preliminary experiences of intralesional immunotherapy in cutaneous metastatic melanoma. Hepatogastroenterology 2002;49(44):335–339.

336. Vaquerano JE, Cadbury P, Treseler P, et al. Regression of in-transit melanoma of the scalp with intralesional recombinant human granulocyte-macrophage colony-stimulating factor. Arch Dermatol 1999;135(10):1276–1277.

337. Si Z, Hersey P, Coates AS. Clinical responses and lymphoid infiltrates in metastatic melanoma following treatment with intralesional GM-CSF. Melanoma Res 1996;6(3):247–255.

338. Dranoff G. GM-CSF-secreting melanoma vaccines. Oncogene 2003;22(20):3188–3192.

339. Spitler LE, Grossbard ML, Ernstoff MS, et al. Adjuvant therapy of stage III and IV malignant melanoma using granulocyte-macrophage colony-stimulating factor. J Clin Oncol 2000;18(8):1614–1621.

340. Daud AI, Mirza N, Lenox B, et al. Phenotypic and functional analysis of dendritic cells and clinical outcome in patients with high-risk melanoma treated with adjuvant granulocyte macrophage colony-stimulating factor. J Clin Oncol 2008;26(19):3235–3241.

341. Atkins MB, Lotze MT, Dutcher JP, et al. High-dose recombinant interleukin 2 therapy for patients with metastatic melanoma: analysis of 270 patients treated between 1985 and 1993. J Clin Oncol 1999;17(7):2105–2116.

342. Scheibenbogen C, Keilholz U, Mytilineos J, et al. HLA class I alleles and responsiveness of melanoma to immunotherapy with interferon-alpha (IFN-alpha) and interleukin-2 (IL-2). Melanoma Res 1994;4(3):191–194.

343. Tartour E, Blay JY, Dorval T, et al. Predictors of clinical response to interleukin-2–based immunotherapy in melanoma patients: a French multiinstitutional study. J Clin Oncol 1996;14(5):1697–1703.

344. Atkins MB, Mier JW, Parkinson DR, et al. Hypothyroidism after treatment with interleukin-2 and lymphokine-activated killer cells. N Engl J Med 1988;318(24):1557–1563.

345. Phan GQ, Touloukian CE, Yang JC, et al. Immunization of patients with metastatic melanoma using both class I- and class II-restricted peptides from melanoma-associated antigens. J Immunother 2003;26(4):349–356.

346. Rosenberg SA, White DE. Vitiligo in patients with melanoma: normal tissue antigens can be targets for cancer immunotherapy. J Immunother Emphasis Tumor Immunol 1996;19(1):81–84.

347. Wang E, Miller LD, Ohnmacht GA, et al. Prospective molecular profiling of melanoma metastases suggests classifiers of immune responsiveness. Cancer Res 2002;62(13):3581–3586.

348. Sabatino M, Kim-Schulze S, Panelli MC, et al. Serum vascular endothelial growth factor and fibronectin predict clinical response to high-dose interleukin-2 therapy. J Clin Oncol 2009;27(16):2645–2652.

349. Liu D, O'Day SJ, Yang D, et al. Impact of gene polymorphisms on clinical outcome for stage IV melanoma patients treated with biochemotherapy: an exploratory study. Clin Cancer Res 2005;11(3):1237–1246.

350. Garcia-Hernandez ML, Hernandez-Pando R, Gariglio P, et al. Interleukin-10 promotes B16-melanoma growth by inhibition of macrophage functions and induction of tumour and vascular cell proliferation. Immunology 2002;105(2):231–243.

351. Huang S, Xie K, Bucana CD, et al. Interleukin 10 suppresses tumor growth and metastasis of human melanoma cells: potential inhibition of angiogenesis. Clin Cancer Res 1996;2(12):1969–1979.

352. Howell WM, Turner SJ, Bateman AC, et al. IL-10 promoter polymorphisms influence tumour development in cutaneous malignant melanoma. Genes Immun 2001;2(1):25–31.

353. Atkins M, Garnick M. Renal Neoplasia. In: Benner B, ed. The Kidney. Philadelphia, PA: WB Saunders Co., 2000:1844–1868.

354. Upton MP, Parker RA, Youmans A, et al. Histologic predictors of renal cell carcinoma response to interleukin-2-based therapy. J Immunother 2005;28(5):488–495.

355. Atkins M, Regan M, McDermott D, et al. Carbonic anhydrase IX expression predicts outcome of interleukin 2 therapy for renal cancer. Clin Cancer Res 2005;11(10):3714–3721.

356. Bui MH, Seligson D, Han KR, et al. Carbonic anhydrase IX is an independent predictor of survival in advanced renal clear cell carcinoma: implications for prognosis and therapy. Clin Cancer Res 2003;9(2):802–811.

357. Dunn GP, Old LJ, Schreiber RD. The immunobiology of cancer immunosurveillance and immunoediting. Immunity 2004;21(2):137–148.

358. Rivoltini L, Carrabba M, Huber V, et al. Immunity to cancer: attack and escape in T lymphocyte-tumor cell interaction. Immunol Rev 2002;188:97–113.

359. De Paola F, Ridolfi R, Riccobon A, et al. Restored T-cell activation mechanisms in human tumour-infiltrating lymphocytes from melanomas and colorectal carcinomas after exposure to interleukin-2. Br J Cancer 2003;88(2):320–326.

360. Bukowski RM, Rayman P, Uzzo R, et al. Signal transduction abnormalities in T lymphocytes from patients with advanced renal carcinoma: clinical relevance and effects of cytokine therapy. Clin Cancer Res 1998;4(10):2337–2347.

361. Piancatelli D, Romano P, Sebastiani P, et al. Local expression of cytokines in human colorectal carcinoma: evidence of specific interleukin-6 gene expression. J Immunother 1999;22(1):25–32.

362. Lissoni P, Barni S, Ardizzoia A, et al. Correlation between pretreatment serum levels of neopterin and response to interleukin-2 immunotherapy in cancer patients. J Biol Regul Homeost Agents 1995;9(1):21–23.

363. Chen CK, Wu MY, Chao KH, et al. T lymphocytes and cytokine production in ascitic fluid of ovarian malignancies. J Formos Med Assoc 1999;98(1):24–30.

364. Nemunaitis J, Fong T, Shabe P, et al. Comparison of serum interleukin-10 (IL-10) levels between normal volunteers and patients with advanced melanoma. Cancer Invest 2001;19(3):239–247.

365. Chen Q, Daniel V, Maher DW, et al. Production of IL-10 by melanoma cells: examination of its role in immunosuppression mediated by melanoma. Int J Cancer 1994;56(5):755–760.

366. Kim R, Emi M, Tanabe K, et al. Tumor-driven evolution of immunosuppressive networks during malignant progression. Cancer Res 2006;66(11):5527–5536.

367. Prendergast GC, Metz R, Muller AJ. IDO recruits Tregs in melanoma. Cell Cycle 2009;8(12):1818–1819.

368. Witkiewicz AK, Costantino CL, Metz R, et al. Genotyping and expression analysis of IDO2 in human pancreatic cancer: a novel, active target. J Am Coll Surg 2009;208(5):781–787; discussion 787–789.

369. Cesana GC, DeRaffele G, Cohen S, et al. Characterization of CD4+CD25+ regulatory T cells in patients treated with high-dose interleukin-2 for metastatic melanoma or renal cell carcinoma. J Clin Oncol 2006;24(7):1169–1177.

370. van der Vliet HJ, Koon HB, Yue SC, et al. Effects of the administration of high-dose interleukin-2 on immunoregulatory cell subsets in patients with advanced melanoma and renal cell cancer. Clin Cancer Res 2007;13(7):2100–2108.

371. Barnett B, Zou W, Bremer C, et al. Depleting CD4+ CD25+ Regulatory T-cells improves immunity in cancer-bearing patients. In Proceedings of AACR, 2004.

372. Vieweg J, Su Z, Dannuli J. Enhancement of antitumor immunity following depletion of CD+CD25+ regulatory T-cells. In Proceedings of ASCO, 2004.

373. Rasku MA, Clem AL, Telang S, et al. Transient T cell depletion causes regression of melanoma metastases. J Transl Med 2008;6:12.

374. Attia P, Maker AV, Haworth LR, et al. Inability of a fusion protein of IL-2 and diphtheria toxin (Denileukin Diftitox, DAB389IL-2, ONTAK) to eliminate regulatory T lymphocytes in patients with melanoma. J Immunother 2005;28(6):582–592.

375. Phan GQ, Yang JC, Sherry RM, et al. Cancer regression and autoimmunity induced by cytotoxic T lymphocyte-associated antigen 4 blockade in patients with metastatic melanoma. Proc Natl Acad Sci USA 2003;100(14):8372–8377.

376. Reuben JM, Lee BN, Li C, et al. Biologic and immunomodulatory events after CTLA-4 blockade with ticilimumab in patients with advanced malignant melanoma. Cancer 2006;106(11):2437–2444.

377. Ribas A, Camacho LH, Lopez-Berestein G, et al. Antitumor activity in melanoma and anti-self responses in a phase I trial with the anti-cytotoxic T lymphocyte-associated antigen 4 monoclonal antibody CP-675,206. J Clin Oncol 2005;23(35):8968–8977.

378. Maker AV, Phan GQ, Attia P, et al. Tumor regression and autoimmunity in patients treated with cytotoxic T lymphocyte-associated antigen 4 blockade and interleukin 2: a phase I/II study. Ann Surg Oncol 2005;12(12):1005–1016.

to be poorly predictive of human responses to specific antigens or vaccine approaches. Thus, practical issues of dose, schedule, and route of administration and biological questions related to optimal vaccination approach, for example, type of adjuvant, vector delivery, or type of DC, will likely need to be determined in humans. Addressing these issues in patients is complicated by the broad array of antigens and vaccination approaches, the heterogeneity of patient populations, and the lack of validated biological end points correlating to antitumor activity.

Prior studies of cancer vaccines and other immunotherapy agents suggest that the time required for evolution of an effective antitumor immune response may be prolonged, and tumor progression may actually precede control of tumor growth or tumor regression. Although the concept remains controversial, stabilization of disease or slowing of tumor growth, rather than tumor regression, may be a beneficial consequence of the anticancer immune response. In some cases, enlargement of lesions on scans may reflect inflammatory responses, or persistent lesions may not harbor active tumor. Induced immune responses could also influence the outcome to subsequent chemotherapy or signaling antagonists. These potential beneficial effects of a vaccine may not be detected in standard phase 2 clinical trials, and the benefit of treatment may be missed in trials if treatment is stopped too early or if the wrong clinical end point is used, for example, if median progression-free survival rather than OS is the primary end point. Future trials may need to be designed with greater focus on OS and with novel designs that permit assessment of delayed effects of vaccines.

References

1. Van der Bruggen P, Traversari C, Chomez P, et al. A gene encoding an antigen recognized by cytolytic T lymphocytes on a human melanoma. Science 1991;254:1643–1647.
2. Lutz MB, Suri RM, Niimi M, et al. Immature dendritic cells generated with low doses of GM-CSF in the absence of IL-4 are maturation resistant and prolong allograft survival in vivo. Eur J Immunol 2000;30:1813–1822.
3. Banchereau J, Steinman RM. Dendritic cells and the control of immunity. Nature 1998;392:245–252.
4. Lotze MT. Getting to the source: dendritic cells as therapeutic reagents for the treatment of patients with cancer. Ann Surg 1997;226:1–5.
5. Lutz MB, Kukutsch N, Ogilvie AL, et al. An advanced culture method for generating large quantities of highly pure dendritic cells from mouse bone marrow. J Immunol 1999;223:77–92.
6. Dranoff G, Jaffee E, Lazenby A, et al. Vaccination with irradiated tumor cells engineered to secrete murine granulocyte-macrophage colony-stimulating factor stimulates potent, specific, and long-lasting anti-tumor immunity. Proc Natl Acad Sci U S A 1993;90:3539–3943.
7. Walunas TL, Lenschow DJ, Bakker CY, et al. CTLA-4 can function as a negative regulator of T cell activation. Immunity 1994;1:405–413.
8. Krummel MF, Allison JP. CD28 and CTLA-4 have opposing effects on the response of T cells to stimulation. J Exp Med 1995;182:459–465.
9. Chambers CA, Allison JP. Costimulatory regulation of T cell function. Curr Opin Cell Biol 1999;11:203–210.
10. Hodge JW, Sabzevari H, Yafal AG, et al. A triad of costimulatory molecules synergize to amplify T-cell activation. Cancer Res 1999;59:5800–5807.
11. Hsueh EC, Essner R, Foshag LJ, et al. Prolonged survival after complete resection of disseminated melanoma and active immunotherapy with a therapeutic cancer vaccine. J Clin Oncol 2002;20:4549–4954.
12. Morton DL, Hsueh EC, Essner R, et al. Prolonged survival of patients receiving active immunotherapy with Canvaxin therapeutic polyvalent vaccine after complete resection of melanoma metastatic to regional lymph nodes. Ann Surg 2002;236:438–448.
13. Udono H, Srivastava PK. Comparison of tumor-specific immunogenicities of stress-induced proteins gp96, hsp90, and hsp70. J Immunol 1994;152:5398–5403.
14. Wood C, Srivastava P, Bukowski R, et al. An adjuvant autologous therapeutic vaccine (SHPPC-96; vitespen) versus observation alone for patients at high risk of recurrence after nephrectomy for renal cell carcinoma: a multicentre, open-label, randomized phase III trial. Lancet 2008;372:145–154.
15. Testori A, Richards J, Whitman E, et al. Phase III comparison of vitespen, an autologous tumor-derived heat shock protein gp96 peptide complex vaccine, with physician's choice of treatment for stage IV melanoma: the C-100-21 study group. J Clin Oncol 2008;26:955–962.
16. Jonasch E, Wood C, Tamboli P, et al. Vaccination of metastatic renal cell carcinoma patients with autologous tumour-derived vitespen vaccine: clinical findings. Br J Cancer 2008;98:1336–1341.
17. Jaffee EM, Hruban RH, Biedrzycki B, et al. Novel allogeneic granulocyte-macrophage colony-stimulating factor-secreting tumor vaccine for pancreatic cancer: a phase I trial of safety and immune activation. J Clin Oncol 2001;19:145–156.
18. Laheru D, Lutz E, Burke J, et al. Allogeneic granulocyte macrophage colony-stimulating factor-secreting tumor immunotherapy alone or in sequence with cyclophosphamide for metastatic pancreatic cancer: a pilot study of safety, feasibility, and immune activation. Clin Cancer Res 2008;14:1455–1463.
19. Ercolini AM, Ladle BH, Manning EA, et al. Recruitment of latent pools of high avidity CD8$^+$ T cells to the antitumor immune response. J Exp Med 2005;201:1591–1602.
20. Nemunaitis M, Sterman D, Jablons D, et al. Granulocyte-macrophage colony-stimulating factor gene-modified autologous tumor vaccines in non-small-cell lung cancer. J Natl Cancer Inst 2004;96:326–331.
21. Nemunaitis J, Jahan T, Ross H, et al. Phase 1/2 trial of autologous tumor mixed with an allogeneic GVAX vaccine in advanced-stage non-small-cell lung cancer. Cancer Gene Ther 2006;13:555–562.
22. Higano CS, Corman JM, Smith DC, et al. Phase 1/2 dose-escalation study of a GM-SCF-secreting, allogeneic, cellular immunotherapy for metastatic hormone-refractory prostate cancer. Cancer 2008;113:975–984.
23. Fonseca C, Soiffer R, Ho V, et al. Protein disulfide isomerases are antibody targets during immune-mediated tumor destruction. Blood 2009;113:1681–1688.
24. Jinushi M, Hodi FS, Dranoff G. Enhancing the clinical activity of granulocyte-macrophage colony-stimulating factor-secreting tumor cell vaccines. Immunol Rev 2008;222:287–298.
25. Small EJ, Schellhammer PF, Higano CS, et al. Placebo-controlled phase III trial of immunologic therapy with Sipuleucel-T (APC8015) in patients with metastatic, asymptomatic hormone refractory prostate cancer. J Clin Oncol 2006;24:3089–3094.
26. Schadendorf D, Uqurel S, Schuler-Thurner B, et al. Dacarbazine (DTIC) versus vaccination with autologous peptide-pulsed dendritic cells (DC) in first-line treatment of patients with metastatic melanoma: a randomized phase III trial of the DC study group of the DeCOG. Ann Oncol 2006;17:563–570.
27. Tanaka F, Haraguchi N, Isikawa K, et al. Potential role of dendritic cell vaccination with MAGE peptides in gastrointestinal carcinomas. Oncol Rep 2008;20:1111–1116.
28. Avigan DE, Vasir B, George DJ, et al. Phase I/II study of vaccination with electrofused allogeneic dendritic cells/autologous tumor-derived cells in patients with stage IV renal cell carcinoma. J Immunother 2007;30:749–761.
29. Avigan D, Vasir B, Gong J, et al. Fusion cell vaccination of patients with metastatic breast and renal cancer induces immunological and clinical responses. Clin Cancer Res 2004;10:4699–4708.
30. Brown RD, Pope B, Murray A, et al. Dendritic cells from patients with myeloma are numerically normal but functionally defective as they fail to up-regulate CD80 (B7-1) expression after huCD40LT stimulation because of inhibition by transforming growth factor-beta1 and interleukin-10. Blood 2001;98:2992–2998.
31. Berntsen A, Trepiakas R, Wenandy L, et al. Therapeutic dendritic cell vaccination of patients with metastatic renal cell carcinoma: a clinical phase 1/2 trial. J Immunother 2008;31:771–780.
32. Svane IM, Pederson AE, Nikolajsen K, et al. Alterations in p53-specific T cells and other lymphocyte subsets in breast cancer patients during vaccination with p53-peptide loaded dendritic cells and low-dose interleukin-2. Vaccine 2008;26:4716–4724.

33. Yamazaki S, Iyoda T, Tarbell K, et al. Direct expansion of functional CD25+CD4+ regulatory T cells by antigen-processing dendritic cells. J Exp Med 2003;198:235–247.

34. Di Nicola M, Zappasodi R, Carlo-Stella C, et al. Vaccination with autologous tumor-loaded dendritic cells induces clinical and immunologic responses in indolent B-cell lymphoma patients with relapsed and measurable disease: a pilot study. Blood 2009;113:18–27.

35. Yang ZZ, Novak AJ, Stenson MJ, et al. Intratumoral CD4+CD25+ regulatory T-cell-mediated suppression of infiltrating CD4+ T cells in B-cell non-Hodgkin lymphoma. Blood 2006;107:3639–3646.

36. Mittal S, Marshall NA, Duncan L, et al. Local and systemic induction of CD4+CD25+ regulatory T-cell population by non-Hodgkin lymphoma. Blood 2008;111:5359–5370.

37. Colombo MP, Piconese S. Regulatory-T-cell inhibition versus depletion: the right choice in cancer immunotherapy. Nat Rev Cancer 2007;7:880–887.

38. Palmer DH, Midgley RS, Mirza N, et al. A phase II study of adoptive immunotherapy using dendritic cells pulsed with tumor lysate in patients with hepatocellular carcinoma. Hepatology 2009;49:124–132.

39. Ulmer JB, Donnelly JJ, Parker SE, et al. Heterologous protection against influenza by injection of DNA encoding a viral protein. Science 1993;259:1745–1749.

40. Fu TM, Ulmer JB, Caulfield MJ, et al. Priming of cytotoxic T lymphocytes by DNA vaccines: requirement for professional antigen presenting cells and evidence for antigen transfer from myocytes. Mol Med 1997;3:362–371.

41. Trimble CL, Shiwen P, Ferdynand K, et al. A phase I trial of a human papillomavirus DNA vaccine for HPV16+ cervical intraepithelial neoplasia 2/3. Clin Cancer Res 2009;15:361–367.

42. Trimble CL, Piantadosi S, Gravitt P, et al. Spontaneous regression of high-grade cervical dysplasia: effects of human papillomavirus type and HLA phenotype. Clin Cancer Res 2005;11:4717–4723.

43. Harari, A, Bart PA, Stohr W, et al. An HIV-1 clade C DNA prime, NYVAC boost vaccine regimen induces reliable, polyfunctional, and long-lasting T cell responses. J Exp Med 2008;205:63–77.

44. Selby M, Goldbeck C, Pertile T, et al. Enhancement of DNA vaccine potency by electroporation in vivo. J Biotechnol 2000;83:147–152.

45. Widera G, Austin M, Rabussay D, et al. Increased DNA vaccine delivery and immunogenicity by electroporation in vivo. J Immunol 2000;164:4635–4640.

46. Zucchelli S, Capone S, Fattori E, et al. Enhancing B- and T-cell immune response to a hepatitis C virus E2 DNA vaccine by intramuscular electrical gene transfer. J Virol 2000;74:11598–11607.

47. Quaglino E, Mastini C, Iezzi M, et al. Electroporated DNA vaccine clears away multifocal mammary carcinomas in HER2/neu transgenic mice. Cancer Res 2004;64:2858–2864.

48. Roos AK, Moreno S, Leder C, et al. Enhancement of cellular immune response to a prostate cancer DNA vaccine by intradermal electroporation. Mol Ther 2006;13:320–327.

49. Souders NC, Sewell DA, Pan ZK, et al. Listeria-based vaccines can overcome tolerance by expanding low avidity CD8+ T cells capable of eradicating a solid tumor in a transgenic mouse model of cancer. Cancer Immun 2007;7:2.

50. Bijker MS, Melief CJ, Offringa R, et al. Design and development of synthetic peptide vaccines: past, present, and future. Expert Rev Vaccines 2007;6:591–603.

51. Kim JW, Hung CF, Juang J, et al. Comparison of HPC DNA vaccines employing intracellular targeting strategies. Gene Ther 2004;11:1011–1018.

52. Ji H, Wang TL, Chen CH, et al. Targeting human papillomavirus type 16 E7 to the endosomal/lysosomal compartment enhances the antitumor immunity of DNA vaccines against E7-expressing tumors. Hum Gene Ther 1999;10:2727–2740.

53. Gulley JL, Arlen PM, Tsang KY, et al. Pilot study of vaccinia with recombinant CEA-MUC-1-TRICOM poxviral-based vaccines in patients with metastatic carcinoma. Clin Cancer Res 2008;14:3060–3069.

54. Madan R, Gulley J, Duhut W, et al. Overall survival (OS) analysis of a phase II study using a pox viral-based vaccine, PSA-TRICOME, in the treatment of metastatic, castrate-resistant prostate cancer (mCPRC): implications for clinical trial design [abstract]. J Clin Oncol 2008;16:3005.

55. Mohebtash M, Madan R, Arlen P, et al. Phase I trial of targeted therapy with PSA-TRICOM vaccine and ipilimumab in patients with metastatic castration-resistant prostate cancer [abstract]. ASCO Genitourinary Cancers Symposium, Orlando, FL, 2009:184.

56. Kaufman HL, Lenz HJ, Marshall J, et al. Combination chemotherapy and ALVAC-CEA/B7.1 vaccine in patients with metastatic colorectal cancer. Clin Cancer Res 2008;14:4843–4849.

57. Morse MA, Hobeika AC, Osada T, et al. Depletion of human regulatory T cells specifically enhances antigen-specific immune responses to cancer vaccines. Blood 2008;112:610–618.

58. Smith FO, Downey SG, Klapper JA, et al. Treatment of metastatic melanoma using interleukin-2 alone or in conjunction with vaccines. Clin Cancer Res 2008;14:5610–5618.

59. Nicholaou T, Ebert L, Davis ID, et al. Directions in the immune targeting of cancer: lessons learned from the cancer-testis Ag NY-ESO-1. Immunol Cell Biol 2006;84:303–317.

60. Adams S, O'Neill DW, Nonaka D, et al. Immunization of malignant melanoma patients with full-length NY-ESO-1 protein using Toll-like receptor 7 agonist imiquimod as vaccine adjuvant. J Immunol 2008;181:776–784.

61. Davis ID, Chen W, Jackson H, et al. Recombinant NY-ESO-1 protein with ISCOMATRIX adjuvant induces broad integrated antibody and CD4+ and CD8+ T cell responses in humans. Proc Natl Acad Sci U S A 2004;101:10697–10702.

62. Nicholaou T, Ebert LM, Davis ID, et al. Regulatory T-cell-mediated attenuation of T-cell responses to the NY-ESO-1 ISCOMATRIX vaccine in patients with advanced malignant melanoma. Clin Cancer Res 2009;15:2166–2173.

63. Scheibenbogen C, Letsch A, Thiel E, et al. CD8 T-cell responses to Wilms tumor gene product WT1 and proteinase 3 in patients with acute myeloid leukemia. Blood 2002;100:2132–2137.

64. Gilmore R, Xue SA, Holler A, et al. Detection of Wilms' tumor antigen-specific CTL in tumor-draining lymph nodes of patients with early breast cancer. Clin Cancer Res 2006;12:34–42.

65. Rezvani K, Brenchley JM, Price DA, et al. T-cell responses directed against multiple HLA-A*0201-restricted epitopes derived from Wilms' tumor 1 protein in patients with leukemia and healthy donors: identification, quantification, and characterization. Clin Cancer Res 2005;11:8799–8807.

66. Qazilbash MH, Wieder E, Rios R, et al. Vaccination with the PR1 leukemia-associated antigen can induce complete remission in patients with myeloid leukemia [abstract]. ASH Annual Meeting Abstracts 2004;104:259.

67. Mailander V, Scheibenbogen C, Savani BN, et al. Complete remission in a patient with recurrent acute myeloid leukemia induced by vaccination with WT1 peptide in the absence of hematological or renal toxicity. Leukemia 2004;18:165–166.

68. Rezvani K, Yong AS, Mielke S, et al. Leukemia-associated antigen-specific T-cell responses following combined PR1 and WT1 peptide vaccination in patients with myeloid malignancies. Blood 2008;111:236–242.

69. Barve M, Bender J, Senzer N, et al. Induction of immune responses and clinical efficacy in a phase II trial if IDM-2101, a 10-epitope cytotoxic T-lymphocyte vaccine, in metastatic non-small cell lung cancer. J Clin Oncol 2008;26:4418–4425.

70. Bolonaki I, Kotsakis A, Papadimitraki E, et al. Vaccination of patients with advanced non-small-cell lung cancer with an optimized cryptic human telomerase reverse transcriptase peptide. J Clin Oncol 2007;25:2727–2734.

71. Giaccone G, Debruyne C, Felip E, et al. Phase III study of adjuvant vaccination with Bec2/bacilli Calmette-Guerin in responding patients with limited-disease small-cell lung cancer (European organization for research and treatment of cancer 08971-08971B; silva study). J Clin Oncol 2005;23:6854–6864.

72. Bottomley A, Debruyne C, Felip E, et al. symptom and quality of life results of an international randomized phase III study of adjuvant vaccination with Bec2/BCG in responding patients with limited disease small-cell lung cancer. Eur J Cancer 2008;44:2178–2184.

73. Van Oers MH, Klasa R, Marcus RE, et al. Rituximab maintenance improves clinical outcome of relapse/resistant follicular non-Hodgkn's lymphoma, both in patients with and without rituximab during induction: results of a prospective randomized phase III intergroup trial. Blood 2006;108:3295–3301.

74. Longo DL. Idiotype vaccination in follicular lymphoma: knocking on the doorway to cure. J Natl Cancer Inst 2006;98:1263–1265.

75. Inoges S, Rodriguez-Calvillo M, Zabalgui N, et al. Clinical benefit associated with idiotypic vaccination in patients with follicular lymphoma. J Natl Cancer Inst 2006;98:1292–1301.

76. Hung CF, Ma B, Monie A, et al. Therapeutic human papillomavirus vaccines: current clinical trials and future directions. Expert Opin Biol Ther 2008;8:421–439.

77. Kenter GG, Welters MJ, Valentijn AR, et al. Phase I immunotherapeutic trial with long peptides spanning the E6 and E7 sequences of high-risk human papillomavirus 16 in end-stage cervical cancer patients shows low toxicity and robust immunogenicity. Clin Cancer Res 2008;14:169–177.

78. Toubaji A, Achtar M, Provenzano M, et al. Pilot study of mutant ras peptide-based vaccine as an adjuvant treatment in pancreatic and colorectal cancers. Cancer Immunol Immunother 2008;57:1413–1420.

79. Morse MA, Hobeika A, Osada T, et al. Long term disease-free survival and T cell and antibody responses in women with high-risk Her2+ breast cancer following vaccination against Her2. J Transl Med 2007;5:42.

80. Heimberger AB, Sampson JH. The PEPvIII-KLH (CDX-110) vaccine in glioblastoma multiforme patients. Expert Opin Biol Ther 2009;9:1087–1098.

81. Sampson JH, Archer GE, Mitchell DA, et al. An epidermal growth factor receptor variant III-targeted vaccine is safe and immunogenic in patients with glioblastoma multiforme. Mol Cancer Ther 2009;10:2773–2779.

82. Heimberger AB, Hussain SF, Aldape K, et al. Tumor-specific peptide vaccination in newly-diagnosed patients with GBM [abstract]. J Clin Oncol 2006;24:18S.

83. Sampson JH, Aldape KD, Gilbert MR, et al. Temozolomide as a vaccine adjuvant in GBM. [abstract]. J Clin Oncol 2007;25(185):2020.

84. Jordan JT, Sun WH, Hussain SF, et al. Preferential migration of regulatory T cells mediated by glioma-secreted chemokines can be blocked with chemotherapy. Cancer Immunol Immunother 2008;57:123–131.

85. Suntharalingam G, Perry MR, Ward S, et al. Cytokine storm in a phase I trial of the anti-CD28 monoclonal antibody TGN1412. N Engl J Med 2006;355:1018–1028.

86. Melero I, Shuford WW, Newby SA, et al. Monoclonal antibodies against the 4-1BB T cell activation molecule eradicate established tumors. Nat Med 1997;3:682–685.

87. Wilcox RA, Flies DB, Zhu G, et al. Provision of antigen and CD137 signaling breaks immunologic tolerance, promoting regression of poorly immunogenic tumors. J Clin Invest 2002;109:651–659.

88. Ito F, Li Q, Shreiner AB, et al. Anti-CD137 monoclonal antibody administration augments the antitumor efficacy of dendritic cell-based vaccines. Cancer Res 2004;64:8411–8419.

89. Weinberg AD, Rivera MM, Prell R, et al. Engagement of the OX-40 receptor in vivo enhances antitumor immunity. J Immunol 2000;164:2160–2169.

90. Melero I, Hervas-Stubbs S, Glennie M, et al. Immunostimulatory monoclonal antibodies for cancer therapy. Nat Rev Cancer 2007;7:95–106.

91. Peggs KS, Quezada SA, Allison JP. Cell intrinsic mechanisms of T-cell inhibition and application to cancer therapy. Immunol Rev 2008;224:141–165.

92. Maker AV, Attia P, Rosenberg SA. Analysis of the cellular mechanism of antitumor responses and autoimmunity in patients treated with CTLA-4. J Immunol 2005;175:7746–7754.

93. Van Elsas A, Hurwitz AA, Allison JP. Combination immunotherapy of B16 melanoma using anti-cytotoxic T lymphocyte-associated T lymphocyte-associated antigen 4 (CTLA-4) and granulocyte/macrophage colony-stimulating factor (GM-CSF)-producing vaccines induces rejection of subcutaneous and metastatic tumors accompanied by autoimmune depigmentation. J Exp Med 1999;190:355–366.

94. Hurwitz AA, Foster BA, Kwon ED, et al. Combination immunotherapy of primary prostate cancer in a transgenic mouse model using CTLA-4 blockade. Cancer Res 2000;60:2444–2448.

95. Phan GQ, Yang JC, Sherry RM, et al. Cancer regression and autoimmunity induced by cytotoxic T lymphocyte-associated antigen 4 blockade in patients with metastatic melanoma. Proc Natl Acad Sci U S A 2003;100:8372–8377.

96. Beck KE, Blansfield JA, Tran KQ, et al. Enterocolitis in patients with cancer after antibody blockade of cytotoxic T-lymphocyte-associated antigen 4. J Clin Oncol 2006;24:2283–2289.

97. Oble DA, Mino-Kenudson M, Goldsmith J, et al. α-CTLA-4 mAb-associated panenteritis, a histologic and immunohistologic analysis. Am J Surg Pathol 2008;32:1130–1137.

98. Read S, Greenwald R, Izcue A, et al. Blockade of CTLA-4 on CD4+CD25+ regulatory T cells abrogates their function in vivo. J Immunol 2006;177:4376–4383.

99. Attia P, Phan GQ, Maker AV, et al. Autoimmunity correlates with tumor regression in patients with metastatic melanoma treated with anti-cytotoxic T-lymphocyte antigen-4. J Clin Oncol 2005;23:6043–6053.

100. Hodi FS, Mihm MC, Soiffer RJ, et al. Biologic activity of cytotoxic T lymphocyte-associated antigen 4 antibody blockade in previously vaccinated metastatic melanoma and ovarian cancer patients. Proc Natl Acad Sci U S A 2003;100:4712–4717.

101. Hodi FS, Butler M, Oble DA, et al. Immunologic and clinical effects of antibody blockade of cytotoxic T lymphocyte-associated antigen 4 win previously vaccinated cancer patients. Proc Natl Acad Sci U S A 2008;105:3005–3010.

102. Quezada SA, Peggs KS, Curran MA, et al. CTLA4 blockade and GM-CSF combination immunotherapy alters the intratumoral balance of effector and regulatory T cells. J Clin Invest 2006;116:1935–1945.

103. Fife BT, Bluestone JA. Control of peripheral T-cell tolerance and autoimmunity via the CTLA-4 and PD-1 pathways. Immunol Rev 2008;224:166–182.

104. Berger R, Rotem-Yehudar R, Slama G, et al. Phase I safety and pharmacokinetic study of CT-011, a humanized antibody interacting with PD-1, in patients with advanced hematologic malignancies. Clin Cancer Res 2008;14:3044–3051.

105. Luft T, Jefford M, Leutjens P, et al. IL-1β enhances CD40 ligand-mediated cytokine secretion by human dendritic cells (DC): a mechanism for T cell-independent DC activation. J Immunol 2002;168:713–722.

105. Wierda WG, Cantwell MJ, Woods SJ, et al. CD40-ligand (CD154) gene therapy for chronic lymphocytic leukemia. Blood 2000;96:2917–2924.

106. Hirano A, Longo DL, Taub DD, et al. Inhibition of human breast carcinoma growth by a soluble recombinant human CD40 ligand. Blood 1999;93:2999–3007.

107. Von Leoprechting A, van der Bruggen P, Pahl HL, et al. Stimulation of CD40 on immunogenic human malignant melanomas augments their cytotoxic T lymphocyte-mediated lysis of induces apoptosis. Cancer Res 1999;59:1287–1294.

108. Vonderheide RH, Dutcher JP, Anderson JE, et al. Phase I study of recombinant human CD40 ligand in cancer patients. J Clin Oncol 2001;19:3280–3287.

109. Uno T, Takeda K, Kojima Y, et al. Eradication of established tumors in mice by a combination antibody-based therapy. Nat Med 2006;12:693–698.

Adoptive Cellular Therapies

Cassian Yee

Experiments performed more than 30 years ago, demonstrating that malignant cells could be eradicated in tumor-bearing mice following the transfer of splenocytes from an immune mouse, ignited the imagination of immunologists and oncologists who could observe for the first time that a tangible, measurable component—this bolus of immune cells—under appropriate conditions was necessary and sufficient to eliminate cancer in tumor-bearing hosts. Since that time, immunotherapy investigators have weathered numerous failures and obstacles attempting to recapitulate this success in patients with advanced malignancies, most notably metastatic melanoma. With the advent of molecular tools to dissect the immune response and a greater understanding of the extrinsic and intrinsic signals governing a productive T-cell response to cancer, the development of strategies to enrich, expand, and manipulate tumor-reactive T cells ex vivo has led to a renaissance in the field of adoptive cellular therapy.

In this chapter, early studies in adoptive therapy are first described and following this, two major sections are presented: strategies developed to elicit antigen-specific T cells in vitro and the clinical trials exploiting these strategies for the treatment of patients with cancer.

Early Studies

The field of adoptive therapy involves the use of in vitro–expanded immune effector cells. Early on, the availability of clinical-grade, recombinant interleukin-2 (IL-2), a lymphokine for natural killer (NK) cells and T cells, led to clinical trials using peripheral blood lymphocytes exposed to high doses of IL-2 to expand "activated killer" cells, that is, lymphokine-activated killer (LAK) cells. This approach has now been largely abandoned in favor of tumor-infiltrating lymphocytes or TILs when it was discovered that single cell suspensions of lymphocytes could be collected from tumor samples, expanded with IL-2, and generated as an antitumor response in murine models that was 50 to 100 times more effective on a percell basis than LAK cells. TIL therapy accompanied by high-dose IL-2 initially demonstrated a 50% response rate in patients with metastatic melanoma, but subsequent studies yielded a response rate of 22%.[1] Randomized clinical trials using the TIL regimen in patients with stage III renal cancer and melanoma revealed no differences in overall survival compared with IL-2 alone[2,3]; however, the subset of patients with Stage III melanoma and no more than one involved lymph node experienced a statistically significant increase in overall survival, a result that was confirmed in a

follow-up report 7 years later.[4] Taken together, these early results suggested that the therapeutic advantage in using TIL for adoptive therapy was marginalized in patients with increasing tumor burden (more advanced stage III disease or stage IV disease). Without the ability to more clearly define the tumor-rejecting T-cell population among the heterogeneous TIL product, the target antigens recognized mechanisms of immune resistance, and the means to overcome them, further advances in the field would be limited. Defining these parameters would require the development of strategies to generate antigen-specific T cells for adoptive therapy.

Generation of Antigen-Specific T Cells for Adoptive Therapy

The isolation and expansion of T cells require first that tumor-associated antigens recognized by T cells be identified. Following this, in vitro conditions to enrich for a population of antigen-specific T cells are presented. These T cells may be derived from the extant repertoire (*endogenous specificity*) (Fig 33-1) or genetically engineered to express the antigen-specific receptor of interest (*redirected specificity*).

Tumor Antigens Recognized by T Cells

The first human tumor antigen *defined* by T-cell recognition was identified by Thierry Boon and colleagues at the Ludwig Institute almost 20 years ago. A T-cell clone was generated that recognized an autologous melanoma cell line. The cDNA library of the tumor line was transfected into antigen-presenting cells (APCs) expressing the restricting allele and screened using the tumor-reactive T-cell clone. The cDNA of target cells sensitized to lysis by the antigen-specific T cell was recovered and sequenced. By this method, the first human T cell–defined tumor antigen was found to be MAGE-A1.[5,6] It was later discovered that in addition to the MAGE-A1 antigen, a number of MAGE-like antigens, including GAGE, BAGE, LAGE, NY-ESO-1, and SSX-1, were also recognized by tumor-reactive T cells. Based on their restricted tissue expression, that is, tumor cells and germinal cells such as testis, fetal ovary, and placenta, these antigens were grouped together into the family of "cancer-testis" or CT antigens.[7] There are now known to be over 80 CT antigens, several of which are immunogenic to T cells and are expressed in a wide variety of solid and liquid tumors including lung cancer, colorectal cancer, breast cancer, ovarian cancer, and leukemia.

Using a similar approach, the melanoma-associated antigens, tyrosinase, gp100, and MART-1, were also identified as T-cell target antigens.[8–10] In this case, their association with pigmentation pathways

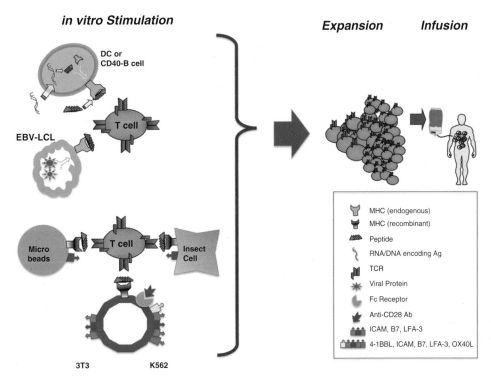

found in normal melanocytes represented the first examples of nonmutated "differentiation" antigens serving as immunologic targets for human T cells.[11] Since then, other "differentiation" antigens for prostate cancer (PSMA, Kallikrein), colorectal cancer (CEA), and breast cancer (NY-BR-1, mammoglobin) have been identified. Along with differentiation antigens, other nonmutated self-proteins that are found to be over-expressed in tumor cells include Her-2-neu (breast cancer), adipophilin (renal cancer), mesothelin (ovarian cancer, pancreatic cancer), and more "universally" expressed antigens that confer a survival advantage to tumor cells, such as, survivin, telomerase, and WT-1.

Mutations in genes associated with tumorigenesis, such as those responsible for cell cycling (the cyclin-dependent kinase, CDK4), delivery of mitogenic signals (B-RAF), and apoptosis (CASP-8), represent attractive targets for immunotherapy because of the decreased likelihood for antigen-loss tumor variants developing. Unfortunately, most of these mutations are not highly prevalent among most tumors and appear to exhibit low immunogenicity.

T cells recognize peptide fragments of target antigens presented by self-MHC molecules on the surface of tumor or APCs such as dendritic cells (DCs), B cells, and monocytes. Those peptide fragments recognized by T cells in the context of the MHC complex are the result of internal processing by proteasomes (class I–restricted epitopes) or lyso/phagosome-associated enzymes (class II–restricted epitopes) followed by binding to their respective MHC complexes and surface presentation. The identification of epitopes recognized by

tumor-reactive T cells has been a focus of considerable research since such epitope peptides can be used to elicit antigen-specific T cells and track T-cell responses and are amenable to clinical use as readily available GMP grade reagents to sort and collect antigen-specific T cells. For class I–restricted epitopes designed to elicit CD8 T-cell responses, these epitopes are generally nine to ten amino acids in length; for class II–restricted epitopes eliciting CD4 T-cell responses, the epitopes can be 14 to over 20 amino acids long since class II alleles are less stringent and can accommodate overhanging flanking regions.

In cases where a tumor-reactive antigen-specific T-cell clone has been isolated, such a clone can be used to probe overlapping peptides to identify the minimal epitope sequence. For common alleles, the target epitope may be deduced using algorithms that predict the sequence on the basis of consensus motifs based on known binding preferences as well as the predilection of the proteasome for certain cleavage sites. On occasion, splice variants, excision of intervening sequences, and even sequence reversal during antigen processing can lead to unexpected surface presentation of the cognate epitope.[12] Often, the definitive sequence can only be deduced by eluting peptides from surface MHC and subjecting the mix to mass spectrometry.

However, when the tumor-associated epitope is nonmutant, as is frequently the case, the naturally occurring peptide ligand may not engender robust and sustained antitumor CTL responses.[13,14] This is a result of immune tolerance mechanisms that suppress or eliminate high-avidity autoreactive T cells.[15] What remains is a low frequency of tumor-specific T cells or T cells that bear low-avidity T-cell receptors for the cognate tumor antigen.[16-19] One method to activate and mobilize these rare and low-avidity tumor-specific T cells uses superagonist altered peptide ligands (APL)[20,21] that deviate from the native peptide sequence by one or more amino acids, to allow for enhanced binding to the restricting MHC molecule[20,21] or favorable interaction with the T-cell receptor (TCR) of a given tumor-specific T-cell subset. While, superagonist APLs have been identified that generate tumor-reactive T cells and have even been used to elicit desired immune responses in clinical studies,[22,23] a comprehensive method for identifying superagonist ligands remains to be developed. Furthermore, the use of APLs must address the potential drawbacks, including cross-reactivity, of the induced T cell not only to the wild-type epitope but also to undesirable autoimmune targets and the possibility that APL-induced responses respond with lower avidity to endogenous target antigens. One advantage of adoptive therapy in this respect is the ability to choose *ex vivo* from among the population of APL-induced T cells that satisfy these criteria by screening *against* those that recognize normal tissue targets and selecting for those that recognize endogenously expressed tumor target antigens with high avidity.

Endogenous Specificity: Generating Antigen-Specific T Cells from Existing Repertoire

The in vitro isolation and expansion of antigen-specific T cells for adoptive therapy are in essence a recapitulation of the in vivo events of priming and expansion and involve at least four components: An effector population (source of T cells), stimulator cell, TCR ligand, and T-cell growth factor (i.e., lymphokines such as IL-2) (Table 33-1).

Naturally Occurring Antigen-Presenting Cells as Stimulator Cells

Although DCs, under specific conditions, can be tolerogenic, they are generally considered "professional" APCs with specialized stimulatory features, for example, their capacity to up-regulate expression of costimulatory ligands, and Th1-type cytokines such as IL-12. They represent a robust in vitro stimulator population. In one embodiment, an enriched population of DCs can be generated by treatment of adherent mononuclear cells with GM-CSF and IL-4. Following maturation with an immunomodulatory cocktail or conditioned media, DCs can then be loaded with peptide, transfected with RNA or expression plasmid or transduced with recombinant viral vectors expressing the target antigen of interest. When cocultivated with autologous T cells, and a source of cytokines such as IL-2, antigen-specific T cells can be expanded in vitro for downstream applications. Other approaches for generating human dendritic cells include the use of cytokines such as IL-15[24,25], toll receptor (TLR) agonists, or CD40 to enhance DC function and the addition of FLT3 ligand to expand DCs in vitro or in vivo prior to peripheral blood mononuclear cell harvest.[22,26]

A more readily available source of autologous APCs has also been developed using CD40 ligand to activate and facilitate long-term growth of human B cells.[27] These CD40-activated B cells express high levels of costimulatory molecules and when transfected with the target antigen of interest or epitope peptide serve as robust APCs in vivo and in vitro. Furthermore, CD40 activation of malignant B cells can render them effective APCs and provide a direct means of stimulating leukemia-reactive CD4 and CD8 T cells.[28]

Whatever the source, when stimulator cells are cocultivated with autologous T cells, in vitro expansion of antigen-specific cells

	TABLE **33.1**	*Generating antigen-specific T cells for adoptive therapy from endogenous repertoire*			

Effector	Source of effector	Stimulator cell	TCR ligand	Growth signal
TIL	Infiltrating lymphocytes from tumor	Tumor cells, in situ APCs	Tumor antigen	IL-2 (high dose) required in vitro and in vivo
Antigen specific T-cell lines and clones	T cells from peripheral blood	Autologous DCs, monocytes, CD40-B cells	Peptide, RNA-/DNA-transfected gene product	IL-2
		Artificial APCs (insect cells, K562, beads)	Peptide, RNA-/DNA-transfected gene product, pMHC complex	IL-2, costimulatory receptors
EBV-specific T cells	T cells from peripheral blood	EBV-B cells, peptide, transduced APCs	EBV-B cells, peptides, adenoviral transgene	IL-2 or none

Infiltrating lymphocytes harvested from tumor sites (TIL) are stimulated by in situ tumor cells and APCs cross-presenting tumor antigens; TILs are expanded with high-dose IL-2 in vitro and require high-dose IL-2 in vivo to maintain survival. Antigen-specific T-cell lines and clones are generated by cocultivation with stimulator cells displaying the TCR ligand in the form of APCs pulsed with peptide, APCs expressing RNA- or DNA-transfected gene product, or artificial APCs decorated with pMHC complex. In the case of EBV-specific T cells, autologous EBV-transformed B cells (LCL) that express the immunodominant viral antigens (e.g., EBNA3) for treatment of PTLD serve as effective APCs; generation of T cells recognizing less immunogenic EBV-associated epitopes for the treatment of HD and NPC is stimulated with APCs infected with adenoviral vectors expressing subdominant epitopes (e.g., LMP2). Artificial APCs can be decorated with peptide-MHC complexes (pMHC) to elicit antigen-specific T cells and costimulatory receptors to facilitate T-cell activation and propagation.

requires a γ-chain receptor cytokine, such as IL-2, and iterative cycles of in vitro restimulation. In contrast to more nonspecific strategies for expanding effectors such as LAK and TIL where high doses of IL-2 (upwards of 6,000 U/mL) are required, low doses of IL-2 (10 to 50 U/mL) are generally sufficient to induce antigen-driven expansion due to the up-regulation of high-affinity IL-2Rα coreceptor following TCR engagement. Other γ-chain receptor cytokines, such as IL-7 and IL-15, can also be used to augment expansion and have been shown to augment a population of memory effector cells. The addition of IL-21 is unique in its capacity to generate antigen-specific T cells displaying elevated levels of CD28 and, in some cases, CD62L, with effector function, and may represent a central memory–like helper-independent CD8$^+$ T cells with features of arrested differentiation and enhanced replicative potential.[29]

Artificial Antigen-Presenting Cells as Stimulator Cells

The use of artificial APCs addresses some of the obstacles to using autologous mononuclear cells by providing a convenient *ex vivo* source of stimulator cells, a product that is more likely to be uniform in its physical and functional properties and the flexibility of expressing desired antigen-specific and/or costimulatory receptors.

Mouse fibroblast (3T3) lines and insect cells (*D. melanogaster*) can be engineered to express the appropriate HLA (usually the prevalent HLA-A2 allele that presents many of the known tumor-associated antigenic epitopes) as well as costimulatory receptors, B7.1, ICAM-1, and LFA-3, found to be necessary for optimal CD8 T-cell stimulation.[30] Pulsed with the desired peptide, these APCs could be used to generate human antigen-specific CTL responses in vitro. Using HLA-A2+ insect cells expressing B7.1 and ICAM, Mitchell et al.[31] were able to enrich for and expand tyrosinase-specific CTL from peripheral blood of patients with metastatic melanoma to more than 10^9 cells in the presence of IL-2 and IL-7 for use in a clinical trial of adoptive therapy.

The human NK-susceptible chronic myeloid leukemia (CML) cell line, K562, has also been explored for use as an artificial APC. In the absence of MHC expression, it can be used as a "blank" slate for decorating with the desired TCR ligand and costimulatory molecules. June et al. stably transduced Fc receptors to allow for display of anti-CD3 and anti-CD28 antibodies. When 4-1BBL (CD137L) was coexpressed, optimal, nonspecific in vitro expansion of T cells was achieved. By transfecting K562 with the relevant HLA allele and pulsing with the desired epitope peptide, tumor-associated antigen-specific CD8$^+$ T cells could be reliably generated in vitro.[32] Engineering aAPCs to express γ-chain receptor cytokines, such as IL-21, led to further enhancement in the qualitative and quantitative expansion of antigen-specific CTL.[33]

Acellular products used as artificial APCs include magnetic beads, liposomes, and exosomes. Magnetic beads covalently linked to anti-CD3 and anti-CD28 provide a means to rapidly expand a population of polyclonal T cells and have been used in a number of clinical trials: anti-CD3–/anti-CD28–activated donor lymphocyte infusions (DLI) have led to increased responses posttransplant for CML, non-Hodgkin's lymphoma (NHL), and myeloma[34–36] compared to untreated DLI. For generating antigen-specific T cells, class I and class II Ig dimers can be attached to the beads to permit exogenous loading of peptides for in vitro stimulation and, as a vaccine reagent, for in vivo expansion of adoptively transferred CTL.[37]

Ex Vivo Selection and Expansion

By whatever means a population of antigen-specific T cells is generated, the question facing immunotherapy investigators is whether the population will require further expansion or in vitro selection before infusion. For some antigens, by virtue of a preexisting high endogenous frequency[38] or an elevated frequency that might be predicted in patients due to a concomitant serologic response,[39] application of the above methods to generate antigen-specific T cells in culture may be sufficient to produce a population with adequate antitumor activity. Further expansion may involve the use of ligands or agonist antibodies to TCR (CD3) and/or costimulatory receptors (CD28, 4-1BB, etc.) coupled with irradiated feeder cells and cytokines. In some cases, the population of T cells can be expanded from 100- to 1,000-fold over 2 to 3 weeks.[40–42]

If selection is desirable, then reagents to nondestructively identify antigen-specific T cells, for example, peptide-MHC multimers, can be used together with a separation method (i.e., flow cytometric cell sorting). Since the natural ligand for the TCR, the peptide-MHC complex, cannot be used singly as a staining reagent for antigen-specific T cells because of its high dissociation rate, multimerizing pMHC complex to a fluorophore-conjugated molecule in a method first pioneered by the Davis lab permits a robust and sensitive means for not only detecting antigen-specific T cells (in a nondestructive manner) but also for isolating tumor-reactive T cells for downstream analysis or adoptive therapy.[43,44] Later developments in this field include the novel use of Ig fragments to multimerize pMHC complexes for ex vivo detection,[45] (and as described above, for in vitro as well as in vivo stimulation) and the creation of class II tetramers to identify and select for antigen-specific CD4 T cells.[46] Global approaches to the selection of antigen-specific T cells exploit functional antigen-driven properties such as cytokine production and surface marker up-regulation. A bispecific antibody binding to a constitutively expressed T-cell surface marker (e.g., CD45) linked to an antibody that captures a secreted cytokine, such as IFN-γ, permits selection of viable antigen-activated IFN-γ+ T cells when a second detection antibody to IFN-γ is used.[47] Alternatively, among surface markers that are up-regulated during antigen recognition (CD25, CD69, 4-1BB/CD137), CD137 surface up-regulation correlates most strongly with TCR ligation and can be used to identify and sort for antigen-specific CD8 T cells.[48]

Redirected Specificity: T-Cell Receptor and Chimeric Antigen Receptor Gene Therapy

Factors limiting the application of adoptive T-cell therapy to a broader pool of patients and diseases include the difficulty in reproducibly isolating high-affinity T cells recognizing tumor-associated antigens and the time and resource-intensive process required to generate such cells. These obstacles may be addressed by genetically modifying T cells to express the cognate TCR or a chimeric antibody receptor (CAR) comprised of the extracellular variable chains recognizing antigen fused to a cytoplasmic T cell signaling domain (usually the TCR zeta chain). TCR and CAR gene therapy enable targeting a wider range of tumor-rejection antigens as well as a means to rapidly produce effector cells for adoptive transfer.[49,50]

TCR Gene Therapy

For TCR gene therapy, a T-cell clone of desired specificity and high affinity for the presented target epitope must first be isolated so that its TCR α- and β-chains can be sequenced and cloned into viral vectors for transgene expression.[51] However, forced expression of specific TCR α- and β-chains in T cells can present mispairing opportunities with the endogenous TCR chains. This can lead to decreased expression of the properly paired chains and lower surface levels of functional TCRs on gene-modified T cells, as well as the possibility that mispaired α- and β-chains can give rise to TCRs recognizing undesired autoimmune targets. To reduce mispairing with endogenous chains, the constant region domains of the transferred TCR α- and β- chains can be substituted with their murine counterparts, thereby eliminating pairing with any human constant regions expressed by endogenous chains.[52] Other strategies include disulfide linkage of the expressed TCR by the addition of a cysteine residue in the α- and β- chain constant domains,[53] the engineering of "knob-in-hole" interaction,[54] fusing of the α- and β- chains directly to CD3 zeta, and silencing of endogenous TCR.[55,56]

In addition to the increased flexibility in antigen targeting that TCR gene therapy offers, functional avidity may be achieved by enhancing TCR mobility[57] or TCR affinity. For the latter, TCR gene sequences were mutagenized and screened using yeast or phage display technology to identify sequences that increase affinity by three logs or more (equivalent to that seen with antibody-antigen interactions).[58,59] While increased TCR affinity has been associated with increased functional T-cell avidity for tumor targets, at least one study has demonstrated that this is not necessarily the case as other factors, such as downstream signaling events may attenuate functional avidity.[60] Strategically, this may be addressed by modulating T cell signaling pathways in a manner that decreases the activation threshold, the functional equivalent of enhancing T-cell avidity; T cells engineered to down-regulate expression of Cbl-b or SHP-1 display enhanced efficacy when transferred into tumor-bearing mice. Augmenting target interaction to such a degree allows for a robust response to the desired tumor-associated antigens but also warrants heightened awareness of the autoimmune consequences of targeting "over-expressed" self-antigens.

Target antigen redirection with either TCR or CAR gene therapy will require a means to ensure efficient delivery to effector cells. This is usually achieved through the use of retroviral or lentiviral vectors. Retroviral vectors are more commonly available and well suited for large-scale production. However, their propensity to integrate near transcriptional start sites can lead to the potential for insertional mutagenesis[61]; in addition, quiescent T cells do not maintain expression of retrovirally driven transgenes which can be a problem since ligation of the TCR is required to initiate the process of cell cycling. Lentiviral vectors hold several advantages in this regard; they have a lowered likelihood of insertional mutagenesis and an increased infection and expression efficiency among quiescent T cells. A nonviral strategy that utilizes transposon technology has been shown to be highly efficient (>40%) in transfecting resting primary T cells and is potentially scalable for clinical use.[62] Ultimately, the choice of a delivery vector will depend on reproducibility of high-efficiency transfection and cognate TCR function, as well as regulatory and safety considerations including integration site bias and transgene copy number.

Once transfected, a high level of transgene expression and translation in human T cells must be achieved. For viral vectors, empirical studies demonstrate that promoters such as MSCV U3, EF-1 alpha, and SSFV offer favorable transcriptional profiles, especially when combined with other elements, for example, a nuclear translocation

sequence, codon optimization, and strategies that enhance RNA stabilization.[55] Persistence of expression in quiescent and activated cells must also be evaluated when comparing among these different delivery vectors and flanking sequences.

Chimeric Antibody Receptor

CARs are comprised of an extracellular portion, the variable fragment (scFv) of a tumor-antigen specific antibody coupled to an intracellular domain delivering a T-cell activation signal (CD3 zeta). These CARs allow the targeting of surface proteins, generally with much higher affinity than TCRs (in the nanomolar vs micromolar range), and, in an MHC-unrestricted fashion, activate effector function through the intracellular signaling domain.[63] CARs have been developed targeting antigens expressed by several epithelial tumors[64]; however, first-generation CARs signaling through CD3 zeta alone are relatively short lived with limited proliferative capacity. In clinical trials, first-generation CARs for the treatment of neuroblastoma targeting CD171,[65] B-cell lymphomas targeting CD20,[66] ovarian cancer targeting the folate receptor[67], and renal cell cancer targeting carbonic anhydrase[68] have provided modest responses limited by short duration of in vivo persistence and an absent second signal.

Subsequent generations incorporated dual and triple signaling domains fused to the antibody receptor so that costimulatory signals such as CD137, ICOS, CD28, and OX40[69] could be delivered solely through antibody engagement without requiring tumors to express the corresponding ligand on its cell surface. These double and triple fusion receptors exhibited increased IL-2 production, enhanced proliferative capacity, and in vivo effector function.

Adoptive T Cell Therapy for the Treatment of Malignant Diseases

Hematopoietic Malignancies

Allogeneic hematopoietic stem cell transplantation (HSCT) represents the earliest evidence of T cell–mediated antitumor immunity in humans when studies documented that a graft versus leukemia (GVL) effect was greatest in patients developing graft versus host disease (GVHD) and weakest in those receiving T cell–depleted marrow cells.[70] This observation was ultimately exploited in the development of nonmyeloablative HSCT as a means of eliminating regimen-related toxicities of host conditioning by establishing donor T-cell chimerism to mediate engraftment and eradicate residual leukemic cells.[71] DLI early on were shown to be instrumental in mediating a GVL effect and remain in use as effective therapy for specific indications in the allogeneic transplant setting.

Donor Lymphocyte Infusions

DLI can induce durable complete remissions in the majority of patients (60% to 75%) with CML relapsing after allogeneic stem cell transplantation and for a subset of patients relapsing with acute lymphoblastic leukemia, lymphoma, and myeloma although results were somewhat less encouraging.[72–75] Strategies to augment DLI for posttransplant relapse include the use of anti-CD3/CD28 beads to activate T cells before transfer.[36] By comparison to standard DLI, activated donor lymphocytes were significantly more effective against acute leukemias and lymphoma (>50% long-term remissions), without excessive GVHD. For patients receiving cord blood transplants, anti-CD3/CD28 provides a feasible means to expand the small cord blood T-cell population for DLI.[76,77] For patients with myeloma receiving an allogeneic HSCT, immunizing the donor against patient-specific myeloma idiotype, which was predicted by preclinical studies in murine models to enhance transferred immunity, has shown promising results in clinical trials.[78–80]

In the autologous setting, ex vivo activation with anti-CD3 and anti-CD28 antibodies led to accelerated lymphoid reconstitution following ablative conditioning in patients with NHL and myeloma. In the latter trial, antigen-specific T cells were primed in vivo with a pneumococcal vaccine before transplant conditioning, harvested by apheresis and expanded ex vivo for infusion posttransplant. Rapid recovery of vaccine-specific memory responses in these patients and encouraging results from this study provide the basis for future trial designs incorporating vaccine and adoptive therapy.[35]

Antigen-Specific T Cell Therapy of Leukemia

The antileukemic response following a matched allogeneic HSCT can be attributed in part to donor T-cell responses against recipient minor histocompatibility antigens (mHAg). Minor antigens are peptides encoded by polymorphic genes that differ between the donor and recipient tissues and are presented on the cell surface by MHC class I and II molecules. MHAg can elicit CD8+ and CD4+ T-cell responses that initiate and maintain both GVHD and the GVL effect. Much current research is motivated by the hypothesis that selective targeting of mHAg expressed only on recipient normal and malignant hematopoietic cells will mediate an antileukemic effect without triggering or exacerbating GVHD. Since the first mHAgs, H-Y/SMCY[81,82] and HA-2,[81] were identified in 1995, at least 30 different genes have been shown to encode mHAgs, and the total number is likely to be much higher. Several of the mHAgs that have been identified to date are selectively expressed in hematopoietic cells, suggesting that therapy targeting these antigens could selectively enhance GVL activity without inducing GVHD. In some cases, these antigens have been shown to be expressed on leukemic stem cells, a finding based on studies demonstrating functional eradication of the leukemia-initiating cell in the NOD/SCID transplant model.[83,84] Aberrant expression of some minor antigens has also been seen in solid tumor malignancies[85,86] and may account for tumor regression observed after allogeneic HSCT.[87]

In the first-in-human use of adoptively transferred donor-derived T-cell clones targeting tissue-restricted minor antigens for the treatment of patients with relapsing leukemia after allogeneic HSCT, five of seven patients with recurrent leukemia achieved a complete but transient response to therapy. The most significant toxicity observed was pulmonary toxicity, which was thought to be attributable in at least one instance to shared minor antigen expression in lung epithelium. In vivo persistence of transferred T-cell clones was relatively short lived (21 days), and strategies to extend survival of adoptively transferred cells will be required to prolong the duration of clinical response.

The antileukemic response following a matched allogeneic HSCT can be attributed to T cell–mediated targeting of mHAg. These minor antigens originate from gene polymorphisms that differ between the donor and recipient tissues and represent highly immunogenic targets for induction of GVHD and GVL effects. By selectively targeting mHAg expressed only in recipient normal

and malignant hematopoietic cells, an antileukemic effect can be achieved while sparing the patient from GVHD. The approximately 30 mHAgs that have been discovered so far are divided between autosomal and Y chromosome–encoded antigens.[88] The majority of autosomally encoded minor antigens (and even some H-Y antigens that are suboptimally presented) exhibit restricted expression to hematopoietic tissues and may serve as suitable targets for T cell therapy in the posttransplant recipient.[89]

In the autologous setting, T cell therapy is being developed against a number of leukemia-associated antigens (LAA), WT-1,[90–92] PRAME,[93,94] PR3,[92,95–97] HNE,[98,99] as well as several cancer-testis antigens. In spite of the relatively rare and weakly avid endogenous T-cell responses to these self-proteins, the feasibility of generating leukemia-reactive antigen-specific T cells has been established using peptide-pulsed APCs in vitro[99–101], and for WT-1, it has been translated to early-phase clinical studies of adoptive therapy.

Adoptive therapy represents an attractive modality for the treatment of leukemic recurrence following allogeneic HSCT if early disease detection and timely generation of minor antigen-specific T cells can be achieved. Concurrent immunosuppressive therapy for treatment of GVHD can impair antitumor immune response, and strategies to render T cells resistant to calcineurin inhibitors (FK6506 and cyclosporine A [CSA]) and steroids are being developed.[102–104]

EBV-Associated Malignancies

Viral-associated malignancies appear more commonly in immunodeficient hosts in the form of HPV-associated squamous cancers, Kaposi's (HHV-8), EBV-posttransplant lymphoproliferative disease (PTLD), or EBV-associated lymphomas but are also seen in immunocompetent individuals developing nasopharyngeal carcinoma (NPC), Hodgkin's disease (HD), and Merkel cell cancer. Among these, the EBV-associated malignancies (PTLD, HD, and NPC) have received the most attention in cellular immunotherapy because EBV-reactive T cells can be collected from donors or generated in vitro and, when adoptively transferred, mediate significant clinical responses.

EBV-Associated Posttransplant Lymphoproliferative Disease

The earliest of these studies treating patients with EBV-PTLD demonstrated that an infusion of lymphocytes from an EBV+ donor mediated tumor regression in all patients developing PTLD after allogeneic HSCT.[105] A larger study evaluated 39 patients who were at high risk for the development of PTLD having received T cell–depleted marrow stem cells. Adoptively transferred donor-derived gene-marked EBV-specific CTLs generated following in vitro stimulation with EBV-transformed lymphoblastoid cell lines (LCL) were found to persist for up to 3 years and effect a 2 to 4 $\log_{10}$ decrease in viral DNA titers. As immunoprophylaxis, none of the 39 patients developed PTLD compared with an expected incidence of more than 11% in case-control analysis. A follow-up multi-institutional study of 114 patients, demonstrated an immunoprophylactic efficacy of 100% and therapeutic efficacy of more than 80% when treating established disease.[106]

For PTLD arising after solid organ transplantation (SOT), adoptive transfer of *autologous* EBV-specific T cells was also highly effective in preventing disease occurrence in all patients and was accompanied by several $\log_{10}$ reductions in EBV DNA titers.[107–109] When administered therapeutically, autologous EBV-reactive CTL induced tumor regression in anecdotal reports. Due to the 2- to 3-month period of in vitro culture required to generate an autologous EBV-reactive line, a bank of allogeneic EBV-specific CTL was established for timely treatment of 31 patients diagnosed with PTLD following SOT. Among this poor prognosis population, complete responses were seen in 14 patients and a partial response in an additional 3 patients. Response correlated with the proportion of CD4 T cells in the cell product and the proximity of HLA matching with donor CTL.

For EBV-associated malignancies such as nasopharyngeal cancer and HD where disease occurs in immunocompetent individuals, these tumors are less immunogenic, and in contrast to PTLD where the immunodominant EBNA3 protein is commonly expressed, only a limited set of less immunogenic viral antigens, such as EBNA1, LMP1, and LMP2, can be targeted. Nevertheless, when EBV-LCLs are used as stimulator cells, a measurable proportion of CTL recognizing subdominant antigens can be elicited and have been used successfully for adoptive therapy of NPC and HD.[110,111] For NPC, durable partial and complete responses, accompanied by a decrease in EBV DNA load, have been observed among those with low tumor burden.[110,112] However, unlike PTLD, in NPC, limited or no in vivo expansion of EBV-specific CTL was observed following adoptive transfer. The addition of anti-CD45 monoclonal antibody as lymphodepleting conditioning regimen yielded a transient lymphopenia, elevation in the homeostatic cytokine, IL-15, and an average 2.8-fold increase in the frequency of EBV-specific CTL, accompanied by a complete response in one patient and disease stabilization in two of eight patients.

In HD, clinical responses in several trials of adoptive therapy using EBV-specific CTL have been reported in patients with advanced or recurrent HD.[113] Patients with the highest likelihood of responding to therapy were those presenting at earlier stage of disease or with low tumor burden.[111,114] In a cohort of patients in remission but at high risk for relapse, autologous CTL administered as maintenance therapy was effective in sustaining durable remission.[115]

One limitation to the use of LCL to stimulate EBV-specific CTL for HD and NPC has been the relatively low frequency of T cells that can be generated in vitro against the less immunogenic viral proteins such as LMP2 expressed in tumor cells. The identification of conserved epitopes of LMP2 provides one means of enriching for the population of tumor-reactive CTL[116,117]; a more comprehensive approach can be achieved using autologous DCs engineered to express LMP2 using an adenoviral vector. When transferred into patients with HD, LMP2-specific CTL expanded several-fold in vivo and mediated significant clinical responses including maintenance of remission in nine of ten high-risk patients and complete clinical remission in four of six patients with refractory disease.

Strategies to address tumor-associated factors limiting the efficacy of adoptive therapy in patients with HD have included the development of methods to render T cells resistant to immunosuppressive factors such as TGF-β, restoration of IL-7 responsiveness, and enhancing targeting and homing of T cells to tumor sites by engineering expression of anti-CD30 CAR and CCR4.[118–120] As these tumor immune evasive features are shared among other solid tumors, discoveries made using this robust model targeting viral-associated malignancies have broad implications for adoptive therapy of cancer in general.

Melanoma

Clinical experience with adoptive cellular therapy has been most extensive in melanoma, initially for the reason that few therapeutic options were available for a tumor that demonstrated responsiveness to immunomodulation with IL-2 and IFN-α. Continued interest was prompted by the discovery of T cell–defined antigens and the development of methods to reliably isolate and expand melanoma-reactive effector cells.

Lymphokine-Activated Killer cells

LAK cells generated by treating peripheral blood lymphocytes with IL-2 were the earliest form of adoptive cellular therapy. Phase I studies demonstrated objective clinical responses but only when LAK cells were given with high-dose IL-2.[121–123] A prospective randomized trial comparing high-dose IL-2 versus high-dose IL-2, lymphocytapheresis, and LAK administration in patients with metastatic cancer (largely melanoma and renal cell carcinoma) revealed a trend toward improved overall survival among the melanoma group for patients treated with both IL-2 and LAK cells compared to IL-2 alone, but this was not statistically significant.[124]

When TILs were found to have greater potency against tumors in murine models[125,126] (see below), attention shifted toward TIL-based adoptive immunotherapy trials.

Tumor-Infiltrating Lymphocytes

Effector cells harvested at tumor sites and expanded in vitro were found to have greater potency against tumors in murine models than LAK cells.[125,126] TILs cultured from tumor fragments[127] could be expanded ex vivo with high doses of IL-2 (6,000 U/mL) and used for adoptive cellular therapy. Among the first 20 patients with metastatic melanoma treated with TIL and high-dose IL-2, half of the patients experienced an objective response including one complete response.[128] In a follow-up report describing a total of 86 metastatic melanoma patients treated with 145 courses of TILs, 34% of patients achieved an objective response (CR or PR). Five patients had durable complete responses.[129]

In one of the few randomized studies performed in adoptive therapy, TILs were used as adjuvant therapy in patients with stage III melanoma.[4] Patients were assigned to receive either TIL plus IL-2 for 2 months or IL-2 alone. Eighty-eight patients were enrolled in the study. Although no significant difference in overall survival was observed, a significant difference was seen in the subset of patients with involvement of only one involved lymph node.

Modifications to the TIL protocol in the manner of in vitro expansion and the use of lymphodepleting conditioning regimens have led to a series of clinically successful trials in T cell therapy by the Rosenberg group at the National Cancer Institute (NCI). TIL cultures with superior antitumor activity following IL-2 treatment in vitro were expanded with a protocol adapted from the "Rapid Expansion Method" (REM) previously developed by Riddell and Greenberg for expanding T-cell clones, involving the use of a TCR trigger (anti-CD3 antibody), irradiated feeder cells, and lymphokine support (IL-2).[130] Numbers sufficient for adoptive transfer (up to 10^{11}) could be achieved in 6 to 8 weeks; a closed system has been developed to expedite the process. The cultures grew in as little as 5 weeks and typically between 6 and 8 weeks.

For both antigen-specific effectors and LAK cells or TIL, preinfusion lymphodepletion whether by cyclophosphamide administration[126] or sublethal irradiation[131] has been shown to be critical for tumor eradication in animal models. It was clearly demonstrated in a seminal study that suppressor cells (later identified as regulatory T cells) played a role in mice bearing the cyclophosphamide-resistant lymphoma (L5178Y) where complete tumor regression was observed only when the combination of cyclophosphamide and tumor-sensitized T cells was administered.[132] The Surgery Branch of the NCI was one of the first groups to combine a high-dose lymphodepletion regimen with adoptive cellular therapy.[133,134] Patients received up to 60 mg/kg of cyclophosphamide in addition to fludarabine before adoptive transfer of autologous TILs and supported in vivo by a course of high-dose IL-2. Among the 35 patients, more than 50% (18 patients) experienced objective responses including 3 CRs at least one of which was durable for over 2 years. Patients had clones persisting for weeks and in some cases even months after TIL infusion.[135,134] However, as a consequence of the coadministered high-dose IL-2 and cytokine milieu accompanying reactivation of infused TIL in the setting of lymphodepletion, serious life-threatening toxicities attributed to cytokine-induced vascular leak syndrome were observed, including respiratory failure and hypotension. Replacement of the immune repertoire with adoptively transferred oligoclonal T cells was effective in inducing tumor regression but also led to immune compromise and, in some cases, opportunistic infections and lymphoproliferative disease. The development of serious autoimmune toxicities including skin rash, vitiligo, and uveitis (treatable with topical glucocorticoids) were consistent with shared melanocyte antigen expression among normal tissues.

Investigators postulated that more intensive conditioning regimens would yield higher response rates[136]; hence, total body irradiation (TBI) was added to cyclophosphamide and fludarabine. A nonmyeloablative dose of 2 Gy failed to improve response rates, while a myeloablative regimen incorporating 12 Gy TBI and coadministration of CD34+ hematopoietic stem cells achieved historically superior rates of > 70%.[134] These results, while highly significant, represent only the select population of patients with advanced melanoma who are able to tolerate life-threatening toxicities associated with a myeloablative HSCT and high-dose IL-2, have undergone fewer lines of prior therapy than patients receiving nonmyeloablative regimens, and present with accessible tumor from which TIL can be cultivated. The durability of these responses and reproducibility of such a dramatically improved response rate remain to be evaluated in multi-institution–based Phase II and III randomized trials.

The results of these studies nevertheless raise important questions: What are the extrinsic factors contributing to the long-term persistence of transferred T cells, the role of lipopolysaccharide (LPS) arising from bacterial translocation, the contribution of homeostatic cytokines, and the elimination of suppressor components? What intrinsic factors represented by differentiation or phenotypic features can be used to identify, from among the heterogeneous TIL population, the effector cell responsible for melanoma eradication and long-term immunoprotection?

Although, phenotypically, the TIL population is comprised of IL-2–responding CD8, CD4, as well as NK and NKT cells,[22,137,138] it is believed that the antigen-specific T cells are dominant contributors to the antitumor effect. Dissecting the reasons for success or failure would require a more uniform population of antigen-specific T cells for adoptive therapy.

Antigen-Specific T Cells

The identification of class I– and, later, class II–restricted epitopes for melanoma antigens enabled the development of methods to generate antigen-specific CD8 and CD4 T cells in vitro for clinical trials.

At least 4 groups have utilized methods described above to isolate and expand antigen-specific CD8 T cells for adoptive therapy. Mitchell et al. used insect cells transduced with HLA-A2, CD80, to generate cultures of tyrosinase-specific CTL. Up to 5×10^8 T cells (10% to 30% of these being tyrosinase specific) were administered. In the absence of IL-2, transferred T cells were short lived and only modest clinical responses were observed. Conventional APCs (dendritic cells) pulsed with peptides of melanocyte-associated antigens were used by several groups to generate antigen-specific T cells for clinical trials. Using CD8 T-cell clones against gp100, MART1 or tyrosinase antigens expanded to 10^{10} cells/m² the Seattle group demonstrated for the first time that a uniform population of T cells persist in vivo in response to low-dose IL-2, traffic to antigen-positive sites in tumor and skin, elicit autoimmune and tumor-specific responses, and mediate clinically relevant responses (one third of patients experiencing CR, PR, or disease stabilization for up to 11 months in patients with progressive metastatic disease). Using unselected, melanoma-reactive cultured adoptively transferred MART-1–specific T cells, Mackensen et al. also achieved favorable clinical responses in three of ten patients with refractory metastatic disease and observed adoptive T cells homing to tumor sites as well as evidence of antigen-loss tumor variants suggesting an effective epitope-specific immune response.[139]

Conditioning regimens can also influence the in vivo persistence of adoptively transferred CTL clones. In one study, adoptively transferred CD8+ CTL clones infused following a regimen of dacarbazine persisted for more than 30 days postinfusion and produced a response rate of 43% in patients with metastatic melanoma.[4] To define a well tolerated conditioning regimen, Yee et al. evaluated, in sequential fashion, the influence of fludarabine lymphodepletion, using the identical CD8 T-cell clone administered first without and then with conditioning. A rise in serum IL-15 accompanying a threefold increase in in vivo persistence was observed among transferred clones following fludarabine compared with no conditioning. However, clinical responses were not substantially improved over previous studies, a result that may be attributable to the rebound increase in the proportion of FOXP3+ regulatory T cells arising after lymphocyte reconstitution.

In a corollary study, the nonmyeloablative regimen of high-dose cyclophosphamide (4 g/m²) as single-agent conditioning before the adoptive transfer of antigen-specific CD8 T-cell clones followed by low-dose IL-2 was evaluated and found to be well tolerated with no complications arising from the 7- to 10-day period of leukopenia yet was capable of achieving T-cell frequencies of 1% to 3% more than 12 months after infusion. Four of six patients with refractory metastatic melanoma on this study experienced tumor regression including one patient with a durable complete response and four with partial or stable responses.

CD4 T Cell Therapy

CD4 T cells play a central role not only in priming a CD8 response but also in the effector phase of cellular immunity by (a) mediating tumor killing directly against class II+ tumor targets or indirectly against class II–tumors following recognition of cross-presenting class II+ APCs and activation of nonspecific effectors such as macrophages or eosinophils[81–85]; (b) supporting the survival of transferred CD8+ CTL via lymphokines and other signals following antigen encounter[83,86–90]; and (c) maintaining CD8 effector function in vivo.[91,92]

The presence of CD4 T cells in EBV-reactive cell products appears to favor the in vivo persistence of CD8 T cells and induction of antitumor responses in patients with PTLD,[140] while, for melanoma patients, the cocultivated CD4 T cells in TIL cultures[141] and polyclonally expanded antigen-specific CTL[139] may provide a helper response to accompanying CD8 T cells.

The identification of a number of class II–restricted epitopes (e.g., tyrosinase, NY-ESO-1, MAGE-1)[142] afforded the opportunity to evaluate helper CD4 T-cell responses in patients with metastatic melanoma first in vaccine studies and subsequently in a first-in-human clinical trial using antigen-specific CD4 T cells in nine patients. NY-ESO-1 or tyrosinase-specific Th1-type CD4 T-cell clones were used to treat refractory metastatic melanoma at doses of up to 10^{10} cells/m^2. T-cell frequencies as high as 3% were observed for up to 2 months. Four patients experienced a partial response or disease stabilization and one patient had a durable complete response of greater than 3 years. In some patients, induction of endogenous responses to nontargeted antigens was also observed (i.e., "antigen-spreading") and may have contributed to a more complete response.[143] Antigen-spreading, whereby uptake and processing of killed tumor cells by APCs can result in cross-presentation of nontargeted antigens and broadening of a focused response, has been observed in previous preclinical and clinical vaccine studies and represents one strategy to circumvent the outgrowth of antigen-loss tumor variants.[144–147]

TCR and CAR Gene Therapy of Melanoma

Early studies demonstrated that redirecting T-cell specificity to melanoma and other tumor-associated antigens was feasible in human lymphocytes.[51,55,148,149] The first clinical trial evaluating genetically modified lymphocytes targeting melanoma was performed by Rosenberg and colleagues at the NCI. Evidence of tumor regression was observed, but limitations to the use of first generation vectors were apparent and may have been responsible for inefficiency of expression, mispairing with endogenous chains, and low TCR affinity. In a second trial performed by the same group at NCI, retroviral vectors encoding high-affinity TCR targeting MART-1 and gp100 antigens demonstrated improved response rates of up to 30% and augmented on-target autoimmune toxicity validating the in vivo potency of high-affinity receptors.[71,150]

Strategies to Enhance Adoptive T Cell Therapy

Clinical studies of adoptive therapy provide clear evidence of T cell–mediated tumor regression but also reveal limitations to achieving a durable complete response. These limitations are discussed below

as translational opportunities designed to enhance the persistence of adoptively transferred T cells and circumvent tumor resistance to T-cell immunity.

Augmenting In Vivo Persistence

In murine studies and clinical trials of adoptive therapy, long-lived T-cell responses demonstrate a strong correlation with tumor regression.[151,152] Antitumor responses following adoptive therapy are associated with T-cell expression of biological markers of enhanced survival such as maintenance of telomere length[153] and up-regulation of CD28 or CD27 in clonally persistent T cells both in vitro and in vivo. While transfer of CD4 T cells alone[143] or in combination with CD8 CTL facilitates tumor eradication by providing helper function to CTL,[152] CTL with helper-independent or enhanced replicative properties can also be effective. Efforts include engineering constitutive expression of γ-chain receptor cytokines, IL-2[154] or IL-15[155,156], telomerase enzyme[157,158], and antiapoptotic genes (Bcl-2 and Bcl-XL)[159,160] While these approaches were successful, and in some cases to the extent of immortalization, delivering proliferative signals in an antigen-driven fashion using a chimeric cytokine receptor or costimulatory fusion constructs would be more effective and minimize safety concerns.[161–164]

An alternative means of augmenting in vivo persistence involves the in vitro selection of T cells with enhanced replicative capacity. It was demonstrated in a nonhuman primate model that antigen-specific effector T cells generated from a selected central memory pool of T cells (T_{CM}, phenotypically defined as CD45RO+, CD62L+)[165] persisted significantly longer in vivo than those derived from effector memory cells (T_{EM}, CD45RO+, CD62L−) and migrated preferentially to anatomic memory compartments.[166] Studies performed in a TCR-transgenic mouse model of melanoma (p-mel) suggested that "early" antigen-specific effector cells were more effective than "late" effectors in mediating tumor regression[167] and further, that naïve T cells were superior to T_{CM} in treating established tumor. Translating these results to clinical trials could be achieved by TCR or CAR gene transfer into the desired effector population.

Other approaches that exploit the intrinsic capacity of T cells to a proliferative advantage include the use of IL-21 or Wnt modulators to arrest differentiation, thus yielding a population of central-memory–like, helper-independent, CD28+ effector cells,[168] and the use of the extant EBV-specific T cell pool present in most individuals as host cells for redirected antigen specificity (retargeting to a tumor-associated antigen). In this latter case, in vivo engagement of the native EBV-specific TCR contributed to its superior in vivo persistence and antitumor efficacy when compared to *unselected* host T cells redirected to the same tumor-associated antigen.[69] In this approach, the host EBV-infected cell serves as an in vivo stimulator cell and optimally activates the dual receptor T cell. The concept of in vivo reactivation can be applied to conventional T cells by coadministering a tumor antigen vaccine. Preclinical studies in a murine model demonstrate that in certain cases, vaccine treatment following adoptive therapy was essential for eradicating established tumor,[169] a model which supports a combined modality approach and borne out in at least one clinical study demonstrating the effectiveness of a postinfusion vaccine in boosting a transferred T-cell response.[35]

Circumventing Mechanisms of Immune Escape

The existence of regulatory or suppressor T cells was predicted more than 30 years ago in murine models and they have only recently been phenotypically defined in humans. One type of regulatory cell, the CD4$^+$ Treg, plays a critical role in suppressing the endogenous antitumor immune response, and eliminating these regulatory cells can lead to enhanced tumor immunity.

In humans, CD4 regulatory T cells (Treg) that comprise 5% to 10% of all CD4 cells in peripheral blood have been found to be elevated in cancer-bearing individuals and are phenotypically characterized as CD4$^+$ cells constitutively expressing high levels of surface CD25, GITR, and CTLA4 and low levels of CD127. Treg CD4 cells can be further distinguished by expression of the forkhead transcription factor, FOXP3[21], that plays a fundamental role in their development. Strategies to deplete Tregs in vivo include the use of lymphodepleting reagents such as cyclophosphamide, but more selective depletion can be achieved by targeting CD25 or GITR (Fig. 33-2).

Myeloid-derived suppressor cells (MDSC) have become an increasingly important consideration in tumor immunity and represent a heterogeneous population of myeloid cells with potent T cell suppressive function. They appear to act in part by depleting L-arginine (required for arginine-dependent T-cell proliferation), through arginase and inducible nitric oxide synthase activity, the latter leading to synthesis of nitric oxide (NO), which also contributes to T-cell effector suppression. Specific pharmacologic inhibitors can significantly reduce Arg-1 and NOS-2 expression in MDSC.

Soluble factors in the tumor microenvironment, such as TGF-β, IL-10, and metabolites generated by indoleamine 2,3-dioxygenase (IDO), can suppress the effector T-cell response. These mechanisms can be addressed by rendering T cells resistant to TGF-beta by genetic modification, anti–IL-10 therapy, and metabolic inhibitors of IDO activity.

Finally, up-regulation of checkpoint inhibitors in T-cell proliferation, designed to prevent overexuberant cell-mediated responses, can also inhibit T-cell antitumor activity. Antibodies that intervene in the CTLA4-B7 and PD1-PDL1 pathways are being used in clinical trials as single agents to significant positive effect and represent a rational choice for combined therapy with adoptively transferred T cells as a means of releasing the "brake" on autoreactive antitumor T cells and decreasing the threshold for inducing nontargeted endogenous T-cell responses (antigen-spreading).

Conclusions

Clinical studies of adoptive T cell therapy have produced unprecedented success in the treatment of patients with advanced disease that is often refractory to conventional therapy. As an approach that can be effective in chemo- and radio-resistant disease and that offers the potential for long-term immunoprotection, adoptive therapy remains an attractive modality. However, limitations to adoptive cellular therapy must be addressed before it can be accepted as a feasible treatment option in clinical practice. These goals include establishing a reliable protocol for generating tumor-reactive, highly persistent, effector population in a timely,

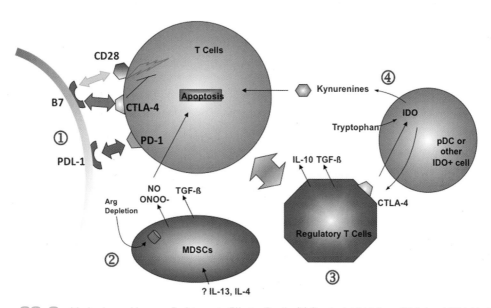

FIGURE 33-2   Mechanisms of Immune Resistance to Effector T cells. (**1**) Checkpoint inhibitors, CTLA-4 and PD-1 block T-cell response. CTLA-4 surface expression is up-regulated following T-cell activation, competes for B7-CD28 interaction, and inhibits CD28 signaling. PDL-1 binds to PD-1 on T cells and inhibits T-cell proliferation and function. Antibodies to CTLA4, PD-1, and PDL-1 block T-cell inhibition and enhance the autoimmune as well as antitumor immune response. (**2**) MDSCs inhibit T-cell function through local arginine depletion secondary to arginase and nitric oxide synthase activity and release of peroxynitrite and TGF-beta. COX-2 inhibitors and PDE-5 block MDSC activity. T cells engineered to express dominant negative TGF-beta receptor are resistant to TGF-beta. (**3**) Regulatory CD4 T cells (Treg) inhibit effector function through cell-cell contact, release of inhibitory IL-10 and TGF-beta, as well as IDO induction in nearby DCs via CTLA-4. Depletion of Treg cells may be achieved using antibodies to CD25 or to GITR and an IL-2-toxin conjugate that binds to CD25 (IL-2Rα). (**4**) Plasmacytoid DCs and other IDO-positive cells metabolize tryptophan to kynurenines that induce T-cell apoptosis. IDO mediates positive reciprocal effect on Tregs. 1-MT, a tryptophan analog, blocks IDO activity.

accessible, and reproducible manner and administering the effector cells in the context of the appropriate clinical setting, patient conditioning, and immunomodulatory support accompanied by the judicious application of a comprehensive strategy to monitor the immunologic consequences of the transferred T-cell response and the tumor response to immunosurveillance.

Underpinning these translational objectives will be the need to capitalize on advances in understanding basic aspects of T-cell biology and mechanisms of tumor immune resistance, which will continue to provide a rich source of innovation to this field.

References

1. Schwartentruber DJ, Hom SS, Dadmarz R. In vitro predictors of therapeutic response in melanoma patients receiving tumor-infiltrating lymphocytes and interleukin-2. J Clin Oncol 1994;12:1475–1483.

2. Figlin RA, Thompson JA, Bukowski RM, et al. Multicenter, randomized, phase III trial of CD8(+) tumor-infiltrating lymphocytes in combination with recombinant interleukin-2 in metastatic renal cell carcinoma. J Clin Oncol 1999;17:2521–2529.

3. Dreno B, Nguyen JM, Khammari A, et al. Randomized trial of adoptive transfer of melanoma tumor-infiltrating lymphocytes as adjuvant therapy for stage III melanoma. Cancer Immunol Immunother 2002;51:539–546.

4. Khammari A, Nguyen JM, Pandolfino MC, et al. Long-term follow-up of patients treated by adoptive transfer of melanoma tumor-infiltrating lymphocytes as adjuvant therapy for stage III melanoma. Cancer Immunol Immunother 2007;56:1853–1860.

5. Van Der Bruggen P, Zhang Y, Chaux P, et al. Tumor-specific shared antigenic peptides recognized by human T cells. Immunol Rev 2002;188:51–64.

6. van der Bruggen P, Traversari C, Chomez P, et al. A gene encoding an antigen recognized by cytolytic T lymphocytes on a human melanoma. Science 1991;254:1643–1647.

7. Scanlan MJ, Simpson AJ, Old LJ. The cancer/testis genes: review, standardization, and commentary. Cancer Immun 2004;4:1.

8. Coulie PG, Brichard V, Van Pel A, et al. A new gene coding for a differentiation antigen recognized by autologous cytolytic T lymphocytes on HLA-A2 melanomas [see comments]. J Exp Med 1994;180:35–42.

9. Kawakami Y, Eliyahu S, Delgado CH, et al. Identification of a human melanoma antigen recognized by tumor-infiltrating lymphocytes associated with in vivo tumor rejection. Proc Natl Acad Sci U S A 1994;91:6458–6462.

10. Kawakami Y, Eliyahu S, Delgado CH, et al. Cloning of the gene coding for a shared human melanoma antigen recognized by autologous T cells infiltrating into tumor. Proc Natl Acad Sciences U S A 1994;91:3515–3519.

11. Van den Eynde BJ, van der Bruggen P. T cell defined tumor antigens. Curr Opin Immunol 1997;9:684–693.

12. Warren EH, Vigneron NJ, Gavin MA, et al. An antigen produced by splicing of noncontiguous peptides in the reverse order. Science 2006;313:1444–1447.

13. Dunn GP, Old LJ, Schreiber RD. The immunobiology of cancer immunosurveillance and immunoediting. Immunity 2004;21:137–148.

14. Hou Y, Kavanagh B, Fong L. Distinct CD8+ T cell repertoires primed with agonist and native peptides derived from a tumor-associated antigen. J Immunol 2008;180:1526–1534.

15. Kazansky DB. Intrathymic selection: new insight into tumor immunology. Adv Exp Med Biol 2007;601:133–144.

16. McMahan RH, Slansky JE. Mobilizing the low-avidity T cell repertoire to kill tumors. Semin Cancer Biol 2007;17:317–329.

17. Morgan DJ, Kreuwel HT, Fleck S, et al. Activation of low avidity CTL specific for a self epitope results in tumor rejection but not autoimmunity. J Immunol 1998;160:643–651.

18. Ohashi PS, Oehen S, Buerki K, et al. Ablation of "tolerance" and induction of diabetes by virus infection in viral antigen transgenic mice. Cell 1991;65:305–317.

19. Zehn D, Bevan MJ. T cells with low avidity for a tissue-restricted antigen routinely evade central and peripheral tolerance and cause autoimmunity. Immunity 2006;25:261–270.

20. Chen JL, Dunbar PR, Gileadi U, et al. Identification of NY-ESO-1 peptide analogues capable of improved stimulation of tumor-reactive CTL. J Immunol 2000;165:948–955.

21. Valmori D, Fonteneau JF, Lizana CM, et al. Enhanced generation of specific tumor-reactive CTL in vitro by selected Melan-A/MART-1 immunodominant peptide analogues. J Immunol 1998;160:1750–1758.

22. Fong L, Hou Y, Rivas A, et al. Altered peptide ligand vaccination with Flt3 ligand expanded dendritic cells for tumor immunotherapy. Proc Natl Acad Sci U S A 2001;98:8809–8814.

23. Rivoltini L, Kawakami Y, Sakaguchi K, et al. Induction of tumor-reactive CTL from peripheral blood and tumor-infiltrating lymphocytes of melanoma patients by in vitro stimulation with an immunodominant peptide of the human melanoma antigen MART-1. J Immunol 1995;154:2257–2265.

24. Dubsky P, Saito H, Leogier M, et al. IL-15-induced human DC efficiently prime melanoma-specific naive CD8+ T cells to differentiate into CTL. Eur J Immunol 2007;37:1678–1690.

25. Mohamadzadeh M, Berard F, Essert G, et al. Interleukin 15 skews monocyte differentiation into dendritic cells with features of Langerhans cells. J Exp Med 2001;194:1013–1020.

26. Davis ID, Chen Q, Morris L, et al. Blood dendritic cells generated with Flt3 ligand and CD40 ligand prime CD8+ T cells efficiently in cancer patients. J Immunother 2006;29:499–511.

27. von Bergwelt-Baildon MS, Vonderheide RH, Maecker B, et al. Human primary and memory cytotoxic T lymphocyte responses are efficiently induced by means of CD40-activated B cells as antigen-presenting cells: potential for clinical application. Blood 2002;99:3319–3325.

28. Buhmann R, Nolte A, Westhaus D, et al. CD40-activated B-cell chronic lymphocytic leukemia cells for tumor immunotherapy: stimulation of allogeneic versus autologous T cells generates different types of effector cells. Blood 1999;93:1992–2002.

29. Li Y, Bleakley M, Yee C. IL-21 Influences the frequency, phenotype, and affinity of the antigen-specific CD8 T cell response. J Immunol 2005;175:2261–2269.

30. Latouche JB, Sadelain M. Induction of human cytotoxic T lymphocytes by artificial antigen-presenting cells. Nat Biotechnol 2000;18:405–409.

31. Mitchell MS. Phase I trial of adoptive immunotherapy with cytolytic T lymphocytes immunized against a tyrosinase epitope. J Clin Oncol 2002;20:1075–1086.

32. Butler MO, Lee JS, Ansen S, et al. Long-lived antitumor CD8+ lymphocytes for adoptive therapy generated using an artificial antigen-presenting cell. Clin Cancer Res 2007;13:1857–1867.

33. Ansen S, Butler MO, Berezovskaya A, et al. Dissociation of its opposing immunologic effects is critical for the optimization of antitumor CD8+ T-cell responses induced by interleukin 21. Clin Cancer Res 2008;14:6125–6136.

34. Rapoport AP, Stadtmauer EA, Aqui N, et al. Rapid immune recovery and graft-versus-host disease-like engraftment syndrome following adoptive transfer of Costimulated autologous T cells. Clin Cancer Res 2009;15:4499–4507.

35. Rapoport AP, Stadtmauer EA, Aqui N, et al. Restoration of immunity in lymphopenic individuals with cancer by vaccination and adoptive T-cell transfer. Nat Med 2005;11:1230–1237.

36. Porter DL, Levine BL, Bunin N, et al. A phase 1 trial of donor lymphocyte infusions expanded and activated ex vivo via CD3/CD28 costimulation. Blood 2006;107:1325–1331.

37. Ugel S, Zoso A, De Santo C, et al. In vivo administration of artificial antigen-presenting cells activates low-avidity T cells for treatment of cancer. Cancer Res 2009;69:9376–9384.

38. Pittet MJ, Valmori D, Dunbar PR, et al. High frequencies of naive Melan-A/MART-1-specific CD8(+) T cells in a large proportion of human histocompatibility leukocyte antigen (HLA)-A2 individuals. J Exp Med 1999;190:705–715.

39. Jager E, Chen YT, Drijfhout JW, et al. Simultaneous humoral and cellular immune response against cancer-testis antigen NY-ESO-1: definition of human histocompatibility leukocyte antigen (HLA)-A2-binding peptide epitopes. J Exp Med 1998;187:265–270.

40. Yee C, Thompson JA, Byrd D, et al. Adoptive T cell therapy using antigen-specific CD8+ T cell clones for the treatment of patients with metastatic melanoma: in vivo persistence, migration, and antitumor effect of transferred T cells. Proc Natl Acad Sci U S A 2002;99:16168–16173.

41. Riddell SR, Greenberg PD. The use of anti-CD3 and anti-CD28 monoclonal antibodies to clone and expand human antigen-specific T cells. J Immunol Meth 1990;128:189–201.

42. Thomas AK, Maus MV, Shalaby WS, et al. A cell-based artificial antigen-presenting cell coated with anti-CD3 and CD28 antibodies enables rapid expansion and long-term growth of CD4 T lymphocytes. Clin Immunol 2002;105:259–272.

43. Altman JD, Moss PAH, Goulder PJR, et al. Phenotypic analysis of antigen-specific T lymphocytes [published erratum appears in Science 1998 Jun 19;280(5371):1821]. Science 1996;274:94–96.

44. Yee C, Savage PA, Lee PP, et al. Isolation of high avidity melanoma-reactive CTL from heterogeneous populations using peptide-MHC tetramers. J Immunol 1999;162:2227–2234.

45. Schneck JP. Monitoring antigen-specific T cells using MHC-Ig dimers. Immunol Invest 2000;29:163–169.

46. Novak EJ, Liu AW, Nepom GT, et al. MHC class II tetramers identify peptide-specific human CD4(+) T cells proliferating in response to influenza A antigen [see comments]. J Clin Invest 1999;104:R63–R67.

47. Becker C, Pohla H, Frankenberger B, et al. Adoptive tumor therapy with T lymphocytes enriched through an IFN-gamma capture assay. Nat Med 2001;7:1159–1162.

48. Wolfl M, Kuball J, Ho WY, et al. Activation-induced expression of CD137 permits detection, isolation, and expansion of the full repertoire of CD8+ T cells responding to antigen without requiring knowledge of epitope specificities. Blood 2007;110:201–210.

49. Duval L, Schmidt H, Kaltoft K, et al. Adoptive transfer of allogeneic cytotoxic T lymphocytes equipped with a HLA-A2 restricted MART-1 T-cell receptor: a phase I trial in metastatic melanoma. Clin Cancer Res 2006;12:1229–1236.

50. Morgan RA, Dudley ME, Wunderlich JR, et al. Cancer regression in patients after transfer of genetically engineered lymphocytes. Science 2006;314:126–129.

51. Clay TM, Custer MC, Sachs J, et al. Efficient transfer of a tumor antigen-reactive TCR to human peripheral blood lymphocytes confers anti-tumor reactivity. J Immunol 1999;163:507–513.

52. Cohen CJ, Zhao Y, Zheng Z, et al. Enhanced antitumor activity of murine-human hybrid T-cell receptor (TCR) in human lymphocytes is associated with improved pairing and TCR/CD3 stability. Cancer Res 2006;66:8878–8886.

53. Kuball J, Dossett ML, Wolfl M, et al. Facilitating matched pairing and expression of TCR chains introduced into human T cells. Blood 2007;109:2331–2338.

54. Voss RH, Willemsen RA, Kuball J, et al. Molecular design of the Calpha-beta interface favors specific pairing of introduced TCR alphabeta in human T cells. J Immunol 2008;180:391–401.

55. Schmitt TM, Ragnarsson GB, Greenberg PD. T cell receptor gene therapy for cancer. Hum Gene Ther 2009;20(11):1240–1248.

56. Okamoto S, Mineno J, Ikeda H, et al. Improved expression and reactivity of transduced tumor-specific TCRs in human lymphocytes by specific silencing of endogenous TCR. Cancer Res 2009;69:9003–9011.

57. Kuball J, Hauptrock B, Malina V, et al. Increasing functional avidity of TCR-redirected T cells by removing defined N-glycosylation sites in the TCR constant domain. J Exp Med 2009;206:463–475.

58. Holler PD, Holman PO, Shusta EV, et al. In vitro evolution of a T cell receptor with high affinity for peptide/MHC. Proc Natl Acad Sci U S A 2000;97:5387–5392.

59. Kessels HW. Immunotherapy through TCR gene transfer. [see comments.]. Nat Immunol 2001;2:957–961.

60. Moore TV, Lyons GE, Brasic N, et al. Relationship between CD8-dependent antigen recognition, T cell functional avidity, and tumor cell recognition. Cancer Immunol Immunother 2009;58:719–728.

61. Deichmann A, Hacein-Bey-Abina S, Schmidt M, et al. Vector integration is nonrandom and clustered and influences the fate of lymphopoiesis in SCID-X1 gene therapy. J Clin Invest 2007;117:2225–2232.

62. Peng PD, Cohen CJ, Yang S, et al. Efficient nonviral Sleeping Beauty transposon-based TCR gene transfer to peripheral blood lymphocytes confers antigen-specific antitumor reactivity. Gene Ther 2009;16:1042–1049.

63. Eshhar Z, Waks T, Gross G, et al. Specific activation and targeting of cytotoxic lymphocytes through chimeric single chains consisting of antibody-binding domains and the gamma or zeta subunits of the immunoglobulin and T-cell receptors. Proc Natl Acad Sci U S A 1993;90:720–724.

64. Berry LJ, Moeller M, Darcy PK. Adoptive immunotherapy for cancer: the next generation of gene-engineered immune cells. Tissue Antigens 2009;74:277–289.

65. Park JR, Digiusto DL, Slovak M, et al. Adoptive transfer of chimeric antigen receptor re-directed cytolytic T lymphocyte clones in patients with neuroblastoma. Mol Ther 2007;15:825–833.

66. Till BG, Jensen MC, Wang J, et al. Adoptive immunotherapy for indolent non-Hodgkin lymphoma and mantle cell lymphoma using genetically modified autologous CD20-specific T cells. Blood 2008;112:2261–2271.

67. Kershaw MH, Westwood JA, Parker LL, et al. A phase I study on adoptive immunotherapy using gene-modified T cells for ovarian cancer. Clin Cancer Res 2006;12:6106–6115.

68. Lamers CH, Sleijfer S, Vulto AG, et al. Treatment of metastatic renal cell carcinoma with autologous T-lymphocytes genetically retargeted against carbonic anhydrase IX: first clinical experience. J Clin Oncol 2006;24:e20–e22.

69. Pule MA, Savoldo B, Myers GD, et al. Virus-specific T cells engineered to coexpress tumor-specific receptors: persistence and antitumor activity in individuals with neuroblastoma. Nat Med 2008;14:1264–1270.

70. Weiden PL, Sullivan KM, Flournoy N, et al. Antileukemic effect of chronic graft-versus-host disease: contribution to improved survival after allogeneic marrow transplantation. N Engl J Med 1981;304:1529–1533.

71. Johnson LA, Morgan RA, Dudley ME, et al. Gene therapy with human and mouse T-cell receptors mediates cancer regression and targets normal tissues expressing cognate antigen. Blood 2009;114:535–546.

72. Dazzi F, Szydlo RM, Cross NC, et al. Durability of responses following donor lymphocyte infusions for patients who relapse after allogeneic stem cell transplantation for chronic myeloid leukemia. Blood 2000;96:2712–2716.

73. Kolb HJ, Mittermuller J, Clemm C, et al. Donor leukocyte transfusions for treatment of recurrent chronic myelogenous leukemia in marrow transplant patients. Blood 1990;76:2462–2465.

74. Soiffer RJ, Alyea EP, Hochberg E, et al. Randomized trial of CD8+ T-cell depletion in the prevention of graft-versus-host disease associated with donor lymphocyte infusion. Biol Blood Marrow Transplant 2002;8:625–632.

75. Verdonck LF, Lokhorst HM, Dekker AW, et al. Graft-versus-myeloma effect in two cases. Lancet 1996;347:800–801.

76. Okas M, Gertow J, Uzunel M, et al. Clinical expansion of cord blood-derived T cells for use as donor lymphocyte infusion after cord blood transplantation. J Immunother 2010;33:96–105.

77. Mazur MA, Davis CC, Szabolcs P. Ex vivo expansion and Th1/Tc1 maturation of umbilical cord blood T cells by CD3/CD28 costimulation. Biol Blood Marrow Transplant 2008;14:1190–1196.

78. Kwak LW, Taub DD, Duffey PL, et al. Transfer of myeloma idiotype-specific immunity from an actively immunised marrow donor. Lancet 1995;345:1016–1020.

79. Neelapu SS, Munshi NC, Jagannath S, et al. Tumor antigen immunization of sibling stem cell transplant donors in multiple myeloma. Bone Marrow Transplant 2005;36:315–323.

80. Kwak LW, Pennington R, Longo DL. Active immunization of murine allogeneic bone marrow transplant donors with B-cell tumor-derived idiotype: a strategy for enhancing the specific antitumor effect of marrow grafts. Blood 1996;87:3053–3060.

81. den Haan JM, Sherman NE, Blokland E, et al. Identification of a graft versus host disease-associated human minor histocompatibility antigen. Science 1995;268:1476–1480.

82. Wang W, Meadows LR, den Haan JM, et al. Human H-Y: a male-specific histocompatibility antigen derived from the SMCY protein. Science 1995;269:1588–1590.

83. Rosinski KV, Fujii N, Mito JK, et al. DDX3Y encodes a class I MHC-restricted H-Y antigen that is expressed in leukemic stem cells. Blood 2008;111:4817–4826.

84. Bonnet D, Warren EH, Greenberg PD, et al. CD8(+) minor histocompatibility antigen-specific cytotoxic T lymphocyte clones eliminate human acute myeloid leukemia stem cells. Proc Natl Acad Sci U S A 1999;96:8639–8644.

85. Miyazaki M, Akatsuka Y, Nishida T, et al. Potential limitations in using minor histocompatibility antigen-specific cytotoxic T cells for targeting solid tumor cells. Clin Immunol 2003;107:198–201.

86. Klein CA, Wilke M, Pool J, et al. The hematopoietic system-specific minor histocompatibility antigen HA-1 shows aberrant expression in epithelial cancer cells. J Exp Med 2002;196:359–368.

87. Tykodi SS, Fujii N, Vigneron N, et al. C19 or f48 encodes a minor histocompatibility antigen recognized by CD8+ cytotoxic T cells from renal cell carcinoma patients. Clin Cancer Res 2008;14:5260–5269.

88. Spierings E. Minor histocompatibility antigens: targets for tumour therapy and transplant tolerance. Int J Immunogenet 2008;35:363–366.

89. Warren EH, Fujii N, Akatsuka Y, et al. Therapy of relapsed leukemia after allogeneic hematopoietic cell transplant with T cells specific for minor histocompatibility antigens. Blood 2010;115(19):3869–3878.

90. Bergmann L, Miething C, Maurer U, et al. High levels of Wilms' tumor gene (wt1) mRNA in acute myeloid leukemias are associated with a worse long-term outcome. Blood 1997;90:1217–1225.

91. Ohminami H, Yasukawa M, Fujita S. HLA class I-restricted lysis of leukemia cells by a CD8(+) cytotoxic T-lymphocyte clone specific for WT1 peptide. Blood 2000;95:286–293.

92. Scheibenbogen C, Letsch A, Thiel E, et al. CD8 T-cell responses to Wilms tumor gene product WT1 and proteinase 3 in patients with acute myeloid leukemia. Blood 2002;100:2132–2137.

93. van Baren N, Chambost H, Ferrant A, et al. PRAME, a gene encoding an antigen recognized on a human melanoma by cytolytic T cells, is expressed in acute leukaemia cells. Br J Haematol 1998;102:1376–1379.

94. Kessler JH, Beekman NJ, Bres-Vloemans SA, et al. Efficient identification of novel HLA-A(*)0201-presented cytotoxic T lymphocyte epitopes in the widely expressed tumor antigen PRAME by proteasome-mediated digestion analysis. J Exp Med 2001;193:73–88.

95. Molldrem JJ, Clave E, Jiang YZ, et al. Cytotoxic T lymphocytes specific for a nonpolymorphic proteinase 3 peptide preferentially inhibit chronic myeloid leukemia colony-forming units. Blood 1997;90:2529–2534.

96. Rezvani K, Grube M, Brenchley JM, et al. Functional leukemia-associated antigen-specific memory CD8+ T cells exist in healthy individuals and in patients with chronic myelogenous leukemia before and after stem cell transplantation. Blood 2003;102:2892–2900.

97. Yong AS, Rezvani K, Savani BN, et al. High PR3 or ELA2 expression by CD34+ cells in advanced-phase chronic myeloid leukemia is associated with improved outcome following allogeneic stem cell transplantation and may improve PR1 peptide-driven graft-versus-leukemia effects. Blood 2007;110:770–775.

98. Fouret P, du Bois RM, Bernaudin JF, et al. Expression of the neutrophil elastase gene during human bone marrow cell differentiation. J Exp Med 1989;169:833–845.

99. Fujiwara H, El Ouriaghli F, Grube M, et al. Identification and in vitro expansion of CD4+ and CD8+ T cells specific for human neutrophil elastase. Blood 2004;103:3076–3083.

100. Weber G, Karbach J, Kuci S, et al. WT1 peptide-specific T cells generated from peripheral blood of healthy donors: possible implications for adoptive immunotherapy after allogeneic stem cell transplantation. Leukemia 2009;23:1634–1642.

101. Ho WY, Nguyen HN, Wolfl M, et al. In vitro methods for generating CD8+ T-cell clones for immunotherapy from the naive repertoire. J Immunol Methods 2006;310:40–52.

102. Brewin J, Mancao C, Straathof K, et al. Generation of EBV-specific cytotoxic T cells that are resistant to calcineurin inhibitors for the treatment of posttransplantation lymphoproliferative disease. Blood 2009;114:4792–4803.

103. De Angelis B, Dotti G, Quintarelli C, et al. Generation of Epstein-Barr virus-specific cytotoxic T lymphocytes resistant to the immunosuppressive drug tacrolimus (FK506). Blood 2009;114:4784–4791.

104. Berger C, Turtle CJ, Jensen MC, et al. Adoptive transfer of virus-specific and tumor-specific T cell immunity. Curr Opin Immunol 2009;21:224–232.

105. Papadopoulos EB, Ladanyi M, Emanuel D, et al. Infusions of donor leukocytes to treat Epstein-Barr virus-associated lymphoproliferative disorders after allogeneic bone marrow transplantation. N Engl J Med 1994;330:1185–1191.

106. Heslop HE, Slobod KS, Pule MA, et al. Long-term outcome of EBV-specific T-cell infusions to prevent or treat EBV-related lymphoproliferative disease in transplant recipients. Blood 2010;115:925–935.

107. Savoldo B, Goss JA, Hammer MM, et al. Treatment of solid organ transplant recipients with autologous Epstein Barr virus-specific cytotoxic T lymphocytes (CTLs). Blood 2006;108:2942–2949.

108. Comoli P, Labirio M, Basso S, et al. Infusion of autologous Epstein-Barr virus (EBV)-specific cytotoxic T cells for prevention of EBV-related lymphoproliferative disorder in solid organ transplant recipients with evidence of active virus replication. Blood 2002;99:2592–2598.

109. Sherritt MA, Bharadwaj M, Burrows JM, et al. Reconstitution of the latent T-lymphocyte response to Epstein-Barr virus is coincident with long-term recovery from posttransplant lymphoma after adoptive immunotherapy. Transplantation 2003;75:1556–1560.

110. Straathof KC, Bollard CM, Popat U, et al. Treatment of nasopharyngeal carcinoma with Epstein-Barr virus–specific T lymphocytes. Blood 2005;105:1898–1904.

111. Rooney CM, Bollard C, Huls MH, et al. Immunotherapy for Hodgkin's disease. Ann Hematol 2002;81(Suppl 2):S39–S42.

112. Comoli P, Pedrazzoli P, Maccario R, et al. Cell therapy of stage IV nasopharyngeal carcinoma with autologous Epstein-Barr virus-targeted cytotoxic T lymphocytes. J Clin Oncol 2005;23:8942–8949.

113. Bollard CM, Aguilar L, Straathof KC, et al. Cytotoxic T lymphocyte therapy for Epstein-Barr virus+ Hodgkin's disease. J Exp Med 2004;200:1623–1633.

114. Roskrow MA, Suzuki N, Gan Y, et al. Epstein-Barr virus (EBV)-specific cytotoxic T lymphocytes for the treatment of patients with EBV-positive relapsed Hodgkin's disease. Blood 1998;91:2925–2934.

115. Bollard CM, Gottschalk S, Leen AM, et al. Complete responses of relapsed lymphoma following genetic modification of tumor-antigen presenting cells and T-lymphocyte transfer. Blood 2007;110:2838–2845.

116. Lee SP, Tierney RJ, Thomas WA, et al. Conserved CTL epitopes within EBV latent membrane protein 2: a potential target for CTL-based tumor therapy. J Immunol 1997;158:3325–3334.

117. Sing AP, Ambinder RF, Hong DJ, et al. Isolation of Epstein-Barr virus (EBV)-specific cytotoxic T lymphocytes that lyse Reed-Sternberg cells: implications for immune-mediated therapy of EBV+ Hodgkin's disease. Blood 1997;89:1978–1986.

118. Di Stasi A, De Angelis B, Rooney CM, et al. T lymphocytes coexpressing CCR4 and a chimeric antigen receptor targeting CD30 have improved homing and antitumor activity in a Hodgkin tumor model. Blood 2009;113:6392–6402.

119. Vera JF, Hoyos V, Savoldo B, et al. Genetic manipulation of tumor-specific cytotoxic T lymphocytes to restore responsiveness to IL-7. Mol Ther 2009;17:880–888.

120. Foster AE, Dotti G, Lu A, et al. Antitumor activity of EBV-specific T lymphocytes transduced with a dominant negative TGF-beta receptor. J Immunother 2008;31:500–505.

121. Rosenberg SA, Lotze MT, Muul LM, et al. Observations on the systemic administration of autologous lymphokine-activated killer cells and recombinant interleukin-2 to patients with metastatic cancer. N Engl J Med 1985;313:1485–1492.

122. Rosenberg SA, Lotze MT, Muul LM, et al. A progress report on the treatment of 157 patients with advanced cancer using lymphokine-activated killer cells and interleukin-2 or high-dose interleukin-2 alone. N Engl J Med 1987;316:889–897.

123. Dillman RO, Oldham RK, Tauer KW, et al. Continuous interleukin-2 and lymphokine-activated killer cells for advanced cancer: a National Biotherapy Study Group trial. J Clin Oncol 1991;9:1233–1240.

124. Rosenberg SA, Lotze MT, Yang JC, et al. Prospective randomized trial of high-dose interleukin-2 alone or in conjunction with lymphokine-activated killer cells for the treatment of patients with advanced cancer. J Natl Cancer Inst 1993;85:622–632.

125. Spiess PJ, Yang JC, Rosenberg SA. In vivo antitumor activity of tumor-infiltrating lymphocytes expanded in recombinant interleukin-2. J Natl Cancer Inst 1987;79:1067–1075.

126. Rosenberg SA, Spiess P, Lafreniere R. A new approach to the adoptive immunotherapy of cancer with tumor-infiltrating lymphocytes. Science 1986;233:1318–1321.

127. Yron I, Wood TA Jr, Spiess PJ, et al. In vitro growth of murine T cells. V. The isolation and growth of lymphoid cells infiltrating syngeneic solid tumors. J Immunol 1980;125:238–245.

128. Rosenberg SA, Packard BS, Aebersold PM, et al. Use of tumor-infiltrating lymphocytes and interleukin-2 in the immunotherapy of patients with metastatic melanoma. A preliminary report. N Engl J Med 1988;319: 1676–1680.

129. Rosenberg SA, Yannelli JR, Yang JC, et al. Treatment of patients with metastatic melanoma with autologous tumor-infiltrating lymphocytes and interleukin 2. J Natl Cancer Inst 1994;86:1159–1166.

130. Crossland KD, Lee VK, Chen W, et al. T cells from tumor-immune mice nonspecifically expanded in vitro with anti-CD3 plus IL-2 retain specific function in vitro and can eradicate disseminated leukemia in vivo. J Immunol 1991;146:4414–4420.

131. Mule JJ, Shu S, Rosenberg SA. The anti-tumor efficacy of lymphokine-activated killer cells and recombinant interleukin 2 in vivo. J Immunol 1985;135:646–652.

132. Awwad M, North RJ. Cyclophosphamide (Cy)-facilitated adoptive immunotherapy of a Cy-resistant tumour. Evidence that Cy permits the expression of adoptive T-cell mediated immunity by removing suppressor T cells rather than by reducing tumour burden. Immunology 1988;65:87–92.

133. Dudley ME, Wunderlich JR, Yang JC, et al. Adoptive cell transfer therapy following non-myeloablative but lymphodepleting chemotherapy for the treatment of patients with refractory metastatic melanoma. J Clin Oncol 2005;23:2346–2357.

134. Dudley ME, Yang JC, Sherry R, et al. Adoptive cell therapy for patients with metastatic melanoma: evaluation of intensive myeloablative chemoradiation preparative regimens. J Clin Oncol 2008;26:5233–5239.

135. Dudley ME, Wunderlich JR, Yang JC, et al. A phase I study of nonmyeloablative chemotherapy and adoptive transfer of autologous tumor antigen-specific T lymphocytes in patients with metastatic melanoma. J Immunother 2002;25:243–251.

136. Wrzesinski C, Paulos CM, Kaiser A, et al. Increased intensity lymphodepletion enhances tumor treatment efficacy of adoptively transferred tumor-specific T cells. J Immunother 2010;33:1–7.

137. Topalian SL, Muul LM, Solomon D. Expansion of human tumor infiltrating lymphocytes for use in immunotherapy trials.. J Immunol Methods 1987;102:127–141.

138. Schleypen JS, Baur N, Kammerer R, et al. Cytotoxic markers and frequency predict functional capacity of natural killer cells infiltrating renal cell carcinoma. Clin Cancer Res 2006;12:718–725.

139. Mackensen A, Meidenbauer N, Vogl S, et al. Phase I study of adoptive T-cell therapy using antigen-specific CD8+ T cells for the treatment of patients with metastatic melanoma. J Clin Oncol 2006;24:5060–5069.

140. Hanley PJ, Cruz CR, Savoldo B, et al. Functionally active virus-specific T cells that target CMV, adenovirus, and EBV can be expanded from naive T-cell populations in cord blood and will target a range of viral epitopes. Blood 2009;114:1958–1967.

141. Sun JC, Bevan MJ. Defective CD8 T cell memory following acute infection without CD4 T cell help. Science 2003;300:339–342.

142. Topalian SL, Gonzales MI, Parkhurst M, et al. Melanoma-specific CD4+ T cells recognize nonmutated HLA-DR-restricted tyrosinase epitopes. J Exp Med 1996;183:1965–1971.

143. Hunder NN, Wallen H, Cao J, et al. Treatment of metastatic melanoma with autologous CD4+ T cells against NY-ESO-1. N Engl J Med 2008;358:2698–2703.

144. Boon T, Van Pel A. Teratocarcinoma cell variants rejected by syngeneic mice: protection of mice immunized with these variants against other variants and against the original malignant cell line. Proc Natl Acad Sci U S A 1978;75:1519–1523.

145. Lally KM, Mocellin S, Ohnmacht GA, et al. Unmasking cryptic epitopes after loss of immunodominant tumor antigen expression through epitope spreading. Int J Cancer 2001;93:841–847.

146. el-Shami K, Tirosh B, Bar-Haim E, et al. MHC class I-restricted epitope spreading in the context of tumor rejection following vaccination with a single immunodominant CTL epitope. Eur J Immunol 1999;29:3295–3301.

147. Brossart P, Wirths S, Stuhler G, et al. Induction of cytotoxic T-lymphocyte responses in vivo after vaccinations with peptide-pulsed dendritic cells. Blood 2000;96:3102–3108.

148. Stanislawski T, Voss RH, Lotz C, et al. Circumventing tolerance to a human MDM2-derived tumor antigen by TCR gene transfer. Nat Immunol 2001;2:962–970.

149. Rossig C, Bollard CM, Nuchtern JG, et al. Targeting of G(D2)-positive tumor cells by human T lymphocytes engineered to express chimeric T-cell receptor genes. Int J Cancer 2001;94:228–236.

150. Johnson LA, Heemskerk B, Powell DJ Jr, et al. Gene transfer of tumor-reactive TCR confers both high avidity and tumor reactivity to nonreactive peripheral blood mononuclear cells and tumor-infiltrating lymphocytes. J Immunol 2006;177:6548–6559.

151. Robbins PF, Dudley ME, Wunderlich J, et al. Cutting edge: persistence of transferred lymphocyte clonotypes correlates with cancer regression in patients receiving cell transfer therapy. J Immunol 2004;173:7125–7130.

152. Greenberg PD. Adoptive T cell therapy of tumors: mechanisms operative in the recognition and elimination of tumor cells. Adv Immunol 1991;49: 281–355.

153. Zhou J, Shen X, Huang J, et al. Telomere length of transferred lymphocytes correlates with in vivo persistence and tumor regression in melanoma patients receiving cell transfer therapy. J Immunol 2005;175: 7046–7052.

154. Heemskerk B, Liu K, Dudley ME, et al. Adoptive cell therapy for patients with melanoma, using tumor-infiltrating lymphocytes genetically engineered to secrete interleukin-2. Hum Gene Ther 2008;19:496–510.

155. Hsu C, Hughes MS, Zheng Z, et al. Primary human T lymphocytes engineered with a codon-optimized IL-15 gene resist cytokine withdrawal-induced apoptosis and persist long-term in the absence of exogenous cytokine. J Immunol 2005;175:7226–7234.

156. Hsu C, Jones SA, Cohen CJ, et al. Cytokine-independent growth and clonal expansion of a primary human CD8+ T-cell clone following retroviral transduction with the IL-15 gene. Blood 2007;109:5168–5177.

157. Migliaccio M, Amacker M, Just T, et al. Ectopic human telomerase catalytic subunit expression maintains telomere length but is not sufficient for CD8+ T lymphocyte immortalization. J Immunol 2000;165:4978–4984.

158. Hooijberg E, Ruizendaal JJ, Snijders PJ, et al. Immortalization of human CD8+ T cell clones by ectopic expression of telomerase reverse transcriptase. J Immunol 2000;165:4239–4245.

159. Charo J, Finkelstein SE, Grewal N, et al. Bcl-2 overexpression enhances tumor-specific T-cell survival. Cancer Res 2005;65:2001–2008.

160. Eaton D, Gilham DE, O'Neill A, et al. Retroviral transduction of human peripheral blood lymphocytes with Bcl-X(L) promotes in vitro lymphocyte survival in pro-apoptotic conditions. Gene Ther 2002;9:527–535.

161. Wang J, Jensen M, Lin Y, et al. Optimizing adoptive polyclonal T cell immunotherapy of lymphomas, using a chimeric T cell receptor possessing CD28 and CD137 costimulatory domains. Hum Gene Ther 2007;18:712–725.

162. Cheng LE, Ohlen C, Nelson BH, et al. Enhanced signaling through the IL-2 receptor in CD8+ T cells regulated by antigen recognition results in preferential proliferation and expansion of responding CD8+ T cells rather than promotion of cell death. Proc Natl Acad Sci U S A 2002;99:3001–3006.

163. Topp MS, Riddell SR, Akatsuka Y, et al. Restoration of CD28 expression in CD28- CD8+ memory effector T cells reconstitutes antigen-induced IL-2 production. J Exp Med 2003;198:947–955.

164. Sadelain M, Brentjens R, Riviere I. The promise and potential pitfalls of chimeric antigen receptors. Curr Opin Immunol 2009;21:215–223.

165. Sallusto F, Lenig D, Forster R, et al. Two subsets of memory T lymphocytes with distinct homing potentials and effector functions. Nature 1999;401:708–712.

166. Berger C, Jensen MC, Lansdorp PM, et al. Adoptive transfer of effector CD8+ T cells derived from central memory cells establishes persistent T cell memory in primates. J Clin Invest 2008;118:294–305.

167. Gattinoni L, Klebanoff CA, Palmer DC, et al. Acquisition of full effector function in vitro paradoxically impairs the in vivo antitumor efficacy of adoptively transferred CD8+ T cells. J Clin Invest 2005;115:1616–1626.

168. Dossett ML, Teague RM, Schmitt TM, et al. Adoptive immunotherapy of disseminated leukemia with TCR-transduced, CD8+ T cells expressing a known endogenous TCR. Mol Ther 2009;17:742–749.

169. Overwijk WW. Breaking tolerance in cancer immunotherapy: time to ACT. Curr Opin Immunol 2005;17:187–194.

Thalidomide and Its Analogs in the Treatment of Hematologic Malignancies, Including Multiple Myeloma, and Solid Tumors

Jacob Laubach, Constantine S. Mitsiades, Teru Hideshima, Kenneth C. Anderson, and Paul Richardson

Thalidomide was originally developed in the 1950s for the treatment of pregnancy-associated morning sickness. However, its extensive over-the-counter marketing in Europe was marked by the tragic consequences of teratogenecity,[1] which triggered its subsequent withdrawal from the market.[2,3] The teratogenic properties of thalidomide raised among oncologists the hypothesis that the potent inhibitory effects of this drug on growing fetal tissues, combined with the pathophysiologic similarities linking tumor biology and fetal development, might be redirected toward applications in cancer treatment.[4] In fact, in the early 1960s at least two clinical trials of thalidomide for patients with advanced cancers were reported.[5,6] In one of these trials, thalidomide was administered at daily doses of 300 to 2,000 mg in 71 patients with various types of cancers. No objective clinical responses were observed, except for resolution of a pulmonary metastasis in a patient with renal cell carcinoma (RCC).[5] In the second trial, 21 patients with various types of advanced cancer (including two patients with multiple myeloma [MM]) received thalidomide at 600 to 2,000 mg daily doses, which led to palliation of symptoms in approximately one third of patients, while 2 patients had minimal slowing of their tumor's growth.[6] However, these results were not deemed sufficiently encouraging to warrant further clinical development efforts.

Thalidomide was therefore not pursued further as a potential anticancer drug for several decades. In the meantime, the drug gradually emerged as a therapeutic agent for a range of medical conditions, on the basis of anecdotal clinical evidence and converging research that suggested potential beneficial pharmacoimmunologic effects.[7] Thalidomide gained renewed attention as an effective treatment of severe erythema nodosum leprosum (ENL),[8,9] Behcet's disease,[10] graft-versus-host disease (GVHD),[11] and oral ulcers and wasting associated with HIV infection.[12,13] This reemergence of thalidomide was reflected by its Food and Drug Administration (FDA) approval in 1998 for the short-term treatment of cutaneous manifestations of moderate to severe ENL, together with its use as maintenance therapy to prevent recurrence of cutaneous ENL.[7] This FDA approval was of critical importance for the clinical applications of thalidomide not only because the drug has since become a treatment of choice for ENL but also because the approval allowed for off-label uses of this medication in other disease states in which the immunomodulatory and antiangiogenic properties of thalidomide might be beneficial.[7,14,15] To prevent any occurrence of teratogenic effects, thalidomide is now administered under strict guidelines to prevent fetal exposure to this medication.[14]

The interest in thalidomide as an anticancer drug was rekindled in the 1990s with the realization that tumor-associated vasculature is an important therapeutic target in a broad range of neoplasias and that thalidomide possesses substantial antiangiogenic properties in a wide range of in vivo and in vitro models of neovascularization.[16-24] Indeed, thalidomide inhibited angiogenesis induced by basic fibroblast growth factor (bFGF) in the rabbit cornea micropocket assay or by vascular endothelial growth factor (VEGF) in a murine model of corneal vascularization.[20,25] Based on these data from D'Amato, Folkman et al. as well as the fact that thalidomide is transformed to active metabolites with antiangiogenic activity in humans,[26] thalidomide was evaluated for the treatment of various neoplasias.[27-31] Of particular note was the well-chronicled decision to test thalidomide, at the suggestion of an especially enlightened wife of an MM patient, in a compassionate use study of three patients with advanced MM at the University of Arkansas. The encouraging evidence of clinical activity in two of these three patients led to a larger phase II effort,[32] which confirmed the clinical activity of thalidomide against MM, and was followed by extensive clinical trials of thalidomide-based therapy for MM worldwide, as well as other applications in a broad range of other hematologic malignancies and solid tumors. Despite progress in its use and the fact that thalidomide is not associated with the classical pattern of toxicities seen with conventional DNA- or microtubule-targeting chemotherapeutics, this drug is not devoid of adverse effects. This realization led to development of thalidomide analogs that retain the clinical activity of thalidomide, without some of its prominent side effects.

In this chapter, we present a comprehensive review of the pharmacology of thalidomide and its analogs, a description of preclinical studies that illuminate the complex mechanisms of the action of thalidomide, and an overview of clinical trials involving thalidomide and its analogs in MM, other hematologic malignancies, solid tumors, and other cancer-related applications.

Mechanism of Action of Thalidomide and Analogs

Although it was originally hypothesized that the teratogenic and antitumor effects of thalidomide may have a common underlying mechanistic denominator, such as the antiangiogenic effect, the precise mechanisms responsible for the clinical activity of thalidomide have not been established. This can be attributed to a number of factors: (a) the preclinical in vitro and in vivo studies of thalidomide necessary to dissect its mechanisms of action are difficult to perform and interpret because of the enantiomeric interconversion and spontaneous cleavage of the drug to multiple metabolites in vivo,[33] many of which have been incompletely characterized; (b) the in vivo activity of thalidomide likely requires metabolic activation by the liver, a finding that may account at least in part for the discordance between the modest, at best, activity of thalidomide in in vitro assays of antitumor activity[26,34] and its potent in vivo effect; (c) a complex series of metabolic, immunologic, and antiangiogenic actions have emerged from preclinical studies; their possible relevance to anticancer therapy in humans is difficult to discern; (d) the chemical structure of thalidomide does not offer readily recognizable clues regarding possible intracellular molecular targets that might explain its clinical activity or profile of adverse events; and (e) the species-specific differences in the metabolism and other pharmacokinetic properties of thalidomide complicate the extrapolation of in vivo data from many animal models to the clinical setting in humans.[25]

A wealth of mechanistic information has been acquired in MM, mainly because this is the disease setting in which thalidomide has demonstrated its most impressive clinical activity. Despite the modest activity of thalidomide in antitumor assays in vitro,[35] this drug is currently considered to confer its in vivo anti-MM effects via at least four distinct, but potentially complementary, actions: (a) direct antiproliferative/proapoptotic antitumor effect,[35] probably mediated by one or more of its in vivo metabolites[36]; (b) indirect targeting of tumor cells by abrogation of protective effects conferred to MM tumor cells by bone marrow stromal cells (BMSCs) via paracrine or autocrine secretion of cytokines and growth factor or via cell adhesion molecule mediated interactions[35]; (c) antiangiogenic effects; and (d) immunomodulatory effects, which contribute to enhanced antitumor immune response.[37]

Direct Antitumor Activity

The notion that thalidomide possesses direct antitumor effects in MM and other diseases is inferred from preclinical and clinical studies. Although the in vitro effect of thalidomide on proliferation and viability of MM cells is relatively modest,[35] thalidomide derivatives, such as lenalidomide (Revlimid, CC-5013), and pomalidomoide (CC-4047, Actimid),[35,36] have far more potent in vitro antiproliferative and proapoptotic properties than the parent compound. These effects were assayed in the absence of any other cell type (e.g., stromal, endothelial, or liver cells), which could facilitate either thalidomide metabolism or indirect effects on targets other than the tumor cells themselves.[35,36] Therefore, the fact that at least some of the known in vivo thalidomide metabolites can have in vitro activity against tumor cells suggests that thalidomide may confer direct in vivo antiproliferative/proapoptotic effects via its metabolites. The precise mechanism(s) for this direct

effect remain(s) under investigation. Cell cycle analyses, by propidium iodide staining, of thalidomide- and lenalidomide-treated MM cell lines indicate G_0/G_1 growth arrest, subsequently followed by increased sub-G1 peak, consistent with apoptosis and induction of cell death.[35]

Interestingly, clinically relevant concentrations of thalidomide derivatives, such as lenalidomide and pomalidomide, trigger suppression of the transcriptional activity of NF-κB in MM cells.[36] NF-κB is well established as an important protective responder to DNA damage. It suppresses apoptosis by promoting the expression of intracellular antiapoptotic molecules, including the caspase inhibitors FLIP, XIAP, cIAP-2 or the antiapoptotic Bcl-2 family member A1/Bfl-1.[38-40] Thalidomide thus may exert its in vivo effects, at least in part, by inhibition of NF-κB signaling in cells. It is also conceivable that because NF-κB protects cells from the proapoptotic effects of steroids or cytotoxic chemotherapeutics,[36,38-40] the synergy of thalidomide and its analogs in concert with dexamethasone or cytotoxic chemotherapeutics may result from suppression of NF-κB.[41-48]

Stroma-Tumor Interactions

Thalidomide and its derivatives modulate the adhesive interactions of MM cells with BMSCs.[49] MM cells adhere to BMSCs and trigger their secretion of proliferative/antiapoptotic cytokines (e.g., interleukin [IL]-6).[50-52] This event is mainly paracrine, is mediated by transcriptional activation of NF-kB in BMSCs,[51] and dampens the sensitivity of MM cells to dexamethasone or cytotoxic chemotherapy.[53] Thalidomide/IMiD blocks this MM-stromal paracrine interaction, significantly inhibits proliferation, and lessens drug resistance of MM cells in the BM microenvironment.

Inhibition of Cytokine Production and Antiangiogenic Action

Thalidomide also inhibits TNF-α production, while leaving the patient's immune system otherwise intact.[54] Thus, thalidomide is useful in various inflammatory disorders characterized by increased TNF-α secretion, such as ENL, mycobacterium tuberculosis infection, GVHD, and cancer- and HIV-related cachexia.

The precise mechanism mediating thalidomide-induced inhibition of TNF-α activity is not fully understood, but is apparently distinct from those of other TNF-α inhibitors, such as pentoxifylline and dexamethasone.[55,56] Thalidomide may accelerate the degradation of TNF-α mRNA, thereby substantially (but not necessarily completely) suppressing the production of TNF-α protein.[55,57] Interestingly, thalidomide can decrease the binding of the transcription factor NF-kB to its consensus DNA-binding sites, which include not only the actual TNF-α gene[58] but also other genes modulated by TNF-α, in an NF-κB-dependent fashion.[36] Even the antiangiogenic properties of thalidomide may be mediated, at least in part, by inhibition of TNF-α signaling, in view of the proangiogenic effects of TNF-α itself.[20] However, the absence of a major effect of TNF-α in experimental models of angiogenesis and the inability of (at least some) potent TNFα inhibitors to directly influence angiogenesis suggest that thalidomide's antiangiogenic effects cannot be attributed to TNF-α inhibition alone.[20,25]

Thalidomide and its analogs suppress the production of cytokines that regulate tumor cell proliferation and osteoclast function,

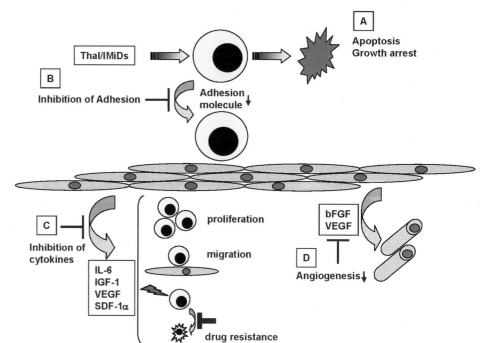

FIGURE 34-1 Antitumor activity of Thal/IMiDs in the bone marrow (BM) milieu. Thal/IMiDs **(A)** induce G1 growth arrest and/or apoptosis in MM cell lines and patient cells resistant to conventional chemotherapy; **(B)** inhibit MM cell adhesion to BM stem cells (SCs); **(C)** decrease cytokine production and sequelae; **(D)** decrease angiogenesis, in the BM microenvironment.

including IL-6, IL-1β, IL-10, and TNF-α.[59] Thalidomide also decreases the secretion of VEGF, IL-6,[60] and bFGF by MM and/or BM stromal cells. These mechanisms are summarized in Figures 34-1 and 34-2. While characterizing the mechanism underlying the teratogenic effects of thalidomide, D'Amato et al. observed its antiangiogenic properties,[20,25] which involved inhibition of the proangiogenic effects of β-FGF and/or VEGF.[20,25,61] Further in vitro studies have suggested that the metabolites, and not the parent compound, are responsible for the antiangiogenic effect of thalidomide.[62]

Immunomodulation

The precise effect of thalidomide on immune effector cells, for example, different subpopulations of lymphocytes, has not been consistent in studies published to date.[63–65] Although thalidomide may not directly suppress lymphocyte proliferation,[49] evidence suggests that it stimulates T-cell responses to tumor and may inhibit

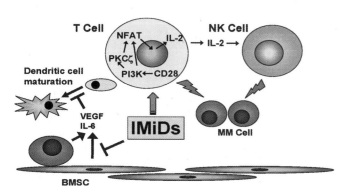

FIGURE 34-2 Mechanisms of action of IMiDs in augmentation of host immune response. IMiDs augment differentiation of dendritic cells (DC) by inhibiting secretion of IL-6 and VEGF from multiple myeloma (MM) or bone marrow stem cells (BMSCs). IMiDs also stimulate natural killer (NK) cell activity by triggering IL-2 secretion from T-cells mediated by CD28/PI3-K/NF-AT2 (nuclear factor of activated T cells) signaling pathway. (Please see Color Insert.)

proliferation of already stimulated lymphocytes.[64,66–69] Thalidomide modifies the expression patterns of cell adhesion molecules on leukocytes, inhibits neutrophil chemotaxis, and inhibits TNF-α signaling and IL-12 production, enhances synthesis of IL-2, and inhibits IL-6.[8,49,54,70–72] Of particular relevance to MM, thalidomide and its analogs augment natural killer (NK) cell-mediated cytotoxicity in MM.[37] Thalidomide and IMiDs do not induce T-cell proliferation alone, but act as costimulators to trigger proliferation of anti–CD3-stimulated T cells from MM patients, accompanied by an increase in interferon-γ and IL-12 secretion. Importantly, treatment of patient peripheral blood mononuclear cells (PBMCs) with thalidomide or IMiDs triggered their lysis of autologous MM cells. Furthermore, in MM patients, thalidomide stimulated an increase in circulating CD3-CD56$^+$ NK cells.[37]

Pharmacology of Thalidomide

Thalidomide or α-N\{phthalimido\} glutarimide ($C_{13}O_4N_2H_9$) (gram molecular weight of 258.2)[73] is a glutamic acid derivative, which contains two amide rings and a single chiral center (Fig. 34-3).[73] The key features for thalidomine are shown in Table 34-1. The currently available formulation of thalidomide consists, at physiologic pH, of a nonpolar racemic mixture of S(−) and R(+) isomers, which are cell membrane permeable.[73,74] The S isomer has been associated with the teratogenicity of thalidomide, while the R isomer has been linked with the sedative properties of the drug.[25,74,75] Because of rapid interconversion of these two isomers at physiologic pH in vivo, efforts to generate formulations of only the R isomer have failed to neutralize the teratogenic potential of thalidomide.[74,76]

Pharmacokinetics

Pharmacokinetic studies of thalidomide in humans have been limited by the lack of suitable intravenous formulations due to

metastatic spread of solid tumors,[120] and the evidence that increased BM blood vessel formation parallels the progression of hematologic malignancies.[32,117,119,121–123]

Vacca and colleagues reported that the extent of BM angiogenesis correlates with the labeling index of BM plasma cells, as well as disease activity in patients with MM,[117] a finding consistent with subsequent studies confirming extensive BM vascularization in MM.[32,119,122,123] They also observed that a poor prognosis correlates with elevated levels of angiogenic cytokines, such as bFGF and VEGF, and increased BM levels of mast cells, which secrete a variety of angiogenic factors.[117,119,122,123] Collectively, these observations provided a rationale for use of antiangiogenic drugs to treat MM and other hematologic neoplasias

Thalidomide in Relapsed and Refractory MM

Thalidomide therapy for advanced refractory MM was initiated after initial experience in three patients treated at the University of Arkansas, Little Rock. This prompted a phase II study of single-agent thalidomide in 84 patients with relapsed and refractory MM.[32] In this heavily pretreated patient population, 76 of 84 (90%) enrolled patients had relapsed after receiving high-dose chemotherapy; 42% harbored MM tumor cells with deletion of chromosome 13, a cytogenetic abnormality associated with unfavorable prognosis in patients receiving cytotoxic chemotherapy-based regimens[32,124]; 21% of patients had greater than 50% infiltration of their BM by malignant plasma cells; and 15% of them had a plasma cell labeling index greater than 1%, which signifies increased proliferative rate of the malignant plasma cells.

The primary endpoint of this trial was paraprotein response, and additional endpoints included time to response, time to disease progression (TTP), event-free survival (EFS), overall survival (OS), and improvement in other laboratory parameters. Single-agent thalidomide was administered for a median of 80 days (range, 2 to 465), at a starting dose of 200 mg at nighttime, with subsequent dose escalations by 200 mg every 2 weeks, to a maximum of 800 mg. Most patients received thalidomide daily doses up to 400 mg (86%), with fewer attaining 600 mg/d (68%) and 800 mg/d (55%). Response was defined as ≥25% reduction in serum or urine levels of paraprotein and was seen in 27 patients (32%). The paraprotein level in serum or urine decreased by ≥90% in eight patients, and the median time to response was approximately 2 months. In 78% of responding patients, decreases in plasma cell infiltration of BM and increased hemoglobin values were observed. BM microvascular density was not significantly decreased, even among those who responded to treatment.

In the initial experience with thalidomide therapy in MM, adverse events were reported to be generally mild to moderate and with increasing incidence at higher dose levels. Constipation was frequent but manageable with administration of laxatives. Peripheral neuropathy was reported by 12% of patients receiving 200 mg daily doses. However, the frequency of neuropathy was higher (28%) among patients receiving 800 mg daily. Other mild to moderate side effects included weakness, fatigue, and somnolence, which were reported by 34% of patients receiving 200 mg daily and 43% of those treated at the 800-mg dose level. More severe adverse events were infrequent (occurring in ≤10% of patients), and hematologic effects were rare. Overall, nine patients discontinued

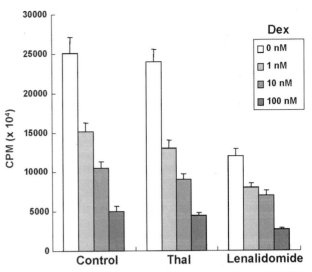

Figure 34-4 Dex augments Thal/IMiDs-induced growth inhibition in MM. MM.1S cells were treated with DMSO control, Thal (1 μM), and IMiD2 (1 μM) in the presence of different concentration of Dex for 48 hours. Cell growth was assessed by [³H]-thymidine uptake.

thalidomide due to drug intolerance. One responding patient died suddenly on day 37 of treatment, most likely due to sepsis, but a possible relationship to thalidomide could not be ruled out. The incidence of myelosuppression was low, with significant leucopenia, anemia and/or thrombocytopenia occurring in less than 5% of patients. After 12 months of follow-up, Kaplan-Meier estimates of the mean EFS and OS for all patients were 22% and 58%, respectively.

Subsequent studies from other centers confirmed that thalidomide is active in MM. In a phase II trial at the MD Anderson Cancer Center, thalidomide was administered in 43 evaluable patients with MM resistant to conventional therapies.[125] Eleven of 43 patients (26%) achieved partial response or better, defined by ≥50% reduction of serum M-protein and/or ≥75% reduction of Bence Jones protein.

The significant clinical activity of single-agent thalidomide in refractory and relapsed MM provided the impetus for trials of combinations of thalidomide with chemotherapy and dexamethasone in view of their nonoverlapping toxicities and different mechanisms of action (Fig. 34-4). Initial clinical experience with thalidomide in conjunction with dexamethasone, cyclophosphamide, etoposide, and cisplatin (DCEP) demonstrated an ability to induce complete responses (CRs) in patients with plasma cell leukemia and MM.[126] Low-dose thalidomide in combination with dexamethasone and also in combination with clarithromycin was shown to be active in relapsed disease in a number of studies,[46] although the effect of clarithromycin appears to involve a change in the metabolism of dexamethasone.

Thalidomide in Newly Diagnosed MM, Transplant Ineligible

In addition to its role in the management of relapsed MM, thalidomide is effective in newly diagnosed MM. Several randomized studies comparing a previous standard of care in MM, melphalan and prednisone (MP), to thalidomide plus MP (MPT) demonstrated the superiority of the three-drug combination.[127–130]

Thalidomide in Newly Diagnosed MM, Transplant Eligible

In the treatment of transplant eligible patients, melphalan-containing induction therapy is avoided due to the toxic effect of melphalan on stem cells. Thalidomide and dexamethasone (TD) represents a good option in this context. In a phase III study involving 470 patients with previously untreated MM, TD was superior to dexamethasone alone with respect to both ORR (63% versus 46%, $P <$ 0.001) and TTP (median 22.6 versus 6.5 months, $P < 0.001$).[131] At the time of publication, there was no difference in OS. High-grade toxicity was more common in the TD group, particularly venous thromboembolic events such as deep vein thrombosis (DVT) and pulmonary embolism (PE). Because of the lower incidence of thromboembolic events in the setting of thalidomide monotherapy, it is conceivable that thalidomide and its metabolites cause a modest increase in the degree of therapy-associated hypercoagulability, which is significantly enhanced when the drug is combined with other potentially prothrombotic antiangiogenic agents.[99]

Thalidomide Maintenance Therapy Following Stem Cell Transplantation

Finally, thalidomide has a role in post-autologous stem cell transplant (ASCT) maintenance therapy for selected patients. Thalidomide maintenance therapy has been evaluated in several randomized trials.[132–134] In each of these four studies, patients who received thalidomide-containing maintenance therapy experienced a longer progression-free interval than those who did not receive maintenance. Moreover, a benefit in terms of OS was observed in three of the four studies. However, several caveats are important to consider when considering thalidomide maintenance following ASCT. In the study by Attal et al., the benefit of thalidomide maintenance therapy was observed in patients who failed to achieve at least a very good partial remission (VGPR) with induction and ASCT.[132] In the study by Barlogie and colleagues, moreover, the median survival following relapse was shorter among patients who received thalidomide as part of therapy.[133] Lastly, the cumulative toxicities associated with maintenance thalidomide, particularly peripheral neuropathy, are an important concern and must be considered in decisions regarding this form of therapy.

Lenalidomide

Rationale for Its Use in MM

As underscored by previous discussion, while the introduction of thalidomide-based therapies improved response rates as well as progression-free survival and OS in patients with MM, the agent is associated with significant adverse events (sedation, neuropathy). These toxicities can generally be managed through preemptive dose reductions (or other components of combination therapies), careful patient selection, and comprehensive monitoring of patients. At the same time, however, experience with thalidomide-associated toxicities stimulated the development of new, related compounds with significant anti-MM activity but improved tolerability.[110]

The original efforts to develop thalidomide analogs yielded two classes of derivatives, the phosphodiesterase type 4 inhibitors, which inhibit TNF-α signaling but have little effect on T-cell activation (the so-called selective cytokine inhibitory drugs or SelCids), and another group of nonphosphodiesterase type 4 inhibitors known as IMiDs, which not only inhibit TNFα but also markedly stimulate T-cell proliferation and interferon gamma production.

Lenalidomide in Relapsed MM

The IMiDs, including lenalidomide, exhibit greater potency than thalidomide in preclinical evaluation. On this basis, phase I, II, and III studies of lenalidomide were performed in patients with relapsed or refractory MM, with favorable clinical results.[110] In 24 evaluable patients (median age 57 years; range, 40 to 71 years) with relapsed and refractory relapsed MM included in a phase I dose escalation study, no dose-limiting toxicity (DLT) was observed in patients treated at any dose level (5 to 50 mg/d) within the first 28 days. However, grade 3 myelosuppression developed after day 28 in all 13 patients at the 50 mg/d dose level. In 12 patients, dose reduction to 25 mg/d was well tolerated and was therefore considered to represent the maximal tolerated dose (MTD). Importantly, no significant somnolence, constipation, or neuropathy was seen in any cohort of that study. Best responses of at least 25% reduction in paraprotein occurred in 17 (71%) of 24 patients (90% confidence interval [CI], 52% to 85%), including 11 (46%) patients who had received prior thalidomide. Stable disease (<25% reduction in paraprotein) was observed in an additional 2 (8%) patients. Therefore, 17 (71%) of 24 patients (90% CI, 52% to 85%) demonstrated benefit from treatment with lenalidomide.[110]

These encouraging results provided the stimulus for additional studies of lenalidomide in MM. A phase II multicenter randomized controlled open-label study was conducted comparing oral lenalidomide at either 30 mg once daily or 15 mg twice daily for a total of six cycles, each comprising 3 weeks on therapy and 1 week off lenalidomide. The trial demonstrated that the 30-mg once daily dose is better tolerated than the twice daily regimen and, when administered as a part of a 3 weeks on followed by 1 week off schedule, is highly active and well tolerated, with a response rate of approximately 35% and a manageable adverse event profile. In patients in whom dexamethasone was added to the IMiD, responses were seen in about 40% of cases.

This was followed by two international phase III studies of lenalidomide in relapsed MM, the North American MM-009 and the European/Israeli/Australian MM-010 study.[107,108] In both studies, patients were randomized to either placebo or lenalidomide 25 mg days 1 to 21 of a 28-day cycle. All patients received dexamethasone 40 mg days 1 to 4, 9 to 12, and 17 to 20 during the first four cycles and on days 1 to 4 of subsequent cycles. Median TTP, the primary endpoint of the study, was superior with lenalidomide-dexamethasone (LD) as compared to dexamethasone in both studies. Moreover, LD resulted in higher overall and CR rates, as well as improvement in OS. These results provided the impetus for approval of lenalidomide in relapsed MM by both the FDA and the European Medicines Agency (EMEA).

Lenalidomide in Newly Diagnosed MM

In addition to its use in relapsed MM, lenalidomide has been evaluated in newly diagnosed disease. In a large, randomized phase III study, 445 patients with previously untreated MM received lenalidomide 25 mg days 1 to 21 of each 28-day cycle and either high-dose dexamethasone (LD) (40 mg days 1 to 4, 9 to 12, and 17 to 20) or low-dose dexamethasone (Ld) (40 mg days 1, 8, 15, and 22).[135] Although response rates were superior with LD, significantly higher 1-year OS was observed in the Ld arm (96% versus 87%, $P = 0.0002$). The OS advantage with Ld presumably occurred as a result of heightened toxicity in association with higher doses of corticosteroid, particular venous thromboembolic events and serious infections.

Other lenalidomide-containing regimens are also being evaluated as front-line therapy in MM. In particular melphalan, prednisone, and lenalidomide (MPL) have been evaluated in elderly, transplant ineligible MM patients. In a phase I study, melphalan 0.18 mg/kg days 1 to 4, prednisone 2 mg/kg days 1 to 4, and lenalidomide 10 mg days 1 to 21 of each 28-day cycle was established as the MTD.[136] The most common grade 3/4 toxicities were neutropenia and thrombocytopenia. This regimen is currently being evaluated in a phase III study comparing MPL to MP.

Pomalidomide

Finally, a second immunomodulatory thalidomide derivative, pomalidomide, or CC-4047, has been evaluated in early phase clinical trials in MM. In a phase I dose-escalation study conducted in 24 patients with relapsed and relapsed/refractory MM patients, the MTD was identified as 2 mg daily.[137] Neutropenia was the major DLT and was observed in 58% of patients. Grade 3 DVT was seen in 4 (16%) of 24 patients. Other side effects were mild and included rash, neuropathy, constipation, edema, and hypotension. Importantly, treatment resulted in minor responses (>25% reduction in paraprotein) or better in two thirds of patients, with 4 (16%) of 24 assessable patients achieving a CR. Pomalidomide administration was associated with T-cell activation, with increased RO expression on CD4$^+$ and CD8$^+$ cells and a concomitant fall in resting CD45RO$^+$ cells seen. Moreover, there were significant increases in serum levels of serum IL-2 receptor and IL-12, possibly indicating activation of T cells.[137]

In a phase II study, pomalidomide 2 mg was administered days 1 to 28 of each 28-day cycle in combination with dexamethasone 40 mg weekly on days 1, 8, 15, and 22 to 60 patients with relapsed MM.[138] The ORR was 63%, with 33% of patients achieving a VGPR or better. Moreover, the ORR was 40% among lenalidomide-refractory patients, 37% among thalidomide-refractory patients, and 60% among those refractory to bortezomib.

Clinical Studies of Thalidomide and Its Derivatives in Other Hematologic Neoplasias

Other Plasma Cell Dyscrasias

The encouraging clinical results seen with thalidomide and its analogs in MM raised the possibility that MM is more thalidomide-responsive than other neoplasias because of characteristics intrinsic to the plasma cell lineage. This also suggested by extension that thalidomide may also be active against other plasma cell dyscrasias, including Waldenström' macroglobulinemia (WM). Indeed,

single-agent thalidomide, administered in the context of a small phase II study, led to a 25% response rate in WM,[139] while a combination of low-dose thalidomide (200 mg daily), dexamethasone (40 mg once weekly), and clarithromycin (500 mg bid) showed activity.[42] Lenalidomide in conjunction with rituximab was subsequently evaluated in WM.[140] However, the regimen unexpectedly led to clinically significant anemia in 13 of 16 patients enrolled and response to therapy was inferior to that historically seen with thalidomide-containing regimens.

> In primary systemic amyloidosis, a phase I/II trial of single-agent thalidomide showed hematologic improvement in 5 of 11 patients and disease stabilization in 3 patients.[141] However, as in other reports, substantial toxicities were observed, especially at higher doses of thalidomide.[142] In contrast to experience with the agent in WM, lenalidomide therapy in AL amyloidosis has generated encouraging results in early phase clinical trials. In a phase II study involving patients with AL amyloidosis, lenalidomide 15 mg daily days 1 to 21 of a 28-day cycle produced an ORR of 60% and a CR rate of 24%.[143]

Myelodysplastic Syndromes

The increased angiogenesis noted in BM biopsies of at least some cases of MDS provided the original basis for evaluation of thalidomide in MDS. Bertolini et al. reported clinical responses in two of five thalidomide-treated MDS patients, with concomitant decreases in bFGF and VEGF in responding patients.[144] In larger studies of 83, 30, and 34 MDS patients, hematologic improvement (e.g., transfusion independence) was observed in approximately 30% of evaluable patients for the first two trials and in 19 of 29 (65%) patients in the third trial.[145–147] Higher platelet counts and lower blast percentage at baseline appeared to be associated with a higher probability of response to thalidomide.

Additional studies documented normalization of counts, with cytogenetic responses, in three thalidomide-treated patients with MDS.[148] However, improvement in nonerythroid lineages was not commonly seen[145] and dose escalation beyond 200 mg daily led to cumulative neurological toxicity, without necessarily conferring better hematological responses. Indeed, the North Central Cancer Treatment Group study N998B evaluated the tolerance and activity of an alternate thalidomide schedule of 200 mg daily with escalation to a maximum daily dose of 1,000 mg and observed extensive early patient withdrawal from the study (after a median of 2.5 months) due to toxicity.[149] The combination of darbepoetin with thalidomide in patients with MDS was associated with increased thromboembolic events in a small study.[150] However, when tolerated, prolonged drug treatment appeared necessary to maximize hematological benefit, since the median time to erythroid response was 16 weeks (range, 12 to 20 weeks), with an erythropoietic response rate of 29% among the patients who completed the minimum 12 weeks of thalidomide treatment in one of the large MDS studies.[145] Subsequent institutional studies confirmed the ability of thalidomide to lower transfusion requirements. Given the necessity for prolonged administration, its use was best suited for treatment of patients with lower risk disease.[146,151,152]

The encouraging clinical experience with thalidomide in MDS, as well as the favorable profile of manageable side effects of thalidomide analogs in MM, provided a strong rationale for evaluating lenalidomide in MDS patients.[153,154] Furthermore, lenalidomide inhibits the VEGF-induced trophic response of myeloblasts and endothelial cells, while augmenting heterotypic adhesion of hematopoietic progenitors to BM stroma to promote sustained growth arrest and preferential extinction of myelodysplastic clones.[155] In an early study involving 25 MDS patients with symptomatic or transfusion-dependent anemia who completed 8 or more weeks of treatment with lenalidomide, 16 (62%) patients experienced an erythroid response according to International Working Group (IWG) criteria, with 12 patients experiencing sustained transfusion independence or a 2 g/dL or greater rise in hemoglobin levels.[153,154] Improvement in hematopoietic function was better among patients with low-risk or int-1–risk MDS, with 15 of 21 (71%) experiencing hematological benefit. Erythroid responses to lenalidomide were associated with complete or partial (>50%) reduction in the proportion of abnormal metaphases in 9 of 13 informative patients, as well as improved primitive progenitor outgrowth, and reduced grade of cytological dysplasia. Myeloid and platelet toxicity was dose limiting but occurred at all dose levels depending upon cumulative drug exposure, necessitating either dose reduction or treatment interruption. These preliminary data suggested that lenalidomide represented a promising oral agent in MDS patients.

Subsequent investigation demonstrated that lenalidomide is particularly effective among MDS patients with chromosome 5q deletion. In a pivotal study involving 148 patients with 5q-MDS who received lenalidomide 10 mg daily days 1 to 21 or daily in a 28-day cycle, the need for red blood cell transfusion decreased in 76% of patients and transfusions were no longer necessary in 67%.[156] Complete resolution of cytogenetic abnormalities occurred in 36% of patients. Therapy was well tolerated, with neutropenia and thrombocytopenia being the most common high-grade toxicities. These impressive results have been confirmed in other studies of lenalidomide in MDS with 5q deletion.[157] Lenalidomide thus now represents a standard of care for individuals with low-risk and int-1–risk MDS with 5q deletion.

Primary Myelofibrosis

The increased microvascular density in the BM of patients with primary myelofibrosis (MF)[158] also prompted evaluation of thalidomide in this clinical setting. Several studies have shown[159–163] that thalidomide offers, in variable percentages of patients, improvement in hematologic parameters, including increased platelet counts and hemoglobin levels, decreases in spleen size (though usually of moderate degree), increased BM megakaryopoiesis, as well as decreased BM angiogenesis.[159] Interestingly, however, some of the patients treated with 200 to 400 mg/d developed significant myeloproliferative reactions, including marked leucocytosis and thrombocytosis,[161,162] the precise etiology of which is not known. Other studies of thalidomide in primary MF showed among a portion of patients improvement in hemoglobin levels, decreased transfusion requirements, increased platelet counts among, and a decrease in spleen size.[164,165] On the other hand, more than 60% of patients discontinued the drug within 6 months of starting thalidomide therapy due to side effects and almost 20% of patients had myeloproliferative reactions with leukocytosis and/or thrombocytosis. However, thalidomide appeared to maintain its clinical activity in primary MF even when daily thalidomide dose was reduced to as low as 50 mg, while most

of the side effects appeared to occur at higher doses, suggesting that lower dosing may improve the therapeutic ratio. Furthermore, it appears that combination of low-dose thalidomide (50 mg daily) with oral prednisone (starting at 0.5 mg/kg/d and tapered over 3 months) is not only well tolerated but also leads to durable objective responses, including improvement in anemia, thrombocytopenia, or spleen size in some patients.[166,167]

Lenalidomide in combination with prednisone appears to be active in this disease entity. In a study involving 40 patients with MF who received lenalidomide 10 mg daily days 1 to 21 of a 28-day cycle for six cycles, the rate of partial response by IWG for Myelofibrosis Research and Treatment (IWG-MRT) was 7.5% and of clinical response, 23%.[168] Anemia and splenomegaly improved in 30% and 42% of patients, respectively. Based on a randomized phase II study, pomalidomide too appears to be active in the setting of primary MF.[162]

Acute Myelogenous Leukemia

The use of thalidomide in acute leukemias was based not only on the putative antiangiogenic effects of this drug and the increased microvascular density of BM of leukemic patients[24] but also on in vitro data suggesting that thalidomide or its derivatives can trigger differentiation or cell death in leukemia cell lines.[169] A phase I/II dose-escalation trial of acute myeloid leukemia (AML) patients showed that thalidomide (200 to 400 mg daily for at least 1 month) led to greater than 50% reduction of blasts in BM with improvement in peripheral blood counts, for a median response duration of 3 months (range 1 to 8 months).[151,152] Responses were associated with significant decrease in microvascular density and plasma bFGF levels.[38–40,151,152] Low-dose thalidomide plus 5-azacytidine has been assessed in the treatment of AML arising from prior MDS, with evidence of activity for the combination in this setting.[145]

With respect to lenalidomide in AML, several case reports have suggested that the agent possesses some activity in this setting.[170,171] At present, however, there is insufficient basis for use of thalidomide and/or lenalidomide in AML outside the context of a clinical trial.

Chronic Lymphocytic Leukemia

Lenalidomide has shown promising activity in the treatment of chronic lymphocytic leukemia (CLL). It has been suggested that the mechanism of antitumor activity induced by lenalidomide in CLL is similar to those characterized in MM, although a direct proapoptotic effect has not been observed in CLL.[172] The activity of single-agent lenalidomide in relapsed and refractory CLL has been demonstrated in several clinical trials, with ORR on the order of 30%.[173] Lenalidomide is used with caution in this disease, however, as it has been associated with the previously mentioned tumor flare syndrome characterized by fever, rash, and rapid lymph node enlargement and at times with tumor lysis. This phenomenon is associated with up-regulation of the costimulatory molecule CD80 on tumor cells and a pronounced increase in T-cell activation.[174] Hydration and allopurinol are indicated in CLL, as well as dose reduction.

Non-Hodgkin's Lymphoma

Similar to other hematologic neoplasias, and despite their ready access to the general circulation, neoplastic lesions of non-Hodgkin's lymphoma (NHL) are also supported by increased microvascular density, while increased serum levels

139. Dimopoulos MA, et al. Treatment of Waldenstrom's macroglobulinemia with single-agent thalidomide or with the combination of clarithromycin, thalidomide and dexamethasone. Semin Oncol 2003;30:265–269.

140. Treon SP, et al. Lenalidomide and rituximab in Waldenstrom's macroglobulinemia. Clin Cancer Res 2009;15:355–360.

141. Seldin DC, et al. Tolerability and efficacy of thalidomide for the treatment of patients with light chain-associated (AL) amyloidosis. Clin Lymphoma 2003;3:241–246.

142. Dispenzieri A, et al. Poor tolerance to high doses of thalidomide in patients with primary systemic amyloidosis. Amyloid 2003;10:257–261.

143. Sanchorawala V, et al. Lenalidomide and dexamethasone in the treatment of AL amyloidosis: results of a phase 2 trial. Blood 2007;109:492–496.

144. Bertolini F, et al. Thalidomide in multiple myeloma, myelodysplastic syndromes and histiocytosis. Analysis of clinical results and of surrogate angiogenesis markers. Ann Oncol 2001;12:987–990.

145. Raza A, et al. Thalidomide produces transfusion independence in long-standing refractory anemias of patients with myelodysplastic syndromes. Blood 2001;98:958–965.

146. Zorat F, et al. The clinical and biological effects of thalidomide in patients with myelodysplastic syndromes. Br J Haematol 2001;115:881–894.

147. Strupp C, et al. Thalidomide for the treatment of patients with myelodysplastic syndromes. Leukemia 2002;16:1–6.

148. Strupp C, Hildebrandt B, Germing U, et al. Cytogenetic response to thalidomide treatment in three patients with myelodysplastic syndrome. Leukemia 2003;17:1200–1202.

149. Moreno-Aspitia A, Geyer S, Li CY, et al. N998B: multicenter phase II trial of thalidomide (Thal) in adult patients with myelodysplastic syndromes (MDS). Blood, 2002;112(11):96a.

150. Steurer M, Sudmeier I, Stauder R, et al. Thromboembolic events in patients with myelodysplastic syndrome receiving thalidomide in combination with darbepoietin-alpha. Br J Haematol 2003;121:101–103.

151. Steins MB, et al. Thalidomide for the treatment of acute myeloid leukemia. Leuk Lymphoma 2003;44:1489–1493.

152. Steins MB, et al. Efficacy and safety of thalidomide in patients with acute myeloid leukemia. Blood 2002;99:834–839.

153. List AF. New approaches to the treatment of myelodysplasia. Oncologist 2002;7(Suppl 1):39–49.

154. List AF, et al. High erythropoietic remitting activity of the immunomodulatory thalidomide analog, CC5013, in patients with myelodysplastic syndrome (MDS). Blood 2002;100:96a.

155. List AF, Tate W, Glinsmann-Gibson BJ, et al. The immunomodulatory thalidomide analog, CC5013, inhibits trophic response to VEGF in AML cells by abolishing cytokine-induced PI3-kinase/Akt activation. Blood 2002;100:139a.

156. List AF, et al. Efficacy of lenalidomide in myelodysplastic syndrome. N Engl J Med 2005;352:549–557.

157. List AF, et al. Lenalidomide in the myelodysplastic syndrome with chromosome 5q deletion. N Engl J Med 2006;355:1456–1465.

158. Mesa RA, Hanson CA, Rajkumar SV, et al. Evaluation and clinical correlations of bone marrow angiogenesis in myelofibrosis with myeloid metaplasia. Blood 2000;96:3374–3380.

159. Elliott MA, et al. Thalidomide treatment in myelofibrosis with myeloid metaplasia. Br J Haematol 2002;117:288–296.

160. Piccaluga PP, et al. Clinical efficacy and antiangiogenic activity of thalidomide in myelofibrosis with myeloid metaplasia. A pilot study. Leukemia 2002;16:1609–1614.

161. Barosi G, et al. Safety and efficacy of thalidomide in patients with myelofibrosis with myeloid metaplasia. Br J Haematol 2001;114:78–83.

162. Tefferi A, Elliot MA. Serious myeloproliferative reactions associated with the use of thalidomide in myelofibrosis with myeloid metaplasia. Blood 2000;96:4007.

163. Marchetti M, et al. Low-dose thalidomide ameliorates cytopenias and splenomegaly in myelofibrosis with myeloid metaplasia: a phase II trial. J Clin Oncol 2004;22:424–431.

164. Merup M, et al. Negligible clinical effects of thalidomide in patients with myelofibrosis with myeloid metaplasia. Med Oncol 2002;19:79–86.

165. Giovanni B, et al. Thalidomide in myelofibrosis with myeloid metaplasia: a pooled-analysis of individual patient data from five studies. Leuk Lymphoma 2002;43:2301–2307.

166. Mesa RA, et al. A phase 2 trial of combination low-dose thalidomide and prednisone for the treatment of myelofibrosis with myeloid metaplasia. Blood 2003;101:2534–2541.

167. Mesa RA, Elliott MA, Schroeder G, et al. Durable responses to thalidomide-based drug therapy for myelofibrosis with myeloid metaplasia. Mayo Clin Proc 2004;79:883–889.

168. Quintas-Cardama A, et al. Lenalidomide plus prednisone results in durable clinical, histopathologic, and molecular responses in patients with myelofibrosis. J Clin Oncol 2009;27:4760–4766.

169. Hatfill SJ, Fester ED, de Beer DP, et al. Induction of morphological differentiation in the human leukemic cell line K562 by exposure to thalidomide metabolites. Leuk Res 1991;15:129–136.

170. Basile FG. Durable clinical and cytogenetic remission in an elderly patient with relapsed acute myeloid leukemia treated with low-dose lenalidomide. Leuk Lymphoma 2009;50:653–655.

171. Penarrubia MJ, Silvestre LA, Conde J, et al. Hematologic and cytogenetic response to lenalidomide in de novo acute myeloid leukemia with chromosome 5q deletion. Leuk Res 2009;33:e8–e9.

172. Chanan-Khan AA, Cheson BD. Lenalidomide for the treatment of B-cell malignancies. J Clin Oncol 2008;26:1544–1552.

173. Chanan-Khan A, et al. Clinical efficacy of lenalidomide in patients with relapsed or refractory chronic lymphocytic leukemia: results of a phase II study. J Clin Oncol 2006;24:5343–5349.

174. Aue G, et al. Lenalidomide-induced upregulation of CD80 on tumor cells correlates with T-cell activation, the rapid onset of a cytokine release syndrome and leukemic cell clearance in chronic lymphocytic leukemia. Haematologica 2009;94:1266–1273.

175. Vacca A, Ribatti D, Roncali L, et al. Angiogenesis in B cell lymphoproliferative diseases. Biological and clinical studies. Leuk Lymphoma 1995;20:27–38.

176. Bertolini F, et al. Angiogenic growth factors and endostatin in non-Hodgkin's lymphoma. Br J Haematol 1999;106:504–509.

177. Pro B, et al. Thalidomide for patients with recurrent lymphoma. Cancer 2004;100:1186–1189.

178. Strupp C, Aivado M, Germing U, et al. Angioimmunoblastic lymphadenopathy (AILD) may respond to thalidomide treatment: two case reports. Leuk Lymphoma 2002;43:133–137.

179. Wilson EA, Jobanputra S, Jackson R, et al. Response to thalidomide in chemotherapy-resistant mantle cell lymphoma: a case report. Br J Haematol 2002;119:128–130.

180. Witzig TE, et al. Lenalidomide oral monotherapy produces durable responses in relapsed or refractory indolent non-Hodgkin's Lymphoma. J Clin Oncol 2009;27:5404–5409.

181. Fife K, Howard MR, Gracie F, et al. Activity of thalidomide in AIDS-related Kaposi's sarcoma and correlation with HHV8 titre. Int J STD AIDS 1998;9:751–755.

182. Abramson N, Stokes PK, Luke M, et al. Ovarian and papillary-serous peritoneal carcinoma: pilot study with thalidomide. J Clin Oncol 2002;20:1147–1149.

183. Little RF, et al. Activity of thalidomide in AIDS-related Kaposi's sarcoma. J Clin Oncol 2000;18:2593–2602.

184. de Medeiros BC, et al. Kaposi's sarcoma following allogeneic hematopoietic stem cell transplantation for chronic myelogenous leukemia. Acta Haematol 2000;104:115–118.

185. Kim WY, Kaelin WG. Role of VHL gene mutation in human cancer. J Clin Oncol 2004;22:4991–5004.

186. Motzer RJ, et al. Phase II trial of thalidomide for patients with advanced renal cell carcinoma. J Clin Oncol 2002;20:302–306.

187. Stebbing J, et al. The treatment of advanced renal cell cancer with high-dose oral thalidomide. Br J Cancer 2001;85:953–958.

188. Daliani DD, et al. A pilot study of thalidomide in patients with progressive metastatic renal cell carcinoma. Cancer 2002;95:758–765.

189. Escudier B, et al. Phase II trial of thalidomide in renal-cell carcinoma. Ann Oncol 2002;13:1029–1035.

190. Minor DR, et al. A phase II study of thalidomide in advanced metastatic renal cell carcinoma. Invest New Drugs 2002;20:389–393.

191. Amato R, Schell J, Thompson N, et al. Phase II study of thalidomide + interleukin-2 (IL-2) in patients with metastatic renal cell carcinoma (MRCC). Proc Am Soc Clin Oncol. 2003;378a.

192. Olencki, T. et al. Phase I trial of thalidomide and interleukin-2 in patients with metastatic renal cell carcinoma. Invest New Drugs 2006;24:321–326.

193. Nathan PD, Gore ME, Eisen TG. Unexpected toxicity of combination thalidomide and interferon alpha-2a treatment in metastatic renal cell carcinoma. J Clin Oncol 2002;20:1429–1430.

194. Harshman LC, Li M, Srinivas S. The combination of thalidomide and capecitabine in metastatic renal cell carcinoma–is not the answer. Am J Clin Oncol 2008;31:417–423.

195. Margulis V, et al. Randomized trial of adjuvant thalidomide versus observation in patients with completely resected high-risk renal cell carcinoma. Urology 2009;73:337–341.

196. Gaziev D, Galimberti M, Lucarelli G, et al. Chronic graft-versus-host disease: is there an alternative to the conventional treatment? Bone Marrow Transplant 2000;25:689–696.

197. Vogelsang GB, et al. Thalidomide for the treatment of chronic graft-versus-host disease. N Engl J Med 1992;326:1055–1058.

198. Heney D, et al. Thalidomide treatment for chronic graft-versus-host disease. Br J Haematol 1991;78:23–27.

199. Rovelli A, et al. The role of thalidomide in the treatment of refractory chronic graft-versus-host disease following bone marrow transplantation in children. Bone Marrow Transplant 1998;21:577–581.

200. Browne PV, et al. Response to thalidomide therapy in refractory chronic graft-versus-host disease. Bone Marrow Transplant 2000;26:865–869.

Section V
Hormonal Therapy

Hormonal Therapy of Breast Cancer

Beverly Moy and Paul E. Goss

Hormonal therapy plays a critical role in the prevention and treatment of breast cancer at all stages of its pathogenesis.[1] This chapter provides an understanding of (a) estrogen synthesis and metabolism, (b) the endocrine regulation of these processes, (c) the molecular basis of estrogen signaling through the estrogen receptor (ER), (d) the response of cancer cells to the modulation of ER signaling, (e) the pharmacology of hormonal therapeutics, and (f) hormonal therapy resistance.

Estrogen Structure, Biosynthesis, Transport, and Metabolism

Structure of Estrogen

Estrogens are steroids containing a hydrated four-ring structure (cyclopentane-perhydro-phenanthrene), in which a five-sided cyclopentane ring (designated the D ring) is attached to three six-sided phenanthrene rings (designated the A, B, and C rings) (Figs. 35-1 and 35-2).

The three endogenous estrogens are estradiol, estrone, and estriol. Estradiol and estrone can be formed directly by aromatization of testosterone and androstenedione, respectively. Estradiol can also be readily formed from estrone and is the principally active estrogen (Fig. 35-3).[2-5] The common and systematic names of selected steroidal hormones and their structures are shown in Figure 35-2.[2-5] The physiologic effects of estrogens are summarized in Table 35-1.

Estrogen Biosynthesis

Estrogen biosynthesis begins from cholesterol. Cytochrome P-450 enzymes convert cholesterol to different steroid hormones via alteration of side chains on the molecule.[6] The final step in estrogen synthesis is aromatization, which is catalyzed by the P-450 aromatase monooxygenase enzyme complex.[6,7] The hormonal regulation of the CYP19 gene on chromosome 15, which spans 120 kb,

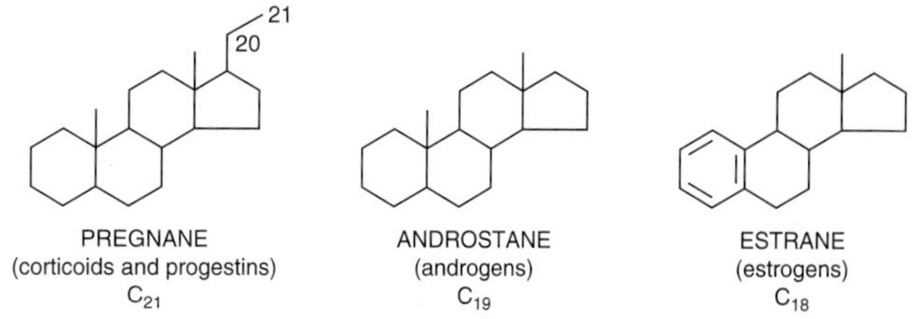

FIGURE **35-2** The structure and names of the five major steroid hormones. (Trivial name is followed by systematic.) Cortisol, 4-pregnen-11β,17α, 21-triol-3,20-dione; aldosterone, 4-pregnen-11β,21-diol-18-al-3,20-dione; progesterone, 4-pregnen-3,20-dione; testosterone, 4-androsten-17β-ol-3-one; estradiol, 1,3,5(10)-estratrien-3,17β-diol.

is intricate, primarily due to a complex and tissue specific promoter structure, with regulatory elements targeted by gonadotropins, glucocorticoids, growth factors, cytokines, and the intracellular signaling molecule cAMP.[8-11]

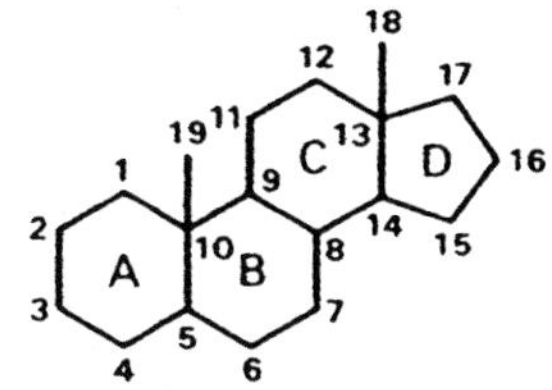

In premenopausal women, estrogens are predominantly produced by the ovaries. By contrast, in postmenopausal women, estrogens are instead formed from the extragonadal conversion of ovarian and adrenal androgens via aromatase. Androgens from the ovaries and adrenal glands are released into circulation and converted to estrogens in tissues with aromatase activity, including adipose tissue and muscle.[12]

Estrogen Transport

Estrogens circulate in the bloodstream predominantly bound to albumin and steroid-binding globulins. The estrogens and androgens are transported via testosterone and estradiol–binding globulin or sex steroid–binding globulin.[13] The unbound, or free, hormone, which makes up only 2% to 3% of total circulating estrogens, enters the cell by diffusion through the cell membrane.[6] Once inside the cell, estrogens bind to the ER, thereby starting a complex series of signaling events in the target cell. Local estrogen synthesis within tissues such as the breast may also act as a paracrine factor.[14]

The Estrogen Receptor

ER Structure

The ER is a member of the nuclear hormone receptor superfamily that includes the progesterone receptor (PgR), androgen receptor (AR), glucocorticoid receptor (GR), and mineralocorticoid

FIGURE **35-1** The structure and numbering of the cyclopentaneperhydrophenanthrene nucleus.

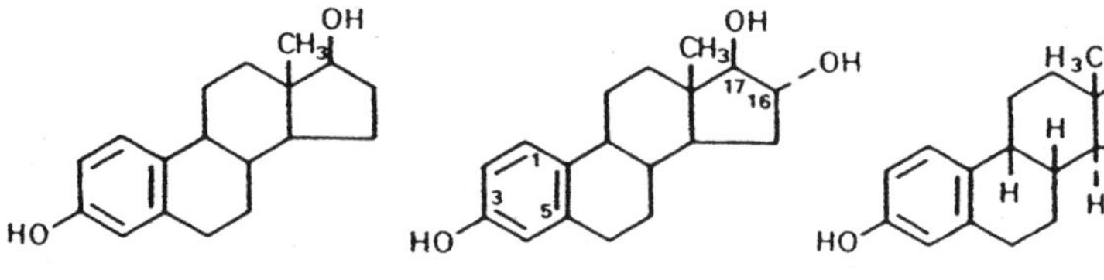

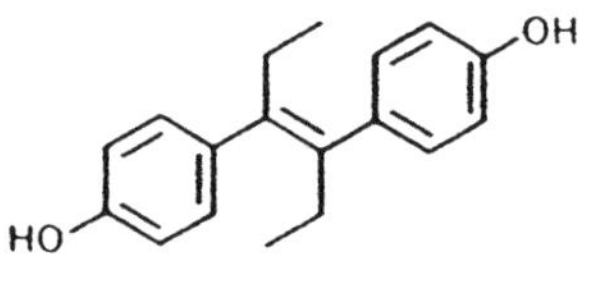

FIGURE **35-3** Endogenous and synthetic estrogens.

receptor. This receptor family also includes receptors for nonsteroidal nuclear hormones such as the retinoids, vitamin D or deltanoids, and thyroid hormones.

The ER, like most nuclear hormone receptors, operates as a ligand-dependent transcription factor that binds to DNA at estrogen response elements (EREs) to direct changes in gene expression in response to hormone binding.[6,15] The ER protein structure includes six domains, designated A to E (Fig. 35-4). Estradiol binds to the ligand-binding site in the E domain. The E domain also mediates ER dimerization, with assistance from residues in domain C. The sequence-specific DNA-binding function resides in domain C. Domain D contains a nuclear localization signal required for transfer of the ER from the cytoplasm to the nucleus. Sequences that promote transcription, or activation functions (AFs), are present in domains A and B (AF1) and domain E (AF2). The basic structure and functional components of steroid hormones follow the same pattern, with a hormone-binding site, a dimerization domain, transactivation domain(s), and a nuclear localization signal.[16]

ER Subtypes: ERα and ERβ

The first identified ER, now known as "ERα," was discovered in the late 1960s, and the gene was cloned in 1986. The second ER, named "ERβ," was first reported in 1996[17] and has provided

TABLE

35.1 *Physiologic effects of estrogens*

Growth and maintenance of female genitalia
Pubertal expression of female secondary sex characteristics
Breast enlargement
Increase in size and pigmentation of nipple and areolae
Molding of body contour with alteration of subcutaneous fat deposition
Promotion of female psyche formation
Alteration in skin texture
Maintenance of pregnancy (in concert with progestins)
Sodium retention

a further layer of complexity to our understanding of estrogen-regulated gene expression.[18] Furthermore, each subtype of ER exists in several isoforms. At the amino acid level, ERα and ERβ are highly homologous in the DNA-binding domain (96%), but the homology in the ligand-binding domain (LBD) is only 58%. This structural comparison suggests that the two subtypes would recognize and bind to similar DNA sites. However, the differences in the LBD suggest that responses to different ligands may be more distinct than anticipated from primary sequence analysis.[19]

There is no consensus on the clinical significance of ERβ since many different studies have conflicting findings. However, breast cancers that coexpress ERα and ERβ tend to be node-positive and of a higher grade than tumors that express ERα alone[20] ERβ-expressing tumors tend to be PgR-negative.[21] These correlations suggest an adverse effect of ERβ expression on prognosis. Other work, on the other hand, suggests that decreased levels of ERβ may be associated with more aggressive clinical behavior.[18]

Classical ER Signal Transduction

Ligand-Dependent ER Signaling

The well-described classical ER signaling pathway is illustrated in Figure 35-5. Estrogens bind to the LBD of the ER, leading to the release of the receptor from heat shock protein 90. This ligand binding is then followed by phosphorylation of the receptor at specific serine residues, ER dimerization, and then sequence-specific DNA binding to a sequence referred to as an "estrogen response element". In the presence of estrogen, messenger RNA (mRNA) transcription is promoted through AF2. Residues in AF1 also promote transcription, although the function of AF1 does not require the presence of estrogen.[22] The consensus DNA-binding sites for each of the nuclear hormones are illustrated in Figure 35-6. While the ER binds most strongly to the ERE consensus sequence, it is also capable of promoting transcription through sequences that have only partial homology to a classic ERE. In these cases, nearby response elements for other transcription factors (e.g., SP-1) contribute to ER activity.[22–24] The characteristics of the target gene promoter are critical to the specific nuclear actions of the activated ER. Other factors that are critical are the structure of the

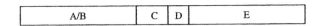

A/B   AF-1 transactivation domain
C   DNA Binding and homodimerization domain
D   NLS and HSP90 binding domain
E   AF-2 transactivation domain

% amino acid homology in relation to GR

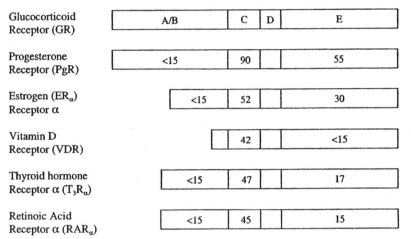

	A/B	C	D	E
Glucocorticoid Receptor (GR)	A/B	C	D	E
Progesterone Receptor (PgR)	<15	90		55
Estrogen (ER$_\alpha$) Receptor α	<15	52		30
Vitamin D Receptor (VDR)		42		<15
Thyroid hormone Receptor α (T$_3$R$_\alpha$)	<15	47		17
Retinoic Acid Receptor α (RAR$_\alpha$)	<15	45		15

FIGURE 35-4 Examples of amino acid homology between nuclear hormone receptors. A/B, activation function 1 transactivation domain; C, DNA-binding and homodimerization domain; D, nuclear localization signal and heat-shock protein 90-binding domain; E, activation function 2 transaction domain.

bound ligand and the balance of coactivators and corepressors associated with the ER-ligand complex. In addition, ERα and ERβ can either homodimerize or heterodimerize, and this has an impact on their activity at the DNA-binding site.[25]

ER Coactivators and Corepressors

Ligand-bound receptors interact with a family of "coactivator" and "corepressor" proteins that are sensitive to the conformational

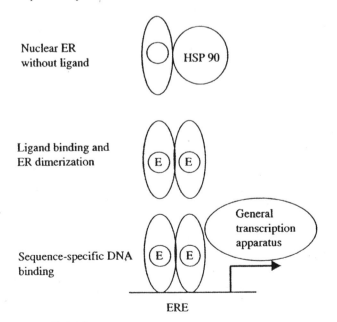

FIGURE 35-5 Simplified operational details of nuclear hormone action, using the estrogen receptor as an example. E, estrogen-occupied ligand-binding site; ER, estrogen receptor; ERE, estrogen response element; HSP, heat-shock protein.

changes that occur in the LBD of each receptor. These coregulatory proteins interact with the ER to either increase or decrease transcriptional activity at a promoter site. One key mechanism for the coactivator and corepressor modulation of ER transcription likely involves histone acetylation and methylation.[26] In addition to alteration of chromatin structure and histone acetylation, coactivators may also promote interactions between the nuclear hormone receptor and the basal transcriptional machinery to activate gene transcription.[27] Corepressors have the opposite function and negatively regulate transcription via recruitment of histone deacetylases.[28]

In general, coactivators and corepressors appear to be expressed at similar levels in many different tissues, suggesting that the responses to estrogen agonists and antagonists are not determined simply by the relative abundance of these cofactors. Instead, it appears that differential regulation of coactivator activity occurs through other signal transduction pathways.[26]

Nonclassical ER Signal Transduction

ER Activation by Other Signal Transduction Pathways

In addition to classical ER signaling, other ER signaling pathways have been described (Fig. 35-7). Nuclear hormones are not simply receptors for lipid-soluble hormones, but are also critical signaling targets for protein phosphorylation–dependent second messenger pathways.[29] These nuclear hormone receptors crosstalk with growth factor pathways that determine the ultimate cellular responses to a complex set of extracellular signals.

TR, ER, RAR receptors

8bp core motif

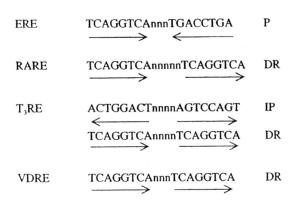

GR, PgR, AR

Core motif: AGAACA

Flanking sequences around the core motif of AR and GR may contribute to receptor specificity

FIGURE **35-6** *Consensus core response element motifs for nuclear hormone receptors. AR, androgen receptor; ARE, androgen receptor response element; DR, direct repeat; ER, estrogen receptor; ERE, estrogen response element; GR, glucocorticoid receptor; GRE, glucocorticoid response element; IP, inverted palindrome; n, any nucleotide; P, palindrome; PgR, progesterone receptor; PRE, progesterone receptor response element; RAR, retinoic acid receptor; RARE, retinoic acid receptor response element; T_3RE, triiodothyronine receptor response element; VDRE, vitamin D receptor response element.*

ER expression and function are strongly influenced by growth factor signaling (Fig. 35-7B). As a result, ER expression levels correlate with distinct patterns of growth factor receptor overexpression. For example, when ErbB2 or EGFR is activated in experimental systems, ER expression is suppressed. This suggests that EGFR and ErbB2 signaling can bypass the requirement for estrogen for breast cancer cell growth and drive breast cancer cells into an ER-negative, endocrine therapy-resistant state.[30]

In other circumstances, EGFR and ErbB2 signaling can activate the ER in an estrogen-independent manner. Signaling of these growth factors through the mitogen-activated protein kinase (MAPK) cascade leads to phosphorylation of the Ser118 residue in the ERα AF1 domain.[31,32] This, in turn, leads to recruitment of coactivators, allowing ligand-independent gene transcription by the ER.[30,33] As discussed in the "Hormonal Resistance" section, insights into the cross talk between the ER and other signal transduction pathways provide a potential strategy for novel therapeutic combinations as well as an approach to new predictive tests for endocrine therapy sensitivity.

Tamoxifen: The First Selective Estrogen Receptor Modulator

High doses of estrogen had long been recognized as effective treatment for estrogen receptor-positive (ER+) breast cancer but serious side effects such as thromboembolism prompted the development of alternative strategies.[34] The antiestrogen tamoxifen, a nonsteroidal triphenylethylene synthesized in 1966, was first developed as an oral contraceptive but paradoxically was found to induce ovulation. Activity in metastatic breast cancer was first described in the early 1970s.[35] Since then, tamoxifen has become a prototype drug for the hormonal treatment of ER+ breast cancer, with use in prevention and treatment of all stages of the disease. Tamoxifen rapidly became the drug of choice for advanced disease, with response rates ranging from 16% to 56%.[36–38] It became the preferred drug not because it proved better than contemporary alternatives but because it was safe and well tolerated. Tamoxifen's tolerability was one of the chief reasons for its success in adjuvant and prevention trials, as patients are able to take it for prolonged periods of time with acceptable levels of toxicity.[35,39–41] To date, tamoxifen is the only hormonal agent approved not only for the treatment of invasive breast cancer in the early and advanced settings but also for the prevention of breast cancer and treatment of ductal carcinoma in situ. Widespread use of tamoxifen has likely contributed to the recent decline in breast cancer mortality observed in high-incidence Western countries.[42]

In addition to its generally antagonist effects on the breast, tamoxifen has estrogen agonist effects on other organs including the endometrium,[43–45] the coagulation system,[46,47] bone,[48,49] and liver.[50,51] Therefore, tamoxifen is correctly described as a selective estrogen receptor modulator (SERM) with organ-specific mixed agonist and antagonist effects. The agonist properties of tamoxifen are illustrated occasionally in advanced breast cancer when "flare reactions," withdrawal responses, and the experimental demonstration of breast tumor growth stimulated by tamoxifen are evidence that tamoxifen can operate as an agonist in breast tissue under certain circumstances.

Clinical Use

Tamoxifen is used for the treatment of ER+ invasive breast cancer in the neoadjuvant, adjuvant, and metastatic settings. Tamoxifen is also used in the treatment of ductal carcinoma in situ and for breast cancer prevention in high-risk patients.

Tamoxifen Metabolism and Pharmacokinetics

The metabolism of tamoxifen is complex.[52] Ten major metabolites have been identified in patient's sera.[53–55] The most abundant plasma metabolite of tamoxifen is *N*-desmethyltamoxifen.[56] Metabolism of tamoxifen is mediated in the liver by cytochrome P-450–dependent oxidases. The metabolites are excreted largely in the bile as conjugates; tamoxifen dose does need to be reduced in the presence of renal dysfunction.[57] There is increasing evidence that endoxifen (4-hydroxy-*N*-desmethyltamoxifen), a second metabolite of tamoxifen, is most responsible for tamoxifen activity.

The initial plasma half-life of tamoxifen ranges from 4 to 14 hours, with a secondary half-life of approximately 7 days.[52,57,60,66]

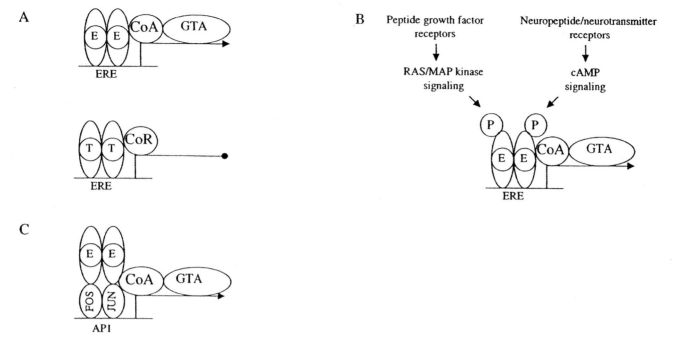

FIGURE **35-7** More complex models of estrogen receptor (ER) models. **A.** Estrogen (E) promotes coactivator (CoA) interactions that activate the general transcription apparatus (GTA). Tamoxifen (T) promotes corepressor (CoR) interactions that prevent activation of the general transcription apparatus. **B.** Estrogen receptor is phosphorylated by protein kinases activated by growth factors and neurotransmitters. **C.** ER interacts with other DNA-binding transcription factors to modulate the transcription of genes that do not possess an ERE. cAMP, cyclic adenosine monophosphate; ERE, estrogen response element; MAP, mitogen-activated protein kinase; P, phosphate.

Steady-state concentrations of tamoxifen are achieved after 4 to 16 weeks of treatment.[66] While the half-life of endoxifen has not been reported, the biologic half-life of the metabolite N-desmethyltamoxifen is 14 days, with a steady-state concentration reached at 8 weeks. These long half-lives reflect the high level of plasma binding to protein (>99%) and enterohepatic recirculation.[66] Only free tamoxifen or metabolites can bind to ERs. Tamoxifen persists in the plasma of patients for at least 6 weeks after discontinuation of treatment.[67] Because of the long plasma half-life of tamoxifen, at least 4 weeks are required to reach steady-state levels in plasma. A thorough analysis indicated that a single dose of 20 mg a day is the most appropriate approach to tamoxifen administration.[67] Because most tamoxifen is bound to serum proteins, tamoxifen is present in low concentrations in the cerebrospinal fluid,[68] suggesting that the response to tamoxifen is likely to be poor in leptomeningeal disease and central nervous system metastasis.

Drug Interactions

The CYP3A family is responsible for N-demethylation of tamoxifen (Fig. 35-8). Many other drugs are substrates for this enzyme family, such as erythromycin, nifedipine, cyclosporine, testosterone, diltiazem, and cortisol. The combination of tamoxifen with any of these drugs could potentially interfere with tamoxifen metabolism.[69]

CYP2D6, which is commonly involved in drug hydroxylation, is the major CYP isoform responsible for the generation of the metabolites 4-hydroxytamoxifen and endoxifen from tamoxifen.[70] As discussed in the "Hormonal Resistance" section, a pilot clinical trial of 12 breast cancer patients on adjuvant tamoxifen observed that plasma concentrations of endoxifen appeared to be influenced by the patient's CYP2D6 genotype.[71] The plasma concentrations of endoxifen were significantly lower in patients who were carriers of nonfunctional CYP2D6 allelic variants compared with those who had two functional wild-type alleles.[71]

The activity of CYP2D6 is also reduced by serotonin selective reuptake inhibitor (SSRI) antidepressants.[71,72] In view of the widespread use of SSRIs in patients with a history of breast cancer, a detailed study was done to determine their effects on tamoxifen metabolites.[73] Levels of 4-hydroxy-N-desmethyltamoxifen, a metabolite generated via CYP3A4 and CYP2D6 activity, were 64% lower in women taking SSRIs. Other studies also showed that plasma endoxifen concentrations were lower in patients who were also taking the SSRI paroxetine.[73] While the clinical significance of these findings is unclear, it is possible that the common combination of tamoxifen and SSRIs may alter clinical results.

Tamoxifen also lowers plasma levels of the aromatase inhibitor letrozole, indicating that at standard doses these two agents should not be administered together.[74] Medroxyprogesterone acetate has also been found to alter the metabolism of tamoxifen.[75] Reports of an interaction between warfarin and tamoxifen have prompted the manufacturer to list concurrent warfarin use as a contraindication.[76] Supratherapeutic effects of warfarin have been reported in patients also receiving tamoxifen; however, the number of cases studied is small. The mechanism of this interaction is likely inhibition of hepatic metabolism of warfarin by tamoxifen. Therefore, close monitoring of coagulation indices is warranted when warfarin and tamoxifen are prescribed together.[76]

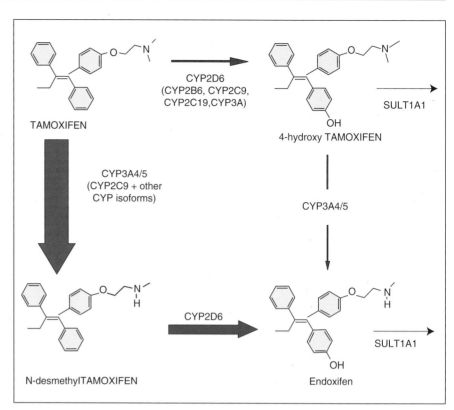

Figure **35-8** Selected transformation pathways of tamoxifen and the main CYP enzymes involved. The relative contribution of each pathway to the overall oxidation of tamoxifen is shown by the thickness of the *arrow.*

Tamoxifen Side Effects

Although tamoxifen remains a standard hormonal therapy for early-stage and advanced breast cancer, important side effects should be considered. The tamoxifen chemoprevention trial, National Surgical Adjuvant Breast Project (NSABP) P1, established one of the most comprehensive sources of information on tamoxifen toxicity because the true incidence of tamoxifen side effects was not obscured by tumor-related medical problems.[77] In NSABP P1, the excess incidence of serious adverse events (pulmonary embolus, deep venous thrombosis, cerebrovascular accident, cataract, and endometrial cancer) for patients receiving tamoxifen therapy was five to six events per 1,000 patient-years of treatment. Other side effects of tamoxifen included hot flashes, nausea, and vaginal discharge. Depression is also commonly considered a side effect of tamoxifen, although there was no clear evidence of this association for women who received tamoxifen or placebo in NSABP P1. In summary, tamoxifen is usually well tolerated and safe and serious side effects occur in no more than 1 in 200 patients annually.

Ophthalmologic Side Effects

Tamoxifen retinopathy, with macular edema and loss of visual acuity, was first reported in patients receiving 120 to 160 mg/d. Three of the four originally reported patients also had corneal opacities.[78] The retinal lesions are superficial, white, refractile bodies 3 to 10 μm in diameter in the macula and 30 to 35 μm in diameter in the paramacular tissues, and they occur in the nerve fiber layer, suggesting that they are products of axonal degeneration.[79] Additional cases have been described among patients receiving 30 to 180 mg/d.[80] Other ophthalmologic findings reported include optic neuritis, macular edema, crystalline macular deposits with reduced

visual acuity, intraretinal crystals with noncystoid macular edema, refractile deposits in the paramacular areas with progressive retinal pigment atrophy, bilateral optic disc edema with visual impairment and retinal hemorrhages, tapetoretinal degeneration, and two cases of superior ophthalmic vein thrombosis.[80–83] It is worth emphasizing that, in the chemoprevention study, the only significant optic toxicity at increased incidence compared with placebo was cataract formation.[77]

Thrombosis

The increased risk of thrombosis associated with tamoxifen therapy may be initiated by decreased levels of antithrombin III levels. Enck and Rios found a decreased functional activity of antithrombin III in 42% of tamoxifen-treated patients.[46] Others found reduced antithrombin III and protein C levels in women taking tamoxifen.[84] The incidence of venous thrombosis in this study was 5.62%, compared with 0% in controls. In the P1 prevention trial, the average annual rates of stroke, pulmonary embolism, and deep venous thrombosis per 1,000 women were increased by 0.53, 0.46, and 0.50 cases, respectively.[77] The NSABP B-14 study reported thromboembolic events in 12 patients (0.9%), with one fatal pulmonary embolus, compared with two thromboemboli (0.2%) in controls,[85] a rate similar to that occurring in the P1 prevention trial.[77] In the P1 trial, tamoxifen-related thrombotic events were more likely to occur in patients with higher body mass index but not with factor V Leiden or prothrombin gene mutations.[86]

Hematologic Side Effects

Thrombocytopenia occurs in 5% of patients and is usually transient, resolving after the 1st week of treatment. Leukopenia is less frequent and is also transient.[87] The mechanism of these side effects is unclear.

Lipoprotein Effects

Changes in serum lipoproteins in patients taking tamoxifen are indicative of an estrogenic agonist effect: an increase in total triglycerides, a decrease in total cholesterol, an increase in low-density lipoprotein (LDL) triglycerides, and a decrease in LDL cholesterol. Many studies substantiate the effect of tamoxifen on lowering total cholesterol and, in most cases, LDL cholesterol and apolipoprotein B.[88–90] Despite these potentially favorable effects, there was no evidence of an improvement in the rate of cardiovascular mortality in either the Oxford meta-analysis[43] of tamoxifen trials or the P1 prevention trial.[77] It is possible that beneficial effects of improved lipoprotein levels induced by tamoxifen are counteracted in part by increased incidence of thromboembolism.

Hepatic Toxicity

Tamoxifen has been associated with various hepatic abnormalities, including cholestasis, jaundice, peliosis hepatitis, and hepatitis. Carcinogenicity studies in rats reveal hepatocellular carcinoma in dosages ranging from 5 to 35 mg/kg/d.[91] A dose of 20 to 40 mg given to humans is 5- to 10-fold lower than the rat dose range of 5 mg/kg, and an increase in hepatocellular carcinoma in humans taking tamoxifen has not been reported. This is significant because tamoxifen metabolites form adducts with DNA and could be mutagenic and carcinogenic.[92]

Bone Side Effects

The positive effect of tamoxifen on bone mineral content in postmenopausal women can be considered an advantageous side effect due to its estrogen agonistic activity.[93,94] In the P1 study, a nonsignificant decrease in fracture rate was documented.[77] In premenopausal women, bone mineral density is decreased, possibly because in a high-estrogen environment, tamoxifen may operate predominantly as an antagonist.[93,95]

Gynecologic Side Effects

A change in the duration of menses or heaviness of flow, and an increased incidence of ovarian cysts may occur. A small increase in endometrial cancer occurs, but screening for endometrial cancer is complicated by tamoxifen-induced benign endometrial hyperplasia and polyp formation. The risk of endometrial cancer relates to age and duration of tamoxifen treatment. In the original Swedish report, the highest frequency occurred among those treated for 5 years and the Swedish patients received the high dose of 40 mg daily.[96] Of 17 tamoxifen-related endometrial cancers, 16 were grade 1 or 2, although three patients died from their endometrial cancer.[96] A case-control study found that exposure to tamoxifen interacts with other risk factors for endometrial cancer such as a history of hormone replacement therapy and higher body mass index.[97]

In addition to endometrial cancer, the risk of uterine sarcoma, a very rare malignancy, is also increased by tamoxifen. Data from six NSABP trials in which over 17,000 women were randomized to tamoxifen or placebo shows that the rate of uterine sarcoma was increased to 0.17 per 1,000 years in women taking tamoxifen versus 0 per 1,000 years in those taking placebo.[98]

Recommendations for gynecologic follow-up of patients taking tamoxifen have varied from observation to yearly vaginal ultrasound to yearly endometrial biopsy, with no solid data supporting any of these approaches. Yearly pelvic examinations and rapid investigation of postmenopausal bleeding, but not radiologic or biopsy screening, are currently recommended.

Pregnancy

Given the possible teratogenicity of tamoxifen, women should use mechanical contraception while on the drug. Of 50 pregnancies on the file at AstraZeneca Pharmaceuticals in women taking tamoxifen, there were 19 normal births, 8 terminated pregnancies, 13 unknown outcomes, and 10 infants with a fetal and neonatal disorder, 2 of whom had craniofacial defects. Yet in another report, 85 women taking tamoxifen for prevention of breast cancer became pregnant; none of these pregnancies resulted in fetal abnormalities.[99] Another case of an infant born with ambiguous genitalia after in utero exposure through 20 weeks has also been reported.[100] The evidence for the teratogenicity of tamoxifen is primarily derived from animal studies, in which reproductive organ abnormalities and increased susceptibility to carcinogens were found.[101] Nevertheless, tamoxifen is contraindicated in women who are pregnant or planning pregnancy.

Male Breast Cancer

There have been case reports of impotence[102] and of nocturnal priapism[103] in male breast cancer patients receiving tamoxifen. Another series reported a decrease in libido in 29.2% of male breast cancer patients.[104] Impotence has been studied in men treated with tamoxifen for male infertility. One paper reports a loss of libido in four cases (9%),[105] whereas studies that reported an increase in testosterone levels with tamoxifen did not report an increase in impotence.[106] These data suggest that tamoxifen has minimal effect on sexual function and is probably not the cause of impotence.

Flare Reactions and Withdrawal Responses

Tamoxifen has been characterized as having both estrogen agonist and antagonist actions. These functions are also tissue and perhaps tumor specific. Tamoxifen's agonist effects on the endometrium, bones, and clotting profile have been described. On the breast its antagonist actions are manifest by anti–breast cancer effects. In patients with advanced breast cancer tamoxifen's occasional paradoxical effects are manifest by the phenomena of a clinical flare and a drug withdrawal response. A clinical flare reaction is characterized by a dramatic increase in bone pain and an increase in the size and number of metastatic skin nodules with erythema.[107] Typically, symptoms occur from 2 days to 3 weeks after starting treatment and can be accompanied by hypercalcemia, which occurs in approximately 5% of patients.[108] Tumor regression may occur as the reaction subsides.[109]

Other SERMs

Background

The structures of other SERMs and antiestrogens are provided in Figure 35.9. Alternative antiestrogens with a modified mixed agonist and antagonist profile have been evaluated with an eye toward developing drugs that are antiestrogenic in the breast and endometrium but retain beneficial effects on bone mineralization. However, although ideal SERMs may represent a small advance in terms of safety, they are not necessarily more efficacious. In general, antiestrogens that

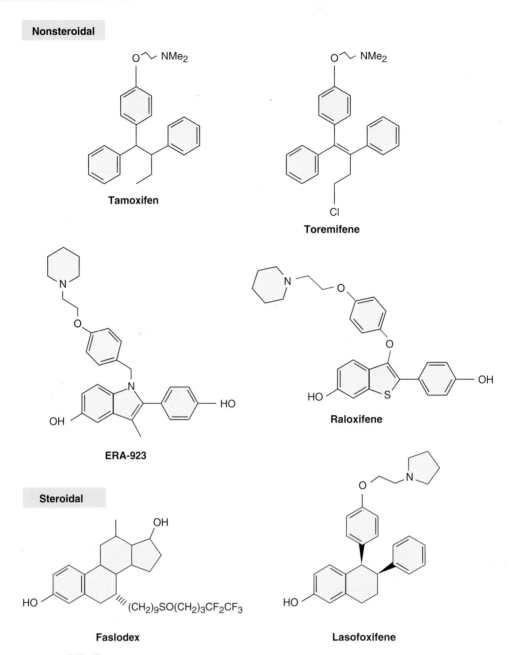

FIGURE 35-9   Antiestrogens. SERM, selective estrogen receptor modulator.

exhibit a mixed agonist and antagonist profile, even if modified in a way that improves tissue-specific toxicities, are likely to exhibit resistance and toxicity profiles that overlap those of tamoxifen.[110] This may be because any antiestrogen that triggers ER dimerization and DNA binding is prone to the same coactivator-based resistance mechanisms that may limit the activity of tamoxifen.

Raloxifene

Raloxifene [6-hydroxy-2-(4-hydroxyphenyl)-benzo[b]thien-3-yl]–[4-[2-(1-piperidinyl) ethoxy] phenyl] is the first approved drug to exhibit a "modified" SERM profile; however, the first approved indication for raloxifene was osteoporosis, not breast cancer.[111] An early evaluation of activity in tamoxifen-resistant breast cancer was disappointing.[112] Consequently, raloxifene is not used for the treatment of either early-stage or advanced breast cancer. However,

raloxifene has been approved in the breast cancer prevention setting.[113] The NSABP-P2 prevention trial demonstrated that in women at high risk for developing breast cancer, raloxifene is as effective as tamoxifen in reducing the risk of invasive breast cancer and has a lower risk of thromboembolic events, endometrial cancer, and cataracts.[114] It is important to note that raloxifene has a nonstatistically significant higher risk of noninvasive (in situ) breast cancer compared to tamoxifen, raising the possibility that it may not be as effective in long-term prevention of invasive cancer.

Mechanism of Action

While raloxifene has agonist and antagonist activity similar to tamoxifen in breast tissue and bones, its nil or only very mild agonist effect on the endometrium results in no or very mild increase in endometrial cancer risk, a distinct advantage over tamoxifen. Raloxifene is a benzothiophene with a structure that includes a flexible "hinge" region. This modification results in a nearly orthogonal orientation of its side chains. This is markedly different from tamoxifen, which has a rigid triphenylethylene structure.[115] Although both drugs bind to the ER, their structural differences lead to dissimilar conformations of the ER-ligand complex.[116] In the Ishikawa endometrial carcinoma cell line, tamoxifen, but not raloxifene, induces recruitment of coactivators SRC-1, AIB1, and CBP to the c-Myc and IGF-1 promoters.[117] This recruitment of coactivators is critical to tamoxifen's transactivating ability and agonist activity in the endometrium. The comparative inability of raloxifene to assemble this coactivator complex may account for its lower agonist activity in the endometrium.

Clinical Use

Raloxifene is indicated for breast cancer prevention in postmenopausal women at high risk for developing breast cancer.

Pharmacology and Metabolism

Raloxifene binds to the ER with a K_d of about 50 pmol/L, which is comparable to the value for estradiol.[118] The drug is given at 60 mg/d, and after oral administration it is rapidly absorbed, reaching its maximal concentration in about 30 minutes.[119] While absorption is 60%, first-pass metabolism limits the drug's bioavailability to 2%. After absorption, raloxifene is distributed widely throughout the body and is bound to plasma proteins, including albumin. The half-life of the drug is 27.7 hours.[120]

Metabolism of raloxifene, as mentioned, is primarily via first-pass glucuronidation. The agent does not appear to be metabolized by the CYP enzyme systems, and there are no other known metabolites.[120] Elimination occurs primarily through bile and feces, with just a small amount found in the urine.

Drug Interactions

Cholestyramine causes a 60% reduction in raloxifene absorption and enterohepatic circulation.[120] Unlike tamoxifen, raloxifene has a minor interaction with warfarin, with just a 10% decrease in prothrombin time. Concomitant therapy with ampicillin reduced the raloxifene peak concentration by 28%, which was felt to be clinically insignificant.[120]

Skeletal Effects

Raloxifene has been demonstrated to have estrogen agonist activity in bone in both animal models and in clinical trials. The multiple outcomes of raloxifene evaluation (MORE) study enrolled 7,705 women with osteoporosis to determine if the drug could decrease the rate of fractures.[121] While vertebral fractures were reduced by 30%, nonvertebral fractures were not significantly different. However, bone mineral density was increased in both the spine and femoral neck.

Endometrial Effects

Unlike estrogen and tamoxifen, raloxifene does not have stimulatory activity in the uterus. In the mature rats, uterine weight and endothelial height were unchanged with raloxifene exposure.[122] However, in the more sensitive immature rat uterine assay, raloxifene is agonistic but less so than tamoxifen. Clinically, raloxifene does not promote uterine proliferation.[122] The 4-year update of the MORE trial confirmed that the rates of vaginal bleeding and endometrial cancer in patients taking raloxifene are the same as that in those on placebo.[123]

Cardiovascular Effects

Raloxifene has estrogen agonist effects on lipid metabolism, with reduction of serum cholesterol levels by 70% in postmenopausal rat models.[122] In clinical trials, raloxifene reduces serum LDL, fibrinogen, lipoprotein (a), homocysteine, and C-reactive protein. Unlike tamoxifen, however, raloxifene does not affect triglycerides or high-density lipoprotein (HDL). While these findings could argue for a possible cardiovascular protective effect, this has not been demonstrated in clinical study.[122] In the MORE trial, there was no difference between arms in cardiovascular events or cerebrovascular events in the overall cohort; however, subgroup analysis with multiple comparisons revealed that women with increased cardiovascular risk had a relative risk reduction in cardiac events of 40% when taking raloxifene.[120] The randomized placebo-controlled RUTH (Raloxifene Use for the Heart) trial failed to show any benefit of raloxifene in the prevention of coronary heart disease but, in fact, increased the incidence of blood clots and death from stroke, possibly related to its hypercoagulable effects.[124,125]

Other Side Effects

Other major symptoms provoked by raloxifene compared to placebo in the MORE trial included hot flashes (9.7% versus 6.4%), leg cramps (5.5% versus 1.9%), and thromboembolic events (1.4% versus 0.47%).[121] Some reports suggest that the increased risk of thromboembolic events is similar to that seen with tamoxifen and is perhaps the side effect of most concern when the drug is used in clinical practice. However, in the NSABP P2 prevention trial, thromboembolic events occurred significantly less often in patients treated with raloxifene compared with tamoxifen.[114] Raloxifene has been demonstrated to be teratogenic in animal studies.[115]

Toremifene

Toremifene is approved in the United States as an alternative to tamoxifen for first-line treatment of advanced ER+ breast cancer.[126] Toremifene has antiestrogenic activity similar to that of tamoxifen.[127] The drug acts as almost a pure antiestrogen in rats and is partially agonistic in mice. Unlike tamoxifen, however, this drug has no hepatocarcinogenicity or DNA adduct-forming ability in rats.[127] It was hoped, therefore, that toremifene would provide a safer SERM for long-term use, such as in the adjuvant setting, although studies comparing the two drugs have shown no clear advantage over tamoxifen. As a result, toremifene's use in the clinic has been somewhat limited. The major CYP-mediated metabolites of toremifene are N-demethyl-toremifene and 4-hydroxytoremifene. The mean terminal half-life of toremifene and these metabolites is from 5 to 6 days.[128] The side effects are similar to those of tamoxifen, with hot flashes being the most common. Toremifene is cross-resistant with tamoxifen and should not be used in tamoxifen-resistant disease.[127]

Fulvestrant: A Pure Antiestrogen

Background

Given the finding that resistance to tamoxifen may sometimes be due to its partial agonist effects, pure antiestrogens without agonist activity were developed as hormonal agents. Fulvestrant, the only approved pure antiestrogen, is a 7α-alkylamide analog of 17β-estradiol (Fig. 35.9). This drug is also often called a "selective estrogen receptor down-regulator", because it has been demonstrated to decrease the level of ER protein in the cell.[128]

Mechanism of Action

Fulvestrant is a steroidal antiestrogen that acts in a distinctly different manner than the SERMs. The drug binds the ER, like SERMs, but its long, bulky alkylamide side chain at the 7α position interferes with ER function. Crystallographic and fluorescence energy transfer studies of the drug indicate that it binds to ERα and promotes receptor dimerization (but less potently than SERMS), suggesting that its downstream effects may lie at the level of interaction of the drug-ER complex with coactivators and/or corepressors.[129] The result is that the ER cannot bind DNA and is eliminated more rapidly via proteosome degradation, leading to a marked reduction in ER protein levels.[129,130] In this way, fulvestrant completely blocks ER-mediated gene transcription completely. In vitro, this results in inhibition of tamoxifen-resistant breast cancer cell lines by fulvestrant. In addition, the drug has no growth stimulatory effect in a tamoxifen-stimulated MCF-7 breast cancer xenograft model.[129] In primate studies, fulvestrant also acts as a pure antiestrogen outside of the breast, with complete inhibition of estrogen stimulation of uterine tissue.[131]

The antiproliferative effects of fulvestrant may be augmented by its ability to suppress insulin-like growth factor receptor signaling. This appears to occur both in vitro and in animal models. Finally, fulvestrant also has activity as an aromatase inhibitor, although it is not known how much this property contributes to the clinical activity of the drug.[132]

The effects of fulvestrant on ER, PgR, proliferation, and apoptosis have been examined in benign endometrial tissue and malignant breast tissue. When fulvestrant was given for a week before hysterectomy, it was found to decrease a Ki67-based proliferation assay; however, ER and PgR levels were not affected. By contrast, short-term exposure to fulvestrant before breast surgery decreased ER and PgR expression, proliferation, and increased apoptosis.[133,134] These data suggest that, as in the case of other antiestrogens, there may be differences in the action of fulvestrant at different organ sites.

While current experience with fulvestrant in breast cancer is limited to postmenopausal women, there have been trials with benign gynecologic conditions that demonstrate its antiestrogenic properties in premenopausal women.[135]

Clinical Use

Fulvestrant is used in the treatment of postmenopausal women with ER+ metastatic breast cancer, following progression on tamoxifen or an aromatase inhibitor.

Pharmacology

In vitro, fulvestrant has an ER-binding affinity 100-fold greater than that of tamoxifen.[130] Because the drug is not reliably absorbed orally, it is formulated as a monthly depot intramuscular injection. With this preparation, peak levels of fulvestrant occur at a median of 8 to 9 days after dosing and decline thereafter, but the levels remain above the projected therapeutic threshold at day 28. In pharmacokinetic studies, the area under the curve (AUC) was 140 micrograms × day/Liter in the first month and 208 micrograms

× day/Liter after 6 months, suggesting drug accumulation.[136] Because a single injection of the 5-mL volume can be difficult in some patients, the drug is often given as two 2.5-mL injections; this alternative method of delivery has no effect on the pharmacokinetics of the drug.[137] Recently completed and ongoing clinical trials are currently addressing the key issue of whether fulvestrant would be more effective if given as a loading dose with larger doses on day 1 and/or additional doses at day 14.

Metabolism

While published data on the metabolism of fulvestrant are sparse, the drug is known to undergo oxidation, hydroxylation, and conjugation with glucuronic acid and/or sulphate in the liver, with negligible renal excretion. The half-life of the drug is approximately 40 days.[138]

Side Effects

In preclinical studies, fulvestrant has been reported to cause decreased bone mineral density in adult female rats, suggesting that osteoporosis might be a side effect.[139] Preclinical data suggests that fulvestrant may have decreased ocular effects compared with tamoxifen; however, large randomized trials would be required to determine differences in this rare complication.[140]

The frequency of hot flashes with fulvestrant in clinical trials has been similar to the frequency with aromatase inhibitors, with the exception of one trial that compared fulvestrant and tamoxifen in the metastatic setting and found decreased hot flashes with fulvestrant.[141] These side effects are often not accurately collected without a hot flash. No other side effects in this trial were statistically different between the two drugs.

In early clinical studies, fulvestrant did not cause a change in sex hormone–binding globulin, prolactin, or serum lipids. In addition, there was no increase in endometrial thickness in patients undergoing hysterectomy.[136] In more recent clinical trials for metastatic breast cancer, fulvestrant has been well tolerated, with hot flashes and gastrointestinal disturbances as the most common adverse events. Tolerability was similar between fulvestrant and anastrozole in two phase III trials with a treatment-related withdrawal rate of 2.5%.[130]

Fulvestrant in Premenopausal Women

While breast cancer trials with fulvestrant have focused on postmenopausal women, the drug has also been used in premenopausal women with uterine fibroids and endometriosis. In these studies, fulvestrant had pure antagonizing effects in endometrial tissue.[130]

Aromatase Inhibitors

Aromatase Background

Postmenopausal Estrogen

The therapeutic effect of reducing estrogen levels for patients with breast cancer was originally restricted to patients with functioning ovaries. However, postmenopausal women produce significant amounts of estrogen through aromatization of circulating adrenal androgens in peripheral normal tissues, such as fat, muscle, liver, and the epithelial and stromal components of the breast.[142,143] Peripheral aromatization is increased in certain medical conditions, including obesity, hepatic disease, and hyperthyroidism, but is independent of pituitary hormone secretion. The relative proportion of estrogens synthesized in extragonadal sites increases with age, and eventually nonovarian estrogens predominate in the circulation.[144]

Intratumoral Aromatase

Aromatase is a key enzyme responsible for the biosynthesis of estrogens. It catalyzes the conversion of testosterone to estradiol. Expression of aromatase in the breast led to the hypothesis that local synthesis of estrogens contributes to breast cancer growth in postmenopausal women.[145,146] In support of this theory, the decline in estrogen concentrations after menopause is less marked in breast tissue than in plasma due to a combination of aromatase activity and to a lesser extent preferential estrogen uptake from the circulation.[53] Furthermore, aromatase activity has been shown to correlate with a marker of breast cancer cell proliferation, and quadrants of the breast bearing a breast cancer have more aromatase expression than those not bearing tumors.[147]

Development of Aromatase Inhibitors

Steroidal Versus Nonsteroidal

Two distinct solutions evolved to the problem of designing potent, specific, and safe aromatase inhibitors.[148] One strategy was to develop "steroidal" aromatase inhibitors that are resistant to aromatase action and that bind aromatase and block conversion of androgenic substrates (Type 1 inhibitors). An alternative was to develop a family of "nonsteroidal" inhibitors that disrupt the aromatase active site by coordinating within the heme complex without affecting the steroid binding sites of other steroidogenic enzymes (Type 2 inhibitors). Both approaches led to the successful introduction of potent and specific aromatase inhibitors into clinical practice.

Early Aromatase Inhibitors

In 1973, Griffiths et al.[149] first demonstrated the activity of aminoglutethimide, an inhibitor of cholesterol conversion to pregnenolone in the treatment of metastatic breast cancer. Subsequently, it was appreciated that inhibition of aromatase, rather than suppression of general steroidogenesis, was key to the therapeutic action of aminoglutethimide.[150,151] Although the drug has well-documented efficacy in the metastatic setting, its side effect profile is troublesome. Aminoglutethimide inhibits the formation of corticosteroids by blocking P-450 enzymes involved in cholesterol side chain cleavage.[152] This lack of specificity exposes patients to the risk of glucocorticoid deficiency. Furthermore, other troublesome side effects include rash, nausea, somnolence, and blood dyscrasias.[152,153]

These observations provided a strong rationale for the development of more potent and selective aromatase inhibitors. While second-generation aromatase inhibitors, such as fadrozole and formestane, had improved potency and selectivity, the third-generation aromatase inhibitors provided superior clinical results and rendered both aminoglutethimide and the second-generation drugs obsolete in breast cancer therapeutics.

Exemestane: Steroidal Aromatase Inhibitor

Background

Exemestane, an androstenedione derivative, exhibits tight or even irreversible binding to the aromatase active site.[154] The compound

is therefore considered a "mechanism-based" or "suicide" inhibitor because it permanently inactivates aromatase.

Clinical Use

Exemestane is used in the adjuvant setting for postmenopausal women with ER+ breast cancer following 2 to 3 years of tamoxifen treatment. Exemestane is also indicated for postmenopausal women with metastatic ER+ breast cancer following progression on tamoxifen.

Pharmacology

Exemestane (Fig. 35.10) has potent aromatase activity with a K^i of 26 nM and no cholesterol side chain cleavage (desmolase) or 5-reductase activity. An oral dose is rapidly absorbed, and peak plasma concentrations are reached within 2 hours of administration. The absorption of exemestane is enhanced by high-fat foods, and it is recommended that the drug be taken after eating.[155] Plasma concentrations fall below the limit of detection 4 hours later (for the approved 25-mg dose), although inhibition of the enzyme persists for at least 5 days.[155] Steady-state levels are achieved within 7 days with daily dosing, and the time to maximal estradiol suppression is 3 to 7 days.[156] The smallest that maximally suppressed of plasma estrone, estradiol, and estrone sulfate and urinary estrone and estradiol was 25 mg, now the recommended daily dosage. This dosage inactivates peripheral aromatase by 98% and reduces basal plasma estrone, estradiol, and estrone sulphate levels by 85% to 95% in postmenopausal women.[157] Other endocrine parameters, such as cortisol, aldosterone, dehydroepiandrosterones, 17-OH-progesterone, follicle-stimulating hormone (FSH), and LH, are not significantly affected by 25 mg of exemestane.[158]

Metabolism

Exemestane is extensively metabolized, with rapid oxidation of the methylene group at position 6 and reduction of the 17-keto group, along with subsequent formation of many secondary metabolites. The drug is excreted in both the urine and feces. As a consequence, clearance is affected by both renal and hepatic insufficiency, with threefold elevations in the AUC under either condition. Metabolism occurs through CYP3A4 and aldoketoreductases.[156,159] While exemestane does not bind to the ER and only weakly binds to the AR, with an affinity of 0.28% relative to DHT, the binding affinity of the 17-dihydrometabolite for AR is 100 times that of the parent compound.[160] As a result, there is slight androgenic activity in the rat with this drug. A screen of potential metabolites for aromatase activity did not reveal any compounds with inhibitory activity greater than exemestane.[161]

Toxicities

In clinical studies, exemestane has been well tolerated and has had a treatment-related discontinuation rate of less than 3%.[159] At high doses in rat studies, exemestane has been observed to have androgenic effects. Similarly, at high doses in clinical trials, androgenic side effects, including hypertrichosis, hair loss, hoarseness, and acne, have been reported in 4% of patients.[159] Other reported side effects include hot flashes, increased sweating, and nausea.

With all aromatase inhibitors, bone loss is a significant concern. However, the androgenic properties of exemestane metabolites

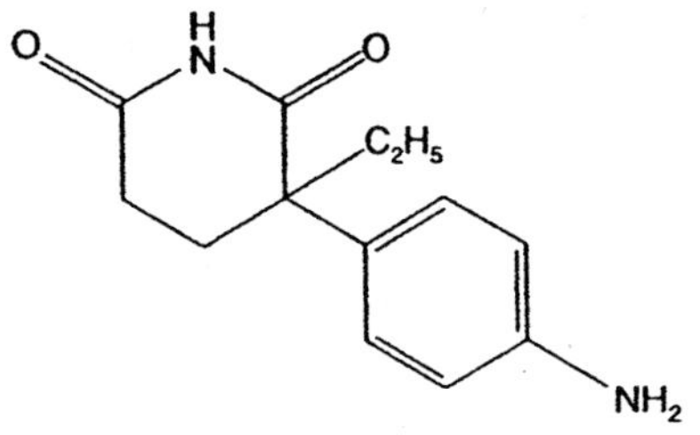

Aminoglutethimide

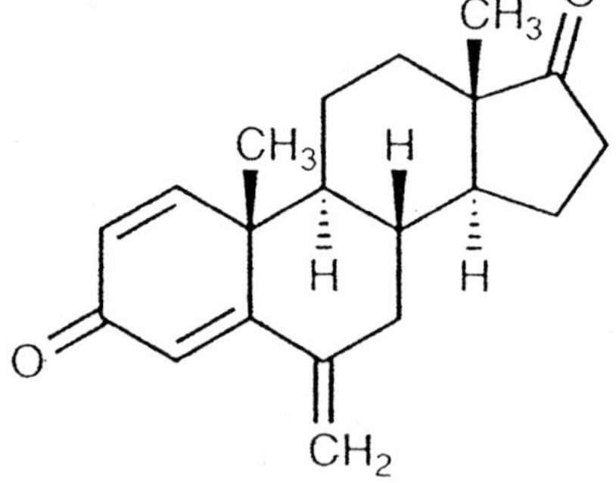

Exemestane

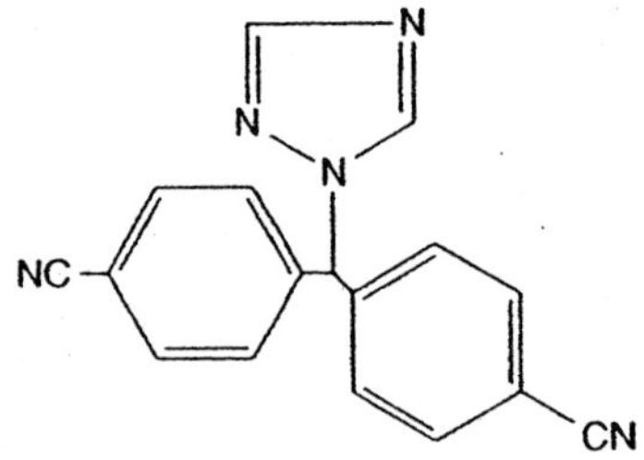

Letrozole

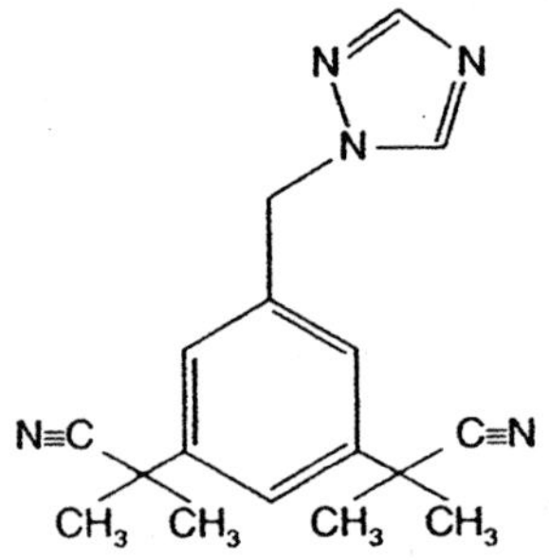

Anastrozole

FIGURE **35-10** Aromatase inhibitors.

might mitigate this effect. In ovariectomized rat studies, exemestane treatment provided protection from bone loss in comparison with untreated animals.[162] Initial studies in postmenopausal women using bone turnover biomarkers suggest that exemestane has a significantly smaller negative impact on bone formation and bone resorption than letrozole.[163] Despite these findings, results of the Intergroup Exemestane Study (IES) showed that postmenopausal patients on exemestane experience more osteoporosis than those on tamoxifen.[164] This may in large part due to improvement in BMD with tamoxifen rather than loss with exemestane. BMD profiles suggest an early mild decrease in exemestane-treated women with stabilization thereafter. Cessation of exemestane with recovery of estrogen levels results in approximate return to placebo-controlled levels within 12 to 24 months after stopping treatment.[165]

Other side effects that were increased in the exemestane group in the IES trial included visual disturbances, arthralgia, and diarrhea. Conversely, patients on tamoxifen experienced more gynecologic symptoms, vaginal bleeding, thromboembolic disease, and cramps.[164]

Drug Interactions

Given that exemestane is extensively metabolized by CYP3A4, interference with other drugs that induce or inhibit this P-450 enzyme may occur. Interestingly, however, ketoconazole does not significantly influence the pharmacokinetics of exemestane, suggesting that with CYP3A4 inhibition exemestane may be metabolized via a different route, or that renal excretion may compensate.[156]

Exemestane has mild androgenic activity, which may exert antitumor effects independent of its aromatase inhibitory action. Other advantages are its irreversible inhibition of aromatase, its better toxicity profile, and improved quality of life. This hypothesis is being tested in a large ongoing adjuvant breast cancer trial, NCIC CTG MA27, results of which are anticipated in 2010.

Nonsteroidal Aromatase Inhibitors

The nonsteroidal approach to aromatase inhibition has yielded two compounds widely applied in the clinic today, anastrozole and letrozole (Fig. 35.10).[166]

in hormonal resistance.[212] Overexpression of another coactivator, NCoA1, similarly increases tamoxifen's agonist activity, indicating a role in tamoxifen resistance.[213]

Conversely, decreased activity of corepressors has also been implicated as a mechanism of resistance. In a mouse model of tamoxifen resistance, NCoR1 levels were decreased.[206] Together, these findings suggest that alteration of the coactivator-corepressor balance can result in conversion of tamoxifen from an antagonist to an agonist.

Growth Factor Signaling Pathways

As previously discussed, ER function is strongly influenced by peptide growth factor signaling, including EGFR, ErbB2, and IGF-1-R, that leads to stimulation of ER activity in the absence of estrogen. These mitogenic pathways are often elevated in nonresponsive tumors that exhibit either primary or acquired resistance, which may lead to downstream activation of kinases that phosphorylate the ER and/or ER coregulators.[214–216] In this way, these growth factor pathways can allow the ER to function in the absence of ligand.

EGF has been shown to mimic the effect of estrogens on uterine cell proliferation in ovariectomized mice, and tumors overexpressing EGFR are less likely to be sensitive to hormonal therapy.[214] Similar results have been demonstrated with overexpression of ErbB2.[214] Several groups have evaluated response to hormonal therapy with respect to ErbB2 tumor status or circulating ErbB2 levels.[217–219] These studies have found a markedly decreased response to hormones in patients with ErbB2-overexpressing tumors.

Recently, the paired box 2 gene product (PAX2) has been identified as a crucial mediator of ER cross talk with ErbB2.[220] PAX2 and the ER coactivator AIB-1/SRC-3 compete for binding and regulation of ErbB2 transcription. This suggests an intrinsic transcriptional link between tumors driven by ER and those driven by ErbB2. PAX2 may be a primary determinant of tamoxifen response in breast cancer cells.

Additionally, the expression and activation of the Ras/Raf-1/MAPK pathway play an important role in the development and progression of cancer. An analysis of breast tumors showed that expression and activation of the Ras pathway were associated with loss of benefit from treatment with tamoxifen but not chemotherapy.[221] This finding is consistent with other studies of the Ras pathway in lung and colon cancer. Patients with a polymorphism of TC21, a member of the Ras superfamily, had higher recurrence rates on tamoxifen.[222]

CYP2D6 Metabolism on Tamoxifen Resistance

As discussed earlier, tamoxifen is biotransformed to the potent antiestrogen, endoxifen, by the CYP2D6 enzyme. Evidence suggests that endoxifen is most responsible for tamoxifen activity. Endoxifen has equivalent potency in vitro to 4-hydroxytamoxifen in ERα and ERβ binding,[223] in suppression of ER-dependent human breast cancer cell line proliferation,[224] and in global ER-responsive gene expression.[225] In women chronically receiving tamoxifen, plasma endoxifen stead-state concentrations are on average—6 to 10 times higher than 4-hydroxytamoxifen.[71,73]

Endoxifen concentrations are directly related to CYP2D6 genetic variation and inhibition of the enzyme system. CYP2D6 genetic variation has been shown to be associated with a higher risk of relapse and a lower incidence of moderate to severe hot flashes in women taking tamoxifen.[226] Women homozygous for the most common allele associated with the CYP2D6 poor metabolizer phenotype appeared to have shorter relapse-free survival. Similarly, in a prospective tamoxifen trial, coadminstration of CYP2D6 significantly reduced mean plasma endoxifen concentrations.[73]

Based on the results of these small but provocative studies, some clinicians choose to perform CYP2D6 gene testing for postmenopausal women about to begin tamoxifen therapy. If the gene testing reveals a CYP2D6 poor metabolizer phenotype, an aromatase inhibitor is often considered as an alternative to tamoxifen. When possible, coadministration of tamoxifen and CYP2D6 inhibitors may be avoided. It is worth emphasizing, however, that there are no prospective data supporting these approaches. Toremifene, which has been shown to be equivalent in terms of efficacy to tamoxifen, is not metabolized by the CYP2D6 enzyme, suggesting the possibility of using this agent in patients who are slow or ultraslow activators of tamoxifen.

Genetic Profiling Studies of Hormonal Resistance

Gene expression analysis and molecular profiling are increasingly used to predict the likelihood of a therapeutic response. Several investigators have used these approaches on tumor samples to develop gene signatures to predict clinical response to hormonal therapy. For example, genome-wide microarray analysis of tumors from women treated with adjuvant tamoxifen discovered that homeobox 13 (HOXB13)/interleukin-17B receptor (IL17BR) gene ratio is an independent predictor of tamoxifen response.[227] As previously discussed, genetic variation in CYP2D6 is also associated with tamoxifen resistance. In an effort to use these genetic markers toward individualized therapy, an index composed of both inherited CYP2D6 and tumor HOXB13/IL17BR has been developed and identifies patients with varying degrees of resistance to tamoxifen.[228]

While gene expression profiling has provided insight into pathways that may contribute to hormonal therapy resistance, there are many challenges associated with this approach. Independent validation studies are often difficult, given the complexity of multiple expression array platforms and technologies. Statistical analysis of these data is also very complex and the risk of excluding biologically relevant genes is significant. Nonetheless, gene expression profiling holds great promise in furthering our understanding of drug resistance.

Strategies to Combat Hormonal Resistance

There has been remarkable growth in the number of hormone therapies available for the treatment of breast cancer. With more hormonal options, the clinical efficacy of hormonal therapy has improved; however, the improvement has been incremental in nature. Our increasing understanding of the molecular basis of hormonal resistance has led to the possibility of using combinations of hormonal agents with new signal transduction inhibitors for the treatment of breast cancer. The inhibition of multiple growth pathways simultaneously could potentially combat the redundancy and cross talk of growth signals, thereby providing effective, well-tolerated therapy.

Future Directions

With the advent of advanced techniques, such as DNA microarrays and proteomic technologies, the characterization of different types of tumors will continue to make major strides. With regard to hormonal therapy, significant achievements have already been made. Several groups have demonstrated that supervised cluster analysis of DNA microarray data allows identification of a set of genes that can distinguish between ER-positive and ER-negative breast tumors.[229,230] The marked difference in the gene expression profile of these breast cancer subtypes suggests the possibility of distinct precursor cells. Interestingly, only a small number of genes that discriminate between ER-positive and ER-negative tumors are involved in ER signaling.[231]

Further subclassification of breast tumors will continue. Given that resistance to hormonal agents does not entirely overlap, further work with other agents will likely show different resistance and sensitivity patterns associated with various hormonal therapies. This will undoubtedly help define how to use different hormonal agents. Furthermore, as signal transduction inhibitors are tested in combination with hormonal therapy, DNA microarrays will be critical in determining which targeted drug cocktail to use against a specific tumor.

In addition to predicting the ER status of tumors and their response to therapy, gene expression profiling has the potential to help elucidate which signaling pathways are critical in tumors and thus provide strategies to improve treatment. It is important to note that, with DNA microarray analysis, the delineation of differences in signaling pathways between tumors is only inferential. While these advanced analytic procedures can help generate hypotheses, the findings from these studies still require testing with more traditional laboratory techniques. A number of laboratories have identified and characterized changes in gene expression that occur with various hormonal agents.[232,233] Ontology mapping, whereby genes are classified into various functional categories, has been helpful in describing major cellular events. However, constructing a detailed and integrated picture of differences in signaling pathways will require further work. Proteomic technologies, which are beginning to allow large-scale interrogation of signaling pathways, will be critical in achieving this goal. Integration of these technologies into clinical trial design is essential.

The determination of predictive biomarkers for targeted therapy is currently a major goal in the oncology community. Interestingly, the use of hormonal therapy for ER/PR-positive breast cancer provides the oldest paradigm for this approach. In addition, this history gives a glimpse of the promise and limitations of targeted therapy. Hormonal resistance remains a problem that we are only beginning to address in the clinic. Finally, classical endocrine therapy continues to evolve with ongoing clinical investigation into the optimal endocrine agent, duration of therapy, and scheduling of therapy. However, with the development of new technologies and new drugs, hormonal therapy can be a foundation on which to build more effectively tailored and targeted treatments.

References

1. Love RR, Philips J. Oophorectomy for breast cancer: history revisited. J Natl Cancer Inst 2002;94:1433–1434.
2. IUPAC Commission on the Nomenclature of Organic Chemistry (CNOC) and IUPAC-IUB Commission on Biochemical Nomenclature (CBN). The nomenclature of steroids: revised tentative rules. Eur J Biochem 1969;10:1–19.
3. Briggs MJ. Steroid Biochemistry and Pharmacology. London: Academic Press, 1970.
4. Brotherton J. Sex Hormone Pharmacology. London: Academic Press, 1976.
5. Briggs MJ, Christie GA. Advances in Steroid Biochemistry and Pharmacology. London: Academic Press, 1977.
6. Gruber CJ, Tschugguel W, Schneeberger C, et al. Production and actions of estrogens. N Engl J Med 2002;346:340–352.
7. Brodie A. Aromatase inhibitors in breast cancer. Trends Endocrinol Metab 2002;13:61–65.
8. Chen SA, Besman MJ, Sparkes RS, et al. Human aromatase: cDNA cloning, Southern blot analysis, and assignment of the gene to chromosome 15. DNA 1988;7:27–38.
9. Agarwal VR, Bulun SE, Leitch M, et al. Use of alternative promoters to express the aromatase cytochrome P450 (CYP19) gene in breast adipose tissues of cancer-free and breast cancer patients. J Clin Endocrinol Metab 1996;81:3843–3849.
10. Santner SJ, Pauley RJ, Tait L, et al. Aromatase activity and expression in breast cancer and benign breast tissue stromal cells. J Clin Endocrinol Metab 1997;82:200–208.
11. Zhou D, Clarke P, Wang J, et al. Identification of a promoter that controls aromatase expression in human breast cancer and adipose stromal cells. J Biol Chem 1996;271:15194–15202.
12. Grodin JM, Siiteri PK, MacDonald PC. Source of estrogen production in postmenopausal women. J Clin Endocrinol Metab 1973;36:207–214.
13. Simpson ER. Sources of estrogen and their importance. J Steroid Biochem Mol Biol 2003;86:225–230.
14. Kutsky RJ. Estradiol. Handbook of Vitamins, Minerals, and Hormones. New York: Van Nostrand Reinhold, 1981:415.
15. Evans RM. The steroid and thyroid hormone receptor superfamily. Science 1988;240:889–895.
16. Shao W, Brown M. Advances in estrogen receptor biology: prospects for improvements in targeted breast cancer therapy. Breast Cancer Res 2004;6:39–52.
17. Yang NN, Venugopalan M, Hardikar S, et al. Identification of an estrogen response element activated by metabolites of 17beta-estradiol and raloxifene. Science 1996;273:1222–1225.
18. Speirs V, Carder PJ, Lane S, et al. Oestrogen receptor beta: what it means for patients with breast cancer. Lancet Oncol 2004;5:174–181.
19. Barkhem T, Carlsson B, Nilsson Y, et al. Differential response of estrogen receptor alpha and estrogen receptor beta to partial estrogen agonists/antagonists. Mol Pharmacol 1998;54:105–112.
20. Saunders FJ. Effects of norethynodrel combined with mestranol on the offspring when administered during pregnancy and lactation in rats. Endocrinology 1967;80:447–452.
21. Williams MT, Clark MR, Ling WY. Role of cyclic AMP in the action of luteinizing hormone on steroidogenesis in the corpus luteum. In: George WJ, Ignarro L, eds. Advances in Cyclic Nucleotide Research. Vol. 9. New York: Raven Press, 1978:573.
22. Weihua Z, Andersson S, Cheng G, et al. Update on estrogen signaling. FEBS Lett 2003;546:17–24.
23. Krege JH, Hodgin JB, Couse JF, et al. Generation and reproductive phenotypes of mice lacking estrogen receptor beta. Proc Natl Acad Sci U S A 1998;95:15677–15682.
24. Porter W, Wang F, Wang W, et al. Role of estrogen receptor/Sp1 complexes in estrogen-induced heat shock protein 27 gene expression. Mol Endocrinol 1996;10:1371–1378.
25. Pace P, Taylor J, Suntharalingam S, et al. Human estrogen receptor beta binds DNA in a manner similar to and dimerizes with estrogen receptor alpha. J Biol Chem 1997;272:25832–25838.

26. McDonnell DP, Norris JD. Connections and regulation of the human estrogen receptor. Science 2002;296:1642–1644.

27. Shao W, Brown M. Advances in estrogen receptor biology: prospects for improvements in targeted breast cancer therapy. Breast Cancer Res 2004;6:39–52.

28. Beato M, Candau R, Chavez S, et al. Interaction of steroid hormone receptors with transcription factors involves chromatin remodelling. J Steroid Biochem Mol Biol 1996;56:47–59.

29. Lannigan DA. Estrogen receptor phosphorylation. Steroids 2003;68:1–9.

30. El-Ashry D, Miller DL, Kharbanda S, et al. Constitutive Raf-1 kinase activity in breast cancer cells induces both estrogen-independent growth and apoptosis. Oncogene 1997;15:423–435.

31. Kato S, Masuhiro Y, Watanabe M, et al. Molecular mechanism of a cross-talk between oestrogen and growth factor signalling pathways. Genes Cells 2000;5:593–601.

32. Kato S, Endoh H, Masuhiro Y, et al. Activation of the estrogen receptor through phosphorylation by mitogen-activated protein kinase. Science 1995;270:1491–1494.

33. Mueller H, Kueng W, Schoumacher F, et al. Selective regulation of steroid receptor expression in MCF-7 breast cancer cells by a novel member of the heregulin family. Biochem Biophys Res Commun 1995;217:1271–1278.

34. Ingle JN, Ahmann DL, Green SJ, et al. Randomized clinical trial of diethylstilbestrol versus tamoxifen in postmenopausal women with advanced breast cancer. N Engl J Med 1981;304:16–21.

35. Furr BJ, Jordan VC. The pharmacology and clinical uses of tamoxifen. Pharmacol Ther 1984;25:127–205.

36. Osborne CK. Tamoxifen in the treatment of breast cancer. N Engl J Med 1998;339:1609–1618.

37. Morgan LR Jr, Schein PS, Woolley PV, et al. Therapeutic use of tamoxifen in advanced breast cancer: correlation with biochemical parameters. Cancer Treat Rep 1976;60:1437–1443.

38. Rose C, Mouridsen HT. Treatment of advanced breast cancer with tamoxifen. Recent Results Cancer Res 1984;91:230–242.

39. Early Breast Cancer Trialists' Collaborative Group. Tamoxifen for early breast cancer: an overview of the randomised trials. Lancet 1998;351:1451–1467.

40. Ingle JN, Krook JE, Green SJ, et al. Randomized trial of bilateral oophorectomy versus tamoxifen in premenopausal women with metastatic breast cancer. J Clin Oncol 1986;4:178–185.

41. Muss HB, Case LD, Atkins JN, et al. Tamoxifen versus high-dose oral medroxyprogesterone acetate as initial endocrine therapy for patients with metastatic breast cancer: a Piedmont Oncology Association study. J Clin Oncol 1994;12:1630–1638.

42. Hermon C, Beral V. Breast cancer mortality rates are levelling off or beginning to decline in many western countries: analysis of time trends, age-cohort and age-period models of breast cancer mortality in 20 countries. Br J Cancer 1996;73:955–960.

43. Jordan VC, Assikis VJ. Endometrial carcinoma and tamoxifen: clearing up a controversy. Clin Cancer Res 1995;1:467–472.

44. Uziely B, Lewin A, Brufman G, et al. The effect of tamoxifen on the endometrium. Breast Cancer Res Treat 1993;26:101–105.

45. Kavak ZN, Binoz S, Ceyhan N, et al. The effect of tamoxifen on the endometrium, serum lipids and hypothalamus pituitary axis in the postmenopausal breast cancer patient. Acta Obstet Gynecol Scand 2000;79:604–607.

46. Enck RE, Rios CN. Tamoxifen treatment of metastatic breast cancer and antithrombin III levels. Cancer 1984;53:2607–2609.

47. Love RR, Surawicz TS, Williams EC. Antithrombin III level, fibrinogen level, and platelet count changes with adjuvant tamoxifen therapy. Arch Intern Med 1992;152:317–320.

48. Barakat RR. The effect of tamoxifen on the endometrium. Oncology (Huntingt) 1995;9:129–134; discussion 139–140, 142.

49. Barni S, Lissoni P, Tancini G, et al. Effects of one-year adjuvant treatment with tamoxifen on bone mineral density in postmenopausal breast cancer women. Tumori 1996;82:65–67.

50. Schapira DV, Kumar NB, Lyman GH. Serum cholesterol reduction with tamoxifen. Breast Cancer Res Treat 1990;17:3–7.

51. Love RR, Newcomb PA, Wiebe DA, et al. Effects of tamoxifen therapy on lipid and lipoprotein levels in postmenopausal patients with node-negative breast cancer. J Natl Cancer Inst 1990;82:1327–1332.

52. Fromson JM, Pearson S, Bramah S. The metabolism of tamoxifen (I.C.I. 46,474), I: in laboratory animals. Xenobiotica 1973;3:693–709.

53. Lyman SD, Jordan VC. Metabolism of nonsteroidal antiestrogens. In: Jordan VC, ed. Estrogen/Antiestrogen Action and Breast Cancer Therapy. Madison: University of Wisconsin Press, 1986.

54. Bain RR, Jordan VC. Identification of a new metabolite of tamoxifen in patient serum during breast cancer therapy. Biochem Pharmacol 1983;32:373–375.

55. Robinson SP, Jordan VC. Metabolism of antihormonal anticancer agents. In: International Encyclopedia of Pharmacology and Therapeutics. Oxford: Pergamon Press, 1994.

56. Adam HK, Douglas EJ, Kemp JV. The metabolism of tamoxifen in human. Biochem Pharmacol 1979;28:145–147.

57. Fromson JM, Pearson S, Bramah S. The metabolism of tamoxifen (I.C.I. 46,474), II: in female patients. Xenobiotica 1973;3:711–714.

58. Sutherland CM, Sternson LA, Muchmore JH, et al. Effect of impaired renal function on tamoxifen. J Surg Oncol 1984;27:222–223.

59. Fabian C, Tilzer L, Sternson L. Comparative binding affinities of tamoxifen, 4-hydroxytamoxifen, and desmethyltamoxifen for estrogen receptors isolated from human breast carcinoma: correlation with blood levels in patients with metastatic breast cancer. Biopharm Drug Dispos 1981;2:381–390.

60. Fabian C, Sternson L, El-Serafi M, et al. Clinical pharmacology of tamoxifen in patients with breast cancer: correlation with clinical data. Cancer 1981;48:876–882.

61. Nicholson RI, Syne JS, Daniel CP, et al. The binding of tamoxifen to oestrogen receptor proteins under equilibrium and non-equilibrium conditions. Eur J Cancer 1979;15:317–329.

62. Wakeling AE, Slater SR. Estrogen-receptor binding and biologic activity of tamoxifen and its metabolites. Cancer Treat Rep 1980;64:741–744.

63. Daniel CP, Gaskell SJ, Bishop H, et al. Determination of tamoxifen and an hydroxylated metabolite in plasma from patients with advanced breast cancer using gas chromatography-mass spectrometry. J Endocrinol 1979;83:401–408.

64. Daniel P, Gaskell SJ, Bishop H, et al. Determination of tamoxifen and biologically active metabolites in human breast tumours and plasma. Eur J Cancer Clin Oncol 1981;17:1183–1189.

65. Kemp JV, Adam HK, Wakeling AE, et al. Identification and biological activity of tamoxifen metabolites in human serum. Biochem Pharmacol 1983;32:2045–2052.

66. Fabian C, Sternson L, El-Serafi M, et al. Clinical pharmacology of tamoxifen in patients with breast cancer: correlation with clinical data. Cancer 1981;48:876–882.

67. Fabian C, Sternson L, Barnett M. Clinical pharmacology of tamoxifen in patients with breast cancer: comparison of traditional and loading dose schedules. Cancer Treat Rep 1980;64:765–773.

68. Noguchi S, Miyauchi K, Imaoka S, et al. Inability of tamoxifen to penetrate into cerebrospinal fluid. Breast Cancer Res Treat 1988;12:317–318.

69. Jacolot F, Simon I, Dreano Y, et al. Identification of the cytochrome P450 IIIA family as the enzymes involved in the N-demethylation of tamoxifen in human liver microsomes. Biochem Pharmacol 1991;41:1911–1919.

70. Desta Z, Ward BA, Soukhova NV, et al. Comprehensive evaluation of tamoxifen sequential biotransformation by the human cytochrome P450 system in vitro: prominent roles for CYP3A AND CYP2D6. J Pharmacol Exp Ther 2004;310:1062–1075.

71. Stearns V, Johnson MD, Rae JM, et al. Active tamoxifen metabolite plasma concentrations after coadminstration of tamoxifen and the selective serotonin reuptake inhibitor paroxetine. J Natl Cancer Inst 2003;95:1758–1764.

72. Crewe HK, Lennard MS, Tucker GT, et al. The effect of selective serotonin re-uptake inhibitors on cytochrome P4502D6 (CYP2D6) activity in human liver microsomes. Br J Clin Pharmacol 1992;34:262–265.

73. Jin Y, Desta Z, Stearns V, et al. CYP2D6 genotype, antidepressant use and tamoxifen metabolism during adjuvant breast cancer treatment. J Natl Cancer Inst 2005;97:30–39.

74. Dowsett M, Pfister C, Johnston SR, et al. Impact of tamoxifen on the pharmacokinetics and endocrine effects of the aromatase inhibitor letrozole in postmenopausal women with breast cancer. Clin Cancer Res 1999;5:2338–2343.

75. Reid AD, Horobin JM, Newman EL, et al. Tamoxifen metabolism is altered by simultaneous administration of medroxyprogesterone acetate in breast cancer patients. Breast Cancer Res Treat 1992;22:153–156.

76. Fogarty PF, Rick ME, Swain SM. Tamoxifen and thrombosis: current clinical observations and treatment guidelines. In: Devita VT, Hellman S, Rosenberg SA, eds. Cancer: Principles and Practice of Oncology. 6th ed. Philadelphia: Lippincott Williams & Wilkins, 2002.

77. Fisher B, Costantino JP, Wickerham DL, et al. Tamoxifen for prevention of breast cancer: report of the National Surgical Adjuvant Breast and Bowel Project P-1 Study. J Natl Cancer Inst 1998;90:1371–1388.

78. Kaiser-Kupfer MI, Lippman ME. Tamoxifen retinopathy. Cancer Treat Rep 1978;62:315–320.

79. Kaiser-Kupfer MI, Kupfer C, Rodrigues MM. Tamoxifen retinopathy: a clinicopathologic report. Ophthalmology 1981;88:89–93.

80. McKeown CA, Swartz M, Blom J, et al. Tamoxifen retinopathy. Br J Ophthalmol 1981;65:177–179.

81. Gerner EW. Low-dose tamoxifen retinopathy. Can J Ophthalmol 1992;27:358.

82. Griffiths MF. Tamoxifen retinopathy at low dosage. Am J Ophthalmol 1987;104:185–186.

83. Bentley CR, Davies G, Aclimandos WA. Tamoxifen retinopathy: a rare but serious complication. Br Med J 1992;304:495–496.

84. Pemberton KD, Melissari E, Kakkar VV. The influence of tamoxifen in vivo on the main natural anticoagulants and fibrinolysis. Blood Coagul Fibrinolysis 1993;4:935–942.

85. Fisher B, Costantino J, Redmond C, et al. A randomized clinical trial evaluating tamoxifen in the treatment of patients with node-negative breast cancer who have estrogen-receptor–positive tumors. N Engl J Med 1989;320:479–484.

86. Abramson N, Costantino, JP, Garber JE, et al. Effect of Factor V Leiden and prothrombin G20210–>A mutations on thromboembolic risk in the national surgical adjuvant breast and bowel project breast cancer prevention trial. J Natl Cancer Inst 2006;98:904–910.

87. Henderson ICI, et al., eds. Endocrine therapy in metastatic breast cancer. In: al HJRe, ed. Breast Diseases. Philadelphia: JB Lippincott, 1991:559.

88. Bruning PF, Bonfrer JM, Hart AA, et al. Tamoxifen, serum lipoproteins and cardiovascular risk. Br J Cancer 1988;58:497–499.

89. Ingram D. Tamoxifen use, oestrogen binding and serum lipids in postmenopausal women with breast cancer. Aust N Z J Surg 1990;60:673–675.

90. Jones AL, Powles TJ, Treleaven JG, et al. Haemostatic changes and thromboembolic risk during tamoxifen therapy in normal women. Br J Cancer 1992;66:744–747.

91. Gau TC. Letter to Physicians. Pasadena, CA: Stuart Pharmaceuticals, 1987.

92. Pathak DN, Bodell WJ. DNA adduct formation by tamoxifen with rat and human liver microsomal activation systems. Carcinogenesis 1994;15:529–532.

93. Turken S, Siris E, Seldin D, et al. Effects of tamoxifen on spinal bone density in women with breast cancer. J Natl Cancer Inst 1989;81:1086–1088.

94. Fornander T, Rutqvist LE, Sjoberg HE, et al. Long-term adjuvant tamoxifen in early breast cancer: effect on bone mineral density in postmenopausal women. J Clin Oncol 1990;8:1019–1024.

95. Gotfredsen A, Christiansen C, Palshof T. The effect of tamoxifen on bone mineral content in premenopausal women with breast cancer. Cancer 1984;53:853–857.

96. Kedar RP, Bourne TH, Powles TJ, et al. Effects of tamoxifen on uterus and ovaries of postmenopausal women in a randomised breast cancer prevention trial. Lancet 1994;343:1318–1321.

97. Bernstein L, Deapen D, Cerhan JR, et al. Tamoxifen therapy for breast cancer and endometrial cancer risk. J Natl Cancer Inst 1999;91:1654–1662.

98. Wysowski DK, Honig SF, Beitz J. Uterine sarcoma associated with tamoxifen use. N Engl J Med 2002;346:1832–1833.

99. Cullins SL, Pridjian G, Sutherland CM. Goldenhar's syndrome associated with tamoxifen given to the mother during gestation. JAMA 1994;271:1905–1906.

100. Woo JC, Yu T, Hurd TC. Breast cancer in pregnancy: a literature review. Arch Surg 2003;138:91–98; discussion 99.

101. Halakivi-Clarke L, Cho E, Onojafe I, et al. Maternal exposure to tamoxifen during pregnancy increases carcinogen-induced mammary tumorigenesis among female rat offspring. Clin Cancer Res 2000;6:305–308.

102. Collinson MP, Hamilton DA, Tyrrell CJ. Two case reports of tamoxifen as a cause of impotence in male subjects with carcinoma of the breast. Breast Cancer Res 1998;2:48–49.

103. Fernando IN, Tobias JS. Priapism in patients on tamoxifen. Lancet 1989;1:436.

104. Anelli TF, Anelli A, Tran KN, et al. Tamoxifen administration is associated with a high rate of treatment-limiting symptoms in male breast cancer patients. Cancer 1994;74:74–77.

105. Traub AI, Thompson W. The effect of tamoxifen on spermatogenesis in subfertile men. Andrologia 1981;13:486–490.

106. Gooren LJ. Androgen levels and sex functions in testosterone-treated hypogonadal men. Arch Sex Behav 1987;16:463–473.

107. Plotkin D, Lechner JJ, Jung WE, et al. Tamoxifen flare in advanced breast cancer. JAMA 1978;240:2644–2646.

108. Beex L, Pieters G, Smals A, et al. Tamoxifen versus ethinyl estradiol in the treatment of postmenopausal women with advanced breast cancer. Cancer Treat Rep 1981;65:179–185.

109. Howell A, Dodwell DJ, Anderson H, et al. Response after withdrawal of tamoxifen and progestogens in advanced breast cancer. Ann Oncol 1992;3(8):611–617.

110. O'Regan RM, Cisneros A, England GM, et al. Effects of the antiestrogens tamoxifen, toremifene, and ICI 182,780 on endometrial cancer growth. J Natl Cancer Inst 1998;90:1552–1558.

111. Lufkin EG, Whitaker MD, Nickelsen T, et al. Treatment of established postmenopausal osteoporosis with raloxifene: a randomized trial. J Bone Miner Res 1998;13:1747–1754.

112. Buzdar AU, Marcus C, Holmes F, et al. Phase II evaluation of Ly156758 in metastatic breast cancer. Oncology 1988;45:344–345.

113. Ettinger B, Black DM, Mitlak BH, et al. Reduction of vertebral fracture risk in postmenopausal women with osteoporosis treated with raloxifene: results from a 3-year randomized clinical trial. Multiple Outcomes of Raloxifene Evaluation (MORE) Investigators. JAMA 1999;282:637–645.

114. Vogel VG, Costantino JP, Wickerham DL, et al. Effects of tamoxifen vs. raloxifene on the risk of developing invasive breast cancer and other disease outcomes. The NSABP study of tamoxifen and raloxifene (STAR) P-2 trial. JAMA 2006;295:2727–2741.

115. Goldstein SR, Siddhanti S, Ciaccia AV, et al. A pharmacological review of selective oestrogen receptor modulators. Hum Reprod Update 2000;6:212–224.

116. Wijayaratne AL, Nagel SC, Paige LA, et al. Comparative analyses of mechanistic differences among antiestrogens. Endocrinology 1999;140:5828–5840.

117. Shang Y, Brown M. Molecular determinants for the tissue specificity of SERMs. Science 2002;295:2465–2468.

118. Glasebrook A, Phillips DL, Sluka JP. Multiple binding sites for the antiestrogen raloxifene. J Bone Miner Res 1993;1(Suppl):268.

119. Morello KC, Wurz GT, DeGregorio MW. Pharmacokinetics of selective estrogen receptor modulators. Clin Pharmacokinet 2003;42:361–372.

120. Snyder KR, Sparano N, Malinowski JM. Raloxifene hydrochloride. Am J Health Syst Pharm 2000;57:1669–1675; quiz 1676–1678.

121. Cummings SR, Eckert S, Krueger KA, et al. The effect of raloxifene on risk of breast cancer in postmenopausal women: results from the MORE randomized trial. Multiple Outcomes of Raloxifene Evaluation. JAMA 1999;281:2189–2197.

122. Hochner-Celnikier D. Pharmacokinetics of raloxifene and its clinical application. Eur J Obstet Gynecol Reprod Biol 1999;85:23–29.

123. Cauley JA, Norton L, Lippman ME, et al. Continued breast cancer risk reduction in postmenopausal women treated with raloxifene: 4-year results from the MORE trial. Multiple Outcomes of Raloxifene Evaluation. Breast Cancer Res Treat 2001;65:125–134.

124. Barrett-Connor E, Mosca L, Collins P, et al. Effects of raloxifene on cardiovascular events and breast cancer in postmenopausal women. N Engl J Med 2006;355:125–137.

125. Grady D, Cauley JA, Geiger MJ, et al. Reduced incidence of invasive breast cancer with raloxifene among women at increased coronary risk. J Natl Cancer Inst 2008;100:854–861.

126. Vogel CL. Phase II and III clinical trials of toremifene for metastatic breast cancer. Oncology (Huntingt) 1998;12:9–13.

127. Wiseman LR, Goa KL. Toremifene: a review of its pharmacological properties and clinical efficacy in the management of advanced breast cancer. Drugs 1997;54:141–160.

128. Wiebe VJ, Benz CC, Shemano I, et al. Pharmacokinetics of toremifene and its metabolites in patients with advanced breast cancer. Cancer Chemother Pharmacol 1990;25:247–251.

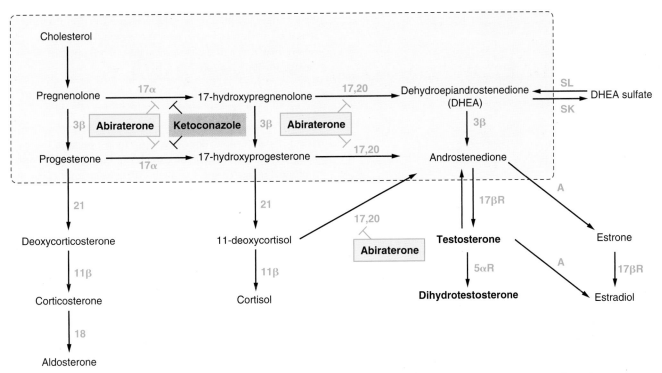

FIGURE **36-1**   Steroid synthesis pathways. The enclosed area contains the pathways used by the adrenal glands and gonads. Enzymes are labeled in *red*. Steps inhibited by ketoconazole and abiraterone are indicated. Enzymes: 17α: 17α-hydroxylase (CYP17); 17,20: C-17,20-lyase (also CYP17); 3β: 3β-hydroxysteroid dehydrogenase; 21: 21-hydroxylase; 11β: 11β-hydroxylase; 18: aldosterone synthase; 17βR: 17β-reductase; 5αR: 5α-reductase; A: aromatase; SULT, sulfotransferase; STS, sulfatase.

member of the nuclear hormone receptor superfamily and is a ligand-dependent transcription factor. AR is comprised of 919 amino acids, with characteristic domains of a nuclear receptor, including ligand- and DNA-binding domains and a long N-terminal transactivation domain that is capable of binding to the C terminus

and autoregulating AR activity. AR signaling is regulated by negative feedback on *AR* gene transcription. Castration results in increased *AR* transcription.[14]

Two polymorphic trinucleotide repeat segments exist in the transactivation domain of AR, (CAG)$_n$ and (GGN)$_n$.[15] CAG repeat length

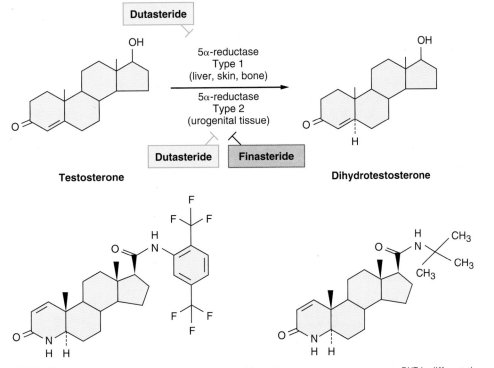

FIGURE **36-2**   The action of 5α-reductase. Two isoforms of 5α-reductase convert testosterone to DHT in different tissues. The 5α-reductase inhibitor dutasteride can inhibit both isoforms, whereas finasteride can only inhibit type 2.

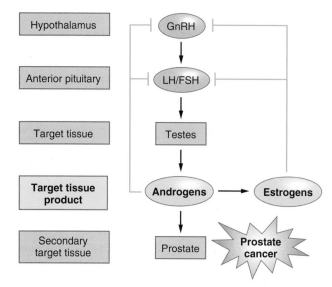

FIGURE **36-3**   The hypothalamic-pituitary-testicular axis. GnRH is secreted from the hypothalamus and induces release of LH and FSH from the pituitary gland. LH stimulates testosterone synthesis from testicular Leydig cells. Testosterone promotes prostate gland development and stimulates prostate cancer cell growth. Testosterone can be converted to estrogens. Androgens and estrogens can inhibit hypothalamic GnRH pulse frequency and pituitary LH production by negative feedback.

and AR mRNA and protein expression are inversely correlated,[16] whereas GGN length and AR transcriptional activity are positively correlated.[17] Increased long-term androgen stimulation due to CAG or GGN repeat lengths is postulated to lead to increased proliferation and subsequently higher rates of somatic mutations. However, numerous large genetic association studies have reported conflicting results; therefore, there is no clear association between these *AR* polymorphisms and prostate cancer risk.[18–22]

AR Signaling

AR is sequestered in the cytoplasm by chaperone proteins such as heat shock proteins. Upon ligand binding, AR is released from the chaperone proteins and can translocate to the nucleus. AR binds in a homodimeric conformation to DNA sequences known as androgen-response elements (AREs), which can vary substantially in different gene promoters (reviewed in Gelmann[14]).

In addition to ligand-stimulated activation of AR, increased AR signaling may occur via growth factor receptors such as HER2,[23,24] IL-6R,[25] EGFR, and IGF-1R.[26] In experimental systems, overexpression of these growth factor receptor tyrosine kinases led to enhanced AR signaling, via downstream activation of growth and survival pathways mediated by AKT, ERK, and STAT. The contribution of purported ligand-independent AR activation to disease progression in prostate cancer patients is unknown.

AR also binds to cytoplasmic proteins such as the tyrosine kinases SRC and Ack1. Ligand-bound AR binds and activates SRC and downstream effectors including ERK. SRC can also phosphorylate and potentiate AR activity via the AR SH3 domain.[27] In the setting of hormone therapy for prostate cancer, SRC may thereby sensitize AR to subphysiologic levels of androgens.[28] Ack1 is a kinase downstream of EGFR/HER2 signaling and also targets AR

for tyrosine phosphorylation and activation.[29] The mechanisms of activation of AR via growth factor receptor and cytoplasmic tyrosine kinases may occur in the castrate state and are putative targets for therapeutic intervention.

Mechanisms of Resistance to Hormone Therapy

While response to hormone therapy is nearly universal, resistance to hormonal manipulations develops in most men. In the castrate state, AR signaling despite low circulating androgen levels supports continued prostate cancer growth. AR signaling may occur due to androgens produced from nongonadal sources, AR gene mutations, AR gene amplification, or ligand-independent activation via growth factor receptor or cytoplasmic tyrosine kinases (as described above).

Nongonadal sources of androgens include the adrenal glands and the prostate cancer cells themselves. Adrenal-produced androstenedione is converted to testosterone in peripheral tissues and tumors.[30] Intratumoral de novo androgen synthesis may also provide sufficient androgen for AR-driven cell proliferation.[31]

Numerous somatic missense mutations have been detected in the *AR* gene in human prostate cancer tissues, cell lines, and xenografts. Primary prostate tumors or metastatic deposits examined prior to initiation of therapy exhibit a range in *AR* mutation frequency from 8% to 44%.[32,33] *AR* mutation frequency in metastases of patients who have progressed despite hormone therapy ranges from 18% to 50%.[34,35] Treatment with antiandrogens favors the selection of recurrent cancer with mutant AR.[35]

Most *AR* gene mutations in prostate cancer cluster in three regions, the ligand-binding domain (LBD), a region flanking the ligand-dependent transactivation function-2 domain (AF-2), and the boundary of the hinge region and the LBD.[36] Mutations in these regions may contribute to altered androgen signaling and disease progression in the context of hormone therapy in patients. Mutations in the LBD can broaden the spectrum of AR agonists to include other steroid hormones such as estrogen, progesterone, and glucocorticoids, as well as antiandrogens.[34,35,37,38] Mutations flanking the AF-2 region increase AR stability and sensitivity to very low levels of DHT[39]; the enhanced AR signaling may also result from altered p160 coactivator interaction with AF-2.[36] Mutations near the hinge region have enhanced transactivation activity, potentially due to a reduction in binding to nuclear corepressors.[40]

Amplification of *AR* may reflect a distinct adaptation of prostate cancer cells to castrate levels of circulating androgens. *AR* amplification occurs in recurrent tumors from 30% of patients with metastatic disease but is not present in the corresponding untreated primary tumors of the same patients.[41] Amplification of *AR* can also occur in patients being treated with AR antagonists; in these patients, testosterone levels are typically above normal.[35,42] Together, these findings reflect the critical importance of AR signaling for growth and survival of cancer cells throughout the clinical course of prostate cancer.

Chemoprevention of Prostate Cancer

Prostate cancer is the most common malignancy for men in the United States, with an estimated 192,280 new diagnoses in 2009.[43]

Strategies for prostate cancer prevention in healthy men are based on evidence that androgens influence prostate cancer development. Drugs that target 5α-reductase reduce androgen levels in the prostate. *Finasteride* (PROSCAR) inhibits type 2 5α-reductase, whereas *dutasteride* (AVODART) inhibits both isoenzymes of 5α-reductase (see Fig. 36-2). Two randomized, placebo-controlled trials were designed to measure the effect of a 5α-reductase inhibitor on prostate cancer incidence. The Prostate Cancer Prevention Trial randomized 18,882 healthy men over age 55 with a normal rectal examination and a PSA less than 3.0 ng/mL to daily finasteride or placebo.[44] Finasteride was associated with a significant 24.8% reduction in prostate cancer prevalence over the 7-year study period. However, high-grade prostate cancer was more frequently diagnosed in the finasteride group (6.4% versus 5.1%; $P = 0.005$). The uncertainty of increased high-grade cancers associated with finasteride has led to limited adoption of finasteride as a chemoprevention agent.[45] A randomized, placebo-controlled study of dutasteride in 8,200 healthy men aged 50 to 75 but with higher PSA levels (2.5 to 10 ng/mL) revealed a 22.4% reduction in prostate cancer prevalence over 4 years, with no difference in high-grade tumors.[46,47] These results were presented in 2009; the impact on chemoprevention and future prostate cancer incidence is as yet unknown.

Approaches to Hormone Therapy

Hormone therapy for prostate cancer includes the following options:

(a) Bilateral orchiectomy (surgical castration)
(b) GnRH agonists (medical castration, alternatively termed LH-RH agonists)
(c) GnRH antagonists
(d) Antiandrogens
(e) Estrogens
(f) Inhibitors of steroidogenesis
(g) Combined androgen blockade (CAB)

The efficacy of each treatment approach for metastatic prostate cancer is described herein. These approaches have not been directly compared in one large trial. A systematic review of various forms of monotherapy (including orchiectomy, GnRH agonists, estrogens, antiandrogens) involving over 6,600 patients in 24 randomized controlled trials (RCTs) suggested that survival is equivalent among these therapies.[48] In addition to its use in metastatic prostate cancer, hormone therapy has an important cytoreductive role when used prior to (neoadjuvant) and concurrently with radiation therapy for locally advanced prostate cancer.[49,50]

Bilateral Orchiectomy

Bilateral orchiectomy is the standard against which other forms of hormone therapy are compared. Orchiectomy is a relatively simple, cost-effective procedure with minor surgical risks.[51] Serum testosterone levels decrease rapidly to castrate levels (<20 ng/mL) after surgery,[52] with concomitant improvements in bone pain and other symptoms such as spinal cord compression.[2] The use of orchiectomy as initial hormone therapy has largely been supplanted by medical castration (described below). However, orchiectomy remains a useful alternative for patients in whom an immediate decrease in testosterone is necessary, such as pending spinal cord compression, or in whom costs or adherence to medical therapy may be an issue. In many countries, bilateral orchiectomy remains the standard of care for initial hormone therapy of metastatic prostate cancer.

The endocrine side effects of orchiectomy include vasoactive symptoms (hot flushes), weight gain, mood lability, fatigue, gynecomastia, cognitive changes, impotence, loss of libido, osteopenia, and dyslipidemia.[51] The psychological impact of orchiectomy is an important consideration for men considering surgical versus medical castration. In a study of 159 men with metastatic prostate cancer who were provided with standard information regarding the costs, benefits, and risks of either orchiectomy or monthly GnRH agonist therapy, only 22% selected orchiectomy.[53]

Gonadotropin-Releasing Hormone Agonists

Medical castration was first reported in 1982.[54] In the United States, the most common form of ADT involves chemical suppression of the pituitary gland with GnRH agonists. Synthetic GnRH analogs have greater receptor affinity and reduced susceptibility to enzymatic degradation than the naturally occurring GnRH molecule and are 100-fold more potent (see Fig. 36-4).[55] GnRH agonists bind to GnRH

Agonists
GnRH:
pyroGlu-His-Trp-Ser-Tyr-Gly-Leu-Arg-Pro-Gly-NH2

Goserelin:
pyroGlu-His-Trp-Ser-Tyr-D-Ser(tBu)-Leu-Arg-Pro-Azgly-NH2

Leuprolide:
5-oxo-Pro-His-Trp-Ser-Tyr-D-Leu-Leu-Arg-N-ethyl-Prolinamide

Triptorelin:
pyroGlu-His-Trp-Ser-Tyr-D-Trp-Leu-Arg-Pro-Gly-NH2

Antagonists
Abarelix:
Ac-D-Nal-D-Cpa-D-Pal-Ser-Tyr(N-Me)-D-Asn-Leu-Lys(iPr)-Pro-D-Ala-NH2

Degarelix:
Ac-D-Nal-D-Cpa-D-Pal-Ser-Aph (L-hydroorotyl)-D-Aph (carbamoyl)-Leu-Lys(iPr)-Pro-D-Ala-NH2

FIGURE **36-4** GnRH agonists and antagonists. GnRH agonists and antagonists are structurally modified peptides. Ac, acetyl; Aph, 4-amino phenylalanine; Arg, arginine; Azgly, azaglycyl; Cpa, chlorophenylalanyl; D-Nal, 3-(2-naphthyl)-D-alanyl; Glu, glutamate; Gly, glycine; His, histidine; Leu, leucine; Pal, 3-pyridylalanyl; Pro, proline; Ser, serine; tBu, tert-butyl; Trp, tryptophan; Tyr, tyrosine.

receptors on pituitary gonadotropin-producing cells, causing an initial release of both LH and FSH, and a subsequent increase in testosterone production from testicular Leydig cells. After approximately 1 week of therapy, GnRH receptors are down-regulated on the gonadotropin-producing cells, causing a decline in the pituitary response.[56] The fall in serum LH leads to a decrease in testosterone production to castrate levels, within 3 to 4 weeks of the first treatment. Subsequent treatments maintain testosterone at castrate levels.[57]

During the transient rise in LH, the resultant testosterone surge may induce an acute stimulation of prostate cancer growth and a "flare" of symptoms from metastatic deposits. Patients may experience an increase in bone pain or obstructive bladder symptoms, lasting for 2 to 3 weeks.[58] A placebo-controlled trial demonstrated that 2 to 4 weeks of antiandrogen therapy with a GnRH agonist can counteract this flare phenomenon.[59]

Current depot forms of GnRH agonists are the result of progressive improvements in drug development. GnRH agonists in common use include *leuprolide* (LUPRON), *goserelin* (ZOLADEX), *triptorelin* (TRELSTAR), and *buserelin* (SUPREFACT; not available in the United States) (Table 36-1). Long-acting preparations of both leuprolide and goserelin are available in doses that are approved for 3-, 4-, and 6-month administrations.

Common side effects of GnRH agonists include vasomotor flushing, loss of libido, impotence, gynecomastia, fatigue, anemia, weight gain, decreased insulin sensitivity, altered lipid profiles, osteoporosis and fractures, and loss of muscle mass.[60] The spectrum of side effects of GnRH agonists is distinct from the metabolic syndrome.[61] The risk of fracture is a significant contributor to morbidity associated with ADT. Observational studies of the Surveillance, Epidemiology, and End Results (SEER) program and Medicare data ($n = 50,613$) revealed a significantly increased number of fractures in men on ADT (19.4% versus 12.6% for those not receiving ADT, $P < 0.001$).[62] Skeletal-related events due to ADT, including fractures, may be significantly mitigated by bisphosphonate therapy, such as *zoledronic acid* (ZOMETA),[63] or inhibitors of osteoclast activation, such as *denosumab*.[64]

Importantly, large observational studies of prostate cancer patients from SEER-Medicare data ($n = 73,196$)[65] and the Veterans Healthcare Administration data ($n = 37,443$)[66] have demonstrated associations between GnRH agonist therapy and incident diabetes and cardiovascular disease. GnRH agonist therapy was associated with statistically significantly increased risks of incident diabetes (adjusted hazard ratio [aHR] = 1.28), incident coronary heart disease (aHR = 1.19), myocardial infarction (12.8 events per 1,000 person-years for GnRH agonist therapy versus 7.3 for no ADT; aHR 1.28), sudden cardiac death (aHR = 1.35), and stroke (aHR = 1.22).[66] Despite these observations, there is no convincing evidence that ADT is associated with increased cardiovascular mortality (reviewed in Saylor and Smith[60]). Careful evaluation of risks and benefits of ADT for an individual patient is of paramount importance. Prospective studies of these issues of survivorship, as well as effective management strategies of potential complications, are important future considerations.

TABLE

36.1 *Key features of GnRH agonists*

Mechanism of action	Inhibition of LH secretion, with resultant decrease in testosterone to castrate levels
Onset of action	After an initial increase, testosterone falls to castrate levels in 2–4 wk
Pharmacokinetics	Leuprolide, $t_{1/2}$: 3 h
	Goserelin, $t_{1/2}$: 4 h
	Triptorelin, $t_{1/2}$: 3 h
Elimination	Metabolized to smaller peptides, eliminated by liver and kidneys
Drug interactions	None known
Toxicity	Vasomotor flushing
	Impotence
	Loss of libido
	Local irritation at injection site
	Gynecomastia and mastodynia
	Disease flare
	Weight gain
	Loss of lean muscle mass (sarcopenia)
	Anemia
	Osteoporosis, osteopenia, and fractures
	Diabetes mellitus
	Altered lipid profiles
	Coronary heart disease, myocardial infarction, sudden cardiac death
	Stroke
Precautions	(1) Transient increases in testosterone may cause disease flare; administer with 2–4 wk of antiandrogen therapy
	(2) No dose adjustments for renal impairment or moderate hepatic impairment; pharmacokinetics in severe hepatic impairment have not been determined

GnRH Agonists Versus Orchiectomy

Medical castration compared with surgical castration offers the possibility of reversibility of hypogonadal symptoms upon cessation of therapy and improved psychological tolerance. The GnRH agonists leuprolide and goserelin have been compared with orchiectomy in randomized trials. A meta-analysis of ten randomized trials involving 1,908 patients comparing a GnRH agonist with orchiectomy found equivalence in overall survival, progression-related outcomes, and time to treatment failure.[48,67–70] The 2-year survival hazard ratio with GnRH agonists compared with orchiectomy was 1.26 (95% CI, 0.92 to 1.39).[48] Although no trials have directly compared the GnRH agonists, the meta-analysis found no evidence of a difference in efficacy among the GnRH agonists leuprolide, goserelin, or buserelin.[48]

Despite the high price of GnRH agonists versus the one-time procedure of orchiectomy, GnRH agonists are given to the majority of American prostate cancer patients for initial ADT.[53,71] The American Society of Clinical Oncology (ASCO) guidelines from 2004 and updated in 2007 maintain the recommendation of GnRH agonists or bilateral orchiectomy as first-line initial hormone therapy.[51,71]

Gonadotropin-Releasing Hormone Antagonists

GnRH antagonists have been developed to suppress testosterone while avoiding the flare phenomenon of GnRH agonists (see Fig. 36-4). Other than avoidance of the initial flare, GnRH antagonist therapy offers no apparent advantage compared with GnRH agonists. The first available GnRH antagonist, *abarelix* (PLENAXIS), rapidly achieves medical castration.[72] However, local reactions and anaphylaxis have discouraged its clinical acceptance and have led to its withdrawal from the market. A second GnRH antagonist, *degarelix* (FIRMAGON), is not associated with systemic allergic reactions and is approved for prostate cancer in the United States.[73]

Antiandrogens (AR Antagonists)

Antiandrogens bind to the AR and competitively inhibit ligand binding and consequent AR translocation from the cytoplasm to the nucleus. Unlike surgical or medical castration, antiandrogen monotherapy does not decrease LH production; therefore, testosterone levels are normal or increased. Men treated with antiandrogen monotherapy maintain some degree of potency and libido and do not have the same spectrum of side effects seen with castration.

Antiandrogens, when compared with GnRH agonists, cause more gynecomastia, mastodynia, and hepatotoxicity, but less bone loss and vasomotor flushing.[74] Antiandrogens are well tolerated and are associated with PSA responses in 20% to 50% of previously untreated patients (median duration, 3 to 6 months).[75]

Currently, antiandrogen monotherapy is not indicated as first-line treatment for patients with advanced prostate cancer. Numerous studies have examined the effectiveness of antiandrogens compared with surgical castration, GnRH agonists, or diethylstilbesterol (DES) treatment. A meta-analysis of eight trials indicated that nonsteroidal antiandrogens had equivalent overall survival relative to castration, although the association between nonsteroidal antiandrogens and decreased survival approached statistical significance.[48] Antiandrogens are most commonly used in clinical practice to prevent the initial flare reaction to GnRH agonists, as secondary hormone therapy, or in CAB.

From a structural standpoint, antiandrogens are classified as steroidal, including *cyproterone* (ANDROCUR) and *megestrol*, or nonsteroidal, including *flutamide* (EULEXIN, others), *bicalutamide* (CASODEX), and *nilutamide* (NILANDRON) (Fig. 36-5; Table 36-2). The steroidal antiandrogens are rarely used. The antiandrogens are taken orally.

Cyproterone is associated with liver toxicity and has inferior efficacy compared with other forms of ADT.[76,77] In a phase III study, cyproterone was inferior to medical castration with goserelin in delaying time to progression.[77] On this basis, cyproterone is not approved in the United States for treatment of men with metastatic prostate cancer, although it is used in Europe.

Flutamide has a half-life of 5 hours and is therefore given as a 250-mg dose every 8 hours. It is metabolized in the liver by CYP1A2 to the major active metabolite, hydroxyflutamide, which has a half-life of 9.5 hours, and to at least five other minor metabolites.[78,79] The common side effects include diarrhea, breast tenderness, and nipple tenderness. Less commonly, nausea, vomiting, and hepatotoxicity occur.[80,81] Hepatotoxicity is uncommon (3 per 10,000 patients) but can be fatal, and therefore, flutamide administration should include close monitoring of serum aminotransferases.[80,81]

Bicalutamide has a serum half-life of 5 to 6 days and is taken once daily at a dose of 50 mg/d when given with a GnRH agonist. Bicalutamide is well tolerated at higher doses with rare additional side effects. Similar to flutamide, breast tenderness and gynecomastia occur in over half of treated men.[82,83] Bicalutamide is a racemate with antiandrogenic activity almost exclusive to the (R)-enantiomer. Whereas (S)-bicalutamide is rapidly metabolized by glucuronidation, (R)-bicalutamide is thought to be metabolized by both hepatic CYP3A4 activity and hydroxylation followed by glucuronidation. (R)-bicalutamide metabolites are eliminated in bile and urine. The elimination half-life of bicalutamide is increased in severe hepatic insufficiency and is unchanged in renal insufficiency.[84]

Bicalutamide is as effective as flutamide in terms of PSA response, objective response, and QOL, with less diarrhea and hepatotoxicity.[85] Daily bicalutamide (either low or high dose) is significantly

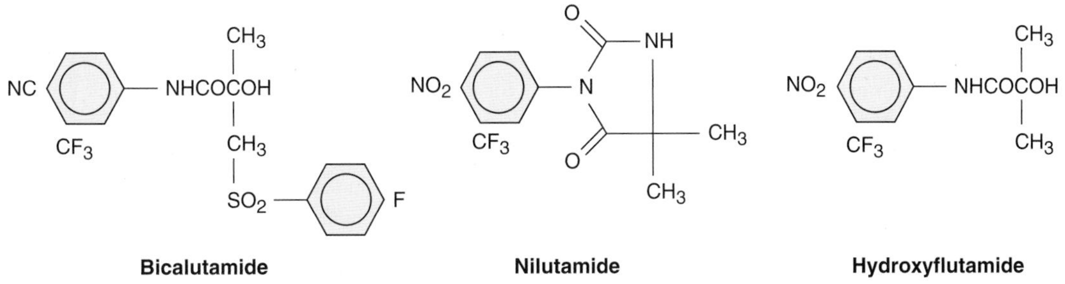

Bicalutamide **Nilutamide** **Hydroxyflutamide**

FIGURE **36-5** The nonsteroidal antiandrogens.

36.2 Key features of nonsteroidal antiandrogens

	Flutamide	Bicalutamide	Nilutamide
Typical dosing	250 mg every 8 h	50 mg daily	150 mg daily
$t_{1/2}$	Parent drug, 5 h	5–6 d	45 h
	Hydroxyflutamide, 9.5 h		
Metabolism	CYP1A2	(a) CYP3A4	CYP2C19
		(b) Hydroxylation then glucuronidation	
Elimination	Urine	Bile and urine	Urine
Drug interactions	May displace warfarin from protein-binding sites and lead to prolonged prothrombin times	May displace warfarin from protein-binding sites and lead to prolonged prothrombin times	May increased plasma levels of phenytoin and theophylline
Toxicity	Diarrhea	Vasomotor instability	Nausea
	Gynecomastia	Gynecomastia	Alcohol intolerance
	Mastodynia	Mastodynia	Diminished ocular adaptation to darkness
	Rare fatal hepatotoxicity		Rare interstitial pneumonitis
Precautions	Monitor liver function	Elimination is increased in severe hepatic insufficiency	Least favorable toxicity profile

inferior compared with surgical or medical castration.[86,87] Although the ease of administration and favorable toxicity are attractive, concerns about inferior survival have limited the use of bicalutamide monotherapy. Neither bicalutamide nor flutamide is approved as monotherapy at any dose for treatment of prostate cancer in the United States, and they are thus most commonly used in combination with GnRH agonists.

Nilutamide is a second-generation antiandrogen with an elimination half-life of 45 hours, allowing once-daily administration at 150 mg/d.[88] Common side effects include mild nausea, alcohol intolerance (5% to 20%), and diminished ocular adaptation to darkness (25% to 40%); rarely, interstitial pneumonitis occurs.[89,90] It is metabolized in the liver by CYP2C19 to at least five products that are all excreted in the urine.[91] Nilutamide appears to offer no benefit over the first-generation drugs above and has the least favorable toxicity profile.[92]

Are Antiandrogens as Effective as Castration?

The different antiandrogens have not been directly compared in a clinical trial. One meta-analysis of eight trials involving 2,717 patients examined the effectiveness of antiandrogens compared with castration, GnRH agonist, or DES.[48] Three studies examined flutamide[93–96] and five studies used bicalutamide.[97–101] One study with flutamide[95] and two studies on bicalutamide[98,101] found statistically significant longer survival in the control arms; no significant survival difference was seen in the other five studies. Overall, the nonsteroidal antiandrogens had equivalent overall survival relative to orchiectomy, although the association between nonsteroidal antiandrogens and decreased survival approached statistical significance (HR 1.22, 95% CI 0.99 to 1.40).[48] Current ASCO guidelines suggest that nonsteroidal antiandrogen monotherapy be discussed but should not be offered.[71]

Estrogens

High estrogen levels can reduce testosterone to castrate levels in 1 to 2 weeks via negative feedback on the hypothalamic-pituitary axis. Estrogen may also compete with androgens for steroid hormone receptors and may thereby exert a cytotoxic effect on prostate cancer cells.[102] Numerous estrogenic compounds have been tested in prostate cancer. Estrogens cause a hypercoagulable state and increase cardiovascular mortality (including increased myocardial infarctions, strokes, and pulmonary emboli) in prostate cancer patients and are not considered standard treatment options.[103] One benefit is that estrogens prevent bone loss.[104]

Most early studies on the use of estrogens used *DES* and were conducted between 1960 and 1975 by the Veterans Administration Cooperative Urological Research Group (VACURG). Two studies compared orchiectomy to different doses of DES to placebo.[103,105,106] DES was as effective as orchiectomy for metastatic prostate cancer but was associated with an increase in cardiovascular events, including myocardial infarction, cerebrovascular accident, and pulmonary embolism; men who received placebo lived longer than men receiving DES, due to higher rates of noncancer deaths in the DES groups.[105–109] The emerging availability of GnRH agonists led to the marked decline in the use of DES. Due to its cardiovascular toxicity and unacceptable mortality at any dose level, DES is not indicated for prostate cancer treatment and is not available in North America for that purpose.

Other estrogens: Other synthetic oral estrogens have similar associated cardiovascular toxicity of DES, but without the efficacy. These compounds include conjugated estrogens (PREMARIN), *ethinyl estradiol* (ESTINYL), *medroxyprogesterone acetate* (PROVERA), and *chlorotrianisene* (TACE). Premarin (1.25 mg three times daily) is approved for metastatic prostate cancer in the United States. In a randomized phase II study of 45 men with castration-resistant prostate cancer who received Premarin either once or three times daily along with 1 mg of daily warfarin, 25% of men on the higher dose achieved at least a 50% decrease in serum PSA. Only three patients in the entire group had a venous thromboembolic event.[110]

Oral estrogens are associated with elevated serum levels of coagulation factor VII and decreased levels of antithrombin III, which may account for their hypercoagulable complications.[111] Parenteral or transdermal estrogens avoid first-pass portal circulation, and indeed, parenteral polyestradiol phosphate was associated with a decreased level of antithrombin III, but no change in factor VII.[111] Transdermal estradiol was associated with castrate levels of testosterone and a biochemical response in all patients of a 20-patient study, without significant cardiovascular toxicity after a median follow-up of 15 months.[112] Intramuscular estrogen has also been attempted; a recent randomized study of parenteral estrogen versus CAB demonstrated equivalent disease control and survival, but significantly more nonfatal cardiovascular events.[113]

Inhibitors of Steroidogenesis

In the castrate state, nongonadal sources of androgens may support continued prostate cancer growth (see the above section on "Mechanisms of Resistance to Hormone Therapy"). Inhibitors of steroidogenesis may be effective secondary hormone manipulations to further lower circulating or intratumoral androgen levels.

Ketoconazole, an oral antifungal agent, interrupts the synthesis of an essential fungal membrane sterol. Ketoconazole inhibits both testicular and adrenal steroidogenesis by blocking cytochrome P450 enzymes, primarily CYP17 (17α-hydroxylase) (see Fig. 36-1). Ketoconazole is typically administered as secondary hormone therapy, to reduce adrenal androgen synthesis in castration-resistant prostate cancer.[114] Ketoconazole causes significant diarrhea and hepatic enzyme elevations, limiting its use as initial hormone therapy. Consequent poor patient adherence deters from its efficacy. Ketoconazole is given in doses of 200 mg or 400 mg three times daily. Hydrocortisone supplementation is coadministered to compensate for inhibition of adrenal steroidogenesis at the 400-mg dose level. High-dose ketoconazole plus corticosteroids demonstrates PSA declines for 27% to 63% of patients with CRPC. Lower doses may have comparable activity with less toxicity.[115]

Abiraterone is an irreversible inhibitor of both 17α-hydroxylase and C-17,20-lyase CYP17 activity, with greater potency and selectivity compared with ketoconazole (see Fig. 36-1). The parent compound, abiraterone acetate, is orally bioavailable, and has been well tolerated in castration-resistant prostate cancer patients as secondary hormone therapy in phase I and II studies.[116,117] With continuous administration, abiraterone increased adenocorticotrophic hormone (ACTH) levels, resulting in mineralocorticoid excess. Therefore, abiraterone acetate is administered with daily low-dose glucocorticoids, such as prednisone. Ongoing phase III trials will evaluate the efficacy and appropriate timing of abiraterone therapy for prostate cancer patients.

Combined Androgen Blockade

CAB requires administration of ADT with an antiandrogen. The theoretical advantage is that the GnRH agonist will deplete testicular androgens, while the antiandrogen component competes at the receptor with residual androgens made by the adrenal glands or by the cancer cells. CAB provides maximal relief of androgen stimulation. However, the benefit of CAB over ADT monotherapy is controversial. Numerous large trials have compared CAB with ADT monotherapy, with variable results (selected studies are summarized in Table 36-3).[5,6,118-125] Notably, the largest studies, Intergroup 0105[6] and Intergroup 0036[5], were performed by the same group and demonstrated conflicting results. Several meta-analyses of these trials suggest a benefit for CAB in 5-year survival but not at earlier time points.[126-128] Toxicity and costs associated with CAB are higher.[129] Current ASCO guidelines suggest that CAB should be discussed, with the emphasis that there may be a gain in overall survival at the cost of higher toxicity.[71]

TABLE

36.3 *Selected larger studies examining CAB versus ADT monotherapy*

Study	Intervention (n)	Median overall survival	P
INTOO36[5]	Leuprolide + flutamide (303)	35.6 mo	0.035
	Leuprolide + placebo (300)	28.3 mo	
International Anandron Study Group[118]	Orchiectomy + nilutamide (225)	27.3 mo	0.0326
	Orchiectomy + placebo (232)	23.6 mo	
EORTC 30853[119]	Goserelin + flutamide (149)	34.4 mo	0.02
	Orchiectomy (148)	27.1 mo	
INTO105[6]	Orchiectomy + flutamide (700)	33.5 mo	0.16
	Orchiectomy + placebo (687)	29.9 mo	
International Prostate Cancer Study Group[130]	Goserelin + flutamide (293)	3.3 y	0.172
	Goserelin (293)	3.2 y	
DAPROCA 86[124]	Goserelin + flutamide (129)	22.7 mo	0.49
	Orchiectomy (133)	27.6 mo	

Future Directions

Despite decades since the 1941 discovery of the role of androgens in prostate cancer growth, optimal hormonal control of advanced prostate cancer remains an area of active investigation. New agents such as abiraterone (above) are targeting specific steps in steroidogenesis. Other agents in development target the AR or other proteins involved in AR activation and signaling, such as the SRC cytoplasmic tyrosine kinase. The effectiveness and appropriate therapeutic use of such agents are the subject of ongoing clinical trials.

Advances in technologies including gene expression profiling, whole transcriptome sequencing, and capture of circulating tumor cells from peripheral blood may allow the development of predictive biomarkers of response to current and future therapies. Indeed, tailoring of a patient's therapy based on AR mutation, amplification, or dominant signaling pathways represents a prime opportunity for improvement in hormonal control of metastatic prostate cancer.

References

1. Huggins C, Hodges CV. Studies on prostatic cancer: I. The effects of castration, of estrogen, and of androgen injection on serum phosphatases in metastatic carcinoma of the prostate. Cancer Res 1941;1:293–297.
2. Huggins C, Stevens RE, Hodges CV. Studies on prostatic cancer: II. The effects of castration on advanced carcinoma of the prostate gland. Arch Surg 1941;43:209–233.
3. Sharifi N, Gulley JL, Dahut WL. Androgen deprivation therapy for prostate cancer. JAMA 2005;294:238–244.
4. Walsh PC, Deweese TL, Eisenberger MA. A structured debate: immediate versus deferred androgen suppression in prostate cancer–evidence for deferred treatment. J Urol 2001;166:508–516.
5. Crawford ED, Eisenberger MA, McLeod DG, et al. A controlled trial of leuprolide with and without flutamide in prostatic carcinoma. N Engl J Med 1989;321:419–424.
6. Eisenberger MA, Blumenstein BA, Crawford ED, et al. Bilateral orchiectomy with or without flutamide for metastatic prostate cancer. N Engl J Med 1998;339:1036–1042.
7. Petrylak DP, Tangen CM, Hussain MHA, et al. Docetaxel and estramustine compared with mitoxantrone and prednisone for advanced refractory prostate cancer. N Engl J Med 2004;351:1513–1520.
8. Tannock IF, de Wit R, Berry WR, et al. Docetaxel plus prednisone or mitoxantrone plus prednisone for advanced prostate cancer. N Engl J Med 2004; 351:1502–1512.
9. Miller WL. Molecular biology of steroid hormone synthesis. Endocr Rev 1988;9:295–318.
10. Russell DW, Wilson JD: Steroid 5alpha-reductase: two genes/two enzymes. Annu Rev Biochem 1994;63:25–61.
11. Bilezikian JP, Morishima A, Bell J, et al. Increased bone mass as a result of estrogen therapy in a man with aromatase deficiency. N Engl J Med 1998; 339:599–603.
12. Hayes FJ, Seminara SB, DeCruz S, et al. Aromatase inhibition in the human male reveals a hypothalamic site of estrogen feedback. J Clin Endocrinol Metab 2000;85:3027–3035.
13. Yeh S, Tsai M-Y, Xu Q, et al. Generation and characterization of androgen receptor knockout (ARKO) mice: An in vivo model for the study of androgen functions in selective tissues. Proc Natl Acad Sci USA 2002;99:13498–13503.
14. Gelmann EP. Molecular biology of the androgen receptor. J Clin Oncol 2002;20:3001–3015.
15. Mononen N, Schleutker J. Polymorphisms in genes involved in androgen pathways as risk factors for prostate cancer. J Urol 2009;181:1541–1549.
16. Chamberlain NL, Driver ED, Miesfeld RL. The length and location of CAG trinucleotide repeats in the androgen receptor N-terminal domain affect transactivation function. Nucl Acids Res 1994;22:3181–3186.
17. Brockschmidt FF, Nothen MM, Hillmer AM. The two most common alleles of the coding GGN repeat in the androgen receptor gene cause differences in protein function. J Mol Endocrinol 2007;39:1–8.
18. Zeegers MP, Kiemeney LALM, Nieder AM, et al. How strong is the association between CAG and GGN repeat length polymorphisms in the androgen receptor gene and prostate cancer risk? Cancer Epidemiol Biomarkers Prev 2004;13:1765–1771.
19. Lindström S, Zheng SL, Wiklund F, et al. Systematic replication study of reported genetic associations in prostate cancer: Strong support for genetic variation in the androgen pathway. Prostate 2006;66:1729–1743.
20. Freedman ML, Pearce CL, Penney KL, et al. Systematic evaluation of genetic variation at the androgen receptor locus and risk of prostate cancer in a multiethnic cohort study. Am J Hum Genet 2005;76:82–90.
21. Chang B-l, Zheng S, Hawkins G, et al. Polymorphic GGC repeats in the androgen receptor gene are associated with hereditary and sporadic prostate cancer risk. Human Genet 2002;110:122–129.
22. Miller EA, Stanford JL, Hsu L, et al. Polymorphic repeats in the androgen receptor gene in high-risk sibships. Prostate 2001;48:200–205.
23. Mellinghoff IK, Vivanco I, Kwon A, et al. HER2/neu kinase-dependent modulation of androgen receptor function through effects on DNA binding and stability. Cancer Cell 2004;6:517–527.
24. Craft N, Shostak Y, Carey M, et al. A mechanism for hormone-independent prostate cancer through modulation of androgen receptor signaling by the HER-2/neu tyrosine kinase. Nat Med 1999;5:280–285.
25. Hobisch A, Eder IE, Putz T, et al. Interleukin-6 regulates prostate-specific protein expression in prostate carcinoma cells by activation of the androgen receptor. Cancer Res 1998;58:4640–4645.
26. Culig Z, Hobisch A, Cronauer MV, et al. Androgen receptor activation in prostatic tumor cell lines by insulin-like growth factor-I, keratinocyte growth factor, and epidermal growth factor. Cancer Res 1994;54:5474–5478.
27. Kousteni S, Bellido T, Plotkin LI, et al. Nongenotropic, sex-nonspecific signaling through the estrogen or androgen receptors: dissociation from transcriptional activity. Cell 2001;104:719–730.
28. Guo Z, Dai B, Jiang T, et al. Regulation of androgen receptor activity by tyrosine phosphorylation. Cancer Cell 2006;10:309–319.
29. Mahajan NP, Liu Y, Majumder S, et al. Activated Cdc42-associated kinase Ack1 promotes prostate cancer progression via androgen receptor tyrosine phosphorylation. Proc Natl Acad Sci USA 2007;104:8438–8443.
30. Stanbrough M, Bubley GJ, Ross K, et al. Increased expression of genes converting adrenal androgens to testosterone in androgen-independent prostate cancer. Cancer Res 2006;66:2815–2825.
31. Montgomery RB, Mostaghel EA, Vessella R, et al. Maintenance of intratumoral androgens in metastatic prostate cancer: a mechanism for castration-resistant tumor growth. Cancer Res 2008;68:4447–4454.
32. Marcelli M, Ittmann M, Mariani S, et al. Androgen receptor mutations in prostate cancer. Cancer Res 2000;60:944–949.
33. Tilley WD, Buchanan G, Hickey TE, et al. Mutations in the androgen receptor gene are associated with progression of human prostate cancer to androgen independence, 1996;2:277–285.
34. Taplin M-E, Bubley GJ, Shuster TD, et al. Mutation of the androgen-receptor gene in metastatic androgen-independent prostate cancer. N Engl J Med 1995;332:1393–1398.
35. Taplin M-E, Bubley GJ, Ko Y-J, et al. Selection for androgen receptor mutations in prostate cancers treated with androgen antagonist. Cancer Res 1999;59:2511–2515.
36. Buchanan G, Greenberg NM, Scher HI, et al. Collocation of androgen receptor gene mutations in prostate cancer. Clin Cancer Res 2001;7:1273–1281.
37. Veldscholte J, Ris-Stalpers C, Kuiper GGJM, et al. A mutation in the ligand binding domain of the androgen receptor of human LNCaP cells affects steroid binding characteristics and response to anti-androgens. Biochem Biophys Res Commun 1990;173:534–540.
38. Zhao X-Y, Malloy PJ, Krishnan AV, et al. Glucocorticoids can promote androgen-independent growth of prostate cancer cells through a mutated androgen receptor. Nat Med 2000;6:703–706.
39. Gregory CW, Johnson RT Jr, Mohler JL, et al. Androgen receptor stabilization in recurrent prostate cancer is associated with hypersensitivity to low androgen. Cancer Res 2001;61:2892–2898.

40. Buchanan G, Yang M, Harris JM, et al. Mutations at the boundary of the hinge and ligand binding domain of the androgen receptor confer increased transactivation function. Mol Endocrinol 2001;15:46–56.

41. Visakorpi T, Hyytinen E, Koivisto P, et al. In vivo amplification of the androgen receptor gene and progression of human prostate cancer. Nat Genet 1995;9:401–406.

42. Palmberg C, Koivisto P, Hyytinen E, et al. Androgen receptor gene amplication in a recurrent prostate cancer after monotherapy with the nonsteroidal potent antiandrogen Casodex (bicalutamide) with a subsequent favorable response to maximal androgen blockade. Eur Urol 1997;31:216–219.

43. Jemal A, Siegel R, Ward E, et al. Cancer statistics, 2009. CA Cancer J Clin 2009;59:225–249.

44. Thompson IM, Goodman PJ, Tangen CM, et al. The influence of finasteride on the development of prostate cancer. N Engl J Med 2003;349: 215–224.

45. Kramer BS, Hagerty KL, Justman S, et al. Use of 5-{alpha}-reductase inhibitors for prostate cancer chemoprevention: American Society of Clinical Oncology/American Urological Association 2008 Clinical Practice Guideline. J Clin Oncol 2009;27:1502–1516.

46. Andriole G, Bostwick D, Brawley O, et al. Chemoprevention of prostate cancer in men at high risk: rationale and design of the reduction by dutasteride of prostate cancer events (REDUCE) trial. J Urol 2004;172: 1314–1317.

47. Andriole G, Bostwick D, Brawley O, et al. further analyses from the REDUCE prostate cancer risk reduction trial. J Urol 2009;181:555.

48. Seidenfeld J, Samson DJ, Hasselblad V, et al. Single-therapy androgen suppression in men with advanced prostate cancer: a systematic review and meta-analysis. Ann Intern Med 2000;132:566–577.

49. Pilepich MV, Winter K, John MJ, et al. Phase III Radiation Therapy Oncology Group (RTOG) trial 86–10 of androgen deprivation adjuvant to definitive radiotherapy in locally advanced carcinoma of the prostate. Int J Radiat Oncol Biol Phys 2001;50:1243–1252.

50. Roach M III, DeSilvio M, Lawton C, et al. Phase III trial comparing whole-pelvic versus prostate-only radiotherapy and neoadjuvant versus adjuvant combined androgen suppression: Radiation Therapy Oncology Group 9413. J Clin Oncol 2003;21:1904–1911.

51. Loblaw DA, Mendelson DS, Talcott JA, et al. American Society of Clinical Oncology recommendations for the initial hormonal management of androgen-sensitive metastatic, recurrent, or progressive prostate cancer. J Clin Oncol 2004;22:2927–2941.

52. Oefelein MG, Feng A, Scolieri MJ, et al. Reassessment of the definition of castrate levels of testosterone: implications for clinical decision making. Urology 2000;56:1021–1024.

53. Cassileth BR, Soloway MS, Vogelzang NJ, et al. Patients' choice of treatment in stage D prostate cancer. Urology 1989;33:57–62.

54. Tolis G, Ackman D, Stellos A, et al. Tumor growth inhibition in patients with prostatic carcinoma treated with luteinizing hormone-releasing hormone agonists. Proc Natl Acad Sci USA 1982;79:1658–1662.

55. Schally AV, Coy DH, Arimura A. LH-RH agonists and antagonists. Int J Gynaecol Obstet 1980;18:318–324.

56. Conn PM, Crowley WFJ. Gonadotropin-releasing hormone and its analogues. N Engl J Med 1991;324:93–103.

57. Limonta P, Montagnani Marelli M, Moretti RM. LHRH analogues as anti-cancer agents: pituitary and extrapituitary sites of action. Expert Opin Investig Drugs 2001;10:709–720.

58. Waxman J, Man A, Hendry WF, et al. Importance of early tumour exacerbation in patients treated with long acting analogues of gonadotrophin releasing hormone for advanced prostatic cancer. Br Med J (Clin Red Ed) 1985;291:1387–1388.

59. Kuhn JM, Billebaud T, Navratil H, et al. Prevention of the transient adverse effects of a gonadotropin-releasing hormone analogue (buserelin) in metastatic prostatic carcinoma by administration of an antiandrogen (nilutamide). N Engl J Med 1989;321:413–418.

60. Saylor PJ, Smith MR. Metabolic complications of androgen deprivation therapy for prostate cancer. J Urol 2009;181:1998–2008.

61. Smith MR. Treament-related diabetes and cardiovascular disease in prostate cancer survivors. Ann Oncol 2008;19:vii86–vii90.

62. Shahinian VB, Kuo Y-F, Freeman JL, et al. Risk of fracture after androgen deprivation for prostate cancer. N Engl J Med 2005;352:154–164.

63. Saad F, Gleason DM, Murray R, et al. A randomized, placebo-controlled trial of zoledronic acid in patients with hormone-refractory metastatic prostate carcinoma. J Natl Cancer Inst 2002;94:1458–1468.

64. Smith MR, Egerdie B, Toriz NH, et al. Denosumab in men receiving androgen-deprivation therapy for prostate cancer. N Engl J Med 2009;361:745–755.

65. Keating NL, O'Malley AJ, Smith MR. Diabetes and cardiovascular disease during androgen deprivation therapy for prostate cancer. J Clin Oncol 2006;24:4448–4456.

66. Keating NL, O'Malley AJ, Freedland SJ, et al. Diabetes and cardiovascular disease during androgen deprivation therapy: observational study of veterans with prostate cancer. J Natl Cancer Inst 2010;102:39–46.

67. The Leuprolide Study Group. Leuprolide versus diethylstilbestrol for metastatic prostate cancer. N Engl J Med 1984;311:1281–1286.

68. Vogelzang NJ, Chodak GW, Soloway MS, et al. Goserelin versus orchiectomy in the treatment of advanced prostate cancer: final results of a randomized trial. Urology 1995;46:220–226.

69. Turkes AO, Peeling WB, Griffiths K. Treatment of patients with advanced cancer of the prostate: phase III trial, zoladex against castration; a study of the British Prostate Group. J Steroid Biochem 1987;27:543–549.

70. Kaisary AV, Tyrrell CJ, Peeling WB, et al. Comparison of LHRH analogue (Zoladex) with orchiectomy in patients with metastatic prostatic carcinoma. Br J Urol 1991;67:502–508.

71. Loblaw DA, Virgo KS, Nam R, et al. Initial hormonal management of androgen-sensitive metastatic, recurrent, or progressive prostate cancer: 2007 Update of an American Society of Clinical Oncology Practice Guideline. J Clin Oncol 2007;25:1596–1605.

72. Trachtenberg J, Gittleman M, Steidle C, et al. A phase 3, multicenter, open label, randomized study of abarelix versus leuprolide plus daily antiandrogen in men with prostate cancer. J Urol 2002;167: 1670–1674.

73. Klotz L, Boccon-Gibod L, Shore ND, et al. The efficacy and safety of degarelix: a 12-month, comparative, randomized, open-label, parallel-group phase III study in patients with prostate cancer. BJU Int 2008;102:1531–1538.

74. McLeod DG. Tolerability of nonsteroidal antiandrogens in the treatment of advanced prostate cancer. Oncologist 1997;2:18–27.

75. Nakabayashi M, Regan MM, Lifsey D, et al. Efficacy of nilutamide as secondary hormonal therapy in androgen-independent prostate cancer. BJU Int 2005;96:783–786.

76. Schroder FH, Collette L, de Reijke TM, et al. Prostate cancer treated by anti-androgens: is sexual function preserved? Br J Cancer 1999;82:283–290.

77. Thorpe SC, Azmatullah S, Fellows GJ, et al. A prospective, randomised study to compare goserelin acetate (Zoladex) versus cyproterone acetate (Cyprostat) versus a combination of the two in the treatment of metastatic prostatic carcinoma. Eur Urol 1996;29:47–54.

78. Luo S, Martel C, Chen C, et al. Daily dosing with flutamide or casodex exerts maximal antiandrogenic activity. Urology 1997;50:913–919.

79. Shet MS, McPhaul M, Fisher CW, et al. Metabolism of the antiandrogenic drug (Flutamide) by human CYP1A2. Drug Metab Dispos 1997;25: 1298–1303.

80. Wysowski DK, Fourcroy JL: Flutamide hepatotoxicity. J Urol 1996;155: 209–212.

81. Wysowski DK, Freiman JP, Tourtelot JB, et al. Fatal and nonfatal hepatotoxicity associated with flutamide. Ann Intern Med 1993;118:860–864.

82. Kolvenbag GJ, Furr BJ. Bicalutamide ('Casodex') development: from theory to therapy. Cancer J Sci Am 1997;3:192–203.

83. Iversen P, Tyrrell CJ, Kaisary AV, et al. Bicalutamide monotherapy compared with castration in patients with nonmetastatic locally advanced prostate cancer: 6.3 years of followup. J Urol 2000;164:1579–1582.

84. Cockshott ID. Bicalutamide: clinical pharmacokinetics and metabolism. Clin Pharmacokinet 2004;43:855–878.

85. Schellhammer PF. Combined androgen blockade for the treatment of metastatic cancer of the prostate. Urology 1996;47:622–628.

86. Bales GT, Chodak GW. A controlled trial of bicalutamide versus castration in patients with advanced prostate cancer. Urology 1996;47:38–43.

87. Tyrrell CJ, Kaisary AV, Iversen P, et al. A randomised comparison of 'Casodex'TM (Bicalutamide) 150 mg monotherapy versus castration in the treatment of metastatic and locally advanced prostate cancer. Eur Urol 1998;33:447–456.

88. Mahler C, Verhelst J, denis L: Clinical pharmacokinetics of the antiandrogens and their efficacy in prostate cancer. Clinical Pharmacokinet 1998;34:405–417.

89. Decensi AU, Boccardo F, Guarneri D, et al. Monotherapy with nilutamide, a pure nonsteroidal antiandrogen, in untreated patients with metastatic carcinoma of the prostate. The Italian Prostatic Cancer Project. J Urol 1991;146:377–378.

90. Pfitzenmeyer P, Foucher P, Piard F, et al. Nilutamide pneumonitis: a report on eight patients. Thorax 1992;47:622–627.

91. Creaven PJ, Pendyala L, Tremblay D. Pharmacokinetics and metabolism of nilutamide. Urology 1991;37:13–19.

92. Dole EJ, Holdsworth MT. Nilutamide: an antiandrogen for the treatment of prostate cancer. Ann Pharmacother 1997;31:65–75.

93. Lund F, Rasmussen F. Flutamide versus stilboestrol in the management of advanced prostatic cancer. A controlled prospective study. Br J Urol 1988;61:140–142.

94. Koutsilieris M, Tolis G. Long-term follow-up of patients with advanced prostatic carcinoma treated with either buserelin (HOE 766) or orchiectomy: classification of variables associated with disease outcome. Prostate 1985;7:31–39.

95. Chang A, Yeap B, Davis T, et al. Double-blind, randomized study of primary hormonal treatment of stage D2 prostate carcinoma: flutamide versus diethylstilbestrol. J Clin Oncol 1996;14:2250–2257.

96. Boccon-Gibod L, Fournier G, Bottet P, et al. Flutamide versus orchidectomy in the treatment of metastatic prostate carcinoma. Eur Urol 1997;32:391–395.

97. Iversen P, Tyrrell CJ, Kaisary AV, et al. Casodex (bicalutamide) 150-mg monotherapy compared with castration in patients with previously untreated nonmetastatic prostate cancer: results from two multicenter randomized trials at a median follow-up of 4 years. Urology 1998;51:389–396.

98. Iversen P. Update of monotherapy trials with the new anti-androgen, Casodex (ICI 176,334). International Casodex Investigators. Eur Urol 1994;26:5–9.

99. Chodak G, Sharifi R, Kasimis B, et al. Single-agent therapy with bicalutamide: A comparison with medical or surgical castration in the treatment of advanced prostate carcinoma. Urology 1995;46:849–855.

100. Kaisary AV, Tyrrell CJ, Beacock C, et al. A randomised comparison of monotherapy with Casodex 50 mg daily and castration in the treatment of metastatic prostate carcinoma. Casodex Study Group. Eur Urol 1995;28:215–222.

101. Iversen P, Tveter K, Varenhorst E. Randomised study of Casodex 50 MG monotherapy vs orchidectomy in the treatment of metastatic prostate cancer. The Scandinavian Casodex Cooperative Group. Scand J Urol Nephrol 1996;30:93–98.

102. Landstrom M, Damber JE, Bergh A. Estrogen treatment postpones the castration-induced dedifferentiation of Dunning R3327-PAP prostatic adenocarcinoma. Prostate 1994;25:10–18.

103. Byar DP, Corle DK. Hormone therapy for prostate cancer: results of the Veterans Administration Cooperative Urological Research Group studies. NCI Monogr 1988;7:165–170.

104. Scherr D, Pitts WRJ, Vaugh EDJ. Diethylstilbesterol revisited: androgen deprivation, osteoporosis and prostate cancer. J Urol 2002;167:535–538.

105. Byar DP. The Veterans Administration Cooperative Urological Research Group's studies of cancer of the prostate. Cancer 1973;32:1126–1130.

106. The Veterans Administration Co-operative Urological Research Group. Treatment and survival of patients with cancer of the prostate. Surg Gynecol Obstet 1967;124:1011–1017.

107. Bailar JCR, Byar DP. Estrogen treatment for cancer of the prostate. Early results with 3 doses of diethylstilbestrol and placebo. Cancer 1970;26:257–261.

108. Waymont B, Lynch TH, Dunn JA, et al. Phase III randomised study of zoladex versus stilboestrol in the treatment of advanced prostate cancer. Br J Urol 1992;69:614–620.

109. de Voogt HJ, Smith PH, Pavone-Macaluso M, et al. Cardiovascular side effects of diethylstilbestrol, cyproterone acetate, medroxyprogesterone acetate and estramustine phosphate used for the treatment of advanced prostatic cancer: results from European Organization for Research on Treatment of Cancer trials 30761 and 30762. J Urol 1986;135:303–307.

110. Pomerantz M, Manola J, Taplin M-E, et al. Phase II study of low dose and high dose conjugated estrogen for androgen independent prostate cancer. J Urol 2007;177:2146–2150.

111. Mikkola AKK, Ruutu ML, Aro JLV, et al. Parenteral polyoestradiol phosphate vs orchidectomy in the treatment of advanced prostatic cancer. Efficacy and cardiovascular complications: a 2-year follow-up report of a national, prospective prostatic cancer study. Br J Urol 1998;82:63–68.

112. Ockrim JL, Lalani EN, Laniado ME, et al. Transdermal estradiol therapy for advanced prostate cancer—forward to the past? J Urol 2003;169:1735–1737.

113. Hedlund PO, Damber J-E, Hagerman I, et al. Parenteral estrogen versus combined androgen deprivation in the treatment of metastatic prostatic cancer: Part 2. Final evaluation of the Scandinavian Prostatic Cancer Group (SPCG) Study No. 5. Scand J Urol Nephrol 2008;42:220–229.

114. Small EJ, Halabi S, Dawson NA, et al. Antiandrogen withdrawal alone or in combination with ketoconazole in androgen-independent prostate cancer patients: a phase III trial (CALGB 9583). J Clin Oncol 2004;22:1025–1033.

115. Harris KA, Weinberg V, Bok RA, et al. Low dose ketoconazole with replacement doses of hydrocortisone in patients with progressive androgen independent prostate cancer. J Urol 2002;168:542–545.

116. Attard G, Reid AHM, Yap TA, et al. Phase I clinical trial of a selective inhibitor of CYP17, abiraterone acetate, confirms that castration-resistant prostate cancer commonly remains hormone driven. J Clin Oncol 2008;26:4563–4571.

117. Attard G, Reid AHM, A'Hern R, et al. Selective inhibition of CYP17 with abiraterone acetate is highly active in the treatment of castration-resistant prostate cancer. J Clin Oncol 2009;27:3742–3748.

118. Dijkman GA, Janknegt RA, De Reijke TM, et al. Long-term efficacy and safety of nilutamide plus castration in advanced prostate cancer, and the significance of early prostate specific antigen normalization. J Urol 1997;158:160–163.

119. Denis LJ, Moura JLCd, Bono A, et al. Goserelin acetate and flutamide versus bilateral orchiectomy: a phase III EORTC trial (30853). Urology 1993;42:119–129.

120. Denis LJ, Keuppens F, Smith PH, et al. Maximal androgen blockade: final analysis of EORTC phase III trial 30853. Eur Urol 1998;33:144–151.

121. Akaza H, Yamaguchi A, Matsuda T, et al: Superior anti-tumor efficacy of bicalutamide 80 mg in combination with a luteinizing hormone-releasing hormone (LHRH) agonist versus LHRH agonist monotherapy as first-line treatment for advanced prostate cancer: interim results of a randomized study in Japanese patients. Jpn J Clin Oncol 2004;34:20–28.

122. Usami M, Akaza H, Arai Y, et al. Bicalutamide 80 mg combined with a luteinizing hormone-releasing hormone agonist (LHRH-A) versus LHRH-A monotherapy in advanced prostate cancer: findings from a phase III randomized, double-blind, multicenter trial in Japanese patients. Prostate Cancer Prostatic Dis 2007;10:194–201.

123. Boccardo F, Rubagotti A, Barichello M, et al. Bicalutamide monotherapy versus flutamide plus goserelin in prostate cancer patients: results of an Italian prostate cancer project study. J Clin Oncol 1999;17:2027.

124. Iversen P, Rasmussen F, Klarskov P, et al. Long-term results of Danish Prostatic Cancer Group trial 86. Goserelin Acetate plus flutamide versus orchiectomy in advanced prostate cancer. Cancer 1993;72:3851–3854.

125. Beland G, Elhilali M, Fradet Y, et al. Total androgen ablation: Canadian experience. Urol Clin North Am 1991;18:75–82.

126. Prostate Cancer Trialists' Collaborative Group. Maximum androgen blockade in advanced prostate cancer: an overview of the randomised trials. Lancet 2000;355:1491–1498.

127. Schmitt B, Bennett C, Seidenfeld J, et al. Maximal androgen blockade for advanced prostate cancer. Cochrane Database Syst Rev 2000;2:CD001526.

128. Samson DJ, Seidenfeld J, Schmitt B, et al. Systematic review and meta-analysis of monotherapy compared with combined androgen blockade for patients with advanced prostate carcinoma. Cancer 2002;95:361–376.

129. Bayoumi AM, Brown AD, Garber AM. Cost-effectiveness of androgen suppression therapies in advanced prostate cancer. J Natl Cancer Inst 2000;92:1731–1739.

130. Tyrrell CJ, Altwein JE, Klippel F, et al. Comparison of an LH-RH analogue (Goeserelin Acetate, 'Zoladex') with combined androgen blockade in advanced prostate cancer: final survival results of an international multicentre randomized-trial. International Prostate Cancer Study Group. Eur Urol 2000;37:205–211.

Section VI
Supportive Care

Drug Therapy of Pain in Cancer Patients

Paul A. Glare

Cancer Pain Management and Choice of Drugs

Epidemiology of Pain in Patients with Cancer

Pain is one of the most feared consequences of cancer. However, approximately one third of patients with advanced cancer never experience any pain. The incidence of pain varies with the primary site, affecting more than 80% patient with primary tumors of bone, cervix, or head and neck, but less than 20% patients with leukemia or lymphoma.[1] Before diagnosis, cancer patients often present with pain that then resolves with treatment.

Approximately one third of ambulatory patients with cancer on chemotherapy have pain.[2-3] Two thirds of patients with advanced cancer have pain, and up to 90% of patients with terminal cancer have pain.[1] Pain is also noted in about one third of cancer survivors. Cancer pain is not a single entity. Patients with cancer often have multiple concurrent pains; in one survey of patients with advanced cancer, 20% had only one pain, while one-third had four or more pains.[4]

There are many ways to classify these various cancer pains and this determines the optimal treatment. One classification is based on etiology: pain may be due to the tumor, may be a side effect of cancer treatments, including the newer targeted therapies, may be secondary to cancer-related debility, or may be secondary to some unrelated painful comorbidity. The prevalence of each depends on the setting (Table 37-1).[5-6]

A second classification of cancer pain, by onset/duration, divides it into acute pain and chronic pain. Most pain due to the tumor is chronic; acute pain in the cancer patient is typically secondary to diagnostic procedures (e.g., bone marrow biopsy, post-LP head-

ache), therapeutic interventions (e.g., mucositis pain, postsurgical pain), or a cancer-associated complication (e.g., DVT, pulmonary embolus). Most of these acute pains are transient and predictable. The key to cancer pain assessment is to identify the underlying mechanism. Lists of acute and chronic cancer pain syndromes have been developed. This simple acute/chronic dichotomy can be problematic in practice. Some neoplasm-related pain can have an acute onset (e.g., pathological fracture of a vertebra) but then persists unless effective treatment of the underlying lesion is provided. Many people with chronic cancer-related pain also experience intermittent, acute flares of pain that can occur even though they are taking analgesic medications on a fixed schedule for pain control. These flares of pain are called breakthrough pain (BTP) because the pain "breaks through" the regular pain medication. Depending on the setting (ambulatory advanced cancer through hospice), approximately one half to two thirds of patients with chronic cancer-related pain also experience episodes of BTP.[7-8] BTP is serious because it is associated with more severe and frequent background pain, more pain-related functional impairment, and worse mood. BTP is of two types: incident pain, which breaks through otherwise adequate analgesia during the dosing interval, and end-of-dosage failure pain, that emerges toward the end of the dosing interval. Incident pain can be frequent or rare and can be predictable or unpredictable. It is usually somatic but can also be visceral or neuropathic. Dosage failure pain is usually consistent and predictable.

Lastly, pain in cancer pain can be classified according to its pathophysiology; cancer pain shares many neuropathophysiological pathways with noncancer pain. Traditionally, this classification has incorporated nociceptive pain (normal transmission of

TABLE

37.1 *Prevalence of cancer pain by etiology, in different settings[5-6]*

Setting	Tumor related (%)	Treatment related (%)	Debility related (%)	Unrelated (%)
MSKCC outpatient, 1989[5]	62	25	—	10
MSKCC outpatient, 2009	67	20	5	10
MSKCC hospitalized, 1989[5]	78	19	—	3
British inpatient hospice[6]	67	5	6	22

noxious stimuli from the periphery to the brain via an intact nervous system), neuropathic pain (pain arising from nerve damage in the absence of a peripheral noxious stimulus), and idiopathic pain (no noxious stimulus, intact nervous system).[9–10] The central nervous system (CNS) may also contribute. For example, nociceptive pain due to peripheral inflammation can develop a central neuropathic component due to changes in the dorsal horn of the spinal cord.[11] Also, cancer has unique pain states not seen in noncancer pain (e.g., cancer-induced bone pain, cancer- and chemotherapy-induced peripheral neuropathy)[12–14] that have therapeutic implications.

Assessment of Pain in the Cancer Patient

A comprehensive assessment of the patient is the key to the optimal treatment of cancer pain, aiming to identify the underlying pain mechanism (in effect combining all three of the classifications above) and the psychosocial factors that are influencing the pain experience. Poor assessment has been identified as the principal barrier to effective pain management.[15] However, it may take an extended period of time to determine the precise cause of the pain, as more information about the patient and his/her disease comes to light. Analgesia should not be withheld during the assessment. Alleviating pain is a dominant priority in medical care and will make investigation of the cause of the pain easier. An eight-step approach is advocated (Table 37-2):[16]

(a) The clinician must ask the patient if he or she is in pain and use the patient self-report of severity as the guide to treatment; absence of altered vital signs or behavior should not be used as indicator that the patient's pain reports are false, either in children or adults.[17]

(b) The detailed pain history should include onset and temporal pattern, location, description, intensity, aggravating and relieving factors, and impact on function and should include efficacy of any previous treatments. The description is important as the quality of the pain is used to determine the type of pain, for example, burning, shooting, and tingling indicating neuropathic.[18] Ideally, a pain assessment tool such as numerical rating scale or even the Brief Pain Inventory should be used.[19] Electronic symptom assessment tools are becoming available.

(c) A history of substance abuse is becoming increasingly relevant, especially in cancer survivors.

TABLE

37.2 Eight-step approach to cancer pain management

1. Believe the patient's pain complaints
2. Take a detailed pain history and assess the severity of the pain
3. Include a substance abuse history
4. Perform a careful physical examination
5. Order and personally review any diagnostic tests
6. Consider pharmacological and nonpharmacological approaches to pain syndromes
7. Assess the psychological state of the patient
8. Assess the level of pain control afterward

(d) The painful area should be carefully examined to determine if palpation or manipulation of the site produces pain. The neurological aspect of the physical examination is emphasized so that syndromes such as spinal cord compression or base of skull metastases are not overlooked.[18] Common sites of pain referral (e.g. shoulder pain from subdiaphragmatic lesions) should be kept in mind when performing the examination.

(e) Appropriate diagnostic tests should be performed to determine the cause of pain and extent of disease and to correlate this information with the findings on the history and physical exam to ensure that the appropriate areas of the body have been imaged and that the abnormalities found explain the patient's pain. As pain may be the harbinger of tumor progression, imaging may need to be repeated.

(f) The clinician needs to be familiar with the common cancer pain syndromes (e.g. epidural disease, plexopathies) in order to facilitate identification of the cause so that treatment can be initiated and morbidity (e.g. paraplegia due to cord compression) prevented or minimized. As identifying a treatable cause is only relevant in patients amenable to further anticancer therapy, investigations may be less appropriate in patients with far advanced cancer on hospice or best supportive care.

(g) Unlike the chronic nonmalignant pain patient, a physical basis for pain can usually be identified in the cancer patient. However, anxiety, depression, and other distress are more common in cancer patients than in the general population, so the psychosocial assessment is very important and should emphasize the effect of pain on patient, the family, and any caregiver and should address cognitive, meaning and social aspects of the pain. Identify pathological anxiety or depression that requires specific treatment. Extreme suffering and anguish may present as uncontrollable pain; a "narrative" approach to the cancer pain history will enable the physician to better understand the link between nociception, pain behavior and coping styles, and suffering in the individual patient.[20]

(h) Subsequent assessment is also required and should evaluate the effectiveness of management. If pain is unrelieved, determine whether the cause is related to the progression of disease, a new cause of pain, or inadequate treatment. These eight steps of the "initial" assessment should be repeated with each new report of pain.

The assessment of BTP requires specific mention. The characteristics of BTP vary from person to person, including the duration of the breakthrough episode and possible causes. Generally, BTP is transient, lasting seconds to minutes, but may occasionally be present for hours, and often occurs several times a day. BTP can happen unexpectedly for no obvious reason, or it may be triggered by a specific activity, like coughing, moving, or going to the bathroom. Importantly, the cause of the BTP may not be the same as that of the baseline chronic pain. For all these reasons, BTP needs as thorough clinical evaluation (proportional to prognosis) as the baseline pain it relates to: site, radiation, intensity, aggravating/relieving factors; physical exam; and investigations. Pharmacological management is the mainstay of treatment, but as this usually involves taking stronger opioids often on multiple times throughout out the day, the inconvenience and toxicity of extra doses suggest that treatment of the underlying cause (e.g., radiotherapy, surgery) should be aggressively pursued, if the treatment is available and the prognosis is appropriate.

Initiating Treatment: The WHO Ladder and the Correct Use of Morphine

Having identified the cause of the pain and the psychosocial factors contributing to the pain-related distress and behavior, individualized multimodal treatment can be instituted. In some cases, anticancer therapy (surgery, radiation, or chemotherapy) can be applied, with either curative or palliative intent, to remove the noxious stimulus and eliminate the pain. However, in many cases, pain is due to advanced, progressive disease and no further treatment options are available; provision of analgesia becomes the main focus of treatment. Even if anticancer treatment is available, analgesia should be provided while it is being scheduled and taking effect. Delivery of effective anticancer therapy can be interfered with when the patient is in pain. The use of anticancer therapy does not preclude the use of analgesics.

Analgesic drugs are the mainstay of cancer pain treatment and fall into three groups, the nonopioids—aspirin, acetaminophen, or nonsteroidal anti-inflammatory drugs (NSAIDs), the weak opioids, and the strong opioids. Coanalgesic drugs are often used as opioid-sparing agents to reduce toxicity or when pain is incompletely responsive to single-agent opioids. The sequential use of analgesics of increasing potency according to the severity of the pain was proposed in the early 1980s by the World Health Organization (WHO)[16] and is often referred to as the WHO Analgesic Ladder. According to these guidelines, a trial of opioid therapy should be given to all cancer patients with pain of moderate or greater severity. Some 30 years on, authorities continue to widely endorse the guiding principle behind the ladder, that analgesic selection should be primarily determined by the severity of the pain.[21-24] But the ladder is not without its critics; a systematic review has criticized the evidence for the efficacy of the ladder.[25] The eight studies included in the review were case series,[26-33] precluding meta-analysis. While each study claimed efficacy of greater than 70%, numerous methodological problems were noted including no information on conditions in which the pain was assessed; two were retrospective; two had short or variable follow-up periods; and three had high withdrawal rates. The review concluded that the evidence provided was insufficient to estimate the efficacy of the ladder. Another study has also challenged the efficacy of the ladder.[34]

Current cancer pain guidelines recommend that patients with mild pain should receive an NSAID or acetaminophen.[22,35] The choice of drug is based on a risk/benefit analysis for individual patients. Much of the evidence for NSAIDs comes from the noncancer pain literature. A systematic review of the safety and efficacy of NSAIDs in cancer pain included 25 studies of both single and repeated dosing of various agents.[36] Single-dose studies found NSAIDs to be roughly equivalent to 5 to 10 mg IM morphine. Some evidence suggested a dose-response effect with a ceiling effect to analgesia. A lack of comparable studies precluded testing whether NSAIDs are particularly effective for malignant bone pain.

Weak opioids (e.g., codeine, hydrocodone, tramadol, propoxyphene) are recommended by the WHO Ladder for moderately severe pain, or mild pain persisting despite treatment with a nonopioid. However, the need for weak opioids is controversial as low dose formulations of strong opioids have been used for the management of mild-moderate pain and may be more effective than weak opioids.[34] Consequently, many experts now advocate skipping the second step of the Ladder and using strong opioids for all cancer pain of moderate intensity or greater.[21,23,37-38] Whether weak opioids alone or in combination with nonopioids are more effective than nonopioids alone has also been controversial. While the efficacy achieved by single doses of weak opioids such as codeine is poor, multiple doses may perform better. At therapeutic doses, no evidence suggests that one opioid is better than another for mild to moderate pain.[39] Tramadol is an opioid with additional effects on the monoaminergic system.[40] At therapeutic doses, its analgesic effect is similar to that of an opioid for mild to moderate pain in combination with a nonopioid.[41-42] The extent to which the dose can be titrated is limited; at doses just above the normal therapeutic dose, tramadol can cause convulsions and it produces serious psychiatric reactions at therapeutic doses in some patients.[40] For these reasons, tramadol offers little advantage over other opioids for mild to moderate pain in patients with advanced cancer.

Meperidine, once the opioid of choice for many physicians, has no place in the modern management of cancer pain. It is no more effective than morphine at treating biliary or renal pain, and its low potency, short duration of action, and unique toxicity (i.e., seizures, delirium, other neuropsychological effects) relative to other available opioid analgesics have led to its declining use. Several countries, including Australia, have put severe limits on its use or curtailed it outright. Nevertheless, some physicians continue to use it as a first-line analgesic, and it is found on the WHO Essential Drug list.

Strong opioids are the mainstay of the management of moderate to severe cancer pain. While opioids have been used as analgesics for centuries, it is only recently that a systematic review has concluded that oral morphine is effective for cancer pain.[43] Although numerous strong opioids are FDA-approved for cancer pain management, morphine remains the drug of first choice,[21] for the following reasons:

(a) the majority of patients tolerate morphine well
(b) it is usually effective, dose titration to a suitable level of analgesia usually being achievable
(c) for long-term use, the oral route is preferable to parenteral or rectal
(d) a wide variety of oral formulations are available, allowing flexibility of dosing intervals
(e) other opioids have less long-term safety data.

Alternative opioids such as hydromorphone, oxycodone, fentanyl, methadone, oxymorphone, and levorphanol should be used when titration of morphine results in dose-limiting side effects.

The principles for the correct use of morphine are shown in Table 37-3 and are based on published guidelines.[21,44] Studies in the 1970s showed that oral morphine was as effective as parenteral morphine, but more had to be given (approximately triple the intravenous [IV] dose with repeated administration) because it undergoes extensive first-pass hepatic metabolism. In patients with chronic cancer pain, oral morphine should be given on a regular scheduled basis, around the clock, to keep pain under control and prevent peaks and troughs in blood levels. The starting dose of oral morphine depends on whether or not the patient was opioid naïve or

TABLE

37.3 *Ten principles for the correct use of morphine in chronic cancer pain*

1. Administer by mouth
2. Administer around the clock not PRN
3. Start immediate-release morphine and titrate up dose
4. Change to sustained-release morphine when dose is stable
5. Continue immediate-release morphine for rescue dosing (breakthrough pain)
6. Anticipate and prevent side effects, especially constipation
7. Know that the oral:parenteral equipotency ratio is 3:1
8. Reduce dose in renal failure because of accumulation of the active metabolite morphine-6-glucuronide
9. Know how and when to use opioid rotation
10. Educate patient and family about morphine

progressing from a weak opioid. Naïve patients should be started on 5 mg of immediate release (IR) morphine and tolerant patients on 10 mg, given q4h plus PRN (as necessary). The dose is titrated up in 50% to 100% increments every 12 to 24 hours until the pain is controlled. Using this approach, respiratory depression and excessive sedation almost never occur. Once the pain is controlled, the patient should be converted to a sustained release (SR) formulation to improve adherence (calculate total daily dose with IR, divide by two, and administer as SR bid; a supply of IR needs to be available for rescue dosing in cases of BTP). The rescue dose for oral pain medicines is usually one twelfth to one sixth of the total daily dose. It is important to anticipate the common side effects of morphine,

especially constipation, and prescribe prophylactic laxatives. Nausea is less common and usually self-limiting; prophylactic antiemetics are not usually needed.

The SR morphine dose needs to be reviewed regularly and may need titration upward if progression of disease is causing increasing pain. In some patients, the noxious stimulus is eliminated in which case the dose needs to be reduced,[45-46] tapering by 25% to 50% or less, every 2 to 3 days. When tapering, educate the patient about possible withdrawal symptoms and give suggestions for abating those symptoms. The dose also needs to be reduced if renal failure occurs, as the active metabolite, morphine-6-glucuronide, accumulates (presenting with respiratory depression and/or neurotoxicity: drowsiness, confusion, myoclonic twitching).[47-48] It is recommended that morphine and codeine are avoided in renal failure/dialysis patients; hydromorphone or oxycodone are used with caution and close monitoring; and that methadone and fentanyl/sufentanil appear to be safe to use.[49] The "safe" drugs in renal failure are also the least dialyzable.

If patients develop dose-limiting side effects, rotation to another strong opioid may enable a dose increase because of interindividual variation in side effects for the various opioids. On making the switch, the opioid dose may need to be decreased because cross-tolerance between the opioids is limited (see Section on "Opioid Rotation"). It is important to know the relative potency ratios of the alternatives to morphine—all are more potent, between 1.5 and 100 times (see Table 37-4).[50] Cost issues are also pertinent as patients may not have insurance coverage for them.

In many patients with advanced cancer, parenteral opioids are needed at some stage in the course of their illness, either because of a pain crisis or because they are unable to swallow. If patients are hospitalized, the IV route is used; in hospice patients, the subcutaneous (SC) route is used. IM injections should be avoided.

TABLE

37.4 *Opioid equianalgesic table*

Drug	IV	PO	Duration	Comment
Morphine	10	30–60	3–4 h	Standard for comparison; Multiple routes available
Hydromorphone	1.5	7.5	3–4 h	Multiple routes; available in HP form (10 mg/mL)
Oxycodone	—	30	3–4 h	Often 5 mg combined with ASA or acetaminophen; long-acting available; short-acting comes in tablet or elixir
Fentanyl	[b]	[b]	[b]	
Methadone[a]	10	20	6–8 h	May accumulate due to long half-life and result in delayed toxicities. Carefully monitor during titration
Oxymorphone	1	10(PR)	3–4 h	
Levorphanol[a]	2	4	4–6 h	May accumulate due to long half-life and result in delayed toxicities during initial dosing or increased dosing
Codeine	130	200	3–4 h	Metabolized to morphine; often combined with acetaminophen
Hydrocodone	—	30	3–4 h	Oral formulation only in combination with acetaminophen

Equivalency of various opioid analgesics to 10 mg of IV morphine
[a]Due to the long half-life, much lower doses will be needed for ATC dosing.
[b]Fentanyl 100 µg/h (IV or TD) is equivalent to MS 4 mg IV/h or PO MS 200 mg/24h.

liver. However, the remainder is absorbed as its pharmacologically active metabolite, salicylate. The NSAIDs are extensively bound to plasma proteins, but the clinical significance of interactions between NSAIDs due to displacement from plasma proteins is not known. A two-compartment open model describes the disposition of the NSAIDs. Both the volume of distribution and clearance of NSAIDs are low, the volume of distribution being below 0.2 1/kg and clearance below 200 mL/min in most cases.[159] NSAIDs are inactivated by hepatic metabolism. Little of the NSAIDs are excreted unchanged in urine. Naproxen has nonlinear kinetics with accumulation less than predicted at high doses. Because of interindividual differences in pharmacokinetics, dosage regimens of NSAIDs should be individualized. Short-acting agents such as ibuprofen may be safer with regard to GI toxicity than long-acting agents such as naproxen or celecoxib. NSAIDs are usually categorized as less potent than opioids, but ketorolac is a potent nonselective NSAID available parenterally, 30 mg IV is equivalent to 10 mg IV morphine, which carries an FDA "black box warning" that it is appropriate only for short-term use (<5 days) at doses not exceeding 120 mg IV because of the increased risk of serious adverse effects (thrombotic events, renal impairment, bleeding). The two main toxicities associated with NSAIDs are GI and renal. These are dose-dependent and can result in peptic ulceration and rarely acute renal failure. While it was hoped that this COX-2 selectivity would reduce GI adverse drug reactions (ADRs), little conclusive evidence suggests this is true in the case of celecoxib (rofecoxib had been shown to produce significantly fewer GI ADRs compared to naproxen before being withdrawn). The VIGOR and APPROVe trials showed an increased risk of cardiovascular events (heart attack or stroke) with rofecoxib, resulting in its worldwide withdrawal.[160-161] A meta-analysis of all trials comparing NSAIDs concluded that selective COX 2 inhibitors are associated with a moderate increase in the risk of vascular events, as are high-dose regimens of the nonselective NSAIDs ibuprofen and diclofenac (but not high-dose naproxen).[162] High-dose celecoxib (200 to 400 mg bid) is also associated with increased cardiac risk.[163] The main drug interactions occur with anticoagulants (increased of GI bleeding; protein displacement of warfarin), diuretics, anticonvulsants, and lithium.

Acetaminophen

The mechanism of action of acetaminophen is becoming clearer. While it inhibits cyclooxygenase in the CNS—not peripherally—it is now believed to provide analgesia by increasing endogenous cannabinoid levels.[164] Acetaminophen has also been shown to inhibit the COX-3 isoenzyme, but this is not believed to be clinically relevant in humans.[165] It has good oral bioavailability, but a short half-life requiring frequent administration. It is metabolized in the liver, the majority of the dose being conjugated with 10% metabolized by CYP 1A2 and 2E1; it has toxic metabolites. It is excreted in urine, only 5% to 10% unchanged. Its metabolites accumulate in renal failure, so dose should be reduced in renal failure. While it has a much more benign side effect profile than NSAIDs, renewed concerns have emerged about hepatotoxicity with long-term use; patients with hepatic impairment or malnutrition are at increased risk. Doses of greater than 1300 mg/d are associated with increased INR in patients on warfarin (Coumadin).[166] Many weak opioids are in compound formulations with acetaminophen including codeine, hydrocodone, and tramadol, as well as oxycodone.

Coanalgesics

Antidepressants

The exact mechanism of action of the analgesic effects of these agents is unknown but has been attributed to enhancement of the endogenous pain inhibiting pathways in the brain stem through inhibition of reuptake of norepinephrine and serotonin. Amitriptyline's pain-relieving properties are mediated by a recruitment of the endogenous opioid system acting through delta-opioid receptors.[167] Additionally, all antidepressants including the SSRIs will ameliorate psychological distress, an effect that can contribute to the relief of cancer pain. All antidepressants carry a FDA black box warning fabout suicide risk.

Amitriptyline is well absorbed orally, but bioavailability is only 30% to 60%, due to first-pass hepatic metabolism. It is highly protein bound.[168] Elimination half-life varies between 10 and 50 hours, typically 15 hours. Extensively metabolized in the liver through CYP 2D6, 1A2, and 2C19 to nortriptyline,[168] just as active as amitriptyline, and excreted in the urine. The main side effects are anticholinergic (orthostatic hypotension, sedation, blurred vision, dry mouth, constipation). It is contraindicated in patients taking monoamine oxidase inhibitors. Nilotinib inhibits the metabolism of amitriptyline. No dose adjustment is needed in hepatic or renal impairment although caution is advised in liver impairment. The initial dose for pain management is 0.1 mg/kg orally QHS, titrated slowly over 2 to 3 weeks to a maximum of 150 mg/d. It is licensed for use in pediatrics and caution is needed in adults less than 25 years of age.

Nortriptyline is well absorbed orally. It is highly protein bound. Elimination half-life varies between 18 and 44 hours. Nortriptyline is metabolized in the liver by CYP 2D6; poor metabolizers might experience more adverse effects, so a lower dosage is often necessary in these individuals. Nortriptyline is less problematic than amitriptyline in terms of drug interactions, being only a weak CYP450 2D6 inhibitor. It is excreted in urine primarily and feces. The main side effects are anticholinergic but milder than amitriptyline. Nortriptyline is also contraindicated in patients taking monoamine oxidase (MAO) inhibitors. It also interacts with nilotinib. No dose adjustment is needed in hepatic or renal impairment although caution is advised in liver impairment. The initial dose for pain management is 0.1 mg/kg orally QHS, titrated slowly over 2 to 3 weeks to a maximum of 150 mg/d. It is licensed for use in pediatrics and caution needed in adults less than 25.

Venlafaxine is well absorbed orally and has a bioavailability of close to 50%. Its elimination half-life is 5 hours, being extensively metabolized in the liver through CYP 2D6 to desvenlafaxine, just as active as the parent compound and now commercially available, with a half-life of 11 hours. Venlafaxine is excreted unchanged in urine. The main side effects are headache, nausea, insomnia, and sexual dysfunction. Hypertension occurs in 5%. The drug is normally a stimulant, although some patients report bothersome sedation. It carries a black box warning for suicide risk. Venlafaxine is contraindicated in patients taking phenothiazines or haloperidol. It is a weak inhibitor of CYP 2D6. Coadministration with sunitinib may result in QT prolongation. Coadministration with fentanyl may cause the serotonin syndrome. The dose should be decreased in patients with hepatic or renal insufficiency. The effective dose for pain management is 75 mg bid or tid. Extended release forms are available. Doses should be tapered to avoid withdrawal syndrome. It is not licensed for use in pediatrics and caution is needed in adults less than 25 years of age.

Duloxetine has a rapid onset (within a week), is well absorbed orally, and has a bioavailability of close to 50%. The half-life is approximately 12 hours, being extensively metabolized in the liver through CYP 2D6 and 1A2. Duloxetine is usually not sedative (20%); the commonest side effects are nausea, insomnia, and dizziness. It is contraindicated in patients taking phenothiazines or haloperidol. It is a moderate inhibitor of CYP 2D6 but has no documented interactions with common chemotherapeutic agents. The drug is contraindicated in patients with hepatic insufficiency and should be avoided when estimated glomerular filtration rate (EGFR) is less than 30. The dose is 60 mg daily, increased in 30 mg increments to a maximum 120 mg/d. It is not licensed for use in pediatrics and caution is needed in adults less than 25 years of age. Tablets cannot be crushed, cut, or chewed.

Anticonvulsants

The mechanism of action of gabapentin and pregabalin does not involve GABA, as their names might suggest, but rather they bind to the $\alpha_2\delta$-1 subunit on voltage-gated calcium channels on neurons in the spinal cord to inhibit calcium influx and prevent release of neurotransmitters.

Gabapentin is well absorbed orally and has a bioavailability of 33% to 60%, depending on the dose. Protein binding is less than 5%. The half-life is 5 to 7 hours; it is not metabolized by the liver, but is excreted unchanged in the urine. Toxicities include dizziness, drowsiness, and pedal edema. Gabapentin has few documented interactions, and none with chemotherapeutic agents. The dose needs to be reduced when EGFR is less than 30. No dose adjustment is required in hepatic insufficiency. The dose is 300 mg tid initially titrated to 600 to 900 mg tid over 9 days. Pharmacokinetics are not linear, the plasma concentration increasing disproportionately to the dose. It is licensed for use in pediatrics. Abrupt withdrawal should be avoided.

Pregabalin is similar in many respects to gabapentin. It is well absorbed orally and has a bioavailability of greater than 90%. The half-life is also 5 to 7 hours. It also does not undergo metabolism in humans and is excreted unchanged in the urine. Toxicity profile is similar to gabapentin: dizziness, drowsiness, and pedal edema being commonest. It also has few documented interactions, and none with chemotherapeutic agents. The dose needs to be reduced when EGFR is less than 60. No dose adjustment is required in hepatic insufficiency The dose is 75 mg bid or tid and can be titrated to 150 mg tid if not effective at lower dose. It is licensed for use in pediatrics. Abrupt withdrawal should be avoided.

References

1. Twycross RG, Lack SA. Symptom control in far advanced cancer: pain relief. London, UK: Pitman, 1983.
2. Jacox A, Carr DB, Payne R. New clinical-practice guidelines for the management of pain in patients with cancer. N Engl J Med 1994;330:651–655.
3. Cleeland CS, Gonin R, Hatfield AK, et al. Pain and its treatment in outpatients with metastatic cancer. N Engl J Med 1994;330:592–596.
4. Twycross RG, Lack SA. Therapeutics in terminal cancer. Edinburgh, UK: Churchill Livingstone, 1990.
5. Foley KM. Pain assessment and cancer pain syndromes. In: Doyle D, Hanks GWC, MacDonald N, eds. Oxford Textbook of Palliative Medicine, 1st ed. Oxford, UK: Oxford University Press, 1993:148–165.
6. Twycross RG, Fairfield S. Pain in far-advanced cancer. Pain 1982;14:303–310.
7. Portenoy RK, Hagen NA. Breakthrough pain: definition, prevalence and characteristics. Pain 1990;41:273–281.
8. Portenoy RK, Payne D, Jacobsen P. Breakthrough pain: characteristics and impact in patients with cancer pain. Pain 1999;81:129–134.
9. Portenoy RK. Cancer pain: pathophysiology and syndromes. Lancet 1992;339:1026–1031.
10. Besson JM. The neurobiology of pain. Lancet 1999;353:1610–1615.
11. Dickenson AH. Central acute pain mechanisms. Ann Med 1995;27:223–227.
12. Honore P, Schwei J, Rogers SD, et al. Cellular and neurochemical remodeling of the spinal cord in bone cancer pain. Prog Brain Res 2000;129:389–397.
13. Shimoyama M, Tanaka K, Hasue F, et al. A mouse model of neuropathic cancer pain. Pain 2002;99:167–174.
14. Mantyh PW, Clohisy DR, Koltzenburg M, et al. Molecular mechanisms of cancer pain. Nat Rev Cancer 2002;2:201–209.
15. Von Roenn JH, Cleeland CS, Gonin R, et al. Physician attitudes and practice in cancer pain management. A survey from the Eastern Cooperative Oncology Group. Ann Intern Med 1993;119:121–126.
16. World Health Organization. Cancer pain relief and palliative care. Geneva, Switzerland: World Health Organization, 1990.
17. Beyer JE, McGrath PJ, Berde CB. Discordance between self-report and behavioral pain measures in children aged 3–7 years after surgery. J Pain Symptom Manage 1990;5:350–356.
18. Elliott K, Foley KM. Neurologic pain syndromes in patients with cancer. Neurol Clin 1989;7:333–360.
19. Daut RL, Cleeland CS, Flanery RC. Development of the Wisconsin Brief Pain Questionnaire to assess pain in cancer and other diseases. Pain 1983;17:197–210.
20. Lickiss JN. Approaching cancer pain relief. Eur J Pain 2001;5(Suppl A):5–14.
21. Hanks GW, Conno F, Cherny N, et al. Morphine and alternative opioids in cancer pain: the EAPC recommendations. Br J Cancer 2001;84:587–593.
22. Scottish Intercollegiate Guidelines Network (SIGN). Cancer pain guidelines. Edinburgh, UK: SIGN, 2000.
23. Benedetti C, Brock C, Cleeland C, et al. NCCN practice guidelines for cancer pain. Oncology (Williston Park) 2000;14:135–150.
24. Hanks G, Cherny NI, Fallon M. Opioid analgesic therapy. In: Doyle D, Hanks G, Cherny N, et al., eds. Oxford Textbook of Palliative Medicine, 3rd ed. Oxford, UK: Oxford University Press, 2004:318–321.
25. Jadad AR, Browman GP. The WHO analgesic ladder for cancer pain management. Stepping up the quality of its evaluation. JAMA 1995;274:1870–1873.
26. Ventafridda V, Tamburini M, Caraceni A, et al. A validation study of the WHO method for cancer pain relief. Cancer 1987;59:850–856.
27. Walker VA, Hoskin PJ, Hanks GW, et al. Evaluation of WHO analgesic guidelines for cancer pain in a hospital-based palliative care unit. J Pain Symptom Manage 1988;3:145–149.
28. Goisis A, Gorini M, Ratti R, et al. Application of a WHO protocol on medical therapy for oncologic pain in an internal medicine hospital.. Tumori 1989;75:470–472.
29. Ventafridda V, Caraceni A, Gamba A. Field-testing of the WHO guidelines for cancer pain relief. In: Foley KM, Bonica JJ, Ventafridda V, et al., eds. Second International Congress on Cancer Pain. Advances in Pain Research and Therapy. New York, NY: Raven Press, 1990:451–464.
30. Takeda F. Japan's WHO cancer pain relief program. In: Foley KM, Bonica JJ, Ventafridda V, et al., eds. Second International Congress on Cancer Pain. Advances in Pain Research and Therapy.. New York, NY: Raven Press, 1990:475–483.
31. Wenk R, Diaz C, Echeverria M, et al. Argentina's WHO Cancer Pain Relief Program: a patient care model. J Pain Symptom Manage 1991;6:40–43.
32. Siguan SS, Damole AA, Mejarito AG. Results of cancer pain treatment at Southern Islands Medical Center, Cebu, Philippines. Philippine J Surg Specialties 1992;47:173–176.

33. Zech DF, Grond S, Lynch J, et al. Validation of World Health Organization Guidelines for cancer pain relief: a 10-year prospective study. Pain 1995;63:65–76.

34. Marinangeli F, Ciccozzi A, Leonardis M, et al. Use of strong opioids in advanced cancer pain: a randomized trial. J Pain Symptom Manage 2004;27:409–416.

35. Jacox A, Carr DB, Payne R. Management of cancer pain. Clinical Practice Guideline No. 9, AHPCR, 1994.

36. Eisenberg E, Berkey CS, Carr DB, et al. Efficacy and safety of nonsteroidal antiinflammatory drugs for cancer pain: a meta-analysis. J Clin Oncol 1994;12:2756–2765.

37. Cleary JF. Cancer pain management. Cancer Control 2000;7:120–131.

38. Walsh D. Pharmacological management of cancer pain. Semin Oncol 2000;27:45–63.

39. De Conno F, Ripamonti C, Sbanotto A, et al. A clinical study on the use of codeine, oxycodone, dextropropoxyphene, buprenorphine, and pentazocine in cancer pain. J Pain Symptom Manage 1991;6:423–427.

40. Tramadol—a new analgesic. Drug Ther Bull 1994;32:85–87.

41. Wilder-Smith CH, Schimke J, Osterwalder B, et al. Oral tramadol, a mu-opioid agonist and monoamine reuptake-blocker, and morphine for strong cancer-related pain. Ann Oncol 1994;5:141–146.

42. Leppart W. Analgesic efficacy of oral tramadol and morphine administered orally in the treatment of cancer pain. Nowotwory 2001;51:257–266.

43. Wiffen PJ, McQuay HJ. Oral morphine for cancer pain. Cochrane Database Syst Rev 2007;CD003868.

44. Expert Working Group of the European Association for Palliative Care. Morphine in cancer pain: modes of administration. Br Med J 1996;312:823–826.

45. Hanks GW, Twycross RG, Lloyd JW. Unexpected complication of successful nerve block. Morphine induced respiratory depression precipitated by removal of severe pain. Anaesthesia 1981;36:37–39.

46. Broadbent A, Glare P. Neurotoxicity from chronic opioid therapy after successful palliative treatment for painful bone metastases. J Pain Symptom Manage 2005;29:520–524.

47. Hagen NA, Foley KM, Cerbone DJ, et al. Chronic nausea and morphine-6-glucuronide. J Pain Symptom Manage 1991;6:125–128.

48. Osborne R, Joel S, Slevin M. Morphine intoxication in renal failure; the role of morphine-6-glucuronide. Br Med J (Clin Res Ed) 1986;293:1101.

49. Dean M. Opioids in renal failure and dialysis patients. J Pain Symptom Manage 2004;28:497–504.

50. Indelicato RA, Portenoy RK. Opioid rotation in the management of refractory cancer pain. J Clin Oncol 2002;20:348–352.

51. Smith TJ, Staats PS, Deer T, et al. Randomized clinical trial of an implantable drug delivery system compared with comprehensive medical management for refractory cancer pain: impact on pain, drug-related toxicity, and survival. J Clin Oncol 2002;20:4040–4049.

52. Wells N, Johnson RL, Wujcik D. Development of a short version of the Barriers Questionnaire. J Pain Symptom Manage 1998;15:294–298.

53. Cherny N, Ripamonti C, Pereira J, et al. Strategies to manage the adverse effects of oral morphine: an evidence-based report. J Clin Oncol 2001;19:2542–2554.

54. Bruera E, Palmer JL, Bosnjak S, et al. Methadone versus morphine as a first-line strong opioid for cancer pain: a randomized, double-blind study. J Clin Oncol 2004;22:185–192.

55. Hardy JR, Quigley C, Ross JR. Opioid rotation. In: Davis MP, Glare P, Quigley C, et al., eds. Opioids in Cancer Pain, 2nd ed. Oxford, UK: Oxford University Press, 2009:301–312.

56. Cherny NJ, Chang V, Frager G, et al. Opioid pharmacotherapy in the management of cancer pain: a survey of strategies used by pain physicians for the selection of analgesic drugs and routes of administration. Cancer 1995;76:1283–1293.

57. Kirsh KL, Casper D, Haley MC, et al. Opioid use in drug and alcohol abuse. In: Walsh D, ed. Palliative Medicine. Philadelphia, PA: Saunders, 2008:1416–1421.

58. Cancer Pain Assessment and Treatment Curriculum Guidelines. The Ad Hoc Committee on Cancer Pain of the American Society of Clinical Oncology. J Clin Oncol 1992;10:1976–1982.

59. Cicero TJ, Surratt H, Inciardi JA, et al. Relationship between therapeutic use and abuse of opioid analgesics in rural, suburban, and urban locations in the United States. Pharmacoepidemiol Drug Saf 2007;16:827–840.

60. Butler SF, Benoit C, Budman SH, et al. Development and validation of an Opioid Attractiveness Scale: a novel measure of the attractiveness of opioid products to potential abusers. Harm Reduct J 2006;3:5.

61. Sellers EM, Schuller R, Romach MK, et al. Relative abuse potential of opioid formulations in Canada: a structured field study. J Opioid Manag 2006;2:219–227.

62. Bostrom E, Simonsson US, Hammarlund-Udenaes M. In vivo blood-brain barrier transport of oxycodone in the rat: indications for active influx and implications for pharmacokinetics/pharmacodynamics. Drug Metab Dispos 2006;34:1624–1631.

63. Bostrom E, Hammarlund-Udenaes M, Simonsson US. Blood-brain barrier transport helps to explain discrepancies in in vivo potency between oxycodone and morphine. Anesthesiology 2008;108:495–505.

64. McGeeney BE. Adjuvant agents in cancer pain. Clin J Pain 2008;24(Suppl 10):S14–S20.

65. Samad TA, Moore KA, Sapirstein A, et al. Interleukin-1beta-mediated induction of Cox-2 in the CNS contributes to inflammatory pain hypersensitivity. Nature 2001;410:471–475.

66. Mukherjee D. Selective cyclooxygenase-2 (COX-2) inhibitors and potential risk of cardiovascular events. Biochem Pharmacol 2002;63:817–821.

67. Brune K, Hinz B. Non-steroidal anti-inflammatory drugs. In: Walsh D, ed. Palliative Medicine. Philadelphia, PA: Saunders, 2008:740–745.

68. Stockler M, Vardy J, Pillai A, et al. Acetaminophen (paracetamol) improves pain and well-being in people with advanced cancer already receiving a strong opioid regimen: a randomized, double-blind, placebo-controlled cross-over trial. J Clin Oncol 2004;22:3389–3394.

69. Resine T, Pasternak G. Opioid analgesics and antagonists. In: Gilman AG, Hardman JG, Limbird LE, eds. Goodman & Gilman's the Pharmacological Basis of Therapeutics, 9th ed. New York, NY: McGraw-Hill, 1996:1026–1038.

70. Abernethy AP, Currow DC, Frith P, et al. Randomised, double blind, placebo controlled crossover trial of sustained release morphine for the management of refractory dyspnoea. Br Med J 2003;327:523–528.

71. Allard P, Lamontagne C, Bernard P, et al. How effective are supplementary doses of opioids for dyspnea in terminally ill cancer patients? A randomized continuous sequential clinical trial. J Pain Symptom Manage 1999;17:256–265.

72. Mazzocato C, Buclin T, Rapin CH. The effects of morphine on dyspnea and ventilatory function in elderly patients with advanced cancer: a randomized double-blind controlled trial. Ann Oncol 1999;10:1511–1514.

73. Bruera E, MacEachern T, Ripamonti C, et al. Subcutaneous morphine for dyspnea in cancer patients. Ann Intern Med 1993;119:906–907.

74. Cohen MH, Anderson AJ, Krasnow SH, et al. Continuous intravenous infusion of morphine for severe dyspnea. South Med J 1991;84:229–234.

75. Boyd KJ, Kelly M. Oral morphine as symptomatic treatment of dyspnoea in patients with advanced cancer. Palliat Med 1997;11:277–281.

76. Reyes-Gibby CC, Shete S, Rakvag T, et al. Exploring joint effects of genes and the clinical efficacy of morphine for cancer pain: OPRM1 and COMT gene. Pain 2007;130:25–30.

77. Ross JR, Rutter D, Welsh K, et al. Clinical response to morphine in cancer patients and genetic variation in candidate genes. Pharmacogenomics J 2005;5:324–336.

78. Sawe J, Dahlstrom B, Paalzow L, et al. Morphine kinetics in cancer patients. Clin Pharmacol Ther 1981;30:629–635.

79. Hoskin PJ, Hanks GW, Aherne GW, et al. The bioavailability and pharmacokinetics of morphine after intravenous, oral and buccal administration in healthy volunteers. Br J Clin Pharmacol 1989;27:499–505.

80. Gourlay GK, Plummer JL, Cherry DA, et al. The reproducibility of bioavailability of oral morphine from solution under fed and fasted conditions. J Pain Symptom Manage 1991;6:431–436.

81. Vater M, Smith G, Aherne GW, et al. Pharmacokinetics and analgesic effect of slow-release oral morphine sulphate in volunteers. Br J Anaesth 1984;56:821–827.

82. Savarese JJ, Goldenheim PD, Thomas GB, et al. Steady-state pharmacokinetics of controlled release oral morphine sulphate in healthy subjects. Clin Pharmacokinet 1986;11:505–510.

83. Poulain P, Hoskin PJ, Hanks GW, et al. Relative bioavailability of controlled release morphine tablets (MST continus) in cancer patients. Br J Anaesth 1988;61:569–574.

84. Gourlay GK, Cherry DA, Onley MM, et al. Pharmacokinetics and pharmacodynamics of twenty-four hour Kapanol compared to twelve-hourly MS Contin in the treatment of severe cancer pain..Pain 1997;69:295–302.

85. Max MB, Inturrisi CE, Kaiko RF, et al. Epidural and intrathecal opiates: cerebrospinal fluid and plasma profiles in patients with chronic cancer pain. Clin Pharmacol Ther 1985;38:631–641.

86. Sawe J, Kager L, Svensson Eng JO, et al. Oral morphine in cancer patients: in vivo kinetics and in vitro hepatic glucuronidation. Br J Clin Pharmacol 1985;19:495–501.

87. Benyhe S. Morphine: new aspects in the study of an ancient compound. Life Sci 1994;55:969–979.

88. Hasselstrom J, Svensson JO, Sawe J, et al. Disposition and analgesic effects of systemic morphine, morphine-6-glucuronide and normorphine in rat. Pharmacol Toxicol 1996;79:40–46.

89. Mazoit JX, Sandouk P, Zetlaoui P, et al. Pharmacokinetics of unchanged morphine in normal and cirrhotic subjects. Anesth Analg 1987;66:293–298.

90. Sandouk P, Serrie A, Scherrmann JM, et al. Presence of morphine metabolites in human cerebrospinal fluid after intracerebroventricular administration of morphine. Eur J Drug Metab Pharmacokinet 1991;3:166–171.

91. Smith MT, Wright AW, Williams BE, et al. Cerebrospinal fluid and plasma concentrations of morphine, morphine-3-glucuronide, and morphine-6-glucuronide in patients before and after initiation of intracerebroventricular morphine for cancer pain management. Anesth Analg 1999;88:109–116.

92. Coffman BL, Rios GR, King CD, et al. Human UGT2B7 catalyzes morphine glucuronidation. Drug Metab Dispos 1997;25:1–4.

93. Paul D, Standifer KM, Inturrisi CE, et al. Pharmacological characterization of morphine-6 beta-glucuronide, a very potent morphine metabolite. J Pharmacol Exp Ther 1989;251:477–483.

94. Shimomura K, Kamata O, Ueki S, et al. Analgesic effect of morphine glucuronides. Tohoku J Exp Med 1971;105:45–52.

95. Pasternak GW, Bodnar RJ, Clark JA, et al. Morphine-6-glucuronide, a potent mu agonist. Life Sci 1987;41:2845–2849.

96. Osborne R, Thompson P, Joel S, et al. The analgesic activity of morphine-6-glucuronide. Br J Clin Pharmacol 1992;34:130–138.

97. Portenoy RK, Thaler HT, Inturrisi CE, et al. The metabolite morphine-6-glucuronide contributes to the analgesia produced by morphine infusion in patients with pain and normal renal function. Clin Pharmacol Ther 1992;51:422–431.

98. Lotsch J, Weiss M, Ahne G, et al. Pharmacokinetic modeling of M6G formation after oral administration of morphine in healthy volunteers. Anesthesiology 1999;90:1026–1038.

99. Penson RT, Joel SP, Bakhshi K, et al. Randomized placebo-controlled trial of the activity of the morphine glucuronides. Clin Pharmacol Ther 2000;68:667–676.

100. McQuay HJ, Carroll D, Faura CC, et al. Oral morphine in cancer pain: influences on morphine and metabolite concentration. Clin Pharmacol Ther 1990;48:236–244.

101. Hanks GW. Morphine pharmacokinetics and analgesia after oral administration. Postgrad Med J 1991;67(Suppl 2):S60–S63.

102. Smith MT, Watt JA, Cramond T. Morphine-3-glucuronide—a potent antagonist of morphine analgesia. Life Sci 1990;47:579–585.

103. Gong QL, Hedner J, Bjorkman R, et al. Morphine-3-glucuronide may functionally antagonize morphine-6-glucuronide induced antinociception and ventilatory depression in the rat. Pain 1992;48:249–255.

104. Yaksh TL, Harty GJ. Pharmacology of the allodynia in rats evoked by high dose intrathecal morphine. J Pharmacol Exp Ther 1988;244:501–507.

105. Labella FS, Pinsky C, Havlicek V. Morphine derivatives with diminished opiate receptor potency show enhanced central excitatory activity. Brain Res 1979;174:263–271.

106. Zhou HH, Sheller JR, Nu H, et al. Ethnic differences in response to morphine. Clin Pharmacol Ther 1993;54:507–513.

107. Holthe M, Rakvag TN, Klepstad P, et al. Sequence variations in the UDP-glucuronosyltransferase 2B7 (UGT2B7) gene: identification of 10 novel single nucleotide polymorphisms (SNPs) and analysis of their relevance to morphine glucuronidation in cancer patients. Pharmacogenomics J 2003;3:17–26.

108. Osborne R, Joel S, Trew D, et al. Morphine and metabolite behavior after different routes of morphine administration: demonstration of the importance of the active metabolite morphine-6-glucuronide. Clin Pharmacol Ther 1990;47:12–19.

109. Andersen G, Christrup L, Sjogren P. Relationships among morphine metabolism, pain and side effects during long-term treatment: an update. J Pain Symptom Manage 2003;25:74–91.

110. Penson RT, Joel SP, Gloyne A, et al. Morphine analgesia in cancer pain: role of the glucuronides. J Opioid Manag 2005;1:83–90.

111. Quigley C, Joel S, Patel N, et al. Plasma concentrations of morphine, morphine-6-glucuronide and morphine-3-glucuronide and their relationship with analgesia and side effects in patients with cancer-related pain. Palliat Med 2003;17:185–190.

112. Glare PA, Walsh TD, Pippenger CE. Normorphine, a neurotoxic metabolite? Lancet 1990;335:725–726.

113. Chen XY, Zhao LM, Zhong DF. A novel metabolic pathway of morphine: formation of morphine glucosides in cancer patients. Br J Clin Pharmacol 2003;55:570–578.

114. Sawe J, Svensson JO, Rane A. Morphine metabolism in cancer patients on increasing oral doses–no evidence for autoinduction or dose-dependence. Br J Clin Pharmacol 1983;16:85–93.

115. Hanks GW, Hanna M, Finlay I, et al. Efficacy and pharmacokinetics of a new controlled-release morphine sulfate 200-mg tablet. J Pain Symptom Manage 1995;10:6–12.

116. Klepstad P, Kaasa S, Jystad A, et al. Immediate- or sustained-release morphine for dose finding during start of morphine to cancer patients: a randomized, double-blind trial. Pain 2003;101:193–198.

117. Houde RW, Wallenstein S, Beaver WT. Clinical measurement of pain. In: Stevens G, ed. Analgesics. New York, NY: Academic Press, 1965: 75–122.

118. Hanks GW, Hoskin PJ, Aherne GW, et al. Explanation for potency of repeated oral doses of morphine? Lancet 1987;2:723–725.

119. Twycross RG. The therapeutic equivalence of oral and subcutaneous/intramuscular morphine sulphate in cancer patients. J Palliat Care 1988;4:67–68.

120. Max MB, Payne R. Principles of analgesic use in terminal cancer. In: Max MB, Payne R, eds. Principles of Analgesic Use in the Treatment of Acute Pain and Cancer Pain. New York, NY: American Pain Society, 1992.

121. Ventafridda V, Ripamonti C, De Conno F, et al. Antidepressants increase bioavailability of morphine in cancer patients. Lancet 1987;1:1204.

122. Shoji A, Toda M, Suzuki K, et al. Insufficient effectiveness of 5-hydroxytryptamine-3 receptor antagonists due to oral morphine administration in patients with cisplatin-induced emesis. J Clin Oncol 1999;17:1926–1930.

123. Gear RW, Miaskowski C, Heller PH, et al. Benzodiazepine mediated antagonism of opioid analgesia. Pain 1997;71:25–29.

124. Palliative Care, version 1. Therapeutic Guidelines. North Melbourne, Therapeutic Guidelines Ltd, 2001: 280–281.

125. Glare P, Walsh D, Sheehan D. The adverse effects of morphine: a prospective survey of common symptoms during repeted dosing for chronic cancer pain. Am J Hosp Palliat Care 2006;23:229–235.

126. Borgbjerg FM, Nielsen K, Franks J. Experimental pain stimulates respiration and attenuates morphine-induced respiratory depression: a controlled study in human volunteers. Pain 1996;64:123–128.

127. Fallon MT, Hanks GW. Morphine, constipation and performance status in advanced cancer patients. Palliat Med 1999;13:159–160.

128. Bennett M, Cresswell H. Factors influencing constipation in advanced cancer patients: a prospective study of opioid dose, dantron dose and physical functioning. Palliat Med 2003;17:418–422.

129. Sykes NP. A volunteer model for the comparison of laxatives in opioid-related constipation. J Pain Symptom Manage 1996;11:363–369.

130. Thomas J, Karver S, Cooney GA, et al. Methylnaltrexone for opioid-induced constipation in advanced illness. N Engl J Med 2008;358:2332–2343.

131. Mercadante S, Ferrera P, Villari P, et al. Hyperalgesia: an emerging iatrogenic syndrome. J Pain Symptom Manage 2003;26:769–775.

132. O'Neill B, Fallon M. ABC of palliative care. Principles of palliative care and pain control. Br Med J 1997;315:801–804.

133. Morita T, Takigawa C, Onishi H, et al. Opioid rotation from morphine to fentanyl in delirious cancer patients: an open-label trial. J Pain Symptom Manage 2005;30:96–103.

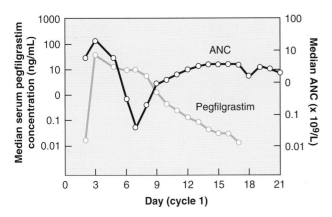

FIGURE 38-2 Pegfilgrastim serum concentrations and absolute neutrophil count (ANC) in patients with breast cancer who received pegfilgrastim as an adjunct to chemotherapy. (Adapted from Green MD, Koelbl H, Baselga J, et al. A randomized double-blind multicenter phase III study of fixed-dose single-administration pegfilgrastim versus daily filgrastim in patients receiving myelosuppressive chemotherapy. Ann Oncol 2003;14:29–35.)

neutrophils, macrophages, monocytes, and eosinophils enhancing phagocytosis. Recombinant GM-CSF is available as sargramostim (yeast derived) and molgramostim (*Escherichia coli* derived) and is approved by the US Food and Drug Administration (FDA) for use in acute myeloid leukemia (AML), autologous and allogeneic hematopoietic stem cell transplantation (SCT), and stem cell mobilization. It is used experimentally as a vaccine adjuvant.

GM-CSF augments the survival and proliferation of cells in the granulocytic and macrophage lineages as well as maintains megakaryocyte progenitors at high concentrations. Increases in granulocyte life span and metabolic functional activity have been noted in vitro. Other alterations of cellular function by GM-CSF include inhibition of neutrophil migration to sterile inflammatory fields.[15] GM-CSF is a potent stimulator (in vitro and in vivo) of dendritic cells, which are important initiators of primary immune responses.[16] Fever and fluid retention are frequently reported in patients receiving GM-CSF particularly when prepared in *E. coli*.

The Erythropoiesis-Stimulating Agents

The glycoprotein hormone, erythropoietin (EPO), is the primary regulator of red cell production. The erythropoiesis-stimulating agents (ESAs) available in the United States include epoetin alfa and the hyperglycosylated recombinant EPO, darbepoetin alfa. EPO illustrates how glycosylation can alter the pharmacologic properties of a molecule. Glycoproteins require terminal sialic acid residues on the oligosaccharides to protect against proteolytic attack.[17] Darbepoetin results from mutagenesis of the gene encoding ESA adding two N-glycosylation sites yielding a 23% increase in molecular weight and a threefold increase in circulation time through protection from metabolic degradation.[18,19] The therapeutic effects of the ESAs include induction, proliferation, and differentiation of erythroid progenitors. The primary effects of EPO are on the erythroid lineage; however, it may also play a role in the stimulation of early multipotent progenitors.[20]

Multiple factors may account for anemia in patients with cancer including disease stage, radiation and chemotherapy, and renal toxicity since endogenous EPO is mainly produced in the peritubular

interstitial cells and regulated by an oxygen sensor. Inappropriately low as well as high EPO concentrations have been reported following chemotherapy due in part to paradoxical elevations of endogenous EPO concentrations immediately following chemotherapy.[21-23] Since the efficacy of EPO is dependent on adequate iron stores, treatment with intravenous iron has been shown to improve the hemoglobin response in cancer patients treated with recombinant EPO.[24]

The Thrombopoietic Agents

The hematopoietic stem cell gives rise to the early common myeloid progenitor, which then leads to the megakaryocyte-erythroid (MK) progenitor that can then lead to either erythroid or megakaryocyte progenitors. Two to five thousand platelets are released from each mature megakaryocyte regulated by various cytokines working in concert. Stem cell factor or c-kit ligand and IL-3 act at early stages and stimulate proliferation and differentiation of progenitor cells into the MK lineage. Thrombopoietin (TPO) has broad activity, stimulating growth and maturation of MK progenitor cells into mature megakaryocytes. In a normal state, 10^{11} platelets are produced daily, with platelets lasting about 8 to 9 days in the circulation.[25]

IL-11 has been shown to synergistically act with early- and later-acting cytokines in various stages of hematopoiesis including megakaryopoiesis, perhaps interacting at a later stage than TPO. Preclinical and in vitro studies indicate that IL-11 directly stimulates megakaryocytes. Oprelvekin (recombinant IL-11) was the first cytokine to reach the market for the prevention of chemotherapy-induced thrombocytopenia. Early clinical trials in patients with cancer demonstrated an ability to increase steady-state platelet counts and to reduce the risk of chemotherapy-induced thrombocytopenia.[26,27]

TPO was initially identified in 1994 and is the primary regulator of thrombopoiesis while also stimulating platelet adhesion and aggregation.[28-30] TPO is a 332-amino acid glycoprotein with an amino domain essential for thrombopoietic activity and a carboxy domain that increases the half-life. TPO is produced primarily in the liver, and its effects are mediated through the TPO receptor on megakaryocytes and platelets with TPO levels regulated primarily by the amount of receptors available for binding.[31] The unbound TPO regulates megakaryocytopoiesis. TPO levels are high in cases of thrombocytopenia due to decreased production while the levels are not sufficiently elevated with increased destruction such as in immune thrombocytopenic purpura (ITP) probably due to the high turnover of TPO with the platelets and their c-Mpl receptors.[25] Recombinant human TPO is identical to endogenous TPO and increases platelet counts in a dose-dependent fashion.[32] While no neutralizing antibodies have been identified, serial bone marrow biopsies from patients treated with TPO demonstrated hypercellularity, megakaryocytic hyperplasia, and reticulin fibrosis, which resolved within 3 months after rhTPO was stopped.[28] Pegylated recombinant human megakaryocyte growth and development factor (PEG-rHuMGDF) consists of the receptor-binding domain of TPO bound to a polyethylene glycol moiety.[33] Although early trials showed improvement in the time to platelet recovery and decreased need for platelet transfusions in cancer patients undergoing high-dose chemotherapy, thrombocytopenia associated with cross-reacting antibody formation that neutralized physiologic TPO occurred in 13 of 325 healthy volunteers and 4 of 650 oncology patients receiving as few as two doses of PEG-rHuMGDF.[34] Therefore, alternative TPO agonists have been sought, lacking any sequence homology with endogenous TPO. These new agents include TPO peptide mimetics, nonpeptide mimetics, and agonist antibodies.[35]

Romiplostim was the first TPO receptor agonist to receive regulatory approval by the US FDA for treatment of thrombocytopenia in patients with chronic ITP poorly responsive to glucocorticoids, immunoglobulins, or splenectomy. The peptide mimetic, romiplostim, is a recombinant fusion protein with two identical subunits consisting of a peptide with two TPO-binding domains covalently bound to the Fc domain of a human IgG molecule.[36] The rationale for the use of TPO agonists in ITP is based on the observation that serum TPO levels are inappropriately normal or low in the majority of patients with an apparent defect in platelet production due to immune destruction of platelet precursors.[37] Alternatively, eltrombopag is a small molecule biarylhydrazone representing a selective nonpeptide agonist of the TPO receptor that results in receptor phosphorylation and activation of cytoplasmic tyrosine kinases and signal transducers of transcription. Eltrombopag promotes proliferation and differentiation of marrow stem cells into committed megakaryocyte precursors in a dose-dependent fashion. Preclinical data demonstrated that this agent has good oral bioavailability with consistent increases in platelet counts following daily oral administration.[38]

Clinical Application of the Hematopoietic Growth Factors in Oncology

Granulocyte Colony-Stimulating Factor

Solid Tumor and Lymphoma

The CSFs are the only biological agents used in clinical practice to reduce the risk of neutropenic complications and to maintain chemotherapy dose intensity.[39] Primary prophylaxis with G-CSF starting within 3 to 5 days of the initial cycle of chemotherapy is based on evidence that the risk of neutropenic complications including FN is greatest during the first cycle of chemotherapy.[40–42] Multiple randomized controlled trials (RCTs) of primary prophylaxis with G-CSF have been reported in a variety of malignancies and treatment regimens.[43] Filgrastim is approved by the US FDA to decrease the incidence of infection, as manifested by FN, in patients with nonmyeloid malignancies receiving myelosuppressive anticancer drugs associated with a significant incidence (>20%) of FN.

Pegfilgrastim

FDA approval of pegfilgrastim was based on two phase III RCTs using filgrastim as an active control due to rates of myelosuppression of 40% associated with the chemotherapy regimen utilized without G-CSF support.[44] While otherwise identical, the pegfilgrastim dose was weight based at 100 μg/kg in one trial[45] and fixed dose at 6 mg in the other[46] (Fig. 38-3). Patients received either a single injection of pegfilgrastim starting 24 hours after chemotherapy followed by daily placebo or daily filgrastim 5 μg/kg until neutrophil recovery or a maximum of 14 days. While equivalent for the duration of severe neutropenia, the incidence of FN was lower in patients who received pegfilgrastim. Combined treatment effect from both

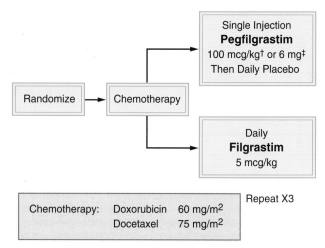

FIGURE   38-3   Design of pegfilgrastim phase III randomized trials in patients receiving chemotherapy for stage II to IV breast cancer. [†]Holmes FA, Jones SE, O'Shaughnessy J, et al. Comparable efficacy and safety profiles of once-per-cycle pegfilgrastim and daily injection filgrastim in chemotherapy-induced neutropenia: a multicenter dose-finding study in women with breast cancer. Ann Oncol 2002;13:903–909; [‡]Green MD, Koelbl H, Baselga J, et al. A randomized double-blind multicenter phase III study of fixed-dose single-administration pegfilgrastim versus daily filgrastim in patients receiving myelosuppressive chemotherapy. Ann Oncol 2003;14:29–35.

studies demonstrated additional relative risk reduction for FN with pegfilgrastim of 44% (95% confidence interval [CI]: 11% to 65%) (P = 0.015).[8] The largest RCT of G-CSF reported to date compared pegfilgrastim to placebo in 928 women with breast cancer receiving docetaxel 100 mg/m² every 3 weeks for four cycles.[47] Patients receiving pegfilgrastim experienced a lower incidence of FN (1% versus 17%; P < 0.001), FN-related hospitalization (1% versus 14%, P < 0.001), and IV antibiotics (2% versus 10%; P < 0.001) than placebo control subjects. Pegfilgrastim is approved by the US FDA to decrease the incidence of infection, as manifested by FN, in patients with nonmyeloid malignancies receiving myelosuppressive anticancer drugs associated with an incidence of FN of 17% or greater risk. The recommended dose is 6 mg single SC injection 24 hours after administration of chemotherapy and not <14 days before the next scheduled chemotherapy cycle.

Systematic Review of Randomized Controlled Trials

The systematic review of RCTs of primary prophylaxis with G-CSF in patients with solid tumors and lymphoma reported a relative risk for FN with G-CSF prophylaxis of 0.54 (95% CI: 0.43 to 0.67) (P < 0.0001) (Fig. 38-4).[43] Likewise, the summary relative risk for infection-related mortality and early all-cause mortality with G-CSF was 0.55 (95% CI: 0.33 to 0.90) (P = 0.018) and 0.60 (95% CI: 0.43 to 0.83) (P = 0.002) (Fig. 38-4), respectively. Finally, median relative dose intensity (RDI) among control subjects was 88.5% compared to 95.5% in patients receiving G-CSF in these trials. Increasing the RDI of chemotherapy utilizing abbreviated treatment schedules (dose dense) with G-CSF support has improved clinical outcomes.[48–50] Administration of filgrastim prophylaxis only after the development of afebrile neutropenia does not reduce the risk or duration of infection compared to placebo.[51] Despite no RCTs directly evaluating the use of the CSFs as secondary prophylaxis only following neutropenic complications, RCTs permitting a crossover of control patients after experiencing FN have dem-

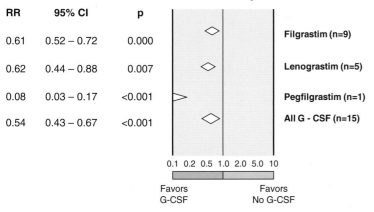

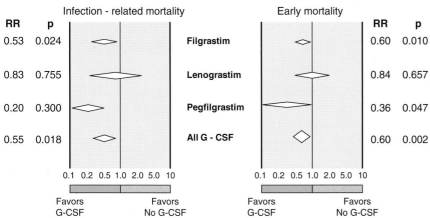

FIGURE **38-4** Forest plots of summary results from a meta-analysis of RCTs of G-CSF prophylaxis in solid tumor and lymphoma patients receiving systemic chemotherapy with or without prophylactic G-CSF including filgrastim, lenograstim, or pegfilgrastim. **Top** figure displays reported rates of FN. (Kuderer NM, Dale DC, Crawford J, et al. Impact of primary prophylaxis with G-CSF on febrile neutropenia and mortality in adult cancer patients receiving chemotherapy: a systematic review. J Clin Oncol 2007;25:3158–3167.) **Bottom graphs** reflect results for infection-related mortality and all-cause early mortality reported across trials.

onstrated a decrease in the risk and duration of FN in subsequent cycles.[43] Finally, a meta-analysis of RCTs of the CSFs as adjunct to empiric antibiotics in treatment of FN reported a reduction in the duration of neutropenia and hospitalization and a borderline reduction in infection-related mortality but not overall mortality.[52]

Clinical Practice Guidelines

Clinical practice guidelines for the use of myeloid growth factors in patients receiving cancer chemotherapy have been developed by three major professional organizations[39,53,54] (Table 38-3). Consistent recommendations across these guidelines include primary prophylaxis with the CSFs when the risk of FN is 20% or greater. All three guidelines also recommend consideration of prophylactic use of myeloid growth factors with regimens reporting lower risk of FN in cancer patients with additional individual risk factors for neutropenic complications including older age, poor performance status, and major comorbidities. Age is a risk factor for FN with the greatest increase in risk in the first cycle of therapy.[41,42] Risk factors for FN in elderly patients include cancer type, prior chemotherapy, planned chemotherapy dose intensity ≥85% of standard dosing, anthracycline- or platinum-based chemotherapy, and elevated blood urea nitrogen or alkaline phosphatase.[55] The effectiveness of G-CSF in reducing the risk of neutropenic complications in older patients is well established.[56–59] An RCT of primary versus secondary prophylaxis in older patients revealed significantly fewer episodes of FN, hospitalization for FN, as well as dose reductions and delays among those receiving primary prophylaxis.[60]

Acute Leukemia and Myelodysplastic Syndrome

The CSFs have been used after induction chemotherapy, priming before induction chemotherapy, and after consolidation chemotherapy in patients with AML. The use of CSFs before chemotherapy as priming therapy to increase the proportion of blasts in growth phase has provided mixed results.[61] Most studies of CSF use after induction therapy have demonstrated a shortening of neutropenia and hospitalization but only a single study demonstrated a survival benefit in older patients receiving GM-CSF.[62] CSF use after AML consolidation therapy has been shown to ameliorate the severity and duration of neutropenia.[63,64] In patients with acute lymphocytic leukemia (ALL), the CSFs shorten the duration of neutropenia and are recommended after initial induction and postremission chemotherapy.[65–68]

Stem Cell Transplantation

The CSFs are commonly used in SCT either for mobilization of peripheral blood progenitor cells (PBPCs) to allow enhanced stem cell collection or after autologous SCT to decrease the duration of neutropenia.[69–75] G-CSF alone or following myelosuppressive chemotherapy is commonly used to enhance in vivo production of PBPCs for SCT. G-CSF may also be administered for several days before SCT to enhance numbers of PBPCs for subsequent reinfusion.[76–78] Pegfilgrastim is capable of enhancing efficient mobilization of PBPCs when given after salvage therapy with ifosfamide, epirubicin, and etoposide.[79] Pegfilgrastim-mobilized stem cells

TABLE

38.3   *Summary of primary prophylaxis recommendations*

Setting/indication	√ Recommended	X Not recommended
General circumstances	Febrile neutropenia risk in the range of 20% or higher	
Special circumstances	Clinical factors dictate use	
Secondary prophylaxis	Based on chemotherapy reaction among other factors	
Therapy of afebrile neutropenia		Not to be used routinely
Therapy of febrile neuropenia	If high risk for complications or poor clinical outcomes	Not to be used routinely as adjunctive treatment with antibiotic therapy
Acute myeloid leukemia	Following induction therapy, patients >55 y old most likely to benefit after the completion of consolidation chemotherapy	Not to be used for priming effects
Myelodysplastic syndrome		Intermittent administration for a subset of patients with severe neutropenia and recurrent infection
Acute lymphoblastic leukemia	After the completion of initial chemotherapy or first postremission course	
Radiotherapy	Consider if receiving radiation therapy alone and prolonged delays are expected	Avoid in patients receiving concomitant chemotherapy and radiation therapy
Older patients	If ≥65 y old with diffuse aggressive lymphoma and treated with curative chemotherapy	
Pediatric population	For the primary prophylaxis of pediatric patients with a likelihood of febrile neutropenia and the secondary prophylaxis or therapy for high-risk patients	G-CSF use in children with acute leukemia should be considered carefully

Smith TJ, Khatcheressian J, Lyman GH, et al. 2006 update of recommendations for the use of white blood cell growth factors: an evidence-based clinical practice guideline. J Clin Oncol 2006;24:3187–3205.
ASCO white blood cell growth factor guidelines update summary.

induce rapid multilineage hematopoietic recovery when reinfused. While mobilization kinetics are similar to that of filgrastim, pegfilgrastim is associated with earlier leukocyte recovery and peak levels of CD34[+] cells.[80] The feasibility of pegfilgrastim mobilization regimens has been demonstrated in several malignancies.[81–83]

G-CSF administered after autologous PBPC reinfusion appears to aid engraftment.[70,84–87] G-CSF administered following high-dose chemotherapy and autologous SCT accelerates neutrophil recovery.[88–91] While the duration of FN is reduced, the proportion of patients with FN is not substantially altered. Pegfilgrastim appears to be at least as effective as filgrastim when administered post-SCT with pegfilgrastim treatment resulting in a lower incidence and shorter duration of FN.[92] The use of the CSFs following allogeneic SCT remains controversial. In a retrospective study of patients with AML undergoing allogeneic SCT, CSF support was associated with higher rate of graft versus host disease (GVHD), transplantation-related mortality, and lower disease-free and overall survival.[93] Alternatively, a meta-analysis of RCTs of CSFs following allogeneic SCT demonstrated more rapid neutrophil engraftment, shorter durations of hospitalization and intravenous antibiotic use, and lower 100-day transplant-related mortality in patients treated with CSF ($P = 0.046$).[94]

Toxicity and Safety

The CSFs are generally well tolerated with mild to moderate bone pain in approximately 20% to 30% of patients representing the most common side effect.[43] Splenomegaly, splenic rupture, and thrombocytopenia have been rarely reported with CSF use in the setting of stem cell mobilization. Reversible laboratory abnormalities include leukocytosis and elevation of uric acid, alkaline phosphatase, and lactate dehydrogenase. The safety experience with pegfilgrastim is similar to that with filgrastim with the most common adverse event being bone pain. Retrospective analyses performed for each of the two randomized phase III studies of pegfilgrastim versus filgrastim showed no statistically significant differences in incidence, severity, or duration of bone pain.[11,46] Despite label restrictions, pegfilgrastim may also be safely used to support dose-dense regimens.[45,95,96]

The presence of G-CSF receptors on the surface of myeloid leukemic cells has led to concern about an increased risk of AML or myelodysplastic syndrome (MDS) in patients receiving G-CSF. Using SEER-Medicare data, Hershman reported a hazard ratio (HR) of 2.14 (95% CI: 1.12 to 4.08) in elderly women with early-stage breast cancer who received adjuvant chemotherapy supported by G-CSF or GM-CSF.[97] The interpretation of retrospective studies is complicated by their post hoc analysis, limited ability to identify confounding factors, and the recognized leukemogenicity of ionizing radiation and many commonly used chemotherapeutic agents. The ability of G-CSF to sustain or increase either dose intensity or cumulative chemotherapy dose further confounds any influence of G-CSF on the risk of AML or MDS. In a meta-analysis of 25 RCTs of G-CSF–supported chemotherapy with at least 2 years of follow-up, AML/MDS was reported in 22 control and 43 G-CSF–treated patients with estimated relative risk of 1.92 (1.19 to 3.07; $P = 0.007$) with an absolute risk increase of 4/1,000.[98] At the same time, the relative risk for all-cause mortality across all trials was 0.897 (0.857 to 0.938; $P < 0.0001$) with an absolute reduction of 34 deaths per 1,000 patients. It remains impossible to separate any risk associated with the growth factor from that of the known increased risk of AML or MDS associated with chemotherapy.

Granulocyte-Macrophage Colony-Stimulating Factor

Acute Myeloid Leukemia

In a large phase III placebo-controlled study in elderly patients with AML, sargramostim enhanced neutrophil recovery, reduced infections, and led to longer survival.[62] In a randomized placebo-controlled study, 240 older patients with AML received molgramostim during and after induction chemotherapy resulting in shorter time to neutrophil recovery and improved disease-free survival than controls.[99]

High-Dose Therapy with Stem Cell Support

Randomized placebo-controlled clinical trials involving GM-CSF have also been conducted in the setting of high-dose chemotherapy with SCT demonstrating accelerated neutrophil recovery when bone marrow alone is used as the sole stem cell source.[100–109] GM-CSF therapy has shown no significant effect on the incidence or severity of GVHD in patients receiving allogeneic transplants.

Priming of Peripheral Blood Progenitor Cells

A number of clinical trials have found GM-CSF alone or following chemotherapy useful in priming PBPCs for subsequent leukapheresis.[77,110–113] GM-CSF–primed PBPCs following cytotoxic chemotherapy with autologous marrow rescue are associated with significantly improved myeloid and platelet recovery compared to controls.[114] Filgrastim and molgramostim appear to produce similar yields of PBPCs more rapidly when used in conjunction with chemotherapy for priming.[115]

Toxicity and Safety

Fever and fluid retention are often reported with GM-CSF.[116] More fever, dyspnea, fluid retention, myalgias, and bone pain are seen with E. coli–derived GM-CSF.[116] Dose-related adverse effects with GM-CSF include capillary leak syndrome, central vein thrombosis, and hypotension. Effects seen over a variety of doses include fever, pleuritis, myalgia, bone pain, pulmonary infiltrates, rash, and thrombophlebitis. Some patients have experienced a syndrome of transient hypoxia and hypotension following the first dose but not subsequent doses of GM-CSF.[117] GM-CSF is a known inducer of other endogenous cytokines, which are thought to account for at least some of the adverse effects. The simultaneous administration of GM-CSF and cycle-specific chemotherapy or radiation therapy has worsened myelosuppression.[118,119]

Erythropoiesis-Stimulating Agents

The clinical and economic impact of anemia in cancer patients receiving chemotherapy has been extensively studied.[120,121] In randomized placebo-controlled trials carried out in anemic cancer patients receiving chemotherapy, both epoetin alfa[122–126] and darbepoetin alfa[127,128] increase hemoglobin levels and reduce red cell transfusion rates. Pooled analysis of trials comparing early intervention to delayed treatment with epoetin alfa or darbepoetin alfa suggested that the former resulted in less severe anemia and greater reductions in transfusion requirements than delayed intervention.[129] Response to EPO is unlikely in the setting of physiologically elevated EPO levels.

Dose and Schedules

Despite early studies suggesting that subcutaneous dosing epoetin alfa three times per week provided better erythropoietic response than dosing once weekly,[130] a large open-label weekly epoetin alfa regimen in cancer patients demonstrated efficacy.[131] Therefore, the most common regimen in current use for cancer patients is 40,000 units per week administered subcutaneously. Although darbepoetin alfa was initially approved as a once-weekly injection, subsequent data support dosing at 200 μg subcutaneously every 2 weeks or 500 μg every 3 weeks.

Toxicity and Safety

While these agents are generally well tolerated, safety concerns have emerged that should be considered by the patient and clinician in any decision to initiate an ESA in patients with cancer. Placebo-controlled RCTs of the ESAs have suggested that some cancer patients receiving these agents experience worse outcomes.[132,133] A systematic review and meta-analysis of RCTs of epoetin alfa and beta and darbepoetin alfa conducted under the auspices of the Cochrane Collaboration confirmed that treatment with these agents significantly reduced the need for red blood cell transfusions and improved hematologic response. However, across these trials, treatment with epoetin or darbepoetin increased the risk of thromboembolic events (relative risk [RR] = 1.67, 95% CI = 1.35 to 2.06). Although not reaching statistical significance, concern was raised whether epoetin or darbepoetin might have an adverse impact on overall survival (hazard ratio [HR] = 1.08, 95% CI = 0.99 to 1.180).[134,135] The capacity of EPO to protect hypoxic cells against apoptosis is being tested in the setting of stroke and heart attack to limit infarct size. Concerns have been raised that EPO may also protect hypoxic tumor cells from death. An updated review by the same group subsequently reported a borderline increase in overall mortality in all studies of ESAs in cancer patients (RR = 1.06; 95% CI: 1.00 to 1.12)[136] (Fig. 38-5). Although a nonsignificant trend toward increased mortality was observed in studies of ESA in support of cancer chemotherapy (RR = 1.10; 95% CI: 0.98 to 1.24), this was most apparent in trials administering the ESAs outside of guideline-recommended starting and target hemoglobin levels[135] (Fig. 38-5). In most randomized trials of ESAs in patients with cancer, no difference in survival has been observed. An individual patient data meta-analysis from all randomized double-blind placebo-controlled trials of darbepoetin alfa in patients with chemotherapy-induced anemia has been conducted demonstrating no decrease in progression-free mortality (HR = 0.93; 95% CI: 0.84 to 1.04) or overall mortality (HR = 0.97; 95% CI: 0.85 to 1.1).[137] Nevertheless, an increase of thromboembolic events was confirmed with the ESAs in this setting. Data review by the US FDA resulted in black box warnings severely

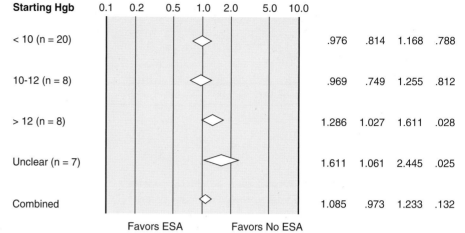

Meta-analysis of Overall Mortality for Cancer Patients Epoetin/Darbepoetin versus standard care

Starting Hgb				
< 10 (n = 20)	.976	.814	1.168	.788
10-12 (n = 8)	.969	.749	1.255	.812
> 12 (n = 8)	1.286	1.027	1.611	.028
Unclear (n = 7)	1.611	1.061	2.445	.025
Combined	1.085	.973	1.233	.132

FIGURE 38-5 Forest plot of summary results of overall mortality among RCTs of epoetin alfa and darbepoetin alfa in cancer patients receiving systemic chemotherapy stratified by reported starting hemoglobin. Derived from Bohlius J, Wilson J, Seidenfeld J, et al. Recombinant human erythropoietins and cancer patients: updated meta-analysis of 57 studies including 9353 patients. J Natl Cancer Inst 2006;98:708–714.

limiting the clinical use of these agents in cancer patients. These warnings stipulate that the ESAs shortened overall survival and/or increased the risk of tumor progression in some clinical studies in patients with breast, head and neck, lymphoid, non–small cell lung, and cervical cancers. To decrease these risks, as well as the risk of serious cardiovascular and thrombovascular events, the lowest dose needed to avoid red blood cell transfusions is recommended and only for treatment of anemia due to concomitant myelosuppressive chemotherapy. Accordingly, the FDA states that the ESAs are not indicated for patients receiving myelosuppressive therapy when the anticipated outcome is cure. Finally, discontinuation of an ESA following the completion of a chemotherapy course is encouraged.

Clinical Practice Guidelines

Current clinical practice guidelines from the American Society of Clinical Oncology and the American Society of Hematology for the use of the ESAs for chemotherapy-induced anemia recommend initiation of an ESA to increase the hemoglobin and decrease transfusion requirements as hemoglobin levels approach or fall below 10 g/dL.[138] In addition, ESA treatment continues to be recommended for patients with low-risk myelodysplasia. The guidelines also recommend monitoring iron stores and supplementing iron intake for ESA-treated patients. Alternatively, guidelines for the use of the ESAs for the management of chemotherapy-induced anemia from the National Comprehensive Cancer Network limit their use to symptomatic patients being treated for noncurative intent.[139] The use of ESAs to treat anemia due to cancer chemotherapy reduces the incidence of red cell transfusions (which have well-defined risks) and the symptoms of anemia. Although the ESAs are generally well tolerated, they have risks including an increase in venous thrombosis. The impact of the ESAs on tumor progression and survival are poorly understood; however, the uncertainty about tumor protection shifts the assessment of risk-to-benefit ratio in favor of blood transfusion rather than ESAs to treat anemia in patients with curable malignancies.

Thrombopoietic Agents

Interleukin 11

A small randomized placebo-controlled evaluation of IL-11 for secondary prophylaxis of thrombocytopenia in cancer patients previously transfused for chemotherapy-induced thrombocytopenia reported subsequent platelet transfusion requirements in 90% and 72% placebo and IL-11–treated patients, respectively.[140] Administration of IL-11 did not appear to alter platelet recovery or transfusion requirements in patients with breast cancer enrolled in a randomized placebo-controlled study following high-dose chemotherapy and infusion with G-CSF–primed PBPCs.[141] Constitutional symptoms such as myalgia, arthralgia, and fatigue were the dose-limiting toxicities in dose-finding trials. Approximately 60% of patients treated with IL-11 experience edema though secondary to sodium retention. Atrial arrhythmias, tachycardia, conjunctival injection, and worsening of effusions can also occur.

Thrombopoietic Agents

Clinical studies of recombinant TPO were initially conducted with either the full-length glycosylated TPO molecule (rTPO, Genetech/Pfizer) or a truncated pegylated derivative (rMGDF, Amgen). A small study of rMGDF in cancer patients not receiving chemotherapy demonstrated a dose-dependent increase in platelet counts. Clinically significant increases in platelet counts were evident following 6 days of therapy, with the counts continuing to rise several days after drug discontinuation.[142] Additional studies of recombinant rMGDF in patients with lung cancer and gynecologic cancer demonstrated a significant reduction in platelet recovery time.[143–145] rTPO and rMGDF were generally well tolerated with no evidence of dose-limiting adverse effects although some patients did experience thrombotic events. Clinical development of rMGDF was stopped when a few cancer patients and healthy volunteers demonstrated neutralizing antibodies to TPO that led to thrombocytopenia.

Romiplostim

Romiplostim is approved for use in patients with chronic ITP based on a durable platelet response in two phase III multicenter double-blind randomized placebo-controlled trials in splenectomized and nonsplenectomized patients receiving at least one prior treatment for ITP. Most adverse events were mild to moderate and no significant increase in serious adverse events was reported in the romiplostim arm.[146] Pooled data from these trials have also demonstrated that romiplostim therapy is associated with significant improvements in health-related quality of life.[147] FDA approval was based on the favorable risk-to-benefit profile in patients with chronic ITP. Overall safety data on romiplostim were substantial given the orphan status of the disease, with a total of 308 ITP subjects included in clinical trials and 114 patients receiving romiplostim for 1 year or more. No neutralizing antibodies to TPO were observed despite careful monitoring. Reticulin formation was observed in ten patients although progression to marrow fibrosis was not observed in the two phase III studies. Severe thrombocytopenia following discontinuation of romiplostim was reported in four patients resolving within two weeks. Therefore, approval was accompanied by pharmacovigilance efforts including a Risk Evaluation and Mitigation Strategy (REMS). Several studies in cancer patients receiving chemotherapy are underway in lymphoma and advanced non–small cell lung cancer. Future indications in patients receiving cancer chemotherapy are likely to be limited to high-risk settings such as those with current or recent severe thrombocytopenia. The impact of less severe thrombocytopenia on chemotherapy dose intensity has yet to be adequately explored.

Eltrombopag

Eltrombopag is the first orally absorbed, small-molecule TPO receptor agonist; it was approved by the US FDA for the treatment of thrombocytopenia in patients with chronic ITP with insufficient response to glucocorticoids, immunoglobulins, or splenectomy. The starting dose is 50 mg daily; in the setting of hepatic dysfunction, 25 mg daily is recommended. Approval was based on data from two double-blind placebo-controlled clinical studies along with additional supportive studies.[148,149] A platelet response was observed among 59% and 70% of the patients receiving eltrombopag compared to placebo response rates among 16% and 11%. Major safety findings pertained to a risk for hepatic toxicity, worsening thrombocytopenia with hemorrhage following discontinuation, and reticulin formation in the bone marrow. The FDA approved eltrombopag based upon a favorable risk-to-benefit profile, where the major benefit consisted of a clinically important increase in platelets among patients refractory to prior therapy. Subsequently, a global randomized placebo-controlled trial has also been performed demonstrating a significantly better platelet response for eltrombopag.[150] A reduction in overall bleeding dependent upon platelet response was also observed. In addition, nearly 300 patients have been treated in the extension study with more than 85% achieving and maintaining platelet counts $\geq 50,000/\mu L$ for most of the study period. Although liver toxicities were generally mild and reversible, routine monitoring of liver function is encouraged.[151] Hemorrhage associated with thrombocytopenia following discontinuation of eltrombopag was also observed. The frequency of this complication is unclear since most patients began with low platelet counts.[150] Continued

assessment for safety signals related to any increased risk of thromboembolism or bone marrow reticulin formation continue under a Risk Evaluation and Mitigation Strategy (REMS) permitting approval and utilization of this class of agents while gathering safety data on larger numbers of patients to better estimate the true rate of important adverse events.

References

1. Metcalf D. Studies on colony formation in vitro by mouse bone marrow cells. I. Continuous cluster formation and relation of clusters to colonies. J Cell Physiol 1969;74:323–332.
2. Metcalf D, Foster R. Bone marrow colony-stimulating activity of serum from mice with viral-induced leukemia. J Natl Cancer Inst 1967;39:1235–1245.
3. Clark SC, Kamen R. The human hematopoietic colony-stimulating factors. Science 1987;236:1229–1237.
4. Burgess AW, Metcalf D. Characterization of a serum factor stimulating the differentiation of myelomonocytic leukemic cells. Int J Cancer 1980;26:647–654.
5. Moore MA. G-CSF: its relationship to leukemia differentiation-inducing activity and other hemopoietic regulators. J Cell Physiol Suppl 1982;1:53–64.
6. Bagby G, Heinrich M. Growth factors, cytokines, and the control of hematopoiesis. In: Hoffman R, Shattil SJ, eds. Heamotology Basic Principles and Practice. Philadelphia, PA: Churchill Livingstone, 2000:154–202.
7. Moore M. Colony stimulating factors: basic principles and preclinical studies. In: Rosenberg S, ed. Principles and Practice of the Biologic Therapy of Cancer. Philadelphia, PA: Lippincott Williams & Wilkins, 2000:113–140.
8. Lyman GH. Pegfilgrastim: a granulocyte colony-stimulating factor with sustained duration of action. Expert Opin Biol Ther 2005;5:1635–1646.
9. Kotto-Kome AC, Fox SE, Lu W, et al. Evidence that the granulocyte colony-stimulating factor (G-CSF) receptor plays a role in the pharmacokinetics of G-CSF and PegG-CSF using a G-CSF-R KO model. Pharmacol Res 2004;50:55–58.
10. Yang BB, Lum PK, Hayashi MM, et al. Polyethylene glycol modification of filgrastim results in decreased renal clearance of the protein in rats. J Pharm Sci 2004;93:1367–1373.
11. Holmes FA, Jones SE, O'Shaughnessy J, et al. Comparable efficacy and safety profiles of once-per-cycle pegfilgrastim and daily injection filgrastim in chemotherapy-induced neutropenia: a multicenter dose-finding study in women with breast cancer. Ann Oncol 2002;13:903–909.
12. Molineux G. The design and development of pegfilgrastim (PEG-rmetHuG-CSF, Neulasta). Curr Pharm Des 2004;10:1235–1244.
13. Burgess AW, Camakaris J, Metcalf D. Purification and properties of colony-stimulating factor from mouse lung-conditioned medium. J Biol Chem 1977;252:1998–2003.
14. Gough NM, Gough J, Metcalf D, et al. Molecular cloning of cDNA encoding a murine haematopoietic growth regulator, granulocyte-macrophage colony stimulating factor. Nature 1984;309:763–767.
15. Peters WP, Stuart A, Affronti ML, et al. Neutrophil migration is defective during recombinant human granulocyte-macrophage colony-stimulating factor infusion after autologous bone marrow transplantation in humans. Blood 1988;72:1310–1315.
16. Demir G, Klein HO, Tuzuner N. Low dose daily rhGM-CSF application activates monocytes and dendritic cells in vivo. Leuk Res 2003;27:1105–1108.
17. O'Dwyer PJ, LaCreta FP, Schilder R, et al. Phase I trial of thiotepa in combination with recombinant human granulocyte-macrophage colony-stimulating factor. J Clin Oncol 1992;10:1352–1358.
18. Elliott S, Lorenzini T, Asher S, et al. Enhancement of therapeutic protein in vivo activities through glycoengineering. Nat Biotechnol 2003;21:414–421.
19. Allon M, Kleinman K, Walczyk M, et al. Pharmacokinetics and pharmacodynamics of darbepoetin alfa and epoetin in patients undergoing dialysis. Clin Pharmacol Ther 2002;72:546–555.

20. Jaar B, Baillou C, Viron B, et al. Long-term effects of recombinant human erythropoietin on bone marrow progenitor cells. Nephrol Dial Transplant 1993;8:614–620.

21. Birgegard G, Wide L, Simonsson B. Marked erythropoietin increase before fall in Hb after treatment with cytostatic drugs suggests mechanism other than anaemia for stimulation. Br J Haematol 1989;72:462–466.

22. Smith DH, Goldwasser E, Vokes EE. Serum immunoerythropoietin levels in patients with cancer receiving cisplatin-based chemotherapy. Cancer 1991;68:1101–1105.

23. Schapira L, Antin JH, Ransil BJ, et al. Serum erythropoietin levels in patients receiving intensive chemotherapy and radiotherapy. Blood 1990;76:2354–2359.

24. Auerbach M, Ballard H, Trout JR, et al. Intravenous iron optimizes the response to recombinant human erythropoietin in cancer patients with chemotherapy-related anemia: a multicenter, open-label, randomized trial. J Clin Oncol 2004;22:1301–1307.

25. Deutsch VR, Tomer A. Megakaryocyte development and platelet production. Br J Haematol 2006;134:453–466.

26. Gordon MS, McCaskill-Stevens WJ, Battiato LA, et al. A phase I trial of recombinant human interleukin-11 (neumega rhIL-11 growth factor) in women with breast cancer receiving chemotherapy. Blood 1996;87:3615–3624.

27. Isaacs C, Robert NJ, Bailey FA, et al. Randomized placebo-controlled study of recombinant human interleukin-11 to prevent chemotherapy-induced thrombocytopenia in patients with breast cancer receiving dose-intensive cyclophosphamide and doxorubicin. J Clin Oncol 1997;15:3368–3377.

28. Douglas VK, Tallman MS, Cripe LD, et al. Thrombopoietin administered during induction chemotherapy to patients with acute myeloid leukemia induces transient morphologic changes that may resemble chronic myeloproliferative disorders. Am J Clin Pathol 2002;117:844–850.

29. Vadhan-Raj S. Recombinant human thrombopoietin: clinical experience and in vivo biology. Semin Hematol 1998;35:261–268.

30. Vadhan-Raj S. Clinical experience with recombinant human thrombopoietin in chemotherapy-induced thrombocytopenia. Semin Hematol 2000;37:28–34.

31. Nurden AT, Viallard JF, Nurden P. New-generation drugs that stimulate platelet production in chronic immune thrombocytopenic purpura. Lancet 2009;373:1562–1569.

32. Kuter DJ, Begley CG. Recombinant human thrombopoietin: basic biology and evaluation of clinical studies. Blood 2002;100:3457–3469.

33. Begley CG, Basser RL. Biologic and structural differences of thrombopoietic growth factors. Semin Hematol 2000;37:19–27.

34. Li J, Yang C, Xia Y, et al. Thrombocytopenia caused by the development of antibodies to thrombopoietin. Blood 2001;98:3241–3248.

35. Wright J, Vadhan-Raj S. Thrombocytopenia and thrombopoietic growth factors. In: Lyman GH, Crawford J, eds. Cancer Supportive Care: Advances in Therapeutic Strategies. New York: Informa Healthcare USA, Inc, 2008:135–148.

36. Wang B, Nichol JL, Sullivan JT. Pharmacodynamics and pharmacokinetics of AMG 531, a novel thrombopoietin receptor ligand. Clin Pharmacol Ther 2004;76:628–638.

37. Bussel JB, Kuter DJ, George JN, et al. AMG 531, a thrombopoiesis-stimulating protein, for chronic ITP. N Engl J Med 2006;355:1672–1681.

38. Jenkins JM, Williams D, Deng Y, et al. Phase 1 clinical study of eltrombopag, an oral, nonpeptide thrombopoietin receptor agonist. Blood 2007;109:4739–4741.

39. Smith TJ, Khatcheressian J, Lyman GH, et al. 2006 update of recommendations for the use of white blood cell growth factors: an evidence-based clinical practice guideline. J Clin Oncol 2006;24:3187–3205.

40. Crawford J, Dale DC, Kuderer NM, et al. Risk and timing of neutropenic events in adult cancer patients receiving chemotherapy: the results of a prospective nationwide study of oncology practice. J Natl Compr Canc Netw 2008;6:109–118.

41. Lyman GH, Delgado DJ. Risk and timing of hospitalization for febrile neutropenia in patients receiving CHOP, CHOP-R, or CNOP chemotherapy for intermediate-grade non-Hodgkin lymphoma. Cancer 2003;98:2402–2409.

42. Lyman GH, Morrison VA, Dale DC, et al. Risk of febrile neutropenia among patients with intermediate-grade non-Hodgkin's lymphoma receiving CHOP chemotherapy. Leuk Lymphoma 2003;44:2069–2076.

43. Kuderer NM, Dale DC, Crawford J, et al. Impact of primary prophylaxis with granulocyte colony-stimulating factor on febrile neutropenia and mortality in adult cancer patients receiving chemotherapy: a systematic review. J Clin Oncol 2007;25:3158–3167.

44. Misset JL, Dieras V, Gruia G, et al. Dose-finding study of docetaxel and doxorubicin in first-line treatment of patients with metastatic breast cancer. Ann Oncol 1999;10:553–560.

45. Holmes FA, O'Shaughnessy JA, Vukelja S, et al. Blinded, randomized, multicenter study to evaluate single administration pegfilgrastim once per cycle versus daily filgrastim as an adjunct to chemotherapy in patients with high-risk stage II or stage III/IV breast cancer. J Clin Oncol 2002;20:727–731.

46. Green MD, Koelbl H, Baselga J, et al. A randomized double-blind multicenter phase III study of fixed-dose single-administration pegfilgrastim versus daily filgrastim in patients receiving myelosuppressive chemotherapy. Ann Oncol 2003;14:29–35.

47. Vogel CL, Wojtukiewicz MZ, Carroll RR, et al. First and subsequent cycle use of pegfilgrastim prevents febrile neutropenia in patients with breast cancer: a multicenter, double-blind, placebo-controlled phase III study. J Clin Oncol 2005;23:1178–1184.

48. Citron ML, Berry DA, Cirrincione C, et al. Randomized trial of dose-dense versus conventionally scheduled and sequential versus concurrent combination chemotherapy as postoperative adjuvant treatment of node-positive primary breast cancer: first report of Intergroup Trial C9741/Cancer and Leukemia Group B Trial 9741. J Clin Oncol 2003;21:1431–1439.

49. Pfreundschuh M, Trumper L, Kloess M, et al. Two-weekly or 3-weekly CHOP chemotherapy with or without etoposide for the treatment of elderly patients with aggressive lymphomas: results of the NHL-B2 trial of the DSHNHL. Blood 2004;104:634–641.

50. Pfreundschuh M, Trumper L, Kloess M, et al. Two-weekly or 3-weekly CHOP chemotherapy with or without etoposide for the treatment of young patients with good-prognosis (normal LDH) aggressive lymphomas: results of the NHL-B1 trial of the DSHNHL. Blood 2004;104:626–633.

51. Hartmann LC, Tschetter LK, Habermann TM, et al. Granulocyte colony-stimulating factor in severe chemotherapy-induced afebrile neutropenia. N Engl J Med 1997;336:1776–1780.

52. Clark OA, Lyman GH, Castro AA, et al. Colony-stimulating factors for chemotherapy-induced febrile neutropenia: a meta-analysis of randomized controlled trials. J Clin Oncol 2005;23:4198–4214.

53. Aapro MS, Cameron DA, Pettengell R, et al. EORTC guidelines for the use of granulocyte-colony stimulating factor to reduce the incidence of chemotherapy-induced febrile neutropenia in adult patients with lymphomas and solid tumours. Eur J Cancer 2006;42:2433–2453.

54. Crawford J, Armitage J, Balducci L, et al. Myeloid growth factors. J Natl Compr Canc Netw 2009;7:64–83.

55. Shayne M, Culakova E, Poniewierski MS, et al. Dose intensity and hematologic toxicity in older cancer patients receiving systemic chemotherapy. Cancer 2007;110:1611–1620.

56. Doorduijn JK, van der Holt B, van Imhoff GW, et al. CHOP compared with CHOP plus granulocyte colony-stimulating factor in elderly patients with aggressive non-Hodgkin's lymphoma. J Clin Oncol 2003;21:3041–3050.

57. Lyman GH, Kuderer N, Agboola O, et al. Evidence-based use of colony-stimulating factors in elderly cancer patients. Cancer Control 2003;10:487–499.

58. Osby E, Hagberg H, Kvaloy S, et al. CHOP is superior to CNOP in elderly patients with aggressive lymphoma while outcome is unaffected by filgrastim treatment: results of a Nordic Lymphoma Group randomized trial. Blood 2003;101:3840–3848.

59. Zinzani PL, Pavone E, Storti S, et al. Randomized trial with or without granulocyte colony-stimulating factor as adjunct to induction VNCOP-B treatment of elderly high-grade non-Hodgkin's lymphoma. Blood 1997;89:3974–3979.

60. Balducci L, Al-Halawani H, Charu V, et al. Elderly cancer patients receiving chemotherapy benefit from first-cycle pegfilgrastim. Oncologist 2007;12:1416–1424.

61. Lowenberg B, van Putten W, Theobald M, et al. Effect of priming with granulocyte colony-stimulating factor on the outcome of chemotherapy for acute myeloid leukemia. N Engl J Med 2003;349:743–752.

62. Rowe JM, Andersen JW, Mazza JJ, et al. A randomized placebo-controlled phase III study of granulocyte-macrophage colony-stimulating

factor in adult patients (>55 to 70 years of age) with acute myelogenous leukemia: a study of the Eastern Cooperative Oncology Group (E1490). Blood 1995;86:457–462.

63. Harousseau JL, Witz B, Lioure B, et al. Granulocyte colony-stimulating factor after intensive consolidation chemotherapy in acute myeloid leukemia: results of a randomized trial of the Groupe Ouest-Est Leucemies Aigues Myeloblastiques. J Clin Oncol 2000;18:780–787.

64. Heil G, Hoelzer D, Sanz MA, et al. A randomized, double-blind, placebo-controlled, phase III study of filgrastim in remission induction and consolidation therapy for adults with de novo acute myeloid leukemia. The International Acute Myeloid Leukemia Study Group. Blood 1997;90:4710–4718.

65. Larson RA, Dodge RK, Linker CA, et al. A randomized controlled trial of filgrastim during remission induction and consolidation chemotherapy for adults with acute lymphoblastic leukemia: CALGB study 9111. Blood 1998;92:1556–1564.

66. Laver J, Amylon M, Desai S, et al. Randomized trial of r-metHu granulocyte colony-stimulating factor in an intensive treatment for T-cell leukemia and advanced-stage lymphoblastic lymphoma of childhood: a Pediatric Oncology Group pilot study. J Clin Oncol 1998;16:522–526.

67. Pui CH, Boyett JM, Hughes WT, et al. Human granulocyte colony-stimulating factor after induction chemotherapy in children with acute lymphoblastic leukemia. N Engl J Med 1997;336:1781–1787.

68. Ottmann OG, Hoelzer D, Gracien E, et al. Concomitant granulocyte colony-stimulating factor and induction chemoradiotherapy in adult acute lymphoblastic leukemia: a randomized phase III trial. Blood 1995;86:444–450.

69. D'Hondt L, Emmons RV, Andre M, et al. The administration of 10 microg/kg granulocyte colony-stimulating factor (G-CSF) alone results in a successful peripheral blood stem cell collection when previous mobilization with chemotherapy and hematopoietic growth factor failed. Leuk Lymphoma 1999;34:105–109.

70. Klumpp TR, Mangan KF, Goldberg SL, et al. Granulocyte colony-stimulating factor accelerates neutrophil engraftment following peripheral-blood stem-cell transplantation: a prospective, randomized trial. J Clin Oncol 1995;13:1323–1327.

71. Kroger N, Zander AR. Dose and schedule effect of G-GSF for stem cell mobilization in healthy donors for allogeneic transplantation. Leuk Lymphoma 2002;43:1391–1394.

72. Kroger N, Zeller W, Hassan HT, et al. Successful mobilization of peripheral blood stem cells in heavily pretreated myeloma patients with G-CSF alone. Ann Hematol 1998;76:257–262.

73. Lefrere F, Makke J, Fermand J, et al. Blood stem cell collection using chemotherapy with or without systematic G-CSF: experience in 52 patients with multiple myeloma. Bone Marrow Transplant 1999;24:463–466.

74. Nemunaitis J, Appelbaum F, Singer J. Effect of GM-CSF on circulating granulocyte-monocyte progenitors in autologous bone marrow transplantation. Lancet 1989;2:1405–1406.

75. Spitzer G, Adkins D, Mathews M, et al. Randomized comparison of G-CSF + GM-CSF vs G-CSF alone for mobilization of peripheral blood stem cells: effects on hematopoietic recovery after high-dose chemotherapy. Bone Marrow Transplant 1997;20:921–930.

76. Chao NJ, Schriber JR, Grimes K, et al. Granulocyte colony-stimulating factor "mobilized" peripheral blood progenitor cells accelerate granulocyte and platelet recovery after high-dose chemotherapy. Blood 1993;81:2031–2035.

77. Peters WP, Rosner G, Ross M, et al. Comparative effects of granulocyte-macrophage colony-stimulating factor (GM-CSF) and granulocyte colony-stimulating factor (G-CSF) on priming peripheral blood progenitor cells for use with autologous bone marrow after high-dose chemotherapy. Blood 1993;81:1709–1719.

78. Sheridan WP, Begley CG, Juttner CA, et al. Effect of peripheral-blood progenitor cells mobilised by filgrastim (G-CSF) on platelet recovery after high-dose chemotherapy. Lancet 1992;339:640–644.

79. Isidori A, Tani M, Bonifazi F, et al. Phase II study of a single pegfilgrastim injection as an adjunct to chemotherapy to mobilize stem cells into the peripheral blood of pretreated lymphoma patients. Haematologica 2005;90:225–231.

80. Steidl U, Fenk R, Bruns I, et al. Successful transplantation of peripheral blood stem cells mobilized by chemotherapy and a single dose of pegylated G-CSF in patients with multiple myeloma. Bone Marrow Transplant 2005;35:33–36.

81. Kroschinsky F, Holig K, Poppe-Thiede K, et al. Single-dose pegfilgrastim for the mobilization of allogeneic CD34+ peripheral blood progenitor cells in healthy family and unrelated donors. Haematologica 2005;90:1665–1671.

82. Noga S, Oroszlan M, Hetherington J. Use of pegfilgrastim for autologous peripheral blood stem cell mobilization: comparison to a daily filgrastim regimen. Bone Marrow Transplant 2003;31:S18.

83. Noga SJ, Oroszlan M, Zhang YL. Single dose pegfilgrastim successfully mobilizes optimal numbers of autologous CD34+ cells for peripheral blood stem cell collection [abstract 3262]. Blood 2002;100:826a.

84. Kawano Y, Takaue Y, Mimaya J, et al. Marginal benefit/disadvantage of granulocyte colony-stimulating factor therapy after autologous blood stem cell transplantation in children: results of a prospective randomized trial. The Japanese Cooperative Study Group of PBSCT. Blood 1998;92:4040–4046.

85. Lee SM, Radford JA, Dobson L, et al. Recombinant human granulocyte colony-stimulating factor (filgrastim) following high-dose chemotherapy and peripheral blood progenitor cell rescue in high-grade non-Hodgkin's lymphoma: clinical benefits at no extra cost. Br J Cancer 1998;77:1294–1299.

86. McQuaker IG, Hunter AE, Pacey S, et al. Low-dose filgrastim significantly enhances neutrophil recovery following autologous peripheral-blood stem-cell transplantation in patients with lymphoproliferative disorders: evidence for clinical and economic benefit. J Clin Oncol 1997;15:451–457.

87. Shimazaki C, Oku N, Uchiyama H, et al. Effect of granulocyte colony-stimulating factor on hematopoietic recovery after peripheral blood progenitor cell transplantation. Bone Marrow Transplant 1994;13:271–275.

88. Asano S, Masaoka T, Takaku F. Beneficial effect of recombinant human glycosylated granulocyte colony-stimulating factor in marrow-transplanted patients: results of multicenter phase II–III studies. Transplant Proc 1991;23:1701–1703.

89. Bishop MR, Tarantolo SR, Geller RB, et al. A randomized, double-blind trial of filgrastim (granulocyte colony-stimulating factor) versus placebo following allogeneic blood stem cell transplantation. Blood 2000;96:80–85.

90. Schmitz N, Dreger P, Zander AR, et al. Results of a randomised, controlled, multicentre study of recombinant human granulocyte colony-stimulating factor (filgrastim) in patients with Hodgkin's disease and non-Hodgkin's lymphoma undergoing autologous bone marrow transplantation. Bone Marrow Transplant 1995;15:261–266.

91. Stahel RA, Jost LM, Cerny T, et al. Randomized study of recombinant human granulocyte colony-stimulating factor after high-dose chemotherapy and autologous bone marrow transplantation for high-risk lymphoid malignancies. J Clin Oncol 1994;12:1931–1938.

92. Staber PB, Holub R, Linkesch W, et al. Fixed-dose single administration of Pegfilgrastim vs daily Filgrastim in patients with haematological malignancies undergoing autologous peripheral blood stem cell transplantation. Bone Marrow Transplant 2005;35:889–893.

93. Ringden O, Labopin M, Gorin NC, et al. Treatment with granulocyte colony-stimulating factor after allogeneic bone marrow transplantation for acute leukemia increases the risk of graft-versus-host disease and death: a study from the Acute Leukemia Working Party of the European Group for Blood and Marrow Transplantation. J Clin Oncol 2004;22:416–423.

94. Komrokji RS, Lyman GH. The colony-stimulating factors: use to prevent and treat neutropenia and its complications. Expert Opin Biol Ther 2004;4:1897–1910.

95. Younes A, Fayad L, Romaguera J, et al. Safety and efficacy of once-per-cycle pegfilgrastim in support of ABVD chemotherapy in patients with Hodgkin lymphoma. Eur J Cancer 2006;42:2976–2981.

96. Lopez A, Fernandez de Sevilla A, Castaigne S. Pegfilgrastim supports delivery of CHOP-R chemotherapy administered every 14 days; a randomised phase II study [abstract 3311]. Blood 2004;104:904a–905a.

97. Hershman D, Neugut AI, Jacobson JS, et al. Acute myeloid leukemia or myelodysplastic syndrome following use of granulocyte colony-stimulating factors during breast cancer adjuvant chemotherapy. J Natl Cancer Inst 2007;99:196–205.

98. Lyman GH, Dale DC, Wolff DA, et al. Acute myeloid leukemia or myelodysplastic syndrome in randomized controlled clinical trials of cancer

chemotherapy with granulocyte colony-stimulating factor: a systematic review. J Clin Oncol 2010;28:2914–2924.

99. Witz F, Sadoun A, Perrin MC, et al. A placebo-controlled study of recombinant human granulocyte-macrophage colony-stimulating factor administered during and after induction treatment for de novo acute myelogenous leukemia in elderly patients. Groupe Ouest Est Leucemies Aigues Myeloblastiques (GOELAM). Blood 1998;91:2722–2730.

100. Advani R, Chao NJ, Horning SJ, et al. Granulocyte-macrophage colony-stimulating factor (GM-CSF) as an adjunct to autologous hemopoietic stem cell transplantation for lymphoma. Ann Intern Med 1992;116:183–189.

101. De Witte T, Gratwohl A, Van Der Lely N, et al. Recombinant human granulocyte-macrophage colony-stimulating factor accelerates neutrophil and monocyte recovery after allogeneic T-cell-depleted bone marrow transplantation. Blood 1992;79:1359–1365.

102. Gorin NC, Coiffier B, Hayat M, et al. Recombinant human granulocyte-macrophage colony-stimulating factor after high-dose chemotherapy and autologous bone marrow transplantation with unpurged and purged marrow in non-Hodgkin's lymphoma: a double-blind placebo-controlled trial. Blood 1992;80:1149–1157.

103. Gulati SC, Bennett CL. Granulocyte-macrophage colony-stimulating factor (GM-CSF) as adjunct therapy in relapsed Hodgkin disease. Ann Intern Med 1992;116:177–182.

104. Hiraoka A, Masaoka T, Mizoguchi H, et al. Recombinant human non-glycosylated granulocyte-macrophage colony-stimulating factor in allogeneic bone marrow transplantation: double-blind placebo-controlled phase III clinical trial. Jpn J Clin Oncol 1994;24:205–211.

105. Khwaja A, Linch DC, Goldstone AH, et al. Recombinant human granulocyte-macrophage colony-stimulating factor after autologous bone marrow transplantation for malignant lymphoma: a British National Lymphoma Investigation double-blind, placebo-controlled trial. Br J Haematol 1992;82:317–323.

106. Link H, Boogaerts MA, Carella AM, et al. A controlled trial of recombinant human granulocyte-macrophage colony-stimulating factor after total body irradiation, high-dose chemotherapy, and autologous bone marrow transplantation for acute lymphoblastic leukemia or malignant lymphoma. Blood 1992;80:2188–2195.

107. Nemunaitis J, Rabinowe SN, Singer JW, et al. Recombinant granulocyte-macrophage colony-stimulating factor after autologous bone marrow transplantation for lymphoid cancer. N Engl J Med 1991;324:1773–1778.

108. Nemunaitis J, Rosenfeld CS, Ash R, et al. Phase III randomized, double-blind placebo-controlled trial of rhGM-CSF following allogeneic bone marrow transplantation. Bone Marrow Transplant 1995;15:949–954.

109. Powles R, Smith C, Milan S, et al. Human recombinant GM-CSF in allogeneic bone-marrow transplantation for leukaemia: double-blind, placebo-controlled trial. Lancet 1990;336:1417–1420.

110. Boiron JM, Marit G, Faberes C, et al. Collection of peripheral blood stem cells in multiple myeloma following single high-dose cyclophosphamide with and without recombinant human granulocyte-macrophage colony-stimulating factor (rhGM-CSF). Bone Marrow Transplant 1993;12:49–55.

111. Elias AD, Ayash L, Anderson KC, et al. Mobilization of peripheral blood progenitor cells by chemotherapy and granulocyte-macrophage colony-stimulating factor for hematologic support after high-dose intensification for breast cancer. Blood 1992;79:3036–3044.

112. Huan SD, Hester J, Spitzer G, et al. Influence of mobilized peripheral blood cells on the hematopoietic recovery by autologous marrow and recombinant human granulocyte-macrophage colony-stimulating factor after high-dose cyclophosphamide, etoposide, and cisplatin. Blood 1992;79:3388–3393.

113. Legros M, Fleury J, Bay JO, et al. rhGM-CSF vs placebo following rhGM-CSF-mobilized PBPC transplantation: a phase III double-blind randomized trial. Bone Marrow Transplant 1997;19:209–213.

114. Kritz A, Crown JP, Motzer RJ, et al. Beneficial impact of peripheral blood progenitor cells in patients with metastatic breast cancer treated with high-dose chemotherapy plus granulocyte-macrophage colony-stimulating factor. A randomized trial. Cancer 1993;71:2515–2521.

115. Ballestrero A, Ferrando F, Garuti A, et al. Comparative effects of three cytokine regimens after high-dose cyclophosphamide: granulocyte colony-stimulating factor, granulocyte-macrophage colony-stimulating factor (GM-CSF), and sequential interleukin-3 and GM-CSF. J Clin Oncol 1999;17:1296.

116. Dorr RT. Clinical properties of yeast-derived versus Escherichia coli-derived granulocyte-macrophage colony-stimulating factor. Clin Ther 1993;15:19–29; discussion 18.

117. Lieschke GJ, Cebon J, Morstyn G. Characterization of the clinical effects after the first dose of bacterially synthesized recombinant human granulocyte-macrophage colony-stimulating factor. Blood 1989;74:2634–2643.

118. Bunn PA Jr, Crowley J, Kelly K, et al. Chemoradiotherapy with or without granulocyte-macrophage colony-stimulating factor in the treatment of limited-stage small-cell lung cancer: a prospective phase III randomized study of the Southwest Oncology Group. J Clin Oncol 1995;13:1632–1641.

119. Shaffer DW, Smith LS, Burris HA, et al. A randomized phase I trial of chronic oral etoposide with or without granulocyte-macrophage colony-stimulating factor in patients with advanced malignancies. Cancer Res 1993;53:5929–5933.

120. Groopman JE, Itri LM. Chemotherapy-induced anemia in adults: incidence and treatment. J Natl Cancer Inst 1999;91:1616–1634.

121. Lyman GH, Berndt ER, Kallich JD, et al. The economic burden of anemia in cancer patients receiving chemotherapy. Value Health 2005;8:149–156.

122. Case DC Jr, Bukowski RM, Carey RW, et al. Recombinant human erythropoietin therapy for anemic cancer patients on combination chemotherapy. J Natl Cancer Inst 1993;85:801–806.

123. Henry DH, Abels RI. Recombinant human erythropoietin in the treatment of cancer and chemotherapy-induced anemia: results of double-blind and open-label follow-up studies. Semin Oncol 1994;21:21–28.

124. Littlewood TJ, Bajetta E, Nortier JW, et al. Effects of epoetin alfa on hematologic parameters and quality of life in cancer patients receiving nonplatinum chemotherapy: results of a randomized, double-blind, placebo-controlled trial. J Clin Oncol 2001;19:2865–2874.

125. Razzouk BI, Hord JD, Hockenberry M, et al. Double-blind, placebo-controlled study of quality of life, hematologic end points, and safety of weekly epoetin alfa in children with cancer receiving myelosuppressive chemotherapy. J Clin Oncol 2006;24:3583–3589.

126. Wilkinson PM, Antonopoulos M, Lahousen M, et al. Epoetin alfa in platinum-treated ovarian cancer patients: results of a multinational, multicentre, randomised trial. Br J Cancer 2006;94:947–954.

127. Hedenus M, Adriansson M, San Miguel J, et al. Efficacy and safety of darbepoetin alfa in anaemic patients with lymphoproliferative malignancies: a randomized, double-blind, placebo-controlled study. Br J Haematol 2003;122:394–403.

128. Vansteenkiste J, Pirker R, Massuti B, et al. Double-blind, placebo-controlled, randomized phase III trial of darbepoetin alfa in lung cancer patients receiving chemotherapy. J Natl Cancer Inst 2002;94:1211–1220.

129. Lyman GH, Glaspy J. Are there clinical benefits with early erythropoietic intervention for chemotherapy-induced anemia? A systematic review. Cancer 2006;106:223–233.

130. Cheung WK, Goon BL, Guilfoyle MC, et al. Pharmacokinetics and pharmacodynamics of recombinant human erythropoietin after single and multiple subcutaneous doses to healthy subjects. Clin Pharmacol Ther 1998;64:412–423.

131. Gabrilove JL, Cleeland CS, Livingston RB, et al. Clinical evaluation of once-weekly dosing of epoetin alfa in chemotherapy patients: improvements in hemoglobin and quality of life are similar to three-times-weekly dosing. J Clin Oncol 2001;19:2875–2882.

132. Henke M, Laszig R, Rube C, et al. Erythropoietin to treat head and neck cancer patients with anaemia undergoing radiotherapy: randomised, double-blind, placebo-controlled trial. Lancet 2003;362:1255–1260.

133. Leyland-Jones B. Breast cancer trial with erythropoietin terminated unexpectedly. Lancet Oncol 2003;4:459–460.

134. Bohlius J, Langensiepen S, Schwarzer G, et al. Recombinant human erythropoietin and overall survival in cancer patients: results of a comprehensive meta-analysis. J Natl Cancer Inst 2005;97:489–498.

135. Bohlius J, Wilson J, Seidenfeld J, et al. Recombinant human erythropoietins and cancer patients: updated meta-analysis of 57 studies including 9353 patients. J Natl Cancer Inst 2006;98:708–714.

136. Bohlius J, Schmidlin K, Brillant C, et al. Recombinant human erythropoiesis-stimulating agents and mortality in patients with cancer: a meta-analysis of randomised trials. Lancet 2009;373:1532–1542.

137. Ludwig H, Crawford J, Osterborg A, et al. Pooled analysis of individual patient-level data from all randomized, double-blind, placebo-controlled

trials of darbepoetin alfa in the treatment of patients with chemotherapy-induced anemia. J Clin Oncol 2009;27:2838–2847.

138. Rizzo JD, Somerfield MR, Hagerty KL, et al. Use of epoetin and darbepoetin in patients with cancer: 2007 American Society of Hematology/American Society of Clinical Oncology clinical practice guideline update. Blood 2008;111:25–41.

139. Rodgers GM III, Becker PS, Bennett CL, et al. Cancer- and chemotherapy-induced anemia. J Natl Compr Canc Netw 2008;6:536–564.

140. Tepler I, Elias L, Smith JW II, et al. A randomized placebo-controlled trial of recombinant human interleukin-11 in cancer patients with severe thrombocytopenia due to chemotherapy. Blood 1996;87:3607–3614.

141. Vredenburgh JJ, Hussein A, Fisher D, et al. A randomized trial of recombinant human interleukin-11 following autologous bone marrow transplantation with peripheral blood progenitor cell support in patients with breast cancer. Biol Blood Marrow Transplant 1998;4:134–141.

142. Basser RL, Rasko JE, Clarke K, et al. Thrombopoietic effects of pegylated recombinant human megakaryocyte growth and development factor (PEG-rHuMGDF) in patients with advanced cancer. Lancet 1996;348:1279–1281.

143. Basser RL, Rasko JE, Clarke K, et al. Randomized, blinded, placebo-controlled phase I trial of pegylated recombinant human megakaryocyte growth and development factor with filgrastim after dose-intensive chemotherapy in patients with advanced cancer. Blood 1997;89:3118–3128.

144. Fanucchi M, Glaspy J, Crawford J, et al. Effects of polyethylene glycol-conjugated recombinant human megakaryocyte growth and development factor on platelet counts after chemotherapy for lung cancer. N Engl J Med 1997;336:404–409.

145. Vadhan-Raj S, Murray LJ, Bueso-Ramos C, et al. Stimulation of megakaryocyte and platelet production by a single dose of recombinant human thrombopoietin in patients with cancer. Ann Intern Med 1997;126:673–681.

146. Kuter DJ, Bussel JB, Lyons RM, et al. Efficacy of romiplostim in patients with chronic immune thrombocytopenic purpura: a double-blind randomised controlled trial. Lancet 2008;371:395–403.

147. George JN, Mathias SD, Go RS, et al. Improved quality of life for romiplostim-treated patients with chronic immune thrombocytopenic purpura: results from two randomized, placebo-controlled trials. Br J Haematol 2009;144:409–415.

148. Bussel JB, Cheng G, Saleh MN, et al. Eltrombopag for the treatment of chronic idiopathic thrombocytopenic purpura. N Engl J Med 2007;357:2237–2247.

149. Bussel JB, Provan D, Shamsi T, et al. Effect of eltrombopag on platelet counts and bleeding during treatment of chronic idiopathic thrombocytopenic purpura: a randomised, double-blind, placebo-controlled trial. Lancet 2009;373:641–648.

150. Bussel J. Update on Eltrombopag for ITP. Oncology 2009;23:1177–1178.

151. McHutchison JG, Dusheiko G, Shiffman ML, et al. Eltrombopag for thrombocytopenia in patients with cirrhosis associated with hepatitis C. N Engl J Med 2007;357:2227–2236.

152. Hovgaard D, Mortensen BT, Schifter S, et al. Comparative pharmacokinetics of single-dose administration of mammalian and bacterially-derived recombinant human granulocyte-macrophage colony-stimulating factor. Eur J Haematol 1993;50:32–36.

153. Petros WP, Rabinowitz J, Stuart AR, et al. Disposition of recombinant human granulocyte-macrophage colony-stimulating factor in patients receiving high-dose chemotherapy and autologous bone marrow support. Blood 1992;80:1135–1140.

154. Petros WP, Rabinowitz J, Stuart A, et al. Clinical pharmacology of filgrastim following high-dose chemotherapy and autologous bone marrow transplantation. Clin Cancer Res 1997;3:705–711.

Antinausea Medications

Ian N. Olver

Nausea and vomiting can be symptoms associated with cancer, but it was the introduction of cytotoxic chemotherapy of high emetic potential to treat cancer that stimulated research on the mechanisms of emesis. This has resulted in the introduction of two new classes of antiemetics, namely, the 5 hydroxytryptamine 3 receptor antagonists (5HT3 RA) and the neurokinin 1 receptor antagonists (NK1 RA), which have made a major impact on the control of emesis (Table 39-1).

Three distinct types of emesis are associated with chemotherapy. The most common is postchemotherapy emesis occurring in the 24 hours after chemotherapy.[1] Delayed emesis is thought to commence around 18 hours after treatment and can last for at least 5 days.[2] For patients who experience emesis with chemotherapy, anticipatory emesis can occur with subsequent cycles as a conditioned response.[3]

The most important predictor of acute postchemotherapy emesis is the type, dose, and schedule of the chemotherapy (Table 39-2). Drugs of high emetic potential have a 90% or greater chance of causing emesis if no antiemetic prophylaxis is given.[4] The paradigm example is cisplatin, which when given over an hour at greater than 60 mg/m^2 will cause almost all patients to vomit, and is associated with both acute and delayed emesis. Trials to test new antiemetic

drugs frequently focus on cisplatin-induced emesis. Drugs such as anthracyclines or cyclophosphamide have moderate emetic potential (between 30% and 90% chance of emesis). The combination of these drugs (AC) is of high emetic potential, however.

A number of patient characteristics predict emesis after chemotherapy.[5] Younger patients are more prone to vomiting than older, as are women compared to men. Patients who have previous vomiting with chemotherapy, or motion sickness, or vomiting with pregnancy are more likely to vomit postchemotherapy. Those patients with a prolonged history of heavy alcohol consumption vomit less after chemotherapy.

Nausea and vomiting are among the most distressing side effects of chemotherapy.[6,7] These side effects are also associated with fatigue, anorexia, and insomnia.[8] Doctors and nurses tend to underestimate nausea and vomiting, particularly in the delayed phase, which can lead to undertreatment.[9]

5HT3 Receptor Antagonists

The initial revolution in the control of chemotherapy-induced emesis came with the introduction of a new class of antiemetics, the 5HT3 RAs. The antiemetics previously available, such as the substituted benzamides, the phenothiazines, and butyrophenones, had very limited efficacy against chemotherapy-induced emesis and had unpleasant side effects, including somnolence, depression, dysphoria, and tardive dyskinesia.

Mechanistic studies revealed that chemotherapy causes the release of 5-hydroxtryptamine from the enterochromaffin cells in the small intestine. This 5HT stimulates the vagal afferents that connect to the dorsal brainstem, the nucleus tractus solitarius, and the area postrema (Fig. 39-1). Efferent fibers then go to an area known as the central pattern generator more ventrally in the brain stem, and the vomiting reflex is initiated.[10,11] The area postrema also has direct contact with the blood and cerebrospinal fluid, sitting as it does in the floor of the 4th ventricle, and can also be stimulated via that route.

The first of the 5HT3 RAs, ondansetron, when given in combination with dexamethasone before chemotherapy of high emetic potential achieved control of acute postchemotherapy emesis in over 80% of patients with a rate of around 65% if used as a single agent (Fig. 39-2).[12] The side-effect profile was favorable, with the main toxicities being mild headache, constipation, and transient elevation in liver transaminases. Randomized studies and meta-analyses did not demonstrate differences in the therapeutic effect of ondansetron, granisetron, tropisetron, or dolasetron, although in

TABLE **39.1**	*Classes of antiemetics*
Drug class	**Examples of drugs**
Serotonin RA	Ondansetron, Granisetron, Tropisetron, Dolasetron, Palonosetron
Neurokinin RA	Aprepitant, Fosaprepitant, Casopitant
Dopamine RA	Metoclopramide, Metopimazine, Prochlorperazine, Alizapride, Droperidol, Haloperidol
Glucocorticoids	Dexamethasone, Methylprednisolone
Cannabinoids	Nabilone, Dronabinol
Benzodiazepine	Lorazepam, Olanzepine[a]
Anticholinergics	Scopolamine
Antihistamines	Diphenhydramine
Miscellaneous	Gabapentin, Ginger

[a] Olanzepine is a thienobenzodiazepine acting on multiple receptors.
RA, receptor antagonist.

TABLE

39.2 *Classification of anticancer drugs based on emetogenic potential*

Level 1 (minimal risk, <10%)	Level 2 (low risk, 10%–30%)	Level 3 (moderate risk, 31%–90%)	Level 4 (high risk, >90%)
Bevacizumab	Bortezomib	Carboplatin	Carmustine
Bleomycin	Cetuximab	Cyclophosphamide	Cisplatin
Busulfan	Clofarabine	High-dose Cytarabine (>1 g/m^2)	High-dose Cyclophosphamide (>1.5 g/m^2)
Cladribine	Cytarabine (<100 mg/m^2)	Daunorubicin	Dacarbazine
Fludarabine	Dasatanib	Doxorubicin	Mechlorethamine
Vinblastine	Docetaxel	Epirubicin	Streptozotocin
Vincristine	Etoposide	Idarubicin	
Vinorelbine	Fluorouracil	Ifosfamide	
	Gemcitabine	Imatinib	
	Ibritumomab tiuxetan	Irinotecan	
	Ixabepilone	Oxaliplatin	
	Lapatanib		
	Methotrexate		
	Mitomycin		
	Mitoxantrone		
	Nilotinib		
	Paclitaxel		
	Pemetrexed		
	Procarbazine		
	Sorafenib		
	Sunitinib		
	Temsirolimus		
	Topotecan		
	Tositumumab		
	Trastuzumab		

Jordan's meta-analysis, there were some differences in subset analyses of the granisetron and tropisetron comparison.[13,14]

The 5HT3 RAs are metabolized by the liver through hydroxylation followed by glucuronide or sulfate conjugation. The metabolites do not seem to contribute to antiemetic activity. Currently, the 5HT3 RAs are given by single daily dosing rather than the initial multiple day schedules in the original ondansetron studies.[15] Oral formulations have also been shown to be as effective as the intravenous dosing (Table 39-3).[16]

The clinical trials of the initial 5HT3 RAs such as ondansetron showed that they demonstrated low efficacy for cisplatin-induced delayed emesis.[17] These first-generation 5HT3 RAs only had modest activity for the delayed emesis associated with chemotherapy of moderate emetic potential.[18]

Palonosetron

The initial second-generation 5HT3 RA, palonosetron, has different properties and efficacies than the first-generation 5HT3 RAs (Fig. 39-2). Palonosetron has a mean elimination half-life of approximately 40 hours as compared to 4 to 9 hours with the first-generation 5HT3 RAs, but the same favorable safety profile.[19]

It also exhibits a 30-fold higher binding affinity for the receptor than the first-generation drugs. The binding differs in that whereas ondansetron and granisetron show simple bimolecular binding, palonosetron demonstrates allosteric binding with positive cooperativity to inhibit receptor function over a longer time and triggers either inactivation or internalization of the 5HT3 receptor.[20]

In the early phase studies of palonosetron, the side effects of headache, constipation, and dizziness were similar to other 5HT3 RAs and no cardiac safety issues were noted. Of the first three large phase III trials, two were for chemotherapy of moderate emetic potential, comparing single intravenous doses of palonosetron with ondansetron or dolasetron.[21,22] Gralla et al.[21] found that single-dose palonosetron (0.25 and 0.75 mg) was not inferior to ondansetron (32 mg) for the response of no vomiting, no rescue for acute emesis, and was considered superior in the control of delayed emesis. Also there was a suggestion that nausea was better controlled than with the first-generation 5HT3 RAs.[21] Similarly, Eisenberg et al.[22] demonstrated a similar outcome in the comparison of palonosetron with 100 mg of dolasetron. The third trial compared palonosetron with ondansetron in the prophylaxis of chemotherapy of high

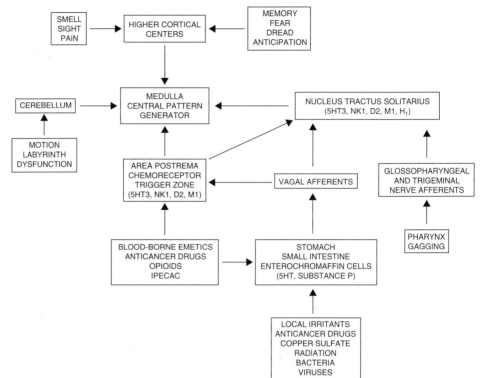

FIGURE **39-1** The emetic response is elicited by signals emanating from a variety of sources including motion, smells, blood-borne toxins, and other signals. These pathways involve a variety of neurotransmitters, including dopamine, acetylcholine, histamine, serotonin (5-hydroxytryptamine), and substance P, among others. Emetic responses can be blocked by agents that interfere with these pathways. Abbreviations: serotonin (5HT); serotonin receptor 3 (5HT3), neurokinin 1 receptor (NK1), dopamine 2 receptor (D2), acetylcholine receptor (M1), histamine 1 receptor (H1).

emetic potential and showed noninferiority for acute, delayed, and overall emesis.[23]

The next step in the assessment of palonosetron was to evaluate it in combination with both dexamethasone and as part of triple prophylactic antiemetic therapy with dexamethasone and an NK1 RA to ascertain whether palonosetron should replace the older

5HT3 RAs in antiemetic regimens with chemotherapy of high or moderate emetic potential.

A pooled analysis of the two studies with chemotherapy of moderate emetic potential had suggested that although the occurrence of acute chemotherapy-induced nausea and vomiting is the strongest predictor of delayed emesis, the efficacy of palonosetron in the

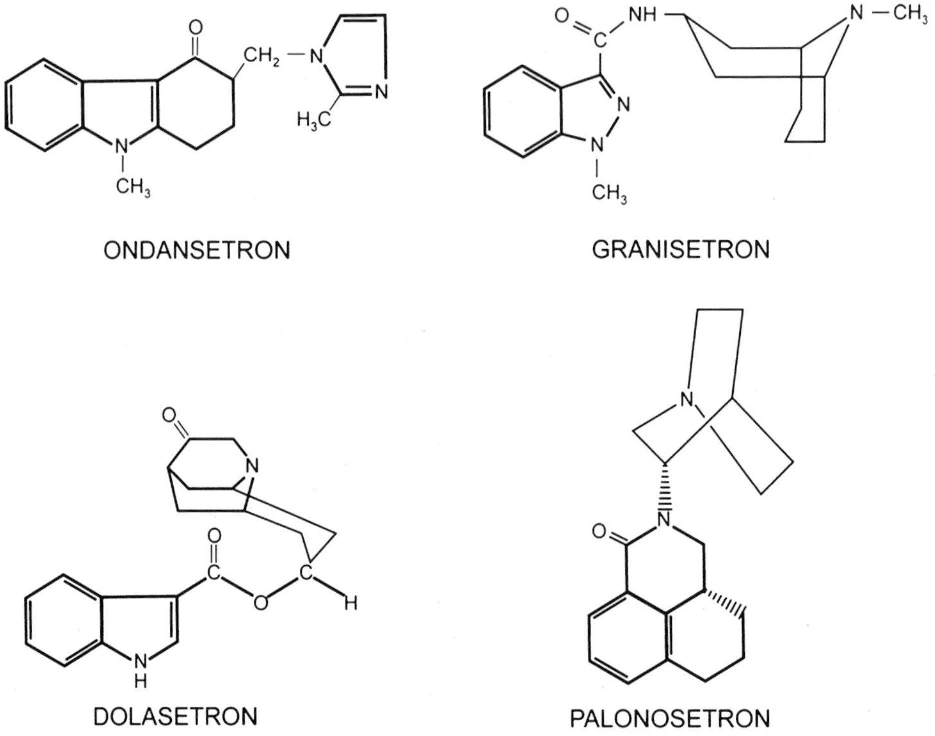

ONDANSETRON

GRANISETRON

FIGURE **39-2** Structure of commonly used 5HT3 RAs.

DOLASETRON

PALONOSETRON

TABLE 39.3 Dosages and plasma terminal half-lives of selected antiemetics

Drug	Dosing	Half-life[a] (hours)
Ondansetron	Oral 24 mg IV 8–32 mg	3–4
Granisetron	Oral 2 mg IV 10 µg/kg	7
Tropisetron	Oral 5 mg IV 5 mg	8
Dolasetron	Oral 100 mg IV 100 mg	7–8
Palonosetron	IV 0.25 mg	40
Aprepitant	Oral 125 mg day 1 80 mg day 2 and 3	9
Fosaprepitant	IV 115 mg	9–13
Casopitant	Single oral 150 mg day 1 IV day 1 90 mg then 50 mg oral days 2 and 3	9–15

[a] Terminal half-life rounded to nearest hour.
IV, intravenous.

delayed phase was not just a carryover effect but directly due to the activity of palonosetron.[24]

Saito et al.[25] compared palonosetron and dexamethasone with granisetron and dexamethasone in 1,114 patients receiving chemotherapy of high emetic potential (including the AC combination). The complete response rate for acute emesis was 75.3% in the palonosetron arm versus 73.3% in the granisetron arm of the study.

Small studies have also shown that palonosetron can be safely administered over multiple days. Einhorn et al.[26] reported giving palonosetron on days 1, 3, and 5 with dexamethasone at different doses and schedules on days 1, 2, 6, 7, and 8 of a 5-day cisplatin regimen for testicular cancer, while Musso et al.[27] used daily palonosetron and dexamethasone through multiple-day chemotherapy regimens in patients with hematological malignancies. In both cases, the regimens were very effective in controlling emesis. Several randomized studies that reported on multiple cycles of chemotherapy with palonosetron without glucocorticoids were analyzed by Cartmell et al.,[28] who found that its efficacy for both acute and delayed postchemotherapy emesis was maintained.

Musso et al.[29] tested palonosetron in combination with dexamethasone in a setting where emesis is particularly difficult to control, that is, patients receiving high-dose chemotherapy before stem cell transplantation. They also gave a further dose for breakthrough emesis at 72 hours. One half of the patients with breakthrough emesis were successfully rescued.

The NK1 Receptor Antagonists

The second major new class of drugs introduced for chemotherapy-induced emesis is the NK1 RAs, which were shown to have efficacy in the delayed phase of emesis when added to a 5HT3 RA and dexamethasone on day 1 and then continued in combination with glucocorticoids. Substance P is a neurotransmitter with a strong affinity for the NK1 receptor. On positron emission tomography scanning, substance P is highly concentrated in areas of the central nervous system such as nucleus tractus solitarius and the area postrema, areas of the brain associated with emesis (Fig. 39-1).[30] The NK1 RAs prevent the binding of substance P to these receptors and, in the ferret model, have activity against both acute and delayed postchemotherapy emesis.[31]

Aprepitant is the first of the NK1 RAs to be marketed and is an oral formulation (Fig. 39-3). It exhibits nonlinear pharmacokinetics and has a bioavailability of 60% to 65%, which is unaffected by food because of its nanoparticle formulation.[32,33] The drug reaches its peak plasma concentration in 4 hours and is 95% protein bound. It is metabolized primarily by the cytochrome P450 3A4 pathway with minor metabolism by cytochrome P450 1A2 and cytochrome P450 2C9.[34] The metabolites are not renally excreted, and it has a terminal half-life of 13 hours. No dosage adjustments are required for moderate hepatic insufficiency, renal disease, age, sex, or race.

Over short-term use, there are many potential drug interactions with aprepitant because it is both a substrate and inhibitor of CYP 3A4. Dexamethasone, as a moderate inhibitor of CYP 3A4, does not change the pharmacokinetics of aprepitant; however, when aprepitant is added to oral dexamethasone, it increases the area under the curve (AUC) of dexamethasone two-fold. Therefore, the dose of dexamethasone should be halved when given with aprepitant.[35] The increase seen in ondansetron AUC when aprepitant is given is not clinically significant and no dose changes are recommended, as is the case with granisetron.[36] No major interactions have been reported with concomitant use of aprepitant with cytotoxic drugs.[37,38] The potential for interactions with intravenous drugs is low, as reflected in studies with docetaxel and vinorelbine, although further data are needed after a report of neurotoxicity when used with ifosfamide.[39] The AUC of ethinyl estradiol was decreased by 40% after 2 weeks dosing with aprepitant, a finding that has led the manufacturers to recommend using alternate contraception, even when using aprepitant in the short-term for antiemetic prophylaxis. Decreases of 15% in the international normalized ratio were reported when aprepitant was given with warfarin and a similar decrease would occur with phenytoin.[40]

The two pivotal trials that led to FDA approval of aprepitant used the dosing schedule of 125 mg on day 1 and then 80 mg on days 2 and 3.[41,42] Ondansetron was given at a dose of 32 mg on day 1 and the dexamethasone dose was 20 mg orally on day 1, then 8 mg twice daily on days 2 to 4 in the control arm, and 8 mg each day with the aprepitant in the experimental arm, with an additional dose on day 4. The dose reduction on the experimental arm was due to the increase in the AUC for dexamethasone when given with aprepitant. Blinding was maintained with placebo aprepitant capsules and dexamethasone tablets.

The combined studies treated 1,099 patients with overall rates of no emesis and no rescue comparing the treatment to the control arm being 52.7% versus 43.3% on one study and 72.7% versus 52.3% on the other, both being highly significant ($P < 0.001$). However, the most impressive result was in the control of the delayed phase of the postchemotherapy emesis, with complete response rates of 67.7% versus 45.8% and 74.4% versus 55.8%, respectively. Fewer patients experienced nausea in the overall and delayed phases, and the efficacy of the triple therapy was maintained over six cycles, a result confirmed in a study to specifically examine control over multiple cycles of chemotherapy.[43] Aprepitant was well tolerated with the main side effects being asthenia, anorexia, and hiccoughs. The outcome also translated into improved quality of life.

A further trial for chemotherapy of high emetic potential had a more intense control arm utilizing 5 days of ondansetron and dexamethasone. Again the aprepitant arm was superior in all phases of emesis with the overall complete response rate if 72% versus 61% ($P = 0.003$).[44]

Warr et al.[45] conducted a trial on 866 women with breast cancer, which included chemotherapy of moderate emetic potential and non-cisplatin combinations such as anthracyclines and cyclophosphamide. They tested triple therapy on day 1 with aprepitant continued on days 2 and 3 against ondansetron and dexamethasone on day 1 with ondansetron continued on days 2 and 3. The rate of no vomiting or rescue over 5 days was better for the aprepitant arm than the control, 51% versus 42%.

In a subsequent study, Rapoport et al.[46] studied a broader range of men and women receiving chemotherapy of moderate emetic potential where 52% were receiving regimens other than AC and compared triple therapy with just ondansetron and dexamethasone. The aprepitant arm was superior irrespective of the regimen, but for the non-AC regimens, no vomiting overall was recorded in 83.2% versus 71.3% of patients and absence of delayed emesis was seen in 84.5% versus 73.9%.

Triple therapy consisting of a 5HT3 RA, dexamethasone, and aprepitant, with a 3-day dosing regimen for aprepitant, became the standard for prophylaxis of emesis for chemotherapy of high or moderate emetic potential. In a small study, palonosetron was the 5HT3 RA in combination with aprepitant and dexamethasone in patients receiving chemotherapy of moderate emetic potential with an 83% response rate.[47]

Fosaprepitant

Fosaprepitant dimeglumine, a water-soluble prodrug of aprepitant, whose antiemetic properties are attributable to aprepitant, is rapidly converted to aprepitant with a plasma half-life of 2.3 minutes and complete conversion within 30 minutes. A dose of 115 mg IV is bioequivalent to aprepitant 125 mg orally.[48]

In the initial clinical development of aprepitant, two of the phase II trials were done with the prodrug L-758298, now called fosaprepitant. In the first, fosaprepitant (60 or 100 mg) was compared to ondansetron 32 mg for patients receiving at least 50 mg/m² cisplatin. There was no difference in the control of acute emesis but in the delayed phase, 70% on fosaprepitant had no emesis compared to 30% receiving ondansetron.[49] The second study investigated combinations of fosaprepitant with dexamethasone on day 1 with or without 4 extra days of aprepitant compared to day 1 of ondansetron and dexamethasone and placebo for 4 days. The ondansetron with dexamethasone best controlled the acute emesis, but fosaprepitant with aprepitant significantly better controlled the delayed emesis (complete response 59% versus 39%; $P < 0.05$).[50]

The efficacy and safety data are just those of aprepitant with the addition of venous irritation at concentrations of 25 mg/mL, or at doses of 50 or 100 mg infused over 30 seconds. The irritation becomes tolerable at concentrations around 1 mg/mL infused over 15 to 30 minutes.[51] Fosaprepitant provides a safe and effective intravenous alternative to oral dosing of aprepitant that can be used on day 1 with other intravenous drugs or when patients are unable to tolerate oral medication.

Casopitant

Several other NK1 RAs are in development, including netupitant, vestipitant, and rolapitant, but casopitant is furthest along in development. Casopitant is a substituted piperidine derivative (Fig. 39-3). It competitively binds to the NK1 receptor. In its oral

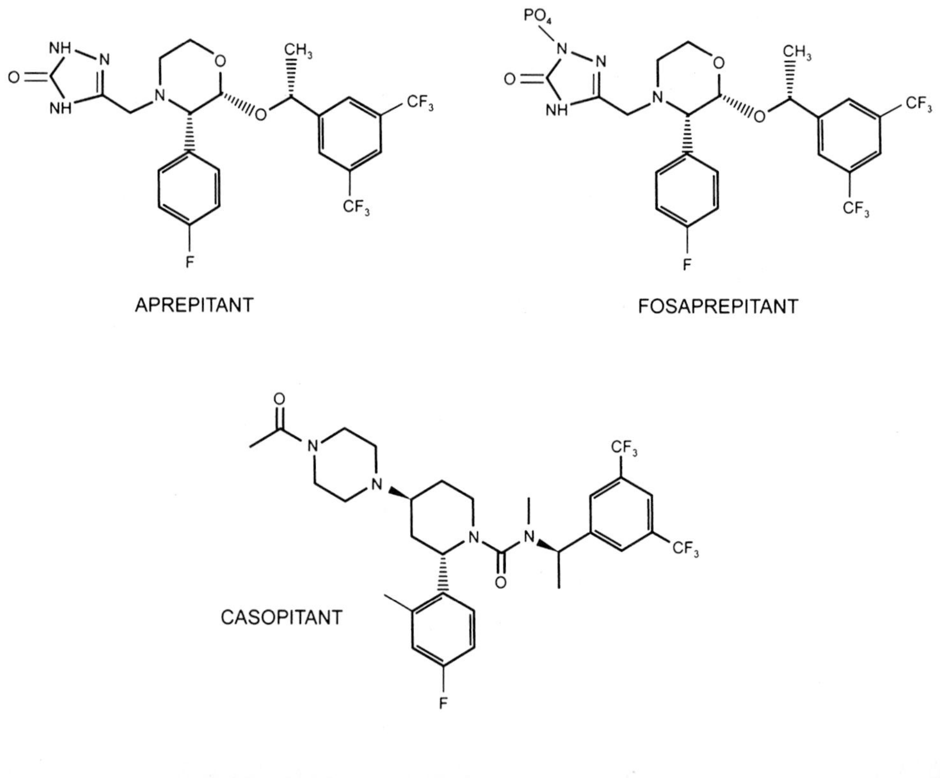

APREPITANT

FOSAPREPITANT

CASOPITANT

Figure **39-3** Structure of NK1 RAs.

formulation, it is rapidly absorbed, with an absorption half-time of less than 17 minutes in all but 30% of the population.[52] It has a plasma half-life of 9 to 15 hours and is 99% protein bound. Body weight influences its volume of distribution. It is metabolized mainly by CYP3A4 and eliminated fecally.

The early phase studies established a similar toxicity profile and drug interactions for casopitant as recorded for aprepitant, and also established the safety of dosing over 3 days. There were two interesting innovations in phase II studies: the exploration of a single higher dose of casopitant on day 1 only and the assessment of rates of nonsignificant nausea (NSN). A double-blinded phase II trial with chemotherapy of moderate emetic potential compared a dexamethasone (8 mg IV day 1) and ondansetron (8 mg twice daily days 1 to 3) control with three arms that added a 3-day regimen of casopitant at three different doses of 50, 100, and 150 mg daily. In addition, two arms explored single day 1 dosing of casopitant (150 mg), one arm also exploring single-day dosing of ondansetron at 16 mg/d.[53] Casopitant significantly increased the control of vomiting in the overall and delayed phases (84.2% for 150 mg versus 69.4% control), but the rates of nausea control did not differ. Day 1 only dosing of casopitant showed rates of control of vomiting similar to the 3-day regimen (79.2%). Similarly, a subset analysis of a phase II study with chemotherapy of high emetic potential that compared a single dose of 150 mg casopitant on day 1 with ondansetron and dexamethasone to ondansetron and dexamethasone with 3 days of aprepitant recorded complete response (CR) rates for 120 hours of 75% and 72%, respectively.[54]

A phase 3 study predominantly in women receiving AC randomly allocated patients to ondansetron and dexamethasone alone, or with either a single oral dose of casopitant on day 1 only, or with 2 further days of oral dosing of 50 mg, or 90 mg IV on day 1 and 50 mg on days 2 and 3.[55] All of the casopitant arms achieved high CR rates over 120 hours (73%, 73%, and 74% versus 59% control; $P < 0.0001$).

With chemotherapy of high emetic potential, the arms were similar; the experimental arms had a single oral dose of casopitant and a 3 day IV, then oral regimen of casopitant added to ondansetron and dexamethasone in an 810-patient study.[56] Again the CR rates in the control group over the first cycle at 66% were significantly worse than the single dose of casopitant at 86% ($P < 0.0001$) and the 3-day intravenous/oral casopitant at 80% ($P = 0.004$). Emesis control was sustained over multiple cycles, and the casopitant was well tolerated.

Glucocorticoids

Dexamethasone and methylprednisolone were among the earliest agents to be used for chemotherapy-induced emesis. Dexamethasone was even shown to be effective in up to 8 of 11 patients receiving cisplatin who had no prior antiemetics and received only multiple doses as a single agent.[57] However, the mechanism of action of glucocorticoids remains unknown. Before the introduction of NK1 RAs, dexamethasone was arguably the best available agent for delayed emesis and is still recommended as a single agent with chemotherapy of low emetic potential.[12,17]

Dexamethasone is mainly prescribed in combinations with 5HT3 RAs and as part of triple therapy with NK1 RAs.[12,15,25,40,41] Following trials of dose ranges, the recommended doses for acute emesis with chemotherapy of moderate and high emetic potential are 8 and 20 mg, respectively, but the optimal dose for delayed emesis is unknown.[58]

Olanzapine

Olanzapine is a thienobenzodiazepine that can act on multiple receptors including dopamine (D1, D2, D3, D4) and the serotonin receptors (5HT2a, 5HT2c, 5HT3, 5HT6) as well as adrenergic, muscarinic, and histamine receptors.[59] Common side effects are weight gain and sedation and impaired glucose tolerance. Its major use is as an oral antipsychotic agent but in early phase trials, it has been found to be active in the prevention of both acute and delayed emesis with chemotherapy of high emetic potential including cisplatin, and chemotherapy of moderate emetic potential including cyclophosphamide, doxorubicin, or irinotecan.

Olanzepine has been used in a phase II trial with granisetron and dexamethasone with high response rates. In a phase II trial of olanzepine in combination with palonosetron and dexamethasone, the complete response rate in eight patients receiving chemotherapy of high emetic potential was 100% with 75% complete response in the delayed phase and 75% complete response overall.[60]

Dopamine Receptor Antagonists

When nausea and vomiting associated with anticancer chemotherapy became a problem, the already existing antiemetic agents used for other types of emesis were tried. These included dopamine antagonists, phenothiazines such as prochlorperazine or metopimazine and substituted benzamides such as metoclopramide and alizapride, or the butyrophenones including droperidol and haloperidol. Domperidone is another dopamine antagonist that also is known to be useful for gastric stasis and was used in this setting. However, all of these drugs had limited efficacy, particularly when highly emetogenic chemotherapy like cisplatin was introduced, for which emesis is a dose-limiting side effect.

Dopamine receptors are known to be in the brain at sites such as the chemoreceptor trigger zone. However, they do not seem to have a major role in chemotherapy-induced emesis. Metoclopramide was known in animal studies to be effective against both centrally and peripherally acting emetic agents. There was some efficacy at low doses, but Gralla[61] showed that very high doses (3 mg/kg) of intravenous metoclopramide were more effective. At high doses, metoclopramide becomes a serotonin antagonist, so this observation is consistent with what is known about the major mechanism of chemotherapy-induced emesis.

Similar studies have been done with prochlorperazine.[62] However, blocking the dopamine receptor causes adverse effects such as extrapyramidal reactions and sedation; with high-dose prochlorperazine, postural hypotension was also an issue. These effects all limit the use of this class of agents clinically. They are now usually only used as rescue medications.

Cannabinoids

Based on anecdotal reports of the antinausea effect of smoking marijuana from patients receiving chemotherapy, oral cannabinoids have been investigated as antiemetic agents. Cannabinoid CB1 receptors are present in the brain stem in areas influencing vomiting, such as the area postrema, nucleus tractus solitarius, and dorsal motor nucleus. CB2 receptors are also found on brain stem neurons, which may mediate cannabinoid effects on nausea and vomiting.[63]

The use of tetrahydrocannabinol was limited by dosing issues associated with variable pharmacokinetics, and the small studies done were difficult to blind because of characteristic side effects. Two synthetic cannabinoids, nabilone and dronabinol, have shown some antiemetic activity when given with chemotherapy of low or moderate emetic potential, but no comparative studies have been done between cannabinoids and the 5HT3 RAs or NK1RAs. The side effects of dysphoric reactions and hypotension are also problematic, particularly with older patients. Given the very favorable therapeutic indices of the newer classes of antiemetics, the interest in cannabinoids as antiemetics has waned.

Adjuvant Antiemetics

Benzodiazepines

Benzodiazepines such as lorazepam have been added to antiemetic regimens to improve the control of emesis. It is both an anxiolytic and has been shown to add antiemetic efficacy when given with conventional antiemetics. One study by Malik et al.[64] showed improvement in antiemesis in both the acute and delayed phases of cisplatin-induced emesis when given in combination with metoclopramide, which may now only be relevant in breakthrough or refractory emesis. It causes sedation, which itself may improve the tolerance for chemotherapy, but it is also associated with retrograde amnesia, which has been shown to reduce anticipatory emesis in subsequent cycles.

Anticholinergics

Scopolamine is an anticholinergic drug that is more often delivered by transdermal patch for motion sickness. It is added to other drugs to control postoperative nausea and vomiting and although not effective as a single agent for the prophylaxis of cisplatin-induced emesis has been added to other antiemetic drugs regimens for chemotherapy-induced emesis. It has been reported as useful in children as part of regimens for refractory or breakthrough vomiting.[65]

Antihistamines

Antihistamines, such as diphenhydramine, have been used in antiemetic regimens for chemotherapy-induced emesis. When given with agents such as metoclopramide they not only acted as antiemetics, but they also had the potential to help relieve the extrapyramidal side effects of metoclopramide. They are now studied mainly as rescue regimens after the first-line therapy is ineffective, whereas in combination they can be part of an effective salvage regimen as reported by Bleicher et al.[66] who combined lorazepam, diphenhydramine, and haloperidol in a transdermal gel.

Nausea

Even with the introduction of the 5HT3 RAs and the NK1 RAs, nausea is not as well controlled as vomiting and is still reported as

a distressing side effect. Many nonpharmacological techniques have been tried for nausea, including acupressure and hypnosis.

Trials have been conducted with nausea as the primary endpoint for drugs including gabapentin and ginger.

Gabapentin

Gabapentin is a gamma aminobutyric acid inhibitor used for epilepsy. Its side effects include dizziness, drowsiness, and peripheral edema. In a small study, gabapentin has been reported to reduce delayed postchemotherapy nausea in patients being treated for breast cancer with a combination of doxorubicin and cyclophosphamide.[67]

Ginger

Ginger (*Zingiber officinale*) is a spice that has been used to treat nausea and vomiting over centuries, particularly pregnancy-associated emesis. In a phase II/III trial, Ryan et al.[68] randomly assigned 644 patients who experienced nausea after any chemotherapy cycle, and were scheduled to receive at least three more cycles, to receive a placebo or three different doses of ginger (0.5, 1.0, and 1.5 g) added to a 5HT3 RA. They took the ginger twice a day in the form of 250-mg capsules for 6 days, starting 3 days before chemotherapy. All doses of ginger significantly reduced nausea ($P = 0.003$), with the largest decreases seen with the two lower doses.

Future Directions for Guidelines for Antiemetics

Evidence-based guidelines for the use of antiemetics are very similar, differing mainly by the timing of their updates. Using the Multinational Association of Supportive Care in Cancer (MASCC) guidelines as an example, where the last consensus meeting was held in June, 2009, some clear principles have emerged for the use of antiemetic drugs.

For chemotherapy of high emetic potential, triple antiemetic prophylaxis with a 5HT3 RA, a NK1 RA, and dexamethasone is the treatment of choice. Studies now suggest that the second-generation 5HT3 RA, palonosetron, should become the recommended serotonin antagonist. The 5HT3 RA is only required on day 1. Intravenous and oral dosing give similar outcomes. Large trials have not investigated therapy for multiple-day chemotherapy, and present practice is to extrapolate from single day recommendations.

The AC regimen, predominantly given to women with breast cancer, has high emetic potential although its two component drugs as single agents are classified as moderately emetogenic. AC should be treated with triple antiemetic prophylaxis like the other regimens of high emetic potential. The NK1 RA of choice may change as more than one drug enters the market and single day 1 dosing may be all that is required.

For regimens of moderate emetic potential, a 5HT3 RA and dexamethasone at 8 mg are recommended but one study suggested the benefit of adding aprepitant. With chemotherapy of low emetic potential, given as a single dose intermittently, a single agent is all that is required. Dexamethasone is the drug most often suggested, but for those who cannot tolerate glucocorticoids, either a single serotonin antagonist or dopamine receptor antagonist will suffice. The emetic potential of oral agents given for prolonged courses, such a capecitabine or imatinib, is largely undefined; therefore, no definitive recommendations for antiemetic therapy can be made. For those drugs with minimal potential for causing emesis, no antiemetic prophylaxis is required.

For radiation-induced emesis, fewer studies exist on which to base recommendations. 5HT3 RAs have been effective for prophylaxis, but some patients still have emesis that is poorly controlled, and it may be appropriate to add dexamethasone. The emetic potential of radiation depends on multiple factors such as the area being irradiated, the size of the field, the dose per fraction, and total dose. Total body radiation and radiation with concomitant chemotherapy are of high emetic potential, while abdominal fields are moderately emetogenic. Certainly, newer agents need to be tested with radiation and the duration of the prophylaxis has to match the duration of the therapy.

An even greater paucity of data is available in children. Certainly, a 5HT3 RA and dexamethasone should be used as prophylaxis before chemotherapy of high or moderate emetic potential. However, some reports of ECG abnormalities in children taking 5HT3 RAs have raised concern. The question of using palonosetron requires further research. The main trial of an NK1 RA was performed in adolescents; thus, aprepitant becomes an option for this group.[69]

Future Development of Antinausea Drugs

Now that vomiting can be controlled in almost 90% patients, the future development of antiemetic agents may focus on nausea as a primary endpoint, where the current antiemetic drugs are less effective. New antiemetics could be developed that target newer opioid, cannabinoid, or peptide YY (PYY) receptor families.

The emergence of gene array technology identifying the genes coding for 5HT3 and NK1 receptors may allow a more rational selection of antiemetic regimens for patients depending on genetic variations detected. Also pharmacogenetic studies identifying cytochrome genotypes may allow specific dosing depending on genetic determinants of drug metabolism rates.

With an increasing number of antiemetic drugs and antiemetic drug combinations, vigilance about the potential for drug interactions will be needed. Examples are the potential interactions between NK1 RAs and other drugs such as cytotoxic agents metabolized by CYP 3A4. A potential interaction between NK1 RAs and abdominal radiation has been raised. Glucocorticoids can also interact with other drugs; they may attenuate cytotoxicity in human glioma cell lines exposed to various chemotherapy agents, or simply have cumulative side effects with prolonged dosing with multiple day cytotoxic therapy. It is also important to be aware of the large number of patients who take alternative or complementary therapies, which may also be metabolized by CYP 3A4 or CYP 2D6, and interact with the antiemetic therapy.

References

1. Andrews PI, Naylor RJ, Joss RA. Neuropharmacology of vomiting and its relevance to anti emetic therapy. Consensus and controversies. Support Care Cancer 1998;6:197–203.
2. Kris MG, Gralla RJ, Clark RA, et al. Incidence, course and severity of delayed nausea and vomiting following the administration of high dose cisplatin. J Clin Oncol 1985;3:1379–1384.
3. Morrow GR. Prevalence and correlates of anticipatory nausea and vomiting in chemotherapy patients. J Natl Cancer Inst 1982;68:585–593.
4. Grunberg SM, Osoba D, Hesketh PJ, et al. Evaluation of new antiemetic agents and definition of antineoplastic agent emetogenicity—an update. Support Care Cancer 2005;13:80–84.
5. Olver IN. The development of future research strategies form reviewing antiemetic trials for chemotherapy induced emesis. Rev Recent Clin Trials 2006;1:61–66.
6. Coates A, Abraham S, Kaye SB, et al. On the receiving end—patient perceptions of the side effects of cancer chemotherapy. Eur J Cancer 1983;19:203—208.
7. De Boer-Dennert M, de Wit R, Schmitz PI, et al. Patient perceptions of side effects of chemotherapy: the influence of 5HT antagonists. Br J Cancer 1997;76:1055–1061.
8. Osoba D, Zee B, Warr D, et al. Effect of postchemotherapy nausea and vomiting on health-related quality of life. The Quality of Life and Symptom Control Committees of the National Cancer Institute of Canada Clinical Trials Group. Support Care Cancer 1997;5:307–313.
9. Grunberg SM, Deuson RR, Mavros P, et al. Incidence of chemotherapy-induced nausea and emesis after modern antiemetics. Cancer 2004;100:2261–2268.
10. du Bois A, Meerpohl HG, Vach W, et al. Course, patterns, and risk-factors for chemotherapy-induced emesis in cisplatin-pretreated patients: a study with ondansetron. Eur J Cancer 1992;28:450–457.
11. Hornby PJ. Central neurocircuitry associated with emesis. Am J Med 2001;111:Suppl 8A:106S–112S.
12. Antiemetic Subcommittee of the Multinational Association of supportive care in Cancer (MASCC). Prevention of chemotherapy and radiotherapy-induced emesis: results of the Perugia Consensus Conference. Ann Oncol 1998;9:1022–1029.
13. del Giglio A, Soares HP, Caparroz C, et al. Granisetron is equivalent to ondansetron for prophylaxis of chemotherapy-induced nausea and vomiting: results of a meta-analysis of randomized controlled trials. Cancer 2000;89:2301–2308.
14. Jordan K, Hinke A, Grothey A, et al. A meta-analysis comparing the efficacy of four 5-HT3-receptor antagonists for acute chemotherapy-induced emesis. Support Care Cancer 2007;15:1023–1033, DOI 10.1007/s00520-006-0186-7.
15. Blackwell CP, Harding SM. The clinical pharmacology of Ondansetron. Eur J Cancer Clin Oncol 1989;25(Suppl 1):S21-4–S25-7.
16. Kris MG, Hesketh PJ, Somerfield MR, et al. American Society of Clinical Oncology guideline for antiemetics in oncology: update 2006. J Clin Oncol 2006;24:2932–2947.
17. Olver I, Paska W, Depierre A, et al. on behalf of the Ondansetron Delayed Emesis Study Group. A multicentre, double-blind study comparing placebo, ondansetron and ondansetron plus dexamethasone for the control of cisplatin-induced delayed emesis. Ann Oncol 1996;7:945–952.
18. Geling O, Eichler H-G. Should 5-hydroxytryptamine-3 receptor antagonists be administered beyond 24 hours after chemotherapy to prevent delayed emesis? Systematic re-evaluation of clinical evidence and drug cost implications. J Clin Oncol 2005;23:1289–1294.
19. Navari RM. Pathogenesis-based treatment of chemotherapy induced nausea and vomiting: two new agents. J Support Oncol 2003;1:89–103.
20. Rojas C, Stathis M, Thomas AG, et al. Palonosetron exhibits unique molecular interactions with the 5-HT3 receptor. Anesth Analg 2008;107:469–478.
21. Gralla R, Lichinitser M, Van Der Vegt S, et al. Palonosetron improves prevention of chemotherapy-induced nausea and vomiting following moderately emetogenic chemotherapy: results of a double-blind randomized phase III trial comparing single doses of palonosetron with ondansetron. Ann Oncol 2003;14:1570–1577.
22. Eisenberg P, Figueroa-Vadillo J, Zamora R, et al. 99–04 Palonosetron Study Group. Improved prevention of moderately emetogenic chemotherapy-induced nausea and vomiting with palonosetron, a pharmacologically novel 5-HT3 receptor antagonist: results of a phase III, single-dose trial versus dolasetron. Cancer 2003;98:2473–2482.

23. Aapro MS, Grunberg SM, Manikhas GM, et al. A phase III, double-blind, randomized trial of palonosetron compared with ondansetron in preventing chemotherapy-induced nausea and vomiting following highly emetogenic chemotherapy. Ann Oncol 2006;9:1441–1449.

24. Grunberg S, Vanden Burgt J, Berry S, et al. Prevention of delayed nausea and vomiting (D-CINV): Carryover effect analysis of pooled data from 2 phase III studies of palonosetron (PALO). J Clin Oncol 2004;22:A8051.

25. Saito M, Aogi K, Sekine I, et al. Palonosetron plus dexamethasone versus granisetron plus dexamethasone for prevention of nausea and vomiting during chemotherapy: a double-blind, double-dummy, randomised, comparative phase III trial. Lancet Oncol 2009;10:115–124.

26. Einhorn LH, Rapoport B, Koeller J, et al. Antiemetic therapy for multiple-day chemotherapy and high-dose chemotherapy with stem cell transplant: review and consensus statement. Support Care Cancer 2005;13:112–116.

27. Musso M, Scalone R, Bonanno V, et al. Palonosetron (Aloxi®) and dexamethasone for the prevention of acute and delayed nausea and vomiting in patients receiving multiple-day chemotherapy. Support Care Cancer 2009;17(Feb):205–209.

28. Cartmell AD, Ferguson S, Yanagihara R, et al. Protection against chemotherapy-induced nausea and vomiting ismaintained over multiple cycles of moderately or highly emetogenic chemotherapy by palonosetron, a potent 5-HT3 receptor antagonist. Proc Am Soc Clin Oncol (Chicago) 2003;May 31–Jun 3:3041.

29. Musso M, Sccalone R, Crescimanno A, et al. Palonosetron and dexamethasone for prevention of nausea and vomiting in patients receiving high-dose chemotherapy with auto-SCT. Bone Marrow Transplant 2010;45(1):123–127.

30. Hargreaves R. Imaging substance P receptors (NKr) in the living human brain using positron emission tomography. J Clin Psychiatry 2002;63(Suppl 11):18–24.

31. Tattersall FD, Rycroft W, Cumberbatch M, et al. The novel NK1 receptor antagonist M K-0869 (L-754,030) and its water soluble phosphoryl prodrug, L-758,298, inhibit acute and delayed cisplatin-induced emesis in ferrets. Neuropharmacology 2000;39:652–663.

32. Merck & Co. Inc. EMEND® (aprepitant)capsules: prescribing information. USA [online]. Available from URL: http://www.merck.com/

33. Olver I, Shelukar S, Thompson KC. Nanomedicines in the treatment of emesis during chemotherapy: focus on aprepitant. Int J Nanomedicine 2007;2:13–18.

34. Sanchez RI, Wang RW, Newton DJ, et al. Cytochrome P450 3A4 is the major enzyme involved in the metabolism of the substance P receptor antagonist aprepitant. Drug Metab Dispos 2004;32:1287–1292.

35. McCrea JB, Majumdar AK, Goldberg MR, et al. Effects of the neurokinin-1 receptor antagonist aprepitant on the pharmacokinetics of dexamethasone and methylprednisolone. Clin Pharmacol Ther 2003;74:17–24.

36. Blum R, Majumdar A, McCrea J, et al. Effects of aprepitant on the pharmacokinetics of ondansetron and granisetron in healthy subjects. Clin Ther 2003;25:1407–1419.

37. Nygren P, Hande K, Petty KJ, et al. Lack of effect of aprepitant on the pharmacokinetics of docetaxel in cancer patients. Cancer Chemother Pharmacol 2005;55:609–616.

38. Loos WJ, de Wit R, Freedman SJ, et al. Aprepitant when added to a standard antiemetic regimen consisting of ondansetron and dexamethasone does not affect vinorelbine pharmacokinetics in cancer patients. Cancer Chemother Pharmacol 2007;59:407–412.

39. Jarkowski A III. Possible contribution of aprepitant to ifosfamide-induced neurotoxicity. Am J Health Syst Pharm 2008;65(23):2229–2231.

40. Depré M, Van Hecken A, Oeyen M, et al. Effect of aprepitant on the pharmacokinetics and pharmacodynamics of warfarin. Eur J Clin Pharmacol 2005;61:34–36.

41. Hesketh PJ, Grunberg SM, Gralla RJ, et al. The oral neurokinin-1 antagonist aprepitant for the prevention of chemotherapy-induced nausea and vomiting: a multinational, randomized, double-blind, placebo-controlled trial in patients receiving high-dose cisplatin – the Aprepitant Protocol 052 Study Group. J Clin Oncol 2003;21:4112–4119.

42. Poli-Bigelli S, Rodrigues-Pereira J, Carides AD, et al. Addition of the neurokinin-1 receptor antagonist aprepitant to standard antiemetic therapy improves control of chemotherapy induced nausea and vomiting: results

from a randomized, double-blind, placebo-controlled trial in Latin America. Cancer 2003;97:3090–3098.

43. de Wit R, Herrstedt J, Rapoport B, et al. Addition of the oral NKl antagonist aprepitant to standard antiemetics provides protection against nausea and vomiting during multiple cycles of cisplatin-based chemotherapy. J Clin Oncol 2003;21:4105–4119.

44. Schmoll HJ, Aapro MS, Poli-Bigelli S, et al. Comparison of an aprepitant regimen with a multiple-day ondansetron regimen, both with dexamethasone, for antiemetic efficacy in high-dose cisplatin treatment. Ann Oncol 2006;17:1000–1006.

45. Warr DG, Hesketh PJ, Gralla RJ, et al. Efficacy and tolerability of aprepitant for the prevention of chemotherapy-induced nausea and vomiting in patients with breast cancer after moderately emetogenic chemotherapy. J Clin Oncol 2005;23:2822–2830.

46. Rapoport BL, Jordan K, Boice JA, et al. Aprepitant for the prevention of chemotherapy-induced nausea and vomiting associated with a broad range of moderately emetogenic chemotherapies and tumor types: a randomized, double-blind study. Support Care Cancer 2010;18(4):423–431.

47. Grote T, Hajdenberg J, Cartmell A, et al. Combination therapy for chemotherapy-induced nausea and vomiting in patients receiving moderately emetogenic chemotherapy: palonosetron, dexamethasone, and aprepitant. J Support Oncol 2006;4:403–408.

48. Hale JJ, Mills SG, MacCoss M, et al. Phosphorated morpholine acetal human neurokinin-1 receptor antagonists as water soluble prodrugs. J Med Chem 2000;43:1234–1241.

49. Cocquyt V, Van Belle S, Reinhardt RR, et al. Comparison of L-758,298 a prodrug for the selective neurokinin-1 antagonist, L-754,030, with ondansetron for the prevention of cisplatin induced emesis. Eur J Cancer 2001;37:835–842.

50. Van Belle S, Lichinister MR, Navari RM, et al. Prevention of cisplatin-induced acute and delayed emesis by the selective neurokinin-1 antagonists, L-758,298 and MK-869: a randomized controlled trial. Cancer 2002;94:3032–3041.

51. Lasseter KC, Gambale J, Jin B, et al. Tolerability of fosaprepitant and bioequivalency to aprepitant in healthy subjects. J Clin Pharmacol 2007;47:834–840.

52. Johnson BM, Hoke JF, Bandekar R, et al. Pharmacokinetics and pharmacodynamics (PK/PD) of casopitant, an NK1 receptor antagonist, in patients undergoing treatment with moderately and highly-emetogenic chemotherapy. Clin Pharmacol Ther 2007;81(Suppl 1):Abs PIII30.

53. Arpornwirat W, Albert I, Hansen VL, et al. Multicenter, randomized, doubleblind, ondansetron (ond)-controlled, dose-ranging, parallel group trial of the neurokinin-1 receptor antagonist (NK-1 RA) casopitant mesylate for chemotherapy-induced nausea/vomiting (CONV) in patients (pts) receiving moderately emetogenic chemotherapy (MEC). J Clin Oncol 2006;24(Suppl):18S–8512.

54. Navari RM. Casopitant, a neurokinin-1 receptor antagonist with antiemetic and antinausea activities. Curr Opin Investig Drugs 2008;9;774–785.

55. Grunberg SM, Aziz Z, Shaharyar A, et al. Phase III results of a novel oral neurokinin-1 (NK-1) receptor antagonist, casopitant: single oral and 3-day oral dosing regimens for chemotherapy-induced nausea and vomiting (CINV) in patients (pts) receiving moderately emetogenic chemotherapy (MEC). J Clin Oncol 2008;26:(Suppl 15);Abs 9540.

56. Grunberg SM, Rolski J, Strausz J, et al. Efficacy and safety of casopitant mesylate, a neurokinin 1 (NK1)-receptor antagonist, in prevention of chemotherapy-induced nausea and vomiting in patients receiving cisplatin-based highly emetogenic chemotherapy: a randomised, double-blind, placebo-controlled trial. Lancet Oncol 2009;10:549–558.

57. Aapro MS, Alberts DS. High-dose dexamethasone for prevention of cisplatin-induced vomting. Cancer Chemother Pharmacol 1981;7:11–14.

58. Hesketh PJ. Chemotherapy-induced nausea and vomiting. N Engl J Med 2008;358:2482–2494.

59. Bymaster FP, Falcone JF, Bauzon D, et al. Potent antagonism of 5-HT3 and 5-HT6 receptors by olanzapine. Eur J Pharmacol 2001;430:341–349.

60. Navari RM, Einhorn LH, Loehrer PJ, et al. A phase II trial of olanzapine, dexamethasone, and palonosetron for the prevention of chemotherapy-induced nausea and vomiting. Support Care Cancer 2007;15:1285–1291.

61. Gralla RJ. Metoclopramide. A review of antiemetic trials. Drugs 1983;25(Suppl 1):63–73.

TABLE

40.5   *Osteoclast-targeted therapy for women diagnosed with breast cancer*

Clinical setting	Goal of treatment	Evidence
Breast cancer with bone metastases	Prevention of skeletal-related events and palliation of pain	Several bisphosphonates have shown benefit. ASCO recommends pamidronate or zoledronic acid every 3–4 wk.[45] Denosumab is under investigation.
Early-stage breast cancer treated definitively but at high risk for relapse	Decreased risk of breast cancer recurrence	Clodronate results have been mixed. Zoledronic acid is promising[46] and is the subject of further trials.
Breast cancer treated with aromatase inhibitor	Decreased risk of fragility fractures	Risedronate,[47] ibandronate,[48] zoledronic acid,[49] and denosumab[3] improve bone mineral density.

In an open-label study in the Netherlands, 161 women with predominantly osteolytic metastases were randomly assigned to receive daily oral pamidronate (300 to 600 mg) or no bisphosphonate.[51] Treatment with pamidronate resulted in a statistically significant 38% reduction in skeletal morbidity. The benefit of treatment appeared to be dose-dependent, although significant gastrointestinal toxicity was observed at the higher dose.

Three randomized studies of intravenous pamidronate therapy have found clinical benefit. The open-label Aredia Multinational Cooperative Group Study (*n* = 295) found that pamidronate (45 mg intravenously every 3 or 4 weeks) significantly increased time to skeletal disease progression in women with progressive bone metastases.[52] The Protocol 18 Aredia Breast Cancer Study (*n* = 372) found that among women receiving hormonal therapy for breast cancer with at least one lytic bone lesion, 2 years of monthly pamidronate significantly reduced the skeletal morbidity rate throughout treatment.[53] The Protocol 19 Aredia Breast Cancer Study (*n* = 380)

found that in women with metastatic breast cancer and at least one lytic bone lesion, up to 2 years of monthly pamidronate significantly delayed the time to first skeletal-related event.[54] None of these three trials detected treatment-related changes in overall survival.

As noted in the section on multiple myeloma, Zometa Protocol 10 was designed to demonstrate that zoledronic acid was not inferior to pamidronate for patients with breast cancer or multiple myeloma.[37] Approximately 1,600 patients with either Durie-Salmon stage III multiple myeloma or advanced breast cancer and at least one bone lesion were randomly assigned to treatment with either 4 or 8 mg of zoledronic acid or 90 mg of pamidronate every 3 to 4 weeks for 12 months.[37] The primary efficacy endpoint was the proportion of patients experiencing at least one skeletal-related event over 13 months. The zoledronic 8-mg group was discontinued because of excess renal toxicity. Overall, the incidence of skeletal-related events, time to first skeletal-related event, and skeletal morbidity rate were similar between the groups. In the subset of

TABLE

40.6   *Major prospective randomized controlled trials of osteoclast-targeted therapy for metastatic breast cancer*

Study	N	Treatment	Result
Canadian[50]	173	Clodronate versus placebo	28% decrease in skeletal events
Netherlands[51]	161	Pamidronate versus no bisphosphonate	38% reduction in skeletal morbidity rate
Aredia Multinational[52]	224	Pamidronate versus no bisphosphonate	48% increase in median time to skeletal progression
Aredia Protocol 18[53]	380	Pamidronate versus placebo	37% reduction in skeletal morbidity rate
Aredia Protocol 19[54]	371	Pamidronate versus placebo	42% reduction in skeletal morbidity rate
Zometa Protocol 10[37]	1,648	Zoledronic acid versus pamidronate	Noninferiority study in breast and myeloma; similar clinical outcomes overall; trend toward better outcomes in breast cancer subset
Japanese[55]	228	Zoledronic acid versus placebo	20% reduction in the percentage of patients who had ≥1 skeletal event (29.8% versus 49.6%)
Ibandronate 4265[56]	466	Ibandronate versus placebo	Significant improvement in SMPR
Oral ibandronate[57]	564	Ibandronate versus placebo	Significant improvement in SMPR
Denosumab[58,59]	255	Denosumab (various schedules) versus IV bisphosphonate	Similar suppression of bone turnover as measured by urinary *N*-telopeptide

1,130 patients with breast cancer, treatment with zoledronic acid was associated with improved outcomes.[60]

Zoledronic acid was notably superior to placebo in a Japanese trial that enrolled 228 women with bone metastases due to breast cancer.[55] After 1 year of treatment with 4 mg zoledronic acid every 4 weeks, women in the treatment group were significantly less likely to experience at least one skeletal-related event (29.8% versus 49.6%, $P = 0.003$).

Three randomized controlled trials evaluated the efficacy of ibandronate in metastatic breast cancer. Together they have demonstrated treatment-related improvements in skeletal morbidity period rate (SMPR), the number of 12-week periods with new skeletal related events. One study ($n = 466$) found significant improvement in SMPR and longer median time to first skeletal-related event (SRE) only at an ibandronate dose of 6 mg.[56] Pooled analysis of the other two studies ($n = 564$) found that oral ibandronate (50 mg/d) caused significant improvement in mean SMPR compared to placebo.[57]

Denosumab has been preliminarily studied for the prevention of skeletal-related events among women with breast cancer metastatic to bone. One study randomized 255 such women to one of five denosumab schedules or to an IV bisphosphonate.[58,59] Suppression of the bone resorption marker urinary *N*-telopeptide and number of skeletal-related events were similar for denosumab and for IV bisphosphonate treatment. An ongoing phase III trial will compare denosumab and zoledronic acid for the prevention of skeletal-related events due to bone metastases in breast cancer. That trial is event-driven and is designed to enroll over 2,000 women.

The ASCO has published clinical practice guidelines for the use of bisphosphonate treatment for women with breast cancer, last updated in 2003.[45] They recommend zoledronic acid (4 mg over 15 minutes) or pamidronate (90 mg over 2 hours) every 3 to 4 weeks for women with plain radiographic evidence of bone destruction. They recommend against the use of pain as an indication for treatment. The authors of the guidelines conclude that bisphosphonates provide a supportive, albeit expensive and non–life-prolonging, benefit to many patients with bone metastases. The authors also conclude that additional information is needed about (1) when to stop therapy, (2) alternative doses or schedules for administration, and (3) how to best coordinate bisphosphonates with other palliative therapies.

Adjuvant Osteoclast-Targeted Therapy

Three randomized controlled trials have evaluated the effect of clodronate on the development of bone metastases in women with high-risk primary breast cancer.

> In one study of 302 women with primary breast cancer and immunohistochemical evidence of tumor cells in the bone marrow, administration of clodronate (1,600 mg by mouth daily for 2 years) initially reduced the incidence of distant metastases by 50% ($P < 0.001$).[61] Osseous and visceral metastases were both significantly lower in the clodronate-treated group than in the control group ($P = 0.003$). These benefits were no longer seen in long-term follow-up. Long-term follow-up did reveal a significant overall survival advantage for those treated with clodronate (40.7% versus 20.4%; $P = 0.04$).[62]
>
> In another study, 1,069 women with operable breast cancer were randomized to receive oral clodronate (1,600 mg/d) or a

placebo for 2 years, starting within 6 months of primary treatment.[63] The primary endpoint was relapse in bone. Clodronate significantly reduced the risk for bone metastases at 2 years and again at 5-year follow-up (51% versus 73%; hazard ratio [HR], 0.692; $P = 0.043$).[64] There was an initially significant reduction in mortality with clodronate. At 5 years, this survival benefit was no longer significant due to multiple analyses (HR of death 0.768; $P = 0.048$). The trend toward survival benefit was stronger among those with stage II and III disease than among those with stage I.

> A third randomized controlled trial failed to demonstrate efficacy of adjuvant clodronate. Two-hundred and ninety-nine women with primary node-positive breast cancer were randomized to clodronate ($n = 149$) or control groups ($n = 150$).[65] Clodronate 1,600 mg daily was given orally for 3 years. The incidence of bone metastases was similar in both groups. Clodronate was associated with greater risk of nonskeletal metastases and shorter disease-free survival.

These three clodronate trials individually produced mixed results. When placebo-controlled clodronate trials involving all stages of breast cancer were combined as a meta-analysis, there was no statistically significant clinical benefit (overall survival, bone metastasis–free survival, or nonskeletal metastasis–free survival) in either the adjuvant or metastatic setting.[66]

The results of the ABCSG-12 trial have raised the possibility that zoledronic acid has activity against breast cancer in tissue other than bone. That large prospective trial enrolled 1,803 premenopausal women who had undergone primary surgery for stage I or II endocrine-responsive breast cancer with fewer than ten positive lymph nodes.[46] Subjects all received ovarian suppression with the gonadotropin releasing harmone (GnRH) agonist goserelin. They were randomized to additionally receive tamoxifen, tamoxifen plus zoledronic acid, anastrozole, or anastrozole plus zoledronic acid. After approximately 4 years of follow-up, disease-free survival was significantly better in the arms that included zoledronic acid (94.0% versus 90.8%; HR for progression 0.64; 95% CI 0.46 to 0.91; $P = 0.01$). Some have questioned the plausibility of these findings (e.g., zoledronic acid reduced the number of contralateral breast cancers). Disease-free survival did not significantly differ between the tamoxifen arms and the anastrozole arms.

Taken together, the data for the use of clodronate treatment of women with early-stage breast cancer are mixed. Initial data in support of the comparatively stronger bisphosphonate zoledronic acid are more promising. Several ongoing large randomized trials are expected to clarify the possible role of adjuvant zoledronic acid in women with early-stage breast cancer.

Prevention of Treatment-Related Fragility Fractures

Drug therapy to lower the risk of fragility fractures is often relevant to women with breast cancer as age and aromatase inhibition are among the factors known to elevate risk. Completed trials in this setting have been powered to detect differences in bone mineral density but not in fracture rates. Clinical trials with several bisphosphonates have demonstrated prevention or reversal of aromatase inhibitor induced loss of bone mineral density (risedronate,[47] ibandronate,[48] and zoledronic acid[49]). Denosumab is emerging as an

TABLE

40.7 *Osteoclast-targeted therapy for men with prostate cancer*

Clinical setting	Goal of treatment	Evidence
Castration-resistant prostate cancer with bone metastases	Prevent or delay skeletal-related events	Zoledronic acid decreases skeletal-related events.[71] Denosumab versus zoledronic acid study ongoing.
Castration-resistant prostate cancer without bone metastases	Prevent or delay the development of metastases	Bisphosphonate trials were negative or closed early. Denosumab under investigation.
Hormone-sensitive prostate cancer with bone metastases	Prevent or delay skeletal disease progression	Clodronate ineffective for primary endpoint but found to improve overall survival. Zoledronic acid under investigation.
Men receiving ADT for prostate cancer and at elevated risk for fragility fractures	Decrease risk of fragility fractures	Multiple bisphosphonates improve bone mineral density. Denosumab[2] and toremifene[72] reduce fracture risk and improve bone mineral density.

additional therapeutic option as it was shown to significantly reduce hip and vertebral fractures in the general population among postmenopausal women with T-scores between −2.5 and −4.0.[1] In a subsequent trial specific to women with breast cancer, 152 women with low bone mass (excluding osteoporosis) and receiving adjuvant aromatase inhibition were randomized to denosumab (60 mg every 6 months) or to placebo. The study was positive as lumbar spine bone mineral density was significantly increased at 12 and 24 months.[3]

Prostate Cancer

Most bone metastases in men with prostate cancer appear osteoblastic by radiographic imaging. Osteolytic and osteoblastic lesions represent two extremes of a spectrum, however, and morphologic studies suggest that most bone metastases from prostate cancer are characterized by both excess bone formation and bone resorption. Pathological acceleration of bone remodeling causes disorganized bone and impaired structural integrity.

Osteoblastic metastases from prostate cancer have increased osteoblast number and activity, increased bone volume, and increased the bone mineralization rate.[67] Osteoclast number and activity are increased in osteoblastic metastases in bone adjacent to metastases and in distant uninvolved bone.[67,68] Biochemical markers of osteoclast activity are elevated in men with osteoblastic metastases from prostate cancer.[69] Although osteoclast activity is increased

in men with prostate cancer, it is unclear whether osteoclast activation precedes bone formation, as in normal bone remodeling, or is secondary to excessive osteoblast activity in the metastases. Markers of osteoclast activity independently predict the risk for subsequent skeletal complications,[70] suggesting that cancer-mediated osteoclast activation accompanies bone metastases and also contributes to the clinical complications of metastatic disease. These observations form the rationale for osteoclast-targeted therapy in men with prostate cancer and blastic bone disease. There are several potential indications for osteoclast-targeted therapy in men with prostate cancer (Table 40-7).

Prevention of Skeletal Events in Castration-Resistant Disease

Three contemporary studies have evaluated the efficacy of bisphosphonates in men with castration-resistant prostate cancer metastatic to bone (Table 40-8). Zoledronic acid is now the standard-of-care for the prevention of skeletal-related events in this clinical setting.

In the zoledronic acid 039 study, 643 men with castration-resistant prostate cancer and asymptomatic/minimally symptomatic bone metastases were assigned randomly to zoledronic acid (4 mg intravenously every 3 weeks) or placebo.[71] All men continued androgen-deprivation therapy (ADT) throughout the study and received additional antineoplastic therapy at the discretion of the investigator. The primary study endpoint was the proportion of men

TABLE

40.8 *Contemporary randomized trials of bisphosphonates for men with castration-resistant metastatic prostate cancer*

Study	N	Treatment	Result
Zometa 039[71]	643	Zoledronic acid versus placebo	Significant decrease in skeletal-related events
Study 032/INT 05[73]	350	Pamidronate versus placebo	No significant difference in pain, analgesic use, or skeletal-related events
NCIC Pr06[74]	204	Mitoxantrone and prednisone ± clodronate	No significant difference in palliative response

who experienced one or more skeletal-related events (pathological fracture, spinal cord compression, surgery or radiation therapy to bone, or change in antineoplastic treatment to treat bone pain). By 15 months, at least one skeletal-related event occurred in 44% of men who received placebo and 33% of men who received zoledronic acid ($P = 0.02$). The median time to first skeletal-related event differed significantly between men who received zoledronic acid and men who received placebo (>420 versus 321 days; $P = 0.01$). The study was not designed to evaluate the effect of zoledronic acid on survival. Median time to death, however, was longer in the zoledronic group than in the placebo group (546 versus 464 days, $P = 0.09$).

The only two other contemporary randomized controlled trials, using a bisphosphonate other than zoledronic acid, for men with castration-resistant prostate cancer were negative. In the National Cancer Institute of Canada Pr06 study, 204 men with castration-resistant prostate cancer and symptomatic bone metastases were assigned randomly to two treatments: mitoxantrone, prednisone, and intravenous clodronate versus mitoxantrone, prednisone, and placebo.[74] The primary study endpoints were pain scores and analgesic use. Pain scores, analgesic use, duration of palliative benefit, and overall survival did not differ significantly between the groups. In a pooled analyses of two multicenter trials, protocol 032 and INT 05, 350 men with castration-resistant prostate cancer and symptomatic bone metastases were assigned randomly to either intravenous pamidronate or placebo every 3 weeks for 27 weeks.[73] The pamidronate and placebo groups were similar with respect to pain scores, analgesic use, proportion of men with at least one skeletal-related event by 27 weeks, and survival.

Prevention of Skeletal Events in Hormone Sensitive Disease

Men treated with ADT for prostate cancer experience accelerated loss of bone density, increased markers of bone resorption, and increased risk of skeletal fractures. Only one study has evaluated the efficacy of bisphosphonates in men receiving initial hormone therapy for metastatic prostate cancer. In the Medical Research Council Pr05 study, 311 men who were starting or responding to primary ADT were assigned randomly to either oral clodronate (2,080 mg/d) or placebo.[75] All the men continued primary ADT. The relative risk of skeletal disease progression or prostate cancer death was lower in the clodronate group, although the difference was not significant. Adverse events were more common among men treated with clodronate. Gastrointestinal problems and elevated serum concentrations of lactate dehydrogenase were the most common adverse events. Long-term follow-up has since revealed a significant overall survival benefit among the men treated with clodronate (8-year overall survival [OS] 22 versus 14%; HR for death 0.77; 95% CI 0.60 to 0.98; $P = 0.03$).[76] In the similar MRC Pr04 trial, clodronate did not produce short- or long-term benefit in men with hormone-sensitive disease without metastases.

The survival benefit seen with long-term follow-up of hormone-sensitive patients treated with clodronate is encouraging. The considerably more potent zoledronic acid is under study in the ongoing CALGB/CTSU 90202 trial that compares early versus standard zoledronic acid treatment for men with prostate cancer metastatic to bone. Men are randomized to start treatment within 3 months of initiation of androgen deprivation or standard initiation upon diagnosis of castration resistance. The primary endpoint is incidence of skeletal-related events.

Applications of Denosumab in Prostate Cancer

Denosumab has been shown to reduce vertebral fracture risk among high-risk men receiving androgen deprivation for prostate cancer and is under evaluation in two ongoing trials for additional clinical settings.

Denosumab is under study for the prevention of skeletal-related events in men with castration-resistant prostate cancer metastatic to bone. As zoledronic acid is standard-of-care in this setting, Amgen protocol 103 randomizes 1,900 men to denosumab or zoledronic acid. Time to first skeletal-related event (pathological fracture, radiation to bone, surgery to bone, or spinal cord compression) is the primary endpoint. The trial is designed to evaluate both noninferiority and superiority.

Denosumab is also under study for the prevention of bone metastases among men with castration-resistant disease that is not yet metastatic to bone. No bisphosphonate has been effective in this setting. Unsuccessful bisphosphonate trials were conducted with clodronate (MRC Pr04) and zoledronic acid (Zometa 704). Amgen protocol 147 randomizes 1,400 men to either denosumab or placebo. Enrollment targets men who are at high risk to develop metastases as reflected by a prostate specific antigen (PSA) doubling time ≤10 months and/or PSA ≥ 8 ng/dL. The primary endpoint is bone metastasis–free survival.

Treatment-Related Fracture Risk

ADT for prostate cancer decreases bone mineral density[77] and is associated with greater risk for clinical fractures.[78,79]

Denosumab has been shown to reduce the risk of clinical fractures in men with increased risk due to age and ADT.[80] Amgen protocol 138 enrolled 1,468 men receiving ADT for prostate cancer and at high risk for fracture due to low bone mineral density, history of fragility fracture, or age ≥70. Subjects were randomized to 3 years of denosumab (60 mg every 6 months) or to placebo. Denosumab reduced the 3-year incidence of new vertebral fractures by 62% ($p = 0.006$) and fractures at any site by 28% ($p = 0.10$), and of multiple fractures at any site by 72% ($p = 0.006$). Bone mineral density was significantly increased at all measured sites (lumbar spine, total hip, and distal radius) at 24 months.[81] Though several bisphosphonates (alendronate,[82] pamidronate,[83,84] zoledronic acid,[85,86] and neridronate[87]) have been shown to improve bone mineral density in this clinical setting, those trials were not adequately powered to demonstrate reduction in fracture risk.

Selective estrogen receptor modulators (raloxifene[88] and toremifene[89]) improve bone mineral density of men receiving androgen deprivation for prostate cancer. Toremifene was studied in a phase III fracture prevention trial. That study enrolled men aged ≥50 years who were treated with androgen deprivation for prostate

2 hours after CVC insertion and continuing for 6 weeks.[130] Venography was performed 6 weeks after randomization and revealed no significant difference in the development of upper limb DVT between the two groups: 14.1% in the patients treated with enoxaparin and 18.0% in the patients treated with placebo.

Two studies compared the use of LMWH with warfarin for the prevention of CVC-related DVT. Fifty-nine patients received 1 mg warfarin or 2,850 IU of nadroparin daily for 90 days. The rate of venographically confirmed upper extremity thrombosis was not statistically different between the two arms: 16.7% in the warfarin arm and 28.6% in the nadroparin group ($P = 0.48$).[12]

In the one recent positive trial, De Cicco et al. randomized 450 patients to 1 mg of warfarin daily for 3 days before and 8 days after CVC insertion or 5,000 IU dalteparin given 2 hours before and daily for 8 days after CVC insertion or no anticoagulation.[63] All patients underwent venography at days 8 and 30 after CVC insertion and then every 2 months until the CVC was removed. Of the 348 analyzed patients, venography-proven CVC-related thrombosis was seen in 22% in the warfarin group, 40% in the dalteparin group, and 53% in the no-treatment group; all comparisons were statistically significant. However, 96% of the CVC-related thrombosis were observed at day 8 and were not occlusive. The rate of occlusive CVC-related thrombosis was not statistically different in the three groups (0.9% warfarin, 3.3% dalteparin, and 1.8% no treatment; $P = 0.40$). Only 5% of the patients in this trial were symptomatic, indicating that studies relying on symptomatic evaluation alone may significantly underestimate the actual CVC-related DVT frequency.

Current Guidelines on Prophylactic Anticoagulation

The majority of the recent prophylactic anticoagulation studies involving both warfarin and LMWH, which are both large and placebo-controlled, fail to show any benefit in reducing the rate of CVC-related DVT. These newer studies prompted the ACCP to change their guidelines in 2004 and the new guidelines have remained in place since. The recently published guidelines from the Eighth ACCP Conference on Antithrombotic Therapy recommend that clinicians not use either prophylactic doses of LMWH or minidose warfarin to prevent catheter-related thrombosis in cancer patients with indwelling catheters.[131]

Future Possibilities in Thrombosis Prevention

Given the recent negative results on low-dose warfarin and LMWH in preventing CVC-related DVT, larger, placebo-controlled studies of these drugs are probably not warranted. It may be more fruitful, instead, to consider other options. One option would be to consider newer antithrombotic agents such as DTIs (e.g., dabigatran, extylate) or the factor Xa inhibitors (e.g., fondaparinux or rivaroxaban). DTIs have some advantages over warfarin in that they are not affected by diet, antibiotics, or inhibitors of the CYP-450 system, such as 5-flurouracil and capecitabine.[132–135] Fondaparinux has recently been approved for prophylaxis and treatment of VTE and is superior to LMWH in terms of efficacy and bleeding rates.[134,136] However, as recent reports suggest, the rate of CVC-related thrombosis in untreated patients appears to be decreasing and may make even an effective prophylactic anticoagulant of limited importance. Moreover, these recent studies have demonstrated that the majority

of CVC-related DVTs occur early, are transient, and nonocclusive. Therefore, a second option would be to focus efforts on identifying a subset of cancer patients who are at high risk of developing clinically significant (symptomatic or occlusive) CVC-related DVT and designing prophylaxis systemic anticoagulation trials for this population.

Late Complications: Infection

Types of Central Venous Catheter-Related Infection

The incidence and mortality associated with catheter-related infections (CRIs) are difficult to ascertain because of the lack of consensus on definitions. The incidence ranges from 2% to 43%[34,38] and the mortality, in bacteremic patients, can be as high as 35%.[137]

Several types of vascular CRIs exist; these include catheter colonization, phlebitis, exit-site infection, tunnel infection, pocket infection, and bloodstream infection.[138–140] The ability to identify each type has important therapeutic implications. Less serious infections, such as an infection at the exit-site, may require only intravenous antibiotics, whereas more serious ones, such as a tunnel infection, may warrant removal and replacement of the catheter.

The seriousness of an infection and the risks associated with it also depend on the type of organism present. Coagulase-negative *Staphylococcus* species are the most common cause of CRIs and the least virulent. *Staphylococcus aureus*, Gram-negative bacilli, and *Candida* species are the next most common and have the potential to cause serious complications.[44,139]

The clinical performance of the patient also has important implications in management decisions and outcome. Immunocompromised or critically ill patients are at significant risk for morbidity and mortality from these infections, and commonly require removal of their catheter.[44,139]

Risks of Central Venous Catheter-Related Infection

Many patient- and catheter-related risk factors are associated with the development of CRIs. Malignancy, AIDS, or neutropenia are a few of the host factors that predispose patients to an increased risk.[138] As discussed in previous sections, the composition of the catheter and the insertion technique confer certain risks. For percutaneous devices, a subclavian approach is thought to be associated with less risk.[38,141] Occlusive plastic dressings, frequent manipulations, and nonsterile techniques increase the risk of infection.

One important identifiable risk factor for CRIs is the presence of thrombosis. This association was first suggested in the early 1980s when a higher rate of bacteremia was discovered in patients with documented CVC thromboses as compared with those without clots.[142] Further studies have confirmed this correlation.[82,90–92,143,144] This finding is not surprising given that, as mentioned earlier, almost all catheters develop a fibrin sheath and almost all fibrin sheaths become colonized with cocci.[47,48,145] To date, none of the anticoagulation studies has shown any reduction in the rate of infection.

Diagnosis of Central Venous Catheter-Related Infection

Techniques to diagnose CRIs can be divided into those that require catheter removal and those that allow it to remain in place. The "role plate, sonification and flushing" methods require removal of the catheter, while the newer approach, the "differential time to positivity" (DTP), involves drawing blood cultures from the central line and peripheral veins simultaneously, and does not require removal.[138,146,147] If the CVC blood culture returns positive 2 hours before the peripheral one, the catheter can be deemed the source with a sensitivity and specificity of 89% and 87%, respectively, for short-term catheters, and 90% and 72%, respectively, for long-term catheters.[148] Once a CRI has been identified, it is important to determine if the infection is confined to the catheter or present in the bloodstream. Catheter-related bloodstream infections (CRBIs) often require further work up to detect the seeding of other tissues, along with the possible development of endocarditis, osteomyelitis, or septic thrombophlebitis.[44,138]

Prevention of Central Venous Catheter-Related Infection

The simplest way to prevent infection is to practice meticulous sterile techniques, not only during the insertion process but also during the maintenance period. Aggressive hand washing by medical personnel is an absolute necessity. A recent study demonstrated that with the use of appropriate hand hygiene, full barrier precautions and chlorhexidine skin antisepsis, avoidance of femoral site for CVC insertion, and removal of the device as soon as it is no longer necessary, the rate of CRBIs decreased from 7.7/1,000 to 1.4/1,000 CVC-days at 18 months of follow-up.[149] Removing the catheter as soon as it is no longer needed is important because the risk of developing a CRBI increases with time. Using adhesive anchoring devices instead of sutures for catheter securement have also dramatically decreased CRBIs. Recognizing the signs and symptoms of localized, systemic, or metastatic infections can help prevent progression.

Besides the patient's skin, another common source of infection is the catheter hub. Disinfecting the hub each time it is accessed can decrease infection risk. New aseptic hub attachments have recently been developed, but their effectiveness needs to be evaluated in future randomized controlled trials.[35,150,151]

Although the use of combined antimicrobial and antiseptic flushes has been shown to significantly decrease the rate of CRBIs,[144] there is great concern that this procedure will promote the development of antibiotic-resistant organisms such as vancomycin-resistant enterococci and/or fungal infections. As a result, the prophylactic antibiotic locks or flushes is not currently recommended.[147,152]

The use of antimicrobial-impregnated catheters, however, is a routine and encouraged practice. Over the past few decades, several randomized trials have consistently shown a decrease in catheter colonization and CRBI. Presently, catheters are impregnated with either chlorhexidine and silver sulfadizine or minocycline and rifampin; both types have been well studied and both show benefit.[2,4,147,153–155] Newer catheters are impregnated not only on the external catheter surface as was commonly done with the first-generation catheters, but also on the internal lumen with the goal of preventing internal colonization.[156] Recent systemic reviews demonstrated the clinical effectiveness of this approach in decreasing CRBIs. Future developments to further decrease infection risk include silver iontophoretic devices, electrically charged catheters, and techniques to limit bacterial adhesion.[26,139]

Treatment of Central Venous Catheter-Related Infection

The most important decision to make when managing CRIs is whether or not to remove the catheter. This assessment depends on the patient, the organism, the extent of the infection, and the type of catheter. Patients diagnosed with uncomplicated CVC-related infections should receive 10 to 14 days of antimicrobial treatments. Patients who are critically ill, suffer from persistent bacteremia, or have metastatic seeding of their infection should have their catheter removed and start appropriate systemic antibiotics.[146] Tunnel or port infections warrant catheter removal. In addition, infections caused by difficult-to-treat organisms (e.g., *S. aureus*), virulent gram-negative infections, or fungal infections, carry a high risk of mortality if not removed. Prompt recognition of a CRI and administration of antibiotics can help decrease morbidity and mortality, especially in critically ill patients.

Conclusion

CVC-related complications are a common clinical problem that may affect nearly half of all cancer patients with CVCs. The mechanical, thrombotic, and infectious complications can result in clinical symptoms, loss of catheter function, postphlebitic syndrome of the upper extremity, PE, high morbidity, and even mortality. Numerous risk factors, both patient- and catheter-related, have been identified and are currently being modified to reduce the rates and types of complications. The two main complications, thrombosis and infection, are unfortunately still occurring at significant rates.

Further efforts to understand and prevent CVC-related complications are of importance. These efforts should include not only assessments of modalities for early diagnosis of complications and assessment of anticoagulant and antibiotic efficacies but also determination of additional risk factors for CVC-related thrombosis and infection, the timing of onset of these complications, the exploration and implementation of newer preventative agents, the optimal duration and types of treatments, and the natural history of these CVC-related complications.

References

1. Darouiche RO, Raad II, Heard SO, et al. A comparison of two antimicrobial-impregnated central venous catheters. Catheter Study Group. N Engl J Med 1999;340:1–8.
2. Falagas ME, Fragoulis K, Bliziotis IA, et al. Rifampicin-impregnated central venous catheters: a meta-analysis of randomized controlled trials. J Antimicrob Chemother 2007;59:359–369.
3. Maki DG, Stolz SM, Wheeler S, et al. Prevention of central venous catheter-related bloodstream infection by use of an antiseptic-impregnated catheter. A randomized, controlled trial. Ann Intern Med 1997;127:257–266.
4. Raad I, Darouiche R, Dupuis J, et al. Central venous catheters coated with minocycline and rifampin for the prevention of catheter-related colonization and bloodstream infections. A randomized, double-blind trial. The Texas Medical Center Catheter Study Group. Ann Intern Med 1997;127:267–274.
5. Bern MM, Lokich JJ, Wallach SR, et al. Very low doses of warfarin can prevent thrombosis in central venous catheters. A randomized prospective trial. Ann Intern Med 1990;112:423–428.
6. Boraks P, Seale J, Price J, et al. Prevention of central venous catheter associated thrombosis using minidose warfarin in patients with haematological malignancies. Br J Haematol 1998;101:483–486.
7. Couban S, Goodyear M, Burnell M, et al. Randomized placebo-controlled study of low-dose warfarin for the prevention of central venous catheter-associated thrombosis in patients with cancer. J Clin Oncol 2005;23:4063–4069.

leukemogenic risk from the use of anthracycline therapy is increased. A population-based cohort of 3,093 women with breast cancer diagnosed were studied for the development of acute leukemia. Women who received chemotherapy and radiation had a SIR for acute leukemia of 28.5, which means that the risk of acute leukemia was increased by more than 28 times compared to women in the general population. A dose-dependent increase in risk was observed in women treated with mitoxantrone, and risk of leukemia was lower in the women receiving anthracyclines.[60] Curtis et al.[61] reviewed the SEER database of 21,708 patients with breast cancer and found an 11.5 RR of developing secondary leukemias in patients treated with alkylating agents with or without radiation therapy as an adjuvant after a median follow-up of 4.2 years. In an attempt to assess the contributions of adjuvant radiotherapy, melphalan, or cyclophosphamide, Curtis et al. also reported a case-control study in a cohort of 82,700 women with breast cancer.[62] Results indicate a 2.4-fold increase in RR of leukemia after radiotherapy alone, a 10-fold increase after chemotherapy alone, and a 17.4-fold increase after a combination of the two. It has been suggested that postmastectomy irradiation increases the risk of lung cancer in smokers, and it is well established that radiation to the breast increases the risk of sarcomas, particularly angiosarcoma.[63-65]

Adjuvant therapy with tamoxifen is now well established to improve relapse-free survival and overall survival in selected patients with breast cancer. In postmenopausal women, tamoxifen treatment leads to endometrial hyperplasia and polyps.[66] Tamoxifen also stimulates the growth of endometrial cancer in vitro.[67] An association is found between tamoxifen and the development of endometrial cancer. An RR of 6.4 was found in a Scandinavian study in which 40 mg/d was used and was continued for 5 years.[68] Other studies using lower tamoxifen dosages and a shorter duration of treatment have reported lower RRs.[69] The NSABP reviewed 2,843 patients randomized to receive 20 mg/d of tamoxifen or placebo in the B-14 study.[70] The RR of endometrial cancer in the tamoxifen-treated group was 7.5, and the overall annual hazard rate for the development of endometrial cancer was 1.6/1,000. More recently in the P-1 trial, 13,207 women who received tamoxifen for 5 years had an RR of developing endometrial cancer of 3.28 compared to placebo; while in the subgroup of women 60 years or older receiving tamoxifen, the RR was 5.33.[71] In a meta-analysis of 32 randomized trials of tamoxifen versus a similar control arm including data from 52,929 patients, there was a significantly increased risk of developing endometrial cancers (RR = 2.7; 95% CI, 1.94 to 3.75) and gastrointestinal cancers (RR = 1.31; 95% CI, 1.01 to 1.69).[72] If the estrogenic effects of tamoxifen cause endometrial cancer, those tumors that develop should be of low grade and have a relatively good prognosis. This assumption has been confirmed in some of the studies reported.[73] Other studies have shown a distribution of grade and stage similar to that seen in nonhormonally induced cancers.[74] In an analysis of 3,457 women with breast cancer, 53 subsequently developed endometrial cancer.[75] Of these women, 15 had received tamoxifen and 38 had not. The number of high-grade cancers increased significantly in the tamoxifen-treated women, who also were more likely to die of their endometrial cancer.

In summary, most studies have demonstrated that adjuvant tamoxifen leads to a higher rate of endometrial cancer, which is dependent in part on dose and duration of therapy. Although tamoxifen induces liver tumors experimentally, there has been no increased incidence of primary liver cancer in the adjuvant breast studies. These tumors could well be missed because any tumor developing in the liver probably would be presumed to be a recurrence of the previous breast cancer.

Patients with Malignant Lymphoma

The incidence of second malignancies among patients with malignant lymphoma was no higher than expected before intensive therapy was initiated.[76] The use of combination chemotherapy and combined radiotherapy and chemotherapy has been associated with a high incidence of second malignancies, specifically AML and solid tumors.[77-81] Many of these patients, however, would not have survived long enough to be exposed to the risk of a second malignancy before the introduction of intensive therapy. The components of MOPP chemotherapy, mechlorethamine hydrochloride, vincristine, procarbazine, and prednisone for Hodgkin's disease, are potent carcinogens in animals.[82] A case-control study of 1,939 patients treated for Hodgkin's disease in the Netherlands assessed factors influencing the development of acute leukemia.[83] The cumulative dose of mechlorethamine was the most important factor. The use of lomustine was also associated with secondary leukemia, as was a requirement for a second course of chemotherapy. Overall, patients receiving chemotherapy had a 40-fold greater risk of leukemia than those receiving radiation therapy alone, whereas the use of combined-modality therapy did not increase the risk of leukemia beyond that seen with chemotherapy.

Although many reports have been concerned with an increased risk of acute leukemia, solid tumors occur more frequently in patients with malignant lymphoma after intensive therapy.[84-87] Three fourths of these are solid tumors, and the remainder are equally divided between leukemia and lymphoma. In a German series of over 1,500 patients with Hodgkin's disease treated with radiation therapy, with or without chemotherapy, from 1940 to 1991, the cumulative risk for malignancy was 1.5%, 4.2%, 9.4%, and 21% at 5, 10, 15, and 20 years, respectively.[88] At the 20-year period, the risk for solid tumors, lymphoma, and leukemia was 19%, 1.9%, and 0.6%, respectively. Three fourths of the solid tumors occurred within the radiation field. In patients receiving both chemotherapy and radiation therapy, the regimen of doxorubicin, bleomycin, vinblastine, and dacarbazine (ABVD) was associated with the highest risk.

In an intergroup trial of ABVD versus MOPP/ABV in 856 patients, secondary malignancies occurred in 18 patients receiving ABVD and 28 receiving MOPP/ABV. Two other patients were initially treated with ABVD but subsequently received MOPP-containing regimens and radiation therapy before developing leukemia.[89] A case-control study that compiled data on 19,046 patients with Hodgkin's disease treated between 1965 and 1994 demonstrated an increased risk of lung cancer for those receiving radiation at doses exceeding 5 Gy. In patients who were treated with alkylating agents and no radiation therapy, the risk of lung cancer was fourfold and the risk increased with the number of cycles administered.[90] The overall risk of second malignancies increased 2.8-fold with intensive chemotherapy. In 885 women treated for Hodgkin's disease from 1961 to 1990, the RR of developing and dying from breast cancer was increased fourfold to fivefold.[84] Although this is primarily the result of mantle irradiation, the concurrent use of chemotherapy further increased the RR. In a British series of 5,519 patients treated for Hodgkin's disease between 1963 and 1993 and followed for development of second malignancy, 27% received only radiotherapy, approximately 40% received both chemotherapy and radiation therapy, and 33% received only chemotherapy. Three hundred and forty-four patients developed a second malignancy (RR of second malignancy, 2.9). The greatest risk was for developing lung cancer, NHL, or leukemia.[91]

Second malignancies after NHL are less well studied. The Groupe d'Etude des Lymphomes de l'Aduite reported a 7-year cumulative incidence rate of 2.75% in 2,837 patients receiving doxorubicin, cyclophosphamide, vindesine, bleomycin, and prednisone (ACVBP). About 64 of the 81 malignancies were solid tumors and 17 were hematologic malignancies. Age was the only risk factor on multivariate analysis. Considering all tumors, there was no increased risk of second cancers; however, in the male population there was an excess of lung cancer and MDS/AML, and in the female population, there was an excess of MDS/AML.[92] Up to 10% of patients with NHL treated with either conventional-dose chemotherapy or high-dose chemotherapy and autologous stem cell transplantation may develop treatment-related MDS/AML within 10 years of primary therapy.[93]

Gastrointestinal Cancer Patients

Analysis of randomized trials of adjuvant methyl-CCNU in the management of patients with gastrointestinal cancers has reinforced the earlier data regarding the leukemogenic potential of this treatment.[4] The results of this analysis indicated that a 12.4 RR of leukemia exists in patients treated with methyl-CCNU. This risk seems to be dose-dependent. The latency period varies from 6 to 69 months and cases may continue to occur beyond that. Because the current data do not suggest a benefit in survival with such therapy, the leukemogenic risk has led to the removal of methyl-CCNU from adjuvant treatment regimens. The most important drug in adjuvant regimens for colorectal cancer is 5-fluorouracil, and it has not been associated with an increased risk of second cancers.

Patients with Testicular Cancer

More than 30 years have passed since cisplatin-based chemotherapy was first used for the treatment of advanced testicular cancer. A large number of patients have been cured with chemotherapy, and reports about the long-term consequences of this therapy are only beginning to appear. In a group of 1,909 patients in The Netherlands diagnosed with testicular cancer between 1971 and 1985, 78 second cancers occurred, or 1.6 times the number expected.[94] In this analysis, radiation therapy was the main contributing factor. In a Norwegian series, the use of chemotherapy plus infradiaphragmatic radiation did increase the RR of second cancers over that seen with infradiaphragmatic radiation alone (RR = 1.3 versus 2.4).[95] The use of cisplatin-containing chemotherapy alone did not appear to increase the risk of a second cancer.

No increases in second cancers have been reported after cisplatin, vinblastine, and bleomycin (PVB) treatment for testicular cancer.[96] Etoposide is now used rather than vinblastine because a randomized trial demonstrated the improved effectiveness of cisplatin, etoposide, and bleomycin over PVB.[97] Among 315 patients at Indiana University receiving etoposide, two cases of acute leukemia (0.63%) occurred.[98] Of 340 patients treated with etoposide at Memorial Sloan-Kettering Cancer Center, two cases of acute leukemia

developed.[99] The overall conclusion of these and other reviews of etoposide use is that the doses in most germ cell cancer protocols slightly increase the risk of acute leukemia, but this increase is acceptable, given the benefits of etoposide-based therapy in this disease.[100]

The largest review of second neoplasms in patients with testicular cancer includes data for almost 29,000 men in 16 different tumor registries.[101] Overall, 1,406 second cancers were identified, yielding an RR of 1.43. The excess number of tumors included leukemias (RR = 3.07 to 5.20), melanoma (RR = 1.69), lymphoma (RR = 1.88), and a variety of gastrointestinal tumors (RR = 1.27 to 2.21). An analysis of the relationship between treatment and these new tumors revealed that the gastrointestinal tumors were associated with radiation therapy, whereas the secondary leukemia was associated with both radiation and chemotherapy.

Patients Receiving High-Dose Therapies

High-dose chemotherapy with autologous bone marrow transplantation (ABMT) or peripheral blood stem cell rescue is used extensively for treating patients with hematologic malignancies. In this setting, very high doses of drugs are given over a short period of time. The specific agents used differ depending on the institution and tumor being treated, but commonly include the oxazaphosphorine nitrogen mustards (cyclophosphamide and ifosfamide), carboplatin, etoposide, or melphalan. The doses delivered with marrow rescue are threefold to sixfold higher than can be given without such support; thus, the total dose of drug delivered is similar to those employed in multiple cycles of conventional regimens. MDS and ANLL have been reported in patients who receive allogeneic, autologous, or peripheral blood transplantation.[102,103] Most patients who have an ABMT, however, also have received other chemotherapy before this procedure, confounding estimation of risk. A review of all 649 patients who received ABMT or peripheral blood stem cell transplantation at the University of Chicago from 1985 to 1997 revealed seven therapy-related cases (1%) of MDS, ALL, or ANLL.[104] These occurred in five patients with Hodgkin's disease, one patient with NHL, and one patient with breast cancer. The median latency period between initial standard-dose treatment of the cancer and development of leukemia/MDS was approximately 5 years, whereas the interval was less than 2 years from the high-dose therapy. In a retrospective analysis of 262 patients undergoing ABMT for NHL at the Dana-Farber Cancer Institute from 1982 to 1991, the overall incidence of posttransplant MDS or AML was 7.6%, with a median onset of 31 months after transplant or 69 months after initial treatment of lymphoma. Variables predicting for development of MDS included prolonged interval between initial treatment and the transplant, a longer duration of exposure to chemotherapy, and radiation therapy before transplant.[105] Both of these studies suggest that conventional chemotherapy before the high-dose therapy was a significant contributing factor. In a situation in which high-dose therapy is given repeatedly, however, the risk of secondary leukemia may become prohibitive. In a series of 86 patients with poor-risk solid tumors treated with repeated high doses of cyclophosphamide/ifosfamide, etoposide, and doxorubicin, the cumulative incidence of treatment-related AML was 8% at 40 months of follow-up.[106] Cytogenetic analysis was consistent with leukemias induced both by alkylators and by etoposide.

The University of Minnesota reported on the development of second malignancies in 3,372 patients who underwent stem cell transplants for various diseases from January 1974 through March 2001. There were 147 posttransplant malignancies in 137 patients; 24 of the malignancies were either nonmelanoma skin cancers or carcinomas in situ. This represented an 8.1-fold increased risk of posttransplant malignancy. For MDS/AML, the cumulative incidence plateaued at 1.4% by 10 years following transplant, but the cumulative incidence of developing a solid tumor did not plateau and was 3.8% at 20 years posttransplant.[107] A higher incidence of solid malignancies was reported by the City of Hope in their analysis of 2,129 patients who had undergone bone marrow transplant for hematologic malignancies. The estimated cumulative probability for developing a solid cancer was 6.1% at 10 years. The risk was particularly elevated for liver cancer with an SIR of 27.7, cancer of the oral cavity with SIR of 17.4, and cervical cancer with SIR of 13.3. Both patients with liver cancer had hepatitis C infection and all patients with squamous cell carcinoma of the skin had chronic graft-versus-host disease. The risk was highest for survivors who were younger than 34 years at the time of transplant. Cancers of the thyroid, liver, and oral cavity occurred primarily in patients who had received total body irradiation (TBI).[108] The development of solid tumors over a prolonged period warrants close long-term monitoring of these patients.

Patients who receive allogeneic transplants also have an increased risk of solid tumors.[103] A large international series of 28,874 patients who received hematopoietic cell transplant between 1964 and 1996 were followed for secondary solid cancer. Overall, there were 189 cases of cancers, including carcinomas in situ and invasive squamous cell carcinomas of the skin. In this cohort, 58% of the patients were less than 30 years old at the time of transplantation, 74% were transplanted for leukemia, and 67% received TBI as part of their conditioning. The risk of developing a solid tumor was 2.5% at 10 years, 5.8% at 15 years, and 8.8% at 20 years.[109]

Patients Receiving Cyclophosphamide or Immunosuppressive Therapy

Bladder toxicity associated with the use of the oxazaphosphorine nitrogen mustards, cyclophosphamide and ifosfamide, has been long recognized.[110] The acute cystitis is likely related to toxic metabolites and can be limited by the concomitant use of mesna. A number of reports have now been published of bladder cancer in patients who received long-term cyclophosphamide therapy.[111,112] The most common situations in which this occurs are in pediatric protocols, in low-grade lymphomas, and in immunosuppressive therapy. A review of a cohort of 6,171 medium-term or long-term survivors of NHL revealed 48 cases of urothelial cancer.[112] Overall, a 4.5-fold increase in risk of bladder cancer was estimated from the use of cyclophosphamide; however, the cumulative dose was critical in determining risk. In patients who received more than 50 g of cyclophosphamide, there is an increase in absolute risk of developing bladder cancer of 7% within 15 years of treatment. The cyclophosphamide is rarely administered as chronic therapy in treating pediatric and adult cancers; however, the risk of secondary urothelial cancer may be an important consideration in decisions about long-term therapy in immunologic diseases.

Cytotoxic agents, such as methotrexate, azathioprine, and cyclophosphamide, are commonly used for immunosuppression in the treatment of rheumatoid arthritis, scleroderma, Wegener's granulomatosis, nephrotic syndrome, and glomerulonephritis, as well as in the control of rejection in renal transplantation.[113-115] Accumulated experience suggests a different mechanism of tumor induction from that observed in patients treated for neoplastic conditions. Patients treated with immunosuppressive agents have a high incidence of malignant lymphomas, often with evidence of the presence of Epstein-Barr virus, and a predilection for primary tumor sites in the brain; this predilection may result from decreased immune surveillance. This state resembles the chronic immunodeficiency of certain inherited disorders, such as Wiskott-Aldrich's syndrome, which is also associated with a high incidence of lymphomas.[116]

Nucleoside analogs are known to be potent immunosuppressors. They have been used in hematologic malignancies such as chronic lymphocytic leukemia (CLL) and hairy cell leukemia (HCL). A retrospective review considered 2,014 patients treated by National Cancer Institute protocols with fludarabine for relapsed or refractory CLL, and 2′-deoxycoformycin (DCF) and 2-chlorodeoxyadenosine (CdA) for HCL. A comparison with the SEER database for the general population indicated an increased incidence of secondary malignancies for fludarabine and 2-CdA. The study concluded that these figures were consistent with an underlying increased risk associated with the diseases themselves, with no appreciable increased risk related to treatment.[117]

Conclusion

Both clinical and laboratory studies have implicated alkylating agents and epipodophyllotoxins as potent carcinogens. Strong evidence exists for carcinogenicity in laboratory systems for the antitumor antibiotics and procarbazine, which translates into increased risk in the clinic. Antimetabolites such as methotrexate, gemcitabine, and cytarabine are much less hazardous, likely because of fewer mutational events occurring in the DNA. Newer agents such as the topoisomerase I inhibitors and the taxanes have not been used for a sufficient duration to allow estimation of any carcinogenic risk. The combined use of chemotherapy and radiotherapy definitely increases the risk of tumor induction. All of this, however, must be interpreted in the context of the need to successfully treat a potentially lethal primary cancer.

The available data suggest that guidelines should be developed in the design, use, and follow-up of chemotherapy (and radiation therapy) for patients with potentially curable diseases. Careful surveillance should be undertaken for secondary neoplasms during long-term follow-up of these patients. An attempt should be made to establish the quantitative risk of neoplasia for any regimen that proves curative, and efforts should be made to limit the use of the more highly carcinogenic agents. Careful prospective and retrospective studies should be aimed at establishing whether a total-dose threshold exists for carcinogenicity of suspected carcinogens in humans and whether modification of the schedule of administration affects this risk. Pharmacogenetic factors may offer further insights into risk factors for second malignancies and help in selection of therapy for patients at increased risk. Despite the development of novel targeted therapies, which appear to have a lower risk of carcinogenicity, the combination of such agents with chemotherapy will still require vigilance.

References

1. Haddow A. Mode of action of chemical carcinogens. Br Med Bull 1947;4:331–342.

2. Lerner HJ. Acute myelogenous leukemia in patients receiving chlorambucil as long-term adjuvant chemotherapy for stage II breast cancer. Cancer Treat Rep 1978;62(8):1135–1138.

3. Fisher B, Rockette H, Fisher ER, et al. Leukemia in breast cancer patients following adjuvant chemotherapy or postoperative radiation: The NSABP experience. J Clin Oncol 1985;3(12):1640–1658.

4. Boice JD, Jr. Second cancer after Hodgkin's disease—the price of success? J Natl Cancer Inst 1993;85:4–5.

5. Kapadia SB, Krause JR, Ellis LD, et al. Induced acute non-lymphocytic leukemia following long-term chemotherapy: a study of 20 cases. Cancer 1980;45(6):1315–1321.

6. Rizzo SC, Ricevuti G, Gamba G, et al. Multimodal treatment in operable breast cancer. Br Med J (Clin Res Ed) 1981;283(6288):437.

7. Miller JA. Carcinogenesis by chemicals: an overview—G. H. A. Clowes memorial lecture. Cancer Res 1970;30(3):559–576.

8. Farber E. Carcinogenesis—cellular evolution as a unifying thread: presidential address. Cancer Res 1973;33(11):2537–2550.

9. Miller EC. Some current perspectives on chemical carcinogenesis in humans and experimental animals: presidential address. Cancer Res 1978;38(6):1479–1496.

10. Pitot HC. The molecular biology of carcinogenesis. Cancer 1993; 72(3 Suppl):962–970.

11. Alban JM, Wild CP, Rollinson S, et al. Polymorphism in glutathione s-transferase P1 is associated with susceptibility to chemotherapy-induced leukemia. Proc Natl Acad Sci U S A 2001;98(20):11592–11597.

12. Kelly KM, Perentesis JP. Polymorphisms of drug metabolizing enzymes and markers of genotoxicity to identify patients with Hodgkin's lymphoma at risk of treatment-related complications. Ann Oncol 2002;13(Suppl 1): 34–39.

13. Hagan CR, Rudin CM. Mobile genetic element activation and genotoxic cancer therapy: potential clinical implications. Am J Pharmacogenomics 2002;2(1):25–35.

14. Mccann J, Ames BN. Discussion paper: the detection of mutagenic metabolites of carcinogens in urine with the salmonella/microsome test. Ann N Y Acad Sci 1975;269:21–25.

15. Mccann J, Choi E, Yamasaki E, et al. Detection of carcinogens as mutagens in the Salmonella/microsome test: assay of 300 chemicals. Proc Natl Acad Sci USA 1975;72(12):5135–5139.

16. Seino Y, Nagao M, Yahagi T, et al. Mutagenicity of several classes of antitumor agents to Salmonella typhimurium Ta98, Ta100, And Ta92. Cancer Res 1978;38(7):2148–2156.

17. Brundrett RB, Colvin M, White EH, et al. Comparison of mutagenicity, antitumor activity, and chemical properties of selected nitrosoureas and nitrosoamides. Cancer Res 1979;39(4):1328–1333.

18. Genther CS, Schoeny RS, Loper JC, et al. Mutagenic studies of folic acid antagonists. Antimicrob Agents Chemother 1977;12(1):84–92.

19. Benedict WF, Baker MS, Haroun L, et al. Mutagenicity of cancer chemotherapeutic agents in the Salmonella/microsome test. Cancer Res 1977;37(7 Pt 1):2209–2213.

20. Lambert B, Ringborg U, Harper E, et al. Sister chromatid exchanges in lymphocyte cultures of patients receiving chemotherapy for malignant disorders. Cancer Treat Rep 1979;62:1413–1419.

21. Lambert B, Ringborg U, Linblad A, et al. The effects of DTIC, melphalan, actinomycin D and CCNU on the frequency of sister chromatid exchanges in peripheral lymphocytes of melanoma patients. In: Jones SE, Salmon S, eds. Adjuvant Therapy of Cancer. New York: Grune & Stratton, 1979:55–62.

22. Ohtsuru M, Ishii Y, Takai S, et al. Sister chromatid exchanges in lymphocytes of cancer patients receiving mitomycin C treatment. Cancer Res 1980;40(2):477–480.

23. Smith MA, Mccaffrey RP, Karp JE. The secondary leukemias: challenges and research directions. J Natl Cancer Inst 1996;88(7):407–418.

24. Bokemeyer C, Schmoll HJ. Secondary neoplasms following treatment of malignant germ cell tumors. J Clin Oncol 1993;11:1703–1709.

25. Van Leeuwen F. Second cancers. In: Devita V Jr, Hellman S, Rosenberg S, eds. Cancer: Principles and Practice of Oncology. Philadelphia, PA: Lippincott, 2001:2939–2964.

26. Travis LB. Therapy-associated solid tumors. Acta Oncol 2002;41(4): 323–333.

27. Makuch R, Simon R. Recommendations for the analysis of the effect of treatment on the development of second malignancies. Cancer 1979;44(1):250–253.

28. Gleevec. [package insert]. Novartis Pharmaceuticals Corp. East Hanover, NJ; 2010.

29. Tucker MA, D'Angio GJ, Boice JD Jr, et al. Bone sarcomas linked to radiotherapy and chemotherapy in children. N Engl J Med 1987;317(10):588–593.

30. Tucker MA, Meadows AT, Boice JD Jr, et al. Leukemia after therapy with alkylating agents for childhood cancer. J Natl Cancer Inst 1987;78(3):459–464.

31. Neglia JP, Friedman DL, Yasui Y, et al. Second malignant neoplasms in five-year survivors of childhood cancer: childhood cancer survivor study. J Natl Cancer Inst 2001;93(8):618–629.

32. Meadows AT, Friedman DL, Neglia JP, et al. Second neoplasms in survivors of childhood cancer: findings from the childhood cancer survivor study cohort. J Clin Oncol 2009;27(14):2356–2362.

33. Jenkinson HC, Hawkins MM, Stiller CA, et al. Long-term population-based risks of second malignant neoplasms after childhood cancer in Britain. Br J Cancer 2004;91(11):1905–1910.

34. Inskip PD, Curtis RE. New malignancies following childhood cancer in the United States, 1973–2002. Int J Cancer 2007;121(10):2233–2240.

35. Olsen JH, Moller T, Anderson H, et al. Lifelong cancer incidence in 47697 patients treated for childhood cancer in the Nordic countries. J Natl Cancer Inst 2009;101(11):806–813.

36. Armstrong GT, Liu Q, Yasui Y, et al. Late mortality among 5-year survivors of childhood cancer: a summary from the Childhood Cancer Survivor Study. J Clin Oncol 2009;27(14):2328–2338.

37. Winick NJ, McKenna RW, Shuster JJ, et al. Secondary acute myeloid leukemia in children with acute lymphoblastic leukemia treated with etoposide. J Clin Oncol 1993;11(2):209–217.

38. Pui CH, Ribeiro RC, Hancock ML, et al. Acute myeloid leukemia in children treated with epipodophyllotoxins for acute lymphoblastic leukemia. N Engl J Med 1991;325(24):1682–1687.

39. Kreissman SG, Gelber RD, Cohen HJ, et al. Incidence of secondary acute myelogenous leukemia after treatment of childhood acute lymphoblastic leukemia. Cancer 1992;70(8):2208–2213.

40. Felix CA. Secondary leukemias induced by topoisomerase-targeted drugs. Biochim Biophys Acta 1998;1400(1–3):233–255.

41. Travis LB, Hill DA, Dores GM, et al. Breast cancer following radiotherapy and chemotherapy among young women with Hodgkin disease. JAMA 2003;290(4):465–475.

42. Horwich A, Swerdlow AJ. Second primary breast cancer after Hodgkin's disease. Br J Cancer 2004;90(2):294–298.

43. Bhatia S, Yasui Y, Robison LL, et al. High risk of subsequent neoplasms continues with extended follow-up of childhood Hodgkin's disease: report from the Late Effects Study Group. J Clin Oncol 2003;21(23):4386–4394.

44. Bagley CM Jr, Young RC, Canellos GP, et al. Treatment of ovarian carcinoma: possibilities for progress. N Engl J Med 1972;287(17):856–862.

45. Einhorn N. Acute leukemia after chemotherapy (melphalan). Cancer 1978;41(2):444–447.

46. Sotrel G, Jafari K, Lash AF, et al. Acute leukemia in advanced ovarian carcinoma after treatment with alkylating agents. Obstet Gynecol 1976;47(1):67s–71s.

47. Morrison J, Yon JL. Acute leukemia following chlorambucil therapy of advanced ovarian and fallopian tube carcinoma. Gynecol Oncol 1978;6(1):115–120.

48. Casciato DA, Scott JL. Acute leukemia following prolonged cytotoxic agent therapy. Medicine (Baltimore) 1979;58(1):32–47.

49. Reimer RR, Hoover R, Fraumeni JF, et al. Acute leukemia after alkylating-agent therapy of ovarian cancer. N Engl J Med 1977;297(4):177–181.

50. Greene MH, Harris EL, Gershenson DM, et al. Melphalan may be a more potent leukemogen than cyclophosphamide. Ann Intern Med 1986; 105(3):360–367.

generally induce longer-lasting oligospermia.[42] As previously described, patients who receive carboplatin-based therapy are more likely to recover spermatogenesis than those who receive cisplatin-based therapy. Other predictors of recovery include normospermia before treatment and less than five cycles of chemotherapy.[23]

High-Dose Chemotherapy and Bone Marrow Transplantation

In general, conditioning regimens involving total body irradiation (TBI) appear to have profound effects on fertility, while gonadal recovery occurs in a portion of patients receiving chemotherapy-only conditioning regimens. The majority of men (61% to 90%) regain spermatogenesis within 3 years after single-agent cyclophosphamide.[43,44] Early studies of busulfan-cyclophosphamide (Bu-Cy) conditioning regimens using 200 mg/kg of cyclophosphamide, reported a low recovery rate of 17%,[43] but more recent studies using a lower dose of cyclophosphamide (120 + 16 mg/kg busulfan) have reported higher rates of recovery, ranging from 50% to 84%.[45] Conditioning regimens combining cyclophosphamide with TBI appear to have profound effects on gonadal function, with only 17% of patients recovering spermatogenesis and never earlier than 4 years posttreatment.[44]

Leydig Cell Dysfunction

Although the effect of chemotherapy on spermatogenesis appears to be the most clinically important, Leydig cell dysfunction may occur as well. While Leydig cells remain morphologically intact after chemotherapy and basal serum LH levels generally remain normal, many patients have been found to have hypersecretion of LH in response to LH-releasing hormone, an indication of sub-clinical Leydig cell dysfunction.[46] The incidence of Leydig cell dysfunction appears to be associated with increasing age and more severe germinal damage.[46,47] Partial recovery of Leydig cell function may occur following treatment, although recovery beyond 5 years is unlikely.[47] The clinical significance of Leydig cell dysfunction is unclear. Complete androgen deficiency is associated with altered body composition, decreased sexual function, hot flushes, excessive sweating, fatigue, anxiety, depression, and reduced bone mineral density (BMD),[48–50] but mild-to-moderate testosterone deficiency has been less well studied and may be associated with sexual dysfunction,[51,52] increased serum cholesterol,[53] and decreased BMD.[54] Men who receive chemotherapy and have mild Leydig cell dysfunction have lower BMD and increased incidence of truncal fat distribution compared with men without Leydig cell dysfunction.[55] Testosterone replacement in men with complete androgen deficiency increases BMD, increases muscle mass, and decreases body fat,[56,57] but further investigation is needed to determine the incidence and clinical significance of mild androgen deficiency, as well as the role of replacement therapy.

Mutagenic Potential of Cancer Chemotherapy

In addition to the effects on fertility and Leydig cell function, cytotoxic treatment may be associated with chromosomal abnormalities in germ cells. These alterations may contribute to posttreatment infertility and may place subsequent generations at risk for carcinogenesis or developmental disorders. Up to 19% of sperm from healthy men have chromosomal alterations.[58] The frequency of structural abnormalities of sperm in cancer patients receiving chemotherapy or radiation has been estimated at up to 40%, with more damage seen in patients who received multiple chemotherapeutic agents and longer durations of therapy.[59,60] It is not clear whether these damaged sperm are able to fertilize eggs. Patients with cancer may also have a higher rate of sperm DNA abnormalities at baseline.[61–63] Animal studies have reported dominant lethal mutations in zygotes after animals were treated with doxorubicin, melphalan, and chlorambucil[64,65] and intrauterine death and developmental and morphologic abnormalities in progeny of animals exposed to gonadotoxic chemotherapy.[66,67] Nonetheless, human epidemiologic studies have failed to show increased developmental abnormalities or carcinogenesis in the offspring of men who received chemotherapy.[68–70] Many clinicians interpret the transgenerational human studies cautiously, and it is reasonable to counsel men about the potential hazards to their future offspring and discuss contraception for 6 months to 1 year after completion of treatment to allow for clearance of potentially affected germ cells from the reproductive tract.[71,72] The absence of transgenerational effects may not apply to offspring conceived by specialized infertility techniques that utilize sperm collected during or soon after chemotherapy, as natural selection at the time of natural fertilization may reduce the likelihood of fertilization by sperm with abnormal chromosomal material.[66,67] Thus, some discourage the use of sperm collection and cyropreservation during cancer treatment.[72]

Assisted Reproductive Techniques for Men

Semen Cryopreservation

Pretreatment sperm banking is presently the only proven means of preserving fertility for men who are to receive combination chemotherapy for cancer. Although pretreatment sperm banking does not guarantee a successful conception in future years, advances in management of male factor infertility have made conception possible for many men. Although approximately 50% of male cancer patients have reduced sperm quality prior to chemotherapy,[24,33,73] particularly men with testicular cancer and Hodgkin's disease,[73–75] the majority of male cancer patients have adequate parameters for sperm storage.[76] Only 12% to 17% of referred male cancer patients are unable to donate sperm for cryopreservation because of severe azoospermia before therapy.[73,75,77] Even with poor semen quality at the time of cryopreservation, many cancer patients are able to conceive using advanced reproductive techniques.[78,79] Therefore, many groups recommend that suboptimal prefreeze sperm analysis should not be used to deny sperm banking, and cryopreservation should be offered to all male patients who have some motile spermatozoa in their sperm sample.[76,78,80,81]

Although the technology of freezing, preserving, and thawing human semen has advanced considerably, ultimate conception rates using preserved semen have been limited by artificial insemination techniques. Classic intrauterine insemination (IUI) of the female partner using thawed spermatozoa was the only insemination technique available for many years. While IUI has been associated with pregnancy rates of 36% to 45% in male cancer patients,[78,82] many male cancer patients have inadequate sperm quantity or quality for this procedure.[83] In vitro fertilization (IVF) can be used with low sperm quantity or when female factors prevent successful IUI. IVF has been associated with higher fertilization rates.[84,85] The newest advance in fertilization technique is intracytoplasmic sperm injection (ICSI), which involves the direct injection of a single spermatozoa into the cytoplasm of an oocyte during IVF. This procedure has revolutionized the treatment of male factor infertility and holds particular promise for azoospermic and oligospermic cancer survivors. Clinical pregnancy rates of 50% have been reported with ICSI among male cancer patients.[82]

Testicular Sperm Extraction

Although the majority of patients are able to have sperm collected before therapy, a proportion of male cancer patients are azoospermic before therapy and therefore unable to undergo standard semen collection or fail to have sperm collected before therapy and find themselves azoospermic after treatment. For these patients, sperm may be obtained through newer technologies such as epididymal aspiration or testicular sperm extraction (TESE). With TESE, testicular biopsy tissue is macerated, centrifuged, and examined for the presence of sperm. Recovery rates with TESE in patients with either complete germinal aplasia or maturation arrest on biopsy have ranged from 45% to 76%, presumably because of adjacent areas of intact spermatogenesis.[86,87] The reported pregnancy rates with TESE and ICSI range from 30% to 40%.[86,87] As this technology is becoming more available, even men with long-standing azoospermia and absent sperm production may be able to father children.

Testicular Germ Cell Transplantation

Testicular germ cell transplantation is an experimental technique that may be available to male cancer patients in the future. Several animal studies have shown that spermatogonial stem cells can repopulate the seminiferous tubules with resumption of spermatogenesis and production of functional spermatozoa, leading to natural live births in the recipient animals.[88–91] Human application has just begun and remains experimental.[89,92] Despite the great interest in testicular germ cell transplantation, there is a theoretical risk of disease transmission, especially in patients with hematologic malignancies. In animal studies, rats that received testicular germ cells from leukemic donors developed leukemia after testicular germ cell transplantation.[93] Tumor cell depletion techniques are currently being developed to address this limitation. One group has successfully sorted leukemia-free germ cells from leukemic mice, transplanted these germ cells, and generated leukemia-free progeny by ICSI.[94] Thus, as techniques are improved and translated to humans, testicular germ cell transplantation may be a viable option for male cancer patients hoping to preserve their reproductive potential.

Chemotherapy Effects in Women

Oogenesis is the process of maturation of the primitive female germ cell to the mature ovum. This process occurs primarily during intrauterine life and involves multiple mitotic divisions to increase the number of germ cells, followed by the beginning of the first meiotic division, which will eventually reduce the diploid chromosome number to half before fertilization. At the time of birth, the oocytes are in the long prophase of their first meiotic division, and they remain in that state until the formation of a mature follicle before ovulation.[95]

In the postnatal ovary, most of the ongoing cellular growth and replication is related to the growth and development of follicles. Primordial follicles develop during gestation and consist of a primary oocyte covered by a layer of mesenchymal cells called granulosa cells. At the time of birth, the ovary may contain 150,000 to 500,000 primordial follicles, many of which subsequently become atretic. From childhood to menopause, follicular growth occurs as a continuous process, with ovulation occurring in a cyclic fashion.[96] The granulosa cells surrounding the primary oocyte proliferate, follicular fluid accumulates, and the ovum completes its first meiotic division to become a secondary oocyte. At this time, the follicle is known as a secondary or graafian follicle. The follicle continues to enlarge until the time of ovulation. Those follicles not undergoing ovulation become atretic and regress. During the reproductive life of a woman, only 300 to 400 oocytes mature and are extruded in the process of ovulation; the remainder undergo some form of atresia.

Assessment of Ovarian Function

The evaluation of chemotherapy effects on ovarian function is hampered by the relative inaccessibility of the ovary to biopsy. There is no readily available direct measurement of the female germ cell population analogous to semen analysis in men. Thus, surrogate markers must be utilized to assess the functional status of the ovary and follicular reserve.[97] Animal studies have shown that chemotherapy decreases the number of follicles, and ovarian fibrosis and follicle destruction have been described in the ovaries of women receiving antineoplastic chemotherapy.[97,98] Drug-induced ovarian failure is associated with low serum levels of estradiol and progesterone, markedly elevated levels of FSH and LH, amenorrhea, and symptoms of estrogen deficiency. Increased serum FSH helps to identify ovarian failure but has not been useful in the early identification of diminished ovarian reserve. Both anti-Mullerian hormone, secreted by the granulosa cells of growing follicles, and inhibin-B, produced by small-growing follicles and involved in the feedback regulation of FSH, are promising markers of ovarian reserve. Transvaginal evaluation of ovarian volume and antral follicle count indirectly measures ovarian reserve, but is limited by wide variations by age and cycle.[97]

Drug Effects on Ovarian Function

The onset and duration of amenorrhea varies with the cytotoxic agent (Table 43-2) and appears to be both dose-related and age-related. Generally, younger patients are able to tolerate larger cumulative drug doses before amenorrhea occurs and have a greater likelihood of resumption of menses when therapy is discontinued. Many chemotherapeutic agents that are toxic to reproductive germ cells in men do not have the same toxicity in women. This is likely because spermatogenesis involves constant cell division, but in women, cell division is intermittent and involves only a small number of primary oocytes with each menstrual cycle.

Alkylating agents are the most frequent cause of ovarian dysfunction among the anticancer drugs. Amenorrhea occurs in at least 50% of premenopausal women receiving 40 to 120 mg of cyclophosphamide daily for an average of 18 months.[99] Studies of the use of adjuvant chemotherapy for the prevention of recurrence of breast cancer suggest that the onset of amenorrhea and the resumption of

TABLE

43.2 Toxicity of single agents to female germ cells

Single-agent drug	References
Drugs highly toxic to female germ cells	
Cyclophosphamide	99, 100, 102, 103, 112
Melphalan	105, 135
Drugs with moderate-to-low toxicity to female germ cells	
Doxorubicin	107, 112, 114, 115
Cisplatin	108–111
Taxanes	113–119
Etoposide/vinca alkaloids	106
Methotrexate	191
5-FU	101, 105

menses are related to the age of the patient during chemotherapy and to the total dose administered.[100] Permanent cessation of menses occurs with adjuvant cyclophosphamide after a mean total dose of 5.2 g in all patients 40 years of age and older. Amenorrhea can occur in women younger than 40 years, but generally only after a mean cyclophosphamide dose of 9.3 g has been administered.[101] The development of amenorrhea also appears to be age-related after adjuvant treatment with cyclophosphamide, methotrexate, and flu-orouracil (CMF).[102] In women younger than 35 years of age, mean time to the onset of amenorrhea is 5.5 months; for women aged 35 to 45 years, the mean time is 2.3 months, and in women older than 45 years, amenorrhea develops very quickly, with a mean onset of 1.0 months. Women who receive intravenous cyclophosphamide before the age of 25 rarely experience permanent amenorrhea. Yet, treatment with cyclosphosphamide in childhood is associated with a lesser likelihood of becoming pregnant.[103]

Although many other chemotherapeutic agents have been evaluated for long-term ovarian toxicity, most evidence comes from studying the effects of combination chemotherapy regimens. Therefore, it is often difficult to determine the contribution of individual agents.[104] A study of single-agent fluorouracil (5-FU) in nine patients with breast cancer found no evidence of ovarian failure.[101] In addition, Fisher et al. found no difference in the incidence of posttherapy amenorrhea in women who received 5-FU and melphalan compared with those who received melphalan alone.[105] A small study evaluating the impact of oral etoposide on ovarian function reported amenorrhea in 41% of patients after a mean cumulative etoposide dose of 5 g.[106] Doxorubicin also does not appear to have profound ovarian ablative effects, although the impact varies by age and dose.[107] Some studies suggest that most women who receive platinum-based chemotherapy have temporary amenorrhea, but resume normal menstrual function.[108,109] Other studies have reported persistent menstrual dysfunction in women after the administration of cisplatin-based therapies.[110,111] Inconsistencies such as these are frequent in the literature describing chemotherapy-induced amenorrhea and may be related to how treatment-related ovarian failure is defined, the duration of follow-up, dose received, and age at administration.

Combination Chemotherapy and Disease-Specific Considerations

Breast Cancer

Age at treatment is the primary factor in predicting chemotherapy-induced amenorrhea in premenopausal women receiving adjuvant chemotherapy for breast cancer. Several studies evaluating a variety of different adjuvant regimens have shown that younger women (<40 years old) have a higher likelihood of resuming their menses and maintaining future fertility.[112] In general, the combination of CMF is the regimen with the highest likelihood of causing premature ovarian failure, with up to 70% of premenopausal women experiencing persistent amenorrhea after adjuvant CMF.[112,113] The likelihood of persistent amenorrhea varies with age; many women who receive CMF before 40 years of age will regain their menses. Yet, the majority of women treated when over 40 years old will experience persistent amenorrhea.[112] Lower overall rates of persistent amenorrhea are noted with doxorubicin or epirubicin-based regimens.[112] Similarly, rates of persistent amenorrhea vary with age. Fifteen to fifty-two percent of women <40 years old who receive anthracycline-based regimens experience persistent amenorrhea, while up to 95% of women greater than 40 years old have persistent amenorrhea.[114,115] The majority of studies suggest no significant differences in rates of persistent amenorrhea with the addition of paclitaxel or docetaxel to anthracycline-based regimens[113,115,116]. Forty-five percent to eighty-five percent of breast cancer patients less than 40 years old who receive adjuvant anthracycline and taxane-based chemotherapy resume menstruation.[114,117] While two studies suggest an association between the use of taxanes with chemotherapy-related amenorrhea in the short term, long-term follow-up failed to establish that the addition of taxanes to anthracycline-based regimens increased rates of persistent amenorrhea.[118,119]

Hodgkin's Disease

The risk of ovarian failure after combination chemotherapy for hematologic malignancies is also clearly related to the age of the patient at the time of treatment. Overall, at least 50% of women treated with MOPP or related regimens become amenorrheic.[120] Apart from age, no clear differences have been noted between those women who become amenorrheic during therapy and those who do not. Among women who received COPP, persistent ovarian failure occurred in 86% of women over 24 years old, but in only 28% of women who were under 24 years old at the time of treatment.[121] Moreover, the time of onset of amenorrhea appears to be age-related; ovarian failure occurs within 1 year of discontinuing therapy in patients over 40 years old, whereas in younger patients, a gradual decrease in frequency of menses following completion of therapy occurs.[120] ABVD chemotherapy is less likely to produce premature ovarian failure, with almost all women regardless of age at treatment regaining normal menses.[122] At least one study has shown that survivors of Hodgkin's lymphoma who received ABVD have equal pregnancy rates as friend or sibling controls.[123] Newer regimens for advanced Hodgkin's disease such as standard or escalated BEACOPP, while very effective, have been associated with ovarian failure in approximately 50% of patients, again with higher rates among those over 30 years old at the time of treatment.[124]

Ovarian Germ Cell Tumors

Although malignant germ cell tumors of the ovary are rare, they principally occur during adolescence and early adulthood. With the advent of cisplatin-based chemotherapy regimens, high cure rates have been obtained, even in the setting of metastatic disease.[108] Fertility-sparing surgery has become the standard of care as removal of the uninvolved ovary does not improve survival.[125] Many patients receive combination chemotherapy, and the regimens used appear to cause relatively little ovarian toxicity. Seventy percent of women regained regular menses after treatment with a variety of regimens containing drugs such as actinomycin D, vincristine, and cyclophosphamide.[126] While many patients experience amenorrhea during therapy, the majority of patients resume normal menstrual periods after cisplatin-based therapy.[108,127,128] In addition, the majority who attempt to conceive children are successful.[128]

High-Dose Chemotherapy and Bone Marrow Transplantation

The risk of treatment-related ovarian failure after high-dose chemotherapy and bone marrow transplant is largely related to age at the time of treatment. Cyclophosphamide-containing preparative regimens for allogeneic bone marrow transplantation induced *reversible* amenorrhea in women younger than 26 years of age, but *permanent* amenorrhea in 67% of women older than 26 years.[129] Similar outcomes have been described with a variety of high-dose chemotherapy regimens followed by autologous bone marrow transplant.[35,130–132] Additionally, TBI may be associated with higher rates of permanent amenorrhea.[130,133] Regimens using TBI cause premature menopause in nearly all patients.[129,134] Although most studies have found that the specific chemotherapy-conditioning regimen did not appear to affect future fertility, Singhal et al. reported a higher pregnancy rate among women who were conditioned with melphalan alone when compared with those who received other conditioning regimens, suggesting that this regimen may be less likely to cause treatment-related ovarian failure.[135] Although bone marrow transplant survivors report lower conception rates than controls, many do conceive, and rates of stillbirth and miscarriage do not appear to be increased.[133]

Estrogen Deficiency

Women who develop premature ovarian failure may also be subject to the physical and emotional disorders that accompany estrogen deficiency. Depressed libido, irritability, sleep disturbances, and poor self-image all occur commonly in women with treatment-related amenorrhea.[136] Hormone replacement therapy may be of considerable benefit to patients with chemotherapy-induced amenorrhea, frequently producing dramatic relief of hot flashes, dyspareunia, and irritability. Hormone replacement can also prevent the early onset of osteoporosis.

Mutagenic Potential of Cancer Chemotherapy in Women

As previously described, the mutagenic potential of cancer chemotherapy remains largely undefined. Most studies suggest no increased incidence of spontaneous abortion or fetal abnormalities in women treated with chemotherapy in comparison with the general population.[137–141] However, some reports suggest an increase in structural congenital cardiac defects, spontaneous abortions, and other congenital anomalies in women previously treated with chemotherapy,[139,142] and larger longitudinal studies may provide additional information regarding risks to subsequent generations. Increased rates of spontaneous abortions, preterm birth, and low birth weight infants have been seen in patients who receive pelvic or spinal radiation, which may explain some of the conflicting data and is clinically relevant for patients who receive multimodality therapy.[104,138]

Assisted Reproductive Techniques for Women

Embryo Cryopreservation

Before the development of embryo cryopreservation, no reliable techniques existed for women who wished to retain the ability to bear children following ovarian ablative chemotherapy. Before initiation of chemotherapy, women may have oocytes harvested and fertilized in vitro with partner or donor sperm. The embryos can be stored in liquid nitrogen and thawed for implantation at a later date when the patient's endometrium has been hormonally prepared. This option has been associated with pregnancy and take-home baby rates of 30% to 35% and 29%, respectively.[143] Unfortunately, although successful, this procedure is not available for many women. First, embryo cryopreservation requires a partner at the time of harvest. Embryo cryopreservation is not an option for prepubertal or pubertal girls. Second, the time involved in ovarian stimulation, monitoring, and oocyte retrieval leads to a delay in beginning cancer treatment, which may compromise outcomes. Additionally, ovarian stimulation increases levels of estradiol, and may be contraindicated in women with hormone-responsive malignancies such as breast cancer.[144,145] For women with breast cancer, an alternative to standard IVF is natural IVF, or oocyte retrieval without hyperstimulation. Unfortunately, unstimulated cycles generally only yield one or two metaphase II eggs. Alternative stimulation programs incorporating letrozole, an aromatase inhibitor, have been evaluated, as they are associated with lower midcycle estradiol levels.[145] While larger prospective evaluation is needed, preliminary studies suggest that "controlled ovarian stimulation" with letrozole does not increase the risk of recurrence in patients with breast cancer.[146,147]

Cryopreservation of Oocytes

Embryo cryopreservation is the standard option, but oocyte cryopreservation could benefit women without a partner at the time of fertility preservation. Embryo cryopreservation became the procedure of choice because embryos survive cryopreservation better than oocytes. With advances in cryopreservation media and procedures, successful oocyte freezing, storage, and thawing have been reported in animals and humans.[104,148] While overall pregnancy and delivery rates (4.7% and 3.1%, respectively) were initially felt to be too low for widespread clinical application, birth rates up to 6% have been reported more recently, and oocyte cryopreservation will likely become a valid reproductive option in the near future.[149]

Ovarian Tissue Cryopreservation and Transplantation

A technique that holds great promise for women anticipating treatment with potentially sterilizing chemotherapy is ovarian autografting. The technique relies on the removal of oocyte-rich ovarian cortical tissue that is then slowly cooled and stored in a cryopreservative. At a later date, the tissue may be thawed and reimplanted near the fallopian tubes for potentially natural ovulation and fertilization. Ovarian tissue cryopreservation and transplantation offer several advantages over oocyte and embryo cryopreservation, including a greater number of immature oocytes, elimination of the need for hormonal stimulation and delays in therapy, and easier cryopreservation and thawing. In addition, ovarian cryopreservation can be offered to prepubertal and pubertal girls and it has the potential to provide an alternative to hormone replacement therapy for patients who develop premature ovarian failure.[150] Although still considered investigational, applications have rapidly developed in humans over the last 10 years.[104] Ovarian tissue has been easily obtained and autotransplanted in women and prepubertal cancer patients via laparoscopy without significant complications.[151,152] Ovarian tissue transplantation has restored ovarian hormonal function and shown evidence of follicular development after transplantation in several patients.[153,154] In addition, pregnancies and at least five live births have been reported,[155–157] although there has been controversy over whether the pregnancies originated from the transplanted ovarian tissue or the native ovary.[156] Despite these successes, this procedure is still in its infancy and concerns include poor graft survival as a result of ischemic-reperfusion injury, the longevity of ovarian tissue grafts, the ability to achieve follicular development within the graft, and malignant disease transmission via the autologous tissue graft. While a small study reported no evidence of Hodgkin's lymphoma in 26 cryopreserved ovarian tissue samples,[158] tumor cells have been identified using highly sensitive markers in at least one chronic myelogenous leukemia (CML) patient undergoing ovarian tissue transplantation.[159] Thus, the risks in cancer patients are unknown and the optimal applications and indications for cryopreserved ovarian grafts are unclear.[160,161] Nonetheless, ovarian tissue transplantation will likely be a viable management option for prepubertal girls and women at high risk for infertility secondary to cytotoxic therapy.

Hormonal Manipulation in Women

Efforts to protect the ovary from the toxic effects of chemotherapy have focused on the use of oral contraceptives and GnRH agonists to induce ovarian suppression. A small preliminary study suggested that ovarian follicles could be protected and normal menses could be preserved by the administration of oral contraceptives during chemotherapy.[162] Larger studies with longer follow-up have failed to demonstrate a protective effect of oral contraceptives,[163] although one study has reported a lower rate of premature ovarian failure after chemotherapy in women with Hodgkin's disease who used oral contraceptives.[124] Thus, further studies are needed to evaluate the role of oral contraceptives in reducing chemotherapy-related infertility.

GnRH analogs have been considered for the protection of female germ cells during the administration of chemotherapy. The goal of this approach is to induce a dormant state in germ cells, suppress cellular replication, and render the cells resistant to the cytotoxic effects of chemotherapy. GnRH analogs appear to partially protect ovarian follicles and fertility in rats and Rhesus monkeys from the damaging effects of cyclophosphamide.[164,165] Several uncontrolled case series and cohort studies have suggested a protective effect of the GnRH agonists on ovarian function in women

undergoing chemotherapy.[104,166] Nonetheless, these effects have not been confirmed in prospective randomized studies, and gonadotropin-releasing hormone (GnRH) agonists are currently not recommended for fertility preservation outside of a clinical trial. Ongoing prospective randomized studies will provide additional information regarding the clinical utility of GnRH agonists.[167]

Chemotherapy Effects in Children

Over 70% of children now survive cancer that is diagnosed and treated in childhood.[168] Because discussion of remission rates, survival rates, and immediate toxicities tend to dominate initial discussions regarding treatment options, consideration of future fertility is a quality of life issue that is often neglected. Many regimens used as treatment for childhood cancer have significant gonadal toxicity. As a result, many survivors experience infertility as adults. Any study of the effects of cytotoxic chemotherapy on gonadal function in children is particularly complex because of the variables introduced by the continuum of sexual development in this patient population. Thus, the effects of chemotherapy can be expected to vary according to when drugs are given and when their effects are evaluated relative to puberty.

Chemotherapy Effects in Boys

Early reports suggested differences in the sensitivity of the prepubertal, pubertal, and adult testis to alkylating-agent chemotherapy, concluding that the prepubertal testis is relatively unaffected by chemotherapy.[169,170] The prepubertal testis may be more tolerant of moderate doses of alkylating agents than is the adult testis, yet a threshold dose does seem to exist, above which germinal epithelial injury will result.[171] Studies of long-term survivors of childhood cancer suggest that alkylating agents and procarbazine have the greatest likelihood of producing permanent azoospermia.[172] Indeed, it appears that MOPP causes permanent gonadal damage in the majority of boys, even in prepubertal boys.[6,173] Rates of long-term azoospermia were lower (37%) among boys who received cisplatin or cisplatin-based regimens and only 16% in those who received nonalkylating agents (doxorubicin, vincristine, MTX, and 6-mercaptopurine).[174] Additionally, male acute lymphocytic leukemia (ALL) survivors showed little impact of treatment on future fertility.[175]

Although future fertility is not the most immediate concern when treating children or adolescent male cancer patients, improved survival rates have led to an increased appreciation for the long-term quality of life effects of chemotherapeutic treatment. For this reason, many authors suggest that clinicians address future infertility before instituting therapy, and some advocate sperm collection and cryopreservation for all peripubertal or postpubertal sexually mature adolescents.[176] Although sperm collection was previously not routinely offered because of a presumption of inadequate collection in adolescent males, the feasibility of sperm cryopreservation in adolescent cancer patients has been confirmed.[176,177] Successful sperm cryopreservation has been reported in more than 80% of male adolescent cancer patients.[176] Epididymal aspiration or testicular biopsy can be employed if adolescent ejaculates are suboptimal. Semen cryopreservation is not an option for prepubertal male cancer patients because the prepubertal testes do not complete spermatogenesis and therefore does not have mature haploid spermatozoa. Prepubertal male cancer patients could potentially benefit from the development of gonadal tissue storage techniques, followed by autotransplant or in vitro maturation, sperm extraction, and ICSI.[178] These techniques are still under investigation, but they may provide prepubertal boys receiving chemotherapy with an opportunity to remain fertile in adulthood.

Chemotherapy Effects in Girls

Early reports suggested no delay in menarche and no interruption of menses in girls treated with single-agent cyclophosphamide.[179] However, damage to the germ cell pool does occur, although clinical manifestations may vary.[137] Ovarian biopsy in girls treated for ALL showed a reduction in the number of follicles and cortical stromal fibrosis, with more severe changes noted in postmenarchal girls.[180] Others have noted absence or inhibition of follicle development after cytotoxic chemotherapy in girls with leukemia and solid tumors.[181,182] As in adult female cancer patients, the degree of gonadal damage depends on the specific cytotoxic agent, the cumulative dose, and the age of the patient at exposure.

Most studies that evaluated ovarian function in girls after exposure to chemotherapy have examined combination regimens. Thus, it is difficult to make definitive conclusions regarding the contribution of individual agents. Nonetheless, the available information is useful to inform patients of the risk of ovarian failure when undergoing treatment for common childhood cancers. Among female pediatric cancer survivors treated for a variety of cancers, the majority (94%) do not develop acute ovarian failure, defined as loss of ovarian function within 5 years of their diagnosis. Risk factors for ovarian failure include ovarian irradiation and exposure to procarbazine (at any age) or cyclophosphamide at ages 13 to 20 years.[183] The majority of young girls who receive therapy for ALL maintain ovarian function and have normal pubertal development.[184,185] However, with long-term follow-up, some patients may later experience premature menopause.[185] The majority of girls who receive combination chemotherapy, including alkylating agents, for Hodgkin's disease will maintain or resume ovarian function, although up to 30% may experience symptomatic ovarian failure and some may require hormone replacement therapy.[186] Preservation of fertility has similarly been noted in a high proportion of long-term survivors of patients with childhood NHL treated with regimens containing cyclophosphamide, vincristine, doxorubicin, and high-dose MTX.[187] However, in one study of prepubertal girls receiving nitrosoureas or procarbazine, or both, for brain tumors, 69% showed biochemical evidence of primary ovarian failure (elevated basal FSH level or abnormal peak FSH response to GnRH stimulation), and only 23% had normal pubertal development and menarche.[188] Likewise, female children who receive high doses of busulfan as part of bone marrow transplant conditioning regimens appear to have high rates of ovarian failure.[189] Similar to adult women, the age at administration may play a role in the risk of ovarian failure. Premenarchal girls experience fewer menstrual irregularities and fewer elevations in gonadotropins than postmenarchal girls, consistent with the theory that younger females have a greater oocyte reserve than older girls.[190] Despite these data, counseling young female cancer patients and their parents regarding the likelihood of future infertility remains difficult, as published experience is limited and long-term follow-up is needed. Even though many girls will have normal pubertal development and menarche, many will likely experience early menopause, potentially limiting their ability to have children by narrowing their window of fertility.[185]

References

1. Walsh PC, Amelar RD. Embryology, anatomy and physiology of the male reproductive system. In: Amelar RD, Dublin L, Walsh PC, eds. Male Infertility. Philadelphia, PA: WB Saunders, 1977:3–32.
2. Clermont Y. Kinetics of spermatogenesis in mammals: seminiferous epithelium cycle and spermatogonial renewal. Physiol Rev 1972;52(1):198–236.
3. Schilsky RL, Sherins RJ. Gonadal dysfunction. In: DeVita VT, Hellman S, Rosenberg SA, eds. Cancer: Principles and Practice of Oncology. Philadelphia, PA: Lippincott, 1982:1713–1717.
4. Bordallo MA, Guimaraes MM, Pessoa CH, et al. Decreased serum inhibin B/FSH ratio as a marker of Sertoli cell function in male survivors after chemotherapy in childhood and adolescence. J Pediatr Endocrinol Metab 2004;17(6):879–887.
5. Meachem SJ, Nieschlag E, Simoni M. Inhibin B in male reproduction: pathophysiology and clinical relevance. Eur J Endocrinol. 2001;145(5):561–571.
6. van Beek RD, Smit M, van den Heuvel-Eibrink MM, et al. Inhibin B is superior to FSH as a serum marker for spermatogenesis in men treated for Hodgkin's lymphoma with chemotherapy during childhood. Hum Reprod 2007;22(12):3215–3222.
7. Mecklenburg RS, Sherins RJ. Gonadotropin response to luteinizing hormone-releasing hormone in men with germinal aplasia. J Clin Endocrinol Metab 1974;38(6):1005–1008.
8. Miller DG. Alkylating agents and human spermatogenesis. JAMA 1971;217(12):1662–1665.
9. Richter P, Calamera JC, Morgenfeld MC, et al. Effect of chlorambucil on spermatogenesis in the human with malignant lymphoma. Cancer 1970;25(5):1026–1030.
10. Cheviakoff S, Calamera JC, Morgenfeld M, et al. Recovery of spermatogenesis in patients with lymphoma after treatment with chlorambucil. J Reprod Fertil 1973;33(1):155–157.
11. Rivkees SA, Crawford JD. The relationship of gonadal activity and chemotherapy-induced gonadal damage. JAMA 1988;259(14):2123–2125.
12. Meistrich ML, Wilson G, Brown BW, et al. Impact of cyclophosphamide on long-term reduction in sperm count in men treated with combination chemotherapy for Ewing and soft tissue sarcomas. Cancer 1992;70(11):2703–2712.
13. DeSantis M, Albrecht W, Holtl W, et al. Impact of cytotoxic treatment on long-term fertility in patients with germ-cell cancer. Int J Cancer 1999;83(6):864–865.
14. Longhi A, Macchiagodena M, Vitali G, et al. Fertility in male patients treated with neoadjuvant chemotherapy for osteosarcoma. J Pediatr Hematol Oncol 2003;25(4):292–296.
15. Williams D, Crofton PM, Levitt G. Does ifosfamide affect gonadal function? Pediatr Blood Cancer 2008;50(2):347–351.
16. Hobbie WL, Ginsberg JP, Ogle SK, et al. Fertility in males treated for Hodgkins disease with COPP/ABV hybrid. Pediatr Blood Cancer 2005;44(2):193–196.
17. Bokemeyer C, Schmoll HJ, van Rhee J, et al. Long-term gonadal toxicity after therapy for Hodgkin's and non-Hodgkin's lymphoma. Ann Hematol 1994;68(3):105–110.
18. Rautonen J, Koskimies AI, Siimes MA. Vincristine is associated with the risk of azoospermia in adult male survivors of childhood malignancies. Eur J Cancer 1992;28A(11):1837–1841.
19. Petersen PM, Hansen SW. The course of long-term toxicity in patients treated with cisplatin-based chemotherapy for non-seminomatous germ-cell cancer. Ann Oncol 1999;10(12):1475–1483.
20. Howell S, Shalet S. Gonadal damage from chemotherapy and radiotherapy. Endocrinol Metab Clin North Am 1998;27(4):927–943.

21. Kopf-Maier P. Effects of carboplatin on the testis. A histological study. Cancer Chemother Pharmacol 1992;29(3):227–235.

22. Reiter WJ, Kratzik C, Brodowicz T, et al. Sperm analysis and serum follicle-stimulating hormone levels before and after adjuvant single-agent carboplatin therapy for clinical stage I seminoma. Urology 1998;52(1):117–119.

23. Lampe H, Horwich A, Norman A, et al. Fertility after chemotherapy for testicular germ cell cancers. J Clin Oncol 1997;15(1):239–245.

24. Chapman RM, Sutcliffe SB, Malpas JS. Male gonadal dysfunction in Hodgkin's disease. A prospective study. JAMA 1981;245(13):1323–1328.

25. Wang C, Ng RP, Chan TK, et al. Effect of combination chemotherapy on pituitary-gonadal function in patients with lymphoma and leukemia. Cancer 1980;45(8):2030–2037.

26. Sherins RJ, DeVita VT Jr. Effect of drug treatment for lymphoma on male reproductive capacity. Studies of men in remission after therapy. Ann Intern Med 1973;79(2):216–220.

27. Dhabhar BN, Malhotra H, Joseph R, et al. Gonadal function in prepubertal boys following treatment for Hodgkin's disease. Am J Pediatr Hematol Oncol 1993;15(3):306–310.

28. Ben Arush MW, Solt I, Lightman A, et al. Male gonadal function in survivors of childhood Hodgkin and non-Hodgkin lymphoma. Pediatr Hematol Oncol 2000;17(3):239–245.

29. Sieniawski M, Reineke T, Nogova L, et al. Fertility in male patients with advanced Hodgkin lymphoma treated with BEACOPP: a report of the German Hodgkin Study Group (GHSG). Blood 2008;111(1):71–76.

30. Shafford EA, Kingston JE, Malpas JS, et al. Testicular function following the treatment of Hodgkin's disease in childhood. Br J Cancer 1993;68(6):1199–1204.

31. Kulkarni SS, Sastry PS, Saikia TK, et al. Gonadal function following ABVD therapy for Hodgkin's disease. Am J Clin Oncol 1997;20(4):354–357.

32. Tal R, Botchan A, Hauser R, et al. Follow-up of sperm concentration and motility in patients with lymphoma. Hum Reprod 2000;15(9):1985–1988.

33. Viviani S, Ragni G, Santoro A, et al. Testicular dysfunction in Hodgkin's disease before and after treatment. Eur J Cancer 1991;27(11):1389–1392.

34. Donaldson SS, Link MP, Weinstein HJ, et al. Final results of a prospective clinical trial with VAMP and low-dose involved-field radiation for children with low-risk Hodgkin's disease. J Clin Oncol 2007;25(3):332–337.

35. Muller U, Stahel RA. Gonadal function after MACOP-B or VACOP-B with or without dose intensification and ABMT in young patients with aggressive non-Hodgkin's lymphoma. Ann Oncol 1993;4(5):399–402.

36. Hansen SW, Berthelsen JG, von der Maase H. Long-term fertility and Leydig cell function in patients treated for germ cell cancer with cisplatin, vinblastine, and bleomycin versus surveillance. J Clin Oncol 1990;8(10):1695–1698.

37. Grossfeld GD, Small EJ. Long-term side effects of treatment for testis cancer. Urol Clin North Am 1998;25(3):503–515.

38. Gandini L, Sgro P, Lombardo F, et al. Effect of chemo- or radiotherapy on sperm parameters of testicular cancer patients. Hum Reprod 2006;21(11):2882–2889.

39. Fossa SD, Aabyholm T, Vespestad S, et al. Semen quality after treatment for testicular cancer. Eur J Urol 1993;23(1):172–176.

40. Kader HA, Rostom AY. Follicle stimulating hormone levels as a predictor of recovery of spermatogenesis following cancer therapy. Clin Oncol (R Coll Radiol) 1991;3(1):37–40.

41. Chakraborti PR, Neave F. Recovery of fertility 14 years following radiotherapy and chemotherapy for testicular tumour. Clin Oncol (R Coll Radiol) 1993;5(4):253–254.

42. Stuart NS, Woodroffe CM, Grundy R, et al. Long-term toxicity of chemotherapy for testicular cancer—the cost of cure. Br J Cancer 1990;61(3):479–484.

43. Sanders JE, Hawley J, Levy W, et al. Pregnancies following high-dose cyclophosphamide with or without high-dose busulfan or total-body irradiation and bone marrow transplantation. Blood 1996;87(7):3045–3052.

44. Anserini P, Chiodi S, Spinelli S, et al. Semen analysis following allogeneic bone marrow transplantation. Additional data for evidence-based counselling. Bone Marrow Transplant 2002;30(7):447–451.

45. Grigg AP, McLachlan R, Zaja J, et al. Reproductive status in long-term bone marrow transplant survivors receiving busulfan-cyclophosphamide (120 mg/kg). Bone Marrow Transplant 2000;26(10):1089–1095.

46. Howell SJ, Radford JA, Ryder WD, et al. Testicular function after cytotoxic chemotherapy: evidence of Leydig cell insufficiency. J Clin Oncol 1999;17(5):1493–1498.

47. Gerl A, Muhlbayer D, Hansmann G, et al. The impact of chemotherapy on Leydig cell function in long term survivors of germ cell tumors. Cancer 2001;91(7):1297–1303.

48. Finkelstein JS, Klibanski A, Neer RM, et al. Osteoporosis in men with idiopathic hypogonadotropic hypogonadism. Ann Intern Med 1987;106(3):354–361.

49. Bagatell CJ, Bremner WJ. Androgens in men—uses and abuses. N Engl J Med 1996;334(11):707–714.

50. Fossa SD, Opjordsmoen S, Haug E. Androgen replacement and quality of life in patients treated for bilateral testicular cancer. Eur J Cancer 1999;35(8):1220–1225.

51. Jonker-Pool G, van Basten JP, Hoekstra HJ, et al. Sexual functioning after treatment for testicular cancer: comparison of treatment modalities. Cancer 1997;80(3):454–464.

52. Howell SJ, Radford JA, Smets EM, et al. Fatigue, sexual function and mood following treatment for haematological malignancy: the impact of mild Leydig cell dysfunction. Br J Cancer 2000;82(4):789–793.

53. Goldberg RB, Rabin D, Alexander AN, et al. Suppression of plasma testosterone leads to an increase in serum total and high density lipoprotein cholesterol and apoproteins A-I and B. J Clin Endocrinol Metab 1985;60(1):203–207.

54. Holmes SJ, Whitehouse RW, Clark ST, et al. Reduced bone mineral density in men following chemotherapy for Hodgkin's disease. Br J Cancer 1994;70(2):371–375.

55. Howell SJ, Radford JA, Adams JE, et al. The impact of mild Leydig cell dysfunction following cytotoxic chemotherapy on bone mineral density (BMD) and body composition. Clin Endocrinol (Oxf) 2000;52(5):609–616.

56. Bhasin S, Storer TW, Berman N, et al. Testosterone replacement increases fat-free mass and muscle size in hypogonadal men. J Clin Endocrinol Metab 1997;82(2):407–413.

57. Katznelson L, Finkelstein JS, Schoenfeld DA, et al. Increase in bone density and lean body mass during testosterone administration in men with acquired hypogonadism. J Clin Endocrinol Metab 1996;81(12):4358–4365.

58. Bischoff FZ, Nguyen DD, Burt KJ, et al. Estimates of aneuploidy using multicolor fluorescence in situ hybridization on human sperm. Cytogenet Cell Genet 1994;66(4):237–243.

59. Genesca A, Miro R, Caballin MR, et al. Sperm chromosome studies in individuals treated for testicular cancer. Hum Reprod 1990;5(3):286–290.

60. Chatterjee R, Haines GA, Perera DM, et al. Testicular and sperm DNA damage after treatment with fludarabine for chronic lymphocytic leukaemia. Hum Reprod 2000;15(4):762–766.

61. O'Flaherty C, Vaisheva F, Hales BF, et al. Characterization of sperm chromatin quality in testicular cancer and Hodgkin's lymphoma patients prior to chemotherapy. Hum Reprod 2008;23(5):1044–1052.

62. Martin RH, Rademaker AW, Leonard NJ. Analysis of chromosomal abnormalities in human sperm after chemotherapy by karyotyping and fluorescence in situ hybridization (FISH). Cancer Genet Cytogen 1995;80(1):29–32.

63. Kobayashi H, Larson K, Sharma RK, et al. DNA damage in patients with untreated cancer as measured by the sperm chromatin structure assay. Fertil Steril 2001;75(3):469–475.

64. Meistrich ML, Goldstein LS, Wyrobek AJ. Long-term infertility and dominant lethal mutations in male mice treated with adriamycin. Mutat Res 1985;152(1):53–65.

65. Generoso WM, Witt KL, Cain KT, et al. Dominant lethal and heritable translocation tests with chlorambucil and melphalan in male mice. Mutat Res 1995;345(3–4):167–180.

66. Brinkworth MH. Paternal transmission of genetic damage: findings in animals and humans. Int J Androl 2000;23(3):123–135.

67. Hales BF, Robaire B. Paternal exposure to drugs and environmental chemicals: effects on progeny outcome. J Androl 2001;22(6):927–936.

68. Lass A, Akagbosu F, Abusheikha N, et al. A programme of semen cryopreservation for patients with malignant disease in a tertiary infertility centre: lessons from 8 years' experience. Hum Reprod 1998;13(11):3256–3261.

69. Lass A, Akagbosu F, Brinsden P. Sperm banking and assisted reproduction treatment for couples following cancer treatment of the male partner. Hum Reprod Update 2001;7(4):370–377.

70. Meistrich ML. Potential genetic risks of using semen collected during chemotherapy. Hum Reprod 1993;8(1):8–10.

71. Morris ID. Sperm DNA damage and cancer treatment. Int J Androl 2002;25(5):255–261.

72. Babosa M, Baki M, Bodrogi I, et al. A study of children, fathered by men treated for testicular cancer, conceived before, during, and after chemotherapy. Med Pediatr Oncol 1994;22(1):33–38.

73. Meistrich ML, Byrne J. Genetic disease in offspring of long-term survivors of childhood and adolescent cancer treated with potentially mutagenic therapies. Am J Hum Genet 2002;70(4):1069–1071.

74. Williams DHt, Karpman E, Sander JC, et al. Pretreatment semen parameters in men with cancer. J Urol 2009;181(2):736–740.

75. Rueffer U, Breuer K, Josting A, et al. Male gonadal dysfunction in patients with Hodgkin's disease prior to treatment. Ann Oncol 2001;12(9):1307–1311.

76. Sankila R, Olsen JH, Anderson H, et al. Risk of cancer among offspring of childhood-cancer survivors. Association of the Nordic Cancer Registries and the Nordic Society of Paediatric Haematology and Oncology. New Engl J Med 1998;338(19):1339–1344.

77. Ragni G, Somigliana E, Restelli L, et al. Sperm banking and rate of assisted reproduction treatment: insights from a 15-year cryopreservation program for male cancer patients. Cancer 2003;97(7):1624–1629.

78. Sanger WG, Olson JH, Sherman JK. Semen cryobanking for men with cancer–criteria change. Fertil Steril 1992;58(5):1024–1027.

79. Tournaye H, Camus M, Bollen N, et al. In vitro fertilization techniques with frozen-thawed sperm: a method for preserving the progenitive potential of Hodgkin patients. Fertil Steril 1991;55(2):443–445.

80. Padron OF, Sharma RK, Thomas AJ Jr, et al. Effects of cancer on spermatozoa quality after cryopreservation: a 12-year experience. Fertil Steril 1997;67(2):326–331.

81. Agarwal A, Shekarriz M, Sidhu RK, et al. Value of clinical diagnosis in predicting the quality of cryopreserved sperm from cancer patients. J Urol 1996;155(3):934–938.

82. Neal MS, Nagel K, Duckworth J, et al. Effectiveness of sperm banking in adolescents and young adults with cancer: a regional experience. Cancer 2007;110(5):1125–1129.

83. Ho PC, Poon IM, Chan SY, et al. Intrauterine insemination is not useful in oligoasthenospermia. Fertil Steril 1989;51(4):682–684.

84. Khalifa E, Oehninger S, Acosta AA, et al. Successful fertilization and pregnancy outcome in in-vitro fertilization using cryopreserved/thawed spermatozoa from patients with malignant diseases. Hum Reprod 1992;7(1):105–108.

85. Rosenlund B, Sjoblom P, Tornblom M, et al. In-vitro fertilization and intra-cytoplasmic sperm injection in the treatment of infertility after testicular cancer. Hum Reprod 1998;13(2):414–418.

86. Tournaye H, Liu J, Nagy PZ, et al. Correlation between testicular histology and outcome after intracytoplasmic sperm injection using testicular spermatozoa. Hum Reprod 1996;11(1):127–132.

87. Chan PT, Palermo GD, Veeck LL, et al. Testicular sperm extraction combined with intracytoplasmic sperm injection in the treatment of men with persistent azoospermia postchemotherapy. Cancer 2001;92(6):1632–1637.

88. Geens M, De Block G, Goossens E, et al. Spermatogonial survival after grafting human testicular tissue to immunodeficient mice. Hum Reprod 2006;21(2):390–396.

89. Brinster RL, Zimmermann JW. Spermatogenesis following male germ-cell transplantation. Proc Natl Acad Sci U S A 1994;91(24):11298–11302.

90. Avarbock MR, Brinster CJ, Brinster RL. Reconstitution of spermatogenesis from frozen spermatogonial stem cells. Nat Med 1996;2(6):693–696.

91. Ogawa T, Dobrinski I, Avarbock MR, et al. Xenogeneic spermatogenesis following transplantation of hamster germ cells to mouse testes. Biol Reprod 1999;60(2):515–521.

92. Brook PF, Radford JA, Shalet SM, et al. Isolation of germ cells from human testicular tissue for low temperature storage and autotransplantation. Fertil Steril 2001;75(2):269–274.

93. Jahnukainen K, Hou M, Petersen C, et al. Intratesticular transplantation of testicular cells from leukemic rats causes transmission of leukemia. Cancer Res 2001;61(2):706–710.

94. Fujita K, Ohta H, Tsujimura A, et al. Transplantation of spermatogonial stem cells isolated from leukemic mice restores fertility without inducing leukemia. J Clin Invest 2005;115(7):1855–1861.

95. Mayer D, Odell WD. Physiology of Reproduction. St. Louis: Mosby, 1971:20–27.

96. Peters H, Byskov AG, Himelstein-Braw R, et al. Follicular growth: the basic event in the mouse and human ovary. J Reprod Fertil 1975;45(3):559–566.

97. Johnston RJ, Wallace WH. Normal ovarian function and assessment of ovarian reserve in the survivor of childhood cancer. Pediatr Blood Cancer 2009;53(2):296–302.

98. Miller JJ III, Williams GF, Leissring JC. Multiple late complications of therapy with cyclophosphamide, including ovarian destruction. Am J Med 1971;50(4):530–535.

99. Warne GL, Fairley KF, Hobbs JB, et al. Cyclophosphamide-induced ovarian failure. New Engl J Med 1973;289(22):1159–1162.

100. Dnistrian AM, Schwartz MK, Fracchia AA, et al. Endocrine consequences of CMF adjuvant therapy in premenopausal and postmenopausal breast cancer patients. Cancer 1983;51(5):803–807.

101. Koyama H, Wada T, Nishizawa Y, et al. Cyclophosphamide-induced ovarian failure and its therapeutic significance in patients with breast cancer. Cancer 1977;39(4):1403–1409.

102. Mehta RR, Beattie CW, Das Gupta TK. Endocrine profile in breast cancer patients receiving chemotherapy. Breast Cancer Res Treat 1992;20(2):125–132.

103. Green DM, Kawashima T, Stovall M, et al. Fertility of female survivors of childhood cancer: a report from the childhood cancer survivor study. J Clin Oncol 2009;27(16):2677–2685.

104. Oktay K, Oktem O. Fertility preservation medicine: a new field in the care of young cancer survivors. Pediatr Blood Cancer 2009;53(2):267–273.

105. Fisher B, Sherman B, Rockette H, et al. 1-phenylalanine mustard (L-PAM) in the management of premenopausal patients with primary breast cancer: lack of association of disease-free survival with depression of ovarian function. National Surgical Adjuvant Project for Breast and Bowel Cancers. Cancer 1979;44(3):847–857.

106. Choo YC, Chan SY, Wong LC, et al. Ovarian dysfunction in patients with gestational trophoblastic neoplasia treated with short intensive courses of etoposide (VP-16-213). Cancer 1985;55(10):2348–2352.

107. Sutton R, Buzdar AU, Hortobagyi GN. Pregnancy and offspring after adjuvant chemotherapy in breast cancer patients. Cancer 1990;65(4):847–850.

108. Low JJ, Perrin LC, Crandon AJ, et al. Conservative surgery to preserve ovarian function in patients with malignant ovarian germ cell tumors. A review of 74 cases. Cancer 2000;89(2):391–398.

109. Meirow D. Reproduction post-chemotherapy in young cancer patients. Mol Cell Endocrinol 2000;169(1–2):123–131.

110. Maneschi F, Benedetti-Panici P, Scambia G, et al. Menstrual and hormone patterns in women treated with high-dose cisplatin and bleomycin. Gynecol Oncol 1994;54(3):345–348.

111. Tangir J, Zelterman D, Ma W, et al. Reproductive function after conservative surgery and chemotherapy for malignant germ cell tumors of the ovary. Obstet Gynecol 2003;101(2):251–257.

112. Bines J, Oleske DM, Cobleigh MA. Ovarian function in premenopausal women treated with adjuvant chemotherapy for breast cancer. J Clin Oncol 1996;14(5):1718–1729.

113. Minisini AM, Menis J, Valent F, et al. Determinants of recovery from amenorrhea in premenopausal breast cancer patients receiving adjuvant chemotherapy in the taxane era. Anticancer Drugs 2009;20(6):503–507.

114. Fornier MN, Modi S, Panageas KS, et al. Incidence of chemotherapy-induced, long-term amenorrhea in patients with breast carcinoma age 40 years and younger after adjuvant anthracycline and taxane. Cancer 2005;104(8):1575–1579.

115. Perez-Fidalgo JA, Rosello S, Garcia-Garre E, et al. Incidence of chemotherapy-induced amenorrhea in hormone-sensitive breast cancer patients: the impact of addition of taxanes to anthracycline-based regimens. Breast Cancer Res Treat 2010;120(1):245–251.

116. Reh A, Oktem O, Oktay K. Impact of breast cancer chemotherapy on ovarian reserve: a prospective observational analysis by menstrual history and ovarian reserve markers. Fertil Steril 2008;90(5):1635–1639.

117. Swain SM, Land SR, Ritter MW, et al. Amenorrhea in premenopausal women on the doxorubicin-and-cyclophosphamide-followed-by-docetaxel arm of NSABP B-30 trial. Breast Cancer Res Treat 2009;113(2):315–320.

118. Tham YL, Sexton K, Weiss H, et al. The rates of chemotherapy-induced amenorrhea in patients treated with adjuvant doxorubicin and cyclophosphamide followed by a taxane. Am J Clin Oncol 2007;30(2):126–132.

119. Han HS, Ro J, Lee KS, et al. Analysis of chemotherapy-induced amenorrhea rates by three different anthracycline and taxane containing regimens for early breast cancer. Breast Cancer Res Treat 2009;115(2):335–342.

120. Clark ST, Radford JA, Crowther D, et al. Gonadal function following chemotherapy for Hodgkin's disease: a comparative study of MVPP and a seven-drug hybrid regimen. J Clin Oncol 1995;13(1):134–139.

121. Kreuser ED, Xiros N, Hetzel WD, et al. Reproductive and endocrine gonadal capacity in patients treated with COPP chemotherapy for Hodgkin's disease. J Cancer Res Clin Oncol 1987;113(3):260–266.

122. Brusamolino E, Baio A, Orlandi E, et al. Long-term events in adult patients with clinical stage IA-IIA nonbulky Hodgkin's lymphoma treated with four cycles of doxorubicin, bleomycin, vinblastine, and dacarbazine and adjuvant radiotherapy: a single-institution 15-year follow-up. Clin Cancer Res 2006;12(21):6487–6493.

123. Hodgson DC, Pintilie M, Gitterman L, et al. Fertility among female Hodgkin lymphoma survivors attempting pregnancy following ABVD chemotherapy. Hematol Oncol 2007;25(1):11–15.

124. Behringer K, Breuer K, Reineke T, et al. Secondary amenorrhea after Hodgkin's lymphoma is influenced by age at treatment, stage of disease, chemotherapy regimen, and the use of oral contraceptives during therapy: a report from the German Hodgkin's Lymphoma Study Group. J Clin Oncol 2005;23(30):7555–7564.

125. Creasman WT, Soper JT. Assessment of the contemporary management of germ cell malignancies of the ovary. Am J Obstet Gynecol 1985;153(8):828–834.

126. Gershenson DM. Menstrual and reproductive function after treatment with combination chemotherapy for malignant ovarian germ cell tumors. J Clin Oncol 1988;6(2):270–275.

127. Zanetta G, Bonazzi C, Cantu M, et al. Survival and reproductive function after treatment of malignant germ cell ovarian tumors. J Clin Oncol 2001;19(4):1015–1020.

128. Gershenson DM, Miller AM, Champion VL, et al. Reproductive and sexual function after platinum-based chemotherapy in long-term ovarian germ cell tumor survivors: a Gynecologic Oncology Group Study. J Clin Oncol 2007;25(19):2792–2797.

129. Sanders JE, Buckner CD, Leonard JM, et al. Late effects on gonadal function of cyclophosphamide, total-body irradiation, and marrow transplantation. Transplantation 1983;36(3):252–255.

130. Schimmer AD, Quatermain M, Imrie K, et al. Ovarian function after autologous bone marrow transplantation. J Clin Oncol 1998;16(7):2359–2363.

131. Hinterberger-Fischer M, Kier P, Kalhs P, et al. Fertility, pregnancies and offspring complications after bone marrow transplantation. Bone Marrow Transplant 1991;7(1):5–9.

132. Salooja N, Chatterjee R, McMillan AK, et al. Successful pregnancies in women following single autotransplant for acute myeloid leukemia with a chemotherapy ablation protocol. Bone Marrow Transplant 1994;13(4):431–435.

133. Carter A, Robison LL, Francisco L, et al. Prevalence of conception and pregnancy outcomes after hematopoietic cell transplantation: report from the Bone Marrow Transplant Survivor Study. Bone Marrow Transplant 2006;37(11):1023–1029.

134. Chatterjee R, Goldstone AH. Gonadal damage and effects on fertility in adult patients with haematological malignancy undergoing stem cell transplantation. Bone Marrow Transplant 1996;17(1):5–11.

135. Singhal S, Powles R, Treleaven J, et al. Melphalan alone prior to allogeneic bone marrow transplantation from HLA-identical sibling donors for hematologic malignancies: alloengraftment with potential preservation of fertility in women. Bone Marrow Transplant 1996;18(6):1049–1055.

136. Schover LR. Premature ovarian failure and its consequences: vasomotor symptoms, sexuality, and fertility. J Clin Oncol 2008;26(5):753–758.

137. Green DM, Sklar CA, Boice JD Jr, et al. Ovarian failure and reproductive outcomes after childhood cancer treatment: results from the Childhood Cancer Survivor Study. J Clin Oncol 2009;27(14):2374–2381.

138. Winther JF, Boice JD Jr, Svendsen AL, et al. Spontaneous abortion in a Danish population-based cohort of childhood cancer survivors. J Clin Oncol 2008;26(26):4340–4346.

139. Green DM, Zevon MA, Lowrie G, et al. Congenital anomalies in children of patients who received chemotherapy for cancer in childhood and adolescence. New Engl J Med 1991;325(3):141–146.

140. Aisner J, Wiernik PH, Pearl P. Pregnancy outcome in patients treated for Hodgkin's disease. J Clin Oncol 1993;11(3):507–512.

141. Dodds L, Marrett LD, Tomkins DJ, et al. Case-control study of congenital anomalies in children of cancer patients. BMJ 1993;307(6897):164–168.

142. Holmes GE, Holmes FF. Pregnancy outcome of patients treated for Hodgkin's disease: a controlled study. Cancer 1978;41(4):1317–1322.

143. Pados G, Camus M, Van Waesberghe L, et al. Oocyte and embryo donation: evaluation of 412 consecutive trials. Hum Reprod 1992;7(8):1111–1117.

144. Blumenfeld Z, Avivi I, Ritter M, et al. Preservation of fertility and ovarian function and minimizing chemotherapy-induced gonadotoxicity in young women. J Soc Gynecol Investig 1999;6(5):229–239.

145. Oktay K, Buyuk E, Davis O, et al. Fertility preservation in breast cancer patients: IVF and embryo cryopreservation after ovarian stimulation with tamoxifen. Hum Reprod 2003;18(1):90–95.

146. Azim AA, Costantini-Ferrando M, Oktay K. Safety of fertility preservation by ovarian stimulation with letrozole and gonadotropins in patients with breast cancer: a prospective controlled study. J Clin Oncol 2008;26(16):2630–2635.

147. Requena A, Herrero J, Landeras J, et al. Use of letrozole in assisted reproduction: a systematic review and meta-analysis. Hum Reprod Update 2008;14(6):571–582.

148. Yang D, Brown SE, Nguyen K, et al. Live birth after the transfer of human embryos developed from cryopreserved oocytes harvested before cancer treatment. Fertil Steril 2007;87(6):1469e1–4.

149. Porcu E, Bazzocchi A, Notarangelo L, et al. Human oocyte cryopreservation in infertility and oncology. Curr Opin Endocrinol Diabetes Obes 2008;15(6):529–535.

150. Fabbri R, Venturoli S, D'Errico A, et al. Ovarian tissue banking and fertility preservation in cancer patients: histological and immunohistochemical evaluation. Gynecol Oncol 2003;89(2):259–266.

151. Poirot CJ, Martelli H, Genestie C, et al. Feasibility of ovarian tissue cryopreservation for prepubertal females with cancer. Pediatr Blood Cancer 2007;49(1):74–78.

152. Meirow D, Baum M, Yaron R, et al. Ovarian tissue cryopreservation in hematologic malignancy: ten years' experience. Leuk Lymphoma 2007;48(8):1569–1576.

153. Radford JA, Lieberman BA, Brison DR, et al. Orthotopic reimplantation of cryopreserved ovarian cortical strips after high-dose chemotherapy for Hodgkin's lymphoma. Lancet 2001;357(9263):1172–1175.

154. Oktay K, Karlikaya G. Ovarian function after transplantation of frozen, banked autologous ovarian tissue. New Engl J Med 2000;342(25):1919.

155. Meirow D. Fertility preservation in cancer patients using stored ovarian tissue: clinical aspects. Curr Opin Endocrinol Diabetes Obes 2008;15(6):536–547.

156. Oktay K. Spontaneous conceptions and live birth after heterotopic ovarian transplantation: is there a germline stem cell connection? Hum Reprod 2006;21(6):1345–1348.

157. Siegel-Itzkovich J. Woman gives birth after receiving transplant of her own ovarian tissue. BMJ 2005;331(7508):70.

158. Seshadri T, Gook D, Lade S, et al. Lack of evidence of disease contamination in ovarian tissue harvested for cryopreservation from patients with Hodgkin lymphoma and analysis of factors predictive of oocyte yield. Br J Cancer 2006;94(7):1007–1010.

159. Meirow D, Hardan I, Dor J, et al. Searching for evidence of disease and malignant cell contamination in ovarian tissue stored from hematologic cancer patients. Hum Reprod 2008;23(5):1007–1013.

160. Seymour JF. Ovarian tissue cryopreservation for cancer patients: who is appropriate? Reprod Fertil Dev 2001;13(1):81–89.

161. Wallace WH, Pritchard J. Livebirth after cryopreserved ovarian tissue autotransplantation. Lancet 2004;364(9451):2093–2094.

162. Chapman RM, Sutcliffe SB. Protection of ovarian function by oral contraceptives in women receiving chemotherapy for Hodgkin's disease. Blood 1981;58(4):849–851.

163. Longhi A, Pignotti E, Versari M, et al. Effect of oral contraceptive on ovarian function in young females undergoing neoadjuvant chemotherapy treatment for osteosarcoma. Oncol Rep 2003;10(1):151–155.

164. Montz FJ, Wolff AJ, Gambone JC. Gonadal protection and fecundity rates in cyclophosphamide-treated rats. Cancer Res 1991;51(8):2124–2126.

165. Ataya K, Rao LV, Lawrence E, et al. Luteinizing hormone-releasing hormone agonist inhibits cyclophosphamide-induced ovarian follicular depletion in rhesus monkeys. Biol Reprod 1995;52(2):365–372.

166. Blumenfeld Z, von Wolff M. GnRH-analogues and oral contraceptives for fertility preservation in women during chemotherapy. Hum Reprod Update 2008;14(6):543–552.

167. Oktay K, Sonmezer M, Oktem O, et al. Absence of conclusive evidence for the safety and efficacy of gonadotropin-releasing hormone analogue treatment in protecting against chemotherapy-induced gonadal injury. Oncologist 2007;12(9):1055–1066.

168. Aslam I, Fishel S, Moore H, et al. Fertility preservation of boys undergoing anti-cancer therapy: a review of the existing situation and prospects for the future. Hum Reprod 2000;15(10):2154–2159.

169. Blatt J, Poplack DG, Sherins RJ. Testicular function in boys after chemotherapy for acute lymphoblastic leukemia. New Engl J Med 1981;304(19):1121–1124.

170. Wallace WH, Shalet SM, Lendon M, et al. Male fertility in long-term survivors of childhood acute lymphoblastic leukaemia. Int J Androl 1991;14(5):312–319.

171. Etteldorf JN, West CD, Pitcock JA, et al. Gonadal function, testicular histology, and meiosis following cyclophosphamide therapy in patients with nephrotic syndrome. J Pediatr 1976;88(2):206–212.

172. van Casteren NJ, van der Linden GH, Hakvoort-Cammel FG, et al. Effect of childhood cancer treatment on fertility markers in adult male long-term survivors. Pediatr Blood Cancer 2009;52(1):108–112.

173. Heikens J, Behrendt H, Adriaanse R, et al. Irreversible gonadal damage in male survivors of pediatric Hodgkin's disease. Cancer 1996;78(9):2020–2024.

174. Kliesch S, Behre HM, Jurgens H, et al. Cryopreservation of semen from adolescent patients with malignancies. Med Pediatr Oncol 1996;26(1):20–27.

175. Byrne J, Fears TR, Mills JL, et al. Fertility of long-term male survivors of acute lymphoblastic leukemia diagnosed during childhood. Pediatr Blood Cancer 2004;42(4):364–372.

176. Bahadur G, Ling KL, Hart R, et al. Semen quality and cryopreservation in adolescent cancer patients. Hum Reprod 2002;17(12):3157–3161.

177. Ried HL, Zietz H, Jaffe N. Cryopreservation of semen from adolescent patients with malignancies. Med Pediatr Oncol 1997;28(4):322–323.

178. Revel A, Revel-Vilk S. Pediatric fertility preservation: is it time to offer testicular tissue cryopreservation? Mol Cell Endocrinol 2008;282(1–2):143–149.

179. De Groot GW, Faiman C, Winter JS. Cyclophosphamide and the prepubertal gonad: a negative report. J Pediatr 1974;84(1):123–125.

180. Marcello MF, Nuciforo G, Romeo R, et al. Structural and ultrastructural study of the ovary in childhood leukemia after successful treatment. Cancer 1990;66(10):2099–2104.

181. Himelstein-Braw R, Peters H, Faber M. Morphological study of the ovaries of leukaemic children. Br J Cancer 1978;38(1):82–87.

182. Nicosia SV, Matus-Ridley M, Meadows AT. Gonadal effects of cancer therapy in girls. Cancer 1985;55(10):2364–2372.

183. Chemaitilly W, Mertens AC, Mitby P, et al. Acute ovarian failure in the childhood cancer survivor study. J Clin Endocrinol Metab 2006;91(5):1723–1728.

184. Wallace WH, Shalet SM, Tetlow LJ, et al. Ovarian function following the treatment of childhood acute lymphoblastic leukaemia. Med Pediatr Oncol 1993;21(5):333–339.

185. Byrne J, Fears TR, Gail MH, et al. Early menopause in long-term survivors of cancer during adolescence. Am J Obstet Gynecol 1992;166(3):788–793.

186. Mackie EJ, Radford M, Shalet SM. Gonadal function following chemotherapy for childhood Hodgkin's disease. Med Pediatr Oncol 1996;27(2):74–78.

187. Haddy TB, Adde MA, McCalla J, et al. Late effects in long-term survivors of high-grade non-Hodgkin's lymphomas. J Clin Oncol 1998;16(6):2070–2079.

188. Clayton PE, Shalet SM, Price DA, et al. Ovarian function following chemotherapy for childhood brain tumours. Med Pediatr Oncol 1989;17(2):92–96.

189. Cicognani A, Pasini A, Pession A, et al. Gonadal function and pubertal development after treatment of a childhood malignancy. J Pediatr Endocrinol Metab 2003;16(Suppl 2):321–326.

190. Couto-Silva AC, Trivin C, Thibaud E, et al. Factors affecting gonadal function after bone marrow transplantation during childhood. Bone Marrow Transplant 2001;28(1):67–75.

191. Shamberger RC, Rosenberg SA, Seipp CA, et al. Effects of high-dose methotrexate and vincristine on ovarian and testicular functions in patients undergoing postoperative adjuvant treatment of osteosarcoma. Cancer Treat Rep 1981;65(9–10):739–746.

Note: Page numbers followed by "f" indicate figures; those followed by "t" indicate tables.

features of
   bifunctional antibodies, 476–477, 476f
   humanized antibodies, 475–476, 476f
   immunoadhesins, 476
fragment definitions, 468t
HAMA response of, 482, 482t, 483
immune activation, 474
immunoglobulin structure, 465–467, 466–467f
limitations of, 465, 488, 488t
modifications of
   binding affinity of engineered antibodies, 475
   cytotoxicity, 475
   immunogenicity, 474–475
naming, 482–483
ontogeny, 467–469, 469f
phagocytosis, 473
pharmacokinetics and pharmacodynamics, 470–471
properties of, 466t
radioimmunotherapy considerations
   choice of radionuclide, 481
   dosimetry, 480
   of radiolabeled, 479–480
receptor blockade of, 473–474
structure of, 466f
as targeted therapy, 465
toxic agents, vector for, 477
toxicity of, 481–482
and trastuzumab, 521–522
and TS detection, 146
vector for radioactivity, 478–479
Monoethylglycinexylidide, 227
Montanide, vaccination, 611
MOPP regimen
   and ABVD, 299–300
   Hodgkin's disease, 9
   infertility
     female, 777
     male, 774, 779
Morphine
   cancer pain, 689–690
   equianalgesic table, 690t
   FDA-approved, 689
   fentanyl, 698
   formulations and dosage strengths, 693t
   hydromorphone, 697
   intravenous, 691, 693–697
   meperidine, 701
   oxycodone, 697
   oxymorphone, 699
   pentazocine, 700
   pharmacodynamics of, 693
   pharmacokinetics of, 693–697
   using principles, 689–690
Mouse models
   ADCC, 472
   antisense oligonucleotides, 539
   dacarbazine, 298, 299
   drug interaction, 369
   human antiglobulin response, 474
   immune modulation, 313

procarbazine, 294, 295t
radioimmunotherapy, 479
thalidomide, 637
6-MP (See 6-Mercaptopurine [6-MP])
mRNA, polyadenylation of, 143
MRP1 (See Multidrug resistance-related protein 1 [MRP1])
MTD regimen, 185
MTX (See Methotrexate [MTX])
Mucositis
   anthracyclines, 370
   from Ara-C, 178
   dactinomycin, 332
   daunorubicin, 370
   doxorubicin, 370
   epipodophyllotoxin, 401
   everolimus, 556
   FdUrd, 151
   from 5-FU, 151, 152
   gastrointestinal toxicity, 151
   irinotecan, 346t
   methylenetetrahydrofolate reductase, 88
   MTX, 124, 125, 127
   from paclitaxel, 240, 244
   sunitinib, 508
   temsirolimus, 556
   thioguanine, 195
   topotecan, 343t
Multidrug resistance-related protein 1 (MRP1), 63
Multifocal leukoencephalopathy, 152
Multiple myeloma
   bisphosphonates for, 735
   bortezomib for, 41, 428–429, 452
   clodronate (Ostac) for, 735
   doxorubicin for, 369
   leukemia, 13
   melphalan for, 269
   osteolytic bone lesions, 735
   pentostatin for, 199
   permeability glycoprotein (Pgp), 224
   rituximab for, 485
   thalidomide for, 632, 638–640
   zoledronic acid for, 738
MuMAb4D5, 517
Musculoskeletal toxicity, tamoxifen, 657
Mutamycin (See Mitomycin C [MMC])
Mutations
   chemotherapy, potential for, 775, 778
   by temozolomide, 302
MVPP regimen, 774
Myelodysplasia (MDS)
   azacytidine analogues, 180
   decitabine, 182, 183
   thalidomide, clinical studies of, 641–642
Myelodysplasia, decitabine, 183
Myeloid-derived suppressor cells (MDSC), 627
Myeloma (See Multiple myeloma)
Myelosuppression
   bleomycin, 329
   carboplatin, 316
   cisplatin, 316
   cladribine, 200

clofarabine, 201
dacarbazine, 298
dactinomycin, 333
etoposide, 403
fludarabine, 198
5-FU, 151
gemcitabine, 185
by ixabepilone, 248
oxaliplatin, 316
by pemetrexed, 130
platinum analogues, 316
procarbazine, 295
6-TG, 196
yondelis, 336
Mylotarg (See Gemtuzumab ozogamicin [Mylotarg])
Myocet (See Doxorubicin [Caelyx, Doxil])

N
N-phosphonoacetyl-l-aspartic acid and 5-FU toxicity, 145
Nalbuphine, 700
Nalidixic acid, 393
Narcotics interactions, procarbazine, 293
National Cancer Institute (NCI)
   cell-based approach to drug screening, 22
   compound libraries, 19–20
   in vivo screening, 23
National Surgical Adjuvant Breast and Bowel Program (NSABP) on tamoxifen, 657
Nausea/vomiting (See also Antinausea medications)
   alklating agents, 282–283
   carboplatin, 316
   cisplatin, 316
   dactinomycin, 333
   decitabine, 182
   estramustine phosphate, 252
   etoposide, 403
   fludarabine, 198
   gastrointestinal toxicity, 283, 289
   from L-ASP, 415
   oxaliplatin, 316
   platinum analogues, 316
   sunitinib, 508
   topotecan, 344
N-desmethyltamoxifen
   for breast cancer, 88
   for renal dysfunction, 654
Nefazodone, 249
Nelarabine
   interactions, 202
   key features of, 202t
   mechanism of action, 202
   pharmacology, 202
   T-cell acute leukemia (T-ALL) and T-cell lymphoblastic lymphoma (T-LBL), 202
   toxicity, 202
Nelfinivar (Viracept), 558
Neoadjuvant chemotherapy, 5